# BLOOD DISEASES OF INFANCY AND CHILDHOOD

# Blood diseases
## OF INFANCY AND CHILDHOOD

**CARL H. SMITH, M.A., M.D.**

Clinical Professor of Pediatrics, Cornell University Medical College, New York, New York; Consulting Pediatrician, The New York Hospital, New York, New York; Beekman-Downtown Hospital, New York; Fitkin Memorial Hospital, Neptune, New Jersey; Misericordia Hospital, Bronx, New York; Staten Island Hospital, Staten Island, New York; St. Joseph's Hospital, Far Rockaway, New York; Roosevelt Hospital, New York, New York; Lenox Hill Hospital, New York, New York; New York Infirmary, New York, New York

*With the editorial assistance of*
**DENIS R. MILLER, M.D.**

Associate Professor of Pediatrics, Cornell University Medical College; Associate Attending Pediatrician, The New York Hospital; Director of Pediatric Hematology, The New York Hospital-Cornell Medical Center; Associate Attending Pediatrician (Hematology), Memorial Hospital, New York, New York

THIRD EDITION

With 175 illustrations
including three color plates

**THE C. V. MOSBY COMPANY**

SAINT LOUIS    1972

THIRD EDITION

Copyright © 1972 by The C. V. Mosby Company

All rights reserved. No part of this book may be reproduced in any manner without written permission of the publisher.

Previous editions copyrighted 1960, 1966

Printed in the United States of America

International Standard Book Number 0-8016-4690-1
Library of Congress Catalog Card Number 70-189079

Distributed in Great Britain by
Henry Kimpton, London

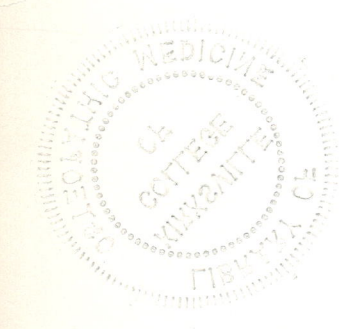

*Affectionately dedicated to my wife*

**MARGARET**

# SPECIAL MESSAGE

When the manuscript was completed for this edition, Dr. Carl H. Smith arranged for his associate, Dr. Denis R. Miller, to assist with the remaining details of preparation. Since Dr. Smith's death, Dr. Miller has devoted much time and effort to follow through on the completion of this work. It is with a deep sense of gratitude that especial thanks are expressed to Dr. Miller not only for his untiring work, but for the kind spirit, deep understanding and humility he has displayed.

It is with profound gratitude that acknowledgment is made to Dr. Virginia C. Canale, whose gracious and generous assistance and cooperation expedited the completion of this book. Special thanks and sincere appreciation are expressed to Dr. Canale.

Deep appreciation and thanks are expressed to Mrs. Marvin Tishcoff for her sincere and unwavering dedication to the various tasks involved in the completion of this edition.

*Margaret B. Smith*

# Preface

In this third edition of *Blood Diseases of Infancy and Childhood* the objectives stated in the Preface of the preceding edition remain unchanged. They are to provide an opportunity to introduce newer developments in pediatric hematology, to revise much of the text in the light of newer concepts, and to review current knowledge in this field. New tables and figures have been added to illustrate these advances. The flood of research data and literature in pediatric hematology and related fields has grown to such proportions that only those contributions were chosen that are relevant to the needs of the medical student, pediatrician, family physician, house staff officer, laboratory technologist, and, in many instances, the pathologist. In recent years the introduction of sophisticated investigational techniques and equipment has resulted in a massive proliferation of knowledge concerning biochemical, physiologic, immunologic, and genetic aspects of blood diseases. To facilitate description and formulation of various entities, their pathogenesis and clinical manifestations, as well as management, the technical complexities of the original publications have been minimized without sacrificing essential information. The bibliography has been greatly expanded to aid the student engaged in an investigative problem and includes over 1200 new references. While recent contributions have been incorporated in the present text, some deletions have been made, and several chapters have been thoroughly revised and reorganized.

Among the topics discussed are the recent studies of 2,3-diphosphoglycerate (2,3-DPG) and its role in determining the affinity of hemoglobin for oxygen. The use of phenobarbital as a means of lowering bilirubin in the management of jaundice of the newborn is described, as well as phototherapy as another measure to prevent the damage of hyperbilirubinemia. In the management of hemolytic anemia resulting from Rh incompatibility, the value of amniocentesis and intrauterine blood transfusion is presented. The injection of Rh antibody in the form of Rh immune globulin into unsensitized Rh-negative postpartum women has been proven to be effective in preventing Rh immunization. Amniocentesis is not only a guide in the management of Rh-hemolytic disease, but also can serve as a diagnostic aid in the prenatal detection and management of certain congenital defects.

The differential diagnosis and etiologic factors in the early and late neonatal periods have been further explored in the light of recent investigations dealing with pigments resulting from hemolysis such as hemopoxin.

Since the infant's diet is usually deficient in iron, iron-fortified milk has been recommended for routine use, together with other carefully selected foods to insure adequate iron intake.

The immunologic implications of blood disorders have their impact in almost every aspect of hematology, including those pertaining to allergic disorders, to the autoimmune hemolytic diseases, to viral interactions, to disorders of immunoglobulin metabolism, in transfusion, and in transplantation procedures.

Transfusion therapy has employed the value of essential blood components, of packed red cells rather than whole blood, the use of frozen-thawed prepared red blood cells, obviating the use of unnecessary plasma infusions. With the use of frozen-thawed prepared red blood cells for transfusion, previous febrile and allergic reactions have been eliminated. In intrauterine transfusions there is the possibility of developing host-versus-graft reaction from the incidental introduction of white blood cells.

The hemolytic anemias have been discussed from the standpoint of three main components of the cell—the membrane, the hemoglobin molecule, and the intracellular enzymes and intermediates of intracellular metabolism—congenital defects of which may have a profoundly adverse effect upon cell function metabolism and survival. Disease is manifested by severe anemia often requiring transfusions. An ever increasing number of red cell enzyme deficiencies have been characterized. These defects result in metabolically abnormal cells and in premature cell death. Recent investigations have demonstrated that the ability of the red cell to perform its various functions is critically dependent upon cell metabolism and that a most important regulator of hemoglobin function (oxygen affinity) and glycolysis (energy production) is 2,3-DPG. It is now possible to pinpoint the large number of enzymopathies and to determine their genetic background and in some instances to determine which will benefit by splenectomy.

The hemoglobinopathies have been dealt with to include investigations of erythrocyte metabolism, survival, organ sequestration, and membrane function. Studies of thalassemia include investigations of the many thalassemia syndromes resulting from deficient alpha, beta, delta, or gamma chain synthesis, as well as an inquiry of the most advantageous treatment with regard to amounts and frequency of blood administration and hemoglobin levels to be achieved. An important group of hemoglobinopathies, the unstable hemoglobin hemolytic anemias or congenital Heinz body anemias have been identified and are caused by amino acid substitutions that alter heme-globin or interchain contacts. Other recently discovered hemoglobinopathies include those associated with increased or decreased oxygen affinity.

Knowledge of the biochemistry and immunology of the leukocyte has been advanced and previously poorly understood diseases associated with increased susceptibility to bacterial diseases have now been related to aberrations of the intricate processes of opsonization, ingestion, and digestion of potentially pathogenic bacteria. One of these, chronic granulomatous disease of childhood, has been related to deficiencies of intracellular enzymes that destroy ingested bacteria.

Recent studies have uncovered a relationship between the Ebstein-Barr virus and infectious mononucleosis and Burkitt's lymphoma.

A vast knowledge has proliferated during the past five years in the field of acute leukemia of childhood. Aided by a greater awareness of the kinetics of leukemic cell proliferation and cell biochemistry, new drugs such as L-asparaginase and cytosine arabinoside and the use of multiple drug combinations have resulted in improved remission rates and prolonged survival in this disease, which less than a quarter of a century ago, before the chemotherapy era, carried a median survival of about four months. Aggressive chemotherapy has effectively decreased the leukemic cell burden. Localized disease, particularly in the central nervous system, has been identified and successfully treated; and supportive therapy, including the use of allopurinol to prevent hyperuricemia, newer antibiotics, and platelet concentrates have in concert prolonged the duration and improved the quality of remission in this disease. The importance of comprehensive support, including the emotional needs of the child, cannot be gainsaid. The eventual complete control, successful treatment, and, hopefully, prevention of leukemia must await further painstaking research efforts.

Improved diagnostic studies, including lymphangiography, the introduction of splenectomy, advanced radiotherapeutic techniques, and new combinations of drugs have improved remission rates and survival in such disorders as Hodgkin's disease. The importance of accurate clinical and pathological staging in determining prognosis has been reviewed. The recognition of an association between immunologic deficiency diseases and lymphoproliferative malignancies has stimulated investigators to redefine the contributions of the reticuloendothelial stimulation and aberrations of lymphoid proliferation and differentiation in these disorders.

The treatment of hemophilia has been aided immensely by the introduction of such new products as cryoprecipitate and amino acid precipitates of purified factor VIII, which when used appropriately have decreased morbidity and permitted children with this disorder to undergo extensive surgery without complications. A modern coagulation scheme, constantly undergoing revision, has been updated to bring into focus the intrinsic and extrinsic systems of coagulation.

The mechanism and etiology of disseminated intravascular coagulation and the laboratory diagnosis and management of this disorder are discussed, as is the fibrinolytic system.

The purpuras are discussed in light of recent advances in platelet metabolism and function. The physiology of the platelet, including platelet adhesiveness, aggregation, and release of thromboplastic materials that initiate clotting are reviewed, and such entities as thrombasthenia and the thrombocytopathy have been given clearer definition and understanding.

Those who have helped immensely in revising and updating this third edition include Drs. Alexander Wiener, Leon Sussman, Julian Schorr, James German, Philip Lanzkowsky, Denis Miller, Virginia Canale, Margaret Hilgartner, Herbert Horowitz, Theo Vats, Richard Silver, George Wantz, Frederick Battaglia, Julius Rutzky, and many others whose generous contributions, photographs, and tables are acknowledged in the text. Mr. Percy W. Brooks, Director of Medical Illustration at Cornell University Medical College, skillfully prepared many of the new illustrations. Miss Denise Berman and Mrs. Bella Mellenhoff provided secretarial assistance, and special praise goes to Mrs. Marvin Tishcoff who typed and retyped much of the manuscript.

Once again, I am particularly grateful to my wife, Margaret, for her encouragement in undertaking another edition. I owe her an enormous debt for her untiring efforts and patience in the multitude of the tasks required in revising the text and index.

*Carl H. Smith*
*April, 1971*

# Contents

**CHAPTER 1**

**Origin and development of blood cells, 1**

    Blood formation in the fetus, 1
    Theories of blood formation, 2
    Embryonic hemoglobin, 2
    Fetal hemoglobin, 3
    Swallowed blood syndrome, 5
    Fetal myoglobin, 9
    Bone marrow at birth, infancy, and childhood, 9

**CHAPTER 2**

**Blood changes during growth—postnatal period, infancy, and childhood, 13**

    Blood changes in the newborn infant, 13
    Physiologic anemia of the newborn infant, 14
    Bone marrow changes, 14
    Blood volume, 15
    Hemoglobin concentration, 15
    Erythrocyte count, 16
    Twin-to-twin transfusion, 17
    Hematocrit percentage (volume of packed red cells), 18
    Size of red cells (MCV) and hemoglobin concentration (MCHC), 18
    Reticulocytes, 18
    Normoblasts, 18
    Platelets, 18
    White blood cells, 19
    Blood of premature infants, 20

**CHAPTER 3**

**Blood dyscrasias in relation to maternal-fetal interaction, 23**

    Hereditary basis of blood diseases—genetic and environmental influences, 23
    Biochemical and genetic aspects, 23
    Blood dyscrasias in relation to congenital anomalies—general principles, 24
    Hematologic aspects of maternal and fetal interaction—placental physiology and defects, 25
    Fetal hemorrhage into the maternal circulation (blood loss from fetal-maternal transfusion), 26
    Bleeding from the placental surface, 27
    Maternal-fetal passage of leukocytes and platelets, 28
    Placental transmission of antibodies and isoagglutinins, 28
    Placental transmission of the L.E. factor, 29
    The gamma globulins, 29
    Plasma proteins in the fetus and newborn infant (immunoglobulin synthesis by the human fetus), 29
    Immunologic relationships, 31
    Transplacental passage of drugs affecting blood elements in the newborn infant, 32

**CHAPTER 4**

**Erythrocytes—general considerations, 37**

    Properties of the erythrocyte, 37
    Hemoglobin components, 41
    Iron content and oxygen capacity, 42
    Heme-heme interaction, 43
    Porphyrins and blood disorders, 44
    Glycogen, 44
    Rouleaux formation and sedimentation, 44
    Electrolyte considerations, 45
    Erythrocyte production, 47
    Normal destruction of erythrocytes, 53
    Fragmentation, 53

**CHAPTER 5**

**Erythrocytes—morphologic abnormalities, 63**

    General considerations, 63
    Abnormalities in size, 63
    Abnormalities in shape, 64
    Miscellaneous changes, 66

**CHAPTER 6**

**Blood groups, 74**

    Blood group antigens, 74
    Definitions of terms in relation to blood groups, 74
    A-B-O blood group system, 76
    Rh-Hr blood group system, 79
    M-N-Ss and P blood group systems, 82
    Other blood group systems, 83
    The sex-linked Xg[a] system, 84
    Gm system—hereditary gamma globulins in man, 84

## CHAPTER 7
### Transfusions in pediatric practice, 89

Introduction, 89
Significant factors in transfusion therapy, 89
Indications for transfusion, 90
Blood volume—plasma, total circulating hemoglobin, and erythrocyte mass, 90
Hemoglobin and hematocrit levels in acute and chronic anemias, 90
Choice and dosage of whole blood, packed erythrocytes, and plasma, 91
Platelet transfusion, 92
Leukocyte transfusion, 94
Transfusions in premature infants, 94
Limitations and hazards of transfusions, 95
Transfusion therapy in hemorrhagic disorders, 100
Intraperitoneal transfusion, 100
Notes on technique and preservation of blood, 100

## CHAPTER 8
### Jaundice—differential diagnosis in the neonatal period, 104

Types of bilirubin, 104
Enzymatic conversion of indirect to direct bilirubin, 104
Jaundice in early neonatal period, 107
　Physiologic jaundice (icterus neonatorum), 107
　Hyperbilirubinemia of the newborn infant unrelated to isoimmunization, 108
　Phenobarbital therapy in neonatal jaundice, 109
　Hyperbilirubinemia in breast-fed infants, 110
　Transient familial neonatal hyperbilirubinemia (Lucey-Driscoll syndrome), 111
　Phototherapy for hyperbilirubinemia, 111
　Relation of vitamin K to hyperbilirubinemia, kernicterus, and hemolytic anemia, 112
　Hereditary spherocytosis, 113
　Hereditary nonspherocytic hemolytic disease, 113
　Elliptocytic (ovalocytic) hemolytic anemia, 114
　Heinz body anemia in newborn infant, 114
　Acute hemolytic anemia related to naphthalene, 114
　Infections in newborn infants, 114
　Cytomegalic inclusion disease, 115
　Congenital toxoplasmosis, 115
　Chronic idiopathic jaundice (Dubin-Johnson type, Dubin-Sprinz disease), 116
Jaundice in later neonatal period, 116
　Prolonged obstructive jaundice, 116
　Obstructive jaundice complicating erythroblastosis—inspissated bile syndrome, 117
　Atresia of bile ducts (congenital obliteration of bile ducts), 118
　Neonatal hepatitis (giant cell hepatitis), 119
　Management of prolonged obstructive jaundice, 120
　Galactosemia, 122
　Congenital familial nonhemolytic jaundice with kernicterus (Crigler-Najjar syndrome), 122
　Familial nonhemolytic jaundice (Gilbert's disease), 123
　Jaundice and carotenemia, 123
　Jaundice due to pyloric stenosis, 124
　Jaundice and hypothyroidism, 124
　Hematomas, 124
　Miscellaneous, 124

## CHAPTER 9
### Erythroblastosis fetalis (hemolytic anemia of the newborn infant)—general considerations, 131

Definition, 131
Pathogenesis, 131
Clinical features, 132
Detection of early jaundice of the newborn infant, 133
Kernicterus, 133
Pathology, 136
Maternal antibodies—prenatal testing, 136
Maternal anti-Rh$_o$ titer, 136
Effect of previous transfusions on the mother, 137
Immunization in the Rh-positive mother and infant, 137
Heterozygous and homozygous status of the husband, 137
Different types of antibodies, 138
Transmission of antibodies, 138
Coombs test (antiglobulin test), 138
Tests with trypsinized cells, 139
Elution, 139
Frequency of blood group factors causing erythroblastosis, 140
Prognostic considerations and family patterns of severity, 141
Laboratory findings—blood, 141
Amniocentesis, 143
Examination of amniotic fluid for genetic defects, 145

## CHAPTER 10
### Erythroblastosis fetalis (hemolytic anemia of the newborn infant)—treatment, 151

Objectives of treatment, 151
Treatment, 151
Prevention, 161
Overall results of treatment of erythroblastosis fetalis, 163
Anemia in the previously treated infant, 163
Anemia in the previously untreated infant, 164
Rupture of the spleen, 164
Management of the infant with erythroblastosis, 164
Treatment of the infant in cardiac failure, 165
Intraperitoneal transfusion of the fetus, 166

Exchange transfusion in physiologic hyperbilirubinemia of the full-term and premature infant, 167
Exchange transfusions as a treatment of poisonings, 169
A-B-O erythroblastosis, 169
Differential diagnosis, 173

## CHAPTER 11
### Anemias—general considerations, 179

Classification, 179
Orientation, 179
Diagnosis, 180
Ferrokinetics and erythrokinetics, 188
General considerations, 188
In the diagnosis of anemias, 189
Principles of treatment, 199
Immunoallergic implications of blood disorders, 199
DNA autosensitivity, 201
Graft-versus-host reaction (runt disease), 201

## CHAPTER 12
### Iron-deficiency anemia, 205

Etiology, 205
Relation of physiologic anemia of the newborn infant to iron-deficiency anemia, 208
Clinical features, 209
Laboratory data, 209
Diagnosis, 211
Treatment, 214
Anemia of the premature infant, 219
Iron transport-serum iron and iron-binding capacity, 220
Iron absorption, 221
Gastroferrin, 224
Iron-binding capacity of plasma in various clinical conditions, 224
Hemosiderosis and hemochromatosis, 227
Transient dysproteinemia (copper deficiency in infants), 229
Exudative enteropathy, 229
Acute iron intoxication, 231
Iron-deficiency anemia in patients with cyanotic congenital heart disease, 232
Refractory hypochromic anemia (sideroachrestic anemia, sideroblastic anemia, hypochromic iron-loading anemia), 232

## CHAPTER 13
### Megaloblastic anemia and related anemias, 242

Vitamin $B_{12}$, 242
Folic acid, 242
Interrelationship of folic acid and vitamin $B_{12}$, 244
Gastrointestinal absorption of folic acid and vitamin $B_{12}$, 244
Diagnosis of the megaloblastic anemias, 245
Megaloblastic anemia of infancy, 246
Etiology, 246
Clinical features, 247
Laboratory findings, 247
Treatment, 248
Prognosis, 248
Juvenile pernicious anemia, 248
Etiology, 248
Clinical manifestations, 250
Laboratory findings, 250
Diagnosis, 251
Course and prognosis, 252
Treatment, 252
Nutritional megaloblastic anemia, 253
Miscellaneous megaloblastic anemias, 254
Megaloblastic anemia with hemolytic anemias, 254
Megaloblastic anemia with malignancies, 254
Megaloblastic anemia of pregnancy, 254
Megaloblastic anemia with hemochromatosis, 254
Megaloblastic anemia with fish tapeworm, 254
Megaloblastic anemia caused by anticonvulsant therapy, 255
Malabsorption syndromes—sprue (tropical), idiopathic steatorrhea (nontropical sprue), and celiac disease, 255
Normoblastic macrocytic anemias, 256

## CHAPTER 14
### Hypoplastic and aplastic anemias, 261

General considerations, 261
Classification, 261
Hypoplastic anemias, 262
Pure red cell anemia, 262
Definition, 262
Pathogenesis, 262
Clinical features, 263
Laboratory findings, 264
Pathologic findings, 264
Diagnosis, 264
Treatment, 265
Prognosis, 266
Acquired hypoplastic anemias, 267
Anemia due to infections, drugs, chemicals, toxins, and autoimmune and allergic states, 267
Aplastic crisis, 267
Anemia resulting from suppressive effect of multiple transfusions on erythropoiesis, 267
Miscellaneous, 267
Aplastic anemia (bone marrow failure, refractory anemia), 267
Definition, 267
Etiology, 268
Congenital or constitutional aplastic anemia, 268
Congenital aplastic anemia with multiple congenital anomalies (Fanconi type), 268
Congenital hypoplastic anemia without associated anomalies, 270
Acquired (secondary) aplastic anemia, 270
Anemia due to antimicrobial and other chemotherapeutic agents, 270
Anemia due to industrial and household chemicals, 271

Anemia due to irradiation, 272
Aplastic anemia following hepatitis, 272
Miscellaneous causes, 273
Features common to congenital and acquired types of aplastic anemia, 273
Pathology, 273
Clinical features, 273
Laboratory findings, 274
Differential diagnosis, 276
Management, 276
Course and prognosis, 283

## CHAPTER 15
## The hemolytic anemias, 290

Definition—general considerations of pathogenesis, 290
Classification, 290
Principal features of increased hemolysis, 291
Folic acid deficiency, 294
Evidence of increased marrow activity, 295
The porphyrias, 296
Additional tests for detecting abnormal hemolysis, 299
Congenital hemolytic syndromes, 302
Hereditary spherocytosis (congenital hemolytic jaundice, congenital hemolytic anemia, spherocytic anemia, chronic acholuric jaundice, chronic familial jaundice), 303
Definition, 303
Inheritance and race, 303
Etiology and pathogenesis, 303
Clinical features, 305
Growth, 306
Laboratory data, 306
Diagnosis, 307
Treatment, 308
Sporadic congenital spherocytosis associated with congenital hypoplastic thrombocytopenia and malformations, 309
Hereditary nonspherocytic hemolytic anemia (atypical familial hemolytic anemia, congenital nonspherocytic anemia), 310
Glucose-6-phosphate dehydrogenase deficiency (G-6-PD deficiency), 311
Pyruvate kinase (PK) deficiency, 313
6-Phosphogluconate dehydrogenase (6-PGD) deficiency, 315
Glutathione reductase (GSSG-R) deficiency, 315
Glutathione (GSH) deficiency, 315
Triosephosphate isomerase (TPI) deficiency, 315
Adenosine triphosphatase (ATPase) deficiency, 315
Hexokinase (HK) deficiency, 315
Glucosephosphate isomerase (GPI) deficiency, 315
Phosphoglycerate kinase (PGK) deficiency, 316
2-3-Diphosphoglycerate mutase (2,3-DPGM) deficiency, 316
Hereditary nonspherocytic hemolytic anemia with an altered phospholipid composition of the erythrocytes, 316
Summary, 316

Hereditary elliptocytosis with hemolytic anemia, 317
Clinical and blood findings, 317
Treatment, 319
Hemolytic anemia due to enzyme deficiency following administration of drugs and other agents, 319
Nonhereditary hemolytic anemia—paroxysmal nocturnal hemoglobinuria (PNH, Marchiafava-Micheli syndrome), 321
Acquired hemolytic anemias, 325
Autoimmune hemolytic anemia (chronic idiopathic autoimmune hemolytic disease, chronic acquired hemolytic anemia), 328
Clinical features, 328
Blood findings, 329
Serologic findings, 329
Pathogenesis, 331
Diagnosis, 332
Treatment, 332
Prognosis, 334
Paroxysmal cold hemoglobinuria, 334
Dysproteinemias, 335
Cryoglobulinemia, 335
Cryofibrinogenemia, 335
Acute acquired hemolytic anemia (Lederer's anemia), 336
Idiopathic paroxysmal myoglobinuria, 336
March hemoglobinuria, 337
Intravascular hemolysis following open heart surgery, 337

## CHAPTER 16
## The hereditary hemoglobinopathies, 353

Methods for determining the hemoglobin types, 353
Designation of hemoglobin types, 356
Structure of the hemoglobin molecule: polypeptide content of globin, 356
Electrophoretic mobility of the individual hemoglobins, 357
Fetal hemoglobin, 359
Hereditary persistence of fetal hemoglobin (the high fetal gene), 359
Primitive hemoglobin (P), 361
Cord blood hemoglobinopathies, 361
Hereditary aspects, 362
Relation of genetic composition to clinical-hematologic variations, 362
Target cells, 363
Syndromes associated with the abnormal hemoglobins, 364
Geographic distribution of the abnormal hemoglobins, 364
Factors involving alteration of oxygen affinity (heme-heme interaction, Bohr effect, and 2,3-diphosphoglycerate), 365
Sickle cell disease, 365
Sickling phenomenon, 366
Pathogenesis, 368
Sickle cell trait, 369
Incidence and geographic distribution, 369
Clinical and laboratory features, 369
Sickling and malaria, 370

Sickle cell (drepanocytic) anemia, 371
    Pathology, 371
    Clinical features, 374
    Skeletal changes, 377
    Blood, 378
    Crises, 378
    Diagnosis, 382
    Treatment, 382
    Prognosis, 384
Thalassemia (Cooley's anemia, Mediterranean anemia, erythroblastic anemia, hereditary leptocytosis), 384
    History, 385
    Nomenclature, 385
    Race and incidence, 385
    Genetic transmission, 386
    Effect of the gene for thalassemia upon other hemoglobins, 387
    Clinical types, 387
    Thalassemia intermedia, 387
    Fetal hemoglobin in patients with thalassemia, 388
    Pathogenesis, 389
    Pathology, 391
    Clinical features, 392
    Growth and maturation, 394
    Skeletal changes, 394
    Blood picture, 397
    Hemosiderosis and hemochromatosis, 404
    Red cell survival, 405
    Diagnosis, 406
    Course and prognosis, 408
    Treatment, 410
Alpha-thalassemia, 413
    Alpha-thalassemia major, 413
    Alpha-thalassemia minor, 413
Hemoglobin H, 414
High hemoglobin F-thalassemia, 416
Homozygous hemoglobin C disease, 416
    Essential features, 416
Hemoglobin C trait, 417
    Hereditary elliptocytosis and hemoglobin C trait, 417
    Hemoglobin C variant with sickling properties, 417
    Hereditary persistence of fetal hemoglobin and hemoglobin C (C-F heterozygotes), 417
Hemoglobin D, 417
Hemoglobin E disease, 418
    Homozygous hemoglobin E disease, 418
    Hemoglobin E trait, 418
Hemoglobin G, 418
    Hemoglobin G trait, 419
    Homozygous hemoglobin G disease, 419
    Hemoglobin G–sickle cell disease, 419
    Hemoglobin G–thalassemia, 419
Hemoglobin I, 419
Hemoglobin J, 419
Hemoglobin M, 420
Miscellaneous abnormal hemoglobins, 420
Sickle cell variants, 421
    Sickle cell thalassemia disease (microdrepanocytic anemia), 421
        Essential features, 421
        Clinical findings, 422
    Sickle cell–hemoglobin C disease, 422
    Sickle cell–hereditary spherocytosis, 424
    Hereditary spherocytosis, sickling, and thalassemia, 424
    Sickle cell–hemoglobin D disease, 424
Thalassemia variants, 424
    Thalassemia–hemoglobin C disease, 424
    Thalassemia–hemoglobin E disease, 426
    Thalassemia and persistent fetal hemoglobin (thal-F heterozygotes), 426
    Thalassemia–Lepore hemoglobin, 426
    Thalassemia trait with simultaneous inheritance of one $A_2$-thalassemia gene and one F-thalassemia gene, 427
Hereditary Heinz body anemias—unstable hemoglobin hemolytic anemias, 428
    Hemoglobin Zürich, 429
    Hemoglobin Köln disease, 430
    Hemoglobin Seattle, 430
    Other unstable hemoglobins, 431
Hemoglobin variants associated with altered oxygen affinity, 431

## CHAPTER 17

## Polycythemia, methemoglobinemia, sulfhemoglobinemia, and miscellaneous anemias, 450

Polycythemia, 450
    Relative polycythemia, 450
    Primary polycythemia (polycythemia vera, erythremia, Vaquez-Osler disease), 450
        Benign familial polycythemia, 450
    Secondary polycythemia (erythrocytosis, erythrocythemia, compensatory polycythemia), 451
Methemoglobinemia, 452
    Pathogenesis, 452
    Congenital (familial) methemoglobinemia, 453
    Congenital methemoglobinemia associated with hemoglobin M, 453
    Drug-induced methemoglobinemia, 453
    Features common to methemoglobinemia, 454
        Diagnosis, 454
        Treatment, 454
    Methemoglobinemia in young infants, 454
Sulfhemoglobinemia, 454
Miscellaneous anemias, 455
    Anemia of chronic renal insufficiency, 455
        Pathogenesis, 455
        Laboratory findings, 456
        Bone marrow, 456
        Diagnosis, 457
        Treatment, 457
    Anemia of infection, 457
        Pathogenesis, 458
        Blood findings and other laboratory data, 458
        Clinical features, 458
        Treatment, 458
    Anemia of acute hemorrhage, 459
        Etiology, 459
        Blood picture, 459
        Clinical features, 459
        Treatment, 459
    Chronic hemorrhagic anemia, 459
        Etiology, 459

Clinical and laboratory features, 459
Treatment, 460
Vitamin deficiencies and anemia, 460
  Vitamin A, 460
  Riboflavin ($B_2$), 460
  Nicotinic acid (niacin), 460
  Pyridoxine (vitamin $B_6$), 460
  Vitamin C and the anemia of scurvy, 461
  Vitamin E deficiency, 462
Anemia of hypothyroidism, 462
Blood changes in lead poisoning, 462

## CHAPTER 18
## Leukocytes—cell types, 469

Growth and multiplication, 469
Chemotactic factors, 469
Glucose-6-phosphate dehydrogenase in leukocytes, 470
Functions—phagocytosis and antibody formation, 470
Chemotaxis and opsonins, 471
Chronic granulomatous disease of childhood, 472
Rebuck skin-window study of leukocytic functions in vivo, 473
Autophagic vacuoles, 474
Muramidase (lysozyme), 474
Erythrophagocytosis, 474
L.E. phenomenon, 475
Life-span of leukocytes, 477
Leukoagglutinins, 478
Types of white cells, 479
  Granulocytic or myeloid series, 479
    Granulopoiesis—maturation compartments, 479
    Myeloblast—differentiation from lymphoblast, 480
    Promyelocytes (progranulocytes) and myelocytes, 481
    Metamyelocyte of juvenile form, 482
    Polymorphonuclear granulocytes, 482
  Lymphocytes, 487
    Small lymphocytes, 488
    Phytohemagglutinin, 488
    Large lymphocytes, 489
    Young lymphocytes (prolymphocytes), 489
    Lymphoblasts, 489
  Monocytes, 489
    Young monocyte (promonocyte), 490
    Monoblasts, 490
    Monocytosis, 491
  Miscellaneous, 491
    Histiocytes, 491
    Plasma cell (plasmacyte), 492
    Türk's cell (Türk irritation cell), 493
    Reider cells, 493
    Auer bodies, 493
Degenerative and toxic cytoplasmic changes, 493
  Amato bodies, 493
  Toxic granules, 495
  Pelger-Huët phenomenon of granulocytes, 495
  Nuclear projections, 496
  Russell bodies, 496
  Hematogones, 496
  Miscellaneous inclusion bodies, 496
  Other lipidoses and related diseases, 500
Cell stains, 500
  Romanowsky stains, 500
  Supravital staining, 500
  Peroxidase stain, 501
  Miscellaneous stains, 501
  Phase contrast microscopy, 501

## CHAPTER 19
## Leukopenia and leukopenic syndromes, 511

Pathogenesis, 511
Tests for bone marrow function, 512
Causes, 512
Treatment, 520

## CHAPTER 20
## Leukocytosis, leukemoid reactions, and lymphocytosis, 524

Leukocytosis, 524
  Physiologic leukocytosis, 524
  Pathologic leukocytosis, 524
Leukemoid reactions, 525
Lymphocytosis, 526
  Acute infectious lymphocytosis, 527
    Definition, 527
    Age, 528
    Etiology, 528
    Epidemiology, 528
    Pathology, 528
    Clinical features, 528
    Incubation period, 529
    Laboratory findings, 529
    Differential diagnosis, 529
    Treatment and prognosis, 532
  Chronic nonspecific infectious lymphocytosis (low-grade fever syndrome), 532
    Clinical picture, 532
    Blood, 533
    Differential diagnosis, 533
    Treatment and prognosis, 534

## CHAPTER 21
## Infectious mononucleosis, 536

Definition, 536
Historical, 536
Pathology, 537
Clinical features, 537
Laboratory findings, 540
Differential diagnosis, 545
Prognosis, 546
Treatment, 546
Recurrences, 547
Febrile postcardiotomy syndromes with splenomegaly and atypical lymphocytes, 547

## CHAPTER 22
## Leukemia—general aspects and clinical features, 551

Classification of leukemia in childhood, 551

Muramidase (lysozyme) in leukemia, 560
Incidence, age distribution, sex, and frequency of types, 560
Epidemiology, 561
Etiology, 562
Chromosomes and leukemia, 566
Glossary of chromosomal terminology, 567
Preleukemic stage of leukemia, 569
Leukemia in the newborn period (congenital leukemia), 570
Spontaneous remissions, 571
Clinical features, 572
Differential diagnosis, 584

CHAPTER 23

Leukemia—treatment, 595

Treatment, 595
Remissions—criteria, 606
Detailed program of treatment, 607
Treatment of acute myeloblastic leukemia, 616
Emotional support, 618
Bone marrow transplantation, 619
Laboratory determinations, 620
Treatment of nervous system involvement, 620
Results of treatment—prognosis for survival, 622

CHAPTER 24

Leukemia—allied disorders, 629

Infrequent types of leukemia, 629
Bone marrow replacement and leukoerythroblastosis, 630
Myelofibrosis, 630
Familial myeloproliferative disease, 631
Osteopetrosis (marble-bone disease), Albers-Schönberg disease), 631
Extramedullary megakaryocytosis and acute megakaryocytic leukemia, 633
Thrombocythemia, 633
Erythremic myelosis (Di Guglielmo's disease), 634
Chloroma and chloroleukemia, 634
Neoplasms of lymphoid tissue (malignant lymphomas), 635

CHAPTER 25

Disorders of the spleen and the reticuloendothelial system, 652

Role of the spleen in blood disorders, 652
Structure of the spleen, 652
Normal functions of the spleen, 652
Splenic aspiration, 655
Adrenaline test in diagnosis of hypersplenic syndromes, 655
Indications for splenectomy, 655
Disorders of the spleen, 656
Splenomegaly, 656
Hypersplenism, 656
Congenital absence of the spleen, 657
Primary splenic neutropenia, 658
Felty's syndrome, 658
Primary splenic panhematopenia, 658
Chronic congestive splenomegaly (Banti's syndrome, portal hypertension, splenic anemia), 658
Etiology and pathogenesis, 658
Collateral circulation, 659
Pathology, 659
Clinical features, 659
Laboratory data, 660
Diagnosis, 660
Course and prognosis, 660
Treatment, 660
Diseases of the reticuloendothelial system, 661
Gaucher's disease, 662
Pathology and pathogenesis, 662
Clinical features, 663
Blood, 666
Heredity, 666
Course and treatment, 666
Niemann-Pick disease, 667
Clinical features, 667
Pathology and pathogenesis, 667
Blood, 668
Heredity, 668
Treatment, 668
Generalized gangliosidosis, 668
Wolman's disease, 668
Letterer-Siwe disease, Hand-Schüller-Christian disease, and eosinophilic granuloma (histiocytosis X), 669
Letterer-Siwe disease (nonlipid reticuloendotheliosis), 669
Pathology, 670
Diagnosis, 670
Blood, 671
Treatment and course, 671
Hand-Schüller-Christian disease, 672
Clinical features, 672
Pathology, 672
Diagnosis, 672
Course, 672
Treatment, 673
Eosinophilic granuloma, 673
Histiocytic medullary reticulosis, 673

CHAPTER 26

Blood coagulation, 681

Normal hemostatic mechanisms, 681
Role of vascular factors, 681
Role of platelets, 681
The blood platelet, 682
Blood coagulation mechanism, 684
Dynamics of coagulation, 691
Natural inhibitors of coagulation, 691
Disorders due to a deficiency of factors required for thromboplastin formation (phase I of coagulation), 692
General consideration of the hemophilias, 692
Classic hemophilia (hemophilia A, factor VIII [AHG] deficiency), 692
Hereditary aspects, 692
Clinical aspects, 694
Hemarthrosis, 694
Management, 695
Treatment of bleeding, 695

## xviii CONTENTS

Treatment of hematuria, 703
Dental extractions, 704
Treatment of hemarthroses, 704
Mild hemophilia, 705
Diagnosis, 705
Roentgenographic findings, 706
Prognosis, 706
Von Willebrand's disease (pseudohemophilia, vascular hemophilia), 706
Christmas disease (factor IX deficiency, hemophilia B, plasma thromboplastin component deficiency, PTC deficiency), 709
Clinical and laboratory features, 710
Treatment, 710
Hemophilia prophylaxis, 711
Plasma thromboplastin antecedent deficiency (factor XI deficiency, PTA deficiency, hemophilia C), 711
Clinical and laboratory features, 711
Treatment, 712
Disorders due to a deficiency of factors required for conversion of prothrombin to thrombin (phase 2 of coagulation), 712
General considerations, 712
Vitamin K–dependent clotting factors, 713
Vitamin K deficiency, 713
Congenital deficiencies, 714
Idiopathic (congenital) hypoprothrombinemia, 714
Congenital deficiency of factor V (parahemophilia, Owren's disease, labile factor deficiency), 714
Congenital factor VII deficiency (stable factor deficiency, proconvertin deficiency, congenital hypoconvertinemia), 715
Bleeding in the newborn, 716
Hemorrhagic disease of the newborn infant (hypoprothrombinemia in the newborn infant), 717
Clinical and laboratory features, 718
Differential diagnosis, 718
Treatment, 719
Factor X deficiency (Stuart-Prower factor deficiency), 720
Factor XII deficiency (Hageman factor deficiency), 720
Multiple defects, 721
Capillary and single coagulation factor deficiency, 721
Multiple factor deficiencies, 721
Disorders due to a deficiency of fibrinogen (phase 3 of coagulation), 721
Congenital afibrinogenemia, 721
Congenital hypofibrinogenemia, 722
Acquired fibrinogen deficiency, 722
Dysfibrinogenemias, 722
Hypofibrinogenemia and other coagulation defects in patients with congenital heart disease: open-heart surgery, 722
Fibrinolysis (fibrinolytic purpura), 723
Laboratory findings in fibrinogen deficiencies, 725
Treatment of the fibrinogen deficiencies, 725
Circulating anticoagulants, 726
Naturally occurring anticoagulants, 726
Acquired anticoagulants, 726

Disseminated intravascular coagulation (DIC, defibrination syndrome, consumption coagulopathy), 727
Tests for anticoagulants, 729
Treatment, 729
Summary of replacement therapy of coagulation disorders, 730
Epistaxis, 731
Procedure for screening potential bleeders, 731
Laboratory investigation of coagulation disorders, 732
General considerations, 732
Screening tests, 733
Significance of routine coagulation tests, 735
Tests for phase 1 of coagulation, 735
Thromboplastin generation test, 736
Mutual correction tests, 739
Comparative value of laboratory tests in detecting thromboplastin deficiency, 739
Prothrombin consumption test, 740
Hageman factor (factor XII) deficiency, 740
Platelet adhesiveness, 741
Aspirin and platelet function, 742
Platelet factor 3 deficiency, 742
Tests for phase 2 of coagulation, 743
Prothrombin complex deficiencies, 743
Prothrombin time (plasma prothrombin time), 743
Combined prothrombin and factor VII (stable factor) deficiency, 744
Stuart-Prower factor (factor X), 744
Tests for phase 3 of coagulation, 744
Fibrinogen deficiencies, 744
FI TEST, 745

### CHAPTER 27

### The purpuras, 760

Classification of purpura, 760
Platelet counts in normal full-term and premature infants, 761
Thrombocytopenia in the newborn, 761
Thrombocytopenic purpuras, 762
Idiopathic thrombocytopenic purpura (ITP, Werlhof's disease, purpura hemorrhagica), 762
Pathogenesis, 762
Pathology, 764
Clinical manifestations, 765
Laboratory data, 768
Diagnosis, 769
Course and prognosis, 770
Treatment, 770
Hereditary thrombocytopenic purpura, 776
Congenital thrombocytopenic purpura, 777
Etiology, 777
Prognosis, 779
Treatment, 779
Thrombocytopenia in fetal rubella, 779
Thrombocytopenia in miscellaneous infections, 780
Thrombocytopenia with renal vein thrombosis, 780
Thrombocytopenia induced by drugs, 780
Aplastic anemia with onset as congenital thrombocytopenic purpura, 782

Chronic hypoplastic thrombocytopenia with depression of megakaryocytes, 782
Thrombocytopenia with absent radius (congenital hypoplastic thrombocytopenia, primary amegakaryocytic thrombocytopenia, phocomelia and congenital hypoplastic thrombocytopenia, myeloid leukemoid reaction, TAR), 782
Thrombotic (thrombohemolytic) thrombocytopenic purpura, 783
  Pathogenesis, 784
  Clinical course and laboratory findings, 784
  Treatment, 785
Wiskott-Aldrich syndrome, 785
  Immunological consideration, 786
Thrombocytopenia following transfusions, 787
Hemolytic-uremic syndrome, 787
  Clinical features, 787
  Pathogenesis, 789
  Etiology, 790
  Pathology, 790
  Prognosis, 791
  Treatment, 791
Cyclic thrombocytopenic purpura related to the menstrual cycle, 792
Hemangioma and thrombopenia (Kasabach-Merritt syndrome), 792

Nonthrombocytopenic purpuras, 793
  Allergic purpura (anaphylactoid purpura, Henoch-Schönlein or Schönlein-Henoch purpura), 793
    Etiology and pathogenesis, 793
    Clinical features, 794
    Laboratory findings, 798
    Diagnosis, 798
    Course and prognosis, 798
    Treatment, 799
  Congenital vascular defects, 800
    Von Willebrand's disease (pseudohemophilia), 800
    Hereditary hemorrhagic telangiectasia (Rendu-Osler-Weber disease), 800
    Ehlers-Danlos syndrome, 801
  Purpura fulminans, 803
    Treatment, 804
  Waterhouse-Friderichsen syndrome, 804
  Idiopathic pulmonary hemosiderosis, 804
    Clinical course, 804
    Prognosis, 806
    Pathology, 806
    Pathogenesis, 807
    Treatment, 807
  Miscellaneous purpuric disorders (nonthrombocytopenic), 807

# Color plates

PLATE 1   **Twin-to-twin transfusion, 18**

PLATE 2   **Atypical lymphocytes in infectious mononucleosis, 542**

PLATE 3   **Diffuse hemorrhagic measles in leukemia, 606**

# BLOOD DISEASES OF INFANCY AND CHILDHOOD

# 1 ORIGIN AND DEVELOPMENT OF BLOOD CELLS

*Blood formation in the fetus.* A review of the essential features of prenatal blood development provides a basis for interpreting postnatal abnormalities of the circulating blood elements, their progenitors, and sites of formation. The designation of prenatal hematopoiesis imparts an implication of continuity to the events occurring in the embryo in the first 2 months and in the fetus in the remainder of gestation. Current emphasis on maternal-fetal relationships, which has shed so much light on other systems, conceivably may clarify the etiology of certain of the blood dyscrasias on the same basis. An understanding of the blood changes in the earlier months of life, furthermore, requires some knowledge of embryonic and fetal blood formation.

*Sites of blood formation.* Blood cells in the embryo arise from the mesenchyme. The first cells produced in the yolk sac become the primitive red corpuscles. Since the mesenchyme is wide-spread throughout the embryo, blood formation begins in multiple sites but eventually becomes specialized in certain organs. With some overlapping, definitive blood centers mainly involving red cell elements appear successively in the yolk sac at the fourth month of gestation.[5] Although the bone marrow makes its appearance in the sixth week of development, it does not become a site of active hematopoiesis until the fourth to fifth month and does not become the exclusive site[5] until 2 to 3 weeks after birth.[28] Until the middle of fetal life the liver is the most actively engaged organ participating in blood formation. It has been stated that the liver as opposed to the marrow represents the principal source of fetal erythrocytes. In this period of hepatic hematopoiesis, fetal hemoglobin is the sole type synthesized. As hematopoiesis wanes in this area, it is assumed by the bone marrow, which exercises this function for the remainder of fetal life. Coincidental activity goes on in the spleen, the lymph nodes, and, to a lesser extent, the thymus.

The bone marrow and spleen provide ideal environments for red cell and hemoglobin formation. In both there are nonanastomosing arterial capillaries emptying into a rich plexus of venous sinusoids. By virtue of sluggish circulation and blood stasis, a relatively high carbon dioxide tension develops, a factor of primary importance in the elaboration of hemoglobin and in formation of the primordial cell.

*Appearance of blood elements.* The mesenchyme is regarded as the essential blood-forming tissue of the embryo, corresponding to fixed connective tissue cells in the adult organism. The hemocytoblast, a derivative of the mesenchyme, is the primitive totipotent cell, the main function of which is involved in hematopoiesis. This early cell, frequently ameboid in embryos, represents the precursor of red blood cells, granular leukocytes, lymphocytes, and megakaryocytes.[22,28]

There are fluctuations in blood cellular elements relative to placental size. The placenta is six times heavier than the fetus at 1 month and only one-seventh the fetal weight at birth.[5] In the smallest fetus studied by Playfair and associates,[47] 1.9 cm. long, 99% of the red cells were nucleated. By 6 cm. (12 weeks) the nucleated counts varied from 10,000 to 100,000 per cubic millimeter and fell steadily thereafter. At term about 0.2% of the red cells were nucleated. Myelocytes were found in the 1.9 cm. fetus and mature granulocytes in a 4.2 cm. fetus. Eosinophils were found in a 6.4 cm. fetus and increased regularly with the size of the fetus (to 17 cm. at 20 weeks). In the 1.9 cm. fetus 57% of the white cells were lymphocytes, in no way distinguishable from normal adult small lymphocytes. They continued to rise with age until in a fetus of about 17 to 22 cm. (20 to 25 weeks) the highest counts were recorded in some over 10,000 per cubic millimeter. Monocytes were found in the smallest fetuses and at all subsequent ages. Proerythroblasts were seen frequently, as well as the bare nuclei suspicious of megakaryocytes.

In another study on the blood of fifty-three human fetuses and newborn infants,[56] the changes in the erythrocyte content and hemoglobin concentration and the pattern of change of the nucleated cell content were analyzed. The erythrocyte content and hemoglobin concentration per unit volume of blood and the packed-cell volume increased throughout development. Between the twelfth and twenty-fifth weeks of gestation, the erythrocyte content per unit volume of blood was more than doubled. The increase in red cells occurred very rapidly during the first half of gestation and thereafter proceeded more gradually until a secondary rapid increase occurred in the third trimester. Nucleated red cells numbered up to 50,000 per cubic millimeter during the twelfth week. They decreased in number until midgestation, when there were only about 1,000 per cubic millimeter of blood. The cells then remained at this level until term. During the first half of gestation there were very few circulating leukocytes. From the tenth to the twenty-fifth week of gestation the lymphocyte count increased rapidly. After the twenty-fifth week the increase proceeded more slowly. The blood contained very few granulocytes before the twenty-sixth week, but at term normal adult values were reached and exceeded.

ERYTHROCYTES. In each area of blood formation the erythroblasts multiply rapidly by mitosis and, as they mature, manifest in sequence the generation of hemoglobin, condensation and subsequent loss of the nucleus, and final entrance into the circulation. In the first 6 weeks of gestation practically all red cells are nucleated. A rapid change to nonnucleated forms occurs during the ninth week and is practically complete by the end of the tenth week.

The very large primitive erythroblasts, representing the first or provisional generation of red cells to appear in the embryo, are replaced by the smaller and more numerous erythroblasts formed in the hepatic period. By the end of the fourth month the primitive cells have entirely disappeared. The fetus triples its red cell mass in the 100 days prior to birth; survival of these young red cells is shorter than that of adult cells.

GRANULOCYTES AND LYMPHOCYTES. Granulocytes, noted initially in the yolk sac and liver, are found in increasing numbers in the fourth month. In the spleen, red cell formation is extremely active initially, but by the fifth month of gestation it gives way to the formation of lymphocytes.[66] In another study[37] it was found that red cells alone were in evidence in the blood for the first 2½ months of intrauterine life. At the end of this time granulocytes made their appearance, with the lymphocytes appearing at the beginning of the fourth month.

MONOCYTES. Although it is still debatable, the origin of monocytes has been relegated to the reticular cells of the reticuloendothelial tissue. From these cells in the liver, lymph nodes, spleen, and marrow, the progenitor of the monocytes, the monoblast, is derived.

PLATELETS. Megakaryocytes are noted in the yolk sac and liver; however, with intensive production of erythroblasts in the liver, granulocytes and, to a lesser extent, megakaryocytes are formed. The latter increase in number as the hepatic period of blood formation becomes more vigorous, but platelet proliferation from megakaryocytes is not active until the bone marrow period.[65] Although platelets appear in the embryo at the same time as megakaryocytes and are derived from them, the origin of the megakaryocytes has been variously traced to hemocytoblasts, reticuloendothelium, are fused histiocyte elements. In extrauterine life evidence has been cited of active platelet formation from megakaryocytes in the lungs as well as the bone marrow.[31]

*Theories of blood formation.* There are two theories as to the origin of blood formation. The monophyletic theory regards the hemocytoblast as the totipotential cell from which all types of blood elements, both red and white, originate. According to the polyphyletic theory, each of the blood cell elements in the peripheral circulation possesses completely differentiated precursors. Myeloblasts are precursors of myelocytes and granulocytes, lymphoblasts of lymphocytes, and monoblasts of monocytes. Reticulocytes and mature erythrocytes are derived from pronormoblasts and the more mature normoblasts. Erythroblasts refer to either megaloblasts or pronormoblasts. The former occur in patients with pernicious anemia. The latter are the progenitors of the normal red cell series. The megakaryoblast and promegakaryocyte are the primitive forms of the mature megakaryocyte.

*Embryonic hemoglobin.* When the blood of early human embryos is studied by electrophoresis, two primitive embryonic hemoglobins are seen.[29,32] They are termed *Gower 1* and *Gower 2*. The Gower hemoglobins contain a unique type of polypeptide chain called the epsilon chain. Gower 1 is the predominant hemoglobin in early embryonic life and has the structure $\epsilon_4$. Gower 2 consists of two alpha chains and two epsilon chains, $a_2 \epsilon_2$. The faster moving fraction is Gower 1. In embryos of 4 to 8 weeks gestation, the Gower hemoglobins predominate but have disappeared by the third month. The concentration of these embryonic hemoglobins is highest in the smallest embryos.

*Fetal hemoglobin.* The earliest evidence of a difference between fetal and maternal hemoglobin was the greater resistance to alkaline denaturation observed in fetal hemoglobin. Fetal hemoglobin constitutes about 45 to 90% of the hemoglobin of the infant at birth and is rapidly replaced within the first year by adult hemoglobin. Normally, about 15% fetal hemoglobin persists to the age of 1 year, 5% to 2 years, and less than 2% after the age of 4 years.[17] It is rarely demonstrable 30 months after birth. Occasionally, a child continues to have small quantities of alkali-resistant hemoglobin as late as 4 years of age.[17]

Thus by the eighth gestational week fetal hemoglobin is the predominant hemoglobin. By the sixth month approximately 90% of the hemoglobin is HbF; after this time a gradual decline occurs. Also by the sixth month small quantities (5 to 10%) of adult hemoglobin are present, increasing steadily and averaging 30% at term (Fig. 1).

The percentage of fetal hemoglobin in cord blood is less variable when determined by chromatography[6] than by the method of alkali denaturation. By chromatography the fetal hemoglobin percentage of full-term infants is relatively narrow—79 to 91%, with an average of 85.5%. In a small number of premature infants born before 37 weeks, the fetal hemoglobin was 91% or greater. As a matter of fact, a value of 91% of fetal hemoglobin is a point that divides the premature from mature infants with few exceptions.

While fetal hemoglobin is found in early fetuses (9 to 13½ weeks) in large concentration, some adult hemoglobin is also present at that time.[26] Adult hemoglobin has even been observed in the 13-week fetus.[60] In a 20-week fetus 94% of the hemoglobin is still the fetal type. Adult hemoglobin[12] appears to increase very slowly with development, and it is not possible to assign any morphologically discrete sites of origin to the two pigments. The change from fetal to adult erythropoiesis is a gradual one and is probably the result of a gene-controlled maturation of the intracellular synthetic mechanism.[26]

Cook and co-workers[19] have shown that, in infants born after more than 34 weeks of gestation, there is an inverse relation between gestational age and percentage of fetal hemoglobin. Most infants born after less than 36 weeks of gestation had more than 90% fetal hemoglobin at birth, and those born after 36 weeks usually had less than 90% at birth. After 34 weeks of gestation the percentage of fetal hemoglobin drops approximately to 3 or 4% per week prenatally, which is similar to the postnatal weekly decrease.

Fetal hemoglobin may occasionally be found in substantial amounts in healthy persons. This condition, referred to as the "hereditary per-

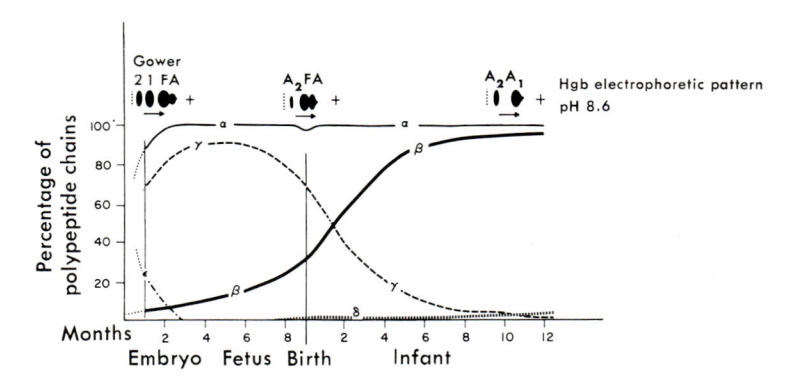

**Fig. 1.** Proportions of the various human polypeptide chains through early life. The hemoglobin electrophoretic pattern typical for each period is also shown. (From Pearson, H. A.: Recent advances in hematology, J. Pediat. 69:466, 1966.)

sistence of fetal hemoglobin" and sometimes as the "high fetal gene," is a specific inherited anomaly manifested throughout life by the presence of large amounts of fetal hemoglobin in the red cells without coexisting anemia or clinical manifestations. Such persons are usually heterozygous for this condition (A-F) and have, on the average, 26% fetal hemoglobin in red cell hemolysates.[18] This anomaly of hemoglobin is apparently caused by a mutant gene that inhibits the synthesis of normal hemoglobins A and $A_2$. First discovered in Nigeria,[24] hereditary persistence of fetal hemoglobin has been encountered in Negroes in Uganda, Jamaica, and the United States, and in a single Causasian family. This anomaly is usually encountered in the heterozygous state, rarely in the homozygous state.[62] It is to be differentiated from other disorders in which fetal hemoglobin may persist in adult life, notably in thalassemia, which it closely resembles. The oxygen dissociation curve is adult in type even when the fetal hemoglobin content is as high as 70%. Characteristically, the distribution of fetal hemoglobin of this type among the red cells is relatively uniform.[57] This remarkably uniform distribution of fetal hemoglobin is unique and is not observed in any other condition in which increased levels of fetal hemoglobin occur, including that present in cord blood. (See Chapter 16 for further discussion of the hereditary persistence of fetal hemoglobin.)

A method has been evolved for differentiating fetal hemoglobin (HbF) from adult hemoglobin (HbA).[36] Exposure of the blood

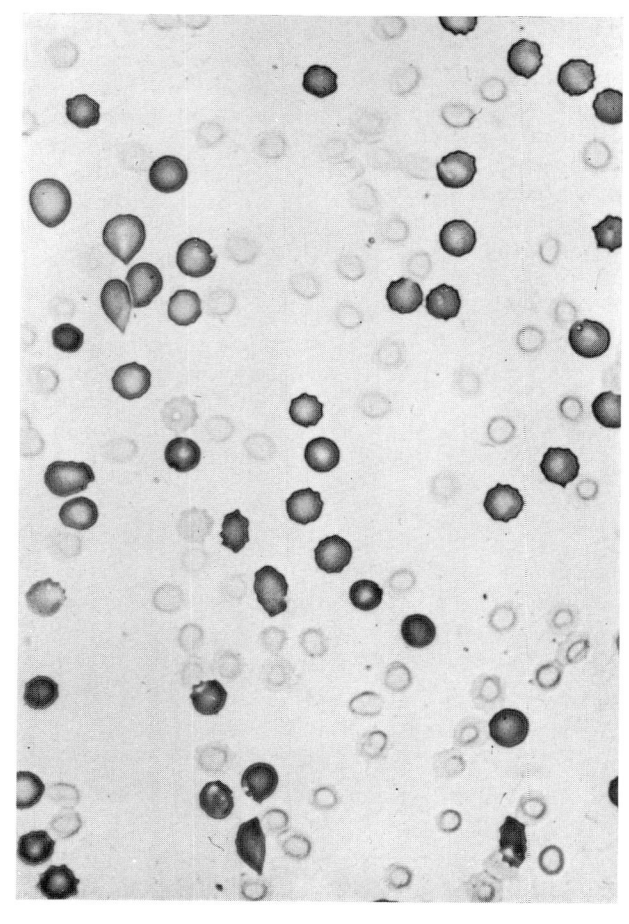

**Fig. 2.** Blood smear prepared from a mixture of adult and cord blood and treated by the acid elution technique (see text). The dark-staining cells contain fetal hemoglobin; the ghostlike cells contain adult hemoglobin. (Courtesy Dr. Alvin Zipursky, Manitoba, Canada.)

smear to citric acid–phosphate buffer results in elution of adult hemoglobin (Fig. 2). Fetal hemoglobin remains in the fetal red cells, which stand out as dark refractile granules. Utilizing this technique, it is observed that there is little change in HbF concentration during the first 4 weeks of life. This is due presumably to the almost total absence of erythrocyte production in the first weeks of life.[67] Erythrocytes containing mostly HbA are produced after 4 weeks of age, resulting in a decrease in the blood concentration of HbF.

All erythropoietic cells have the potential of producing both HbA and HbF. Before birth the production of HbF is favored, whereas after birth HbA is preferentially formed. The HbF concentration in erythrocytes is high at birth, but decreases to low levels by 6 months of age. The amount of HbF relative to that of HbA may vary from cell to cell, with a high value at birth and lower values in the older infant. The stimulus for HbF production is potentially present into adult life. As will be mentioned later (Chapters 3 and 10), in fetal-maternal transfusion during pregnancy and labor this method of differentiating is ideally suited to determine the presence of fetal red cells in the maternal circulation.

Fetal hemoglobin differs characteristically from hemoglobin A. It has four isoleucine residues per molecule, an amino acid notably absent from hemoglobin A.[54] Fetal hemoglobin has two alpha chains and two gamma chains, the latter substituting for the beta chains of normal adult hemoglobin.

The following is Queenan's[49] modification of the Kleihauer-Betke Stain (acid elution).
I. Solutions
  A. 80% ethyl alcohol—prepare each week
  B. Citric acid buffer—once buffer is prepared, it should be refrigerated
    1. Use equal parts of following solutions to give a pH of 3.5
      a. Citric acid monohydrate, 29.294 gm./1,000 ml. $H_2O$
      b. Sodium phosphate dibasic, 17.202 gm./1,000 ml. $H_2O$
    2. Before each use, pH and bacterial growth should be checked
    3. Warm in waterbath to 37° C. before staining
  C. Hematoxylin-Ehrlich (Harleco stain No. 636 X) acid alum solution
  D. 1.5% erythrosin "B" aqueous solution

II. Technique
  A. Make very thin direct smears; control smears consist of part cord and part adult blood
    1. Dry 20 to 30 minutes (not longer)
    2. Do not wash
  B. Fix in alcohol for 5 minutes
    1. Dry for 20 minutes
    2. Do not wash
  C. Immerse in buffer in waterbath of 37° C. for 1 minute
    1. Dry 20 minutes
    2. Do not wash
  D. Stain in hematoxylin for 5 minutes
    1. Wash twice in distilled water
      a. Wash to remove excess stain
      b. Wash for 1 minute
    2. Dry for 20 minutes
  E. Counterstain in erythrosin for 5 minutes
    1. Wash twice in distilled water (as above)
    2. Dry
    3. Fetal blood cells appear as bright purple-pink
    4. Adult blood cells appear as colorless "ghost" cells

*Swallowed blood syndrome.* Blood in stools passed on the second or third day of life may be confused with hemorrhage from the gastrointestinal canal. The blood may be derived from its ingestion during delivery or from a fissure of the mother's nipple. The differentiation between ingested maternal blood and blood of the infant is based on the facts that infant blood contains fetal hemoglobin, which is alkali-resistant, and that maternal blood contains adult hemoglobin, which is promptly changed to alkaline hematin upon the addition of alkali.

The test devised by Apt and Downey[4] to differentiate the two sources of hemoglobin is carried out as follows and is particularly useful only for bright red blood in the stool.

1. One part stool is added to 5 to 10 parts water. A blood-stained diaper may be rinsed, or a grossly bloody stool may be mixed with sufficient water to give a pink supernatant hemoglobin solution.

The authors caution that the stool be grossly bloody (red) and not tarry, for in a tarry stool the oxyhemoglobin has already been converted to hematin.

2. Centrifuge and add 1 ml. 0.25 normal sodium hydroxide (1%) to 5 ml. of supernatant and read. Adult type hemoglobin changes from pink to brown to yellow within 2 min-

utes. A yellow-brown color indicates that the blood is maternal in origin. As a control, perform the test using infant peripheral blood. The fetal hemoglobin solution of infant's blood remains predominantly pink.

*Fetal hemoglobin content as an index of maturity.* The content of fetal hemoglobin has been advanced as an approximate index of maturity, especially in the overmature newborn infant. Cottom[20] observed a close correlation between the percentage of fetal hemoglobin and the period of gestation but not the birth weight. The mean fetal hemoglobin ranged from 90% at 35 weeks of gestation to values below 60% at 42 weeks. A similar observation was made by Abrahamov and associates,[1] who found an average fetal hemoglobin concentration of 85.5% (range, 64.1 to 95%) in the normal control group as compared with an average of 65.1% in the postmature newborn infant (range 54.4 to 76.4%).

Several methods have recently been described to delineate the duration of pregnancy. One method measures the creatinine concentration of amniotic fluid,[63] and the other the percentage of radioactive fetal hemoglobin synthesized by immature red cells in vitro.[10] With the latter method, the ratio of fetal hemoglobin synthesis to total hemoglobin synthesis was significantly higher in growth-retarded infants than in infants who were appropriate in weight for gestational ages.

*Fetal blood and oxygen dissociation.* Fetal blood takes up oxygen at a tension at which it is relinquished by maternal blood, a mechanism of distinct advantage to the fetus. Eastman and associates[23] found that at gas tensions between 25 and 60 mm. Hg fetal blood absorbs oxygen more effectively and that at all gas tensions it releases carbon dioxide more readily than does the blood of the mother. The dissociation curve of fetal blood thus is displaced to the left as compared with that of the pregnant and nonpregnant woman, a circumstance favorable to the uptake of oxygen by the fetus in utero.[42] Barcroft[7,8] suggested that the greater affinity for oxygen of fetal blood than maternal blood depends upon the fetal type of hemoglobin, a type which was thought to acquire oxygen readily and shed it with difficulty. The greater affinity for oxygen is shared by the fetal hemoglobin of other vertebrates, including chickens, rabbits, goats, and sheep.[9]

Although it is true that the fetal type of hemoglobin differs chemically from normal adult hemoglobin (see discussion of fetal hemoglobin), evidence that it is responsible for the fetal type of oxygen dissociation is inconclusive. Prepared hemoglobin solutions from fetal and maternal blood posses similar affinities for oxygen.[3] It has not yet been determined whether fetal hemoglobin residing within the intact erythrocytes absorbs oxygen at low concentrations more effectively than normal blood. The properties ascribed to fetal blood possibly may depend upon factors inherent in the intact red cell in which fetal hemoglobin plays an influential part.

On the other hand, the differences in oxygen uptake in the fetal as compared with the adult red cells may be due to properties in the red cells or plasma exclusive of fetal hemoglobin. It is also conceivable that differences in thickness or thinness of the maternal and fetal red cells may account for the peculiarities of oxygen dissociation and uptake in fetal life. On this basis the maternal red cells, which are thinner than those of the fetus,[66] would promote oxygen transfer to the fetus,[58] where it would be retained because of the greater red cell thickness.

Battaglia and associates[11] have recently offered an explanation for these discrepancies. They showed if red cells of fetal and adult blood are packed and lysed, the oxygen dissociation curve of each is shifted to the left but the difference between adult and fetal blood is maintained. The shift of both adult and fetal blood on lysis can be accounted for by the gradient of pH across the red cell membrane and the loss of this gradient on lysis.

The difference in oxygen affinity between concentrated solutions of adult and fetal hemoglobin produced by lysis of packed red cells disappears on dialysis of these hemoglobin solutions. This work suggested that the adult red cell stroma contains a low molecular weight component that lowers the oxygen affinity of adult hemoglobin.

This puzzle regarding the difference in oxygen affinity between fetal and maternal blood has now been solved with the recent discovery of the function of 2,3 diphosphoglycerate (DPG) present in mammalian red cells.[14-16] This small phosphate molecule functions by complexing hemoglobin in the deoxygenated state, a reaction that inhibits oxygen binding but facilitates its unloading at physiologic oxygen tensions. The reason for the difference in oxygen affinity between fetal and maternal blood lies in the presence of DPG. It has been shown that, although the concentration of DPG in the two types of blood is not significantly different, the affinity of DPG for fetal deoxyhemoglobin is substantially less than for the adult pigment. According to Benesch[13] the DPG which serves as an essential cofactor of the oxygen carrier also confers a lower oxygen affinity on the mother's blood as compared with that of the fetus. These results thus provide a molecular basis for a more expeditious transport of oxygen from mother to fetus.

*Fetal hemoglobin in various pathologic conditions.* Studies of cyanotic patients with congenital heart disease have failed to demonstrate increased quantities of fetal hemoglobin.[25] In many of the hemoglobinopathies large concentrations of fetal hemoglobin are regularly present, notably in thalassemia major, and smaller amounts in aplastic anemia.[51] Fetal hemoglobin is also present in increased amounts in occasional cases of myeloid leukemia, addisonian pernicious anemia, spherocytic anemia, nutritional anemia, refractory normoblastic anemia, and megaloblastic anemia due to folic acid deficiency.[12] Increased levels may rarely be a familial or hereditary disorder. It has been shown that anoxia favors the production of fetal hemoglobin in reticulocytes extracted from cord blood.[2]

*Hematologic changes in $D_1$ trisomy syndrome.* In a 27-month-old child with a $D_1$ trisomy syndrome (malformed ears, hemangiomas, microcephaly, and so on), the fetal hemoglobin concentration was 34 and 35% and the $A_2$-hemoglobin was only 1%.[48] The extra chromosome is a large acrocentric of group 13 to 15. The parents and three siblings had less than 3% hemoglobin F. It was postulated that some environmental and/or genetic mechanism, which normally almost completely represses the activity of the structural gene responsible for hemoglobin F production during the early months of life, did not function in this infant. Possibly, loci for hemoglobin F production lie on the trisomic chromosome.

The polymorphonuclear leukocytes in this infant were also peculiar: the nuclei of these cells were clumped and pyknotic, hypersegmentation was frequent, and, in addition, peculiar hooklike appendages of nuclear chromatin were present. Erythrocyte carbonic anhydrase, as assessed by protein staining after starch gel electrophoresis, was also absent in two neonates with this syndrome and abnormally low in a 13-month-old patient.[27] This enzyme (a zinc protein complex) catalyzes the hydrolysis of carbonic acid to carbon dioxide and water, accelerating the release of carbon dioxide. The $HbA_2$ concentration has been found to be decreased in most of these patients. The decrease was greater than could be accounted for by the fetal hemoglobin that was present. These findings may indicate that the structural genes for carbonic anhydrase and for the delta chain of $HbA_2$ (and hence for the beta chain) are on the same chromosome.

Another patient with the same syndrome was reported by Walzer and colleagues.[61] The fetal hemoglobin was 37.5%, and carbonic anhydrase was lower than in normal newborns. Increased numbers of nuclear projections from the polymorphonuclear neutrophils were also present. The multiple congenital anomalies consisted of sloping forehead, micrognathia, low-set ears, elfin appearance, cleft uvula and tip of tongue, systolic murmur, fingers flexed at all joints, and thumbs overlapping dorsum of the third finger. Chromosomal changes of a D/D translocation "trisomy" were found.

Snodgrass and associates[53] reported seven similar cases of the $D_1$ trisomy syndrome and noted additional anomalies: simian palmar creases, a ventricular septal defect, microphthalmia with hypoplasia of the optic nerves, and aplasia of the skin of the scalp.

Not all cases possess all the criteria of the $D_1$ trisomy syndrome. A 10-year-old girl with this syndrome[40] showed an absence of nuclear projections of the polymorphonuclear neutrophils and a normal concentration of fetal hemoglobin. In other respects of somatic and chromosomal anomalies, this case was similar to cases previously reported.

Wilson and co-workers[64] found that, in Down's syndrome (G trisomy), fetal hemoglobin at birth tends to be lower than normal and persists at this level throughout the first several months of life, in contrast to the $D_1$ trisomy in which fetal hemoglobin is markedly increased. While hemoglobin F is decreased, the $A_2$ hemoglobin tends to be increased. These distinctions between normal infants and those with Down's syndrome disappear at 80 days of life.

*The switch mechanism from fetal to adult hemoglobin.* One of the most puzzling aspects of hemoglobin synthesis is the mechanism by which the switch from fetal to adult hemoglobin synthesis takes place at birth and, to a lesser degree, in late fetal life. Also difficult to explain is its persistence at low or high levels in an occasional adult (hereditary persistence of fetal hemoglobin) and its excessive production in the hemoglobinopathies (for example, thalassemia major) and in stress situations (for example, leukemia, aplastic anemia).

This transfer from fetal protein to adult protein is a dynamic change at the molecular level.[33,44] It will be shown in Chapters 4 and 16 that adult hemoglobin contains four polypeptide chains, two alpha and two beta, and that fetal hemoglobin contains two alpha and two gamma chains. These three polypeptide chains are chemically differentiated. It will be seen that the alpha chain is concerned in both fetal and adult hemoglobin synthesis, while the gamma chain is part of the fetal hemoglobin molecule and the beta chain is part of the adult hemoglobin molecule. Alpha chain production remains constant since it is needed for both fetal and adult hemoglobin production. Gamma chains decrease greatly following birth, dropping to almost zero by the time the infant has reached 6 months, while concurrently there is an increase in beta polypeptide chains of adult hemoglobin type. Practically, this means that the alpha chain gene is turned on all the time and the gene controlling gamma chain production is gradually turned off while the beta chain gene is slowly turned on.[33]

This phenomenon has been explained in more complex fashion on the basis of a system of integrated regulator, operator, and structural genes.[34] It is the structural gene that ultimately carries the information to produce peptide chains of specific amino acid sequences. Such a method of switching from fetal to adult hemoglobin production ensures the adult of adult hemoglobin and the fetus of fetal hemoglobin.[33] The problem not yet solved is why a fetal erythroid cell makes gamma chains and few, if any, beta chains, whereas the opposite is true of the erythroid cell after the human being is 6 months old.

Many of the parallels of human hemoglobin synthesis are based on the scheme for the control of protein synthesis proposed by Jacob and Monod.[34] They state that the synthesis of enzymes in bacteria follows a double genetic control. According to their concept, so-called structural genes determine the molecular organization of protein. They postulated a system of functionally specialized genes, the genetic determinants, designated as regulator and operator genes which control the rate of protein synthesis. This is accomplished through the medium of cytoplasmic components or repressors. The latter can either be inactivated (induction) or activated (repression) by specific metabolites. This regulatory plan seems to operate directly at the level of synthesis by the gene of a short-lived intermediate or messenger, which is associated with ribosomes when protein synthesis takes place. In summary, a "gene," according to these workers, connotes a DNA molecule in which the specific self-replicating structure can be translated through unknown mechanisms into specific structures of a polypeptide chain.

In an adult patient with bronchogenic carcinoma, a macrocytic anemia with ineffective erythropoiesis was associated with 35% fetal hemoglobin.[45] There was no hereditary basis for abnormal hemoglobin synthesis or persistence of hemoglobin F. In this report, two other cases are cited in which reactivation of fetal hemoglobin occurred. The hypothesis offered was that malignant tumor cells may synthesize a substance which directly or indirectly interferes with the control of erythropoiesis so that the stem cells revert to production of fetal erythrocytes.

*Relation of cord blood hemoglobin to fetal oxygen saturation.* The mean umbilical cord hemoglobin obtained by most observers ranges between 15.7 and 17.9 gm. per 100 ml. of blood.[41] The wide spread of hemoglobin values observed by Marks and co-workers,[41] extending from 12 to 22 gm. per 100 ml. of blood (95% range of 13.7 to 20.1 gm.) with a mean value of 16.9 gm., is representative of values noted in most series. Marks and colleagues[41] also showed that, whether an infant is born with a cord hemoglobin as low as 13 gm. or as high as 20 gm., the hemoglobin will be established at a level of about 11 gm. at 2 months of age.

Studies of the cord blood from infants of varying age of fetal maturity have been analyzed from the standpoint of influences acting on the fetus before birth. Several factors particularly have been investigated: the state of oxygen saturation, the hemoglobin concentration, and a possible relationship between the two. Walker and Turnbull[59] found that the hemoglobin level during gestation rose steadily from 9 gm. per 100 ml. in the tenth week to 14 or 15 gm. by the twenty-second to the twenty-fourth week. By the thirty-eighth week the mean value was 15.2 gm., and by the fortieth week it was 16.5 gm. When pregnancy was prolonged, this rise continued. By the forty-third week the mean value was 18.8 gm. They interpreted the increasing hemoglobin value as a response to a falling oxygen supply in the fetus and, furthermore, decided that postmaturity was associated with abnormally high hemoglobin levels.

Marks and associates[41] and Rooth and Sjostedt[50] could find no correlation between cord blood hemoglobin and fetal gestation time. The latter were unable to confirm Walker and Turnbull's[59] findings that there is a continuous decrease in oxygen saturation with advancing pregnancy. They found a constant mean hemoglobin level of 17 gm. per 100 ml. from the fortieth to the forty-third week, and during these 4 weeks there was no correlation between cord blood hemoglobin and the duration of pregnancy. On the other hand, MacKay[39] observed the gradual reduction in the oxygen levels of the cord blood in normal pregnancy as term is approached and passed but no relation to hemoglobin levels.

Cook and co-workers[19] also showed that intrauterine hypoxia in the postmature infant was not associated with an increase in percentage of fetal hemoglobin. On the basis of reticulocyte counts and clinical examination, they suggested that increased total concentrations of hemoglobin observed in the postmature infant with prenatal hypoxia are possibly the result of hemoconcentration rather than an erythropoietic response to lack of oxygen.

Despite these conflicting observations, it may be stated that oxygen saturation in the fetus is decreased but that additional data are required with techniques designed to obtain precise intrauterine fetal measurements. At present, additional causes for the variation in cord hemoglobin levels at birth other than the factor of decreased oxygen saturation alone must be sought.

*Survival time of fetal red cells.* It is of interest that the life-span of fetal red cells, when measured by tagging umbilical cord blood at birth with radioactive chromium,[30] is shorter than that of normal adult red cells. There are studies[55] indicating that this difference in survival rates of the adult and of the newborn red cells as determined by $^{51}Cr$ is only apparent since elution of the isotope from cord blood hemoglobin after dialysis is considerably greater than that from adult hemoglobin. The method of a differential agglutination also demonstrates that the survival of red cells from infants is only slightly less than that from adults.[43] By using $^{51}Cr$-tagged erythrocytes and autotransfusion or heterotransfusion methods, red cell survival of premature and full-term infants was also found at normal adult levels during the first week of life but was reduced at the second and third months.[35]

According to Pearson,[46] the life-span of red cells from newborn infants has been shown to be only two-thirds of that of normal adult red cells. On the basis of the published $^{51}Cr$ data, the life-span of fetal red cells is about 70 days. The precise site of attachment of $^{51}Cr$ is on the beta chains of adult hemoglobin and the gamma chains of fetal hemoglobin. Pearson's studies have shown that the mean red cell survival of fetal red cells is 60 to 80 days.

*Fetal myoglobin.* Human myoglobin may also be separated into fetal and adult types. Fetal human myoglobin (MbF) exhibits a distinct spectroscopic and electrophoretic behavior which is different from that of adult muscle pigment (MbA). The muscles of premature and normal newborn infants contain only MbF, which is gradually replaced by MbA within the first 6 months of life, comparable in sequence to the period of disappearance of fetal red cell hemoglobin from the bloodstream.[52] The purpose and function of both the fetal hemoglobins and myoglobins have not been definitely established.

Myoglobin is a single polypeptide chain of 153 amino acids to which is attached a single heme group.[38] Like hemoglobin, it acts not only by oxidation or reduction of its iron but by becoming oxygenated and deoxygenated. In hemoglobin, as in myoglobin, when oxygen pressure is high an oxygen molecule is attached to the ferrous atom in the center of the heme group. Of the approximately 4 gm. of iron in an adult, 4% resides in myoglobin.

*Bone marrow at birth, infancy, and childhood.* At birth the bone marrow assumes the role of the dominant hematopoietic organ, but the potencies of mesenchymal cells or of their reticular derivatives in the connective tissues for blood formation persist throughout life. In older infants and children, in whom the usual blood sites are strained, as in those with the hereditary hemolytic diseases and leukemia, compensatory hematopoiesis occurs quite readily in the liver and in the spleen.

So active is the demand for blood cell formation that in the infant and young child all the bones are filled with red marrow. Fat appears in the long bones at about 5 to 7 years of age, although incipient changes may occur during infancy. From that time until about the age of 20 years, a gradual retrogression occurs so that active marrow is eventually restricted to the trunk (ribs, sternum, and vertebrae) and proximal portions of the femur and humerus. Red marrow is also found in the clavicles, scapulas, skull, and pelvis.[21] With the appearance of nonfunctioning yellow marrow, a potential reservoir is created for active blood formation in periods of stress.

## REFERENCES

1. Abrahamov, A., Salzberger, M., and Bromberg, M.: Fetal hemoglobin in postmature newborn infants, Amer. J. Clin. Path. 26:146, 1956.
2. Allen, D. W., and Jandl, J.: Factors influencing relative rates of synthesis of adult and fetal hemoglobin in vitro, J. Clin. Invest. 39:1107, 1960.
3. Allen, D. W., Wyman, J., Jr., and Smith, C. A.: The oxygen equilibrium of fetal and adult human hemoglobin, J. Biol. Chem. 203:81, 1953.
4. Apt, L., and Downey, W. S., Jr.: "Melena" neonatorum: the swallowed blood syndrome. A simple test for the differentiation of adult and fetal hemoglobin in bloody stools, J. Pediat. 47:5, 1955.
5. Arey, L. B.: Developmental anatomy—a textbook and laboratory manual of embryology, ed. 6, Philadelphia, 1954, W. B. Saunders Co.
6. Armstrong, D. H., Schroeder, W., and Fenninger, W. D.: A comparison of the percentage of fetal hemoglobin in human umbilical cord blood as determined by chromatography and by alkali denaturation, Blood 22:554, 1963.
7. Barcroft, J.: Conditions of fetal respiration, Lancet 2:1021, 1933.
8. Barcroft, J.: Fetal circulation and respiration, Physiol. Rev. 16:103, 1936.
9. Barcroft, J.: Researches on pre-natal life, vol. 1, Springfield, Ill., 1947, Charles C Thomas, Publisher.
10. Bard, H., Makowski, E. L., Meschia, G., and Battaglia, F. C.: The relative rates of synthesis of hemoglobins A and F in immature red cells of newborn infants, Pediatrics 45:766, 1970.
11. Battaglia, F. C., Hellegers, A. E., Behrman, R. E., and Seeds, A. F.: Correlation of the oxygen dissociation curves of adult and fetal hemoglobin solutions with the $H^+$ ion concentration gradients of adult and fetal red blood cells, J. Pediat. 65:1101, 1964.
12. Beaven, G. H., Ellis, M. J., and White, J. C.: Studies on human foetal haemoglobin. II. Foetal haemoglobin levels in healthy children and adults and in certain haematological disorders, Brit. J. Haemat. 6:201, 1960.
13. Benesch, R.: How do small molecules do great things? New Eng. J. Med. 280:1179, 1969.
14. Benesch, R., and Benesch, R. E.: The effect of organic phosphates from the human erythrocyte on the allosteric properties of hemoglobin, Biochem. Biophys. Res. Commun. 26:167, 1967.
15. Benesch, R., and Benesch, R. E.: Intracellular organic phosphates as regulators of oxygen release by haemoglobin, Nature 221:618, 1969.
16. Chanutin, A., and Curnish, R. R.: Effect of organic and inorganic phosphates on the oxygen equilibrium of human erythrocytes, Arch. Biochem. Biophys. 121:96, 1967.
17. Chernoff, A. I., and Singer, K.: Studies on abnormal hemoglobins; persistence of fetal hemoglobin in erythrocytes of normal children, Pediatrics 9:469, 1952.
18. Conley, C. L., Weatherall, D. J., Richardson, S. N., Shepard, M. K., and Charache, S.: Hereditary persistence of fetal hemoglobin; a study of 79 affected persons in 15 Negro families in Baltimore, Blood 21:261, 1963.
19. Cook, C. D., Brodie, H. R., and Allen, D. W.: Measurement of fetal hemoglobin in newborn infants, Pediatrics 20:272, 1957.
20. Cottom, D. G.: Foetal haemoglobin and postmaturity, J. Obstet. Gynaec. Brit. Comm. 62:945, 1955.
21. Custer, R. P.: An atlas of the blood and bone marrow, Philadelphia, 1949, W. B. Saunders Co.
22. Downey, H.: Handbook of hematology, New York, 1938, Paul B. Hoeber, Inc.
23. Eastman, N. J., Geiling, E. M. K., and DeLawder, A. M.: Foetal blood studies; oxygen and carbon-dioxide dissociation curves of foetal blood, Bull. Johns Hopkins Hosp. 53:246, 1933.
24. Edington, G. M., and Lehmann, H.: Expression of the sickle-cell gene in Africa, Brit. Med. J. 2:1328, 1955.
25. Farrar, J. F., and Blomfield, J.: Alkali-resistant haemoglobin content of blood in congenital heart disease, Brit. J. Haemat. 9:278, 1963.

26. Fraser, I. D., and Raper, A. B.: Observations on the change from foetal to adult erythropoiesis, Arch. Dis. Child. 37:289, 1962.
27. Gerald, P. S., Walzer, S., and Diamond, L. K.: Location of the genetic elements controlling the hematologic changes in the $D_1$ trisomy, Blood 24:836, 1964.
28. Gilmour, J. R.: Normal hemopoiesis in intrauterine and neonatal life, J. Path. Bact. 52:25, 1941.
29. Hecht, F., Motulsky, A. G., Lemire, R. J., and Shepard, T. E.: Predominance of hemoglobin Gower 1 in early human embryonic development, Science 152:91, 1966.
30. Hollingsworth, J. W.: Life span of fetal erythrocytes, J. Lab. Clin. Med. 45:469, 1955.
31. Howell, W. H., and Donahue, D. D.: The production of blood platelets in the lungs, J. Exp. Med. 65:177, 1937.
32. Huehns, E. R., Dance, N., Beaven, G. H., Keil, J. V., Hecht, F., and Motulsky, A. G.: Human embryonic haemoglobin, Nature 201:1095, 1964.
33. Ingram, V. M.: The hemoglobins in genetics and evolution, New York, 1963, Columbia University Press.
34. Jacob, F., and Monod, J.: Genetic regulatory mechanisms in synthesis of proteins, J. Molec. Biol. 3:318, 1961.
35. Kaplan, E.: Studies of red cell survival in early infancy, Amer. J. Dis. Child. 98:603, 1959.
36. Kleihauer, E., Braun, H., and Betke, K.: Demonstration von fetalem Hemoglobin in den Erythrocyten eines Blutausstrichs, Klin. Wchnschr. 35:637, 1957.
37. Knoll, W.: Untersuchungen über embryonale Blutlidung beim Menschen, Ztschr. mikr. Anat. 18:199, 1929.
38. Lehmann, H., and Huntsman, R. G.: Man's haemoglobins; including the haemoglobinopathies and their investigation, Philadelphia, 1966, J. B. Lippincott Co.
39. MacKay, R. B.: Observations on the oxygenation of the foetus in normal and abnormal pregnancy, J. Obstet. Gynaec. Brit. Comm. 64:185, 1957.
40. Marden, P. M., and Yunis, J. J.: Trisomy $D_1$ in a 10-year-old girl. Normal neutrophils and fetal hemoglobin, Amer. J. Dis. Child. 114:662, 1967.
41. Marks, J., Gairdner, D., and Roscoe. J. D.: Blood formation in infancy. III. Cord blood, Arch. Dis. Child. 30:117, 1955.
42. McCarthy, E. F.: Oxygen affinity of human maternal and foetal haemoglobin, J. Physiol. 102:55, 1943.
43. Mollison, P. L.: Blood transfusion in clinical medicine, Springfield, Ill., 1956, Charles C Thomas, Publisher.
44. Neel, J. V.: The hemoglobin gene; a remarkable example of the clustering of related genetic functions on a single mammalian chromosome, Blood 18:769, 1961.
45. Nyman, M., Skölling, R., and Steiner, H.: Acquired macrocytic anemia and hemoglobinopathy—a paraneoplastic manifestation? Amer. J. Med. 48:792, 1970.
46. Pearson, H. A.: Life-span of the fetal red blood cell, J. Pediat. 70:166, 1967.
47. Playfair, J. H. L., Wolfendale, M. R., and Kay, E. H. M.: The leukocytes of peripheral blood in the human fetus, Brit. J. Haemat. 9:336, 1963.
48. Powars, D., Rohde, R., and Graves, D.: Foetal haemoglobin and neutrophil anomaly in the $D_1$-trisomy syndrome, Lancet 1:1363, 1964.
49. Queenan, J. T.: Modern management of the Rh problem, New York, 1967, Harper & Row, Publishers.
50. Rooth, G., and Sjostedt, S.: Haemoglobin in cord blood in normal and prolonged pregnancy, Arch. Dis. Child. 32:91, 1957.
51. Shahidi, N. T., Gerald, P. S., and Diamond, L. K.: Alkali-resistant hemoglobin in aplastic anemia of both acquired and congenital types, New Eng. J. Med. 266:117, 1962.
52. Singer, K., Angelopoulos, B., and Ramot, B.: Studies on human myoglobin. II. Fetal myoglobin; its identification and its replacement by adult myoglobin during infancy, Blood 10:987, 1955.
53. Snodgrass, G. J. A., Butler, L. J., France, M. E., Crome, L., and Russel, A.: The "D" (13-15) trisomy syndrome: an analysis of 7 examples, Arch. Dis. Child. 41:250, 1966.
54. Stein, W. H., Kunkel, H. G., Cole, R. D., Spackman, D. H., and Moore, S.: Observations on the amino acid composition of human hemoglobins, Biochim. Biophys. Acta 24:640, 1957.
55. Suderman, H. J., White, F. D., and Israels, L. G.: Elution of chromium-51 from labeled hemoglobins of human adult and cord blood, Science 126:650, 1957.
56. Thomas, D. B., and Yoffey, J. M.: Human foetal haemopoiesis. I. The cellular composition of foetal blood, Brit. J. Haemat. 8:290, 1962.
57. Thompson, R. B., Mitchner, J. W., and Huisman, T. H. J.: Studies on the fetal hemoglobin in the persistent high HbF anomaly, Blood 18:267, 1961.
58. Valtis, D. J., and Baikie, A. G.: The influence of red cell thickness on the oxygen dissociation curve of blood, Brit. J. Haemat. 1:152, 1955.
59. Walker, J., and Turnbull, E. P. N.: Haemo-

globin and red cells in the human foetus, Lancet **2**:312, 1953.
60. Walker, J., and Turnbull, E. P. N.: Haemoglobin and red cells in the human foetus. III. Foetal and adult haemoglobin, Arch. Dis. Child. **30**:111, 1955.
61. Walzer, S., Gerald, P. S., Breau, G., O'Neill, D., and Diamond, L. K.: Hematologic changes in the $D_1$ trisomy syndrome, Pediatrics **38**:419, 1966.
62. Wheeler, J. T., and Krevans, J. R.: The homozygous state of persistent fetal hemoglobin and the interaction of persistent fetal hemoglobin with thalassemia, Bull. Johns Hopkins Hosp. **109**:217, 1961.
63. White, C. A., Doorenbos, D. E., and Brandbury, J. T.: Role of chemical and cytologic analysis of amniotic fluid in determination of fetal maturity, Amer. J. Obstet. Gynec. **104**:664, 1969.
64. Wilson, M. G., Schroeder, W. A., Graves, D. A., and Kach, Y. D.: Postnatal change of hemoglobins F and A in infants with Down's syndrome (G trisomy), Pediatrics **42**:349, 1968.
65. Windle, W. F.: Physiology of the fetus, Philadelphia, 1940, W. B. Saunders Co.
66. Wintrobe, M. M.: Clinical hematology, Philadelphia, 1956, Lea & Febiger.
67. Zipursky, A., Neelands, P. J., Pollock, J., Chown, B., and Israels, L. G.: The distribution of fetal hemoglobin in the blood of normal children and adults, Pediatrics **30**:262, 1962.

# 2  BLOOD CHANGES DURING GROWTH—
POSTNATAL PERIOD, INFANCY, AND CHILDHOOD

Knowledge of the normal blood values in the growing period is a prerequisite to the interpretation of a particular blood response in infancy and childhood. For this reason the normal changes in hematologic values for each of the developmental periods are included in this discussion. It is recognized that the values to be cited are subject to wide variations, both in each individual and among members of an age group. These values are given as yardsticks based on experience and in terms of which abnormalities of graded severity may be judged and are in general agreement with the data available in standard texts and articles dealing with this subject.*

*Blood changes in the newborn infant.* During the first week of life the decline in hemoglobin and red cells in the peripheral blood is at a minimum. Following this initial stationary period, a definite decline sets in. The postnatal adjustment is characterized by a normal or slightly increased rate of blood destruction accompanied by diminished or stationary hematopoietic activity. During this period the drop in red cells occurs within the limits of normal survival—100 to 120 days or approximately 0.8% per day. The changes are usually orderly and gradual and appear to be directed toward the establishment of hematopoietic equilibrium designed to function at a lower level than exists at birth. Although hemolysis accounts for the fall in hemoglobin and red cells, the continued drop represents a diminished rate of compensatory regeneration. The fall in hemoglobin represents a gradual adjustment to the increased oxygen saturation of the blood which prevails when the lung replaces the placenta as a source of oxygen. Gairdner and co-workers[11] believe that erythrogenesis ceases when the oxygen saturation at birth is elevated from about 65% in the umbilical vein to 95% a few hours after birth. Accordingly, red cell formation is at a minimum until the hemoglobin level reaches 11 to 12 gm. per 100 ml., when regeneration sets in. This regulation by the arterial oxyhemoglobin level implies that during the neonatal period decreases below 11 to 12 gm. per 100 ml. induce hematopoietic activity, whereas elevations above 11 to 12 gm. tend to decrease bone marrow activity. Increased reticulocyte formation can be observed in the anemic infant in the first days of life, presumably from blood loss during delivery or the seepage of blood into the maternal circulation. Neerhout[39] has presented data on the erythrocyte lipid composition of cord blood samples of forty-two healthy, full-term infants. When compared to the erythrocytes of the adult, cord blood erythrocytes showed an increased amount of total lipid, phospholipid, and cholesterol per cell. He suggested that the susceptibility of neonatal erythrocytes to hemolysis in dilute hydrogen peroxide may be related to the increased amount of total lipid in the red cell stroma and therefore a limited ability to detoxify this substance.

Carbonic anhydrase is a zinc metalloenzyme which is important in the physiologic transport of carbon dioxide. Less carbonic anhydrase activity has been found in blood obtained from newborn infants than in that from adults, and even lower enzyme activity in blood from premature infants.[27,44] Results of assay showed that normal full-term newborn infants had approximately 25% of the enzymatic activity of adults. Premature infants without the respiratory distress syndrome averaged 13% of the adult enzyme activity; those with the respiratory distress syndrome averaged 5% of adult activity. The reasons for the decreased blood carbonic anhydrase activity in infants with respiratory distress are not clear. At any rate, if there is insufficient enzyme catalysis, this conversion of bicarbonate to carbon dioxide will be

---
*See references 3, 18, 22, 25, 30, 32, 34, 37, 54-56, and 61.

slowed to the degree that equilibrium will not be attained in the short time that the blood is in the pulmonary capillaries.

Zinc deficiency per se cannot explain the low enzyme activity in infants with this syndrome because these infants have as much zinc as infants without the disease.

Two carbonic anhydrase fractions designated B and C can be readily seen in starch-gel electrophoretic patterns of human red cell lysates stained for proteins.[57] Both isozymes are lower in infancy and reach their adult intensity at the second to third year of life. Enzyme B is markedly reduced in patients with thyrotoxicosis and elevated in hypothyroidism, returning to normal after treatment. Carbonic anhydrase activity is markedly elevated in red cells from patients with megaloblastic anemia secondary to vitamin $B_{12}$ deficiency and is probably elevated in folic acid deficiency.

*Physiologic anemia of the newborn infant.* Physiologic anemia of the newborn infant occurs in the first 2 or 3 months of life when the red cells and hemoglobin drop concurrently and in equal degrees. The erythrocytes are normocytic and normochromic and there is no excessive reticulocytosis. This decline proceeds in an orderly fashion and is not accelerated by hyperhemolysis unless pathologic factors set in. Following this neonatal adjustment, hemoglobin reaches its lowest level at 6 weeks to 2 months of age and remains fairly constant for the remainder of infancy. During the first 2 years of life, the hemoglobin usually ranges from approximately 10 to 12 gm. per 100 ml. of blood.

*Bone marrow changes.* During the first week of life when the decline in hemoglobin and red cells is at a minimum, a marked drop in nucleated red cells occurs in the bone marrow. The lowest levels are reached between the end of the first week and the fourth week of life, with a considerable increase in cells following this period. For example, Shapiro and Bassen[49] found that on the first day of life the percentage of myeloid cells (neutrophils, myelocytes, and myeloblasts) averages 61% and nucleated red cells 32%. On the eighth day the myeloid percentage increases to 77%, whereas the erythroid elements drop sharply to 12%. At about 2 months of age, as the marrow erythroid activity returns, the peripheral blood shows an increase in reticulocytes and a rise in hemoglobin.

Gairdner and co-workers[10] found in the bone marrow of the full-term infant 40% erythroid cells on the first day of life, 15% from 3 to 5 days, 8% from 8 to 10 days, 7% from 26 to 33 days, 15% from 55 to 62 days, and 16% from 82 to 99 days. The total cellularity of the bone marrow averaged 136,000 per cubic millimeter on the first day, 35,000 per cubic millimeter on the ninth day, and 201,000 per cubic millimeter at 3 months.

In Sturgeon's study[51] in five full-term infants between 5 and 13 hours of age, nucleated red cells averaged 36 to 17% between 15 hours to 6 days. Glaser and associates[16] found erythroid values of 32% in the bone marrow on the first and second days, with a gradual drop to 8% on the fifteenth to seventeenth days, after which a rise took place. Stable values of about 23% are reached in the full-term infant by the end of the first month.

Wolman and Dickstein[62] summarized these fluctuations in the full-term infant as follows: On the day of birth nucleated red cells are relatively numerous, ranging from 30 to 65%, falling to 12 to 40% by the seventh day and to 8 to 30% by the fourteenth day, with an average of about 10%. The cells then increase gradually, reaching the normal childhood level of about 20% at 3 to 4 weeks of age.

Lichtenstein and Nordenson[31] observed in a series of sixteen premature infants a similar pattern in the bone marrow. The total number of nucleated red cell elements within the first 24 hours varied from 15 to 45%, from 7 to 33.5% on the second day, from 21 to 22% on the fourth day, and averaged 15% on the fifth day. On the first day the values were usually at maximal levels. They also pointed out that bone marrow preparations from premature infants are usually richer in cells than those of full-term infants. In the premature infant there are also irregularities of maturation of the normoblasts which have been interpreted as evidence of functional insufficiency of the marrow. Alison and Prevot-Pignède[4] give the figure of erythroblasts in bone marrow of premature infants as 50 per 100 white blood cells at birth, dropping to 3 to 5 per 100 white blood cells by the third day. Between the fourth and ninth days there are evidences of a rise, which reaches 20 to 25% at the end of the first month.

In twenty-nine marrow examinations of premature infants, Gairdner and co-workers[12] found no differences in the myelograms of premature and normal infants. By relating the marrow count to the hemoglobin level of the marrow they found that as the hemoglobin drops erythropoiesis increases, although the response is a sluggish one. In general, there is an inverse relationship between the marrow erythroid count and hemoglobin concentration of the blood.

Along the same lines, Kalpaktsoglou and Emery[23]

studied the cellularity of the bone marrow in the neonatal period. Their observations were based on the examination of the fifth rib obtained at necropsy of 144 stillborns and infants. They found a rapid change in cellularity of the hematopoietic tissue from an almost equally mixed myeloid and erythroid picture at birth to a predominantly myeloid picture by the end of the third week after birth. There was an immediate diminution of erythroblasts, the number being halved by the end of the first week. This low level persisted for 4 to 6 weeks and then there was a slow, steady increase so that by the end of the twelfth week the birth level had been regained. The marrow of children over 32 weeks' maturity responded to birth in a way identical to that of children born at term. They also found that the marrow hematopoietic tissue reaches a maximum intrauterine level at about 30 weeks' maturity and remains at this level for the last 10 weeks.

*Blood volume.* The blood volume of the full-term infant at birth is approximately 85 ml. per kilogram and that of the premature infant averages 108 ml., the difference being due mainly to an excess of plasma in the latter.[47] Normal blood volumes of 75 to 80 ml. per kilogram, which are the values in the adult, are reached after the second month. In the treatment of erythroblastosis the blood volume for both full-term and premature infants is calculated on the basis of 85 ml. of blood per kilogram.

Iodinated human albumin was used to measure serial blood volume in twenty-seven normal full-term infants. Usher and associates[53] found the blood volume at the moment of birth was 78 ml. per kilogram, with a venous hematocrit of 48%. When the cord clamping was delayed for 5 minutes, the blood volume increased by 61% to 126 ml. per kilogram. This placental transfusion amounted to 166 ml. for a 3,500 gm. infant, one-fourth of which occurred in the first 15 seconds of birth and one-half within 60 seconds. Stripping of the umbilical cord ten times during the 5 minutes did not increase the volume of the transfusion. During the first 4 hours there was a marked decrease from 126 to 89 ml. per kilogram in the blood volume in infants who received a placental transfusion, due to transudation of one-half of the original plasma volume. The venous hematocrit rose from 48% at birth to 64% by 4 hours. No changes in blood volume occurred in the first 4 hours in those infants in whom placental transfusion was prevented by immediate clamping of the cord.

The red cell volume remained stable during the first 3 days of life in each of the infants. Those who received a placental transfusion maintained a red cell volume about 60% larger than those who had not. Average values at 72 hours for infants who had not received a placental transfusion were 82 ml. per kilogram blood volume, 31 ml. per kilogram red blood cell volume, 51 ml. per kilogram plasma volume, and 44% venous hematocrit. Infants who had received a placental transfusion had average values of 93 ml. per kilogram blood volume, 49 ml. per kilogram red blood cell volume, 44 ml. per kilogram plasma volume, and 60% venous hematocrit.

Confirming these results, Lanzkowsky[29] found that at 3 months of age the mean hemoglobin level in the early-clamped infants was 11.08 gm. per 100 ml. and in those clamped later, 11.09 gm. per 100 ml. The advantages of late clamping of the umbilical cord may conceivably be of importance to the premature infant. At the age of 3 months delayed clamping had no demonstrable benefit to the hemoglobin level.

The placental vessels contain approximately 150 ml. of whole blood, with a range of 50 to 200 ml. In infants of diabetic mothers the residual placental blood volume has been found to be at least twice as large as that of control groups.[26] A transfusion of blood usually takes place within seconds of birth, and approximately 45 ml. of this volume may be accommodated in the pulmonary circulation. A contributory cause of the large residual placental blood volume in infants of diabetic mothers seems to be the late onset of respiration and shallow breathing.

*Hemoglobin concentration.* The cord blood hemoglobin varies approximately between 16.6[13] and 17.1 gm. per 100 ml. of blood.[18] In our laboratory the hemoglobin averaged 16.4 gm. per 100 ml., with a range from 14 to 19 gm. per 100 ml.

Gairdner and associates[13] compared the composition of cord blood at birth with venous blood and concluded that the elevation of the hemoglobin level during the first day of life is due to the shift of fluid (whole plasma) from the circulation and is independent of placental blood transfer. The postnatal rise in hemoglobin and packed cell volume, effected by the shift of fluid from the vascular compartment, takes place within a few minutes after birth and is complete within an hour or two, reaching a value of 19.1 gm. per 100 ml. of hemoglobin (S.D., 2.36) in 1 to 8 hours (as compared with 16.6 gm. in cord blood). The extent to which placental blood transfer contributes to this rise has been controversial.

According to Haselhorst and Allmeling,[20] the average amount of blood in the placental vessels is 105 ml., with a range from 50 to 200 ml. Infants receive varying amounts of this blood, depending upon the time after delivery at which the cord is clamped: 51% of the blood reaches the infant in the first minutes after delivery, 79% in 5 minutes, and 91% in the first 10 minutes. It is usually estimated that the placenta contains a reservoir of 125 to 150 ml. of blood and that delayed clamping may account for the addition of as much as 100 ml. of blood to the circulation of the newborn infant. It is claimed[8] that the increased red cell and hemoglobin mass resulting from late clamping becomes apparent after birth only as the plasma volume is readjusted and equalized. DeMarsh and associates[8] observed that hematocrit values were higher for the infants whose placental blood had been allowed to pass into their circulation at birth, averaging 61% on the first day and 60% on the third day. In those infants who failed to receive placental blood, the hematocrit values averaged 50% on the first day and 51% on the third day, practically the same as the average hematocrit reading of the umbilical cord blood, which was 51%. It seems most likely that the placental transfusion of substantial amounts of blood by late clamping of the cord should be reflected in an elevation in hemoglobin soon after birth. In another study[59] no significant difference was found in erythrocyte values in the neonatal period with respect to the time of clamping unless the cord was deliberately stripped.

Blood samples from heel puncture show a higher concentration of hemoglobin than those from the vein. This may be largely due to the stasis in the peripheral blood of newborn macrocytic red cells. Mollison and Cutbush[36] give the following comparative normal hemoglobin values in newborn infants: with cord blood hemoglobin of 13.6 to 19.6 gm. per 100 ml. the venous blood on the first day increases to 14.5 to 22.5 gm., with corresponding skin prick values of 15.4 to 22.8 gm. These variations are important in the management of erythroblastosis (Chapter 10).

The drop in hemoglobin to 11 gm. per 100 ml. of blood in the first 2 years of life is followed by a gradual rise, reaching a maximum at 14 years of 16 gm. for males and 14 gm. for females, with an average of 15 gm. for both sexes. (See Table 1.)

*Erythrocyte count.* The red cell count is high at birth and averages 5.5 million, with a range from 5 to 6 million per cubic milli-

Table 1. Normal blood values at different ages*

| Age | Hemoglobin (gm./100 ml.) | RBC per cu. mm. | Hematocrit PRCV/100 ml. (means) | MCV ($\mu^3$) | MCH ($\mu\mu g$) | MCHC (gml/100 ml. packed RBC) |
|---|---|---|---|---|---|---|
| Birth (cord values) | 13.6-19.6 | 5.4 | 56.6 | 106 | 38 | 38 |
| 1 day | 21.2 | 5.6 | 56.1 | 106 | 38 | 38 |
| 1 week | 19.6 | 5.3 | 52.7 | 101 | 37 | 37 |
| 2 weeks | 18.0 | 5.1 | 49.6 | 96 | 35 | 36 |
| 3 weeks | 16.6 | 4.9 | 46.6 | 93 | 34 | 36 |
| 4 weeks | 15.6 | 4.7 | 44.6 | 91 | 33 | 35 |
| 2 months | 13.3 | 4.5 | 38.9 | 85 | 30 | 34 |
| 3 months | 12.5 | 4.5 | 38.0 | 84 | 29 | 34 |
| 4 months | 12.4 | 4.5 | 36.5 | 79 | 27 | 34 |
| 6 months | 12.3 | 4.6 | 36.2 | 78 | 27 | 34 |
| 8 months | 12.1 | 4.6 | 35.8 | 77 | 26 | 34 |
| 10 months | 11.9 | 4.6 | 35.5 | 77 | 26 | 34 |
| 1 year | 11.6 | 4.6 | 35.2 | 77 | 25 | 33 |
| 2 years | 11.7 | 4.7 | 35.5 | 78 | 25 | 33 |
| 4 years | 12.6 | 4.7 | 37.1 | 80 | 27 | 34 |
| 6 years | 12.7 | 4.7 | 37.9 | 80 | 27 | 33 |
| 8 years | 12.9 | 4.7 | 38.9 | 80 | 27 | 33 |
| 10-12 years | 13.0 | 4.8 | 39.0 | 80 | 27 | 33 |
| Adult males | 16.0 | 5.4 | 47.0 | 87 | 29 | 34 |
| Adult females | 14.0 | 4.8 | 42.0 | 87 | 29 | 34 |

*These are averages based on standard sources as well as observations made at The New York Hospital—Cornell Medical Center, New York, N.Y. Table compiled by T. Vats, M.D.

meter. The red cells are macrocytic at birth. They range in size from 8 to 9$\mu$ in diameter, decrease to their smallest size of about 5$\mu$ after 3 to 6 months, and rise to adult dimensions of 7.2 to 7.5$\mu$ at 8 months.

The red blood cells average 4.6 million at the end of the first year and 4.8 million at the end of 12 years. At 14 years of age and over males average 5.4 million red cells per cubic millimeter and females average 4.8 million.

Abnormally high erythrocyte values of unknown etiology were reported at birth in an infant with anorexia, lethargy, cyanosis, and convulsions.[63] The clinical signs subsided when blood was withdrawn and replaced with plasma. No congenital abnormalities were found. The etiology of this syndrome is unknown. Three infants were reported[35] with hematocrits between 73 and 80%, hemoglobin levels of 21 to 25 gm. per 100 ml., and over 7 million red cells between 1 and 9 days of age. Evidence was presented to implicate a maternal-fetal transfusion as the cause of plethora in these infants. The blood types of two of the infants differed from those of the mother, and maternal erythrocytes could be demonstrated in the infant's blood by differential agglutination. Ordinarily a fetus might lose blood into the mother and be born anemic, the pressure gradients within the placenta and uterus favoring such a transfer. Conceivably, an anatomic abnormality in the placentas of the infants accounted for the reverse situation—maternal-fetal transfusion. If cardiovascular collapse threatens in the plethoric newborn infant, gradual removal of blood with or without replacement of plasma may be of value.

Gatti and co-workers[15] reported ten infants with transient plethora and cyanosis in the newborn period. The elevated hematocrit and hemoglobin levels consistent with neonatal polycythemia may have been due to excessive transfusion of placental blood at delivery. While spontaneous improvement generally occurs, phlebotomy on occasion has been therapeutically applied, especially in those with cardiorespiratory distress. In these infants moderate cyanosis is a uniform finding.

The suggestion that neonatal plethora might be due to the passage of the maternal cells into the fetal circulation has been discounted by Cohen and Zuelzer.[7] They conclude that the presence of maternal red cells in the fetal circulation reflects unavoidable contamination of cord blood.

*Twin-to-twin transfusion.* In a reported case polycythemia in one twin and anemia in the other occurred in single-ovum twins with hemoglobin values of 25.2 and 3.7 gm. and red cell counts of 7.47 and 1.85 million per cubic millimeter, respectively.[28] This discrepancy was explained on the basis of an arteriovenous shunt between the supposedly separate placental circulations, which resulted in a parabiotic circulatory system. Unequal functioning between the two circulations accounted for the sharp differences in blood levels. In this case withdrawal of blood from the polycythemic infant was followed by an uneventful course. Usually, newborn polycythemic levels drop to normal spontaneously and without ill effect to the infant. In another newborn infant polycythemic levels with a maximum of 7.5 million red cells per cubic millimeter persisted for 6 weeks before a spontaneous drop to 5 million red cells occurred.[50] Erythremia or polycythemia vera is not known to occur in infancy.

The polycythemic twin is subject to the hazards of hemorrhage, venous thrombosis, cardiac failure, pulmonary edema, and hyperbilirubinemia. Phlebotomy has been recommended over a period of hours or days until the concentration of hemoglobin and hematocrit readings reach a reasonable level.[6,21] The anemic twin is treated with small transfusions to combat shock.

In postmortem examination of eleven pairs of twins,[38] hyaline membrane disease was found to be present in both members of four twin pairs. In the recipient twin myocardial hyperplasia involving all the chambers develops with a corresponding increase of muscle about the arteries of both major circulatory beds. In contrast, small hearts and reduced arterial muscle masses found in the anemic twins suggest a relative hypotension in the circulatory beds. In twins with the syndrome the anemic member is on the arterial side and the polycythemic member on the venous side of one or more placental arteriovenous shunts. The polycythemic twins acquire cardiomegaly and an increase of muscle about the pulmonary and systemic arteries, suggesting antenatal hypertension in both circulatory beds. In contrast, the anemic partner shows evidence of hypotension.

In 130 monochorial twin pregnancies studied in one institution, the twin transfusion syndrome was diagnosed nineteen times.[46] In ten instances both twins were lost in the perinatal period, in five only one twin survived, and in four both twins survived. Most of the deaths occurred in utero early in pregnancy. The twin transfusion syndrome was shown to account for a significant number of the fetal and neonatal deaths in twin pregnancies. It was suggested that surviving uniovular twins subjected to twin transfusion in utero have persistent alterations in comparative growth and development. The twin transfusion syndrome appears to be the cause of a large part of the higher case fatality rate noted in monochorial in contrast to dichorial twin gestation. (See Plate 1.)

**Hematocrit percentage (volume of packed red cells).** The hematocrit obtained after centrifugation of a given amount of blood averages 55% at birth, declines to 30% by the second month, increases to 36% at 1 year of age and 40% at 3 years of age, and achieves normal adult values of about 45% for males and 42% for females in adolescence. Normal children occasionally reveal a marked elevation of hematocrit, red cells, and hemoglobin during adolescence. These changes simulating polycythemia are transient and benign, revert to normal in the postadolescent period, and require no treatment.

The cord blood hematocrit value according to various studies ranges from 51.3 to 56.0%.[42] The hematocrit values together with the hemoglobin values show a sharp increase during the first few hours of life, then slowly decrease, so that by the end of the first week of life they approximate the initial cord blood values. According to one study,[58] the hemoglobin value increases by 17 to 20% of the earliest values during the first 2 hours of life, but then drops slightly during the next 2 hours.

Gatti[14] found that the hematocrit levels of the capillary blood in a large group of healthy newborn infants were 62.9% (S.D. = 3.2) and decreased gradually to 53.7% (S.D. = 2.5) by the tenth day of life. It should be understood that capillary blood is more concentrated than venous blood during the first week of life. At 1 week of age the mean capillary hematocrit level was 57.8% (S.D. = 2.4), which was significantly higher than the mean venous hematocrit level of 55.8% (S.D. = 2.0).

**Size of red cells (MCV) and hemoglobin concentration (MCHC).** The red cells are unusually large at birth, with an average in the cord blood of 113 $\mu^3$ and a range of 90 to 124 $\mu^3$.[19] They diminish in size to a value of 69 $\mu^3$ at 1 year of age.[22] The lower limit of normal of 80 $\mu^3$ for children and adults is reached at 4 to 5 years.[19] The adult MCHC of 34% is reached at 4 years of age.

**Reticulocytes.** According to Windle,[60] there are about 90% reticulocytes in the blood of the human fetus at 3 months' gestation and 15 to 30% at 6 months' gestation. The increased number of reticulocytes at birth reflects active red cell formation existing in fetal life.

Reticulocytes number 4 to 6% at birth and remain approximately constant for about 3 days after birth. From the first half of the fourth day to the first half of the sixth day of life there is a pronounced drop. From the sixth to the seventh day there is a further and slower decrease to approximately adult levels (0.5 to 1.5%).[48]

**Normoblasts.** Normoblasts are frequently observed in the normal infant on the first day of life but usually disappear during the first week, in most instances from the third to the fifth day. The average number at birth ranges from 3 to 10 per 100 white blood cells. In the premature infant the number of nucleated cells in the cord blood ranges from 10 to 20 per 100 white blood cells, with higher figures prevailing in the smaller infant. Occasional nucleated red cells will be observed in the peripheral blood of an older infant with acute infection associated with anemia. The presence of normoblasts in the blood of the older infant and child with leukopenia, granulocytopenia, and moderate anemia is indicative of bone marrow embarrassment and, frequently, invasion of the marrow by leukemic cells. With hypoxia and anemia associated with blood loss and hemolytic disease, or in infections such as congenital syphilis, in the occasional case of cytomegalic inclusion disease, and in sepsis, increased numbers of normoblasts appear in the peripheral blood, at birth, and in the neonatal period.

**Platelets.** Variable numbers of platelets have been given for the neonatal period. Some workers have found fewer platelets during the first 48 hours than in older infants. Figures reported at time of birth range from 150,000 to 350,000 per cubic millimeter, with an average of 300,000 at 2 weeks of age. The smaller number of platelets at birth has been attributed to the trauma incident to delivery. The rise in platelets is supposedly slower in the premature infant. The platelets of the newborn baby also show greater variation in size and shape than those in adults, in whom larger platelets are found in appreciable numbers.[52] The adult values of 250,000 to 350,000 per

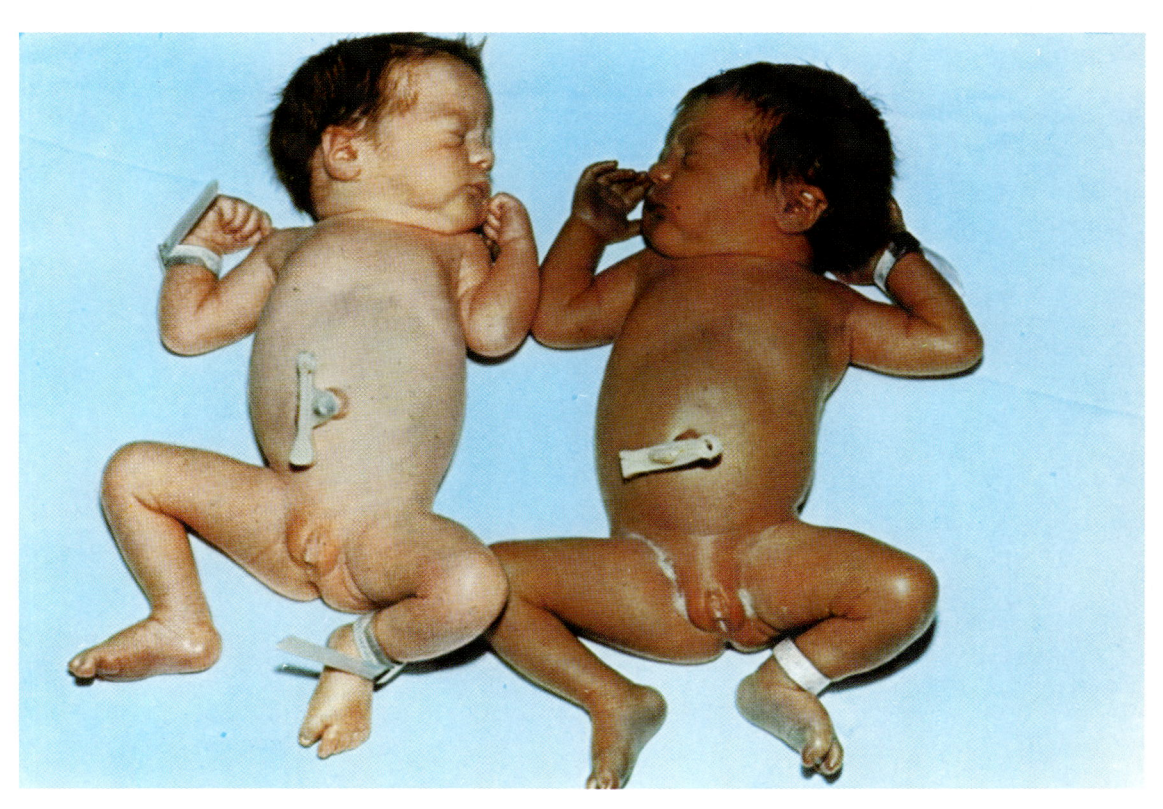

**Plate 1.** Twin-to-twin transfusion. Appearance of twins 6 hours after birth. The color of the plethoric twin became much darker with the development of jaundice. (From Pochedly, C., and Musiker, S.: Twin-to-twin transfusion syndrome. Reproduced from Postgraduate Medicine, Vol. 47, No. 3, March 1970, © McGraw-Hill, Inc.)

cubic millimeter of blood are reached at about 6 months of age.

In a series of 204 platelet counts in 105 normal, full-term, newborn infants, platelet counts of 100,000 to 300,000 were found to be normal for the first 96 hours of life.[2] In twenty-six premature infants[33] in the first 5 days of life, platelets ranged from 31,000 to 197,000 per cubic millimeter. Serial counts in thirteen infants under 1,700 gm. at birth showed a decrease below 50,000 per cubic millimeter by 10 to 20 days of age, with a hemorrhagic tendency in one infant. Large premature infants (over 1,700 gm. at birth) usually showed a prompt rise to 100,000 or more platelets per cubic millimeter by the tenth day.

In two other series platelet counts below 100,000 were extremely unusual and considered to be pathological. Aballi and associates[1] found that in the first 2 days of life platelet counts of the premature infant were somewhat lower than those observed in full-term infants. The differences though statistically significant were not notably marked. A steady rise was generally observed during the first month of life, irrespective of the birth weight. Fogel and co-workers,[9] in another study on seventy-three premature infants with birth weights below 2,200 gm., found that the majority had platelet counts corresponding to adults with a range of 156,000 to 300,000 per cubic millimeter and a mean of 212,000 per cubic millimeter. It seems apparent, until further data to the contrary are available, that significant thrombocytopenia in premature infants should be considered abnormal and possible causes should be sought.[45]

In this connection the syndrome of thrombocytopenia and intestinal bleeding observed in a nursery in Baltimore affected more than 10% of the infant population. Thrombocytopenia did not invariably accompany the bleeding.[24]

*White blood cells.* The total leukocyte count is high at birth, ranging from 9,000 to 38,000 per cubic millimeter during the first 2 days of life, with an average of 22,000 cells at the end of 12 hours.[3] In the first week the white blood count drops to an average of 12,000 per cubic millimeter, with a range of 5,000 to 21,000. At the end of the first year the white blood cell count averages 12,000, with a gradual decline to values of 8,000 to 10,000 by the fourth year. The total white blood cell count at birth tends to be lower in the premature infant than in the full-term infant.

*Neutrophilic leukocytes.* Neutrophilic leukocytes average 60% at birth, with a range from 40 to 80%, and include a small percentage of myelocytes. By the tenth day the average drops to 40%, and then to 30% in the fourth to the sixth month. It remains at this level until the fourth year, when a rise to 40% takes place. In the sixth year there is a rise to 55 to 60%.

*Lymphocytes.* Lymphocytes average 30% at birth and rise to 60% in the fourth to sixth month. These values are maintained until the fourth year, when they drop to 50%. They drop to 40% at the end of the sixth year and to 30% by the eighth year.

*Monocytes.* Monocytes number 6% at birth and, except for a rise to 9% in the second and third weeks, remain at levels of about 5% during infancy and childhood.

*Eosinophils and basophils.* Eosinophils and basophils maintain levels of 2 to 3% and 0.5%, respectively, throughout infancy and childhood.

*Plasma cells.* Plasma cells are large spherical cells with deep blue cytoplasm containing vacuoles of varying size. The nucleus, eccentrically placed, is round or oval, with dense chromatin masses arranged like spokes in a wheel. Plasma cells are not found in the embryo but appear after birth in interstitial, lymphoid, and glandular tissue. Clinical evidence suggests their relationship to immunity because of their presence in patients with subacute and chronic infections. Increased numbers of plasma cells have been noted in patients with infections in whom hyperglobulinemia is found. On the other hand, patients with agammaglobulinemia regularly exhibit a deficiency of plasma cells in hematopoietic centers and in inflammatory exudates.[5,17]

*Summary of white blood cell changes.* Certain approximate values may be designated for comparative purposes. At the end of the second month of life leukocytes total 12,000 per cubic millimeter, with 35% granulocytes and 60% lymphocytes. These values are maintained until the fourth and fifth years, when the total count drops to 8,000 white cells per cubic millimeter and the differential percentage is reversed to 60% granulocytes and 35% lymphocytes. From the sixth to the fourteenth year there is a gradual numerical shift to adult values of 7,000 white blood cells per cubic millimeter, with 65% neutrophilic granulocytes and 30% lymphocytes. Newborn infants with total leukocytes counts at either extreme should be investigated for existing abnormalities. There is evidence that premature infants as compared with full-term infants show higher granulocyte, lower lymphocyte, and lower white blood cell counts.

*Blood of premature infants.* At the end of the decline in the second and third months, the premature infant shows hemoglobin levels of 1 gm. or more (depending upon the birth weight) below the values of 11 gm. for full-term infants and red blood cell counts below the average of 3,800,000 for full-term infants. Thereafter a gradual recovery sets in, with values approximating normal full-term levels at about 1 year of age. The number of platelets may be somewhat lower at birth in the premature infant than in the full-term infant, averaging about 190,000 per cubic millimeter at birth and rising to 300,000 at the sixth month. The total number of white cells may be lower and nucleated red cells may persist for longer periods than in the full-term infant. Polycythemia at birth may be exaggerated in the premature infant as compared with the full-term infant because of differences in the proportion of the volume of blood in the body to that in the placenta. Whereas the amount of blood in the placenta remains fairly constant during the third trimester of pregnancy, that in the body increases steadily. The effect of the transfer of placental blood in the infant after birth therefore would produce a greater relative effect in the premature infant than in the full-term infant, especially when tying of the cord is delayed and the full complement of blood is obtained from this source.

The erythrocytes of the premature infant have a shortened life-span, an increased tendency to form Heinz bodies, higher levels of methemoglobin, and glutathione instability. Experimentally the red cells of premature infants, however, consume more glucose than those of adults. The percentage of glucose metabolized by the pentose phosphate pathway in these infants is as great and often greater than that observed in normal adults and patients with reticulocytosis. Since inadequate generation of triphosphopyridine nucleotide (NADPH or TPNH) is not responsible for the ease with which red cells of the premature develop oxidative denaturation of hemoglobin, the underlying basis for the phenomenon has not yet been demonstrated.[40]

Oski and his associates[43] found that, when glycolysis in the cells of neonates is compared with that observed in a hetergeneous group of patients with comparable reduction in the mean age of their cell population, the glycolytic rate for age of the red cells of the premature infant is actually lower than the rate of the young red cells of older individuals. In other words, these cells do not consume as much glucose as would be expected from cells of a similar young mean cell age. In another paper, Oski and his associates[41] suggest that the erythrocytes produced in utero and perhaps during the first few months of life differ not only in their hemoglobin content but also in many aspects of their enzyme profile. In what way these metabolic characteristics are responsible for the shortened red cell survival is still unknown.

## REFERENCES

1. Aballi, A., Puapondh, Y., and Desposito, F.: Platelet counts in thriving premature babies, Pediatrics 42:685, 1968.
2. Ablin, A. R., Kushner, J. H., Murphy, A., and Zippin, C.: Platelet enumeration in the neonatal period, Pediatrics 28:822, 1961.
3. Albritton, E. C., editor: Standard values in blood; biological data, AF Technical Report No. 6039, 1951.
4. Alison, F., and Prevot-Pignède, J.: L'influence de transfusions de sang sur la moelle osseuse des prematures, Ann. pediat. 35:401, 1959.
5. Barr, D. P.: The function of the plasma cell, Amer. J. Med. 9:277, 1950.
6. Becker, A. H., and Glass, H.: Twin to twin transfusion syndrome, Amer. J. Dis. Child. 106:134, 1963.
7. Cohen, F., and Zuelzer, W. W.: The transplacental passage of maternal erythrocytes into the fetus, Amer. J. Obstet. Gynec. 93:566, 1965.
8. DeMarsh, Q. B., Windle, W. F., and Alt, A. L.: Blood volume of newborn infant in relation to early and late clamping of umbilical cord, Amer. J. Dis. Child. 63:1123, 1942.
9. Fogel, B. J., Arias, D., and Kung, F.: Normal platelet counts in premature infants, J. Pediat. 73:108, 1968.
10. Gairdner, D., Marks, J., and Roscoe, J. D.: Blood formation in infancy. I. The normal bone marrow, Arch. Dis. Child. 27:128, 1952.
11. Gairdner, D., Marks, J., and Roscoe, J. D.: Blood formation in infancy; normal erythropoiesis, Arch. Dis. Child. 27:214, 1952.
12. Gairdner, D., Marks, J., and Roscoe, J. D.: Blood formation in infancy. IV. The early

anaemias of prematurity, Arch. Dis. Child. 30:203, 1955.
13. Gairdner, D., Marks, J., Roscoe, J. D., and Brettell, R. O.: The fluid shift from the vascular compartment immediately after birth, Arch. Dis. Child. 33:489, 1958.
14. Gatti, R. A.: Hematocrit values of capillary blood in the newborn infant, J. Pediat. 70:117, 1967.
15. Gatti, R. A., Muster, A. J., Cole, R. B., and Paul, M. H.: Neonatal polycythemia with transient cyanosis and cardiorespiratory anomalies, J. Pediat. 69:1063, 1966.
16. Glaser, K., Limarzi, L. R., and Poncher, H. G.: Cellular composition of the bone marrow in normal infants and children, Pediatrics 6:789, 1950.
17. Good, R. A.: Agammaglobulinemia, Bull. Univ. Minnesota Hosp. 26:1, 1954.
18. Guest, G. M., and Brown, E. W.: Erythrocytes and hemoglobin of the blood in infancy and childhood; factors in variability, statistical studies, Amer. J. Dis. Child. 93:486, 1957.
19. Guest, G. M., Brown, E. W., and Wing, M.: Erythrocytes and hemoglobin of the blood in infancy and childhood; variability in number, size and hemoglobin content of the erythrocytes during the first five years of life, Amer. J. Dis. Child. 56:529, 1938.
20. Haselhorst, G., and Allmeling, A.: Die Gewichtszunahme von Neugeborenen infolge postnataler Tranfusion, Ztschr. Geburtsh. u. Gynäk. 98:103, 1930.
21. Hodapp, R. V.: The case of the red and white Minnesota twins; intrauterine blood transfer between twins, Journal Lancet 82:413, 1962.
22. Horan, M.: Studies in anemia of infancy and childhood; the hemoglobin, red cell count, and packed cell volume of normal English infants during the first year of life, Arch. Dis. Child. 25:110, 1950.
23. Kalpaktsoglou, P. K., and Emery, J. L.: The effect of birth on the haemopoietic tissue of the human bone marrow; a biological study, Brit. J. Haemat. 11:453, 1965.
24. Kaplan, E., and Klein, S. J.: Thrombocytopenia and intestinal bleeding in premature infants, J. Pediat. 61:17, 1962.
25. Kato, K.: Leucocytes in infancy and childhood, J. Pediat. 7:7, 1935.
26. Kjeldsen, J., and Pederson, J.: Relation of residual placental blood-volume to onset of respiration and respiratory-distress syndrome in infants of diabetic and non-diabetic mothers, Lancet 1:180, 1967.
27. Kleinman, L. I., Petering, H. G., and Suterland, J. M.: Blood carbonic anhydrase activity and zinc concentration in infants with respiratory-distress syndrome, New Eng. J. Med. 277:1157, 1967.
28. Klingberg, W. G., Jones, B., Allen, W. M., and Dempsey, E.: Placental parabiotic circulation of single ovum human twins, Amer. J. Dis. Child. 90:519, 1955.
29. Lanzkowsky, P.: Effects of early and late clamping of umbilical cord on infant's haemoglobin level, Brit. Med. J. 2:1777, 1960.
30. Leichsenring, J. M., Norris, L. M., and Halbert, M. L.: Hemoglobin, red cell count, and mean corpuscular hemoglobin of healthy infants, Amer. J. Dis. Child. 84:27, 1952.
31. Lichtenstein, A., and Nordenson, N. G.: Studies on bone marrow in premature children, Folia haemat. 63:155, 1939.
32. Lippman, H. S.: A morphologic and quantitative study of the blood corpuscles in the new-born period, Amer. J. Dis. Child. 27:473, 1924.
33. Medoff, H. S.: Platelet counts in premature infants, J. Pediat. 64:287, 1964.
34. Merritt, K. K., and Davidson, L. T.: The blood during the first year of life, Amer. J. Dis. Child. 46:990, 1933.
35. Michael, A. F., Jr., and Mauer, A. M.: Maternal-fetal transfusion as a cause of plethora in the neonatal period, Pediatrics 28:458, 1961.
36. Mollison, P. L., and Cutbush, M.: Haemolytic disease of the newborn. In Gairdner, D., editor: Recent advances in pediatrics, New York, 1954, The Blakiston Co.
37. Mugrage, E. R., and Andresen, M. I.: Values for red blood cells of average infants and children, Amer. J. Dis. Child. 51:775, 1936.
38. Naeye, R. L.: Human intrauterine parabiotic syndrome and its complications, New Eng. J. Med. 268:804, 1963.
39. Neerhout, R. C.: Erythrocyte lipids in the neonate, Pediat. Res. 2:172, 1968.
40. Oski, F. A.: Red cell metabolism of the premature infant. II. The pentose phosphate pathway, Pediatrics 39:689, 1967.
41. Oski, F. A., Brigandi, E., and Noble, L.: Red cell metabolism in the newborn infant. V. Glycolytic intermediates and glycolytic enzymes, Pediatrics 44:84, 1969.
42. Oski, F. A., and Naiman, J. L.: Major problems in clinical pediatrics, Volume IV. Hematologic problems in the newborn, Philadelphia, 1966, W. B. Saunders Co.
43. Oski, F. A., Smith, C., and Brigandi, E.: Red cell metabolism in the premature infant. III. Apparent inappropriate glucose consumption for cell age, Pediatrics 41:473, 1968.
44. Pablete, E., Thibeault, D. W., and Auld, P. A. M.: Carbonic anhydrase in the premature, Pediatrics 42:429, 1968.
45. Pearson, H. A.: Thrombocytopenia in pre-

mature infants—physiological or pathological, J. Pediat. **73**:160, 1968.
46. Rausen, A. R., Seki, M., and Strauss, L.: Twin transfusion syndrome; a review of 19 cases studied at one institution, J. Pediat. **66**:613, 1965.
47. Schulman, I., Smith, C. H., and Stern, G. S.: Studies on the anemia of prematurity, Amer. J. Dis. Child. **88**:567, 1954.
48. Seip, M.: The reticulocyte level and the erythrocyte production judged from reticulocyte studies in newborn infants during the first week of life, Acta Paediat. **44**:355, 1955.
49. Shapiro, L. M., and Bassen, F. A.: Sternal marrow changes during the first week of life; correlation with peripheral blood findings, Amer. J. Med. Sci. **202**:341, 1941.
50. Smith, C. H.: Hypoplastic and aplastic anemias of infancy and childhood; with a consideration of the syndrome of nonhemolytic anemia of the newborn, J. Pediat. **43**:457, 1953.
51. Sturgeon, P.: Volumetric and microscopic pattern of bone marrow in normal infants and children. II. Cytologic pattern, Pediatrics **7**:642, 1951.
52. Tocantins, L. M.: Mammalian blood platelet in health and disease, Medicine **17**:155, 1938.
53. Usher, R., Shephard, M., and Lind, J.: The blood volume of the newborn infant and placental transfusion, Acta Paediat. **52**:497, 1963.
54. Washburn, A. H.: Blood cells in healthy young infants; the leukocyte picture during the first three months with special reference to hourly and daily variations, Amer. J. Dis. Child. **47**:993, 1934.
55. Washburn, A. H.: Blood cells in healthy young infants; a comparison of routine and special technics in the differentiation of leukocytes, Amer. J. Dis. Child. **50**:395, 1935.
56. Washburn, A. H.: Blood cells in healthy young infants; a study of 608 differential leukocyte counts, with a final report on 908 total leukocyte counts, Amer. J. Dis. Child. **50**:412, 1935.
57. Weatherall, D. J., and McIntyre, P. A.: Developmental and acquired variations in erythrocyte carbonic anhydrase isozymes, Brit. J. Haemat. **13**:106, 1967.
58. Wegelius, R.: On changes in peripheral blood picture of newborn infant immediately after birth, Acta Paediat. **35**:1, 1948.
59. Whipple, G. A., Sisson, T. R. C., and Lund, C. J.: Delayed ligation of the umbilical cord, Obstet. Gynec. **10**:603, 1957.
60. Windle, W. F.: Development of the blood and changes in the blood picture at birth, J. Pediat. **18**:538, 1941.
61. Wolman, I.: Laboratory applications in clinical pediatrics, New York, 1957, The Blakiston Co.
62. Wolman, I. J., and Dickstein, B.: Clinical applications of bone marrow examination in childhood, Amer. J. Med. Sci. **214**:677, 1947.
63. Wood, J. L.: Plethora in the newborn infant associated with cyanosis and convulsions; a review of postnatal erythropoiesis, J. Pediat. **54**:143, 1959.

# 3 BLOOD DYSCRASIAS IN RELATION TO MATERNAL-FETAL INTERACTION

The pathogenesis and interpretation of many of the blood dyscrasias characteristic of infancy and childhood depend upon a consideration of maternal-fetal relationships, environmental and genetic influences, and normal developmental changes. The problems of diagnosis and therapy often hinge on an understanding of many of the interrelated mechanisms that play a role in the control of the formation and development of blood cells.

*Hereditary basis of blood diseases—genetic and environmental influences.* Many of the blood disorders in the pediatric age group are conditioned by the overlapping influence of heredity and environment. Congenital defects may be genetically determined at the moment of conception or acquired during fetal development due to stress in the mother during critical moments of gestation. Warkany[90,91] postulated that the repeated appearance of defects in a family indicates the influence of a dominant or recessive inheritance of abnormal genes or of the repeated exposure of the developing embryo to the same adverse environmental factors. The majority of developmental defects are caused by a combination of circumstances involving both genetic and environmental factors.[25,26]

*Biochemical and genetic aspects.* In Chapter 4 (under the heading of *Nucleic acid and cellular development*) are outlined some of the pertinent concepts of how genetic chemicals replicate themselves and how they dictate the structure of vital cell proteins. In the present section those details are reviewed which might facilitate the interpretation of the hereditary basis of blood disorders.

The work of Beadle and Tatum[5] established the concept that genes control specific proteins. The genes are segments of DNA arranged in a linear fashion along the chromosome and constitute units of heredity. DNA is visualized as the basis of genetic material and RNA as associated with protein synthesis. It was postulated that DNA carries information through the medium of the nucleotide bases with ribosomes as the site of protein synthesis.[93] The DNA code is translated on to the messenger RNA, which is regarded as the template on the ribosomes on which the protein is synthesized. Protein synthesis involves three species of RNA: (1) messenger RNA is the form in which information contained in the DNA is delivered to the site of protein synthesis, the polyribosomes; (2) transfer RNA; and (3) ribosome RNA, on which the protein is synthesized. Amino acids must be "activated" for assembly into polypeptides. This requires energy, specific enzymes, and a transfer RNA (tRNA). A particular transfer RNA can accept only a specific amino acid, although there are several amino acids for which there is more than one particular transfer RNA.[57]

In the case of erythrocytes, the capacity for protein synthesis persists through the reticulocyte stage, although RNA synthesis occurs predominantly before the polychromatophilic erythroblast stage. No RNA is formed in the reticulocytes.[57]

*Genetic principles.* Since hereditary principles are involved in many of the blood disorders, several basic genetic facts may be reviewed. Every normal human somatic cell contains forty-six chromosomes. Following fertilization the zygote receives two sets of twenty-three chromosomes, one set from each of the parents. Twenty-two of these pairs are known as autosomes. The remaining pair is concerned with sex determination. The normal female has a sex chromosome constitution of XX, while the normal male is XY. The Y chromosome of man appears to carry little specific genetic information other than the determinant for the male phenotype.

The gene may be considered as a small piece or section of chromosome concerned with a specific biochemical function. It has been estimated that the total number of genes in a human being is about 42,000, with at least 2,000 of these on the X chromosome.[71] The genes, like chromosomes, exist in pairs. If a pair of genes are identical, the person is homozygous at this locus. If the two genes of a pair are different, the person is heterozygous for this gene pair. Alternative forms of a gene which may occur at a single gene locus are called allelomorphs or alleles. Thus, an individual with the same allele on each member of the chromosome pair is said to be homozygous for this gene locus. In contrast, an individual with two different alleles at the corresponding gene locus of the chromosome pair is said to be heterozygous for that gene locus or a heterozygote. All the traits or characteristics determined by a gene are probably mediated through the regulation or synthesis of proteins.

A curious imbalance that appears to occur in nature is the possession of two X chromosomes by the female as compared with only one in the male. According to the Lyon hypothesis,[18,54] one of the two X chromosomes is in a tightly coiled or condensed state and is functionally inactive. At some point in embryogenesis one of the X chromosomes is turned off. Thus, only one X chromosome is active in somatic cells of mammals regardless of the number actually present.[75] In females, the inactive X chromosome becomes heteropyknotic and is termed the Barr body—a localized chromatin particle that is Feulgen positive and thus presumably contains deoxyribonucleic acid or DNA.[19] The number of Barr bodies is usually one less than the number of X chromosomes. The buccal mucous membrane is usually examined for the presence of the Barr body. Its absence does not necessarily mean that the individual is a male, but merely that there are not two X chromosomes.

Most patients with Down's syndrome (mongolism) have forty-seven chromosomes.[40,48] The most common abnormality is a trisomy for chromosome 21, that is, the occurrence of three chromosomes of a particular pair instead of two. Nondisjunction of homologous chromosomes in the maternal germ cells is generally considered to be the basic mechanism by which the majority of affected individuals arise. Specifically, this is due to a failure of the two chromosomes of pair 21 to separate during gametogenesis in the mother. An abnormal ovum is produced and, thus, a child with trisomy 21. In some individuals there is an abnormally large chromosome in pair 15 resulting from the translocation of extra chromosome 21 material, also producing Down's syndrome. While the actual chromosome count is the normal forty-six, this still constitutes an overdose of chromosome 21. Mongolism can, therefore, result from either trisomy for chromosome 21 or translocation of chromosomes 13, 14, 15, and 22.[8,77] In the females thus far described, the translocation has been present in otherwise normal mothers as well as in a number of normal relatives.

***Blood dyscrasias in relation to congenital anomalies—general principles.*** A growing body of evidence has been accumulating[4] in support of the association of a variety of disease states in the mother and the occurrence of abnormalities in the offspring. In the elaboration of these concepts more intensive investigation has also been directed toward genetic and familial aspects of a variety of diseases in which many of the blood disorders have been included.

The experimental production of developmental defects has prompted consideration of the origin of anomalies in every system. According to current interpretation, single or coexisting anomalies represent deviations from orderly development induced by a known infection such as rubella or other as yet unidentified agents or states acting upon the pregnant woman and the placenta. If one accepts the principle that for all organs injury is most likely to occur during the stage of active differentiation, the vulnerable period of erythropoiesis would extend from the sixth to the twelfth week, when the liver, spleen, and bone marrow are simultaneously involved in the proliferation of erythroblasts. Chronic thrombocytopenia present from birth may be related to suppression of platelet formation from the second month of fetal life when platelet production becomes evident.[27]

It is thus apparent that the type of deformity depends upon nonspecific noxious influences operating at "developmental moments" corresponding to periods when organs are in their most rapidly proliferating condition. The infrequent association of severe types of hematologic disorders[15,62] with other congenital malformations suggests the relative resistance of hematopoietic tissues in comparison with the vulnerability of other systems during critical periods of development. However, the demonstration of injury to single or multiple cell types in the marrow in combination with other well-defined somatic defects, infrequent as it appears, supports the hypothesis of embryonic hematopoietic disturbances as a causative factor in blood dyscrasias.

Examples of blood dyscrasias associated with congenital anomalies include congenital leukemia and mongolism, hypoplastic-aplastic anemias with skeletal defects (i.e., Fanconi syndrome), sporadic congenital spherocytosis associated with congenital hypoplastic thrombocytopenia and malformations, and congenital factor V (labile factor) deficiency with syndactylism.

*Hematologic aspects of maternal and fetal interaction—placental physiology and defects.* The bulk of the placenta consists of chorionic villi which are exposed to a collection of maternal blood. Fetal and maternal blood are separated from each other by only two layers of cells at the trophoblastic endothelial junction of each villus. The maternal blood constantly circulates between the individual villi, from which it is drained by the decidual sinuses. Microscopic defects or breaks in the villi conceivably could permit leaks of small amounts of fetal blood into the maternal circulation, causing mild to moderate anemia in the newborn infant,[42] as may be observed in Fig. 3.

Maternal arterial blood enters the intervillous space at a pressure of 60 to 70 mm. Hg higher than the already existing pressure in this area and is dissipated by lateral dispersion. On the other hand, the difference between the umbilical arterial blood pressure and that in the intervillous space creates a pressure gradient conductive to the passage of water and metabolites from fetus to mother. It is conceivable that fetal blood may follow a similar course, especially through breaks or infarcts in the villi, resulting in neonatal anemia exclusive of incompatibilities.[55] These observations suggest a mechanism by which an Rh-negative woman

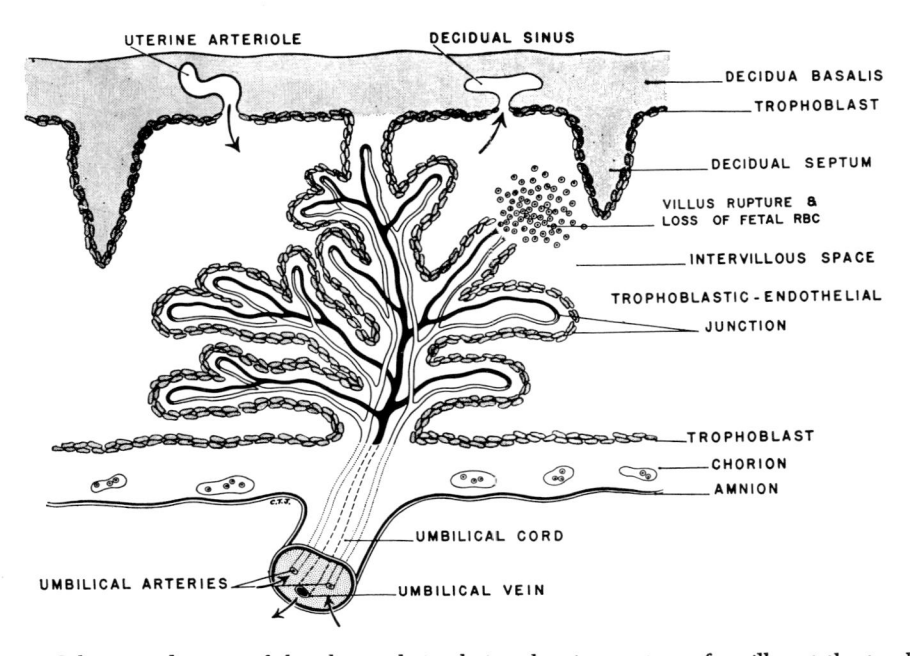

Fig. 3. Schematic diagram of the placental circulation showing rupture of a villus at the trophoblastic endothelial junction, permitting the mixing of fetal and maternal blood and the entrance of fetal red blood cells into the maternal circulation. (Modified from Javert, C. T., and Reiss, C.: Origin and significance of macroscopic intervillous coagulation hematomas [red infarcts] of human placenta, Surg. Gynec. Obstet. 94:257, 1952.)

is sensitized by an Rh-positive fetus (i.e., by the transplacental passage of fetal red blood cells or their products).

*Fetal hemorrhage into the maternal circulation (blood loss from fetal-maternal transfusion).* Wiener[94] was the first to suggest that the fetus can become severely anemic from bleeding into the maternal circulation. This concept was confirmed by Chown,[11,12] who reported a case in which a high concentration of fetal hemoglobin as well as fetal red cells could be found in the maternal blood soon after delivery. This suggested to him that anemia in the infant resulted from bleeding into the maternal circulation. The subsequent disappearance of fetal hemoglobin from the maternal circulation coincided with the disappearance of the infant's D (Rh$_o$) positive cells. It was calculated that approximately 90 to 180 ml. of fetal blood had entered the maternal circulation sometime before birth. Approximately 35 ml. of fetal blood will result in a 2% fetal hemoglobin value in the maternal blood.

When transplacental bleeding from the fetus occurs, appropriate agglutination and serologic tests reveal that the mother has been the recipient of erythrocytes that differ in the A-B-O and Rh-Hr blood groups from her own erythrocytes and that are identical with those of the newborn infant. Also an elevated concentration of bilirubin and fetal hemoglobin in the mother's circulation immediately postpartum and their subsequent disappearance constitute further proof of the passage of fetal blood into the maternal circulation through breaks of varying size in the placental barrier. The finding of increased fetal hemoglobin levels in the mother's blood, which gradually diminish, provides evidence for the leakage of fetal blood when the A-B-O and Rh-Hr blood groups in the fetus and the mother are identical.[70]

Additional evidence for the entrance of fetal antigens into the maternal circulation just before delivery is the reported appearance in group O mothers of immune anti-A antibodies (from A infants) 10 to 20 days after delivery when none had been present at birth.[22]

The loss of fetal blood into the maternal circulation has been described in many reports on the basis of an excess of alkali-resistant hemoglobin and differential agglutination of red cells in maternal blood.[7,30,33,66,79] Iron-deficiency anemia has been reported as one of the complications of occult blood loss due to fetal-maternal transfusion.[59]

Massive transplacental hemorrhage is of sufficient magnitude when in excess of 50 ml.[23] to lead to recognizable blood loss in the fetus. Massive hemorrhage is to be differentiated from smaller hemorrhages that occur, according to one series,[23] in up to 20% of pregnancies and are of no immediate clinical significance to the baby. The diagnosis of transplacental hemorrhage can be readily diagnosed in the maternal circulation by the appearance of red cells containing fetal hemoglobin determined by the method if elution of the fixed smear by citric acid phosphate buffer (p. 5). The most serious drawback of this technique occurs in A-B-O heterospecific pregnancies in which any A-B-O incompatible fetal cells entering the maternal circulation are destroyed almost instantaneously. A negative result in an anemic newborn infant may be attributed to an A-B-O heterospecific pregnancy.

With the use of the same acid elution method (cells containing mostly fetal hemoglobin are dark staining, whereas cells containing primarily hemoglobin A appear ghostlike, p. 5) it was noted that of 1,019 blood specimens of the blood of 384 pregnant and postpartum women, 15.8% contained fetal cells. These were found in each trimester of pregnancy as well as after birth.[97] The volume of cells in the maternal circulation was estimated at 0.1 to 0.2 ml., and only two women received more than 0.5 ml. Transplacental hemorrhage of more than 0.5 ml. was common in deliveries complicated by manual removal of the placenta or cesarean section.

In a study of 622 unselected women compatible with their offspring in the A-B-O system and not sensitized against the Rh factor, the acid elution method and immunofluorescent technique were used to demonstrate fetal erythrocytes in maternal blood.[13] Postpartum fetal erythrocytes were demonstrated in 50% of the mothers. In approximately 10% of the series, large fetal losses estimated to range from 0.5 to 40 ml. were observed. Massive transplacental hemorrhage was detected in nearly 1% of the cases by examination of the maternal blood and usually, but not always, by overt anemia in the fetus. Cohen and her associates[13] estimate that, in the first trimester of pregnancy, between 4 and 10% of normal women have fetal erythrocytes present in the normal smear. They concluded that the intermittent entry of fetal erythrocytes into the maternal circulation in small quantities occurs normally.

It is generally agreed that fetal Rh-positive red cells enter the maternal circulation during labor when the placenta separates from the uterine wall. These cells provide the antigenic stimulus for primary Rh immunization. Their presence in large numbers in the maternal circulation correlated with the development of the Rh antibodies.

With the Kleihauer-Betke technique the total number of fetal red cells counted in 10 minutes, the volume of fetal red cells entering the maternal circulation was less than 0.04 ml. with a fetal count of 1 to 10, 0.04 ml. to 0.1 ml. with a count of 11 to 40; 0.1 ml. to 0.4 ml. with a count of 41 to 100; and greater than 0.4 ml. with a count greater than 100. When fetal red cells were detected postpartum, the incidence of Rh isoimmunization increased fivefold as compared with another whose blood lacked fetal red cells. With a fetal bleed in excess of 0.40 ml. packed cells, 63% of the women developed anti-Rh.

Kleihauer's formula for calculating the volume of fetomaternal hemorrhage has been shown to give reliable results in a biological trial in which samples of cord blood were injected into nineteen patients. According to him, the volume of transplacental hemorrhage can be calculated from the following formula[32]: transplacental hemorrhage = ratio of fetal to adult red cells expressed as a percentage of 50. The population of adult red cells was asumed to be 500,000 in 50 sq. mm. of blood film. The only questionable aspect of this method is the assumption that 50 sq. mm. of blood film will contain 500,000 adult cells. The error of this assumption is unlikely to exceed 15%. If the concentration of scanning 50 sq. mm. of blood film for fetal cells is used, and if the assumption is made that the total adult cell population in 50 sq. mm. is 500,000, the volume of the transplacental hemorrhage is arrived at by dividing the fetal score by 100.

The evidence suggested that fetal bleeding usually began well before the onset of labor. Though labor, under pathologic conditions, may be associated with massive transplacental hemorrhage, it was ordinarily found to be of little or no significance with regard to the passage of fetal red cells into the maternal circulation. Under normal conditions, mechanical factors connected with labor and the use of oxytocics have no significant effect on the passage of fetal cells across the placenta. The placenta is, therefore, rarely, if ever, a completely tight seal, and the intermittent passage of fetal erythrocytes into the maternal circulation in minute quantities during the latter part of pregnancy, according to these workers, appears to be a physiologic event.[13] Fear and Queenan,[24] in a study of 636 obstetrical patients, found significant increases in the number of fetal cells postpartum in patients having manual removal of the placenta, difficult forceps delivery, and cesarean sections.

*Symptomatology and blood findings.* An evaluation of these reports indicates that the leakage of fetal blood into the maternal circulation can occur in small amounts over a prolonged period or may take place in larger amounts shortly before delivery or during labor.

Severe anemia and shock in the immediate postnatal period indicate transplacental hemorrhage from fetus to mother just prior to delivery.[79] Pallor is a significant feature; jaundice is absent. The spleen and liver are not enlarged. Anemia of moderate or severe degree with a hypochromic microcytic blood smear characteristic of iron deficiency may be present. If severe hemorrhage occurs at the time of delivery, the cord blood hemoglobin may be normal due to hemoconcentration. The evidences of anemia become perceptible with later hemodilution. Leukocytosis, reticulocytosis, and nucleated red cells are noted occasionally, but hyperbilirubinemia is unusual in contrast to erythroblastosis.[30]

The mother may experience no symptoms during pregnancy from fetal bleeding into her circulation. When the mother is the recipient of incompatible blood from the fetus the symptomatology is analogous to a transfusion reaction with chills, fever, and hyperbilirubinemia.[11,30]

*Treatment.* Transfusions with packed cells sufficient to bring the hemoglobin to approximately 12 gm. per 100 ml. are advisable in severe anemia. Since the loss of blood implies a decrease of potential iron stores, supplemental oral iron medication is advisable during recovery.

**Bleeding from the placental surface.** A significant number of newborn infants are born anemic not only because of occult hemorrhage from the passage of fetal blood into the maternal circulation but also because of serious fetal blood loss during labor and delivery. In abruptio placentae and placenta previa, bleeding takes place from the placental surface in the area of its attachment to the uterine wall. Blood loss suffered by the mother is shared by by the infant, with resulting posthemorrhagic anemia and shock (asphyxia pallida) and even stillbirth. Similar consequences follow intrauterine rupture or tear of fetal vessels during labor.[60] Exsanguination from rapid blood loss occurs in precipitous deliveries from velamentous insertion of the cord and, less commonly, from rupture of a normal or abnormally short cord.[44,45] Treatment is urgent and consists of clearing the airway and administering oxygen, artifical respiration, and transfusions with packed red cells.

**Pulmonary hemorrhage** in the newborn infant

is commonly recognized by the pathologist but seldom by the clinician. It was postulated by Rowe and Avery[74] that abnormal surface forces may at times produce pulmonary hemorrhage. Some hemorrhage from the upper airway occurs commonly. The association of pulmonary hemorrhage and hyaline membrane disease has been known for many years—possibly elevated surface tension of itself can cause transudation.

*Maternal-fetal passage of leukocytes and platelets.* The transplacental passage of normal red cells, sickle cells,[56] and elliptocytes[36] from mother to fetus has also been observed in the case of leukocytes and platelets. Desai and Creger[19] demonstrated the passage of maternal white cells and platelets to the fetal circulation using quinacrine-labeled maternal blood. They postulated that small numbers of maternal antibody-making cells capable of crossing the placenta could colonize permanently and function immunologically. The recent use of intrauterine transfusion in the management of erythroblastosis fetalis has afforded the opportunity to study the transfer of formed elements of blood from fetus to mother in humans.[20] Leukocytes and platelets labeled by the atabrine fluorescent technique have been demonstrated in the maternal circulation from 30 minutes to 4 hours following intraperitoneal transfusion of the fetus in utero. The peak concentration of labeled cells was observed 2 hours after transfusion. Whether this occurs in normal fetuses, and the mechanism involved, are not yet understood. Studies by Rigby and associates[72] also demonstrated the passage of quinacrine-labeled white cells from a mother with acute myelogenous leukemia across the placenta to the infant's circulation. The infant was born in good condition, although the fate and function of the transmitted cells are still in question.

Further studies have demonstrated that the fetomaternal transfer of lymphocytes is not uncommon and that it can be detected as early as the fourteenth week of gestation.[89] This phenomenon may be a consequence of the transplacental migration of circulating lymphoid cells as well as the leakage of blood. The antenatal diagnosis of a male fetus can be made by karyotypic analysis of lymphocytes in maternal blood. Transfer of fetal lymphocytes to the mother may play a part in the acceptance of the fetus as a homograft. Since lymphocytes contain transplantation antigens thought to be present very early in fetal life, it may be that the transplacental passage of fetal lymphocytes contributes to the acceptance of the fetus during gestation.

*Placental transmission of antibodies and isoagglutinins.* Since, from an anatomic point of view, the maternal and fetal circulations in man are separated by only two layers of cells, placental transmission of a variety of substances, including maternal antibodies, isoagglutinins, plasma proteins, and steroids, is effected in the human infant. Antibodies and gamma globulin are not produced in significant amounts in the fetus of any species under normal conditions. Their presence in the fetus and newborn infant prenatally results from transfer across the placenta from the mother. Postnatally these substances are derived from the ingestation of colostrum and maternal milk.[87] This contrasts with the more difficult transmission in the ruminant, in which there is a complex placental structure (five tissue layers between maternal and fetal circulation at full term of gestation). Therefore, as knowledge of placental function has been extended, it has become increasingly clear that a wide variety of substances, including proteins and red cells, cross the placental barrier into the fetal circulation and also that the rate of transfer is selectively controlled.[16]

While A and B isoagglutinogens can be demonstrated in the fetus in the second and third months,[49,50] isoagglutinins appear later. In a majority of newborn infants isoagglutinins detected in the cord blood diminish in titer or completely disappear. Consideration of the similiarity existing between the blood of the baby and that of the mother with respect to isoagglutinins suggests the passive transfer of isoagglutinins from the maternal into the fetal circulation through the placenta.[80] This process is analogous, for example, to the transplacental passage of anti-Rh antibodies, gamma globulin, diphtheria and tetanus antitoxin, and immune bodies for measles and mumps virus from mother to child.

Antibodies in the newborn infant transferred through the placenta are almost exclusively of the 7S globulin fraction. If the mother has both 7S and 19S (macroglobulins) antibodies in her circulation, only the 7S passes into the infant.[81] At the time of life when gamma globulin decreases, there is an absence of an antibody response to antigenic stimulation. Lymphoid tissue is quantitatively deficient and plasma cells absent from the bone marrow. Immunologic capability develops during the second month, with the appearance of plasma cells in the tissues and their production in response to antigenic stimulation.[10]

The 19S gamma₁ globulins contain Wassermann and heterophil antibodies, some isohemagglutinins, and the major rheumatoid factors. Agammaglobulinemia is a syndrome characterized by a deficiency in the synthesis of the three gamma globulins (less than 25 mg. per 100 ml.) and associated with recurrent grave bacterial infections.[28] The congenital disease is inherited as a sex-linked recessive characteristic and is manifest in males. The normal level of the total gamma globulins is approximately 600 to 1,200 mg. per 100 ml.

*Placental transmission of the L.E. factor.* Cases of systemic lupus erythematosus in pregnancy have been reported in which the L.E. phenomenon has been demonstrated in the newborn infant.[6,9,61] The L.E. factor was present in the cord blood and persisted for approximately 7 weeks after delivery, a period corresponding with the half-life of gamma globulin with which it is identified. (See discussion on L.E. phenomenon, Chapter 18.) The babies remained healthy; this was considered an indication that the L.E. factor is derived by transplacental passage from the mother rather than by an immunologic process developing in utero. The inheritance of systemic lupus erythematosus is rare[29] in comparison with the number of cases in which the factor presumably appears in the newborn infant by passive transfer.

*The gamma globulins.* Gamma globulin was the term given by Tiselius[86] to describe that portion of the serum globulins which migrated most slowly toward the positive electrode in an electrophoretic field at pH 8.6. According to Heremans,[37] the gamma globulins or immunoglobulins are a family of structurally and functionally related glycoprotein molecules with antibody activity. Three major molecular species make up the gamma globulin family. The three immunoglobulins are known as IgG ($\gamma$G), IgA ($\gamma$A), IgM ($\gamma$M). Synonyms for IgG are 7S$\gamma$-globulin; for IgA, 7S$\gamma$-1 globulin; and for IgM, 19S$\gamma$-globulin.

Three groups of gamma globulin of plasma contain antibodies[82]: (1) 7S gamma globulin (IgG), which represents 90% of the total gamma globulin, contains most of the antitoxic, antibacterial, and antiviral antibodies; (2) 19S gamma globulin (IgM) constitutes 10% of the total; and (3) 7S gamma globulin (IgA), the function of which is still unknown. A high proportion of gamma-A globulins is secreted into the tears, saliva, and respiratory and gastrointestinal tracts. A fourth immunoglobulin species has recently been identified and named IgD ($\gamma$D).[82] What may represent still another class of immunoglobulin, that with which reaginic antibody is associated, is designated as IgE ($\gamma$E).[72a]

Structural studies have revealed that the immunoglobulins are composed of two different kinds of polypeptide chains, the H (heavy) and L (light) chains, designated as such on the basis of the molecular weight of these units.

The heavy chains are definitive in structure, amino acid sequence, and biologic function for each class of immunoglobulin, and are represented in the nomenclature by the small Greek letters alpha, mu, and delta. The light chains are common to each of the immunoglobulin classes. These light chains are of two types, kappa and lambda. Only one of these types is represented on any individual antibody molecule.[82]

For the clinician the obvious importance of quantitating the immunoglobulins is for the purpose of attempting to establish the diagnosis of immunoglobulin deficiency disease.

*Plasma proteins in the fetus and newborn infant (immunoglobulin synthesis by the human fetus).* The gamma globulin in the cord blood and in the blood of the newborn baby (600 to 1,200 mg. per 100 ml.) is derived entirely from the maternal circulation by placental passage. Low gamma globulin levels are found in fetal blood until the fourth or fifth month of pregnancy, after which they rise gradually to reach maternal concentrations by the eighth to ninth month. At birth the gamma globulin level in fetal blood is somewhat higher than in maternal blood.[87] The gamma globulin is observed to fall steadily in the first month of life, following a simple exponential curve, reaching one-third of the birth value at 1 month of age when it is stabilized.[67] No change occurs between 1 and 3 months of age (300 to 600 mg. per 100 ml.), when the rate of synthesis balances the rate of catabolism. From 3 months of age, levels of gamma globulin rise slowly and progressively and reach adult levels (900 mg. per 100 ml.) at 2 years of age[41] (Fig. 4). According to these calculations, the half-life of gamma globulin is approximately 25 days,[68,69] which is comparable to the 30-day half-life of the Rh antibody molecule which passes through the placenta.[95] This value agrees with the T½

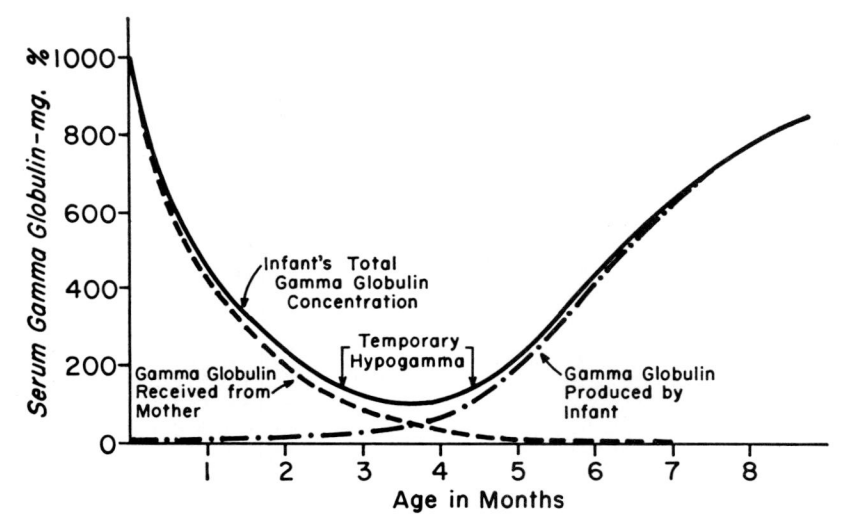

**Fig. 4.** Graph showing levels of gamma globulin in physiologic hypogammaglobulinemia of newborn infants. As level of gamma globulin from mother drops and production by infant begins, there is a temporary drop in gamma globulin concentration. (From Barrett, B., and Volwiler, W.: Agammaglobulinemia and hypoglobulinemia, J.A.M.A. 164:866, 1957.)

values derived from immunochemical determinations after the administration of gamma globulin to agammaglobulinemic patients. Stiehm and co-workers[85] infused patients with agammaglobulinemia with fresh or fresh-frozen plasma and found that the mean half-life of $\gamma G(7S)$, $\gamma M(19S)$, and $\gamma A(7S\text{-}1)$ globulins was 32, 9.6 and 5.9 days, respectively. In newborn infants after exchange transfusion the mean half-life of $\gamma M$ and $\gamma A$ globulins was 7.4 and 4.3 days, respectively.

Dancis and associates[17] have shown that under normal circumstances the placenta does not contribute significantly to the plasma proteins of the fetus. Beginning early in gestation, the fetal liver is capable of synthesizing all plasma proteins with the exception of gamma globulin. Little gamma globulin can be detected in fetal plasma up to 6 months of gestation.[64] It is problematic whether the infant normally synthesizes gamma globulin before the fourth week of extrauterine life. Probably no significant amounts are synthesized before the age of 3 months. (See Table 2.)

Mean values for total serum protein are lower in the cord blood of newborn infants than in their mothers at term. The lowering is a reflection of the lower globulin fraction since the mean value for serum albumin is much higher in the newborn infant than in the mother at term. After birth the level of serum globulin falls steadily, reaching its lowest level at 3 to 4 months of age and then rising to adult levels by 7 to 11 months of age.[65]

While all maternal $\gamma A$ and virtually all $\gamma M$ globulins are excluded from the fetus, maternal $\gamma G$ globulin is carried across the placental barrier with great efficiency. Consequently, the detection of $\gamma A$ and $\gamma M$ globulin in umbilical cord blood indicates that the infant was provoked into an antibody response by intrauterine infection. Alford and associates[1] demonstrated that $\gamma M$ antibodies are the first to appear in the response sequence and because elevated concentrations of $\gamma M$ or $\gamma A$ antibodies in cord serum cannot normally be of maternal origin, their presence in cord serum is indicative of intrauterine infection. Normally in pregnancy, the human placenta does not actively transport immune gamma M globulin or gamma A globulin from maternal to fetal serum. Serum immunoglobulin elevations can occur some time in utero after infection due to rubella virus, cytomegaloviruses, and *Treponema pallidum*. Therefore, since no transfer of IgM or IgA takes place across the placenta, the postnatal appearance and rise of immunoglobulin reflects exposure to the antigen. The levels of serum immunoglobulin in the infants depended more on the nature of the pathogen, the response to treatment, and the chronicity of intrauterine fetal

Table 2. Immunoglobulin levels in infancy and childhood*

|  | IgG (mg./100 ml.; mean ± 1 S.D. and range) | IgA (mg./100 ml.; mean ± 1 S.D. and range) | IgM (mg./100 ml.; mean ± 1 S.D. and range) |
|---|---|---|---|
| Cord blood | 1086 ± 290 (740 – 1374) | 2 ± 2 (0 – 15) | 14 ± 6 (0 – 22) |
| 1–3 months | 512 ± 152 (280 – 950) | 16 ± 10 (4 – 36) | 28 ± 14 (15 – 86) |
| 4–6 months | 520 ± 180 (240 – 884) | 22 ± 14 (11 – 52) | 36 ± 18 (21 – 74) |
| 7–12 months | 742 ± 226 (281 – 1280) | 54 ± 17 (22 – 112) | 76 ± 27 (36 – 150) |
| 13–24 months | 945 ± 270 (290 – 1300) | 67 ± 19 (9 – 143) | 88 ± 36 (18 – 210) |
| 25–36 months | 1030 ± 152 (546 – 1562) | 89 ± 34 (21 – 196) | 94 ± 23 (43 – 115) |
| 3–5 years | 1150 ± 244 (546 – 1760) | 126 ± 31 (56 – 284) | 87 ± 24 (26 – 121) |
| 6–8 years | 1187 ± 289 (596 – 1744) | 147 ± 35 (56 – 330) | 108 ± 37 (54 – 260) |
| 9–11 years | 1217 ± 261 (744 – 1719) | 146 ± 38 (44 – 208) | 104 ± 46 (27 – 215) |
| 12–16 years | 1248 ± 221 (796 – 1647) | 168 ± 54 (64 – 290) | 96 ± 31 (60 – 140) |
| Adult | 1274 ± 280 (664 – 1825) | 227 ± 53 (59 – 311) | 127 ± 46 (45 – 205) |

*Abstracted from Children are different (No. 11). In Serum proteins, immunoglobulin and their properties in relation to age, Columbus, Ohio, 1967, Ross Laboratories. (From unpublished data by Ellis, E. F., and Robbins, J. B.)

infection than on the severity of clinical illness.

Routine assessment of γM and γA globulin content of umbilical cord serum can be of particular value in detecting infants with subclinical or unusual types of congenitally acquired infection and is particularly useful in identifying those born after inapparent maternal illnesses.

IgM immunoglobulin levels are often elevated in infants in association with congenital and perinatal infections. When these children are identified, specific studies can be conducted to attempt to identify the cause of the immune response.[78]

Recent studies have demonstrated that the normal fetus is not totally immunologically incompetent but does produce small amounts of IgM and IgG as early as 20 weeks of gestation.[88] Although IgA has not been found in normal fetal blood or other tissue, increased levels of IgA and IgM have been demonstrated in infants with congenital infections with protozoal, spirochetal, viral, and bacterial agents.

Cord sera were obtained from 5,006 infants.[63] There were 135 sera with IgM values greater than 20 mg. per 100 ml. Of these, 60% probably were due to a placental leak, 13% were in a questionable category, and 27% were considered to be due to production of abnormal amounts of IgM in utero; 20 mg. per 100 ml. IgM and 5 mg. per 100 ml. IgA were considered the upper limit of normal. Determination of IgM and IgA levels may be valuable as screening tests to discover those infants who have inapparent congenital infections.

According to Allansmith and co-workers,[2] IgM undergoes rapid synthesis in the first week of postnatal life and expands to adult levels by the age of 1 year for boys and 2 years for girls. IgA synthesis begins by 2 to 3 weeks of age, increases slowly, and reaches adult levels by about 12 years. Rapid IgG synthesis probably begins by the first 4 to 6 weeks of life, and adult levels are reached at about 8 years.[2]

*Immunologic relationships.* Immunologic relationships exist in erythroblastosis fetalis, thrombocytopenic purpura, and fetal-maternal leukocyte incompatibility.

*Erythroblastosis fetalis.* The maternal-fetal

relationships in sensitization by antigens of the Rh-positive fetus and in cases of a heterospecific pregnancy of the A, B, and O groups will be dealt with in Chapter 9. They represent important examples of antibody relationships and immunosensitization between maternal and fetal blood.

*Thrombocytopenic purpura in the newborn infant.* Hemorrhagic disease of the newborn infant and congenital thrombocytopenic purpura make their appearance soon after birth and reflect disturbances resulting from maternal-fetal relationships. Thrombocytopenic purpura in the newborn infant may be cited as another example of the influence of maternal suppressing factors on a fetal blood element. This disease affects children whose mothers either have thrombocytopenic purpura or are entirely normal. In the former instance the reduction of platelets in the infant results from the passage across the placental membrane of a circulatory factor which depresses platelet formation in the infant and causes purpura. Platelet autoagglutinins have been found in the blood of the mother and infant. Isoagglutinins for each other's platelets have been found also.[76] These agglutinins disappear from the infant's circulation by the age of 3 months.

Thrombocytopenia in newborns may be due to other causes than isoimmunization from maternal antibodies which are active against both the infant's and the mother's platelets and antibody production in the mother to the infant's platelets. The most common cause is infection. Toxoplasmosis, cytomegalic inclusion disease, herpes simplex, rubella, and septicemia are often associated with marked depletion of platelets. Giant hemangiomas and disseminated intravascular coagulation (DIC) may be associated with thrombocytopenia. DIC may be a more common complication of severely ill newborn infants than is generally realized.[35] Neonatal thrombocytopenia associated with fetal rubella will be dealt with in Chapter 27.

*Fetal-maternal leukocyte incompatibility.* That leukoagglutinins may develop in multitransfused patients has been recognized. Leukoagglutinins are believed to be comparable to antibodies for erythrocytes and platelets. Antigenic differences in human leukocytes are known, and leukoagglutinins have been held responsible for febrile transfusion reactions.[68]

Fetal-maternal incompatibility may induce leukoagglutinin formation in the mother who has had no transfusions when the antigenic factor has been inherited from the father and is absent in the mother.[69]

Transient agranulocytosis has been observed in successive siblings in the neonatal period.[53] Such a circumstance was explained by transplacental isoimmunization of the mother to a leukocyte factor of her infant in a manner analogous to Rh isoimmunization causing hemolytic disease of the newborn infant. In these cases agranulocytosis persisted for 3 to 4 weeks, and in one of the infants it was accompanied by pulmonary infection. The predominance of neutrophilic myelocytes in the bone marrow in these infants may represent either a maturation arrest or a depletion of mature cells because of their increased agglutination and destruction in the peripheral blood.

Two infants born of mothers with chronic neutropenia showed a transitory neutropenia which persisted for 3 weeks.[84] The blood picture in the babies was presumably caused by the transplacental passage of a neutropenic factor. In one case the mother's serum contained a demonstrable leukoagglutinin which could be transferred by transfusion to a normal person. In these patients the bone marrow showed hyperplasia of the granulocytic series with a maturation arrest at the myelocytic stage.

*Transplacental passage of drugs affecting blood elements in the newborn infant.* Several examples may be cited of the passage of drugs through the placenta affecting the blood elements in the newborn infant. In one case report[58] the administration of quinine to induce labor resulted in thrombocytopenia in the mother and infant. The mechanism was based on the transmission of quinine platelet "antibodies" derived from the mother who had originally received the drug in childhood. The parenteral administration of a large dose of a vitamin K analogue (Hykinone) to mothers during labor has also been shown to result in marked hyperbilirubinemia in newborn premature infants, with nervous system involvement in several cases.[52] The increased pigment presumably resulted from the hemolytic effects of the vitamin. In another case[96] the ingestion of mothballs by a mother produced jaundice and hemolytic anemia in her newborn infant. This was attributed to the passage of naphthalene and its derivatives to the infant.

Generally, substances capable of injuring the fetus and newborn infant which have been transmitted by transplacental passage from the mother play a passing role in producing pathologic states. The noxious agent has a limited activity since it cannot be replenished once the maternal source is eliminated, except in circumstances in which it can be conveyed by colostrum or maternal milk.

Cancer chemotherapeutic drugs taken by the mother may injure the fetus. Aminoprotein (and presumably amethoprotein–Methotrexate), in addition to being a potent abortifacient, can induce major fetal abnormalities when administered during the first trimester of pregnancy. Busulfan and 6-mercaptopurine administered in alternating doses throughout pregnancy produced multiple severe fetal abnormalities, although neither drug alone produces major fetal damage.[83] No reports of important fetal abnormalities have been encountered in cases in which chemotherapeutic drugs were used only after the first trimester of pregnancy. Multiple congenital malformations are described in a child whose mother attempted abortion with Aminopterin in the tenth week of gestation.[92]

A variety of other drugs given to the mother such as Dicumarol and its derivatives, salicylates, intravenous fluids, vitamin K analogues, and hypotensive, hemolytic, and antibacterial agents (i.e., sulfonamides, chloramphenicol) will cross the placenta in sufficient concentration and may place the fetus in jeopardy.[14,51] There have also been reports of thrombocytopenia[73] and of Heinz body hemolysis[34] in newborn infants from maternally ingested thiazides.

Hemorrhages have occurred in babies born of epileptic mothers who have had anticonvulsant therapy during pregnancy. In such cases the administration of prophylactic vitamin $K_1$ has been recommended, given at twelve hourly intervals for three doses.[21,46]

The use of anticoagulants in pregnancy presents a special problem because treatment may be complicated by fetal hemorrhage.[81] The vitamin K antagonists have been shown in experimental animals to cross the placenta and to cause fetal hemorrhage.[47] The effect on the fetus of giving coumadin in pregnancy was evaluated in rabbits. When coumadin was given throughout pregnancy the fetuses were stillborn and showed widespread hemorrhages.[38] Fetuses, however, were born alive and without hemorrhage when coumadin was stopped 4 to 5 days before delivery and when delivery was performed by cesarean section at a time when the fetal coagulation defect was severe. It was suggested that the risk of fetal hemorrhage was high only when fetuses with a severe coagulation defect were exposed to the trauma of delivery. The proposal that the increased incidence of fetal hemorrhage occurs only when treatment with vitamin K antagonists is continued until term is in keeping with human experience in a number of clinical observations.[39] It has been suggested that Warfarin (coumadin), if administered in the first 8 weeks of gestation, may have a teratogenic effect.[43] Patients with prosthetic aortic valves in pregnancy have delivered normal infants when these patients did not receive anticoagulants during pregnancy.

## REFERENCES

1. Alford, C. A., Schaefer, J., Blankenship, W. J., Straumfjord, J. V., and Cassidy, G.: A correlative immunologic, microbiologic and clinical approach to the diagnosis of acute and chronic infections in newborn infants, New Eng. J. Med. 277:437, 1967.
2. Allansmith, M., McClellan, B. H., Butterworth, M., and Maloney, J. R.: The development of immunoglobin levels in man, J. Pediat. 72:276, 1968.
3. Barr, M. L., and Bertram, E. G.: Morphological distinction between neurones of male and female; behavior of nucleolar satellite during accelerated nucleoprotein synthesis, Nature 163:676, 1949.
4. Bass, M.: In Dock, W., and Snapper, I., editors: Advances in internal medicine, vol. 5, Chicago, 1952, Year Book Medical Publishers, Inc.
5. Beadle, G. W., and Tatum, E. L.: Genetic control of biochemical reactions in Neurospora, Proc. Nat. Acad. Sci. 27:499, 1941.
6. Berlyne, G. M., Short, I. A., and Vickers, C. F. H.: Placental transmission of the L.E. factor, Lancet 2:15, 1957.
7. Borum, A., Lloyd, H. O., and Talbot, T. R., Jr.: Possible fetal hemorrhage into maternal circulation, J.A.M.A. 164:1087, 1957.
8. Breg, W. R., Miller, O. J., and Schmickel, R. D.: Chromosomal translocation in patients with mongolism and their normal relatives, New Eng. J. Med. 266:345, 1962.
9. Bridge, R. G., and Foley, F. E.: Placental transmission of the lupus erythematosus factor, Amer. J. Med. Sci. 227:1, 1954.

10. Bridges, R. A., Condie, R. M., Zak, S. J., and Good, R. A.: The morphologic basis of antibody formation development during the neonatal period, J Lab. Clin. Med. 53:331, 1959.
11. Chown, B.: Anaemia in a newborn due to the fetus bleeding into the mother's circulation, Lancet 1:1213, 1954.
12. Chown, B.: Anaemias in the newborn other than haemolytic disease, Ped. Clin. N. Amer. 4:371, 1957.
13. Cohen, F., Zuelzer, W. W., Gustafson, D. C., and Evans, M. M.: Mechanisms of isoimmunization. I. The transplacental passage of fetal erythrocytes in homospecific pregnancies, Blood 23:621, 1964.
14. Cohlan, S. Q.: Fetal and neonatal hazards from drugs administered during pregnancy, New York J. Med. 64:493, 1964.
15. Congenital malformations, Pediatrics (supp.) 23:195, 1959.
16. Dancis, J.: The placenta, J. Pediat. 55:85, 1959.
17. Dancis, J., Braverman, N., and Lind, J.: Plasma protein synthesis in the human fetus and placenta, J. Clin. Invest. 36:398, 1957.
18. Davidson, R. G.: The Lyon hypothesis, Pediatrics 65:765, 1964.
19. Desai, R. G., and Creger, W. P.: Materno-fetal passage of leukocytes and platelets in man, Blood 21:665, 1963.
20. Desai, R. G., McCutcheon, E., Little, B., and Driscoll, S. G.: Fetomaternal passage of the leukocytes and platelets in erythroblastosis fetalis, Blood 27:858, 1966.
21. Douglas, H.: Haemorrhage in the newborn, Lancet 1:816, 1966.
22. Dunsford, I.: Proof of fetal antigens entering the maternal circulation, Official Program of the Sixth International Congress of the International Society of Hematology, Boston, 1956, p. 539.
23. Durkin, C. M., and Finn, R.: Foetal haemorrhage into the maternal circulation, Lancet 2:100, 1961.
24. Fear, R. E., and Queenan, J. T.: Factors affecting the transplacental passage of fetal erythrocytes, Obstet. Gynec. (abstract) 29: 444, 1967.
25. Fraser, F. C., and Fainstat, T. D.: Causes of congenital defects; a review, Amer. J. Dis. Child. 82:593, 1951.
26. Fraser, F. C., Walker, B. E., and Trasler, D. G.: Experimental production of congenital cleft palate; genetic and environmental factors, Pediatrics 19:782, 1957.
27. Fruhling, L., Roger, S., and Jobard, P.: L'hématologie normale (tissus et organes hématopoiétiques sang circulant) de l'embryon, du foetus et du nouveau-né humains, Sang 20:267, 1949.
28. Gitlin, D., Rosen, F. S., and Janeway, C. A.: Undue susceptibility to infection, Ped. Clin. N. Amer. 9:405, 1962.
29. Glagov, S., and Gechman, E.: Familial occurrence of disseminated lupus erythematosus, New Eng. J. Med. 255:936, 1956.
30. Goodall, H. B., Graham, F. S., Miller, M. D., and Cameron, C.: Transplacental bleeding from the foetus, J. Clin. Path. 11:251, 1958.
31. Gordon, R. R., and Dean, T.: Foetal deaths from antenatal anticoagulant therapy, Brit. Med. J. 2:719, 1955.
32. Grobbelaar, B. G., and Dunning, E. K.: A method of calculating the volume of transplacental foetal maternal haemorrhage, Brit. J. Haemat. 17:231, 1969.
33. Gunson, H. H.: Neonatal anemia due to fetal hemorrhage into the maternal circulation, Pediatrics 20:3, 1957.
34. Harley, J. D., Robin, H., and Robertson, S. E. J.: Thiazide-induced neonatal haemolysis, Brit. Med. J. 1:696, 1964.
35. Hathaway, W. E., Mull, M. M., and Pechet, G. S.: Disseminated intravascular coagulation in the newborn, Pediatrics 43:233, 1969.
36. Hedenstedt, S., and Naeslund, J.: Investigations of permeability of placenta with help of elliptocytes, Acta Med. Scandinav. (supp.) 170:126, 1946.
37. Heremans, J. F.: Immunochemical studies on protein pathology: immunoglobulin concept, Clin. Chim. Acta 4:639, 1959.
38. Hirsh, J., Cade, J. F., and Gallus, A. S.: Fetal effects of Coumadin administered during pregnancy, Blood 36:623, 1970.
39. Hirsh, J., Cade, J. F., and O'Sullivan, E. F.: Clinical experience with anticoagulant therapy in pregnancy, Brit. Med. J. 1:270, 1970.
40. Jacobs, P. A., Baikie, A. G., Court-Brown, W. M., and Strong, J. A.: The somatic chromosomes in mongolism, Lancet 1:710, 1959.
41. Janeway, C. A., and Gitlin, D.: The gamma globulins. In Levine, S. Z., and others, editors: Advances in pediatrics, vol. 4, Chicago, 1951, Year Book Medical Publishers, Inc., p. 65.
42. Javert, C. T., and Reiss, C.: The origin and significance of macroscopic intervillous coagulation hematomas (red infarcts) of the human placenta, Surg. Gynec. Obstet. 94:257, 1952.
43. Kerber, I. J., Warr, O. S., III, and Richardson, C.: Pregnancy in a patient with a prosthetic mitral valve associated with a fetal anomaly attributed to Warfarin sodium, J.A.M.A. 203:157, 1968.
44. Kirkman, H. N., and Riley, H. D.: Posthem-

orrhagic anemia and shock in the newborn due to hemorrhage during delivery; report of eight cases, Pediatrics 24:92, 1959.
45. Kirkman, H. N., and Riley, H. D.: Posthemorrhagic anemia and shock in the newborn; a review, Pediatrics 24:97, 1959.
46. Kohler, H. G.: Hemorrhage in the newborn of epileptic mothers, Lancet 1:267, 1966.
47. Krauss, A. P., Perlow, A., and Singer, K.: Danger of dicoumarol treatment in pregnancy, J.A.M.A. 139:758, 1949.
48. Lejeune, J., Gautier, M., and Turpin, R.: Etude des chromosomes somatiques de neuf enfants mongoliens, Compt. rend. Acad. sc. 248:1721, 1959.
49. Levine, P.: Serological factors as possible causes in spontaneous abortions, J. Hered. 34:71, 1943.
50. Levine, P., Burnham, L., Katzin, F. M., and Vogel, P.: The role of iso-immunization in the pathogensis of erythroblastosis fetalis, Amer. J. Obstet. Gynec. 42:295, 1941.
51. Lucey, J. F.: Hazards to the newborn infant from drugs administered to the mother, Ped. Clin. N. Amer. 8:413, 1961.
52. Lucey, J. F., and Dolan, R. G.: Injections of vitamin-K compound in mothers and hyperbilirubinemia in the newborn, Pediatrics 22:605, 1958.
53. Luhby, A. L., and Slobody, L. B.: Transient neonatal agranulocytosis in two siblings; transplacental isoimmunization to a leucocyte factor? Amer. J. Dis. Child. 92: 496, 1956.
54. Lyon, M. F.: Gene action in the X-chromosome of the mouse (Mus musculus L.), Nature 190:372, 1961.
55. M. & R. Laboratories: Report of the fifteenth M & R pediatric research conference, 1955, p. 27.
56. Macris, N. T., Hellman, L. M., and Watson, R. J.: Transmission of transfused sickle-trait cells from mother to fetus, Amer. J. Obstet. Gynec. 76:1214, 1958.
57. Marks, P. A.: Thalassemia syndromes: biochemical, genetic and clinical aspects, New Eng. J. Med. 275:1363, 1966.
58. Mauer, A. M., DeVaux, W., and Lahey, M. E.: Neonatal and maternal thrombocytopenic purpura due to quinine, Pediatrics 19:84, 1957.
59. McGovern, J. J., Driscoll, R., DuToit, C. H., Grove-Rasmussen, M., and Bedell, R. F.: Iron-deficiency anemia resulting from fetomaternal transfusion, New Eng. J. Med. 258:1149, 1958.
60. Michaels, J. P.: Intrauterine rupture of fetal vessels during labor, Amer. J. Obstet. Gynec. 70:1251, 1955.
61. Mijer, F., and Olsen, R. N.: Transplacental passage of the L.E. factor, J. Pediat. 52:690, 1958.
62. Miller, H. C., Clifford, S. H., Smith. C. A., Warkany, J., Wilson, J. L., and Yannet, H.: Special report from the committee for the study of congenital malformations of the American Academy of Pediatrics; study of the relation of congenital malformations to maternal rubella and other infections; preliminary report, Pediatrics 3:259, 1949.
63. Miller, M. J., Sunshine, P. J., and Remington, J. S.: Quantitation of cord serum IgM and IgA as a screening procedure to detect congenital infection: results in 5,006 infants, J. Pediat. 75:1287, 1969.
64. Moore, D. H., Martin du Pan, R., and Boxton, C. L.: An electrophoretic study of maternal, fetal and infant sera, Amer. J. Obstet. Gynec. 57:312, 1949.
65. Oberman, J. W., Gregory, K. O., Burke, F. G., Ross, S., and Rice, E. C.: Electrophoretic analysis of serum proteins in infants and children; normal values from birth to adolescence, New Eng. J. Med. 255:743, 1956.
66. O'Connor, W. J., Shields, G., and Schuyler, K.: Anemia of the newborn in association with the appearance of fetal hemoglobin in maternal circulation, Amer. J. Dis. Child. 93:10, 1957 (Abst.).
67. Orlandini, O., Sass-Kortsak, A., and Ebbs, J. H.: Serum gamma globulin levels in normal infants, Pediatrics 16:575, 1955.
68. Payne, R.: The association of febrile transfusion reactions with leuko-agglutinins, Vox Sang 2:233, 1957.
69. Payne, R., and Rolfs, M. R.: Fetomaternal leukocyte incompatibility, J. Clin. Invest. 37:1756, 1958.
70. Pearson, H. A., and Diamond, L. K.: Fetomaternal transfusion, Amer. J. Dis. Child. 97:267, 1959.
71. Review: The Lyon hypothesis: a significant advance in human genetics, Nutr. Rev. 22:68, 1964.
72. Rigby, P. G., Hanson, T. A., and Smith, R. J.: Passage of leukemic cells across the placenta, New Eng. J. Med. 271:124, 1964.
72a. Robbins, J. B.: Structure and biologic activity of immunoglobulin E. In Kagan, B. M., and Stiehm, E. R., editors: Immunologic incompetence, Chicago, 1971, Year Book Medical Publishers, Inc.
73. Rodriguez, S. U., Leikin, S. L., and Hiller, M. C.: Neonatal thrombocytopenia associated with ante-partum administration of thiazide drugs, New Eng. J. Med. 270:881, 1964.
74. Rowe, S., and Avery, M. A.: Massive pulmonary hemorrhage in the newborn. II. Clinical considerations, J. Pediat. 69:12, 1966.

75. Russell, L. B.: Another look at the single-active X hypothesis, N. Y. Acad. Sci. **26**:726, 1964 (series II).
76. Schoen, E. J., King, A. L., and Duane, R. T.: Neonatal thrombocytopenic purpura, Pediatrics **17**:72, 1956.
77. Sergovich, F. R., Soltan, H. C., and Carr, D. H.: Twelve unrelated translocation mongols: cytogenetic, genetic and parental age data, Cytogenetics **3**:34, 1964.
78. Sevette, J. L.: Immunoglobulin determinations for the detection of perinatal infection, J. Pediat. **75**:1111, 1969.
79. Shiller, J. G.: Shock in the newborn caused by transplacental hemorrhage from fetus to mother, Pediatrics **20**:7, 1957.
80. Smith, C. H.: Iso-agglutinins in the newborn with special reference to their placental transmission, Amer. J. Dis. Child. **36**:54, 1928.
81. Smith, R. T.: Immunity in infancy, Ped. Clin. N. Amer. **7**:269, 1960.
82. Smith, R. T.: Human immunoglobulins; a guide to nomenclature and clinical application, Pediatrics **37**:822, 1966.
83. Sokal, J. E., and Lessmann, E. M.: Effects of cancer chemotherapeutic agents on the human fetus, J.A.M.A. **172**:1765, 1960.
84. Stefanini, M., Mele, R. H., and Skinner, D.: Transitory congenital neutropenia; a new syndrome, report of two cases, Amer. J. Med. **25**:749, 1958.
85. Stiehm, S. R., Vaerman, J. P., and Fudenberg, H. H.: Plasma infusions in immunologic deficiency states; metabolic and therapeutic states, Blood **28**:918, 1966.
86. Tiselius, A.: Electrophoresis of serum globulin. II. Electrophoretic analysis of normal and immune sera, Biochem. J. **31**:1464, 1937.
87. Vahlquist, B.: Transfer of antibodies from mother to offspring. In Levine, S. Z., and others, editors: Advances in pediatrics, vol. 10, Chicago, 1958, Year Book Medical Publishers, Inc., p. 305.
88. vanFurth, R., Schvit, H., and Hijmans, W.: The immunological development of the human fetus, J. Exp. Med. **122**:1173, 1965.
89. Walknowska, J., Conte, F. A., and Grumbach, M. M.: Practical and theoretical implication of fetal/maternal lymphocyte transfer, Lancet **1**:1119, 1969.
90. Warkany, J.: Etiology of congenital malformations. In Levine, S. Z., and others, editors: Advances in pediatrics, vol. 2, New York, 1947, Interscience Publishers, Inc., p. 1.
91. Warkany, J.: Congenital anomalies, Pediatrics **7**:607, 1951.
92. Warkany, J., Beaudry, P. H., and Hornstein, S.: Attempted abortion with aminopterin (4-amino-pteroylglutamic acid) malformations of the child, Amer. J. Dis. Child. **97**:274, 1959.
93. Warner, J. R., and Soeiro, R.: The involvement of RNA in protein synthesis, New Eng. J. Med. **276**:563, 1967.
94. Wiener, A. S.: Diagnosis and treatment of anemia of newborn caused by occult placental hemorrhage, Amer. J. Obstet. Gynec. **56**:717, 1948.
95. Wiener, A. S.: The half-life of passively acquired antibody globulin molecules in infants, J. Exp. Med. **94**:213, 1951.
96. Zinkham, W. H., and Childs, B.: A defect of glutathione metabolism in erythrocytes from patients with a naphthalene-induced hemolytic anemia, Pediatrics **22**:461, 1958.
97. Zipursky, A., Pollock, J., Neelands, P., Chown, B., and Israels, L. G.: The transplacental passage of foetal red blood-cells and the pathogenesis of Rh-immunisation during pregnancy, Lancet **2**:489, 1963.

# 4 ERYTHROCYTES—GENERAL CONSIDERATIONS

*Properties of the erythrocyte.* The essential morphologic and physiologic aspects of the erythrocyte are considered in the following discussion.

*Erythron.* The term *erythron* refers to the tissue made up of the circulating red blood cells and their precursors in the bone marrow. It conveys a sense of functional unity to a series of cells ranging from the early erythroblast to the nonnucleated red corpuscles.

*Erythrocyte—structure and function.* Normal human red blood cells are nonnucleated biconcave disks, the primary function of which is the transport of hemoglobin, which represents 34% of their fresh weight. They are structurally adapted for rapid movement throughout the circulation to bring oxygen from the lungs and distribute it rapidly to the tissues through the smallest capillaries. The red cell is thicker at the periphery than in the central portion and possesses an elasticity which facilitates mechanical buffeting and movement through capillaries narrower than its own diameter. Collectively, the red cells offer an extensive surface of approximately 3,000 square meters in the adult to facilitate the absorption and discharge of oxygen and perhaps contribute to the movement of other substances by surface absorption. The outer surface or envelope, which serves as a semipermeable selective membrane in the passage of substances in and out of the cell, is composed principally of lipids consisting of a protein, stromatin, in combination with lecithin and cholesterol. The red cell surface possesses blood group properties, affinities, and specificities involved in hemolysis and agglutination.

In addition to hemoglobin, which constitutes more than 90% of solids, the red cell contains water, protein, liquids, carbohydrates, vitamins, iron, and a group of enzyme systems which maintains the integrity of the cell membrane. In the circulation hemoglobin remains relatively static, whereas other red cell constituents undergo constant physical and chemical changes relating to their metabolism.[39]

*Erythrocyte membrane.* The stroma is the insoluable portion of the erythrocyte which remains after the red cell has been hemolyzed and freed of hemoglobin. The stroma is frequently referred to as a ghost and the chemical composition of the membrane is obtained from this source. The stroma constitutes about 2 to 5% of the wet weight of the erythrocyte. Estimates indicate that 80 to 90% of the weight of the red cell membrane is protein.[36] One of the problems of precise determination is the possible contamination of membrane specimens with hemoglobin. Human erythrocyte lipids[104] consist of approximately 65% phospholipids, 23% cholesterol, 2% cholesterol esters, glycerides, and fatty acids, and 10% other lipids, probably glycolipids.

In cord blood the total red cell membrane lipid is increased[96] due to a proportional rise in both phospholipid and cholesterol despite a plasma environment which is quite low in phospholipid and cholesterol. These deviations from the adult pattern may have adaptive value for intrauterine life but may render the red cell more vulnerable to oxidative damage in postnatal life.[95] The evidence is also increasing that much of the oxygen dissociation characteristics of the fetal red cell is associated with the cell membrane and not merely with the presence of fetal hemoglobin.

The major functions of the red cell membrane are water and electrolyte transport and homestasis. The red cell possesses a number of properties reflecting its membrane structure. It is permeable to water and to a lesser extent to anions but impermeable to hemoglobin and selectively permeable to cations.

The major blood group antigens are mucopolysaccharides in nature. They form an important part of the red cell membrane, and are situated in part or in whole on its external surface.

It is also apparent that hemolysis in vitro indicates a pathologic lesion in the erythrocyte membrane, which permits the escape of hemoglobin.

*Metabolism of the erythrocyte.* The nucleated erythroid cells are capable of most of the metabolic reactions characteristic of nucleated cells of other tissues.[79] They can synthesize deoxyribonucleic acid (DNA) and ribonucleic acid (RNA) required for cellular proliferation. It is during this period in the bone marrow that nearly all the hemoglobin of the cells is synthesized. The reticulocyte is devoid of a nucleus and has little DNA, but it does contain RNA as well as mitochondria. The reticulocyte is capable not only of synthesizing the protoporphyrin but also of incorporating the iron into the protoporphyrin ring to form heme. In the mature erythrocyte there is little or no RNA. With extrusion of its nucleus, the circulating erythrocyte no longer functions as an active respiring tissue and the enzymes of the Krebs cycle and cytochrome system are absent. In the absence of an intact Krebs tricarboxylic acid cycle, the mature erythrocyte must derive its energy primarily from anaerobic glycolysis (Embden-Meyerhof pathway)[97] and from the oxidation of glucose via the hexose monophosphate shunt (Fig. 5). The major substrate glucose is in constant demand since the storage

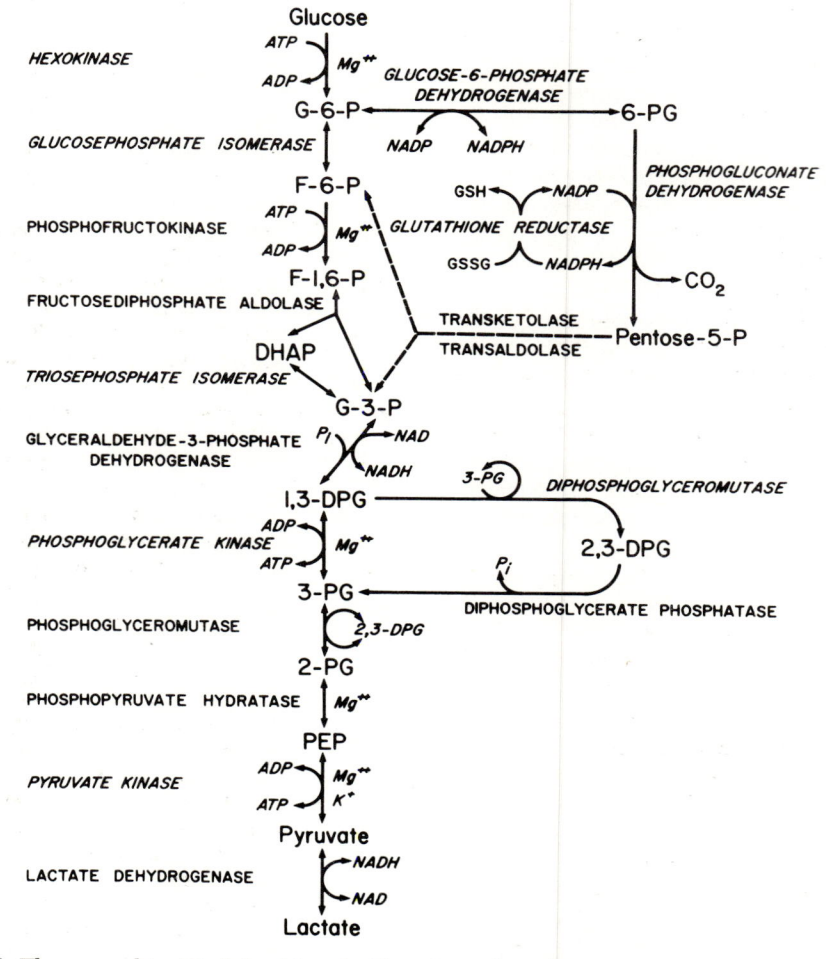

Fig. 5. The anaerobic (Embden-Meyerhoff) and aerobic (hexose monophosphate) pathways of erythrocyte glycolysis. Known enzyme deficiencies associated with hemolytic anemia are indicated in italics. (From Valentine, W. N.: Medical progress: hereditary hemolytic anemias associated with specific erythrocyte enzymopathies, Calif. Med. 108:280, 1968.)

of glycogen is virtually absent. The hexose monophosphate shunt is the active metabolic pathway primarily concerned with the generation of reduced triphosphate nucleotide (TPNH or NADPH), which, in turn, protects hemoglobin, and perhaps other proteins, from oxidative degradation. The enzymes involved in TPNH generation are more active in the erythrocytes of newborn infants than in adult subjects.

Within cells there exists a mechanism whereby the free energy available from oxidative processes may be utilized for those processes requiring free energy. This is accomplished by trapping the free energy through the formation of a special class of phosphate compounds of high energy content. Such an energy-rich phosphate compound is adenosine triphosphate (ATP). This source of metabolic energy is essential for maintenance of the normal composition of the red blood cell and thus for its ability to stabilize its volume and maintain its shape. It will be noted in examination of the Embden-Meyerhof pathway that, for the expenditure of two molecules of adenosine triphosphate (ATP) per molecule of glucose used, the erythrocyte can generate four, a potential gain of two.[68] This ATP can be utilized for various functions, for example, to maintain the high intracellular potassium and low sodium content essential for human erythrocytes against concentration gradients and potassium leaks by means of an ATPase system. ATP can also be utilized for the resynthesis of purine nucleotides and the synthesis of pyridine nucleotides, both essential cofactors in glycolysis. To maintain the lipids of the erythrocyte and to keep the iron of the heme moiety in the ferrous state also require metabolic activity and ATP. A decrease in glycolysis and in the generation of ATP has been shown to be associated with red cell aging and susceptibility to destruction. It is generally considered that destruction of the normal red cell at the end of its life-span is due to failure of one or more essential metabolic activities, as a result of which the cell is unable to produce sufficient energy to maintain its structural integrity. When this occurs, the cell breaks down and is removed from the circulation by the reticuloendothelial tissue.[103,110]

In both the full-term newborn infant and the premature infant the levels of ATP and its precursor, adenosine diphosphate (ADP), are higher than in the adult. In the premature infant the level of the ADP is increased over that in the term infant. The higher values for ATP and ADP, supported by the increased activity of the related enzymes, suggest that the newborn infant's red cells are more active than those of the adult in generating metabolic energy.[49]

Mitochondria have been recognized as the chief centers of cellular respiration in plants and animals. They are cytoplasmic organelles which are the cellular sites of various multienzyme metabolic processes, particularly the citric acid cycle, oxygen-linked respiration, and oxidative phosphorylation. They are present in all blood and lymphoid cells with the exception of the mature erythrocyte, which therefore is unable to carry on these processes. The mitochondrial inner membrane is a specialized structure peculiar to this organelle. Its integrity is essential to the link between respiration and oxidative phosphorylation and adenosine triphosphate (ATP) generation.[52]

It has been pointed out that in addition to the structural proteins there are approximately forty enzymes thus far identified in the human red cell.[142] Among these are the specific enzymes linked with the multiple activities of the red cell in supplying energy from glycolysis. Another example of the mediation of enzymes is the increased susceptibility of the cells to hemolysis caused by primaquine sensitivity due to a low glutathione level of the red cell and a deficiency of glucose-6-phosphate dehydrogenase activity.

Enzyme activity in the erythrocytes of the newborn infant differs in certain respects from that of the adult. Cholinesterase, glyoxalase, carbonic anhydrase, catalase, and methemoglobin reductase are diminished in cord blood. Thus, in certain infants difficulties in preventing excessive methemoglobin formation, rendering them susceptible to methemoglobinemia, may be attributed to a deficiency of methemoglobin reductase.[111] Increased hemolysis in newborn infants may stem from a defect in glutathione stability or from a lack of readily available glucose, despite normal increased levels of glucose-6-phosphate dehydrogenase at this time.[143] The activity of glucose-6-phosphate dehydrogenase, 6-phosphogluconic dehydrogenase, and aldolase is significantly higher in the erythrocytes of full-term infants and to an even greater extent in erythrocytes of premature infants.[48] It is not until the second 6 months that the activities of these enzymes consistently fall within the lower range of adults. Galactose-1-phosphate uridyl transferase is deficient in the red cells from patients with galactosemia. Erythrocyte acetylcholinesterase, a stromal enzyme, is increased in activity in younger red cells and decreased in older ones[13] It is in lesser concentration in normal newborn red cells than in those of adults and reaches the latter values by 3 to 5 months.

Although red cell acid phosphatase has not been very widely studied in pathologic conditions, two rather striking abnormalities have been reported—a significantly increased level of activity in megaloblastic anemia[133] and a markedly decreased level of activity in red cells of individuals with the Caucasian type of glucose-6-phosphate dehydrogenase deficiency.[99] A human polymorphism involving differences in acid phosphatase of red cells has been detected by starch gel electrophoresis, which includes five phenotypes. The acid phosphatase patterns appear to be fully developed at birth.[60,61]

Erythrocytes of the newborn infant are known to lose potassium at a rapid rate during short periods of incubation. Both term and premature infants possess a significantly lower percentage of ouabain-sensitive active transport ATPase than adults or patients with comparable reticulocyte counts.[139] This ATPase deficiency may play a role in the shortened life-span of red cells in the newborn.

The normal red blood cell has a volume of $85\mu^3$ and contains 28 to $30\mu\mu g$ of hemoglobin. The red cells, macrocytic at birth, diminish in size during the neonatal period and reach normal sizes of 7.2 to $7.5\mu$ in diameter by 8 months of age.

*Hemoglobin—structure and function.* Hemoglobin, the coloring matter of erythrocytes, is a conjugate of a pigment (heme) and a protein (globin). The heme component consists of a porphyrin (the union of four pyrrole groups) in combination with iron in the ferrous state. The hemes are pigments which account for the characteristic red color of hemoglobin. The particular porphyrin of hemoglobin is structurally a protoporphyrin. In the synthesis of heme, protoporphyrin is elaborated from the interaction of glycine and "active" succinate.[108] In vitro evidence suggests that the biosynthesis of heme from iron and protoprophyrin is enzyme dependent.[116]

The overall synthesis of heme from glycine and succinate has been studied in immature red blood cells of mammals, especially of birds.[79,83] The enzymes in these cells can be divided into three groups. The first group, which synthesizes succinyl coenzyme A and condenses it with glycine to form delta aminolevulinic acid, is bound to cell particles, presumably mitochondria. The second group is composed of soluable enzymes and converts delta aminolevulinic acid to coproporphyrinogen. The third group converts coproporphyrinogen to protoporphyrin and heme.[83]

Hemoglobin may then be regarded as a ferrous protoporphyrin with the following composition:

$$\text{Protoporphyrin} + \text{Iron} = \text{Heme}$$
$$\text{Heme} + \text{Globin} = \text{Hemoglobin}$$

Heme is also found in myoglobin (muscle hemoglobin) and in the respiratory enzymes such as the cytochromes. The basic function of the heme compounds is to transport oxygen and make it available to the cell. Hemoglobin combines loosely with oxygen to form oxyhemoglobin; this unstable association permits the diffusion of oxygen to tissues for oxidative purposes.

Iron participates as iron porphyrin complexes in reversible oxygenation, as a key part of the respiratory pigments hemoglobin and myoglobin, and in oxidative enzyme systems such as the cytochromes, peroxidases, and catalases. The iron of hemoglobin remains in the ferrous state throughout respiration. Methemoglobin, on the other hand, is the oxidized heme formed from reduced hemoglobin in which the iron is in firm combination in the ferric state and is incapable of functioning as an oxygen carrier. Globin, the protein component of the hemoglobin, is synthesized from the amino acids of destroyed protein and from the globin of effete red blood cells. For the complete synthesis of globin an adequate intake of protein is required.

Oxygen is normally picked up in the lungs from inspired air, bound to hemoglobin, and carried to the tissue capillaries. Here oxygen must be at a pressure sufficiently high to permit it to leave the capillaries and diffuse through the tissues.[55]

The iron of hemoglobin remains permanently in the ferrous state and functions by reversible combination with molecular oxygen. On the other hand, inorganic iron and free heme do not possess the property of reversible combination with molecular iron. The globin part of the hemoglobin molecule amounts to about 95% of the molecular mass. The heme is protected by the surrounding globin molecule so that the ferrous atom is permitted to undergo oxygenation.[75] Oxygen dissociation is said to influence the steady-state of the hemoglobin concentration of the blood. Alterations of the oxygen dissociation curve may be responsible for anemia and polycythemia.[5] Structural mutations involving the hemoglobin molecule may produce shifts in the dissociation curve. These mutations contribute to polycythemia observed in hemoglobin Chesapeake and hemoglobin Yakima (see Chapter 16).

An additional factor in oxygen dissociation is the compound 2,3-diphosphoglycerate (DPG). The central role of this compound in the metabolism and function of most mammalian red cells is receiving increasing attention, particularly in relation to its effect on oxygen binding by hemoglobin. This compound present in human red cells lowers the oxygen affinity and facilitates oxygen unloading because it is preferentially bound to deoxyhemoglobin.[4,5] DPG is a powerful regulator of the oxygen affinity of hemoglobin. Although both ATP (adenosine triphosphate) and 2,3-diphosphoglycerate can decrease the oxygen affinity of hemoglobin, the latter is quantitatively much more important, since its normal concentration in the human red cell is three to four times that of ATP[25] (see Chapter 1).

*Hemoglobin components.* The major component of hemoglobin, $HbA_1$, comprises about 95% of the total pigment. With starch electrophoresis a slow-moving minor component of hemoglobin, $HbA_2$, constitutes approximately 2.5% of normal adult hemoglobin. The latter is increased in most cases of thalassemia minor to about twice the normal value. A fast minor component, $HbA_3$ (with electrophoresis at pH 8.6), may be observed as a forward projection from the major spot of $A_1$. For practical purposes this small fraction is combined with $HbA_1$.

Observations of the rate of glycine uptake into heme and globin during normal red cell maturation indicate that heme and globin are synthesized independently during the development of the mature erythrocyte. Globin appears to be maximally synthesized at a primitive stage of erythrocyte development, whereas heme is maximally synthesized midway in maturation.[93]

Hemoglobin has a molecular weight of approximately 68,000 and is composed of four amino acid chains—two alpha and two beta polypeptide chains—and four heme groups. Each polypeptide chain of molecular weight of 17,000 is combined with a single heme group. The polypeptide chains are differentiated by their N-terminal sequences. The two open ends of the chain are characterized by a free amino acid group at one end and a free carboxyl group at the other[107] (Fig. 6). The first three amino acids of the amino terminal residues of the normal polypeptide chains are as follows: the alpha chain—valine, leucine, and serine; the beta chain—valine, histidine, and leucine; and the gamma chain—glycine, histidine, and phenylalanine. The carboxyl-terminal residues of the alpha chains are serine, lysine, tyrosine, and arginine; for the beta chains, alanine, histidine, lysine, tyrosine, and histidine; and for the gamma chains, serine, serine, arginine, tyrosine, and histidine.[57,115]

The two alpha chains are formed by 141 amino acids and the two beta chains by 146 amino acids each.[57] They are made from nineteen different amino acids. The whole molecule consists, therefore, of 574 amino acids. The two minor components of normal hemoglobin (HbA) are fetal hemoglobin (HbF) and hemoglobin $A_2$ ($HbA_2$). Each possesses two alpha chains identical with those of HbA, but the second pair of peptide chains differ—there are two gamma chains in HbF and two delta chains in $HbA_2$. Both the beta and gamma chains contain 146 amino acids.[115] The gamma and delta chains are chemically differentiated from the beta chains.[90] Furthermore, isoleucine is present in fetal hemoglobin and virtually absent in adult hemoglobin. On the basis of similarities of amino acid sequences, the delta and beta chains are nearly identical and beta and gamma chains are more similar to one another than either is to alpha. Also the delta, beta, and gamma chains share similarities with one another and dissimilarities with the alpha chain.[10]

The alpha and beta subunits of hemoglobin are under control of separate genes. Ingram[62] postulated that a single, primitive, myoglobin-like precursor protein is the evolutionary forerunner of all four types of polypeptide chains. By duplication and translocation, the genes for each of the chains are presumed to have undergone recurrent mutation and have thus come to differ from one another. In the evolutionary scheme of the original alpha chain, the gamma, beta, and finally the delta chains are derived in sequence (alpha ⟶ gamma ⟶ beta ⟶ delta). The structural genes for alpha, beta, gamma, and delta chains of normal hemoglobin are thus remarkably clustered on a single chromosome.[94]

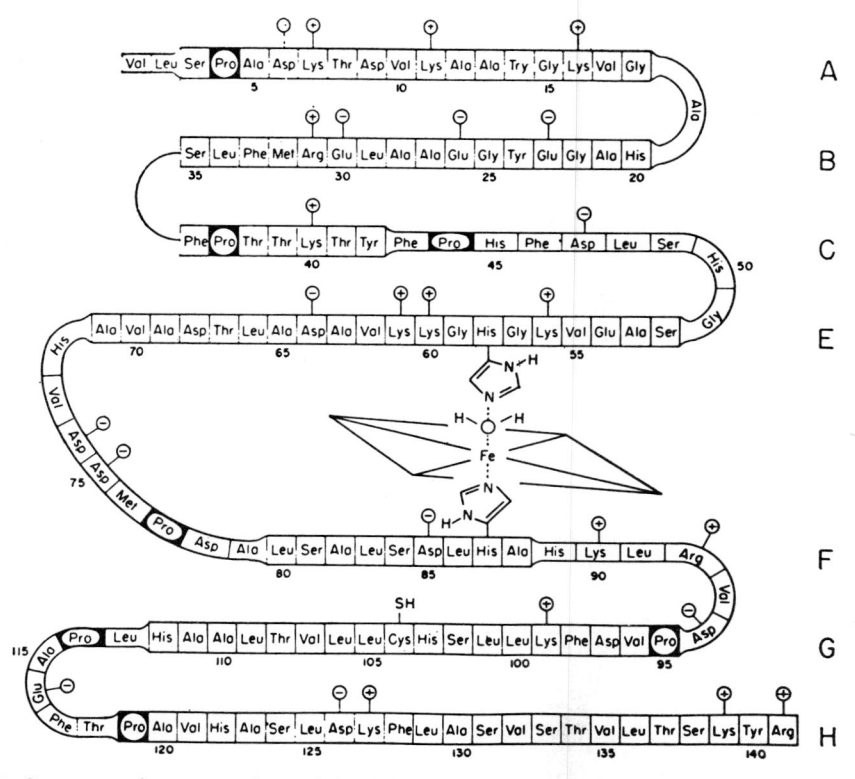

**Fig. 6.** Sequence of amino acids in alpha (above) and beta (see opposite page) peptide chains of normal human hemoglobin. The abbreviations represent amino acid residues of these seventeen amino acids:

| | | |
|---|---|---|
| Ala, alanine | Glu, glutamic acid | His, histidine |
| Gly, glycine | Thr, threonine | Lys, lysine |
| Val, valine | Cys-SH, cysteine | Asp, aspartic acid |
| Leu, leucine | Met, methionine | Ser, serine |
| Pro, proline | Try, tryptophan | Tyr, tyrosine |
| Phe, phenylalanine | Arg, arginine | |

(Courtesy Dr. William Konigsberg, The Rockefeller Institute.)

In rare instances the abnormal hemoglobins contain four identical chains, each with an absence of alpha chains: hemoglobin Bart's is a tetramer containing only four gamma chains, and HbH four beta chains. In cord blood of Negro babies, Hb Bart's occurs frequently in the absence of other hematologic changes.[87]

Most of the abnormal hemoglobins result from point substitutions of single amino acids in one or another polypeptide chain (Chapter 16). For instance, the amino acid alteration characteristic of sickle cell hemoglobin occurs in the beta chain, and both beta chains are so altered. Without an adequate amount of hemoglobin characterizing the hemoglobinopathies, the erythrocyte envelope is inadequately filled, resulting in flat hypochromic cells with a reduced life-span.

*Iron content and oxygen capacity.* Hemoglobin contains 0.335% of iron so that 1 gm. may be said to contain 3.4 mg. of iron. Also, 1 gm. of hemoglobin unites with 1.34 ml. of oxygen. Oxygen capacity depends upon hemoglobin concentration. Since the normal hemoglobin in the older child and adult is approximately 15 gm., the oxygen capacity is therefore 20 ml. per 100 ml. of blood or 20 vol.%. The degree of oxygen saturation of blood is derived from the ratio of oxygen content (19 vol.% in arterial blood) to oxygen capacity and is normally 95%.

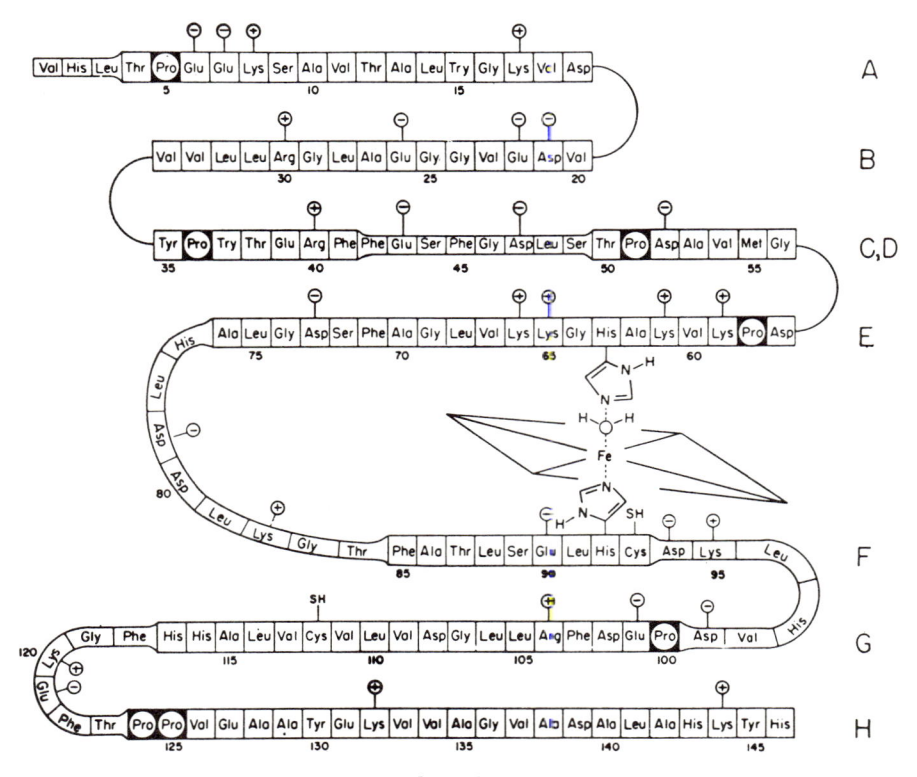

Fig. 6, cont'd. For legend see opposite page.

Cyanosis depends upon the absolute amount of reduced hemoglobin in capillary blood and not upon the content of carbon dioxide. It has been determined that capillary blood must contain at least 5 gm. of hemoglobin per 100 ml. of blood to reveal cyanosis. In severe anemia with values below this level, the amount of reduced hemoglobin will therefore be insufficient to show cyanosis.

The amount of oxygen combining with hemoglobin is regulated by the partial pressure of oxygen ($pO_2$), the partial pressure of carbon dioxide ($pCO_2$), and the pH. The smaller the $pCO_2$ the greater will be the oxygen saturation at a given $pO_2$; conversely, an increase in $pCO_2$ reduces the oxygen saturation. Oxyhemoglobin arriving at the tissues in which the $pCO_2$ is higher gives off oxygen and takes up carbon dioxide; the $pCO_2$, being low, is now able to take up more oxygen.[84]

*Heme-heme interaction.* Briefly stated, heme-heme interaction refers to the process in which the oxygenation of the iron atom of one heme group alters the affinity for oxygen of the other iron atoms in the hemoglobin molecule by enhancing it. Hemoglobin, the oxygen-transporting protein of blood, is composed of two pairs of subunits, the alpha and beta chains. Each subunit contains a single heme which can combine reversibly with oxygen so that each hemoglobin molecule can bind as many as four oxygen molecules. The affinity of hemoglobin for oxygen increases as more oxygen is bound.[120]

It has been determined that the heme is embedded in the globin segment of each molecule as in a pocket. The iron atom of each heme is connected to the amino acid histidine on one side of the globin pocket and to another (distal) histidine on the other side. It is between the iron atom and the distal histidine that the oxygen molecule is introduced when oxygenation of the hemoglobin occurs.[15,75] On oxygenation the units of hemoglobin move closer together and when hemoglobin is reduced they move further apart. The amino acids forming each of the globin molecules possess side chains which are of two types—hydrophilic chains, which interact with water, and hydrophobic side chains, which tend to repel water molecules. Hydrophilic chains are placed exteriorly, while hydrophobic side chains are placed internally in close association with each other. In the formation of binding forces between the internal hydrophobic side chains stability of the globin chain is achieved.[15,75]

The movement of the alpha and beta chains has been well described by Perutz.[101a] It can be deduced from the comparison of the structure by x-ray crystallography of oxy- and deoxyhemoglobin. In oxyhemoglobin the chains are much more closely associated than in deoxyhemoglobin, where they are more apart. This obviously involves the sliding apart of the alpha and beta chains during deoxygenation.

Thus in the heme-heme interaction the oxygenation and deoxygenation of one heme facilitates the oxygenation and deoxygenation of the second, and so on until all four heme groups are oxygenated or deoxygenated. Each heme group has one iron atom capable of combining reversibly with molecular oxygen while remaining in the ferrous state.[101a] The oxygen affinity of a hemoglobin solution rises with the degree of its saturation with oxygen, giving the oxygen equilibrium curve a sigmoidal shape which is attributed to the interaction between the four hemes in one molecule. The configuration change from deoxy- to oxyhemoglobin is transmitted from one chain to the other. If one is changed it helps the next chain to change its shape from deoxy- to oxyhemoglobin, and when two are changed the third one will be even more quickly deoxygenated, and so forth.[74] Deoxyhemoglobin also has a high affinity for certain phosphates present in the red cells, especially for 2,3-diphosphoglycerate, which has been previously discussed.

**Porphyrins and blood disorders.** The porphyrins are red pigments with a pyrrole structure which serve as precursors of protoporphyrins I and III and of their corresponding coproporphyrins. Both coproporphyrins are excreted in excess in urine and stool in certain blood disorders: type I in pernicious anemia, congenital spherocytic anemia, and leukemia and type III in aplastic anemia and Hodgkin's disease and after administration of heavy metals such as lead, mercurials, and arsenicals. The examination of the urine for porphyrins is especially important in lead poisoning. The greatest increases in coproporphyrin excretion occur in this condition, although this may not be a consistent finding. Splenectomy may be followed by diminished porphyrin formation in the bone marrow. Free protoporphyrin normally found in small amounts in erythrocytes is greatly increased in the blood of patients with iron-deficiency anemia and disorders in which utilization of iron in hemoglobin synthesis is interfered with, such as in anemia of infection.

**Glycogen.** At least six types of glycogen storage disease have been described.[121] In the normal erythrocyte, glycogen varies from 123 $\mu$g per gram of hemoglobin in cord blood to 65.6 $\mu$g at 1 year and 57.3 $\mu$g in the adult. Whereas the concentration of glycogen in the erythrocytes was normal in types I and II (classic form of von Gierke's disease and cardiac type, respectively), it is greatly increased in the erythrocytes in type III in which there is a deficiency of the amylo-1,6-glucosidase or debrancher enzyme.

**Rouleaux formation and sedimentation.** In a fresh preparation on a slide, red cells tend to cluster together with their broad surfaces in contact, forming a grouping called rouleaux. The disproportionate thickness and difficulty of approximation of the red cells in congenital spherocytic anemia results in loss of rouleaux formation and represents a diagnostic feature of this disease.

Erythrocytes suspended in plasma or serum settle because their density is greater than the density of the medium. When an erythrocyte suspension is placed in a vertical tube, aggregates form, varying in size from a few cells per aggregate to macroscopic particles. As aggregates settle there is an upward displacement of the plasma. In general, the sedimentation rate increases in proportion to the size of the erythrocyte aggregate. The rate of settling of red cells in a column of blood to which anticoagulant is added is known as the sedimentation rate.[32]

In rheumatic fever, arthritis, tuberculosis, nephritis, sickle cell anemia complicated by infection, and lupus erythematosus, to mention a few disorders in which elevated rates occur, repeated tests are of great value in management. In the final analysis it is recognized that the determination must be interpreted on the basis of clinical judgment. It should also be emphasized that the sedimentation rate is not a specific test. It estimates existing infection and tissue damage. Because of the abnormal shape of sickled red cells rouleaux formation is slow in the face of severe anemia.[12] Only with infection are sedimentation rates elevated in sickle cell anemia.

A variety of methods have been devised, usually with blood samples obtained by venipuncture.[140] When frequent tests are required in a protracted illness, it may be desirable, especially in young children, to employ a micromethod using capillary blood. Such a method has been described which utilizes a macrosedimentation tube of reduced dimensions[122] (Fig. 7).

A micro-erythrocyte sedimentation test utilizing capillary blood has been found especially useful in evaluating the small neonate with sepsis.[31]

Dilute suspensions of red cells cause accelerated rates of sedimentation so that the speed of sedimentation is inversely proportional to the concentration or the volume of red blood cells. Correction for anemia, therefore, seems necessary, but it is generally agreed that the adjusted figure constitutes a rough approximation since overcorrection often occurs. As a matter of fact, the red blood cells of infants and children with iron-deficiency anemia do not sediment with the velocity ascribed to diluted blood.[123] This is apparently due to the retarding influence inherent in the red cells.

In conditions associated with rapid sedimentation the initial phase consists of increased rouleaux formation; the larger the aggregates, the more rapid is the sedimentation rate. Acclerated rates are primarily influenced by increases in fibrinogen and, to a large extent, by globulin in the plasma.

*Electrolyte considerations.* The electrolyte composition of red blood cells is qualitatively similar to that of the plasma, except for the predominance of potassium in the former and sodium in the latter. In the passage of inorganic ions in and out of the cell, the red cell membrane acts as a dynamic rather than as a passive semipermeable structure. The energy for this and other functions of the mammalian cell is derived from the breakdown of glucose into lactic acid and from the presence of nucleotides such as adenosine triphosphate (ATP). In normal metabolic activity of the red cell membrane, a high concentration of potassium is maintained within the cell and sodium is excluded. Sodium and potassium cross the red cell membrane by two processes: passive diffusion or "leak" and active transport or "pumping" action.[97] The active process requiring the expenditure of energy "pumps" potassium into the cell and sodium out of the cell. Under normal circumstances these two rates, "leak" and "pump," are equal so that there is no net change in the internal red cell concentration of sodium and potassium. Details of the "pumping" process are elaborated in other sections of the text (pp. 301 and 303).

In blood stored under refrigeration, glycolytic activity is inhibited and potassium diffuses out of the cells into the plasma and the

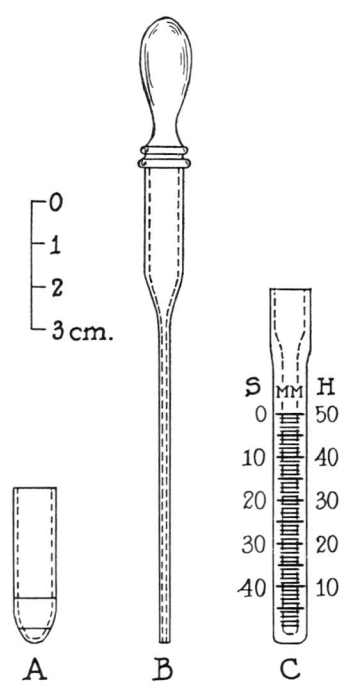

Fig. 7. The receiving tube, **A**, is calibrated at 0.06 ml. and 0.3 ml. Five percent sodium citrate solution is introduced to the lower calibration (0.06 ml.), moistening the sides of the tube as it is pipetted in. Sharp puncture of the fingertip secures a free flow of blood to the upper calibration (0.3 ml.). Blood flows down the side of the tube, being gently mixed in the process. The citrated blood is transferred to the sedimentation tube, **C**, by a simple capillary or Wright pipette, **B**. The normal sedimentation rate in 1 hour ranges from 3 to 13 mm. If heparinized blood is used, the microsedimentation tube is converted to a hematocrit after centrifugation (30 minutes at a speed of 2,500 revolutions per minute). The value is doubled to obtain the percentage of packed red cells.

sodium enters.[132] The accumulation of potassium in the donor plasma is an important consideration in exchange transfusions in erythroblastosis and can conceivably result in increased serum potassium levels in the infant. With normal kidney function, however, this state rarely develops. On the other hand, the too-rapid infusion of hyperkalemic donor blood that is not fully warmed carries the potentiality of untoward toxic effects. Since the metabolic activity is restored by exposure to 37° C. and results in return of the intracellular potassium, the use of fresh warm blood is recommended.[9,85] It has also been found that the ability of stored red cells to regain potassium when they are warmed depends upon the presence of adenosine and that the addition of this substance and glucose is needed for optimal red cell preservation.[23,38]

It has been recognized for many years that, early in their reaction to hemolytic substances, red cells leaked K⁺ and this was accompanied by an influx of Na⁺. The pumping in of K⁺ and the pumping out of Na⁺ are to a large extent linked processes in which the rate of active transport is stimulated by a rise in intracellular Na⁺ or extracellular K⁺.[69]

A clinically important class of compounds having the potential ability to hemolyze red cells rapidly are the hemolysin antibodies that fix complement (C′) and thereby cause lysis in vitro. Agents such as C′ affect permeability markedly by creating large holes in the red cell membrane and are responsible for rapid cell death. These events are illustrated in several hemolytic diseases. The red cells of paroxysmal nocturnal hemoglobinuria (PNH) are unusually sensitive to lysis by complement. In hereditary spherocytosis during periods of metabolic stress, there occurs an abnormal loss of membrane lipid and a concurrent shrinkage of surface area. This disorder appears to be associated with mild increase in permeability in which Na⁺ influx plays a dominant role. In nonspherocytic hemolytic anemia of pyruvate kinase deficiency, a reduction in active transport occurs in which K⁺ loss becomes a dominant event. The red cells from most such patients tend to "leak out" more than they "leak in" as they autohemolyze.[117]

Thus hereditary spherocytosis may result from a mild increase in permeability in which Na⁺ influx plays a dominant role. Nonspherocytic anemia of pyruvate kinase deficiency, on the other hand, appears to arise from a reduction in active transport in which K⁺ loss becomes a dominant event.[69]

For additional details on "pumping action of the red cell," see p. 304.

*Adsorption by the surface of red blood cells.* In the relation between the red cells and their environment, the occurrence of adsorptive phenomena is to be expected. The extensive surface presented by the red blood cells and its intimate contact with a diversity of substances in the plasma provide opportunities for adsorptive processes[124] comparable to those that occur at other interfaces. This function of red blood cells, as yet but little investigated, may account in part for the transport of metabolic, immune, and endocrine products through the bloodstream. The quantity attached to the red blood cell, however, is probably minimal as compared with that free in the plasma, and the substances fixed by the stroma are probably more slowly released than those in the plasma.

It has been demonstrated that erythrocytes are capable of binding bilirubin.[98] This activity is impaired when the erythrocyte is coated with antibody as demonstrated by a positive Coombs test. This binding activity appears to be a physicochemical property of the cell membrane in that it occurs almost instantly. Albumin, a protein known to bind bilirubin, appears capable of competing effectively with the lipid of erthyrocyte membrane for bilirubin binding and removes some from its surface. A reduction of approximately 3 mg.% can occur for each 100 ml. of nonsensitized erythrocytes added to each 100 ml. of serum.

*Osmotic fragility.* Changes in osmotic equilibrium surrounding the red cells influence their size. At a concentration of 0.85% a solution of sodium chloride is isotonic for the red cell, so neither swelling nor shrinkage results. In a medium of hypotonic sodium chloride solution, on the contrary, fluid passes into the cells, increasing their size, and the cells lose their biconcavity and become spherical. As a critical level is reached, more and more of the cells swell, burst, and release hemoglobin. The first trace of hemolysis normally appears when sodium chloride concentration reaches 0.42%, and hemolysis is complete at 0.32 to 0.35% (Chapter 15).

The resistance of the red corpuscles to varying dilutions of hypotonic solution of sodium chloride constitutes an important laboratory procedure in the diagnosis of the anemias and is especially useful in the differentiation of the hemolytic group.[125] The response of blood cells in the fragility test does not necessarily reflect their reaction within the circulating blood, where conditions of isotonicity prevail, but undoubtedly depends upon a number of intrinsic factors which involve the structure and properties of the cell envelope. However, the test constitutes a useful gross index of the relative thickness of the major number of red cells in the sample of blood to be tested. If the red cell envelope is small in relation to its volume, as in the thick red cells or spherocytes of hereditary spherocytosis, the resistance is decreased. Increased resistance to hemolysis is noted when the bulk of red blood cells possess relatively larger surfaces in comparison with their substance, as occurs in the thin red cells of patients with Mediterranean anemia and in patients with iron-deficiency anemia. Sickle cells are also more resistant to hypotonic saline solution than are normal cells.

Studies of the fragility of red blood cells of the newborn infant led to equivocal results varying from decreased[41] to increased resistance. In our laboratory moderately increased resistance has been observed in the cord blood of the full-term infant but is more marked in the premature infant. On the other hand, a slightly increased or normal fragility has been found[1] in the cord blood of the normal newborn infant. In these studies it was noted that the erythrocytes of most children with congenital cyanotic heart disease had only slightly greater fragility than those of normal patients. These purely in vitro studies bear no relation to the shortened life-span of fetal red blood cells when they are tagged with $^{51}$Cr and injected into normal individuals.

The increased resistance of red cells to osmotic lysis in obstructive jaundice is discussed in Chapter 5. In this condition the red cells are flat, have a target appearance on stained smear, and demonstrate an increased cholesterol:phospholipid ratio.

*Mechanical fragility.* Tests on mechanical fragility which evaluate the strength of the red cell membrane by exposing erythrocytes to the trauma of rolling glass beads under prescribed conditions are regarded as more closely simulating physiologic conditions prevailing in the circulation. With this test it was found[42] that erythrocytes of the newborn infant break down more rapidly in the first days of life. This increased mechanical fragility, which falls to normal by the fifth and sixth days, was associated with a rise in serum bilirubin. Although red cells and hemoglobin levels show minimal quantitative fluctuations in the first days of life, it is possible that shifts in plasma volume may obscure the rapid elimination of macrocytic cells existing during this period. According to this concept, physiologic jaundice stems from at least two sources: a hemolytic component and hepatic immaturity. However, current emphasis has been placed on the latter factor as being of major importance.

*Red cell thickness and oxygen dissociation.* It has been demonstrated by animal experiments that thickness of red cells bears a relation to oxygen dissociation. Thus the blood of patients with spherocytic cells was found to be less able to deliver oxygen to the tissues than was blood of normal patients or of patients with anemias in which the red cells were reduced in thickness.[134] Using more definitive technique, Carlsen and Comroe[13a,13b] have shown that gas transport in biconcave discs and in spherocytes induced by in vitro manipulation (heat or hypotonic solutions) was not measurably different.

*Erythrocyte production.* Multiple factors, many of which have specialized functions, enter into the production of red cells.

*Factors required for red cell production.* Normal maturation of erythrocyte precursors requires amino acids, proteins, and the B vitamins, especially pyridoxine, folic acid (pteroylglutamic acid), riboflavin, vitamin $B_{12}$, and the nucleic acid constituents, thymine and thymidine.[22] Of these factors, vitamin $B_{12}$, folic acid, and to a certain extent ascorbic acid are fundamentally involved in the development of the red blood cell. Folic acid participates in red cell maturation only after conversion, largely by ascorbic acid, to its biologically active form, folinic acid or citrovorum factor. Vitamin $B_{12}$ constitutes both the extrinsic factor and the erythrocyte maturation factor. The intrinsic factor from the stomach is necessary for the absorption of vitamin $B_{12}$. Whereas patients with pernicious anemia respond to either folic acid or vitamin $B_{12}$, those with megaloblastic anemia of infancy, in whom similar abnormal cells appear in the bone marrow, usually respond to folic acid alone but rarely to vitamin $B_{12}$. Both folinic acid (or folic acid) and vitamin $B_{12}$ serve as coenzymes in nucleic acid synthesis in the production of thymine and thymidine.

When vitamin $B_{12}$ and folic acid are deficient, purine and thymidine methyl synthesis is impaired, megaloblasts are formed instead of normal erythroblasts, and erythropoiesis is defective.

It is generally accepted that the intrinsic factor is a substance secreted by the normal stomach, rendering it possible for small amounts of vitamin $B_{12}$ present in most normal foods to be absorbed through the ileal mucosa. Vitamin $B_{12}$, in contrast to other nutrients that are absorbed mainly in the upper part of the small intestine, is absorbed principally from the lowest level of the ileum. (The primary site of folic acid absorption is in the jejunum.) The intrinsic factor is probably a glycoprotein or mucopolysaccharide, with a molecular weight of about 50,000 and an end-group conformation similar to that of partly degraded blood group substance.[56] An antibody to the human intrinsic factor exists in the serum of about one-third of adult patients with pernicious anemia, but whether the factor contributes to the pathogenesis of the disease is controversial.

Factors required in red cell (stroma) formation and hemoglobin (heme and globin) synthesis overlap to the extent that the separate consideration of each process is not always feasible. Although the need for minerals applies more particularly to the elaboration of hemoglobin, many of the vitamins and amino acids are involved in both processes. For example, a deficiency in minerals results in both lowered hemoglobin levels and morphologic changes in the red blood cell. Many of the inherited abnormal hemoglobins are associated with the presence of such definitive changes in the erythrocytes as sickle cells and target cells. To overcome the need for a sharp division and to allow for this interrelationship the term *erythropoiesis* is, therefore, frequently employed to cover both processes.

*Humoral regulation of erythropoiesis (erythropoietin).* The physiologic balance between red cell production and destruction which results in a remarkable consistency of number and volume involves the participation of several regulatory mechanisms. These are manifested in the stimulation of erythropoiesis after hemorrhage and after exposure to an atmosphere of reduced oxygen tension.

Bone marrow anoxia provides the primary stimulus for erythropoiesis as evidenced by polycythemia in chronic hypoxic states and the suppression of erythropoiesis when oxygen concentration is increased. It is not yet clear whether anoxia acts directly on the bone marrow or on the organism to produce a stimulating impulse.[46] It is probable that lowered oxygen tension stimulates bone marrow activity by a mediation of a humoral factor, erythropoietin.

Erythropoietin probably acts by stimulating differentiation of primitive undifferentiated mesenchymal cells (stem cells) to erythroid cells (erythroblasts). There are several conflicting theories concerning the role of erythropoietin in the regulation of erythropoiesis. In one,[67] the rate of red cell production is controlled by erythropoietin delivered to the site of red cell production by the plasma. Others[76,77] consider a more complex scheme in which at least two distinct erythropoietins play different roles in promoting this process (thermolabile and thermostable factors). Still others consider that there are regulators other than erythropoietin that affect red cell production; for instance, those that initiate DNA synthesis or cell division, the release of reticulocytes, and the prevention of normoblastic release into the peripheral blood. A feedback mechanism from the peripheral blood cells appears also to be implicated.[130] The in vitro effect of sheep erythropoietin on bone marrow cells indicates that it acts primarily or exclusively on stem cells and does not have a measurable effect on differentiated nucleated red blood cells or reticulocytes. Its main action is to accelerate the rate by which stem cells are differentiated to pronormoblasts.[30]

The ability of the serum and plasma of bled animals to induce a rise of reticulocytes, red blood cells, and hemoglobin when injected into normal animals gives further support to the presence of such a humoral factor. The existence of this factor was originally postulated in 1906 by Carnot and Deflandre,[14] who transfused plasma from a bled animal into an intact animal. Reismann[105] presented the first convincing evidence for the existence of a humoral factor by demonstrating similar hyperplasia of the bone marrow in a pair of parabiotic rats following chronic hypoxia induced in one partner. Erslev and Lavietes[28,29] stimulated further interest in this mechanism by the bioassay of large amounts of plasma from bled rabbits and monkeys which had induced reticulocytosis and other evidences of increased erythropoietic activity of the bone marrow in normal animals.

In the human subject, data have become available compatible with the humoral regulation of erythropoiesis. Plasma filtrates from patients with severe Cooley's anemia were found to stimulate hematopoiesis in intact rats, whereas similar preparations from normal subjects and one patient with chronic hypoplastic anemia were inactive.[102] Gurney and associates reported finding increased erythropoietin (erythrocyte-stimulating factor activity) in the serum of two patients with congenital hypoplastic anemia.[51]

The suppression of erythropoiesis after hypertransfusion[8,26] may indicate the mediation of humoral regulation in response to a lessened need for erythropoiesis. On the other hand, the similar depression of hematopoiesis following multiple transfusions[126] in chronically anemic patients suggests regulation in different ways or degrees from those involved in the normal individual. It appears possible that the physiologic adjustments in the chronically anemic person are such that hemoglobin concentrations which would be considered indicative of severe anemia under ordinary circumstances are, in fact, "normal" for that patient.

The effect of cobalt in increasing the rate of erythropoiesis in man and experimental animals to produce polycythemia has been attributed to bone marrow anoxia as a consequence of a toxic action on one or more enzyme systems. It has been shown that certain of the properties of erythropoietin in plasma of anemic patients are also common to those of the active factor in cobalt plasma, indicating that cobalt enhances red cell production by increasing the formation of erythropoietin.[43]

The actual site where the erythrocyte-stimulating factor is produced has not yet been clearly determined. Emphasis has been placed on the kidney as being directly or indirectly concerned with formation of the factor rather than the hemopoietic or other tissues.[44,66] It seems clear that the kidney produces erythropoietin, but whether it is the sole site awaits further confirmation.[129] That the plasma erythropoietin level is influenced by the functional state of the erythroid tissues of the marrow, as well as the severity of the hypoxic stimulus, is suggested by the high plasma values noted in refractory anemias and the relatively low values in most hemolytic disorders.[128] Erythropoietin is preferably utilized by a hyperplastic rather than an aplastic marrow. The plasma erythropoietin level is, therefore, related to the degree of erythroid activtiy of the marrow. Plasma erythropoietin levels reflect the balance between the erythropoietin produced in response to hypoxia and that utilized by the bone marrow. Any condition that leads to a decrease in bone marrow production of red cells would therefore permit an accumulation of erythropoietin in the plasma by virtue of decreased utilization (Chapter 14).

Significant amounts have been noted in congenital hypoplastic anemia, aplastic anemia, acute lymphoblastic leukemia, and chloramphenicol-induced bone marrow aplasia. In patients with hemolytic conditions associated with erythroid hyperplasia, as Cooley's anemia and sickle cell disease, significant levels of erythropoietin are found; however, they are found less frequently than in patients with the aplastic group of anemias. Low concentrations are observed in patients with uremia and chronic inflammation. The only sources of erythropoietin are the plasma and urine, but therapeutic use is limited until richer exogenous supplies become available. Although cobalt increases endogenous erythropoietin production, its use is handicapped by toxicity.[127]

Thalassemia patients with hemoglobins between 15 and 7 gm. per 100 ml. showed no increased serum erythropoietin activity. Those with hemoglobin concentrations between 7 and 4 gm. per 100 ml. showed increased activity. The rise in erythropoietic activity in both serum and urine was abrupt and increased markedly as the patients' hemoglobin value decreased below 7 gm. per 100 ml. At all hemoglobin levels there was correspondence between serum and urine erythropoietin levels, but serum showed greater erythropoietic activity than the corresponding urine. Only as hemoglobin values decreased below 7 gm.% did patients show an abrupt and marked increase in erythropoietic activity in both serum and urine.[84]

Following birth there is, under normal conditions, an almost immediate improvement in the oxygenation of the blood, and adult levels for oxygen tensions are reached within 3 hours after birth. No erythropoietin is detectable in plasma from normal newborn infants 1 day of age or more, confirming the concept that the decrease in erythropoiesis following birth is due to improved oxygen supply reducing the need for hemoglobin. If the postnatal decrease in erythropoiesis was due to bone marrow failure, one would have expected high erythropoietin levels as found in hypoplastic anemia. The decrease in erythropoiesis is not due to failure of erythropoietin production, since neonates are capable of producing erythropoietin in response to hypoxic stimuli.[53]

On the other hand, measured levels of erythropoietin have been demonstrated in cord blood from infants with hemolytic anemia due to maternal Rh-immunization. In severe cases erythropoietin has also been demonstrated in the amniotic fluid.[34,54] Greatly elevated erythropoietin levels have been found in some infants in the preeclamptic, postmature group and in infants of diabetic mothers.[35] Infants with the highest erythropoietin values showed signs of dysmaturity. Studies show that both anemic and hypoxic infants may demonstrate an increase in erythropoietin content. Erythropoietin appears to be a stimulating factor for red cell production in fetal life, at least in the last 6 months.

Erythropoietin contains a protein or polypeptide containing arginine or lysine and a carbohydrate component containing sialic acid. The latter may protect the active portion of the molecule from excretion or inactivation.[50] A renal factor may also interact with a serum factor, perhaps enzymatically on a serum substrate, to produce more erythropoietin. It has been suggested that the renal factor is not physiologically active unless it interacts with a serum carrier or activator, or that factor may be the enzyme which produced erythropoietin from some serum substrate. The appearance of prompt erythroid differentiation that follows administration of erythropoietin in the hypertransfused mouse, an animal essentially devoid of erythroid precursors, indicates that this is one way in which this hormone acts, namely, to initiate differentiation of a primitive hematopoietic stem cell.[17]

*Renal tumors and erythropoietin.* Certain tumors as well as various types of renal lesions are known to produce polycythemias. Among the renal lesions associated with polythemia are hypernephromas, renal cysts, hydronephrosis, renal adenomata, and Wilms' tumors.

Thurman and his associates[131] reported the first case of Wilms' tumor with polycythemia in an 18-year-old girl. In this case preoperative plasma erythropoietin levels were elevated and subsequently fell to normal when the primary tumor resected. Erythropoietin was found later in a metastatic pulmonary lesion. A second case, this in a 20-month-old boy, was reported[118] with an erythropoietin-producing Wilms' tumor and elevated hemoglobin and hematocrit values. Four months after nephrectomy the blood values were normal and there was no evidence of metastatic disease.

*Ineffective erythropoiesis.* The concept of ineffective erythropoiesis applies to the production of defective erythrocytes, which are destroyed either as precursors of mature cells within the marrow or almost immediately upon release into the peripheral blood.[33,141] This process stands in striking contrast to effective erythropoiesis, which results in the delivery of normal erythrocytes to the circulation. Although occurring normally to slight degree, significant ineffective erythropoiesis is characteristic of a number of anemias in which the bone marrow shows marked erythroblastic hyperplasia with a peripheral anemia—notably thalassemia major. In the case of pernicious anemia, for instance, the total marrow activity may be increased to three times the normal, but only one-third of the cells enter the circulation. The others are presumably defective and are destroyed at birth (ineffective erythropoiesis). In this condition, vitamin $B_{12}$ converts ineffective to effective erythropoiesis.

When glycine 2-$^{14}$C is administered orally, heme, globin, and stercobilin are tagged. Much of the excreted stercobilin is derived from the breakdown of hemoglobin at the end of the life-span of circulating red cells. Isotope appearing in high concentration during the first days after administration, however, may be due to various causes. In thalassemia[47] and in pernicious anemia[79] the early excretion of labeled stercobilin indicates an abnormal degree of premature destruction of red cells or hemoglobin in the marrow resulting from ineffective erythropoiesis.

*Characteristics of primitive blood cells.* Primitive cells of both the red and white cell series possess similar structural characteristics and, in their maturation, reveal many points in common. The early blast forms are large, the cytoplasm is deeply basophilic, the nucleus occupies more space and stains less deeply than the cytoplasm (leptochromatic), the chromatin is finely granular, and one or more nucleoli are present. At this stage, classification is facilitated by comparison with more mature cells with which they are associated by noting morphologic similarities. Maturation is accompanied by the following features: the primitive cell in each series becomes progressively smaller in the content of cytoplasm and nucleus, the basophilia of the cytoplasm lessens, the chromatin becomes more condensed, its original purplish color changes to dark blue, and the nucleoli disappear early. In the red cell the basophilia is replaced by hemoglobin. In the mature granulocyte the cytoplasm becomes faintly pink with specific granulation; in the lymphocyte, a hyaline or sky-blue color; and in the monocyte, a gray-blue with fine reddish blue granules.

*Stages in maturation of red blood cells—general principles.* The normal progression of red cell maturation is based upon intracellular chemical changes. A knowledge of these changes aids in identification of individual cells.

NUCLEIC ACID AND CELLULAR DEVELOPMENT. Cellular growth and multiplication of cells are closely identified with the content of the nucleic acids, ribonucleic acid (RNA) and deoxyribonucleic acid (DNA). Although they occur together, the former predominates in the cytoplasm (especially in the mitochondria) and nucleolus and the latter in the chromatin of the cell nucleus. Deoxyribonucleic acid, present in the nuclear material of all living cells, is generally believed to be the principal component of genes. Rapid growth of all cellular types, especially during mitosis, is accompanied by increased concentrations of the nucleic acids.[45]

DNA is visualized as consisting of two polynucleotide chains forming an interlocking helix about the central axis. Sugar-phosphate backbones make up the lines of the helix, while purines (adenine and guanine) and pyrimidines (cytosine and thymine) point inward toward the center. Much evidence now indicates that genetic information for protein structure is encoded in DNA, whereas the actual assembling of amino acids into proteins occurs in cytoplasmic ribonucleoprotein particles called "ribosomes." Proteins are not synthesized directly on genes, and an intermediate information carrier is required. The latter is generally assumed to be a stable ribonucleic acid (RNA), the RNA of ribosomes. The amino acid sequence along the polypeptide chain of a protein is probably determined by the sequence of the bases along some particular part of the nucleic acid of the genetic material. Since there are twenty common amino acids found in nature, but only four common bases (adenine, guanine, thymine, and cytosine), the sequence of the latter serves in some manner as a code for the sequence of the amino acids.[18] The genetic code, therefore, describes the way in which a sequence of twenty different kinds of amino acids is determined by a sequence of specified bases in DNA. It is highly probable that a specific sequence of only three nucleotide bases controls the insertion of one of the twenty amino acids into a polypeptide chain. The detailed mechanism by which the nuclear DNA code is transferred to messenger RNA, which in turn transmits the genetic information to the protein forming ribosomes, is still under investigation.[59]

BASOPHILIA. Deep basophilia of the cytoplasm characterizes the stem cell and red and white cell precursors at the "blast" level of immaturity. The high content of ribose nucleic acid parallels the maximal cytoplasmic basophilia. The basophilic staining is ascribed to the affinity of nucleic acid in cytoplasm for the basic component (methylene blue) of Wright's stain or other polychromatic stains. In all cell types, basophilia recedes with increasing maturity, and in the red cell its gradual replacement by hemoglobin results in an increased affinity for acid dyes (eosin).

POLYCHROMASIA AND STIPPLING. Admixtures of basophilic substance and hemoglobin in intermediate stages produce polychromatophilia of the cytoplasm. Stippling (punctate basophilia) refers to the fine or coarse bluish violet granules found in the red cells. Stippled cells are noted in a variety of clinical conditions such as lead poisoning and hemolytic and deficiency anemia of varying severity.

ERYTHROPOIESIS. Two types of red cell maturation can be described: the pathologic form associated with a deficiency of hematopoietic or liver principle, megaloblastic erythropoiesis, and the normal process, normoblastic erythropoiesis. The recognition of the various stages in either normal maturation depends upon cell size, staining of the cytoplasm, and nuclear conformation according to the principles already stated. Only those cell types need be included here that are commonly observed in pediatric practice and can be identified by bone marrow aspiration. The difficulties in distinguishing between megaloblasts and early cells of the normoblastic series are confined to two conditions in this age period: megaloblastic anemia of infancy and the rare juvenile pernicious anemia. Other forms of anemia involve the orderly maturation of the normoblastic series. The term *erythroblast* has assumed a comprehensive connotation and includes all nucleated red cells, both normal and pathologic.

After administration of glycine $^{14}C$ and $^{59}Fe$ citrate to normal individuals, it was determined that the maturation time of the normoblast is approximately 5 days and that globin synthesis precedes maximal heme synthesis during maturation of normoblasts. In megaloblastic erythropoiesis, the maturation time of the primitive megaloblast is prolonged. Vitamin $B_{12}$ appears to shorten maturation time also, enhancing globin synthesis in the primitive cell.[92]

*Normal maturation.* It will be noted that in the normal maturation the cytoplasm and nucleus mature simultaneously and synchronously. The stages of normal red cell development and their chief morphologic and staining characteristics may be outlined as follows:

*Pronormoblast (proerythroblast)*
About twice the size of a normal mature erythrocyte. Cytoplasm: narrow-rimmed, deeply basophilic. Nucleus: light purplish, vesicular, granular, slight clumping, one or more nucleoli present.

*Basophilic normoblast (early normoblast or early erythroblast)*
Smaller than pronormoblast. Cytoplasm: basophilic. Nucleus: darker purplish staining, chromatin, clumping more marked, may be cartwheel, nucleoli absent.

*Polychromatic normoblast (intermediate normoblast, late erythroblast)*
Cytoplasm: less basophilic, traces of hemoglobin present. Nucleus: shrunk, more mature, chromatin bluish-black, coarse, clumped; a light area resembling hemoglobin often seen at one pole of the nucleus.

*Orthochromatic normoblast (late normoblast)*
Size somewhat larger than erythroblast. Cytoplasm: almost completely filled with hemoglobin, late forms red staining, eosinophilic. Nucleus: chromatin condensed, dark, homogenous, structureless mass referred to as pyknotic.

*Reticulocytes*
Slightly larger than normal erythrocyte. Nucleus has been extruded. Reticulum or filamentous substance, varying in amounts and arrangements, stains deep blue with brilliant cresyl blue, the smallest amounts seen in those nearly mature. Reticulum is a precipitate material now known to be ribonucleic acid and corresponds to basophilia of cytoplasm and is not related to nuclear remnants, mitochondria, or hemoglobin. In 2 to 5 days, perhaps in less time, reticulocytes mature in circulation and normally number 0.5 to 1.5%. Reticulocytes reflect reactivity of the bone marrow; an increase indicates accelerated hematopoiesis. Reticulocytes show maximal peaks following specific treatment of patients with pernicious anemia and related megaloblastic anemia in 5 to 7 days and following iron therapy in patients with iron-deficiency anemia in 5 to 10 days. Reticulocytes formed during periods of rapid cell production differ from those formed under usual conditions.[119] These are known as stress or shift reticulocytes. These shift reticulocytes are delivered prematurely from the marrow pool into the circulating blood and require 1 to 3 days longer than the normal reticulocytes to lose their reticulum. These immature or shift cells are recognizable through their relatively large size and increased basophilia. The crude reticulocyte percentage so extensively used to indicate erythropoietin activity is dependent not only on the number of reticulocytes in circulation but also on the number of adult cells to which they are related.[58] Appropriate corrections must, therefore, be applied both for variations in the peripheral red blood count and for changes in the maturation process. The shift cells are of greater diameter, contain more reticulum, and are of lower density than the normal reticulocyte. Approximately 25% of the reticulocytes formed are destroyed within 10 days, whereas the remainder have a longer life-span. The ATP (adenosine triphosphate) content of stress reticulocytes is significantly greater than that of normal erythrocytes and returns to normal within 8 days following the peak of reticulocytosis. Reticulocytes are increased in the embryo and high values are found in the newborn infant. Hemoglobin is synthesized in the reticulocytes. With an in vitro system using reticulocyte-rich rabbit red cells incubated with $^{59}Fe$-labeled plasma, $^{59}Fe$ is first associated with particulate matter of the cell (stroma, mitochondria, and microsomes); then it is gradually released to the soluble cytoplasm.[2] On the release from these fractions, $^{59}Fe$ is first associated with nonhemoglobin protein and later incorporated into hemoglobin. It is probable that a suitable concentration of lead allows $^{59}Fe$ to accumulate in stroma but blocks its entry into the nonhemoglobin protein iron phase and into hemoglobin.

*Abnormal maturation (deficiency of the hematopoietic factors—liver, folic acid, and vitamin $B_{12}$).* The cells are abnormally large and the nucleus matures more slowly than cytoplasm.

*Promegaloblasts (erythrogones)*
Regarded by some as common progenitors of both pathologic megaloblasts and of normoblasts; may

be regarded as earlier form of megaloblast; large cell. Cytoplasm: abundant, basophilic. Nucleus: light purplish staining, chromatin open reticular pattern, stippled, no clumping as in pronormoblast, several nucleoli present.

*Megaloblast (basophilic megaloblast)*

Corresponds to promegaloblast. Cytoplasm: more intense dark blue basophilia. Nucleus: no nucleoli, chromatin finely divided.

*Polychromatic megaloblast (intermediate megaloblast)*

Large cell. Cytoplasm: hemoglobin now present and basophilia decreased, resulting in multicolored polychromatophilic cytoplasm. Nucleus: purplish, still finely granular with occasional clumping.

*Orthochromatic megaloblast (late megaloblast)*

Larger than corresponding late normoblast. Cytoplasm: deeply eosinophilic. Nucleus: purplish blue, reduced in size, irregular clumping, but reticular appearance still present, never cartwheel shaped.

*Macrocyte*

Larger than normal erythrocyte which it resembles, measures $9\mu$ or more in diameter.

The megaloblast series, in contrast to corresponding normoblasts, shows less clumping and greater retention of the fine reticulated appearance of the nucleus during maturation, and at each stage is larger than the corresponding normoblast. Cells with partial deficiency of the hematopoietic factor, intermediate in nuclear structure between the megaloblast and normoblast, appear in the bone marrow. With increased deficiency, megaloblasts appear, whereas specific treatment (such as folic acid in infantile megaloblastic anemia) results in differentiation into normoblasts.

Reisner[106] pointed out that the nuclear chromatin particles are more homogeneous in the normoblastic cells as compared with the diffuse, particulate, meshlike chromatin of the megaloblastic cells and that the ratio of "mitotable" (that is, capable of mitosis) to maturing cells is much increased in the latter. Megaloblasts are conceived as red cell precursors with a prolonged resting phase between mitoses, allowing a longer time for the dispersion of the chromatin throughout the nucleus. The conditions most conducive to megaloblastic blood formation are states in which vitamin $B_{12}$ or folic acid is deficient. Normoblastic hematopoiesis results in normal erythrocytes as compared with the oval macrocytes of megaloblastic hematopoiesis. Megaloblasts are found in the bone marrow not only in pernicious anemia and megaloblastic anemia of infancy and of intestinal origin, but also in a number of miscellaneous states in which for various reasons the patient has levels of vitamin $B_{12}$ and folic acid inadequate for the increased demands for hematopoiesis. These include multiple myeloma, hemolytic anemia, idiopathic aplastic anemia, chronic blood loss with superimposed acute hemorrhage, myelofibrosis, erythremic myelosis, advanced cirrhosis of the liver, after anticonvulsant drugs (phenytoin sodium [Dilantin][113] and primidone [Mysoline][40]) and leukemia, in which antifols and 6-mercaptopurine have been used.[106]

The multiple designations given to the same blood cells have led to an attempt to standardize the nomenclature and to provide more precise criteria for identity of each cell type.[16] The recommended terms for the red cell series and a few of their alternates include the following: rubriblast (megaloblast, hemocytoblast), prorubricyte (pronormoblast), rubricyte (basophilic and polychromatic normoblasts), and metarubricyte (orthochromatic normoblast). "Pernicious anemia type" is applied as a qualifying phrase to any cell in this series in which the morphologic changes are those of pernicious anemia.

**Normal destruction of erythrocytes.** The destruction of the red cell is accompanied by a number of phenomena of which those relative to the excretion of bile pigment are among the most important.

*Fragmentation.* Fragmentation is regarded as an important mechanism in the destruction of worn-out red cells.[112] Red cell fragmentation has been defined as loss from the red cell of a piece of membrane which may or may not contain hemoglobin. Weed and Reed[137] describe fragmentation as the formation of a tongue of the red cell in its passage through the capillary bed in general and the spleen in particular and its eventual separation from the red cell. These irregularly shaped fragments are known as schistocytes (see p. 294). With each successive fragmentation the spheroidicity of the cell increases and ultimately the characteristics are altered from those of a deformable body to those of a rigid body. Erythrocytes may fragment earlier if they are subjected to excessive trauma in the circulation[11] such as may result from a malfunctioning prosthetic heart valve or incomplete repair of an intracardiac defect.

While hemolysis in vitro results from a pathologic alteration in the erythrocyte permitting the escape of hemoglobin, hemolysis in vivo is generally regarded as a shortening of the life-span of erythrocytes. The latter is based on such membrane disturbances as changes in permeability, phagocytosis of damaged red cells, and fragmentation. Cellular rigidity and membrane fragmentations are related to a variety of hemolytic disorders. These include the thalassemic disorders, aggregating and unstable hemoglobins, defects of the pentose phosphate shunt, extrinsic mechanical damage, antibody injured cells, hereditary spherocytosis, and disorders involving cellular ATP (adenosine triphosphate) instability.[137]

*Life-span of the red blood cell.* The life-span of the human red cell in the circulation is approximately 120 days, corresponding to a normal rate of replacement of 0.83% per day. The methods used for this determination are based on the Ashby method of differential agglutination,[3] in which the number of transfused group O red cells is determined periodically in the blood of the recipient of another group. The same objective can be achieved with the use of compatible blood for the major blood groups but with differences on the M and N factors. In either case the agglutination of the recipient's blood by appropriate sera permits the counting of the residual unagglutinated cells of the donor. Comparable results for the normal life-span have been obtained and more expeditiously with the use of red cells tagged with an isotope of nitrogen ($^{15}N$), of iron ($^{59}Fe$), or of chromium ($^{51}Cr$).

Radioactive sodium chromate can be satisfactorily employed to measure the circulating red cell mass, blood volume, and red cell survival and to localize the site of red cell destruction.[62,70] The method of labeling red cells by radioactive chromium has replaced the other more elaborate methods. It affords a simple method for studying red cell survival in normal subjects and in patients with various hematologic disturbances. By reinjecting blood that had been mixed with the sodium radiochromate into the circulation of the patient, the longevity of the cells is measured in their natural environment. The chromium taken into the cell becomes firmly attached to the globin portion of the hemoglobin molecule. It has been found that the beta chains of hemoglobin have a greater affinity for chromium than do the alpha chains.[82,100]

The half-life survival of $^{51}Cr$-tagged red cells has been found to average from $26 \pm 2$ days[24] to $33.1 \pm 3.2$ days.[71] When correction is made for the loss of radioactivity by elution from the red cell of 1% per day, the half-life of chromated cells corresponds to the half-life of transfused cells as determined by other methods. A considerably reduced half-life has been noted in many of the intrinsic hemolytic anemias or in blood dyscrasias accompanied by a hemolytic component.[138]

*Life-span of newborn red cells.* Estimates of the life-span of the red cell in premature and full-term infants have not always been in agreement. In one study, fetal red blood cells obtained from the umbilical cord and tagged with $^{51}Cr$ were noted to have a shortened life-span with a half-life of 15 to 23 days as compared with a range of 24 to 35 days in normal adults.[59] The survival of similarly tagged placental red cells also transfused into adult recipients gave a mean half-life of 22.8 days (17 to 28 days) in the full-term infant and 15.8 days (10 to 18 days) in the premature infant, compared with 27.5 days in the adult.[37] Another study[72] demonstrated an essentially normal half-life (25 to 35 days) in full-term infants in the first 5 days of life, whereas in premature infants the half-life was less than 20 days. In the same study, in the third to ninth week of life, the $^{51}Cr$ erythrocyte half-life was 12 to 33 days for eight full-term infants and 12 to 34 days for fourteen premature infants. (See Chapter 1.)

These findings indicated that survival of full-term infants' erythrocytes is usually at adult levels during the first 5 days of life, whereas in the premature infant it is invariably shortened.[72] On the other hand, when $^{15}N$-labeled glycine was fed to premature infants in the first 48 hours of life, the rate of elimination of newly formed tagged erythrocytes was identical with that seen in normal adults similarly treated—120 days.[21] The normal results in these observations, as compared with the shorter red cell life-span of premature infants reported by others, may be due to differences between adult type erythrocytes produced postnatally as compared with red cells of shortened survival produced in utero.

Aging of red blood cells is associated with a decrease in enzyme activity as well as other disturbances of cell metabolism. Normal old red cells are low in glucose-6-phosphate dehydrogenase activity.[144] Erythrocytes nearing the end of their life-span produce less energy in the form of adenosine trisphosphate (ATP) and are more susceptible to the destructive effects of oxidation.[144]

*Normal hemolysis.* With a normal life-span of 120 days, approximately 1% of the red cells leave the circulation daily. Under normal conditions wornout red cells are removed from the circulation by cells of the reticuloendothelial system in the spleen, bone marrow, and liver and, to a lesser extent, in other tissues. The major physiologic method by which red cells are destroyed is by fragmentation caused by the traumatic effects of circulation. Erythrophagocytosis within the spleen and lytic factors present in the plasma and tissues are contributory agents in this physiologic process. Phagocytosis of intact red cells may be observed occasionally in the peripheral blood and bone marrow in patients with erythroblastosis and acute leukemia.

Although phagocytosis and hemolysis may be involved in this process, these factors exert their influence largely in pathologic conditions. Fragmented cells (schistocytes) formed in this manner also result from the wearing out of enzyme systems controlling the integrity of the cell or its membrane. Stagnation in the spleen can also contribute to red cell dissolution by altering the spheroidicity and osmotic fragility.

The destruction of the red blood cell is accompanied by a breakdown of hemoglobin. Following preliminary oxidative opening of the protoporphyrin ring and the formation of a green bile pigment (iron-protein complex), verdohemoglobin, iron is split off. Iron, attached to a beta-1-globulin of the plasma (siderophylin, transferrin), is transported in the bloodstream to the bone marrow for the regeneration of hemoglobin or to the liver, spleen, and other organs where it is deposited in the form of ferritin and, when excessive, hemosiderin.

Important evidence suspicious of a hemolytic process includes the following elements: shortened red cell survival time, increased fecal and urinary urobilinogen excretion, hemoglobinuria, elevation of serum bilirubin, reticulocytosis and polychromatophilia, decreased haptoglobin, increased bone marrow activity, spherocytosis, and splenomegaly.

Attachment of antibody molecules to antigenic sites in the red cell surface does not by itself appear to produce any serious damage to the cell. Red cells acted on by agglutinating antibodies appear to be attached to one another by spicules presumably derived from the red cell membrane, but lysis is not observed. If, however, the attachment of antibody to red cells is followed by activation of complement, membrane lesions may be produced, leading to dissolution of the cell. There is evidence that a single IgM molecule attached to a red cell can activate complement resulting in red cell lysis, but that two adjacent IgG molecules are required.[88]

*Erythrocyte deformability and red cell life-span.* According to Weed,[136] the normal cellular deformability is the most important determinant of red cell life-span in vivo. He defined erythrocyte deformability as "those geometric and physical characteristics which permit a cell whose greater diameter normally exceeds $8\mu$ to pass through $14\mu$ or longer segments of normal capillaries which range from 3 to $12\mu$ in diameter." He also emphasized that, in specialized regions of the microcirculation such as in the bone marrow and within the spleen, red cells must pass through channels of varying length less than $14\mu$ and down to $0.5\mu$ in diameter. Normal erythrocytes will pass easily through channels having a diameter down to $2.9\mu$. The determinants of red cell deformability are the shape factor (surface area to volume ratio) and intrinsic deformability, which is controlled by the state of intracellular hemoglobin. In the former the biconcave shape of the normal erythrocyte, according to Weed,[136] made possible by its excess of surface area to volume, is basic to its ability to deform. In the case of the abnormal hemoglobin there is a predisposposition to undergo intracellular gelation or crystallization as in sickle cell anemia and homozygous hemoglobin C disease. In the case of rigid cells such as sickle cells intracellular fragmentation occurs and shortens their life-span. Heinz body formation associated with abnormalities of the pentose phosphate shunt, unstable hemoglobins, and unbalanced synthesis of globin chains as in the thalassemia syndromes will also result in premature red cell destruction. If sufficient numbers of Heinz bodies are formed within a cell the whole erythrocyte assumes a rigidity, resulting in its removal from the circulation.

*Formation of bilirubin.* Bilirubin is derived from hemoglobin. It is the globin- and iron-free fraction of the hemoglobin molecule. An increased destruction of red cells during hemolysis results in a corresponding increase in bile pigment production. When iron is split off, the compound has been stated to exist for a time as a bilirubin-globin complex. Following the loss of iron, the green bile pigment is formed. The separation of globin and the degradation to bilirubin probably occur in the reticuloendothelial system. Globin enters the body protein pool as amino acids to be utilized in hemoglobin formation.

Bilirubin pigment is formed in the reticuloendothelial elements of the spleen, lymph nodes, bone marrow, liver, and connective tissue (probably with the bone marrow as the most significant site). About 10 to 15% of total bile pigment is derived from precursors other than hemoglobin,[73,80] such as heme not used in the synthesis of hemoglobin, myoglobins, peroxidase, catalase, and cytochromes. Bile pigments in human serum range from 0.5 to 0.8 mg. per 100 ml. of blood, and those in the serum of patients with chronic hemolytic anemias range from 1 to 3 mg., rarely above 5 mg. per 100 ml of blood. When normal bilirubin levels occur in a patient with hemolytic anemia, it is due to the ability of a healthy liver to excrete excess quantities of the pigment. The accumulation of indirect bilirubin in the plasma, as occurs in patients with erythroblastosis and in those in a hemolytic crisis, results from overloading of the liver with products of blood destruction.

London[78,81] includes the following considerations in evaluating the gross bile pigment metabolism: the amount of hemoglobin which is being destroyed daily, the functional capacity of the liver to excrete bilirubin into the bile, the patency of the biliary tree, the functional capacity of intestinal bacteria to reduce bilirubin to the urobilinogens, the functional capacity of the liver to reexcrete urobilinogen, and the threshold of the kidney for the excretion of direct bilirubin.

*Direct and indirect bilirubin.* Two types of bilirubin have been differentiated on the basis of the van den Bergh reaction. The basis of this test is the observation by Ehrlich that the addition of diazo reagent (diazotized sulfanilic acid) to blood plasma or other bile-containing solutions yields a reddish violet color. The immediate evolution of maximum color intensity is termed a direct reaction. If color fails to develop in 1 minute but appears after the addition of alcohol, the reaction is regarded as indirect. No completely satisfactory explanation has been offered for the direct and indirect reactions, although it is now known that the direct reaction depends upon the formation of soluble glucuronides of bilirubin.

The van den Bergh test employs these reactions to distinguish the two types of bilirubin involved in clinical jaundice. If the jaundice results from intrahepatic or extrahepatic obstruction to the passage of bile into the intestine, most of the bilirubin is of the direct-reacting form. This is the 1 minute bilirubin. When jaundice is due to excessive destruction of hemoglobin as in hemolytic anemia, most of the bilirubin is in the indirect-reacting form, that is, the addition of alcohol is essential for color to develop. It is possible that the alcohol catalyzes the transformation of indirect to direct bilirubin so that the diazo reagent will produce the reddish violet color. The total concentration of both types of bilirubin usually ranges from 0.2 to 1.4 mg. per 100 ml., with 0.2 mg. as the upper limit of normal for the direct type.

Klatskin and Bungards[73] have shown that the bulk of bilirubin in serum is bound to albumin irrespective of its behavior in the van den Bergh reaction. They found no evidence that in the breakdown of hemoglobin globin remains attached to its porphyrin fraction to yield indirect-reacting bilirubin. The action of alcohol in facilitating the diazotization of indirect-reacting bilirubin does not depend upon release of bilirubin from its protein complex. This contradicts the former concept that the indirect-reacting bilirubin is attached to alpha globin in contrast to the linkage of direct-reacting bilirubin to serum albumin.

It has also been postulated[91] that the direct bilirubin is a bilirubin-metal complex and that indirect bilirubin represents bilirubin not bound to metal.

Robinson and co-workers[100] studied the formation of early-labeled bile pigment from both glycine-2-[14]C and delta-aminolevulinic acid with congenital nonhemolytic hyperbilirubinemia. They concluded that the initial component of early bilirubin formation is derived from nonerythroid sources such as turnover of nonhemoglobin hemes in the liver and possibly other tissues.

The excretion of bile depends upon the conversion of indirect to direct bilirubin. This process has heretofore been regarded as a function of enzyme systems in the liver which are active in the dissociation of pigment-protein complexes. It has been demonstrated, however, that the water-insoluble indirect bilirubin requires conjugation with glucuronic acid for the formation of water-soluble direct bilirubin which is then capable of excretion in the bile. The terms *bilirubin* and *conjugated bilirubin* have therefore been suggested as substitutes for *indirect bilirubin* and *direct bilirubin,* respectively.[7] According to this concept, indirect bilirubin, being water-insoluble, requires prior addition of alcohol to initiate coupling with the diazo reagent, whereas conjugated bilirubin, being water-soluble, is readily diazotized. The formation of bilirubin glucuronide is mediated by a glucuronyl transferase enzyme system and the delay in its formation accounts for the accumulation of indirect bilirubin in the plasma in jaundice of the newborn infant (Chapter 8). In obstructive jaundice conjugated (direct) bilirubin gains access to the blood and then to urine.[6,114] It is thus understandable that soluble bilirubin glucuronides (direct-reacting bilirubin) can be readily filtered by the kidneys and that relatively insoluble indirect bilirubin is incapable of being filtered. Hence the indirect type of bilirubin does not appear in the urine despite excessive amounts in the blood. Increased excretion of bile by the liver, however, accounts for the excess of urobilinogen in the urine of patients with hemolytic anemia. On the other hand, the soluble direct bilirubin can be excreted by the kidney when it accumulates in the blood as it does in patients with obstructive jaundice and hepatic or duct disease.

*Urobilinogen excretion—an index of hemolysis.* Bile pigment are derived from the breakdown of heme, and the amount found is related almost quantitatively to the hemoglobin produced and destroyed each day. The porphyrin portion of hemoglobin, exclusive of the iron constitutes 3.5% by weight of the hemoglobin molecule. Theoretically, all of the porphyrin of the destroyed hemoglobin is converted to bilirubin. Thus 1 gm. of hemoglobin yields 35 mg. of bilirubin.[19] However, 10 to 15% more than the estimated quantity actually appears each day as urobilinogen.[78,80] The precursors of this additional fraction are some porphyrin, which is synthesized in the liver and not incorporated into red cells, and porphyrin derived from the destruction of hemoproteins other than hemoglobin (myoglobins, cytochromes, catalases, and peroxidases).

The early appearance of labeled stercobilin after the administration of 2-$^{14}$C-labeled glycine may be due not only to destruction of newly formed red cells before reaching the circulation, or to heme formed in excess of globin, but also to the direct synthesis of bilirubin from heme precursors by a shunt mechanism.[65]

Bilirubin is excreted into the bile and passes into the colon, where it is reduced by bacterial action to a group of urobilinogens consisting of mesobilirubinogen and stercobilinogen. Oxidation in the urine and stool results in conversion of colorless urobilinogen to the colored urobilin. A portion of the urobilinogens is excreted in the stools but in large part is reabsorbed from the intestine to reenter the liver in the portal circulation and is then reexcreted in the bile. A few milligrams leave the general circulation to be excreted in the urine.

Quantitative estimates of urobilinogen excretion are an index of hemoglobin breakdown since the bulk of bile pigments stem from this source. It has been estimated that 1 mg. of urobilinogen is derived from approximately 24 mg. of destroyed hemoglobin. Increased hemoglobin destruction is invariably associated with excessive urobilinogen excretion in the feces and usually in the urine. The presence or absence of urobilinogen in the urine largely depends upon the capacity of the liver for reexcretion in the bile. With hepatic damage of dysfunction from overload, reexcretion of urobilinogen is impaired, a spill-over in the blood occurs, and urobilinogen appears in the urine. The normal daily adult excretion of urobilinogen in the feces is 40 to 280 mg.[135]; in the urine it is 0.5 to 3.5 gm. In infants and children the normal daily mean value for fecal urobilinogen ranges from 3.8 mg. under 1 year of age to 45.2 mg. from 10 to 14 years of age; in patients with hemolytic disease it ranges from 15.1 to 205 mg., respectively.[86]

For the formation of bilirubin in the neonate, calculations have been as follows (Pearson).[101] The average 3.4 kilogram neonate has a blood volume of 85 cc. per kilogram and an average hemoglobin of 17 gm.%, making the circulating hemoglobin mass about 49 gm. The life-span of fetal red cells appears to be about 70 days; therefore 1.4% of the circulating red cell mass is hemolyzed each day. About 0.69 gm. of hemoglobin is thus broken down each day. Since each gram of hemoglobin catabolized yields 35 mg. of bilirubin, 24 mg. of bilirubin are formed daily.

*Compensated hemolytic disease.* The processes of blood destruction and formation are normally balanced so that the concentration of hemoglobin and red cells in the circulating blood remains unaltered. In a state of balance, the red cells and hemoglobin destroyed are replaced each day. When blood destruction is increased, bone marrow activity is accelerated, more red cells and hemoglobin are produced, and equilibrium is reestablished. Within limitations, an excessive degree of hemolysis will not result in anemia in a patient with adequately compensating bone marrow activity. According to Crosby and Akeroyd,[20] hemolytic anemia follows only when the average life-span of the red blood cell (normally 120 days) becomes so short that the bone marrow, working at maximum capacity (six to eight times the normal), cannot maintain an adequate output of hemoglobin and red blood cells. They have emphasized the important fact that abnormal hemolysis without anemia is indicative of a completely compensated hemolytic process and that the underlying feature of the hemolytic syndrome is reduced survival of the red cells. When these limits are exceeded and anemia develops, equilibrium may be reestablished at lower levels, depending upon the capacity of the bone marrow to form red cells and the extent of their survival in the circulation.

When the rate of red cell destruction exceeds the rate of red cell production, the red cell volume is lowered and fewer red cells are being destroyed per unit of time. When the red cell volume has been reduced to that point at which the number of red cells being destroyed is equaled by the number of red cells being produced, a new equilibrium is established, resulting in a stable but anemic hemoglobin level.[27] At any one time in a hemolytic disease, a particular hemoglobin value is the resultant of the extent of the hemolytic defect present and the particular capacity of the bone marrow to respond with an increase in hemoglobin synthesis and red cell production.

The concept of compensated hemolytic disease is important in appraising blood conditions in which blood levels appear unduly high in the face of a known hemolytic process. Because of this mechanism, anemia in hereditary spherocytosis (familial hemolytic anemia) may not always be present, and in patients with the trait or mild form of Mediterranean anemia (thalassemia minor) overcompensation accounts for the polycythemia at times in association with elevated hemoglobin levels. Evidences of increased hemolysis can be detected with the aid of appropriate laboratory tests. A significant increase of reticulocytes represents a simple index of compensated hemolytic disease. In erythroblastosis fetalis augmented reticulocyte values with a normal red cell count on the first day of life may indicate increased red cell turnover and the need for close watch in succeeeding days for the development of anemia and jaundice. In crises of sickle cell anemia the hemoglobin level often remains unchanged, but increased reticulocytes reflect compensatory bone marrow activity.

## REFERENCES

1. Adams, F. H., and Cunningham, S. C.: Fragility of red blood cells from newborn infants and children with cyonotic congenital heart disease, J. Pediat. **39**:180, 1951.
2. Allen, D. W., and Jandl, J. H.: Kinetics of intracellular iron in rabbit reticulocytes, Blood **15**:71, 1960.
3. Ashby, W.: Determination of length of life of transfused blood corpuscles in man, J. Exper. Med. **29**:267, 1919.
4. Benesch, R., and Benesch, R. E.: Intracellular organic phosphates as regulators of oxygen release by haemoglobin, Nature **221**:618, 1969.
5. Beutler, E.: "A shift to the left" or "a shift to the right" in the regulation of erythropoiesis, Blood **33**:496, 1969.
6. Billing, B. H., and Lathe, G. H.: The excretion of bilirubin as an ester glucuronide, giving the direct van den Bergh reaction, Biochem. J. **63**:6, 1956.
7. Billing, B. H., and Lathe, G. H.: Bilirubin metabolism in jaundice, Amer. J. Med. **24**:111, 1958.
8. Birkhill, F. R., Maloney, M. A., and Levenson, S. M.: Effect of transfusion polycythemia upon bone marrow activity and erythrocyte survival in man, Blood **6**:1021, 1951.
9. Bolande, R. P., Traisman, H. S., and Philipsborn, H. F., Jr: Electrolyte considerations in exchange transfusions for erythroblastosis fetalis, J. Pediat. **49**:401, 1956.
10. Boyer, S. H.: Proteins, evolution and disease (editorial), Amer. J. Med. **36**:337, 1964.
11. Brain, M. C.: Microangiopathic hemolytic anemia, New Eng. J. Med. **281**:832, 1969.
12. Bunting, H.: Sedimentation rates of sickled and non-sickled cells from patients with sickle cell anemia, Amer. J. Med. Sci. **198**:191, 1939.
13. Burman, D.: Red cell cholinesterase in in-

fancy and childhood, Arch. Dis. Child. **36:** 362, 1961.
13a. Carlsen, E., and Comroe, J. H.: Rate of gas uptake by intact human erythrocytes, Amer. J. Physiol. **187:**590, 1950.
13b. Carlsen, E., and Comroe, J. H.: Rate of uptake of carbon monoxide and of nitric oxide by normal human erythrocytes and experimentally produced spherocytes, J. Gen. Physiol. **42:**83, 1958.
14. Carnot, P., and Deflandre, C.: Sur l'activité hémopoiétique du serum Compt. rend. Acad. sc. **143:**384, 1906.
15. Carrell, R. W., and Lehmann, H.: The unstable haemoglobin haemolytic anaemias, Seminars Hemat. **6:**116, 1969.
16. Condensation of the first two reports of the Committee for Clarification of the Nomenclature of Cells and Diseases of the Blood and Blood-Forming Organs, Blood **4:**89, 1949.
17. Contrera, J. T., and Gordon, A. S.: Erythropoietin: production by a particulate fraction of the kidney. Science **152:**653, 1966.
18. Crick, F. H. C., Barnett, L., Breener, S., and Watt-Tobin, R. J.: General nature of the genetic code for proteins, Nature **192:**1227, 1961.
19. Crosby, W. H.: The hemolytic states, Bull. N. Y. Acad. Med. **30:**27, 1954.
20. Crosby, W. H., and Akeroyd, J. H.: The limit of hemoglobin synthesis in hereditary hemolytic anemia, Amer. J. Med. **13:**273, 1952.
21. Dancis. J., Danoff, S., Zabriskie, J., and Balis, M. E.: Hemoglobin metabolism in the premature infant, J. Pediat. **54:**748, 1959.
22. Dinning, J. S.: Nutritional requirements for blood cell formation in experimental animals, Physiol. Rev. **42:**169, 1962.
23. Donohue, D. M., Finch, C. A., and Gabrio, B. W.: Erythrocyte preservation; the storage of blood with purine nucleosides, J. Clin. Invest. **35:**562, 1956.
24. Donohue, D. M., Motulsky, A. G., Giblett, E. R., Pirsio-Biroli, G., Viranuvatti, V., and Finch, C. A.: The use of chromium as a red-cell tag, Brit. J. Haemat. **1:**249, 1955.
25. Eaton, J. W., and Brewer, G. J.: The relationship between red cell 2,3-diphosphoglycerate and levels of hemoglobin in the human, Proc. Nat. Acad. Sci. **61:**756, 1968.
26. Emlinger, P. J., Huff, R. L., and Oda, J. M.: Depression of red cell iron turnover by transfusion, Proc. Soc. Exper. Biol. Med. **79:**16, 1952.
27. Erlandson, M. E., Schulman, I., Stern, G., and Smith, C. H.: Studies of congenital hemolytic syndromes; rates of destruction and production of erythrocytes in thalassemia, Pediatrics **22:**910, 1958.
28. Erslev, A. J.: Humoral regulation of red cell production, Blood **8:**349, 1953.
29. Erslev, A. J., and Lavietes, P. H.: Observations on the nature of the erythropoietic serum factor, Blood **9:**1055, 1954.
30. Erslev, A. J.: Erythropoietin in vitro. II. Effect on "stem cells," Blood **24:**331, 1964.
31. Evans, H. E., Glass, L., and Mercado, C.: The micro-erythrocyte sedimentation rate in newborn infants, J. Pediat. **76:**449, 1970.
32. Fahraeus, R., Om Hamägglutination en Sarskitt med Hänsyn Till Havandeskapet och möjligheten avatt Diagnostiskt Vtnyttja Densamma, Hygiea **80:**369, 1918.
33. Finch, C. A., Coleman, D. H., Motulsky, A. G., Donohue, D. M., and Reiff, R. H.: Erythrokinetics in pernicious anemia, Blood **11:** 807, 1956.
34. Finne, P. H.: Erythropoietin levels in the amniotic fluid, particularly in Rh-immunized pregnancies, Acta Paediat. Scand. **53:**269, 1964.
35. Finne, P. H.: Erythropoietin levels in cord blood as an indicator of intrauterine hypoxia, Acta Paediat. Scand. **55:**478, 1966.
36. Firkin, B. G., and Wiley, J. S.: The red cell membrane and its disorder. In Brown, E. B., and Moore C. V., editors: Progress in Hematology, New York, 1966, Grune & Stratton.
37. Foconi, S., and Sjölin, S.: Survival of $Cr^{51}$-labelled red cells from newborn infants, Acta Paediat. (supp. 117) **48:**18, 1958.
38. Gabrio, B. W., Donohue, D. M., and Finch, C. A.: Erythrocyte preservation relationship between chemical changes and viability of stored blood treated with adenosine, J. Clin. Invest. **34:**1509, 1955.
39. Gabrio, B. W., Finch, C. A., and Huennekens, F. M.: Erythrocyte preservation; a topic in molecular biochemistry, Blood **11:** 103, 1956.
40. Girdwood, R. H., and Lenman, J. A. R.: Megaloblastic anaemia occurring during primidone therapy, Brit. Med. J. **1:**146, 1956.
41. Goldbloom, A., and Gottlieb, R.: Icterus neonatorum, Amer. J. Dis. Child. **38:**57, 1929.
42. Goldbloom, R. B., Fischer, E., Reinhold, J., and Hsia, D. Y-Y.: Studies on the mechanical fragility of erythrocytes; normal values for infants and children, Blood **8:**165, 1953.
43. Goldwasser, E., Jacobson, L. O., Fried, W., and Plzak, L.: Mechanism of the erythropoietic effect of cobalt, Science **125:**1085, 1957.
44. Gordon, A. S.: Hemopoietine, Physiol. Rev. **39:**1, 1959.
45. Granick, S.: The chemistry and functioning

of the mammalian erythrocyte, Blood 4:404, 1949.
46. Grant, W. C., and Root, W. S.: Fundamental stimulus for erythropoiesis, Physiol. Rev. 4:449, 1952.
47. Grinstein, M., Bannerman, R. M., Vavea, J. D., and Moore, C. V.: Hemoglobin metabolism in thalassemia in vitro studies, Amer. J. Med. 29:18, 1960.
48. Gross, R. T., and Hurwitz, R. E.: The pentose phosphate pathways in human erythrocytes; relationship between age of the subject and enzyme activity, Pediatrics 22:453, 1958.
49. Gross, R. T., Schroeder, E. A., and Brounstein, O.: Energy metabolism in the erythrocytes of premature infants compared to full term newborn infants and adults, Blood 21:755, 1963.
50. Gurney, C. W.: Erythropoietin and erythropoiesis, Ann. Intern. Med. 65:377, 1966.
51. Gurney, C. W., Pierce, M. I., Schrier, S.E., Carson, P. E., and Jacobson, L. O.: The stimulatory effect of "anemic plasma" in congenital hypoplastic anemia, J. Lab. Clin. Med. 50:821, 1957.
52. Hall, D. O., and Palmer, J. M.: Mitochondrial research to-day, Nature 221:717, 1969.
53. Halvorsen, S.: Plasma erythropoietin levels in cord blood and in blood during the first weeks of life, Acta Paediat. 52:425, 1963.
54. Halvorsen, S., and Finne, P. H.: Transfer of erythropoietin to amniotic fluid in Rh-immunized pregnant women, Brit. Med. J. 1:1132, 1963.
55. Harris, J. W.: The red cell, production, metabolism, destruction: normal and abnormal, Cambridge, Massachusetts, 1963, Commonwealth Fund of Harvard University Press.
56. Herbert, V., and Castle, W. B.: Intrinsic factor, New Eng. J. Med. 270:1181, 1964.
57. Hill, R. J., Konigberg, W., Guidotti, G., and Craig, L. C.: Structure of human hemoglobin. I. The separation of the alpha and beta chains and their amino acid composition, J. Biol. Chem. 237:1549, 1962.
58. Helman, R. S., and Finch, C. A.: The misused reticulocytes, Brit. J. Haemat. 17:313, 1969.
59. Hollingworth, J. W.: Life span of fetal erythrocytes, J. Lab. Clin. Med. 45:469, 1955.
60. Hopkinson, D. A., Spencer, N., and Harris, H.: Red cell and phosphatase variants; a new human polymorphism, Nature 199:969, 1963.
61. Hopkinson, D. A., Spencer, N., and Harris, H.: Genetical studies on human red cell acid phosphatase, Amer. J. Human Genet. 16:141, 1964.

62. Hughes-Jones, N. C., and Szur, L.: Determination of the sites of red-cell destruction using $^{51}CR$-labelled cells, Brit. J. Haemat. 3:320, 1957.
63. Ingram, V. M.: Gene evolution and the haemoglobins, Nature 189:704, 1961.
64. Ishikawa, A., and Hammond, G. D.: Erythropoietin in serum and urine in Cooley's anemia, Amer. J. Dis. Child. 102:592, 1961.
65. Israels, L. G., Skanderberg, J., Guyda, H., Zuigg, W., and Zipursky, A.: A study of the early-labelled fraction of bile pigment; the effects of altering erythropoiesis on the incorporation of ($2^{14}$-C) glycine into haem and bilirubin, Brit. J. Haemat. 9:50, 1963.
66. Jacobson, L. O., Goldwasser, E., Fried, W., and Plzak, L.: Role of the kidney in erythropoiesis, Nature 179:633, 1957.
67. Jacobson, L. O., Gurney, C. W., and Goldwasser, E.: The control of erythropoiesis. In Dock, W., and Snapper, I., editors: Advances in internal medicine, vol. 10, Chicago, 1960, Year Book Medical Publishers, Inc.
68. Jaffé, E. R.: Hereditary hemolytic disorders, Bull. N. Y. Acad. Med. 46:397, 1970.
69. Jandl, J. H.: Leaky red cells, Blood 26:367, 1965.
70. Jandl, J. H., Greenberg, M. S., Yonemoto, R. H., and Castle, W. B.: Clinical determination of the sites of red cell sequestration in hemolytic anemias, J. Clin. Invest. 35:842, 1956.
71. Jones, P. N., Weinstein, I. M., Ettinger, R. H., and Capps, R. B.: Decreased red cell survival associated with liver disease; use of radioactive sodium chromate in measurement of red cell survival, Arch. Intern. Med. 95:93, 1955.
72. Kaplan, E., and Hsu, K. S.: Determination of erythrocyte survival in newborn infants by means of $Cr^{51}$-labelled erythrocytes, Pediatrics 27:354, 1961.
73. Klatskin, G., and Bungards, L.: Bilirubin-protein linkages in serum and their relationship to the van den Bergh reaction, J. Clin. Invest. 35:537, 1956.
74. Lehmann, H.: Personal communication.
75. Lehmann, H., and Huntsman, R. G.: Man's haemoglobins, Philadelphia, 1966, J. B. Lippincott Co.
76. Linman, J. W.: Factors controlling hemopoiesis; erythropoietic effects of "anemic plasma," J. Lab. Clin. Med. 59:249, 1962.
77. Linman, J. W., and Bethell, F. W.: Factors controlling erythropoiesis, Springfield, Ill., 1960, Charles C Thomas, Publisher.
78. London, I. M.: Metabolism of hemoglobin and of bile pigment, Bull. Acad. Med. 30:509, 1954.

79. London. I. M.: The metabolism of the erythrocyte, Harvey Lectures Series 56:151, 1961.
80. London, I. M., West, R., Shemin, D., and Rittenberg, D.: On the origin of bile pigment in normal man, J. Biol. Chem. 184:351, 1950.
81. London, I. M., West, R., Shemin, D., and Rittenberg, D.: Porphyrin formation and hemoglobin metabolism in congenital porphyria, J. Biol. Chem. 184:365, 1950.
82. Malcolm, D., Ranney, H. M., and Jacobs, A. S.: Association of radioactive chromium with various components of hemoglobin, Blood 21:8, 1963.
83. Mauzerall, D.: Normal porphyrin metabolism, J. Pediat. 64:5, 1964.
84. Miale, J. B.: Laboratory medicine—hematology, ed. 3, St. Louis, 1967, The C. V. Mosby Co.
85. Miller, G., McCoord, A. B., Joos, H. A., and Clausen, S. W.: Studies of serum electrolyte changes during exchange transfusion, Pediatrics 13:412, 1954.
86. Mills, S. D., and Mason, H. L.: Values for fecal urobilinogen in childhood, Amer. J. Dis. Child. 84:322, 1952.
87. Minnich, V., Cordonnier, J. K., Williams, W. J., and Moore, C. V.: Alpha, beta, and gamma hemoglobin polypeptide chains during the neonatal period with description of a fetal form of hemoglobin D$_a$-St. Louis, Blood 19:137, 1962.
88. Mollison, P. L.: The role of complement in antibody-mediated red-cell destruction, Brit. J. Haemat. 18:249, 1970.
89. Motoulsky, A. G.: Genetic aspects of abnormal hemoglobins. In first inter-American conference on congenital defects, The International Medical Congress, Ltd., Philadelphia, 1963, J. B. Lippincott Co., p. 22.
90. Muller, C. J., and Jonxis, J. H. P.: Identity of haemoglobin A$_2$, Nature 188:949, 1960.
91. Najjar, V. A.: The metabolism of bilirubin, Pediatrics 10:1, 1952.
92. Nathan, D. G., and Gardner, F. H.: Erythroid cell maturation and hemoglobin synthesis in megaloblastic anemia, J. Clin. Invest. 41:1086, 1962.
93. Nathan, D. G., Piomelli, S., and Gardner, F. H.: The synthesis of heme and globin in the maturing human erythroid cell, J. Clin. Invest. 40:940, 1961.
94. Neel, J. V.: The hemoglobin genes; a remarkable example of the clustering of related genetic functions on the single mammalian chromosome, Blood 18:769, 1961.
95. Neerhout, R. C.: Erythrocyte lipids in the neonate, Ped. Res. 2:172, 1968.
96. Neerhout, R. C.: Disorders of the red cell membrane, Clin. Pediat. 7:451, 1968.
97. Oski, F. A.: The metabolism of erythrocytes and its relation to hemolytic anemias in the newborn, Ped. Clin. N. Amer. 12:687, 1965.
98. Oski, F. A., and Naiman, J. L.: Red cell binding of bilirubin, J. Pediat. 63:1034, 1963.
99. Oski, F. A., Shahidi, N. T., and Diamond, L. K.: Erythrocyte acid phosphomonoesterase and glucose-6-phosphate dehydrogenase deficiency in Caucasians, Science 139:409, 1963.
100. Pearson, H. A.: The binding of $Cr^{51}$ to hemoglobins. I. In vitro studies, Blood 22: 218, 1963.
101. Pearson, H. A.: Life-span of the fetal red blood cell, J. Pediat. 70:166, 1967.
101a. Perutz, M. F.: The haemoglobin molecule, Proc. Roy. Soc. 173:113, 1968.
102. Piliero, S. J., Medici, P. T., Pansky, B., Luhby, A. L., and Gordon, A. S.: Erythropoietic stimulating effects of plasma extracts from anemic human subjects, Proc. Soc. Exp. Biol. Med. 93:302, 1956.
103. Prankerd, T. A.: The metabolism of the human erythrocyte; a review, Brit. J. Haemat. 1:131, 1955.
104. Reed, C. L., Swisher, S. N., Marinetti, G. V., and Eden, E. G.: Studies of the lipids of the erythrocyte. I. Quantitative analysis of the lipids of normal human red blood cells, J. Lab. Clin. Med. 56:281, 1960.
105. Reismann, K. R.: Studies on the mechanism of erythropoietic stimulation in parabiotic rats during hypoxia, Blood 5:372, 1950.
106. Reisner, E. H., Jr.: The nature and significance of megaloblastic blood formation, Blood 13:313, 1958.
107. Rhinesmith, H., Schroeder, W., and Martin, N.: The N-terminal sequence of the beta chains of normal adult human hemoglobin, J. Amer. Chem. Soc. 80:3358, 1958.
108. Rimington, C.: Biosynthesis of haemoglobin, Brit. Med. Bull. 15:19, 1959.
109. Robinson, S. H., Lester, R., Crigler, J. F., Jr., and Tsong, M.: Early-labeled peak of bile pigment in man; studies with Glycine-$^{14}$C and delta-aminolevulinic acid-$^3$H, New Eng. J. Med. 277:1323, 1967.
110. Robinson, M. A., Loder, P. B., and de-Gruchy, G. C.: Red-cell metabolism in nonspherocytic congenital haemolytic anaemia, Brit. J. Haemat. 7:327, 1961.
111. Ross, J. D.: Deficient activity of DPNH-dependent methemoglobin diaphorase in cord blood erythrocytes, Blood 21:51, 1963.
112. Rous, P.: Destruction of the red blood corpuscle in health and disease, Physiol. Rev. 3:75, 1923.
113. Ryan, G. M. S., and Forshaw, J. W. B.: Megaloblastic anaemia due to phenytoin sodium, Brit. Med. J. 2:242, 1955.

114. Schmid, R.: Direct-reacting bilirubin, bilirubin glucuronide in serum bile and urine, Science **124**:76, 1956.
115. Schroeder, W. A., Shelton, T. R., Shelton, J. B., Cormick, J., and Jones, R. T.: The amino acid sequence of the gamma chain of human fetal hemoglobin, Biochemistry **2**:992, 1963.
116. Schwartz, H. C., Cartwright, G. E., Smith, E. L., and Wintrobe, M. M.: Studies on the biosynthesis of heme from iron and protoporphyrin, Blood **14**:486, 1959.
117. Selwyn, J. G., and Dacie, J. V.: Autohemolysis and other changes resulting from the incubation in vitro of red cells from patients with congenital hemolytic anemia, Blood **9**:414, 1954.
118. Shalet, M. F., Holder, T. M., and Walters, T. R.: Erythropoietin-producing Wilms' tumor, J. Pediat. **70**:615, 1967.
119. Shojania, A. M., Roland, M., Simovitch, H., Israels, L. G., and Zipursky, A.: Alterations in red cell structure and metabolism associated with rapid blood production; the stress reticulocyte, J. Pediat. **65**:1101, 1964.
120. Shulman, R. G., Ogawa, S., Wuthrick, K., Yamane, T., Peisach, S., and Blumberg, W. E.: The absence of "Heme-heme" interactions in hemoglobin, Science **165**:251, 1969.
121. Sidbury, J. B., Jr., Cornblath, M., Fisher, J., and House, E.: Glycogen in erythrocytes of patients with glycogen storage disease, Pediatrics **27**:103, 1961.
122. Smith, C. H.: Sedimentation rate and red cell volume, Amer. J. Med. Sci. **192**:73, 1936.
123. Smith, C. H.: Sedimentation rate in nutritional anemia of infants and children, Amer. J. Dis. Child. **56**:510, 1938.
124. Smith, C. H.: Adsorption of methylene blue by blood of infants and children; mechanism of reaction and clinical application, Amer. J. Dis. Child. **57**:1223, 1939.
125. Smith, C. H.: Diagnosis of anemias in infancy and childhood, J.A.M.A. **134**:992, 1947.
126. Smith, C. H., Schulman, I., Ando, R. E., and Stern, G.: Studies in Mediterranean (Cooley's) anemia; the suppression of hematopoiesis by transfusions, Blood **10**:707, 1955.
127. Stohlman, F., Jr.: Erythropoietine, Pediatrics **23**:835, 1959.
128. Stohlman, F., Jr.: Observations on physiology of erythropoietin and its role in regulation of red cell production, Ann. N. Y. Acad. Sc. **77**:710, 1959.
129. Stohlman, F., Jr: Erythropoiesis, New Eng. J. Med. **267**:342, 392, 1962.
130. Stohlman, F., Jr., Brecker, G., and Moores, R. R.: Humoral regulation of erythropoiesis VIII. The kinetics of red cell production and the effect of erythropoietin. In Jacobson, L. O., and Doyle, M., editors: Erythropoiesis, New York, 1962, Grune & Stratton, p. 162.
131. Thurman, W. G., Grabstald, H., and Lieberman, P. H.: Elevation of erythropoietin levels in association with Wilms' tumor, Arch. Intern. Med. **117**:280, 1966.
132. Tullis, J. L.: Blood cells and plasma proteins; their state in nature, New York, 1953, Academic Press, Inc., p. 242.
133. Valentine, W. N., Tanaka, K. R., and Fredericks, R. E.: Erythrocyte acid phosphatase in health and disease, Amer. J. Clin. Path. **36**:328, 1961.
134. Valtis, D. J., and Baike, A. G.: The influence of red-cell thickness on the oxygen dissociation curve of blood, Brit. J. Haemat. **1**:152, 1955.
135. Watson, C. J.: Medical progress; bile pigment, New Eng. J. Med. **227**:665, 1942.
136. Weed, R. I.: The Importance of erythrocyte deformability, Amer. J. Med. **49**:147, 1970.
137. Weed, R. I., and Reed, C. F.: Membrane alterations leading to red cell destruction, Amer. J. Med. **41**:681, 1966.
138. Weinstein, I. M., Spurling, C. L., Klein, H., and Necheles, T. E.: Radioactive sodium chromate for the study of survival of red blood cells. III. The abnormal hemoglobin syndrome, Blood **9**:1155, 1954.
139. Whaun, J. M., and Oski, F. A.: Red cell stromal adenosine triphosphatase (ATPase) of newborn infants, Pediat. Res. **3**:105, 1969.
140. Wintrobe, M. M., and Landsberg, J. W.: A standardized technique for the blood sedimentation test, Amer. J. Med. Sci. **189**:102, 1935.
141. Witts, L. J.: Some aspects of the pathology of anaemia. I. Theory of maturation arrest, Brit. Med. J. **2**:325, 1961.
142. Young, L. E.: Hemolytic disorders; some highlights of twenty years of progress, Ann. Intern Med. **49**:1073, 1958.
143. Zinkham, W. H.: An in vitro abnormality of glutathione metabolism in erythrocytes from newborns; mechanism and clinical significance, Pediatrics **23**:18, 1959.
144. Zipursky. A.: Metabolic abnormalities of erythrocytes in the hemolytic anemias, Ped. Clin. N. Amer. **9**:559, 1962.

# 5 ERYTHROCYTES—MORPHOLOGIC ABNORMALITIES

*General considerations.* Of all of the laboratory procedures, the most important for its diagnostic value, yet the simplest, is the examination of the blood smear. Although corroborative evidence from auxiliary sources may be required to establish a final diagnosis, the stained film constitutes a visual representation of the effect on morphology of the factors involved in the pathogenesis of a specific anemia. In describing the changes in the red blood cells it should be pointed out that there are few specific red cells that are indicative of a particular disorder. Target cells, oval cells, hypochromic macrocytes and basophilic stippling, and hypochromic microcytes appear in varying percentages in certain stages of many anemias and therefore cannot be regarded as distinguishing features of a single disease. They are significant with the support of other pertinent information.

Although overlapping occurs and differentation from the normal is often difficult, the following represent the most conspicuous alterations in size, shape, and structural changes and staining peculiarities of the erythrocytes.

*Abnormalities in size.* Following are discussions of abnormalities of size that may be noted in erythrocytes.

*Anisocytosis.* The excessive variation in size of the red cells (average diameter, $7.5\mu$) is termed *anisocytosis*.

*Poikilocytosis.* Marked irregularity in the shape of the red cell is termed *poikilocytosis*. The pear-shaped cell is most commonly found in those patients with anemias in which there is marked variation in size of the cells.

*Microcytes.* Microcytes are cells with diameters of less than $6.5\mu$ and usually characterize the blood smear of the patient with iron-deficiency anemia. Microblasts or microcytic nucleated red cells are increased in the bone marrow of patients with iron deficiency or blood loss. Pointed projections may extend from the cytoplasm. The chromatin of the nucleus is condensed and deeply stained.

*Macrocytes.* Macrocytes are found principally in patients in whom there is a deficiency of liver maturation principle, such as in those with pernicious anemia, or in patients with a deficiency of folic acid, such as in megaloblastic anemia of infancy. They are large cells with a diameter of $8.5\mu$ or more, are thicker than the normocyte, are well filled with hemoglobin, and possess a mean corpuscular volume greater than normal.

*Hypochromic macrocytes.* Hypochromic macrocytes are found in small numbers in the blood of patients with many of the chronic anemias of childhood. They appear in larger numbers in the blood of patients with Mediterranean anemia (thalassemia) of varying grades of severity; they are of special value in the diagnosis of the mild form. Normochromic macrocytes are observed in small numbers in the blood smear of the patient with aplastic anemia in childhood.

*Spherocytes (microspherocytes).* In hereditary spherocytosis the spherical shape of the cells results from a developmental defect which occurs after the erythroblast stage and in which a normal cell volume is enclosed within a greatly diminished surface area. Spherocytes are globular, thick red cells of lessened diameter but usually are normal in volume; hence they are readily hemolyzed in hypotonic solutions of sodium chloride. Since normal red cells become thicker as they take up water, spherocytes, already globular, require less water before hemolysis sets in. Mechanical fragility is also increased. The small, deeply stained spherocytes which characterize hereditary spherocytosis may also be observed in varying degrees in patients with other conditions associated with hemolysis, such as acquired hemolytic anemia and erythroblastosis due to sensitization by the A-B agglutinogens, and less frequently in patients with congenital nonspherocytic hemolytic anemia, leukemia, and conditions of stasis within the spleen and in stored blood. Only the peculiar shape of these cells renders them susceptible to trapping by the spleen.

**Abnormalities in shape.** Another morphologic abnormality of erythrocytes is irregularity of shape.

*Elliptocytosis (ovalocytosis).* Oval or elliptical cells occur typically as a dominant hereditary anomaly in which they constitute from 25 to 90% of all erythrocytes. The cells vary in shape from the rod or elongated forms to the oval shape, all being well filled with hemoglobin. Contrary to sickle cells, these cells cannot be made to sickle in an environment of lowered oxygen tension. Elliptocytosis is usually benign and symptomatic; however, asymptomatic mild compensated anemia and, more rarely, overt hemolytic anemia have been reported as complications in about 15% of the patients.[37]

The average survival of elliptocytes transfused into a normal recipient was found to be about 30 days[25] or 60 days by the Ashby technique[28] in contrast to the normal of 120 days. Measured by sodium chromate ($^{51}Cr$), the survival of the patient's red cells within his own circulation is considerably reduced, with a half-life of 18.5 days as compared with the half-life of normal cells of 33.1 days.[40] In other studies no uniformity of red cell survival was found. The survival was normal in two patients and shortened to 45 days in another, with evidences of hemolysis but no anemia (compensated hemolytic disease).[44] Nucleated red cell precursors show no abnormalities of shape. Elliptical cells occur in smaller numbers in the blood of patients with sickle cell disease[58,68] and in that of the newborn infant.[70] They do not reach their maximum level in the infant until he is 3 to 4 months of age. On the other hand, ovalocytosis may be associated with hemolytic anemia and be accompanied by hyperbilirubinemia soon after birth; in such cases exchange transfusion should be considered.

Oval and elliptical cells are often noted in association with marked anisocytosis and poikilocytosis. It is necessary, therefore, to differentiate symptomatic from hereditary elliptocytosis[44] since oval-shaped cells appear in variable numbers in the blood of patients with Mediterranean anemia (thalassemia), severe iron-deficiency anemia, pernicious anemia, anemia of infection, leukemia, and hereditary nonspherocytic hemolytic disease. Also included is a type of familial hypochromic microcytic anemia with splenomegaly affecting male members.[54] A more extensive discussion of hereditary elliptocytosis appears in Chapter 15.

*Sickle cells (drepanocytes).* The characteristic sickle cells are elongated and narrow with rounded, pointed, or filamentous ends. Although they appear in the stained smears of the severely anemic patient, they are greatly increased in number in sealed wet films with reduced oxygen tension. Reversion to the normal form occurs with exposure to oxygen or carbon monoxide. Frequently in the trait or sicklemia the cells assume a holly-leaf appearance, exhibiting numerous superficial spines. The mature orthochromatic normoblast can be made to sickle slowly, although stained bone marrow smears show no morphologic changes in the nucleated red cells.

The sickling phenomenon is based on the presence of an abnormal form of hemoglobin which can be separated from normal hemoglobin by differences in electrophoretic mobility.[51] This disparity between the two hemoglobins is caused by the globin rather than the heme part of the molecule. The peculiar shape of the erythrocytes has been attributed to the greatly diminished solubility of reduced sickle cell hemoglobin as compared with reduced normal hemoglobin. This results in intracellular crystallization of the hemoglobin[52] and increased viscosity, with tactoid formation resembling sickled erythrocytes.[24] A minimal value of at least 20% of sickle hemoglobin is required to elicit the sickling phenomenon.[61]

Ovalocytosis has been observed in association with the sickle cell trait with evidence of both varieties of cells in the peripheral blood.[17]

*Stomatocytosis.* Lock and co-workers[38] recently reported an unusual erythrocyte abnormality in a mother and daughter. This disorder, termed *stomatocytosis*, is a congenital hemolytic anemia in which the erythrocytes in wet preparations are bowl-shaped rather than biconcave. They are given this name because in stained films they have a linear unstained area across the center instead of the normal circular area of pallor. The osmotic fragility of these cells is greater than normal (as in hereditary spherocytosis), but a characteristic swelling in hypotonic solution suggests an inelasticity of the red cell membrane.

Stomatocytes appeared in the blood of an 18½-year-old patient with hemolytic anemia, jaundice, and splenomegaly. Splenectomy resulted in clinical improvement but did not completely arrest abnormal hemolysis nor alter red cell abnormalities. Osmotic fragility and autohemolysis were greater at 5° C. than at 37° C. There was a decreased concentration of reduced glutathione, although glucose-6-phosphate dehydrogenase was normal.[43]

Stomatocytes were observed in the blood smear of a girl 3 years and 8 months of age who had intermittent jaundice, anemia, reticulocytes of 30%, increased autohemolysis, and grossly enlarged spleen and moderate hepatomegaly.[41] Following splenectomy, reticulocytes were still elevated. The stomatocytes were described on the stained film as red cells in which there was a slit or mouthlike opening into the cell. The cells showed a marked increase in osmotic fragility after incubation for 24 hours at 37° C. Splenectomy did not alter the stomatocytosis although it partially cured the anemia.

In another report,[72] large numbers of stomatocytes were observed in the blood smear of a 3½-year-old child whose anemia dated from infancy. The red cell defect was associated with an abnormality of the cell content of sodium and potassium. Intracellular concentrations of sodium and potassium were 100 mEq. per liter and 40 mEq. per liter, respectively, as compared with the normal of 10 and 95 mEq. per liter of cells, respectively. This discrepancy necessitated excessive cation pump activity to correct the massive cation leak. Like the red cells of hereditary spherocytosis, these cells are abnormally fragile in hypotonic solution. Splenectomy resulted in moderate correction of the anemia with resulting hemoglobin values of 10.0 and 11.0 gm. per 100 ml. and reticulocyte counts of approximately 10%. The parents and one female sibling had normal hemograms and osmotic-fragility tests.

*Target cells.* In target cells hemoglobin is concentrated in the periphery and in the center, producing concentric light and dark zones after staining. The deeply stained central area gives the impression of a bull's eye in a target.[3] Target cells are a variety of leptocytes, or thin cells in which the cell envelope is too large and out of proportion to its meager contents and accounts for the increased osmotic resistance in hypotonic solutions of sodium chloride.

Target cells, originally regarded as diagnostic of Mediterranean anemia (thalassemia), are now known to be nonspecific and are found in increased numbers in many anemic states in infants and children, in patients with obstructive jaundice and hypochromic anemia, following splenectomy, and especially in patients with conditions associated with abnormal hemoglobins. Target cells are present in patients with both mild and severe Mediterranean anemia (usually up to 10%), are further increased in those with sickle cell anemia, and appear in larger numbers in patients with a combination of these diseases (microdrepanocytic or thalassemia-sickle cell disease). These cells are prominent also in the blood of patients with the hemolytic diseases associated with other pathologic hemoglobins. In those with sickle cell–hemoglobin C disease, for instance, they are present to the extent of 40 to 85% of all red cells.[31] It has been suggested that large numbers of target cells in the blood smear indicate the presence of C hemoglobin. Whereas target cells are also increased in patients with hemoglobin E disease, perhaps less than in those with C hemoglobin, few or none of these cells have been noted in reported cases of sickle cell–hemoglobin D disease.[66]

Cooper and Jandl[11] have shown that the red cell membrane accumulates cholesterol in obstructive jaundice as a consequence of the elevated levels of bile salts. In so doing the red cells on stained smear assume the features of target cells. Target cells are the morphologic expression of an increased surface-to-volume ratio, namely, an increase in surface area while the volume remains the same. In acquiring a flattened shape these cells show an increased resistance to osmotic lysis. Such cells are frequently encountered in patients with hepatitis, particularly during the obstructive phase, and are always observed in patients with extrahepatic biliary tract obstruction.

*Leptocytes.* Leptocytes are abnormally thin erythrocytes; some are bowl-shaped and assume the appearance of the target cell following drying and preparation of the film. Leptocytosis refers to a preponderance of leptocytes such as occur in patients with hypochromic microcytic anemia and Mediterranean anemia (thalassemia); the term *hereditary leptocytosis* is an alternative name for the latter disease. Other cells found in the latter condition are non-target cells but are extremely thin, leaflike, and of remarkable transparency.

*Miscellaneous changes.* Miscellaneous morphologic abnormalities in erythrocytes are considered in the following discussions.

*Pocked erythrocytes.* A study of red-cell surface morphologic using interference or contrast microscopy revealed striking morphologic differences in premature and term infants, in infants of various ages, and in normal adults.[27] In normal adults 2.6% of erythrocytes gave the appearance of having small (0.2 to 0.5$\mu$) pits or craters on their surface. By contrast, premature and term infants had a mean of 47.2% and 24.3% pitted cells, respectively, reaching near adult values by 2 months of age in term infants and taking somewhat longer in premature infants. An inverse correlation was observed between birth weight and the number of pitted cells.

The finding of increased numbers of pitted cells in the neonate may reflect reticuloendothelial or splenic hypofunction since this type of cell has so far been observed with such frequency only in patients without a spleen.

Nathan and Gunn,[46] using interference-contrast microscopy, were able to observe crater-like membrane indentations (pits) in two thalassemic patients after splenectomy, noting their absence in splenectomized subjects.

Later it was demonstrated that the indentations seen with interference-contrast microscopy are largely optical illusions which reflect the presence of erythrocyte inclusions and vacuoles beneath the cell membrane. The evidence further suggested that mature normal erythrocytes may continuously form vacuoles and that the majority are removed by the normal spleen.[26]

*Basophilic stippling.* Basophilic stippling or punctate basophilia, already described, applies to the presence of round, fine, or coarse bluish violet or dark blue granules scattered in the cytoplasm of the polychromatophilic red blood cells. They represent regeneration or immaturity of the cell and are sometimes best observed in slightly thicker and moderately overstained blood smears. They are associated with all chronic anemias, leukemia, iron-deficiency anemia, the trait or mild form of Mediterranean anemia (thalassemia), and lead poisoning. They are to be differentiated from the network found in reticulocytes in cresyl blue preparations.

*Hypochromia and hyperchromia.* Hypochromia is observed in cells with a lack of hemoglobin and is represented by an increase in central pallor. Deeply and homogeneously stained red cells lacking central pallor because of complete hemoglobinization are termed *hyperchromic*. A macrocyte with a normal concentration of hemoglobin contains more of this substance than a normocyte only because of its size. Since oversaturation with hemoglobin does not occur, the cell cannot be truly regarded as hyperchromic. Nevertheless, according to common usage, hyperchromic anemias identify conditions in which macrocytes prevail and in which the color index is greater than unity.

*Siderocytes.* Siderocytes are red blood cells containing nonhemoglobin iron particles which are visualized by the Prussian blue method of staining. Sideroblasts are normoblasts containing similar iron inclusions. Both types of cells in the peripheral blood and the bone marrow, respectively, appear in moderate numbers in normal persons. They are increased in those with infection, aplastic and hemolytic anemias and are markedly decreased in those with iron-deficiency anemias.[30] Siderocytes are significantly increased after splenectomy.

The iron-containing granules of siderocytes are to be differentiated from punctate basophilia.[7] Siderotic granules of siderocytes stain with Prussian blue but fail to stain with basophilic dyes. The basophilic stippling in red cells is due to ribonucleic acid—containing granules that fail to give a Prussian blue reaction but stain with basophilic dyes. Granules of punctate basophilia are almost invariably round, regular, and well defined. Iron-positive siderocytic or sideroblastic granules, in contrast, vary in size and shape and are often ill defined. Basophilic and siderotic granules occasionally coexist in the same cell.

Dacie and Mollin[14] describe three types of sideroblasts:

1. Sideroblasts seen in normal bone marrow—iron-containing granules are few in number, difficult to photograph, and are only visible in a population of erythroblasts.

2. Sideroblasts in conditions in which the percentage saturation of transferrin is inceased—such conditions are hemochromatosis and transfusion hemosiderosis in which iron stores have accumulated. This type is also found with excessive hemolysis and where dyshematopoiesis occurs as in megaloblastic anemia or thalassemia. Granules are numerous and diffusely scattered.

3. Sideroblasts in sideroblastic anemia—siderotic granules are larger than normal and many are present. In some cases there is a conspicuous ring or collar around the nucleus. These are the "ring"

or "ring type" sideroblasts. Excessive iron stores, a high-serum iron concentration, and impaired heme synthesis leading to defective iron utilization characterize this condition.

*Pappenheimer bodies.* Pappenheimer bodies are present in red blood cells as single or double granules or dots and appear in largest numbers in the peripheral blood in certain cases of hemolytic anemia following splenectomy.[50] Usually present as a single dot, less commonly as multiple dots, they stain a darker shade of blue than does the filamentous material of reticulocytes. They represent deposits of ferric iron aggregates in mitochondria which lie in close proximity to ribosomes. They stain with Prussian blue and with basophilic dyes. These granules closely resemble the iron-staining granules of the siderocyte. As mentioned, the latter stain with Prussian blue but fail to stain with basophilic dyes.[7]

*Heinz (Heinz-Ehrlich) bodies.* Heinz bodies are moderately sized round or irregularly shaped protein-containing granules lying at or close to the periphery of the red blood cell. They are single or multiple refractile inclusion bodies and are observed after supravital staining with brilliant cresyl blue and methyl violet. The Romanowsky dyes such as Wright's stain obscure their presence. They are easily detected as refractile bodies in unstained wet preparations. These intracellular inclusions have been described as refractile agglomerations of denatured globin, verdohemoglobin, and perhaps stromal material. Heinz bodies represent rather severe intoxication of the red cell[8] and are particularly noticeable in the presence of intrinsic defects within the cell. They are to be differentiated from Howell-Jolly bodies, reticulocytes, and siderotic granules. Not only are Heinz bodies primarily composed of degradation products of hemoglobin, but evidence has also been offered indicating that methemoglobin is an essential stage in the destruction of "intact" hemoglobin.[23]

The presence of Heinz bodies in significant numbers is indicative of injury to the red cells and serves as an index of existing or impending anemia. Sulfonamides, primaquine, phenylhydrazine, naphthalene, phenacetin, and the fava bean associated with red cell destruction are prominent among Heinz-forming compounds.[18] They appear in increased numbers in patients with hemolytic anemias and leukemia, following splenectomy,[59] and in patients with agenesis of the spleen.[20] (See Chapters 8 and 15.) The development of Heinz body anemia in the premature infant reflects the increased susceptibility of the premature infant to the development of these inclusion bodies.

*Howell-Jolly bodies.* Howell-Jolly bodies are small, rounded, densely staining nuclear remnants occurring singly or doubly and are eccentrically placed in the red cell. They stain a reddish blue or dark violet with Wright's stain and are prominent after splenectomy and in many anemias, such as severe iron-deficiency anemia, pernicious anemia, spherocytic anemia, and leukemia. The origin of these bodies has been ascribed to abnormal mitosis in the late megaloblast stage when single chromosomes or groups of chromosomes become detached, fail to be included in the formation of the interphase nucleus, and remain free in the cytoplasm as nuclear remnants.[29]

The presence of target cells, siderocytes, normoblasts, and Howell-Jolly and Heinz bodies in varying combinations in the peripheral blood of a young infant prompts consideration of agenesis of the spleen, especially when associated with serious anomalies of the heart and situs inversus of the abdominal viscera.[10] It has been stated that the diagnosis of asplenia can be made with confidence in infants with congenital cardiac disease who are polycythemic and whose peripheral blood shows numerous Howell-Jolly bodies.[39]

*Cabot rings.* Cabot rings are basophilic rings, circular or twisted into a figure-of-eight, which occur occasionally in red blood cells of patients with hemolytic anemias, untreated pernicious anemia, leukemia, and lead poisoning. They stain reddish purple with Wright's stain. Originally regarded as nuclear remnants, they are now interpreted as an expression of cellular degeneration resulting from the action of hemolytic agents.[56]

The intracellular concentrations of the red blood cell are numerous. Nathan[45] summarizes these as follows, namely, that the red cell is derived from a nucleated precursor filled with the equipment for ferritin and hemoglobin synthesis with bits of nuclei (Howell-Jolly bodies), nuclear membranes (Cabot rings), remnants of ribosomes and RNA (basophilic stippling), ferruginous granules (Pappenheimer bodies), traces of endoplasmic reticulum (reticulocytes), and inclusions of precipitated hemoglobin (Heinz bodies). These concretions are found in developing as well as in newly formed or more mature erythrocytes.

*Crenation.* In blood smears that dry slowly, the red cell envelope becomes exposed to a hypertonic medium which causes wrinkling of the surface with the appearance of a moderate number of knoblike or prickly projections. This process, known as crenation, occurs normally. Three other types of crenated cells have been described which, however, are of pathologic significance.

*Burr cells.* The burr cell is a mature red cell possessing one to several spiny projections along its periphery and represents a type of preformed poikilocyte. Burr cells have been especially noted in persons with conditions with impaired renal function.[57] In the syndrome of hemolytic anemia, thrombocytopenia, and nephropathy (hemolytic-uremic syndrome, red cell fragmentation syndrome), the striking feature is the presence of bizarre poikilocytosis in the peripheral blood, characterized by the presence of many triangular crescentic and burr-shaped cells.[21] The pathogenesis of the red cell defect is thought to be the result of fragmentation occurring within the microcirculation, but it has been pointed out that burr cells are not specific but are commonly present in uremia from any cause[2] and is regarded as a serious prognostic sign. Burr cells appear in infants in connection with toxic hemolytic anemias associated with Heinz body formation.

Burr cells have also been observed in aplastic anemia,[36] after mechanical injury to the red cells,[9] in Laennec's cirrhosis,[60] in pyruvate kinase deficiency,[47,49] and following splenectomy especially for idiopathic thrombocytopenic purpura.[63] Their appearance after splenectomy has been attributed to the absence of the "culling" function of the spleen. The "culling" function[13] describes the unique ability of this organ to scrutinize circulating red cells and remove those which do not meet the requirements for survival. The normal spleen is a particularly effective filter that clears abnormal cells or particles from the circulation.

The burr cells differ from the crenated red cell, which is produced as a result of shrinkage in hypotonic solutions or exposure to lytic agents. The processes in the burr cell are longer and more irregularly spaced and appear more pointed than those in the crenated red cell, which are short, blunt, and more regularly spaced. The sequence of events ending in a burr cell appears to be the formation of a vacuole at the periphery of the red cell that subsequently ruptures through the cell membrane leaving a crater and a deformed erythrocyte.[6]

*Pyknocytes and infantile pyknocytosis.* In the first trimester of life, distorted contracted erythrocytes or burr cells appear in small numbers in normal full-term and premature infants. The percentages range from 0.3 to 1.9% in full-term infants and from 1.3 to 5.6% in premature infants, increasing with age up to at least 2 to 3 months. This type of burr cell staining intensely and having several to many spiny projections resembles spherocytes and is designated as a pyknocyte[67] (Fig. 8). The cells may, however, be associated with an acute severe hemolytic anemia early in life, in which case they may increase up to 50%, and the condition is referred to as infantile pyknocytosis.[67] In some cases this is associated with anemia and no jaundice, whereas in others the hyperbilirubinemia may reach a level to justify exchange transfusion. In a series of twelve cases of infantile pyknocytosis in which the pyknocytes ranged from 4 to 20%, five of the infants, all male, had glucose-6-phosphate dehydrogenase deficiency.[71] Burr cells may appear sporadically at later ages in patients with severe hemolytic anemia.

It has been observed[38] that, in pyknocytosis, both infant's cells and donor cells show a shortened survival, suggesting the presence of an extracorpuscular factor present in the blood of newborn infants. Of seven Mexican-American infants with hyperbilirubinemia associated with infantile pyknocytosis, exchange transfusions were required in two.[1] It is of interest that this procedure did not eliminate this morphologic abnormality and suggested to the author that an extracorpuscular factor was present in the affected infants which caused morphologic changes in the donor erythrocytes.

*Acanthocytosis (acanthrocytosis, Bassen-Kornzweig syndrome).* Acanthocytes (thorny red cells, from the Greek *akantha*, thorn) resemble burr cells but in the stained film look like spherocytes with pseudopods. The projections are large, coarse, and irregularly spaced. These malformed cells were observed in large numbers in the blood of a child with progressive ataxic neuropathy.[62] The differentiation between acanthocytes and burr cells may be difficult and bizarre erythrocytes of an intermediate type have been observed as an in-

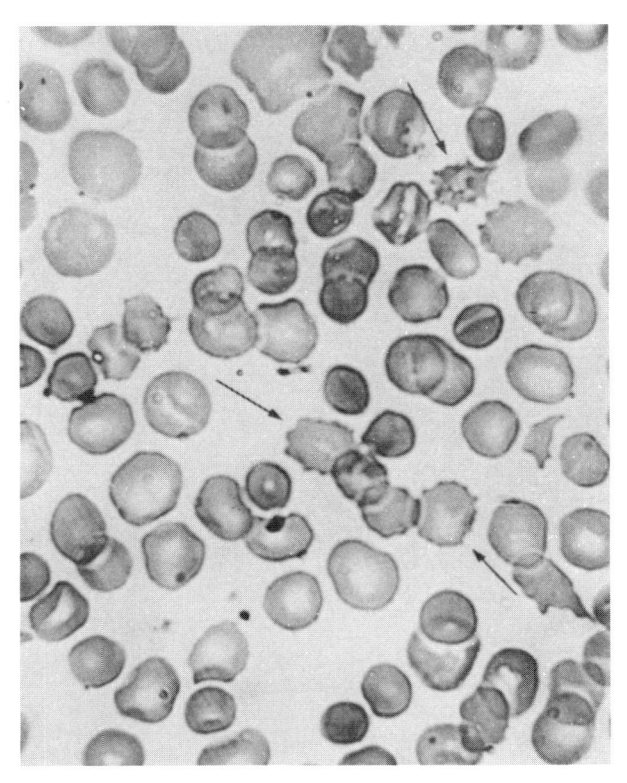

Fig. 8. Blood smear of an infant showing pyknocytes. Arrows point to distorted, irregular, contracted, dense red cells with spiny projections which are commonly found in small numbers in young infants. When present in large numbers, they are associated with hemolytic anemia and jaundice. (×1350.)

herited abnormality in association with retinal pigmentary degeneration.[4,34]

Acanthocytosis has been intensively studied in the few patients suffering with this disease. The basic feature in both the pathogenesis or the deformity of the red cell and the nervous system abnormality is a congenital absence of beta-lipoprotein.[35,42,55] Since beta-lipoprotein is the main lipid-carrying protein of the plasma, its absence results in gross depletion of the various blood lipids. In addition to the striking decrease in plasma lipids, the relative concentration of lecithin is decreased and the relative concentration of sphingomyelin increased in both the plasma and red blood cells.[53] Total lipid and cholesterol are low and no chylomicra appear in the blood after a fat meal. All patients have steatorrhea. The stools are loose, bulky, and fatty. The red cells show acanthocytosis, poikilocytosis, anisocytosis, absence of rouleaux formation, low sedimentation rate, shortened survival in normal recipients, and decreased fragility in hypotonic solutions of sodium chloride. The main features, therefore, include a celiac syndrome with severe impairment of fatty absorption, retardation of the physical and mental growth, progressive ataxic neuropathy, atypical retinitis pigmentosa, acanthocytosis, increased urinary excretion of copper, absence of beta lipoproteins, a very low level of blood cholesterol, phospholipid, and total lipids. The condition manifests itself in homozygotes as a mutant autosomal gene (Fig. 9). Grahn and coworkers[22] found some evidence in patients with alcoholic cirrhosis that a serum factor related to serum albumin appeared to be associated with acanthoid transformation.

Erythrocytes with minimal spurs resembling acanthocytes were observed in a patient with hepatic cirrhosis and hemolytic anemia. The morphologic change was reproduced in nor-

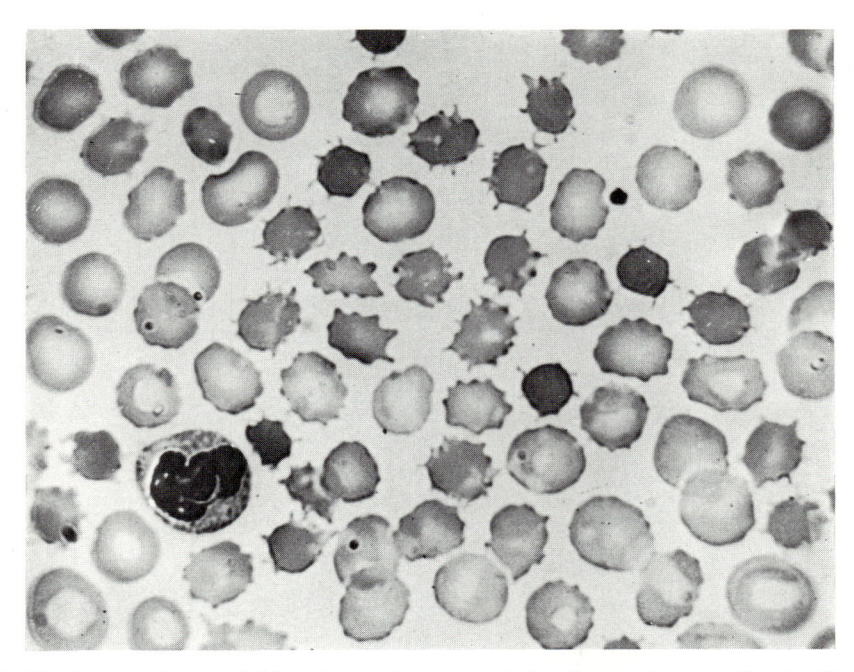

Fig. 9. Blood smear from a child with acanthocytosis. Red cells are almost uniformly distorted. Many possess spiny projections; others have irregularly spaced protuberances. Note small and deeply stained red cells resembling spherocytes with irregularly spaced spines. (×500.)

mal erythrocytes with the patient's plasma, pointing to a factor rendering them susceptible to hemolysis. There was no other evidence of clinical acanthocytosis (Bassen-Kornzweig syndrome).[64] On the other hand, acanthocytes were found in other cases to retain their abnormal shape when incubated in normal serum, and, conversely, the serum of these patients did not convert normal cells into acanthocytes. The abnormality would therefore appear to be inherent in the erythrocyte rather than in the serum.[5]

The neurologic manifestations of these patients indicate the presence of progressive degeneration of the posterior and anterior columns of the spinal cord, the cerebellum, and certain peripheral nerves.[65] This picture of spinocerebellar degeneration often prompts a diagnosis of Friedreich's ataxia. The neurologic features appear in childhood and continue to progress slowly until adulthood. Classically, gait disturbances, ataxia, deep tendon areflexia, hypotonia, and loss of vibratory sense develop. Visual disturbances consist of blurred vision due to macular degeneration. The autopsy findings in one case[65] revealed demyelinating lesions of cerebellar molecular layer. Marked optic macular atrophy was present. The pathogenesis of the neurologic manifestations remains obscure.

Two additional children with this uncommon syndrome have recently been described. One was a 17-month-old Maori child who, in association with acanthocytosis, a-beta-lipoproteinemia, hypocholesterolemia, and steatorrhea, showed impairment of renal function, aminoaciduria, and recurrent pulmonary infections.[5] A 7-year-old boy, the product of consanguineous parents, presented with diarrhea in early infancy and was later found to have a-beta-lipoproteinemia, steatorrhea, acanthocytosis, retinal degenerative changes, and ataxic neuropathy.[19] He was also mentally retarded. It was pointed out that prolonged absence of beta-lipoprotein from the serum may have played a part in the changes found in the erythrocytes, retina, and central nervous system.

A boy of Italian extraction was admitted to the hospital at 5 years of age because of the sudden onset of severe anemia (Hgb. 4.3 gm./100 ml.). Numerous burr cells were found in the blood smear. Neurologic signs and symptoms appeared at 8 years of age. These consisted of broad-based gait, coarse intention tremor, impaired position and vibratory sense, absent tendon reflexes, and positive Romberg test. No retinal changes were noted. Cardiac abnormalities appeared at 10 years of age and included episodes of palpitation, premature ventricular contractions, and bilateral ventricular enlargement. The patient died suddenly of cardiac failure. The prominent features at autopsy were interstitial myocardial fibrosis and long tract degeneration in the spinal cord similar to that seen in fatal cases of Friedreich's ataxia. Excessive deposition of lipochrome pigment in intestinal and cardiac muscle was a prominent feature.[15]

*Vitamin E deficiency and acanthocytosis.* The relation between vitamin E deficiency and structural deformities of the red cell is obscure. In the late anemia of prematurity occuring at 6 to 10 weeks of age attributed to vitamin E deficiency, Oski and Barness[48] noted irregularly contracted and spiculated red cells resembling pyknocytes of infantile pyknocytosis. In patients with acanthocytosis associated with a hereditary defect in beta lipoprotein synthesis, a marked deficiency of vitamin E has been observed.[16,32] Raising the plasma vitamin E to normal levels, however, had no effect on the morphology of the red cell. In another case of spur-shaped erythrocytes in Laennec's cirrhosis, a decrease in the plasma level of vitamin E was not observed and the administration of vitamin E, in vitro, did not correct the abnormal autohemolysis.[60]

*Familial erythroid (congenital dyserythropoietic) multinuclearity.* A familial erythroid anomaly has been observed[69] in which giant-sized erythrocytes, giant plurinuclear red cell precursors, and nucleated red cells with coarse cytoplasmic stippling and karyorrhexis have been found in the bone marrow. Although persons with this anomaly have no symptoms, they have a tendency toward mild anemia with peripheral blood showing anisocytosis, with a tendency toward macrocytosis and poikilocytosis.

Crookston and associates[12] described another type of erythroblastic multinuclearity in which giant-sized erythrocytes (gigantoblasts) were not present. Their five patients (including two sisters) showed an unusual anemia characterized by marked erythroid hyperplasia of the bone marrow, a large proportion of the erythroblasts being binucleated or multinucleated, ineffective erythropoiesis, and a positive acidified-serum test. Unlike in paroxysmal nocturnal hemoglobinuria (PNH), the sugar-water test was always negative in these patients. The lysis of their cells by acidified normal sera indicated their abnormal sensitivity to an agglutinating and complement-binding antibody present in some normal subjects. The disorder is apparently inherited as an autosomal recessive characteristic. Although there is a wide range in the severity of the anemia there is no evidence that it tends to become more severe with time.

## REFERENCES

1. Ackerman, B. D.: Infantile pyknocytosis in Mexican-American infants, Amer. J. Dis. Child. **117**:417, 1969.
2. Aherne, W. A.: The "burr" red-cell and azotaemia, J. Clin. Path. **10**:252, 1957.
3. Barrett, A. M.: Special form of erythrocytes possessing increased resistance to hypotonic saline, J. Path. Bact. **46**:603, 1938.
4. Bassen, F. A., and Kornzweig, A. L.: Malformation of the erythrocytes in a case of atypical retinitis pigmentosa, Blood **5**:381, 1950.
5. Becroft, D. M. O., Costello, J. M., and Scott, P. J.: A-beta-lipoproteinaemia (Bassen-Kornzweig syndrome); report of a case, Arch. Dis. Child. **40**:40, 1965.
6. Bell, R. E.: The origin of "burr" erythrocytes, Brit. J. Haemat. **9**:552, 1963.
7. Beritic, T.: Siderotic granules and granules of punctate basophilia, Brit. J. Haemat. **9**:185, 1963.
8. Bevan, G. H., and White, J. C.: Oxidation of phenylhydrazines in the presence of oxyhemoglobin and the origin of Heinz bodies in erythrocytes, Nature **173**:389, 1954.
9. Brain, M. C., Dacie, J. V., and Hourihane, D. O. B.: Microangiopathic haemolytic anaemia; the possible role of vascular lesions in pathogenesis, Brit. J. Haemat. **8**:358, 1962.
10. Bush, J. A., and Ainger, L. E.: Congenital absence of the spleen with congenital heart disease, Pediatrics **15**:93, 1955.
11. Cooper, R. A., and Jandl, J. H.: Bile salts and cholesterol in the pathogenesis of target cells in obstructive jaundice, J. Clin. Invest. **47**:809, 1968.
12. Crookston, J. H., Crookston, M. C., Burnie, K. L., Franconte, W. H., Dacie, J. V., Davis, J. A., and Lewis, S. M.: Hereditary erythroblastic multinuclearity associated with a positive acidifies-serum test: a type of congenital dyserythropoietic anemia, Brit. J. Haemat. **17**:11, 1969.
13. Crosby, W. H.: Normal functions of the spleen relative to the red cells; a review, Blood **14**:399, 1959.
14. Dacie, J. V., and Mollin, D. L.: Siderocytes, sideroblasts and sideroblastic anemia, Acta Med. Scand. (supp.) **445**:237, 1966.
15. Dische, M. R., and Porro, R. S.: The cardiac lesions in Bassen-Kornsweig syndrome; report

of a case with autopsy findings, Amer. J. Med. **49**:568, 1970.
16. Dodge, J. T., Cohen, G., Kayden, J. H., and Phillips, G. B.: Peroxidative hemolysis of red cells from patients with abetalipoproteinemia (acanthocytosis), J. Clin. Invest. **46**:357, 1967.
17. Fadem, R. S.: Ovalocytosis associated with the sickle cell trait, Blood **4**:505, 1949.
18. Fertman, M. H., and Fertman, M. A.: Toxic anemia and Heinz bodies, Medicine **34**:131, 1955.
19. Forsyth, C. C., Lloyd, J. K., and Fosbrooke, A. S.: A-beta-lipoproteinaemia, Arch. Dis. Child. **40**:47, 1965.
20. Gasser, C., and Willi, H.: Spontane Innenkörperbildung bei Milzagenesie, Helvet. Paediat. Acta **7**:369, 1952.
21. Githens, J. H., and Hathaway, W. E.: Autoimmune hemolytic anemia and the syndrome of hemolytic anemia, thrombocytopenia and nephropathy, Ped. Clin. N. Amer. **9**:619, 1962.
22. Grahn, E. P., Dietz, A. A., Stefani, S. S., and Donnelly, W. J.: Burr cells, hemolytic anemia and cirrhosis, Amer. J. Med. **45**:78, 1968.
23. Harley, J. D., and Mauer, A. M.: Studies on the formation of Heinz bodies. II. The nature and significance of Heinz bodies, Blood **17**:418, 1961.
24. Harris, J. W.: Studies on the destruction of red blood cells; molecular orientation in sickle-cell hemoglobin solutions, Proc. Soc. Exp. Biol. Med. **75**:197, 1950.
25. Hedenstedt, S.: Elliptocyte transfusions as a method in studies on blood destruction, blood volume and peritoneal resorption, Acta Chir. Scandinav. (supp. 128) **95**:1, 1947.
26. Holroyde, C. P., and Gardner, F. H.: Acquisition of autophagic vacuoles by human erythrocytes; physiologic role of the spleen, Blood **36**:566, 1970.
27. Holroyde, C. P., Oski, F. A., and Gardner, F. H.: The "pocked" erythrocyte; red-cell surface alterations in reticuloendothelial immaturity of the neonate, New Eng. J. Med. **281**:516, 1969.
28. Hurley, T. H., and Weisman, R., Jr.: The determination of the survival of transfused red cells by a method of differential hemolysis, J. Clin. Invest. **33**:835, 1954.
29. Hutchinson, H. E., and Ferguson-Smith, M. A.: The significance of Howell-Jolly bodies in red cell precursors, J. Clin. Path. **12**:451, 1959.
30. Kaplan, E., Zuelzer, W. W., and Mouriquand, C.: Sideroblasts; a study of stainable nonhemoglobin iron in marrow normoblasts, Blood **9**:203, 1954.
31. Kaplan, E., Zuelzer, W. W., and Neil, J. V.: Further studies on hemoglobin C; the hematologic effects of hemoglobin C alone and in combination with sickle cell hemoglobin, Blood **8**:735, 1953.
32. Kayden, J. H., and Silber, R.: The role of vitamin E deficiency in the abnormal autohemolysis of acanthocytosis, Trans. Ass. Amer. Physicians **78**:338, 1965.
33. Keimowitz, R., and Desforges, J. F.: Infantile pyknocytosis, New Eng. J. Med. **273**:1152, 1965.
34. Kornzweig, A. L., and Bassen, F. A.: Retinitis pigmentosa, acanthocytosis, and heredodegenerative neuromuscular disease, Arch. Ophthal. **58**:183, 1957.
35. Lamy, F., Frezal, J., Polonovski, J., Druez, G., and Rey, J.: Congenital absence of beta lipoproteins, Pediatrics **31**:277, 1963.
36. Lewis, S. M.: Red-cell abnormalities and haemolysis in aplastic anaemia, Brit. J. Haemat. **8**:322, 1962.
37. Lipton, E. L.: Elliptocytosis with hemolytic anemia; the effects of splenectomy, Pediatrics **15**:67, 1955.
38. Lock, S. P., Smith, R. S., and Hardisty, R. M.: Stomatocytosis; a hereditary red cell anomaly associated with haemolytic anaemia, Brit. J. Haemat. **7**:303, 1961.
39. Lyons, W. S., Hanlon, D. G., Helmholz, H. F., Jr., and Edwards, J. E.: Congenital cardiac disease and asplenia; report of seven cases, Proc. Staff Meet. Mayo Clin. **32**:277, 1957.
40. McBryde, R. R., Hewlett, J. S., and Weisman, R., Jr.: Elliptocytosis; a study of erythrocyte survival using radioactive chromium (CR$^{51}$), Amer. J. Med. Sci. **232**:258, 1956.
41. Meadow, S. R.: Stomatocytosis, Proc. Roy. Soc. Med. **60**:13, 1967.
42. Mier, M., Schwartz, S. O., and Boshea, B.: Acanthrocytosis, pigmentary degeneration of the retina and atoxic neuropathy; a genetically determined syndrome with associated metabolic disorder, Blood **16**:1586, 1960.
43. Miller, G., Townes, P. L., and MacWhinney, J. B.: A new congenital hemolytic anemia with deformed erythrocytes(?"stomatocytes") and remarkable susceptibility of erythrocytes to cold hemolysis in vitro. I. Clinical and hematologic studies, Pediatrics **35**:906, 1965.
44. Motulsky, A. V., Singer, K., Crosby, W. H., and Smith, V.: The life span of the elliptocyte; hereditary elliptocytosis and its relationship to other familial hemolytic diseases, Blood **9**:57, 1954.
45. Nathan, D. G.: Rubbish in the red cell, New Eng. J. Med. **281**:558, 1969
46. Nathan, D. G., and Gunn, R. B.: Thalassemia; consequences of unbalanced hemoglobin synthesis, Amer. J. Med. **41**:815, 1966.
47. Nathan, D. G., Oski, F. A., Sidel, V. W., Gardner, F. H., and Diamond, L. K.: Studies

of erythrocyte spicule formation in haemolytic anaemia, Brit. J. Haemat. 12:385, 1966.
48. Oski, F. A., and Barness, L. A.: Vitamin E deficiency in recognized cause of hemolytic anemia in the premature infant, J. Pediat. 70:211, 1963.
49. Oski, F. A., Nathan, D. G., Sidel, V. W., and Diamond, L. K.: Extreme hemolysis and red cell distortion in erythrocyte kinase deficiency. I. Morphology, erythrokinetics and family enzyme studies, New Eng. J. Med. 270:1023, 1964.
50. Pappenheimer, A. M., Thompson, K. P., Parker, D. D., and Smith, K. E.: Anaemia associated with unidentified erythrocytic inclusions after splenectomy, Quart. J. Med. 14:75, 1945.
51. Fauling, L., Itano, A. H., Singer, S. J., and Wells, J. C.: Sickle-cell anemia, a molecular disease, Science 110:543, 1949.
52. Perutz, M. F., and Mitchison, J. M.: State of haemoglobin in sickle-cell anaemia, Nature 166:677, 1950.
53. Phillips, G. B.: Quantitative chromatographic analysis of plasma and red blood cell lipids in patients with acanthocytosis, J. Lab. Clin. Med. 59:357, 1962.
54. Rundles, R. W., and Falls, H. F.: Hereditary (?sex-linked) anemia, Amer. J. Med. Sci. 211:641, 1946.
55. Salt, H. B., Wolff, O. H., Lloyd, S. K., Fosbrooke, A. S., Cameron, A. H., and Hubble, D. V.: On having no beta-lipoprotein; a syndrome comprising a beta-lipoproteinemia, acanthocytosis and steatorrhea, Lancet 2:325, 1960.
56. Schleicher, E. M.: Origin and nature of the Cabot ring bodies of erythrocytes, J. Lab. Clin. Med. 27:983, 1942.
57. Schwartz, S. O., and Motto, S. A.: The diagnostic significance of "burr" red blood cells, Amer. J. Med. Sci. 218:563, 1949.
58. Scott, R. B., Crawford, R. P., and Jenkins, M.: Incidence of sicklemia in the newborn Negro infant, Amer. J. Dis. Child. 75:842, 1948.
59. Selwyn, J. G.: Heinz bodies in red cells after splenectomy and after phenacetin administration, Brit. J. Haemat. 1:173, 1955.

60. Silber, R., Amorosi, E., Lhowe, J., and Kayden, J. H.: Spur-shaped erythrocytes in Laennec's cirrhosis, New Eng. J. Med. 275:639, 1966.
61. Singer, K., and Fisher, B.: Studies on abnormal hemoglobins, Blood 8:270, 1953.
62. Singer, K., Fisher, B., and Perlstein, M. A.: Acanthrocytosis; a genetic erythrocytic malformation, Blood 7:577, 1952.
63. Smith, C. H., and Khakoo, Y.: Burr cells; classification and effect of splenectomy, J. Pediat. 76:99, 1970.
64. Smith, J. A., Lonergan, E. T., and Sterling, K.: Spur-cell anemia; hemolytic anemia with red cells resembling acanthocytes in alcoholic cirrhosis, New Eng. J. Med. 271:369, 1964.
65. Sobrevilla, L. A., Goodman, M. L., and Kane, C. A.: Demyelinating central nervous system disease, macular atrophy and acanthocytosis (Bassen-Kornzweig syndrome), Amer. J. Med. 37:821, 1964.
66. Sturgeon, P., Itano, H. A., and Bergren, W. R.: Clinical manifestations of inherited abnormal hemoglobins; the interaction of hemoglobin-S with hemoglobin-D, Blood 10:389, 1955.
67. Tuffy, P., Brown, A. K., and Zuelzer, W. W.: Infantile pyknocytosis, a common erythrocyte abnormality of the first trimester, Amer. J. Dis. Child. 98:227, 1959.
68. Watson, J., Stahman, A. W., and Bilello, F. P.: The significance of the paucity of sickle cells in newborn Negro infants, Amer. J. Med. Sci. 215:419, 1948.
69. Wolff, J. A., and von Hofe, F. H.: Familial erythroid multinuclearity, Blood 6:1274, 1951.
70. Wyandt, H., Bancroft, I. M., and Winship, T. O.: Elliptic erythrocytes in man, Arch. Intern. Med. 68:1043, 1941.
71. Zannos-Mariolea, L., Kattamis, C., and Paidoucis, M.: Infantile pyknocytosis and glucose-6-phosphate dehydrogenase deficiency, Brit. J. Haemat. 8:258, 1962.
72. Zarkowsky, H. S., Oski, F. A., Sha'afi, R., Shohet, S. B., and Nathan, D. G.: Congenital hemolytic anemia with high sodium, low potassium red cells. I. Studies of membrane permeability, New Eng. J. Med. 278:573, 1968.

# 6 BLOOD GROUPS

***Blood group antigens.*** Blood group agglutinogens are genetically determined substances on the surfaces of erythrocytes which are present in certain persons and absent in others.[28] The blood group agglutinogen is antigenic and is that portion of the red cell that combines with a specific antibody. Blood group specificity is carried by the mucopolysaccharides.[71] The A-B-O and Rh-Hr blood groups are the most important, clinically.

Naturally occurring antibodies in significant concentration are normally absent in the Rh group and numerous minor blood types and are present in the A-B-O groups. Both the A-B-O and Rh-Hr agglutinogens are antigenic, and if they are introduced into a host in whom they are absent, antibodies may be formed. Each agglutinogen is highly specific and can be differentiated by its behavior with its corresponding antibodies. If cells containing one of these antigens are suspended in serum containing the corresponding antibody, the antibody unites with the antigen with resulting agglutination of the red cells. In certain cases (not Rh) the agglutinated red cells may undergo lysis. The significance of blood group differences stems from hemolytic reactions that may occur when red cells are transfused into recipients with corresponding antibodies within the circulation and during pregnancy when antibodies of maternal origin cross the placenta, combining with fetal red cells. Thus, the blood group systems A-B-O and Rh-Hr are of paramount importance in the pathogenesis of hemolytic transfusion reactions and in erythroblastosis fetalis (hemolytic disease of the fetus and newborn infant).

A, B, and $Rh_o$ (D) antigens on leukocytes have been demonstrated.[5] The presence of the antigens was not related to the secretor status of the leukocyte donor. Incubation of leukocytes from group O blood with plasma of a strong A secretor did not confer A reactivity to the leukocytes. The presence of blood group substances does not, therefore, represent absorption of soluble antigens from plasma of secretors.

***Definitions of terms in relation to blood groups.*** Several terms are frequently employed in the various relationships of the blood groups. These may be defined as follows:

*isoimmunization* the formation of antibodies resulting from the injection of erythrocytes containing specific blood group agglutinogens into other individuals of the *same* species who lack this antigen.

*agglutinogens* substances on the surface of cells (red cells and bacteria) which on combination with a corresponding antibody result in clumping or agglutination of cells.[80]

*blood factors* serologic specificities of red cell agglutinogens. Red cell agglutinogens are characterized by multiple blood factors, and it is possible for each agglutinogen to elicit more than one antibody, as a rule. Multiple tests with different antisera identify the set of blood factors that characterize the agglutinogens. Agglutinogens are designated after the most important blood factor or factors that characterize them.[80] (According to Weiner and Wexler[80] the various Rh factors do not necessarily all represent separate structures on the red cell envelope, but are extrinsic attributes of complex structures—the Rh agglutinogens, each of which is characterized by its own specific set of Rh factors.)

*blood typing* the determination of blood groups with the use of specific antisera; blood specimens are classified into groups or types on the basis of the blood factors or agglutinogens that they contain.

*cross-matching* test for compatibility between the patient's serum and the donor's red cells; this is necessary even when the patient and donor belong to the same blood group because of the presence of subgroups and rare types.

*heteroimmunization* immunization by injection of red cells of one species into members of another species.

*alleles or allelomorphs* alternative forms of genes which occupy the same position on a pair of corresponding chromosomes; each chromosome contains a series of places or loci occupied by different genes.

*homozygous* refers to individuals having identical allelic genes on the two corresponding loci of a pair of chromosomes.

*heterozygous* refers to individuals having two different allelic genes on the two corresponding loci of a pair of chromosomes.

*titer* a measure of the amount of antibody by determining the highest dilution of serum that can visibly agglutinate cells (in this context, erythrocytes).

*heterospecific pregnancy* a pregnancy in which the fetal red cells possess an A or B agglutinogen not present in the mother's cells; also the mother's blood contains an anti-A or an anti-B agglutinin that is incompatible with the A and B agglutinogen in the red blood corpuscles of the fetus.

*phenotypes* the characteristics of an individual apparent by direct observation; thus, blue eyes, tall, short, hemophilia, group O, Rh positive, etc., are all phenotypes.[80]

*genotype* the genetic constitution of an individual for a particular characteristic (in this instance, blood groups). The genotype is transmitted through the germ cells by means of their chromosomes. A normal human being has twenty-three pairs of chromosomes: twenty-two autosomes, with a pair of X's in the female and one X and one Y in the male. The genes of all the known blood group systems, including the Rh-Hr, are carried on one of the autosomes. An X chromosome-linked blood group system Xg has recently been discovered.

*porpositus (proband)* the original member of the family whose blood group (or other presenting physical or mental characteristic) prompted a genetic or hereditary study.

*polymorphism* the occurrence in the same habitat of two or more inherited forms of a species in such proportion that the rarest of them is too common to be kept in existence by recurrent mutations.[7] Intermediates between the forms are not present. In polymorphic traits two or more of the genotypes determining variation of the trait are common in the population. Polymorphisms are thought to arise as a result of selective differences between genotypes. The sickle-cell homozygote develops a severe hemolytic anemia which, under natural conditions, is usually fatal. The heterozygote, however, is at a selective advantage compared to the normal person, apparently because of greater resistance

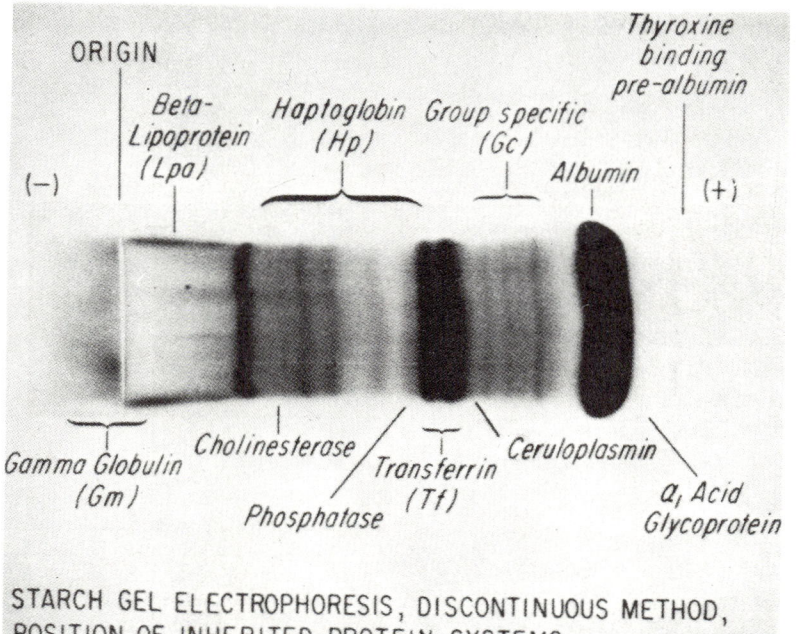

**Fig. 10.** Photograph of starch gel electrophoresis of normal serum to illustrate the position of some of the inherited serum protein systems. (From Blumberg, B. S.: Polymorphisms of the serum proteins and the development of isoprecipitins in transfused patients, Bull. N. Y. Acad. Med. **40**:377, 1964.)

to falciparum malaria and increased fertility. As a consequence of the selection in favor of the heterozygote, the sickle gene is maintained in the populations at high levels despite the elimination of genes due to the death of the homozygotes (balanced polymorphism). As a consequence of disease and environmental forces, as well as other factors, a large number of polymorphisms may exist in a population. Polymorphic traits exist with regard to the A-B-O and other red blood cell types, hemoglobins, glucose-6-phosphate dehydrogenase, and white blood cell and platelet antigens. The polymorphisms of the serum proteins include the haptoglobins, transferrins, gamma globulins, beta-lipoprotein, group-specific substance, serum cholinesterase, and serum esterase (Fig. 10).

**A-B-O blood group system.** The blood of any person falls into one of the four, well-defined major groups, according to the agglutinogens on their red cells. The presence or absence of each of these blood group agglutinogens is detected by their agglutinating reaction with high-titered and specific anti-**A** or anti-**B** serum. Since anti-**A** and anti-**B** are almost invariably present in the blood when the corresponding antigen is absent (Landsteiner's law), except in newborn babies, the validity of these tests may be confirmed by adding inactivated serum from the subject to a suspension of known A and B cells.

*Distribution of A-B-O groups.* In the United States the incidence of each group is as follows: group O, 45%; A, 41%; B, 10%; and AB, 4%.

*Inheritance of A-B-O blood groups.* Inheritance of A-B-O groups depends upon three alleles—*A*, *B*, and *O*. Since an individual inherits an *A*, *B*, or *O* gene from each parent, the pairing of genes in the body determines six possible genotypes: *OO, AA, AO, BB, BO,* and *AB*. The gene *A* occurs in two forms, $A^1$ and $A^2$, the former being dominant and more frequent. About 80% of the persons belonging to group A are included in subgroup $A_1$ and about 20% in subgroup $A_2$. With anti-**A** and anti-**B** typing serums, the four phenotypes O, A, B, and AB may be detected, as shown in Table 3.

The red cells of persons with genotype *AA* and of those with genotype *AO* cannot, however, be differentiated from each other; nor can the red cells of persons with genotype *BB* be differentiated from those with genotype *BO*. It is also not possible to distinguish homozygous *AA* and *BB* cells from heterozygous *AO* and *BO* cells by titration against the corresponding anti-**A** or anti-**B** isoagglutins.

Genes *A* and *B* are dominants and *O* is recessive. Several genetic and medicolegal principles stem from the A-B-O groups. For A or B to be inherited, at least one parent must transmit either an *A* or a *B* gene to the offspring. It is apparent that a child cannot belong to group O if either parent belongs to AB, for at least one dominant gene *A* or *B* must be received from such a parent. Nor can a child be of any group other than O (genotype *OO*) if both parents are group O. Also, a parent belonging to group O cannot have a child who belongs to group AB. It follows that if an individual is typed as AB, his genotype is automatically established as *AB*. Similarly, if he is typed as O, the genotype must be *OO*.

Most blood group antibodies in human serum are gamma globulins with a molecular weight of approximately 160,000 and a sedimentation coefficient of 7S, but some antibodies have a much higher molecular weight (1,000,000) with a sedimentation coefficient of 19S. Incomplete blood group antibodies are normally 7S globulins and agglutinating antibodies usually 19S globulins.[29] Others have found that anti-**A** and anti-**B** antibodies might be composed of either 19S or 7S globulins or a mixture of the two.[17] Wiener[78] pointed out the existence of an additional antibody—anti-**C**—present in group O serum. The existence of such individuals indicates that group O does not merely contain a mixture of anti-**A** and anti-**B** isoagglutinins but also contains a third isoagglutinin, anti-**C**. This isoagglutinin reacts with the red cells of individuals who may therefore be designated as possessing factor **C**. Wiener[78] claims that factor **C** plays an important role in **A-B-O** hemolytic disease of the newborn.

*H substance in red cells.* Group O cells are

**Table 3.** Reaction with the four A-B-O blood groups

| Blood group | Reactions of red cells with | | Isoagglutinins present in serum |
|---|---|---|---|
| | Anti-**A** serum | Anti-**B** serum | |
| O | − | − | Anti-**A**, anti-**B** |
| A | + | − | Anti-**B** |
| B | − | + | Anti-**A** |
| AB | + | + | None |

+ = Agglutination. − = No agglutination.

not inagglutinable since they are clumped by so-called anti-**H** sera. H refers to a basic substance from which the A and B substances are made under the influence of the *A* and *B* genes. H is present in largest quantity in group O and $A_2$ red cells and least in group $A_1B$.[47,70] A large number of reagents of human, animal, and even plant origin (such as extract of *Ulex* seeds), that react with group *O* cells but not with cells belonging to group $A_1B$, have been discovered.

The regular occurrence of **A-B-H** isoagglutinins in the absence of known antigen stimulation probably results from immunization by cross-reacting exogenous material.[57] The presence of material with ABH blood group activity in animals, plants, and bacteria has been amply documented.

According to Marcus,[43] the A-B-H substances purified from secretions are glycoproteins composed of aproximately 80% carbohydrate and 20% amino acids. These substances occur in human tissues and secretions in two forms, water-soluble and alcohol-soluble, and persons with these substances in saliva (secretors) have more water-soluble substances in their tissues than those lacking the substances in saliva (nonsecretors). A-B-H substances are secreted by mucous glands in many organs, including the upper respiratory tract, the gastrointestinal tract from the esophagus through the colon, and the uterine cervix. The synthesis of blood-group substances in superficial glands of the gastric and small intestinal mucosa is regulated by the secretor gene.

Thus the human A-B-H and Lewis blood-group antigens occur in secretions and cell membranes throughout the body. The specific antigenic determinants are oligosaccharide chains, which are linked to a polypeptide backbone in glycoprotein molecules or to sphingosine in glycosphingolipids.

Human milk contains oligosaccharides and macromolecules with Lewis and A-B-H activity and the production of these materials is regulated by the secretor gene.

A rare type of blood called "Bombay," which is characterized by a failure of the red cells to be agglutinated by either anti-**A**, anti-**B**, or anti-**H**, has been described.[6] The serum contains anti-**A**, anti-**B**, and anti-**H**, all active at 37° C., while the saliva is devoid of A-B-O group specific substances. A rare gene, "x," has been postulated for Bombay red cells, which in the homozygous state suppresses the blood group genes from producing A-B-O-specific substances both on the red cells and in the saliva.[39]

*Development of blood groups.* A and B isoagglutinogens can be demonstrated in the fetus in the second and third months of life.[36] Anti-**A** and anti-**B** isoagglutinins found in the cord blood diminished in titer or completely disappear in the first weeks or months of life. That these isoagglutinins have been passively transferred from the mother is evident from the similarity existing between the serum of the newborn infant and that of the mother with respect to isoagglutinins.[58] The isoagglutinins in the newborn infant's serum are, therefore, not the infant's own, but are derived from the mother by filtration through the placenta. In many pregnancies, however, the placenta exerts a definite limiting effect upon the extent to which the maternal agglutinins can enter the baby's circulation.[67] Between 3 and 6 months of age, the child begins to make his own isoagglutinins. The strength of the isoagglutinins rapidly rises and is at its maximum at 5 to 10 years of age; after this there is a gradual fall.[51]

Human A and B antigens in fetal red cells are weaker than those in erythrocytes of infants and adults.[23] The strength of antigen A has been more thoroughly investigated than antigen B. Antigen A increases rapidly during the first months of life up to about 5 months. It then increases at a slower rate until adult values are reached at approximately 2 to 4 years of age.

Naturally occurring antibodies are usually composed of 19S globulin and immune antibodies, usually 7S. The placenta readily transfers 7S gamma globulin but not 19S gamma globulin. Most antibodies which are capable of agglutinating red cells suspended in saline are composed of 19S globulin. Some anti-**A** and anti-**B** are 19S, some are 7S, and some are mixtures. According to Mollison,[47] anti-**A** and anti-**B** isoagglutinins are more commonly composed of 19S gamma globulin but may be composed in part of 7S gamma globulin. When the mother's serum contains only 19S isoagglutinins, none will pass to the infant. On the other hand, when the mother's serum contains a mixture of 19S and 7S isoagglutinins, the 7S component is readily transported across the placenta and the titer of 7S isoagglutinins is similar in mother and child. In the cord blood the isoagglutinins are found only in the fraction which contains 7S gamma globulin.

Thomaidis and co-workers[65] have shown that natural isohemagglutinins in adults with blood group A or B are predominantly of the gamma M-globulin (19S) type, whereas those of adults with blood group O have been predominantly of the gamma G type (7S) or a mixture of gamma M (19S) and gamma G (7S) globulins. It has also been demonstrated that isohemagglutinins may also be associated with gamma A globulins. Neither gamma M nor gamma A globulins cross the placental barrier. Isohemagglutinins were present in 57% of randomly selected newborn infants. The gamma M isoagglutinins detected in thirty-six newborn infants must have been of fetal origin since gamma M globulins are known to be incapable of crossing the placental barrier. Cord blood drawn from 137 randomly selected full-term newborn infants revealed maternal isoagglutinins in ninety-seven, or 57%. Since in a considerable proportion of neonatal sera isoagglutinins were of the gamma M type, it was concluded that most fetuses produce their own isohemagglutinins.

*Secretors and nonsecretors.* Blood factors **A, B,** and **O** (in reality blood group substances A, B, and H) are not restricted to the red cells, since in approximately 80% of human beings they are also present in water-soluble form in the body fluids and in such secretions as saliva, gastric juice, nasal secretion, semen, and amniotic fluid.[73] Persons who have blood group substances present in their secretions are known as "secretors," and those who do not are known as "nonsecretors." The blood group substances (agglutinogens) A and B are stable polysaccharide-amino acid complexes.[11] The classification of a person as a secretor or a nonsecretor is most readily accomplished by testing the saliva, where blood group substances are present in high concentration. It has been shown that almost all nonsecretors of A, B, and H substances have red cells that agglutinate in so-called anti-Le[a] serum. (See discussion of the Lewis group later in this chapter.)

*Universal donor and recipient.* Since the red cells of group O are not agglutinated by anti-**A** or anti-**B,** persons belonging to this group are termed universal donors. However, some group O blood may contain such a high titer of anti-**A** and anti-**B** agglutinins that, despite dilution in the recipient's circulation, the titer may remain sufficiently elevated to cause serious destruction of the recipient's red cells. Generally, such blood is considered safe if the titer is not over 1 to 100. Blood group-specific substances A and B (Witebsky substance) are added to neutralize the anti-**A** and anti-**B** isoagglutinins of group O blood before it is given to persons of other blood groups. One unit (vial) is sufficient to reduce the anti-**A** and anti-**B** in 500 ml. of blood to about one-fourth of its original titer.[10] When group AB blood is not available for AB recipients, experience has shown that low titer group O blood is satisfactory. It has been estimated that the serum of 3% of persons belonging to subgroup $A_1B$ contains anti-**H**.

*Blood chimeras.* A blood chimera, a rare occurrence in the human being, refers to one of nonidentical twins who has in his bloodstream two populations of red cells of different antigenic composition. The term *chimera* (originally a fabulous, fire-spouting monster, part lion, part goat, and part serpent) has been used in botany to denote an individual plant with two or more tissues differing in genetic constitution, such as a graft hybrid.[48] Originally described in cattle,[49] this phenomenon is ascribed to a union of placentas of dizygotic twins at an early stage in embryonic development, allowing the exchange and subsequent grafting of hematopoietic elements. Chimeras may also be produced artificially by transplantation of hematopoietic tissue. Natural chimerism is common in dizygotic cattle twins, but is rare in man.

Human chimeras may be recognized by differential red cell grouping[81] and by the recognition of female polynuclear leukocytes in the blood of the male twin.[15] In the natural human chimeras, in which there is a mixture of group A and group O cells, there are no anti-**A** agglutinins in the serum.[81] In one set of human twins the male twin had 86% group A red cells and 14% O red cells. The female twin had 99% group O and 1% A cells.[8]

Ordinarily, blood group mosaicism of human erythrocyte population is attributed to naturally occurring transplantation of blood and precursors through vascular anastomoses found in utero between fraternal twins. An individual has been reported[83] who was not a twin, yet possessed a predominating group A red cell population and a minor population of group B cells, amounting to approximately 10%. Other divergent characters such as sickling, hemoglobin composition, and secretor status were also found. The findings were interpreted as evidence of double fertilization of a maternal gamete possessing two dissimilar nuclei, representing an egg and its polar body.

Sturgeon and co-workers[63] presented the case of an adult who appeared to be a "blood chimera" as a result of intrauterine transfusion through chorionic vascular anastomoses with undetected twins. The presence of type A, MNS, and O red cells led to the conclusions that the interfetal transplantation of erythropoietic tissue was due most likely to a state of blood chimerism. Unlike other well-documented examples of human blood group chimerism, there was no co-twin. It was postulated that a co-twin had been absorbed in early fetal life.

***Rh-Hr blood group system.*** The discovery of the Rh factor provided an explanation for the cause of transfusion reactions other than those due to the four major blood groups of the A-B-O system described by Landsteiner. In 1940, Landsteiner and Wiener[32] reported their discovery of the Rh factor. They found that when the blood of the rhesus monkey was injected into a rabbit, the serum contained an antibody that not only agglutinated rhesus but human red cells as well. In retrospect, this factor explained a case reported by Levine and Stetson,[40] in which a severe hemolytic reaction occurred in a woman soon after the delivery of her baby.

In 1941 Levine and co-workers[36] proved that the pathogenesis of erythroblastosis was related to the Rh factor.

Wiener and co-workers[79] described two additional factors related to the original rhesus factor of Landsteiner and Wiener. The original factor was then named **Rh**$_o$ and the other, **rh'** and **rh''**. Wiener showed that these three blood factors determine eight types of blood which are inherited by multiple allelic genes. Levine subsequently described factor **hr'** reciprocally related to **rh'**.

Further investigation revealed that the Rh factor was present in 85% of the white population. Persons having this agglutinogen were designated Rh positive, whereas those in whom it was absent were designated Rh negative. In the Negro population in New York City the percentage of Rh positive is 93%, and in the Chinese it is 99%. There are no naturally occurring antibodies to the Rh factor in contrast to the presence of isoantibodies in the A and B groups. The Rh agglutinins may be produced, however, when an Rh-negative person receives Rh-positive blood. This was demonstrated to be the most common cause of intragroup hemolytic transfusion reactions.[75]

The capacity of red cells to react with a given antiserum is based on the presence of a specific antigen in the cell. When one of the Rh antigens cannot be demonstrated, as indicated by a negative reaction with its antiserum, another contrasting or reciprocal antigen (Hr) is often present in its place. Thus, every person inherits one set of three Rh genes or corresponding Hr genes from each parent (this is not strictly so since no reagent has been found for the theoretically possible Hr$_o$ or d).

***C-D-E notations for blood groups and the Fisher-Race concept.*** The Fisher-Race concept[51] postulates the presence of closely linked genes on the same chromosomes that are inherited as a unit. According to the Fisher-Race concept, each gene determines a corresponding antigen, which is identified by a specific antiserum. Following this concept, the Rh-Hr antigens can be fitted into a model based on the existence of three closely linked gene pairs, *C-c*, *D-d*, and *E-e*, with a one-to-one relationship between each gene and its corresponding agglutinogens. The symbols C, c, D, d, E, and e are used for blood antigens detected by appropriate antiserum, the small letters corresponding to the Hr factors. Thus, there are two sets of terminologies in relation to the Rh-Hr system. An allelomorphic relationship exists, therefore, between rh' and hr', Rh$_o$ and Hr$_o$, rh'' and hr'' (C and c, D and d, E and e, respectively). Fisher-Race renamed the factors D (**Rh**$_o$), C (**rh'**), and E (**rh''**) and postulated that since c (**hr'**) existed, so must d (**Hr**$_o$) and e (**hr''**). d (**Hr**$_o$) has not yet been discovered.

According to the Fisher-Race theory, a person inherits three Rh genes from each of his parents—C or c, D or d, E or e. For example, all children of CDe/CDe × cde/cde parentage would be of genotype CDe/cde, having recieved one CDe chromosome from the Rh-positive parent and one cde chromosome from the Rh-negative parent. It is now generally agreed, however, that an Rh gene should be regarded as an entity and that *C*, *D*, and *E* are not separable genes.[47]

***Genetics of Rh-Hr blood types.*** According to Wiener and Wexler,[79] the inheritance of Rh-Hr antigens is determined by a series of allelic genes. Their concept that the inheritance of Rh antigens is determined by a single gene is now held to be correct. They have claimed that the single Rh-Hr gene with a series of alleles at one locus on the chromosome determines the presence of corresponding agglutinogens, each characterized by multiple blood factors. Wiener and Wexler[79] state further that each agglutinogen has not merely one corresponding antibody, but multiple antibodies. Thus, each agglutinogen is characterized by multiple serologic specificities (blood factors). In other words, the gene may be regarded as a unit controlling an agglutinogen that may have multiple blood factor specificities. Recognition of the blood factors is possible by specific antisera. Antibodies define agglutinogens and not genotypes. For example, blood factors **hr'** and **hr"** are present in agglutinogen rh. The agglutinogen is identified by its behavior with available antisera. The cells of an individual with agglutinogen rh then react with anti-**hr'** and anti-**hr"**, but do not react with anti-**Rh$_o$**, anti-**rh'**, and anti-**rh"**. Anti-**hr**, an unusual antibody, identifies a factor **hr** or "little f(ce)."[56] This antibody detects agglutinogens determined by the genes R⁰ and r.

According to the Fisher-Race concept,[51] on the other hand, each Rh blood factor is controlled by an individual gene in a series of pairs of alleles, each at one of three adjacent, closely linked loci on the same chromosome. The Fisher-Race theory and nomenclature, although simpler to many, does not distinguish between agglutinogens and blood factors. It holds that since the determination of allelic characters is a fundamental property of genes, there is no point in removing these allelic characters further than necessary from the gene.[51]

The Rh-Hr factors, as determined by their corresponding antisera, are listed in Table 5. Of those listed, five are most important since no antisera have been found for Hr$_o$ and d. Rh-Hr allelic genes and their corresponding agglutinogens and blood factors, as described by Wiener, and shown in Table 5. The Fisher-Race nomenclature is shown in Tables 4 and 6.

Since the Rh-Hr genes are alleles occupying the same locus or position on corresponding chromosomes, a person must have an Rh antigen or one Hr antigen or both. Thus, Rh testing with specific sera may reveal that the person has either **rh'** or **hr'** (homozygous), or both **rh'** and **hr'** (heterozygous). In accordance with Rh nomenclature, Rh-negative persons (type rh) must be genotype rr and Rh-positive persons may belong to a variety of genotypes, e.g., $R^1r$, $R^1R^2$, $Rh^1R^1$, $R^2r$, etc.

Considering only blood factor **Rh$_o$**, there are three possible genotypes—$R^oR^o$, $R^or$, and rr. If anti-**Hr$_o$** (anti-d) serum were available, all three could be recognized. Since only anti-**Rh$_o$** (anti-D) is available, no distinction can be made between $R^oR^o$ and $R^or$ and both are similarly agglutinated.

**Table 4.** Six basic Rh-Hr factors as determined by their corresponding antisera

| Wiener system | Fisher-Race system |
|---|---|
| **Rh$_o$** | D |
| **rh'** | C |
| **rh"** | E |
| **Hr$_o$**\* | d\* |
| **hr'** | c |
| **hr"** | e |
| **hr** | f(ce) |

\*Postulated, since anti-**Hr$_o$** (d) serum does not exist.

**Table 5.** The eight "standard" Rh allelic genes\*

| Gene | Corresponding agglutinogen | Blood factors present | |
|---|---|---|---|
| r | rh | **hr', hr"**, and **hr** | |
| r' | rh' | **rh'** and **hr"** | **Rh$_o$**-negative agglutinogens |
| r" | rh" | **rh"** and **hr'** | |
| r$^y$ | rh$_y$ | **rh'** and **rh"** | |
| R⁰ | Rh$_o$ | **Rh$_o$, hr', hr"**, and **hr** | |
| R¹ | Rh$_1$ | **Rh$_o$, rh'** and **hr"** | **Rh$_o$**-positive agglutinogens |
| R² | Rh$_2$ | **Rh$_o$, rh"** and **hr'** | |
| R$^z$ | Rh$_z$ | **Rh$_o$, rh'** and **rh"** | |

\*From Wiener, A. S., and Wexler, I. B.: Heredity of the blood groups, New York, 1958, Grune & Stratton, Inc., p. 75. Also see Wiener, A. S., and Wexler, I. B.: An Rh-Hr syllabus. The types and their application, ed. 2, New York, 1963, Grune & Stratton, Inc.

There are three principal Rh factors: **Rh$_o$**, present in approximately 85% of Caucasian people; **rh'**, present in 70%; and **rh"**, present in 30%. The symbol **Rh$_o$** has a capital R to indicate its special serologic and genetic position, whereas **rh'** and **rh"** have a small r to indicate their lesser clinical importance. For some reason the **Rh$_o$** factor is a more potent producer of antibodies than are **rh'**, **rh"**, **hr'**, **hr"**, etc. The rh-negative person is represented by rh since the cells do not react with anti-**Rh$_o$**, anti-**rh'** and anti-**rh"** sera. Testing sera are available for each of the five most important **Rh-Hr** factors. Despite the lack of anti-**Hr$_o$** (anti-d), it is possible to hazard the presence of homozygosity or heterozygosity in a person on the basis of the statistic frequency of the reaction of the subject's cells to the available antisera. The cells of an individual with agglutinogen rh then react with anti-**hr'**, and anti-**hr"** and anti-**hr**, but do not react with anti-**Rh$_o$**, anti-**rh'**, and anti-**rh"**.

For routine clinical use it is sufficient to subdivide patients into Rh positive and Rh negative, according to their reactions with the single anti-**Rh$_o$** (anti-D) serum. By this means it is found that, of all of those who become immunized to Rh whether by transfusion or pregnancy, approximately 99% are **Rh$_o$** negative[47] (some regard the figure nearer 95%).

The Rh-Hr system receives its widest clinical application in erythroblastosis fetalis. **Rh$_o$** (D) is the most antigenic factor and is involved in approximately 93% of the cases of this disease.

The divergent views of Rh-Hr nomenclature of Wiener and Fisher-Race have been summarized by Miale.[46] Wiener distinguishes sharply between the terms "blood factor" and "agglutinogen." The agglutinogen is the substance in or on the erythrocyte, whereas the factor is the serologic specificity characterizing the agglutinogen as manifested by agglutination following the addition of the corresponding antiserum. Hence, an agglutinogen is characterized by more than one blood factor identified by serologic specificity. Each gene in effect determines an agglutinogen, which in turn has more than one factor. The Race-Fischer theory, on the other hand, conceives of a one-to-one relationship between a gene and an antigen. According to Wiener, there is a series of allelic genes, each determining a corresponding agglutinogen having multiple blood factors (serologic specificities). Each agglutinogen is recognized by its many blood factors. Fisher-Race postulates a set of triply linked genes which determine a corresponding set of three antigens on the red cell surface. In recent years close linkage of the genes has been assumed. The Wiener Rh-Hr nomenclature is regarded as a "logical sequence of symbols which leads to a better understanding of this complex blood group system."[64]

Realizing the difficulties of always assigning a specific immune response to a specific blood factor, which is itself part of a complex antigen, Rosenfield and associates[53] have proposed a new Rh nomenclature. Twenty-five different Rh antigenic determinants have been recognized on the basis of the known Rh antisera. Each kind of Rh antisera determines an antigenic property or properties that are inherited as mendelian characters, recognizable irrespective of gene dosage. The numerical order chosen was dictated partly by the order of discovery and partly by usefulness. The array of serologic distinctions is determined by the Rh locus. According to this scheme the most important of the Rh phenotypes are Rh 1 (Rh$_o$ or D), Rh 2 (rh' or C), Rh 3 (rh" or E), Rh 4 (hr' or c), and Rh 5 (hr" or e).

*Rh$_o$ variant* ($\mathfrak{R}h_o$, *D$^u$*). Some blood specimens react weakly with anti-**Rh$_o$** sera. These are said to have an **Rh$_o$** variant (or **D$^u$**) factor and are encountered most often among Negroes. Not infrequently, the reaction with anti-**Rh$_o$** serum can be elicited only by special techniques, notably the antiglobulin method. Its positive Rh character can be recognized by its reaction to high-titered anti-**Rh$_o$** (anti-D) serum and the indirect Coombs test. In the person with **D$^u$** factor, exposure of the blood to immune (incomplete) anti-**Rh$_o$** serum (anti-D serum) will result in agglutination with antiglobulin (Coombs) serum. To avoid overlooking the **Rh$_o$** variant, all blood designated as Rh negative should be subjected to additional

**Table 6.** Fisher-Race linked gene theory

| Gene* | Gene complexes | Corresponding antigens |
|---|---|---|
| r | cde | c, d, e |
| r' | Cde | C, d, e |
| r" | cdE | c, d, E |
| r$^y$ | CdE | C, d, E |
| R$^0$ | cDe | c, D, e |
| R$^1$ | CDe | C, D, e |
| R$^2$ | cDE | c, D, E |
| R$^z$ | CDE | C, D, E |

*For meaning of short notations in this column, see Table 5. Superscript designates genes.

screening by the indirect Coombs test. Such cases can cause confusion since the blood may be classified as either Rh negative or Rh positive, depending on the technique and reagent used. When used as donors, such individuals should be considered Rh positive; as patients they should be considered Rh negative.

**rh$^w$ factor (C$^w$).** The **rh$^w$** factor is an uncommon (2 to 7%) one, and when it is present, it is associated with blood factor **rh'**. Sensitization to the **rh$^w$** (**C$^w$**) factor has been a source of hemolytic transfusion reactions in Rh-positive recipients; e.g., recipient type Rh$_1$, donor type Rh$_1^w$. The **rh$^w$** (anti-**C$^w$**) antibodies result not only from transfusions with rh$^w$ (C$^w$) blood, but also from isoimmunization in pregnancy,[54] causing hemolytic disease of the newborn baby.

**Rh$_{null}$.** Rh$_{null}$ is an extremely rare phenotype lacking all Rh components. In other words, it completely fails to react with all Rh antibodies. Several cases have been reported in the homozygous state. In 1961 Vos and associates[68] reported the first example of blood with no detectable Rh antigen in an Australian aboriginal woman. Her ---/--- condition was interpreted as the absence of a common gene necessary for for the production of some Rh precursor substance. Levine and co-workers[37] described a second example of a phenotype in a white woman with a similar deletion. It was demonstrated that an independent mutant gene prevented the expression of Rh antigens completely in the homozygote and partly in the heterzygote. A third example was reported by Ishimori and Hasekura[26] in a healthy Japanese boy. He gave no reaction with any antisera. The phenotype of the propositus was rh or ---/---. This was the first example of a homozygote of silent Rh alleles or deleted Rh chromosomes.

Since patients with Rh$_{null}$ have no Rh or Hr antigens, transfusions if needed must be carried out with blood which is also Rh$_{null}$ so as to prevent the formation of red cell antibodies.

• • •

In addition to the A-B-O and Rh-Hr blood group systems, there are other red cell antigens of clinical importance, such as Kell and Duffy. Still others (M-N-Ss, P, Lutheran, and Lewis) are rarely, if ever, involved in human disease but are employed in precise identification of the red cell.

**M-N-Ss and P blood group systems.** The M-N-Ss and P blood group systems are rarely involved in intragroup incompatibilities. In addition to their use in the investigation of the cause of obscure transfusion reactions, they provide useful tools in human genetics and, with the major blood groups, help to resolve medicolegal problems of identity and parentage.

The M, N, and P agglutinogens were discovered by Landsteiner and Levine,[31] who used the sera of rabbits immunized with human red cells. After absorption of species agglutinins, the sera agglutinated some samples of human blood but not others. Naturally occurring antibodies against M and N are infrequent in the human being, so that their detection requires the use of rabbit immune sera. Like A and B antigens, M and N are well established in the newborn infant.

Three genotypes occur: *MM*, *MN*, and *NN*. Type *MN* is found in approximately 50% of human beings, M in 30%, and N in about 20%. A few human beings with acquired anti-**M** antibodies have been encountered, but these rarely lead to transfusion reactions or erythroblastosis. N is a much weaker antigen and has only very rarely been responsible for any difficulties.

Severe erythroblastosis due to anti-**M** agglutinins affecting twins has been reported.[61] One child was stillborn and the other responded to exchange transfusions. The maternal serum was found to contain a powerful anti-**M** agglutinin. Two exchange transfusions were required, using group N blood and the infant recovered.

The antigenic factor **S** and related antigen **s** are also present in human blood.[69] Cases of erythroblastosis fetalis and hemolytic transfusion reactions have resulted[9] from antigenic stimulation by anti-**S**. S bears a close genetic relationship[51] to M and N. A number of examples of anti-**S** antibodies occurring spontaneously have been reported, but more commonly they result from immunization.

**Factor U.** The **U** factor was originally described in a patient with a fatal transfusion reaction.[77] This factor is almost universally present in human erythrocytes. The few persons who are negative to this factor possess blood type N or MN.[79] This fact, together with the observation that almost all **U**-negative persons lack **S** and **s**, suggests that **U** belongs to the

M-N-S blood group system. Sensitization to the U factor is extremely rare, and it is of interest that all clinical cases have been reported in Negroes. Of Negroes tested, 1.2% are U-negative; hence, the possibility of sensitization by transfusion.[55]

Blood cells possessing the **P** factor are designated **P+** and those lacking it, **P−**. Naturally occurring anti-**P** agglutinins can be found in a few unselected P-negative persons. Anti-**P** isoimmunization is not known to cause erythroblastosis, but may occasionally cause hemolytic transfusion reactions.

The Donath-Landsteiner antibody of paroxysmal cold hemoglobinuria has the specificity of anti-**P** and reacts with all human red cells except the very rare pp and p$^k$ cells.[82] The reason for this unexpected specificity is unknown.

**Other blood group systems.** The Kell, Duffy, Lewis, Lutheran, and Kidd factors derive their names from the patients involved in cases of erythroblastosis fetalis, transfusion reactions, and from prospective donors.

*Kell groups* (Kk). The Kell (*K*) and Cellano (*k*) genes are alleles with equal dominance. The **Kell** antibody has been responsible for many cases of transfusion reactions and erythroblastosis. In these respects it is secondary in importance only to the antibodies **Rh$_o$ (D), A,** and **B**. On the other hand, the **Cellano (k)** factor, which is the reciprocal of **Kell**, is of minor importance. No naturally occurring **Kell** antibodies have been described.

Two additional factors, **Kp$^a$** and **Kp$^b$**, and their respective antibodies, anti-**Kp$^a$** and anti-**Kp$^b$**, are now recognized as being related to the Kell system.[2,3]

*Sutter blood groups.* An antibody has been described relating to another blood group system—Sutter—whose antigen is referred to as **Js$^a$** and its allele, **Js$^b$**.[18,19] The antigen has been found only in the Negro population, of whom 19% were found to be positive. The antigen has not been detected in Caucasians, Asians, American Indians, or Eskimos.

The allelic antigens Js$^a$ and Js$^b$ have now been found to be related to the Kell system.[62] Apparently the Sutter locus is closely linked to the Kell locus.

*Duffy group* (Fy$^a$ and Fy$^b$). For the Duffy, Lewis, Kidd, and Lutheran systems a combination of two letters is used to indicate the blood group system and the particular gene or antigen is further designated by adding a, b, etc., as a superscript.[47]

The Duffy system (Fy) has been shown to be responsible for hemolytic transfusion reactions, but not, as far as is known, for erythroblastosis fetalis. Fy$^a$ and Fy$^b$ constitute two of the better known alleles of this factor. Anti-**Fy$^a$** antibody is by far the more common of the two.

*Lewis groups* (Le$^a$ and Le$^b$). Only a few cases of hemolytic transfusion reactions have been caused by anti-**Le$^a$**.[45] It is of interest that practically all persons whose red cells are Lewis$^a$ positive are also salivary nonsecretors of **AB** and **H** substances and vice versa. Thus, anti-**Le$^a$** serum can be used for a presumptive test to detect the nonsecretor groups A, B, and O.[21] The Lewis blood groups are characterized by a system of soluble antigens. Unlike antigens of the other blood group systems, Lewis antigens of red cells apparently are acquired by absorption from plasma.[59] The Lewis antigens are present at birth in saliva and serum though they are absent from the red cells.[33,34] Rosenfield and Ohno (cited by Mollison[47]) have also pointed out that "the Lewis phenotype appears as an agglutinable characteristic of the red cells only after a few weeks of life." Red cells of the Lewis group are designated as Le (a+b−), Le (a−b+), Le (a−b−). Apparently Le (a+b+) is not found. It is noteworthy that at different ages red cells demonstrate a variable reactivity with regard to the **Le$^a$** factor. Thus, as many as 80% of infants less than 3 months old have Le (a+) red cells. Among older babies, the percentage of positive reactions is lower. At about 2 years of age retyping shows approximately 20% to be Le (a+), which is the same as the adult type. Le (b+), on the other hand, is rarer in young children than in adults. The adult frequency of around 70% is reached only at about 6 years of age.[51] The interrelations between Lewis and ABH secretor types and methods for their determination have been thoroughly described by Wiener.[74]

*Lutheran group* (Lu$^a$ and Lu$^b$). The Lutheran blood group system, occurring in 6% of the English population, has no clinical importance. The Lutheran antibody has been detected in Lutheran-negative subjects who have received multiple transfusions. This group plays no part in hemolytic transfusion reactions or erythroblastosis.

*Kidd group* (Jk$^a$ and Jk$^b$). Anti-Jk$^a$ was initially described in the blood of a patient who had given birth to an infant with erythroblastosis.[1] This patient had never had a transfusion. There have been few instances recorded in which this antibody was responsible for hemolytic transfusion reactions. The allelomorph **Jk$^b$**, discovered later, occurs even more rarely. The antibodies of the Kidd group are usually detected by the indirect Coombs test, but preliminary application of trypsin to the red cells may be necessary. The Kidd blood system consists of three alleles—*Jk$^a$, Jk$^b$,* and *Jk.* Approximately 25% of the white population is of the genotype *Jk$^a$Jk$^a$,* 50% *Jk$^a$Jk$^b$,* and 25% *Jk$^b$Jk$^b$.*

A few well-documented cases of hemolytic transfusion reactions secondary to anti-**Jk$^a$** have been reported.[30] Two cases of delayed hemolytic reaction due to anti-**Jk$^a$** following the transfusion of apparently compatible blood were described by Rauner and Tanaka.[52a] It has been shown that detection of this blood group may be complement-dependent requiring fresh serum samples and enzyme-treated test cells.

*Antigen I.* Cold agglutinins occurring as weak antibodies on the serum of normal subjects or in much higher titer in the serum of certain patients with acquired hemolytic anemia have recently been shown to have blood group specificity. This antibody has been named anti-**I**. While it may appear as a weak cold autoagglutinin in the serum of subjects without hemolytic anemia and in very occasional normal subjects, its main interest is its occurrence as a powerful cold antibody in the serum of certain patients with acquired hemolytic anemia.[27,66,76]

The red cells of persons reacting weakly at 4° C. and not at 24° C. are designated as "i." The results with anti-**I** and anti-**i** sera show that the red cells of infants at birth are extremely weak in "I" and rich in "i." After birth, this relationship gradually reverses, and by the age of about 18 months, the normal adult relationship of strong "I" and weak "i" becomes established.[44] The decrease in antigen "i" is, therefore, associated with a reciprocal increase in antigen "I." A notable exception occurs in thalassemia major in which there is an increased amount of antigen "i," regardless of age.[20] Red cells of patients with hypoplastic anemia, and many with acute leukemia, also have increased reactivity with anti-**i**. In thalassemia there is no consistent correlation between the amount of fetal hemoglobin and "i" antigen.

*Low incidence antigens ("private" blood group antigens).* Infrequent cases of intragroup immunization to a variety of rare antigens constitute a miscellaneous group known as "family antigens" or "private" blood group antigens.[35] Here the positive or negative reactions are linked solely to members of a particular family. They are usually discovered in the investigation of cases of erythroblastosis fetalis in which the etiology is not accounted for by established blood groups. Of special interest is the Jay antigen (Tj$^a$), now known to belong to the P blood group system.[51] In five married women of childbearing age, each of eighteen pregnancies ended in a miscarriage at 2 to 5 months' gestation.[38]

**The sex-linked Xg$^a$ system.** While all blood group antigens behave as autosomal characters, a new antigen has been described that is sex-linked and therefore controlled by a gene carried on the X chromosome.[42] The antibody is termed anti-**Xg$^a$**; the antigen, Xg$^a$, and the phenotypes Xg (a+) and Xg (a−). The antigen was present in 89% of 188 Caucasian females and in 62% of males. The antigen is well developed at birth and the distribution in the Negro is the same as in the Caucasian.

This antibody defining the antigen was discovered during cross-matching tests on a patient with familial telangiectasia who had received numerous transfusions for severe nosebleeds. The finding of this antibody offers an excellent opportunity for establishing linkage with other genes in the X chromosome and for investigating X chromosome abnormalities.[52] Linkage has already been found between hemophilia and Xg and blood groups, and also for Xg and Christmas disease (PTC, factor IX) and for hemophilia and deutan color blindness.[25]

Markers for X chromosomes in man are already known because of sex-linked inheritance patterns, such as the genes responsible for color blindness, hemophilia A (factor VIII) and B (factor IX), glucose-6-phosphate dehydrogenase deficiency, and blood group Xg$^a$.[42]

**Gm system—*hereditary gamma globulins in man.*** Normal sera can be divided into two groups, Gm (a+) and Gm (a−), by means of an agglutination inhibition reaction involving red cells coated with incomplete anti-$Rh_o$ (anti-D) and rheumatoid sera. Red cells coated with human antibody, to which the rheumatoid arthritis factor and normal serum are added, gave certain results. If there is an inhibition of agglutination, the group is Gm (a+). If agglutination takes place, an inhibitor is lacking and the patient belongs to Gm (a−). Gm (a+) sera thus contain an inhibitor that is not observed in Gm (a−) sera. The anti-$Rh_o$ serum used to coat the red cells should emanate from a Gm (a+) person.[22,60]

At least seven different gamma globulin factors have been defined in man. These factors are determined by genes present at two separate loci, the Gm and Inv loci. In white persons, factors **Gm (a)** and **Gm (b)** are determined by two genes which behave as alternate alleles. The same is true for **Inv (a)** and **Inv (b)** factors.[24]

The sera of children receiving multiple transfusions contain agglutinating antibodies against a **Gm** factor absent in the individual's gamma globulin. In each instance the patient's serum lacks the factors for which the agglutination was specific. It is concluded that these antibodies resulted from the introduction of foreign gamma globulins through multiple transfusions.[2]

The discovery of suitable human gamma globulin factor[22] has led to the identification of genetically determined antigens. More specific information comes from the reductive alkylation of immunoglobulins which breaks the disulfide bonds and results in two subfractions: light chains (L) and heavy chains (H). A single immunoglobulin molecule consists of two heavy chains.[16,72] The main immunoglobulins (IgG, IgA, IgM, and IgD) are differentiated by the structure of the heavy chains. Two allelic expressions are relatively well established. The so-called $G_m$ locus governs the amino acid sequence of the H chain and about twenty variants occur at this locus and are numbered 1 to 20. Another genetic locus has been found to determine the L chain structure and is designated the Inv locus. Variations regulated by this locus are designated **Inv (1)**, **Inv (2)**, and **Inv (3)**.

Following Coombs' and Mourant's observations that anti-Rh was part of the gamma globulins of human serum, Dacie[13] investigated other blood group antibodies as well as the autoantibodies associated with acquired hemolytic anemia. Dacie[13] and Cutbush and associates[12] observed that, when purified gamma globulin was added to certain antihuman globulin sera, the reagents would no longer agglutinate anti-**Rh**—sensitized red cells, but continued to react with anti-**Le**$^a$—sensitized cells.

The addition of a mixture of alpha and beta globulins to these antihuman sera neutralizes the antibody agglutinating the anti-**Le**$^a$ sensitized cells without neutralizing the antibody agglutinating anti-**Rh** sensitized cells. For this reason the Rh antibodies have been termed "gamma globulin antibodies" with most anti-**Kell** sera being similarly classified.

The incomplete forms of these antibodies, normally considered as cold agglutinins (e.g., anti-**Le**$^a$, anti-**Jk**$^a$, anti-**H**, and others), are known as "nongamma globulin" types of antibodies. Dacie[14] observed that certain of the so-called "cold" antibodies could not be demonstrated by the antiglobulin test unless the immune serum was freshly drawn. He believed that serum complement played an important role in the "nongamma globulin" antiglobulin reactions. It has also been shown that gamma globulin type antibodies (anti-**Rh**, anti-**Kell**) do not fix complement. The potentially hemolytic antibodies (i.e., anti-**Lewis**, anti-**Kidd**, etc.) fix large amounts of complement. A broad-spectrum, antihuman serum must contain both components "antigamma" and "antinongamma" (anticomplement) antibodies in optimum proportions.

In sera obtained from 100 patients before and after open-heart surgery and concomitant transfusions, anti-gamma globulin antibodies of one or another variety were noted in thirty-four patients for the first time after the operation and Gm-specific antibodies in fourteen patients.[50]

## REFERENCES

1. Allen, F. H., Diamond, L. K., and Niedziela, B.: A new blood antigen, Nature **167**:482, 1951.
2. Allen, F. H., and Lewis, S. J.: Kp$^a$ (Penney), a new antigen in the Kell blood group system, Vox Sang. **2**:81, 1957.
3. Allen, F. H., Lewis, S. J., and Fudenberg, H.: Studies of anti-**Kp**$^b$, a new antibody in the Kell blood group system, Vox Sang. **8**:1, 1958.
4. Allen, J. C., and Kunkel, H. G.: Antibodies to genetic types of gamma globulin after multiple transfusions, Science **139**:418, 1963.
5. Anderson, R. E., and Walford, R. L.: Direct demonstration of A, B, and $Rh_o$ (D) blood group antigens on human leukocytes, Amer. J. Clin. Path. **40**:239, 1963.
6. Bhende, Y. M., Despande, C. K., Bhatia, H. M., Sanger, R., Race, R. R., Morgan, W. T. J., and Watkins, W. M.: A "new" blood-group

character related to the ABO system, Lancet **1**:903, 1952.
7. Blumberg, B. S.: Polymorphisms of the serum proteins and the development of isoprecipitins in transfused patients, Bull. N. Y. Acad. Med. **40**:377, 1964.
8. Booth, P. B., Plaut, G., James, J. D., Ikin, E. W., Moores, P., Sanger, R., and Race, R. R.: Blood chimerism in a pair of twins, Brit. Med. J. **1**:1456, 1957.
9. Brandes, W. W., Cahan, A. C., and Jack, J. A.: Incompatible transfusion caused by anti-S, J.A.M.A. **156**:836, 1954.
10. Bray, W. E.: Clinical laboratory methods, ed. 5, St. Louis, 1957, The C. V. Mosby Co.
11. Carpenter, P. L.: Immunology and serology, Philadelphia, 1956, W. B. Saunders Co.
12. Cutbush, M., Crawford, H., and Mollison, P. L.: Observations on antihuman globulin sera, Brit. J. Haemat. **1**:410, 1955.
13. Dacie, J. V.: Differences in the behavior of sensitized red cells to agglutination by antiglobulin sera, Lancet **2**:594, 1951.
14. Dacie, J. V.: 'Incomplete' cold antibodies; role of complement in sensitization to antiglobulin serum by potentially hemolytic antibodies, Brit. J. Haemat. **3**:77, 1957.
15. Davidson, W. M., Fowler, J. F., and Smith, D. R.: Sexing the neutrophil leucocytes in nature and artificial chimaeras, Brit. J. Haemat. **4**:231, 1958.
16. Engle, R. L., Jr., and Wallis, L. A.: Immunoglobulins, immune deficiency syndromes, multiple myeloma and related disorders, Springfield, Ill., 1969, Charles C Thomas, Publisher.
17. Fudenberg, H. H., Kunkel, H. G., and Franklin, E. C.: High molecular weight antibodies, Acta Haemat. **10**:522, 1959.
18. Giblett, E. R.: Js, a "new" blood group antigen found in Negroes, Nature **181**:1221, 1958.
19. Giblett, E. R., and Chase, J.: Js[a], a "new" red cell antigen found in Negroes; evidence for an eleventh blood group system; Brit. J. Haemat. **5**:319, 1959.
20. Giblett, E. R., and Crookston, M. C.: Agglutinability of red cells by anti-i in patients with thalassemia major and other haematological disorders, Nature **201**:1138, 1964.
21. Grubb, R.: Correlation between Lewis blood group and secretor character in man, Nature **162**:933, 1948.
22. Grubb, R.: Hereditary gamma globulin groups in man. In Wolstenholme, G. E. W., and O'Connor, C. M., editors: Ciba Foundation Symposium on Biochemistry of Human Genetics, Boston, 1959, Little, Brown & Co., p. 264.
23. Grundbacher, F. J.: Changes in human A antigen of erythrocytes with the individual's age, Nature **204**:192, 1964.

24. Harboe, M., and Osterland, C. K.: Genetically determined structures of immune-globulins. In Grabar, P., and Miescher, P. A., editors: Immunopathology, 3rd International Symposium, Basel, 1963, Benno Schwabe & Co.
25. Harrison, J. F.: Haemophilia, Christmas disease and the Xg blood groups; observations based on the haemophiliacs of Birmingham, Brit. J. Haemat. **10**:115, 1964.
26. Ishimori, T., and Hasekura, H.: A Japanese with no detectable Rh blood group antigen due to silent Rh alleles or deleted chromosomes, Transfusion **7**:84, 1967.
27. Jenkins, W. J., Marsh, W. L., Noades, J., Tippet, P., Sanger, R., and Race, R. R.: The I antigen and antibody, Vox Sang. **5**:97, 1960.
28. Kabat, E. A.: Blood group substances, New York, 1956, Academic Press, Inc.
29. Kekwick, R. A., and Mollison, P. L.: Blood group antibodies associated with the 19S and 7S components of human sera, Vox Sang. **6**:398, 1961.
30. Kronenberg, H., Kooptzoff, O., and Walsh, R. J.: Haemolytic transfusion reaction due to anti-Kidd, Aust. Ann. Med. **7**:34, 1958.
31. Landsteiner, K., and Levine, P.: A new agglutinable factor differentiating individual human bloods; further observations on individual differences of human blood, Proc. Soc. Exp. Biol. Med. **24**:600, 1927.
32. Landsteiner, K., and Wiener, A. S.: An agglutinable factor in human blood recognized by immune sera for rhesus blood, Proc. Soc. Exp. Biol. Med. **43**:223, 1940.
33. Lawler, S. D., and Marshall, R.: Lewis and secretor characters in infancy, Vox Sang. **6**:541, 1961.
34. Lawler, S. D., and Marshall, R.: Significance of the presence of Lewis substances in serum during infancy, Nature **190**:1020, 1961.
35. Levine, P.: A brief review of the newer blood factors, Trans. N. Y. Acad. Sci. **13**:205, 1951.
36. Levine, P., Burnham, L., Katzin, F. M., and Vogel, P.: The role of isoimmunization in the pathogenesis of erythroblastosis fetalis, Amer. J. Obstet. Gynec. **42**:925, 1941.
37. Levine, P., Celano, M. J., Falkowski, F., Chambers, J. W., Hunter, O. B., Jr., and English, C. T.: A second example of ---/--- or $Rh_{null}$ blood, Transfusion **5**:492, 1965.
38. Levine, P., and Koch, E. A.: The rare human isoagglutinin anti-Tj[a] and habitual abortion, Science **120**:239, 1954.
39. Levine, P., Robinson, E., Celano, M., Briggs, O., and Falkinburg, L.: Gene interaction resulting in suppression of blood group substance B, Blood **10**:1100, 1955.
40. Levine, P., and Stetson, R.: An unusual case

of intra-group agglutination, J.A.M.A. **113**: 126, 1939.
41. Levine, P., Vogel, P., and Rosenfield, R. E.: Hemolytic disease of the newborn. In Levine, S. Z., editor: Advances in pediatrics, Chicago, 1953, Year Book Medical Publishers, Inc., p. 97.
42. Mann, J. D., Cahan, A., Gelb, A. G., Fisher, N., Hamper, J. Tippett, P., Sanger, R., and Race, R. R.: A sex-linked blood-group, Lancet **1**:8, 1962.
43. Marcus, D. M.: The ABO and Lewis blood-group system; immunochemistry, genetics and relation to human disease, New Eng. J. Med. **280**:994, 1969.
44. Marsh, W. L.: Anti-i; a cold antibody defining the Ii relationship in human red cells, Brit. J. Haemat. **7**:200, 1961.
45. Matson, G. A., Coe, J., and Swanson, S.: Hemolytic transfusion reaction due to anti-Le$^a$, Blood **10**:1236, 1955.
46. Miale, J. B.: A pathologist's critique of the controversy over blood group serology and nomenclature, Trans. N.Y. Acad. Sci., Series II **29**:887, 1967.
47. Mollison, P. L.: Blood transfusion in clinical medicine, ed. 3, Oxford, England, 1961, Blackwell Scientific Publications.
48. Nicholas, J. W., Jenkins, W. J., and Marsh, W. L.: Human blood chimeras; a study of surviving twins, Brit. Med. J. **1**:1458, 1957.
49. Owen, R. D.: Immunogenetic consequences of vascular anastomosis between bovine twins, Science **102**:400, 1945.
50. Pretty, H. M., Fudenberg, H. H., Perkins, H. A., and Garbode, F.: Anti-γ globulin antibodies after open-heart surgery, Blood **32**:205, 1968.
51. Race, R. R., and Sanger, R.: Blood groups in man, ed. 4, Philadelphia, 1963, F. A. Davis Co.
52. Race, R. R., and Sanger, R.: The X-linked blood group system Xg; work in progress, Acta Haemat. **31**:205, 1964.
52a. Rauner, T. A., and Tanaka, K. R.: Hemolytic transfusion reactions associated with the Kidd antibody (Jk$^a$), New Eng. J. Med. **276**:1486, 1967.
53. Rosenfield, R. E., Allen, F. H., Jr., Swisher, S. N., and Kochwa, S.: A review of Rh serology and presentation of a new terminology, Transfusion **2**:287, 1962.
54. Sacks, M. O., Schultz, C., Dagovitz, L., and Vanecko, M.: Hemolytic disease of the newborn due to the rare blood factor rh$^w$ (C$^w$), Pediatrics **21**:443, 1958.
55. Sampson, C. C., Thomas, C., and Griffin, S.: Isosensitization to the U factor, J.A.M.A. **171**:1203, 1959.
56. Sanger, R., Race, R. R., Rosenfield, R. E., Vogel, P., and Gibbel, N.: Anti-f and the "new" Rh antigen it defines, Proc. Nat. Acad. Sci. **39**:824, 1953.
57. Schiffman, G., and Marcus, D. M.: Chemistry of AHB blood group substances. In Moore, C. V., and Brown, E. B., editors: Progress in hematology, vol. IV, New York, 1964, Grune & Stratton, Inc.
58. Smith, C. H.: Isoagglutinins in the newborn with special reference to their placental transmission, Amer. J. Dis. Child. **36**:54, 1928.
59. Sneath, J. S., and Sneath, P. H. A.: Transformation of the Lewis groups of human red cells, Nature **176**:172, 1955.
60. Steinberg, A. G.: Progress in medical genetics. In Steinberg, A. G.: Progress in the study of genetically determined human gamma globulin types (the Gm and Inv groups), vol. II, New York, 1962, Grune & Stratton, Inc., p. 1.
61. Stone, B., and Marsh, W.: Haemolytic disease of the newborn caused by anti-M, Brit. J. Haemat. **5**:344, 1959.
62. Stroup, M., MacIlroy, M., Walker, R., and Aydelotte, J. V.: Evidence that Sutter belongs to the Kell blood group system, Transfusion **5**:309, 1965.
63. Sturgeon, P., McQuiston, D. T., Sparkes, R., Solomon, J., and Barnett, E. V.: Atypical immunologic tolerance to a human blood group chimera, Blood **33**:507, 1969.
64. Sussman, L. N.: Blood grouping tests, medicolegal uses, Springfield, Ill., 1968, Charles C Thomas, Publisher, p. 54.
65. Thomaidis, T., Agathopoulos, A., and Matsaniotis, N.: Natural isohemagglutinin production by the fetus, J. Pediat. **74**:39, 1969.
66. Tippett, P., Noades, J., Sanger, R., Race, R. R., Sansais, L., Holman, C. A., and Buttimer, R. J.: Further studies of the I antigen and antibody, Vox Sang. **5**:107, 1960.
67. Tovey, C. H.: A study of the protective factors in heterospecific blood group pregnancy and their role in the prevention of haemolytic disease of the newborn, J. Path. Bact. **57**:295, 1945.
68. Vos, G. H., Vos, D., Kirk, R. L., and Sanger, R.: A sample of blood with no detectable Rh antigen, Lancet **1**:14, 1961.
69. Walsh, R. J., and Montgomery, C. M.: A new human iso-agglutinin subdividing the MN blood groups, Nature **160**:504, 1947.
70. Watkins, W. M., and Morgan, W. T. J.: Some observations on the O and H characters of human blood and secretions, Vox Sang. **5**:1, 1955.
71. Watkins, W. M., and Morgan, W. T. J.: Possible genetic pathways for the biosynthesis of blood group polysaccharides, Vox Sang. **4**:97, 1959.
72. Weiser, R. S., Myrik, Q. N., and Pearsall, N.

N.: Fundamentals of immunology for students of medicine and related sciences, Philadelphia, 1969, Lea & Febiger.
73. Wiener, A. S.: Blood groups and transfusion, ed. 3, Springfield, Ill., 1943, Charles C Thomas, Publisher.
74. Wiener, A. S.: Lewis blood types; theoretical implications and practical applications, Amer. J. Clin. Path. 43:388, 1965.
75. Wiener, A. S., and Peters, H. R.: Hemolytic reactions following transfusions of blood of the homologous group, with three cases in which the same agglutinogen was responsible, Ann. Intern. Med. 13:2306, 1940.
76. Wiener, A. S., Unger, L. J., Cohen, I., and Feldman, J.: Type-specific cold auto-antibodies as a cause of acquired hemolytic anemia and hemolytic transfusion reactions; biologic test with bovine red cells, Ann. Intern. Med. 44:221, 1956.
77. Wiener, A. S., Unger, L. J., and Gordon, E. B.: Fatal hemolytic transfusion reaction caused by sensitization to new factor U, J.A.M.A. 153:1444, 1953.
78. Wiener, A. S. and Ward, F. A.: The serological specificity (blood factor) C of the A-B-O groups; theoretical implications and practical applications, Amer. J. Clin. Path. 46:27, 1966.
79. Wiener, A. S., and Wexler, I. B.: Heredity of the blood groups, New York, 1958, Grune & Stratton, Inc.
80. Wiener, A. S., and Wexler, I. B.: An Rh-Hr syllabus. The types and their application, ed. 2, New York, 1963, Grune & Stratton, Inc.
81. Woodruff, M. F. A., Fox, M., Buckton, K. A., and Jacobs, P. M.: The recognition of human blood chimeras, Lancet 1:192, 1962.
82. Worlledge, S. M., and Rousso, C.: Studies on the serology of paroxysmal cold haemoglobinuria (P.C.H.), with special reference to its relationship with the P blood group systems, Vox Sang. 10:293, 1965.
83. Zuelzer, W. W., Beattie, K. M., and Reisman, L. I.: Generalized unbalanced mosaicism attributable to dispermy and probable fertilization of polar body, Amer. J. Human Genet. 16:38, 1964.

# 7 TRANSFUSIONS IN PEDIATRIC PRACTICE*

*Introduction.* The availability of plastic blood collection sets with one or more satellite bags, together with a more accurate appraisal of the need for either whole blood or the separate cellular or noncellular components of blood, have greatly altered transfusion practice. The need will vary for the infant who requires an exchange transfusion, for the child with congenital coagulation disorders, or for the patient with acute leukemia or aplastic anemia, who periodically may require platelets instead of whole blood.

The cellular and noncellular components of blood differ in life-span, in the degree to which they exist in physiologic excess in the circulation or in extravascular depots, in the speed of their return to the circulation after their loss, and finally in the ways in which their survival is affected by the process of blood collection, preservation, or reinfusion.

The life-span of the various cellular components of blood varies greatly, ranging from a span of 1 to 4 months for the red cell to a span measured in days for platelets and granulocytes. The latter two elements are present in large extravascular pools so that, following moderate hemorrhage, the peripheral count may be normal. Of the cellular elements, only red cell replacement is required following moderate or even fairly massive blood loss, assuming the patient has a normally functioning bone marrow.

After mild to moderate blood loss, plasma water is quickly replaced from extravascular sources and plasma volume is maintained after mild to moderate blood loss. It is of interest that, immediately following hemorrhage, hemoglobin and hematocrit values are unchanged. Since each is a measure of the relative volume of red cell mass and plasma water, hemoglobin and hematocrit levels fall only after interstitial fluid enters the circulation. With the plasma water replaced, exogenous albumin administration is unnecessary since the latter is present in abundant supply in intravascular and interstitial pools. Acute blood loss, therefore, does not imply significant hypoalbuminemia. These are factors to be considered in appraising and planning restitution following extensive blood loss.

*Significant factors in transfusion therapy.* The approach to transfusion in the pediatric patient necessitates certain background data in order to evaluate the need of transfusion in relation to the growth period, potential risks, and technicalities of administration. Such data, summarized as follows, also provide a basis for the indications and certain of the limitations of transfusion therapy.

Blood volume—80 ml. per kilogram
Plasma volume—45 ml. per kilogram
Erythrocyte volume—35 ml. per kilogram
Hemoglobin concentration—12 to 13 gm. per 100 ml.
Hematocrit—36%
1 gm. hemoglobin = 3.4 mg. iron
100 ml. transfused whole blood (average) = 50 mg. iron
100 ml. transfused packed cells (average) = 70 mg. iron
500 ml. transfused whole blood (average) = 250 mg. iron

*Dosage for transfusion*
Whole blood
  20 ml. per kilogram when body weight is less than 25 kg.
  Units of 500 ml. when body weight is more than 25 kg.
Packed or sedimented erythrocytes
  15 ml. per kilogram when body weight is less than 20 kg.
  Units of 300 ml. when body weight is more than 20 kg.
Plasma—10 to 15 ml. per kilogram

---

*Quoted in part from Smith, C. H.: Transfusions in pediatric practice; indications and limitations, Pediatrics 17:596, 1956.

***Indications for transfusion.*** The indications for transfusion are listed as follows:

    To restore deficit of hemoglobin and erythrocytes
        Acute and chronic blood loss
        Hemolytic anemias—congenital and acquired
        Defective blood formation
        Preoperative and postoperative
    To restore blood volume
        Shock, burns, trauma
    To supply specific coagulation factors, including platelets
    Miscellaneous
        Infections
        Hypoproteinemia
        Exchange in erythroblastosis
        Poisoning
        Extracorporeal

In pediatric practice the indications usually apply to treatment of patients with blood disorders, infection, and nutritional and deficiency states. In contrast to the situation in the adult, the management of transfusion needs in the child requires the additional appraisal of abnormality in relation to a specific stage of growth and development. For instance, prescribing a hemoglobin level to be achieved by transfusion may not be a simple task in the infant or young child because the optimal value is not fixed but is subject to individual interpretation.

***Blood volume—plasma, total circulating hemoglobin, and erythrocyte mass.*** Comparisons in terms of total hemoglobin and erythrocyte mass permit evaluation of therapeutic procedures or the need for such procedures by eliminating the influence of variations in plasma volume. The determination of total circulating hemoglobin and erythrocyte content, therefore, has come into greater use because it frequently obviates erroneous conclusions drawn from a peripheral blood sample. From the blood volume (80 ml. per kilogram of body weight) and hemoglobin measurements (expressed as grams per 100 ml.), the total circulating hemoglobin mass can be readily determined. In patients in whom transfusions are being considered, periodic estimations of the absolute hemoglobin mass frequently prove more valuable in detecting the early regeneration of hemoglobin than in determining the peripheral hemoglobin concentration. This calculation, which takes into account the factors of growth and hemodilution, has proved helpful in recognizing the initial states of hemoglobin regeneration in the premature infant[48] and in evaluating the hemoglobin level prior to transfusion in the patient with refractory chronic hemolytic anemia such as thalassemia.[50] In erythroblastosis, for instance, transfusions can be postponed in patients with hemoglobin concentrations of 8 gm. per 100 ml. at the fourth to sixth week of life in the so-called convalescent anemic phase,[42] when it is found that the total circulating hemoglobin mass either has stabilized or has begun to rise.

With certain exceptions, a blood volume of 80 ml. per kilogram of body weight applies throughout life. In the newborn infant the value of 85 ml. per kilogram has been found more accurate in calculating the blood volume prior to performing an exchange transfusion. In our experience the blood volume has been found to exceed the normal, with values as high as 104 ml. per kilogram in a small number of patients with sickle cell anemia who were not in crisis. An inordinate increase in plasma volume was responsible for such values. This hemodilution probably accounted for the freedom from disability of these patients since their hemoglobin values were maintained without transfusions at levels of 6 to 7 gm. per 100 ml. In our experience crisis is associated with a sharp decrease in plasma volume, but the amount of hemoglobin undergoes little or no change. In an attempt to restore the expanded precritical plasma volume, whole blood and plasma have been given with moderate success. Increased fluid intake, either orally or parenterally, is a valuable adjunct.

Mollison[38] gives the blood volume of newborn infants as 84.7 ml. per kilogram and for normal adults as 76.6 ml. per kilogram. Others regard 80 ml. per kilogram for the young infant and the values for the older child as follows:
    Blood volume—70 ml. per kilogram
    Plasma volume—40 ml. per kilogram
    Erythrocyte volume—30 ml. per kilogram

***Hemoglobin and hematocrit levels in acute and chronic anemias.*** In the management of severe anemia, the objective in the restoration of a normal level of hemoglobin is different in acute blood loss from that in chronic anemia. In the patient with nonrecurring hemorrhage or in the infant with severe iron deficiency who is too ill to await the effects of specific therapy, a sufficient amount of whole blood or, preferably, packed erythrocytes may be given to achieve hemoglobin levels of 12 to 13 gm. per 100 ml. and a hematocrit of 36%.

The transfusion of packed erythrocytes to the patient with chronic anemia is to be contrasted with the need for rapid transfusion of whole blood to the patient with acute hemorrhage. Provided the cause of acute hemorrhage is corrected, the bone marrow will be adequate to maintain normal blood levels subsequently. In patients with chronic hemorrhagic disorders, completely normal levels of hemoglobin need not be attained with each transfusion if large amounts of blood are required to accomplish this end. A normally functioning bone marrow will eventually raise blood levels to desired values.

The hemoglobin value at which a transfusion is indicated in patients with anemias of the aplastic-hypoplastic group or with chronic hemolytic anemias, such as severe Mediterranean anemia (thalassemia major) and sickle cell anemia, cannot be arbitrarily fixed; rather, it varies with associated signs and symptoms of the individual patient. As a guide to management, patients with the aplastic-hypoplastic and chronic hemolytic anemias usually do not require transfusions until hemoglobin levels decrease to 7 to 7.5 gm. per 100 ml., at which point clinical symptoms usually appear. Whereas blood levels in children with the aplastic-hypoplastic anemias and in those with severe Mediterranean anemia (thalassemia major) tend to decline progressively unless treatment is given, the patient with sickle cell anemia reacts differently. In the latter the need for repeated transfusions is much less urgent because hemoglobin levels usually stabilize in a range between 6 and 7 gm. per 100 ml., without discomfort or interference with activities and regardless of treatment. Although these criteria find general application, the amounts of blood given and the intervals between transfusions require specialized study for each patient.

**Choice and dosage of whole blood, packed erythrocytes, and plasma.** Although the choice and dosage of whole blood, packed erythrocytes, and plasma are frequently clear-cut, they often depend upon the appraisal of factors other than the hemoglobin level and the erythrocyte count. Except for marked blood loss in which the whole blood is perfused, in almost all other situations in which a child with anemia requires transfusion, packed or sedimented red blood cells are employed. The use of packed cells permits restoration of hemoglobin levels with less volume. In addition, febrile or allergic transfusion reactions are significantly less frequent when packed cells are administered rather than whole blood. Finally, there is some evidence suggesting that the incidence of serum hepatitis[31] is significantly less following packed cell transfusions than following whole blood administration.

The volume of blood to be given depends upon the condition of the patient. Generally if there is no underlying or accompanying disease which could predispose to heart failure, 20 to 25 ml. per kilogram may be administered over 1 to 2 hours. The effects of transfusion on cardiovascular dynamics is much the same whether whole blood or packed cells are administered.

Whole blood, plasma, or a combination plays a part in the treatment of dehydration, diarrhea, or protein deficiency. The immunologic support represented by the transfer of circulating antibodies and gamma globulin in combating infection has been replaced by the use of antibiotics.

The precise hemoglobin levels at which a child requires transfusion depends upon a number of factors. A child who has iron deficiency anemia or anemia of prematurity but is otherwise healthy can tolerate hemoglobin levels as low as 5 to 6 gm./100 ml. Since fairly rapid elevation can be expected within a matter of weeks, transfusion of such patients is generally not recommended. Patients with sickle cell disease likewise tolerate lower levels of hemoglobin, and unless there is evidence of respiratory infection or aplastic crisis, transfusion is usually not required. An exception may be the presence of progressive nephritis. Patients with thalassemia major apparently do best if their hemoglobin level is maintained at 10 gm./100 ml. or above.

*Calculation of dosage of blood for simple transfusion.* Mollison[37] suggested a simplified method of calculating the amount of blood required for transfusion. The basic principle is that a hemoglobin concentration of 15 gm./100 ml. corresponds to a red cell volume of 30 ml./Kg. body weight. This constitutes a convenient proportion for the sake of calculation. It implies that a transfusion of 2 ml. of red cells per kilogram of body weight will raise the hemoglobin concentration by 1 gm./100 ml. Citrated blood as supplied by most transfusion services contains approximately one-third its volume of red cells. Thus 6 ml. (3 × 2 ml.) of citrated blood per Kg. of body weight are required to raise the hemoglobin concentration 1 gm./100 ml. For those who prefer to think in terms of pounds for body weight and percent for hemoglobin (100% Hgb. = 14.8 gm./100 ml.) the formula is: 4 ml. citrated blood per pound of body weight are required to raise the hemoglobin concentration by approximately 10%. To allow for nonviable cells, 4.5 ml. per pound will raise the hemoglobin 10%.

The expected change in hemoglobin following transfusion can be calculated as follows:
1. Multiply: Blood volume (70 ml./Kg.) × Hgb. (gm. %) = initial body hemoglobin in grams
2. Calculate grams of hemoglobin transfused (1 unit of packed cells = 60 gm. Hgb.)
3. Add transfused hemoglobin to initial hemoglobin = new total body hemoglobin
4. Divide initial blood volume by 100 into new hemoglobin levels

This equals the new hemoglobin level in gm. %.

In regulating the amounts of blood for transfusion, it should be remembered that citrated (ACD) blood usually has a hematocrit of 32 to 36% as compared with 40 to 50% for whole blood and 60 to 70% for packed erythrocytes, depending upon the amount of supernatant plasma removed in the latter.[37]

*Platelet transfusion.* Platelet transfusion has now reached a point where its effectiveness, particularly in situations where the bone marrow is aplastic or replaced with nonmyeloid elements, is very clear. Whereas fresh whole blood once was the only available means for replacing platelets, in recent years the introduction of plastic blood collection apparatus has made platelet-rich plasma or platelet concentrate available in most communities.

In general, platelets should be transfused to patients who are bleeding and in whom platelet counts are below 60,000/cu. mm. In some treatment centers all patients with platelet counts below 30,000/cu. mm. are given platelet transfusions; however, such a prophylactic approach cannot as yet be advocated. Unless there are other coexisting coagulation factor deficiencies which would require treatment with fresh frozen plasma, platelet transfusions are given in the form of platelet concentrate. Where feasible, the aim is to achieve a level of approximately 100,000 platelets/cu. mm. This can be achieved by the administration of 1 unit of platelet concentrate per 10 pounds of body weight.[2] When platelet-rich plasma is used, the same effect can be achieved with two-thirds the number of units. When infection or high fever is present, the amount necessary may have to be doubled. While it may be desirable to achieve levels of 100,000/cu. mm., experience indicates that smaller transfusions which do not achieve significant elevation of platelet count may produce hemostasis. Because platelets contain specific antigen components akin to blood group factors, patients who receive numerous platelet transfusions may become immunized to platelet group other than their own.

In such circumstances platelets may have to be cross-matched. Aside from these rare occurrences, when platelet concentrates are given, A-B-O blood group may be ignored, and the same is true for Rh type. Occasionally, Rh-negative recipients become immunized to the Rh factor because of the small number of Rh-positive erythrocytes present in platelet concentrates prepared from Rh-positive donors.

Platelets generally survive 1 to 3 days following transfusion, and the platelet count falls by about 50% each 24 hours following transfusion. It must be emphasized that platelet transfusion is recommended primarily for patients in whom the thrombocytopenia has resulted from inadequate production. Survival of platelets in patients with ITP or hypersplenism is usually less than 8 hours. In these conditions platelet transfusion is rarely indicated.

At present platelets, prepared in a refrigerated centrifuge and maintained at 2 to 6° C., should be transfused within 6 hours after collection. Evidence has accumulated recently suggesting that preparation and storage of platelets at 20° C. may yield an equal degree of viability for up to 96 hours.[39] Standard refrigerated storage at 4° C. resulted in a marked shortening of the life-span of platelets labeled with $^{51}$Cr and reinfused into the original donor. Storage at ambient room temperature (22° C.) preserved a normal platelet life-span.

With availability of platelet concentrations, there is a lesser need for other sources of platelets such as platelet-rich plasma. Rarely, fresh platelet-rich plasma collected in plastic bags and administered directly after bleeding may be employed in lieu of platelet concentrates, but the plasma must be group compatible. Blood platelets drawn in this manner have a survival span of approximately 4 to 6 days. In normal subjects platelet survival measures 8 to 11 days. (See Chapter 26.) Occasionally platelet-rich blood from a polycythemic donor has been given by direct transfusion through silicone-coated syringes, thus providing for intact platelets and red blood cells.[52]

The infusion of platelet concentrates prepared as a by-product of ordinary blood banking by means of the plastic-bag system increased the number of circulating platelets in thrombocytopenic patients. The greatest increase usually occurred within 2 hours of infusion. Even with large infusions, the increased platelet count rarely persisted for more than 24 hours.[19] The degree of elevation of platelet counts tended to vary in direct relation to the amount of platelets infused. The increase in platelet levels was smaller than could have been expected on the basis of the number of platelets infused. The occurrence of hemostasis in the absence of sustained elevation of the platelet count is occasionally due to an immediate utilization of the infused platelets. Although the survival of transfused platelets may be reduced on repeated administration, it appears that when the recipients are ill, the survival of platelets is shorter than the theoretic span of their viability. This is probably due to rapid utilization. The undesirable effect of possible antibodies to platelets may be overcome by increasing the dose of platelets in subsequent transfusions.

Adrenocorticotropic hormone (ACTH) and steroids (prednisone, prednisolone, and hydrocortisone) given intravenously also serve as valuable hemostatic agents. This form of therapy is especially indicated in patients with idiopathic thrombocytopenic purpura in the active state, in patients being prepared for splenectomy, and also in controlling hemorrhage in patients with secondary thrombopenic states.

Two isotopic methods using $DF^{32}P$ (di-isopropylfluorophosphate) and $^{51}Cr$, respectively, have been employed in the measurement of platelet life-span. In normal subjects the platelet life-span with the former method is 8 to 9 days;[33] with the latter, the mean life-span in vitro is in the order of 8 to 11 days.[5a] As a general rule, in disease, the platelet life-span is reduced to 4 to 5 days, and with repeated transfusions it may be progressively shortened. Clinically, however, repeated transfusions of platelets often do not result in a decreased life-span since hemostasis appears to be adequately controlled with each administration.

When transfused into normal human subjects, $^{51}Cr$-labeled platelets behave according to a specific pattern.[16] A large proportion of the infused platelets disappear from the bloodstream within 30 minutes and a varying proportion of these returns to the circulation within 24 hours. After return, their subsequent survival is of the order of 8 to 10 days in most subjects. The early disappearance followed by a partial return to the circulation is termed "segregation." There is a temporary adhesion of the infused platelets to vascular endothelium throughout the body, particularly to the rich vascular beds of the liver and lungs. Subsequently they return to the circulation from these sites and from marginated and extravascular platelet reserves.

A prospective controlled study of the frequency of hepatitis following transfusion of commercial pooled plasma stored for at least 6 months in a liquid state at 30 to 32° C. was performed using 5% albumin as a control solution.[44] Twelve of 120 plasma recipients developed hepatitis. Fifty percent of the hepatitis cases were icteric. It has been further recommended that the use of whole, pooled plasma be discouraged and even discontinued unless a clear-cut case can be made for its unique requirements.[14] In addition to the danger of hepatitis, some pools have dangerous levels of anti-A and anti-B even after storage at room temperature for long periods. To avoid the complication of hepatitis, the need for giving a single transfusion has been questioned.

The dosages listed on p. 92 serve as guides for the amount of blood and plasma to be given in a single transfusion. In the case of whole blood and packed erythrocytes the values are calculated to elevate hemoglobin concentration and erythrocyte count in varying degree, depending upon the severity of the anemia but within safe limits of blood volume.

With increasing weight and expanding blood volume, these figures lose their significance, and other criteria are substituted, depending upon the objectives of therapy, such as hemoglobin elevation, cessation of hemorrhage, and clinical improvement. It should be obvious that the older child with chronic anemia who, at irregular periods, receives a single transfusion of 500 ml. of whole blood and lesser amounts of packed erythrocytes cannot be expected to show a significant rise in hemoglobin. The amount of blood is necessarily diluted in a higher blood volume than it is in the smaller child to whom similar amounts may be given. Hence, in determining the rate of survival of donor blood, several transfusions are necessary within a short period of time to raise blood values to normal levels from which the rate of decline may be estimated.

The preoperative transfusion of children with mild anemia has fallen into disrepute. The general anesthesia may be given with safety to most patients whose hemoglobin exceeds 9.5 gm. per 100 ml.[18]

Patients with cyanotic heart disease represent a unique transfusion problem. Their compensatory polycythemia is necessary to provide adequate tissue oxygenation, and in the face of normal or just slightly subnormal hemoglobin levels these patients may suffer cardiorespiratory embarrassment. The indication for transfusion of such children can be best determined by a cardiologist.

In the conduct of an outpatient transfusion clinic for children with chronic anemias—usually thalassemia major, pure red cell anemia, and aplastic anemia—transfusions are given every 2 to 4 weeks. In general, a hemoglobin of 7 to 8 gm. per 100 ml. is an indication for a transfusion. Only packed cells are used for the chronic anemias. Small children are given 10 ml. per kilogram initially, and this may be increased to 12 to 13 ml. per kilogram in order to achieve a transfusion interval of 3 to 4 weeks. The maximum amount given to any patient, regardless of size, is 250 ml. (one unit of packed cells). The patient remains in the clinic until 30 minutes after the transfusion, at which time his temperature is taken and any medication given, if necessary, for fever, chills, or hives (Table 7).

Initially, no premedication is given. If a patient shows evidences of frequent febrile reactions during or after transfusion, he is given aspirin as premedication. If, in spite of this treatment, he continues to develop fever, he will also be given an antihistamine or a steroid for persistent and severe reactions. If a patient develops a reaction during a transfusion, the transfusion is stopped, and the patient is given aspirin or an antihistamine (Adrenalin is kept on hand for emergencies).

**Leukocyte transfusion.** Leukocyte concentrates have been transfused into leukopenic patients with sepsis.[25,49] Unless obtained by plasmapheresis from patients with high count chronic myelogenous leukemia, the concentrates prepared from up to thirty normal blood donations would be used in treating a large child. Recently a leukopheresis apparatus has been introduced.

Febrile, respiratory, and dermatologic reactions to leukocyte transfusions occur. In one series,[49] patients with severe neutropenia received blood from patients with chronic myeloid leukemia. In 50% of the cases the transfusions were followed by disappearance of fever and associated signs of infection and a rise in leukocyte count which was dependent on the establishment of a graft by the transfused cells. The demonstration in the blood of cells carrying the Philadelphia chromosome gave proof of the establishment of a graft by the transfused cells. Usually white cell elevations from leukocyte concentrates are barely detectable, and clinical results are so variable that it is not possible to recommend white cell transfusions at this time.

**Transfusions in premature infants.** In most clinics a conservative policy is followed with regard to transfusions in the healthy premature infant. At the age of 4 to 7 weeks, when the

Table 7. Recommended dosages of aspirin, antihistamine, and prednisone for allergic reactions to multiple transfusions[5]

| | |
|---|---|
| Aspirin | |
| Up to 5 years | 1 grain (60 mg.) per year |
| 5 to 10 years | 10 grains |
| Tripelennamine (Pyribenzamine)* | |
| Up to 5 years | 25 mg. |
| 5 years and over | 25 to 50 mg. |
| Prednisone | 5 to 10 mg. given ½ to 1 hour before transfusion, if previous experience demonstrated difficulties with other medications |

*Other antihistamines may be substituted for Pyribenzamine.

infant's fetal and adult hemoglobin values have decreased to low levels, spontaneous recovery usually begins with the predominant synthesis of the adult type.[48] Administration of transfusions at a time when normal regeneration of hemoglobin is at hand seems unnecessary. Besides the known complications, to give transfusions at this point is to run the risk of depressing inherent bone marrow function.[4,48]

The present trend, as disclosed in a survey,[26] is to give transfusions to only those premature infants whose hemoglobin values have decreased to between 6 and 9 gm. per 100 ml. Our own practice has been to transfuse only those whose hemoglobin concentrations persist at levels of approximately 7 to 8 gm. per 100 ml. in the absence of significant reticulocytosis. Transfusion is employed when there are evidences of infection, anorexia, listlessness, and failure to gain weight. We have found that premature infants rarely need transfusions on the basis of anemia alone. When transfusions are required, either packed erythrocytes or whole blood is given in amounts not to exceed 10 ml. per kilogram of body weight.

**Limitations and hazards of transfusions.** Increased experience and investigation of untoward reactions have provided a greater measure of safety in the administration of transfusions. Of the limitations and hazards included in the following list, the most common are reactions to nonerythroid cellular blood elements and perhaps plasma proteins, serum hepatitis, and circulatory overload.

I. Hemolytic transfusion reactions
  A. Incompatible blood
  B. Intradonor incompatibility in multiple transfusion
II. Nonhemolytic transfusion reactions
  A. Leukocyte or platelet antibodies
  B. Plasma protein antibodies (anti-IgA, anti-Gm, etc.)
III. Transmission of infection
  A. Bacterial contamination
  B. Homologous serum hepatitis
  C. Malaria
  D. Syphilis
  E. EB virus (posttransfusion pseudomononucleosis)
IV. Circulatory overload
V. Suppression of erythropoiesis
VI. Excessive iron deposition
  A. Hemosiderosis
  B. Exogenous hemochromatosis
VII. Antibody formation
VIII. Allergic reactions
IX. Massive transfusion—extracorporeal circulation
X. Air embolism
XI. Electrolyte disturbances
  A. Hyperkalemia
  B. "Citrate intoxication"

*Hemolytic transfusion reactions—rare.* Better methods of crossmatching and routine examination of the prospective recipient's serum for atypical antibodies have made hemolytic transfusion reactions rare. When a hemolytic transfusion reaction occurs, the overwhelming probability is that it has resulted from an error in labeling, or the use of the wrong patient or donor sample for the crossmatch, or the careless administration of a correctly labeled unit of blood to the wrong patient. The mortality from an incompatible transfusion reaction increases with the volume of blood administered. Since most hemolytic reactions cause fever, chills, headache, and backache, and since these signs frequently appear early in the course of the transfusion, careful observation of each patient during the administration of the first 50 ml. of blood is strongly recommended. When a hemolytic transfusion reaction is suspected, the transfusion is stopped, and the blood container plus a freshly drawn specimen from the patient are sent to the blood bank. In patients who have a disease requiring frequent transfusions, fever, hives, and headache are frequently observed. In such instances it may be impossible to distinguish these "allergic" reactions from a hemolytic reaction. When any doubt exists, treatment should be based on the possibility that hemolysis has occurred. When a significant amount of incompatible blood has been administered (over 5 ml./Kg.), shock may develop, requiring supportive measures, including the administration of compatible blood as well as 5% albumin or electrolyte solutions. When evidence of hemoglobinemia is present, and this can quickly be determined by examination of the plasma in a centrifuged capillary pipette, therapy designed to prevent renal shutdown should be instituted immediately.

In a suspected hemolytic transfusion reaction the following features should be looked for:[17] free hemoglobin in plasma (visible if over 50 mg./100 ml.), bilirubinemia, urinary pigments, hemoglobinuria, methemalbuminemia (Schumm's test, see p. 293), reduced haptoglobin levels, and agglutination of the red cells from donor by serum of patient's blood drawn before transfusion. The transfused blood should also be examined for bacteria.

Twenty percent mannitol, (0.2 gm./Kg.) is given intravenously over 3 to 5 minutes. Careful observation of urinary flow during the next hour will determine whether additional mannitol is necessary. If urinary flow is maintained at 1 ml./Kg. per hour, renal shutdown will not occur. As a result of the routine use of mannitol, total anuria resulting from hemolytic transfusion reactions has been almost completely eliminated. When a substantial amount of intravascular hemolysis occurs, there are released into the circulation phospholipids which are capable of instituting intravascular coagulation. When this occurs a generalized hemorrhagic state may supervene. In such instances coagulation studies may reveal low levels of fibrinogen, prothrombin, factor V, and factor VIII, along with moderate to severe thrombocytopenia. Until recently, replacement therapy with fibrinogen and fresh frozen plasma was considered correct therapy. At present, there seems to be good reason for treating these patients with intravenous heparin, 100 units/Kg. every 4 hours, in addition to platelet-rich plasma, 20 ml./Kg. The defibrination is usually of fairly short duration, and with vigorous therapy, death from hemorrhage is rare.

*Nonhemolytic transfusion reactions.* The most frequent type of reaction to transfusion is the development of fever, often accompanied by urticaria. This type of reaction, previously referred to as a "nonspecific" or "allergic" reaction, now appears to be the result of immunization of the recipient to a platelet or leukocyte antigen in the donor blood. Much less frequently these reactions have been ascribed to plasma proteins, particularly the immunoglobulin IgA. While symptomatic therapy with salicylates and antihistamines has been used with some success, recent experience with the use of frozen blood or washed packed red cells indicates that this type of transfusion reaction can be almost completely eliminated.

Untoward signs and symptoms may be unrelated to mismatching of blood but due to causes inherent in the disease for which transfusions are given. In thalassemia, for instance, certain children react constantly with hives and chills during transfusions for reasons that cannot be ascertained. The possibility that frequent blood transfusions may lead to the formation of leukoagglutinins responsible for reactions has led to the recommendation that in such cases blood rendered leukocyte-poor be employed.[11,12,27] A child with the hemolytic-uremic syndrome who, on three occasions, sustained severe transfusion reactions with whole blood or packed cells had no difficulties when washed red cells were substituted. A strict correlation between the presence of leukoagglutinins and the occurrence of transfusion reactions cannot, however, always be demonstrated.[30]

*Transmission of infection.* Hepatitis, syphilis, brucellosis, and cytomegalovirus infection may be transmitted by blood transfusion.[9] Significant bacterial contamination of a unit of blood is a very rare event, inasmuch as these instances often result in a fatality. The transmission of malaria is frequent in endemic areas, and Americans or Europeans returning from these areas are usually proscribed from donating blood except for fractionation.

The spirochete which causes syphilis rarely survives refrigeration, and syphilis transmitted by transfusion is rare. Since spirochetemia often occurs before a positive STS develops, preparation of fresh components such as platelet concentrate may result in transmission of this disease.

Lastly, there has been observed in a significant number of patients who underwent surgical procedures, particularly associated with extracorporeal circulation, and infectious mononucleosis-like syndrome. The possibility that that this may be the result of blood-transmitted infection with cytomegalovirus or the virus associated with Burkitt's lymphoma (EB virus) is presently under consideration.

The most frustrating disorder resulting from transfusion is homologous serum hepatitis. The use of gamma globulin following transfusion to prevent hepatitis received support from a large study by Mirick and associates.[36] They had concluded that the administration of 10 ml. of gamma globulin in the week after blood transfusion and again 1 month later will prevent three-fourths of the cases of icteric posttransfusion hepatitis. Not only is there insufficient gamma globulin available to permit its routine use in the prophylaxis of posttransfusion hepatitis, but some uncertainties exist about the significance of results with this procedure.

Recently the point of view in connection

with hepatitis has changed with evidence that it may be possible to determine the carrier of hepatitis.

Blumberg and his associates[9] detected an antibody in the serum of a transfused hemophilia patient which was clearly different from the lipoprotein precipitins previously found in patients who had received multiple transfusions. The antigen was given the geographic name "Australia antigen" (Au). The Australia antigen (Au) can be readily identified by two well-known laboratory tests: immunodiffusion and complement fixation.[43] Subsequent studies showed the antigen to be extremely rare in the American population. Of interest is its presence in approximately 10% of patients with leukemia. The total absence of the Australia antigen suggests that the presence of the antigen may be of value in the diagnosis of acute leukemia. Changes in red blood cell antigens during the course of leukemia lend indirect support to the hypothesis that the Australia antigen results from rather than precedes the leukemia process, since alterations in ABO specificities have been demonstrated during the course of leukemia.[8,45] Subsequently it became apparent that the Australia antigen (Au) was associated with serum hepatitis (SH) but not viral hepatitis. Blumberg and co-workers[10] then tested the sera of 125 patients who either had or were suspected of having viral hepatitis; of these 20% were positive for Australia antigen (Au). Prince,[43,44] who had assisted with the isolation of Australia antigen (Au) reported an antigen (SH) that was found in the blood of patients with serum hepatitis during the incubation period of the disease. He later identified this antigen as Australia antigen (Au). It seems possible that the presence of Australia antigen (Au) in the serum of an individual identifies that person as a hepatitis carrier and possibly this antigen represents the infectious agent.[10]

It later[32] became clear that the Australia antigen or hepatitis-associated antigen (HAA) and antibody (anti-HAA) were consistently present in serum specimens from patients with MS-2 strain of serum hepatitis (SH) and were not present in MS-1, infectious hepatitis (IH). Hepatitis-associated antigen was detected earlier after a parenteral exposure to SH than after an oral exposure. Antigen appeared 2 weeks to 2 months before the onset of jaundice; it was transient in 65% of patients, but persisted for 4 months to 13 years in 35% of children. The average incubation period of IH (MS-1) was essentially the same following an oral or parenteral exposure (32 to 33 days); in SH (MS-2) it was 65 days after parenteral exposure and 98 days after oral exposure. Gamma globulin consistently neutralized the infectivity of IH (MS-1) serum; in most cases it did not neutralize the infectivity of SH (MS-2) serum.

A study by Embil and associates[23] of cytomegalovirus infection before and after extracorporeal circulation during heart surgery suggested that the infection was acquired during or soon after the operation. The source of infection is not known, but the evidence presented suggested that cytomegalovirus may be transmitted in transfused blood. The reported incidence in children and adults ranges from 3 to 11% of patients perfused during surgery.

*Circulatory overload.* The administration of excessively large quantities of blood or even smaller amounts if given rapidly may precipitate cardiac failure from circulatory overload. In the course of a transfusion or shortly thereafter, precordial pain, dyspnea, cyanosis, and a dry cough are indicative of a rising venous pressure and pulmonary edema. In patients with severe anemia and evidences of congestive heart failure, preliminary digitalization may occasionally be required. Packed or sedimented red cell suspensions are useful whenever it is essential to provide blood with the least possible disturbance to the patient's blood volume. Another expedient to prevent overloading the circulatory system is to give one-half the calculated amount of blood on successive days.

In erythroblastosis death may result from cardiac failure caused by administering more blood than has been removed. Preliminary withdrawal of 30 to 50 ml. of blood from the severely anemic infant may be necessary,[37] or a deficit of even larger amounts (40 to 80 ml.) should be established within a short time after beginning the exchange when venous pressures are excessively high.[1]

*Transfusions and suppression of blood production.* One of the limitations of transfusion that deserves comment and that has as yet received scant attention is its potential depressant effects upon endogenous erythropoiesis and hemoglobin synthesis. That transfusions possess this secondary inhibitory effect was recognized in the treatment of pernicious anemia before the advent of specific therapy and has been confirmed more recently in several studies.[6,15,24,46] Although retardation of hematopoiesis, in minor degree, may accompany a single transfusion, it is overshadowed by the major corrective effects. In the case of multiple transfusions, however, this limiting influence may explain the failure of transfusion to produce an anticipated rise in hemoglobin and erythrocytes in the absence of hemolysis or hemorrhage.

Two sets of observations[50,51] document the thesis that transfusions administered at frequent intervals retard hemoglobin and erythrocyte formation. These data are based on an intensive study of a small group of children with severe Mediterranean anemia (thalassemia major) in whom transfusions could be interrupted following splenectomy. By the methods designed to permit quantitative differentiation between donor and recipient blood and by serial examinations of the total erythrocyte mass and circulating hemoglobin, it was possible to demonstrate that a retarding effect occurred that was most marked from the first to the third week following transfusion. Not until donor blood had been entirely eliminated from the circulation were pretransfusion blood levels restored in the patient. The depressant effect of transfusion was further substantiated by another means. In patients with severe Mediterranean anemia (thalassemia major), the presence of large amounts of fetal hemoglobin provides a biologic tag of endogenous hemoglobin synthesis. Transfusions resulted in a depression of this component which increased sharply as donor cells left the circulation. The diminution in circulating fetal hemoglobin persisted in one patient for the first 7 weeks after transfusion, and in two others the decrease amounted to 50%. Paralleling these observations is a recent report[20] that, in patients with sickle cell anemia who received multiple transfusions, a period of maximum depression of erythropoiesis occurred from the twelfth to the twenty-fifth day, with the percentage of sickle cells decreasing from 100 to 5%. It is therefore advisable to withhold treatment occasionally in patients with chronic anemia to determine innate bone marrow function. In critical periods of growth, such as in the anemia of prematurity, it may be undesirable to interfere with bone marrow function by transfusions. In patients with erythroblastosis it has been suggested[13] that a similar retardation can result from a persistent effort to maintain normal blood levels. These studies suggest the need for a less empirical and more individualized orientation, not only in patients with refractory anemias but also in those with other disease conditions requiring frequent transfusions. The spacing and size of transfusions and blood levels to be attained require constant reexamination and appraisal.

*Transfusions and hemosiderosis.* Studies in iron metabolism have extended into an investigation of "iron overload" or hemosiderosis resulting from repeated transfusions. The total amount of iron in a normal adult approximately 4 to 5 gm., of which 15 to 20% represents the iron reserve stored principally in the liver as ferritin and hemosiderin. In children, storage iron normally represents 8.5 to 10.5 mg. per kilogram of body weight. In states of iron deficiency in infancy, due to inadequate diet and periods of rapid growth, storage depots are taxed and may be depleted. Iron otherwise accumulates and, except for the normal excretion of approximately 1 mg. daily, cannot leave the body except by bleeding. From the list on p. 89 it is apparent that excessive amounts of iron from destroyed erythrocytes become available for storage in patients receiving multiple transfusions (250 mg. of iron in 500 ml. of blood). Under such conditions hemosiderin deposits in normal storage depots increase greatly, and, in addition, accessory sites assume the function of iron storage. Hemosiderosis refers to increased iron stores without tissue damage; hemochromatosis, to the development of tissue damage in persons with prolonged iron excess (Chapter 12). The amount of iron present in organs such as the liver may exceed the amount given by repeated transfusions, indicating excessive absorption of iron from the gastrointestinal tract.[22]

Whether iron from transfused blood actually may produce hemochromatosis is still controversial, but there is evidence that excessive iron storage is potentially injurious.[21] It must be understood that no unequivocal statement can be made as yet to the extent or manner in which tissue siderosis is harmful. Studies in severe Cooley's anemia[22] (thalassemia major) have shown, however, that hemosiderosis and fibrosis frequently coexist although there was no uniformity about the progression.

The development of true hepatic cirrhosis and fibrosis of the pancreas that characterizes hemochromatosis asociated with transfusion hemosiderosis may depend upon the intervention of accessory factors such as continued hypoxia in addition to large iron deposits. Whether iron deposits alone are responsible for the hepatic damage in hemochromatosis is still debatable, but that it is a prerequisite for this pathologic process is more likely.

From these considerations it would seem that the iron derived from an occasional transfusion is harmless. A contrary situation may prevail, however, in the patient receiving multiple transfusions over long periods of time. In view of the risk involved, the most prudent course is to restrict the number of transfusions to the minimum compatible with comfort and moderate activity.

*Antibody formation in the course of multiple transfusions.* Patients who receive large numbers of transfusions for anemia and other causes may develop precipitins in their blood. These precipitins may react in agar gel—double diffusion experiments with specific human serum lipoproteins found in the blood of other individuals. These antibodies have been regarded as antibodies against serum lipoprotein which develop as a result of repeated transfusions. This antilipoprotein isoprecipitin was found in approximately 30% of forty-seven patients with thalassemia who had received transfusions.[7] In the thalassemia group the frequency of antibodies against lipoproteins (29.8%) parallels the frequency of antiwhite blood cell (37%) and antiplatelet antibodies (32.6%), but is considerably greater than that of antierythrocytic antibody (12.8%).

*Allergic reactions.* It has been estimated that about 1 to 5% of blood transfusions are followed by allergic reactions, principally urticaria and, less often, angioneurotic edema and asthma. These reactions are especially frequent in children with refractory anemias requiring multiple transfusions. In our experience such children benefit from oral premedication of an antihistamine and aspirin given 30 minutes before transfusion. Prednisone has been useful in children with a tendency toward hemolytic reactions and in those in whom other medications have proved ineffective in preventing severe febrile and allergic reactions.

Recommended dosages of aspirin, antihistamine, and prednisone for allergic reactions to multiple transfusions are listed in Table 7.

*Massive transfusion.* The administration of large quantities of blood which have been stored for more than a week may result in a decrease in platelet levels or a decrease of the labile coagulation factors. While not a frequent problem, it is well to evaluate the circulating level of these factors in any patient receiving massive transfusion of bank blood. Following extracorporeal circulation using large amounts of nonautologous blood, unexpected decreases in blood volume have been observed. The etiology of this "homologous blood syndrome" is poorly understood.

*Air embolism.* The use of plastic blood containers has almost totally eliminated the possibility of air embolism. Whenever blood or other fluid is being administered under pressure, it is important to normalize the pressure before the bag is completely empty.

*Electrolyte disturbances.* In blood stored under refrigeration the potassium content of red cells decreases and that of the plasma increases, both factors being intensified during prolonged storage. Marked electrocardiographic changes do not occur until the potassium level reaches approximately 8 mEq. per liter.[37] Hyperkalemia induced in patients during exchange transfusions is transient, but the potential risk of toxic effects should be kept in mind. The latter can be minimized by the use of relatively fresh blood, the removal of part of the plasma, and the judicious use of calcium during replacement transfusions with citrated whole blood.[35]

Blood storage and preservation with acid-citrate-dextrose (ACD) solutions are associated with a chemical lesion of the red cell, characterized by interference with intracellular production of organic high-energy phosphates and the accumulation of inorganic phosphate salts.[28] Red cells lose their viability on storage at 5° C., so that only 70% are viable on the twenty-first day.[8] During this period there is also a substantial flow of intracellular potassium from the red cells into the plasma, and a reverse flow takes place for sodium. Thus, potassium rises in the plasma from 7 mEq. per liter on the first day, and sodium decreases from 160 to 153 mEq. per liter in the same period. These changes are accompanied by decreased intracellular potassium and increased sodium, respectively. Patients with heart disease, especially those on digitalis, patients with kidney disease already hyperkalemic, and newborn infants are in situations in which the excess potassium in citrated blood may be harmful. The use of packed cells affords a simple means of avoiding additions to the patient's hyperkalemia.[28] This problem can be obviated by transfusing packed cells alone or resuspended in saline, 5% albumin, or fresh frozen plasma. Whether there is a significant disturbance in electrolyte balance as a result of the rapid administration of ACD blood is a matter of conjecture. Clearly, exchange transfusion of a sick newborn with ACD blood may increase the acidosis usually present in such infants. However, the effect of ACD blood is relatively short-lived, and the need for addition of sodium bicarbonate or THAM (tris-buffer) is not clear.

**Transfusion therapy in hemorrhagic disorders.** The intensive investigations of the hemorrhagic disorders have led to a clear definition of the role of established and newly discovered factors in maintaining hemostasis. With the application of specialized procedures, defects heretofore unknown have been described and appropriate treatment advised. These will be discussed under hemorrhagic diseases in Chapter 26. In general, the patients with hemorrhagic disorders will benefit from fresh whole blood, fresh frozen plasma, or specific blood components until the specific defect is determined.

**Intraperitoneal transfusion.** The recent demonstration of successful intraperitoneal transfusions in the fetus with erythroblastosis fetalis (p. 166) reawakened interest in the possibilities of this technique in infants and children. Prior to the use of superficial veins, intraperitoneal transfusions were common in pediatric practice. In infants with open fontanelles the superior sagittal sinus was also utilized. Despite the perfection of current techniques of blood transfusion, situations arise in which superficial veins are no longer accessible and extensive cutdowns are required. Under these circumstances, especially when transfusions are repeated as in the infant with Cooley's anemia, intraperitoneal transfusions have been successfully performed and advocated as an alternate technique.[40,54] Absorption of blood is more rapid than expected. In one case of Cooley's anemia in an infant 14 months of age, the hemoglobin rose by 22% by the third day, with comparable results on subsequent occasions.[40] In a child with thalassemia major weighing 18 kg. the injection of a small amount of $^{51}$Cr-labeled red cells was followed by an intraperitoneal transfusion of 350 ml. of blood. A lag of 24 hours was noted before any labeled red cells appeared in the circulation, but by the fourth day after transfusion more than 50% were labeled. The rate of increase in hemoglobin concentration agreed well with the rate of labeled cells in the circulation. Despite the reported efficiency and safety of intraperitoneal transfusion, the use of superficial veins should be a primary objective. Conceivably, infection and respiratory embarrassment are possibilities when blood is injected into the peritoneum.[37]

**Notes on technique and preservation of blood.** When siliconized equipment is available, its use is desirable for collection and administration of blood. A 20-gauge by 1-inch needle with a short sharp bevel is used in transfusion of patients in any age group.

In young children who require multiple transfusions, such as those with leukemia or aplastic anemia, suitable superficial veins often eventually become inaccessible or thrombosed. To avoid a cutdown that may be accompanied by persistent oozing, whole blood or plasma can be transfused into the proximal end of the tibia several inches below the tubercles. An appropriate bone marrow needle, usually 18 guage by 1 inch, is inserted into the marrow as for aspiration, and the distal plastic tip of the administration set is placed directly into the marrow needle. The flow is regulated as for intravenous administration, with the plastic bag suspended at a level permitting flow by gravity. Because of the danger of infection, it should be emphasized that this method of administering blood is used only as a last resort.

Acid-citrate-dextrose solution (ACD) is now generally used as an anticoagulant. The inclusion of dextrose in the preservation of blood slows the fall of adenosine triphosphate (ATP), which is involved in the energy-producing mechanism of the red cell and permits it longer survival by maintaining red cell integrity.[53]

During blood storage the leukocytes quickly disintegrate and lose their phagocytic power. The platelets disappear in about 4 days, antihemophilic globulin is progressively decreased[41] (in some instances as much as 10% in the first week and approximately 50% of the initial antihemophilic globulin after 3 weeks' storage), and the prothrombin time is prolonged due to the loss of factor V. The use of plastic bags retards the destruction of platelets. Platelet-rich plasma obtained by this means has become increasingly popular in the treatment of serious bleeding in patients with thrombocytopenic purpura and leukemia.

*Blood preservation.* Maintenance of viability of the red cells in a unit of blood is dependent upon the anticoagulant used, the storage temperature, and the addition of metabolically active constituents to the anticoagulant solution.

The anticoagulant most in use is acid-citrate-dextrose (ACD). Recently, the use of a citrate-phosphate-dextrose solution (CPD) has been approved. The anticoagulant has a higher pH than ACD, and although use within 21 days is recommended, a number of studies have indicated that CPD maintains viability of 70% of the red cells for at least 4 weeks.

Blood may be anticoagulated with heparin; however, this blood must be used within 48 hours because the anticoagulant effect decreases after that time and because there is no glucose added to maintain red cell metabolism. Heparin has been recommended for exchange transfusion in the neonatal period, and for extracorporeal circulation. There are, however, few data to support the contention that heparin is superior to ACD in these situations.

In recent years a number of techniques for freezing red cells have been described. Most of the methods currently in use depend upon the addition of glycerol, which enters the red cells and prevents the formation of ice crystals which would damage the cells. The technique for freezing is relatively simple. At the New York Blood Center, packed red cells are suspended in a glycerol mannitol-saline solution, which results in a 14% glycerol concentration. This mixture is transferred to 500 ml. stainless steel containers, and the blood is frozen in 2 to 3 minutes by immersion in liquid nitrogen at −196° C. When needed for use the cells are thawed rapidly by agitation in a 42° C. water bath. The blood must then be deglycerolized by washing the cells first with mannitol and then twice with saline. The washed cells may be transfused as packed cells, or resuspended in fresh frozen plasma, 5% albumin, or saline. Red cells frozen and stored below −80° C. maintain viability for at least 3 years. The major uses for frozen blood at present include storage of rare blood, storage of autologous blood for autotransfusion, and, because thawed frozen blood is washed thoroughly, for reducing the incidence of febrile transfusion reactions due to platelet or leukocyte antibodies. At The New York Hospital, in a group of children with Cooley's anemia, all of whom had experienced frequent febrile reactions to packed cell transfusions, the use of frozen blood completely eliminated these reactions in over 300 consecutive transfusions.[29,47]

Lastly, it has been observed that the incidence of serum hepatitis following transfusion of frozen blood is exceedingly low, perhaps because the viral particles are removed during the cell washing.

*Transfusion techniques.* The availability of thin-walled scalp vein sets has considerably eased the technical problems associated with starting and maintaining transfusions, particularly in young infants. Although at first limited to scalp vein injections, the fact that the needle and the syringe attachment lid are separated by a length of plastic tubing makes the problems encountered in uncooperative patients much easier to handle. Antecubital veins, scalp veins, and hand veins are all frequently available. When these veins are not available, the external jugular vein is an excellent site. The use of a No. 19 gauge scalp vein needle inserted into an external jugular vein facilitates outpatient transfusion of packed cells in periods of less than 2 hours. Intraperitoneal transfusions and intra-tibial transfusions are still occasionally used, but they are no longer regarded as methods of choice.

## REFERENCES

1. Allen, F. H., Jr., and Diamond, L. K.: Erythroblastosis fetalis including exchange transfusion technic, Boston, 1957, 1958, Little, Brown & Co.
2. Alvarado, J., Djerassi, I., and Farber, S.: Transfusion of fresh, concentrated platelets to children with acute leukemia, J. Pediat. 67: 13, 1965.
3. American Association of Blood Banks: Technical methods and procedures of the American Association of Blood Banks, rev. ed., Chicago, 1960, American Association of Blood Banks.
4. Arthurton, M., O'Brien, D., and Mann, T.: Haemoglobin levels in premature infants, Arch. Dis. Child. 29:38, 1954.
5. Baker, R. J., Moinichen, S. L., and Nyhus, L. M.: Transfusion reaction; a reappraisal of surgical incidence and significance, Ann. Surg. 169:684, 1969.
5a. Baldini, M., Costea, N., and Dameshek, W.: The viability of stored human platelets, Blood 16:1669, 1960.
6. Birkhill, F. R., Maloney, M. A., and Levenson, S. M.: Effect of transfusion polycythemia upon bone marrow activity and erythrocyte survival in man, Blood 6:1021, 1951.
7. Blumberg, B. S., Alter, H. J., Riddell, N. M., and Erlandson, M.: Multiple antigenic specificities of serum lipoproteins detected with sera of transfused patients, Vox Sang. 9:128, 1964.

8. Blumberg, B. S., Alter, H. J., and Visnich, S.: A "new" antigen in leukemia sera, J.A.M.A. **191**:541, 1965.
9. Blumberg, B. S., Sutnick, A. I., and London, W. T.: Hepatitis and leukemia; their relation of Australian antigen, Bull. N. Y. Acad. Med. **44**:1366, 1968.
10. Blumberg, B. S., Sutnick, A. I., and London, W. T.: Australian antigen as a hepatitis virus; variation in host response, Amer. J. Med. **48**:1, 1970.
11. Bridges, J. M., Boyd, D. A., and Nelson, M. G.: Leucocyte antibodies with transfusion reactions, Lancet **2**:223, 1962.
12. Brittingham, T. E., and Chaplin, H., Jr.: Febrile transfusion reaction caused by sensitivity to donor leukocytes and platelets, J.A.M.A. **165**:819, 1957.
13. Cathie, I. A. B.: The treatment of erythroblastosis fetalis, Arch. Dis. Child. **21**:229, 1946.
14. Committee on Plasma and Plasma Substitutes of the Division of Medical Sciences, National Research Council: Editorial—Statement on normal (whole, pooled) human plasma, Transfusion **8**:52, 1968.
15. Dacie, J. V.: Transfusion of saline-washed red cells in nocturnal haemoglobinuria (Marchiafava-Micheli disease), Clin. Sci. **7**:65, 1948.
16. Davey, M. G., and Lander, H.: The behavior of infused human platelets during the first twenty-four hours after infusion, Brit. J. Haemat. **10**:94, 1964.
17. Davidsohn, I., and Stern, K.: Diagnosis of hemolytic transfusion reactions, Amer. J. Clin. Path. **25**:381, 1955.
18. Dietrich, E. B.: Evaluation of blood transfusion therapy, Transfusion **5**:82, 1965.
19. Djerassi, I., Farber, S., and Evans, A. E.: Transfusions of fresh platelet concentrates to patients with secondary thrombocytopenia, New Eng. J. Med. **268**:221, 1963.
20. Donegan, C. C., Jr., MacIlwaine, W. A., and Leavell, B. S.: Hematologic studies on patients with sickle cell anemia following multiple transfusions, Amer. J. Med. **17**:29, 1954.
21. Dubin, I. N.: Idiopathic hemochromatosis and transfusion siderosis; a review, Amer. J. Clin. Path. **25**:514, 1955.
22. Ellis, J. T., Schulman, I., and Smith, C. H.: Generalized siderosis with fibrosis of liver and pancreas in Cooley's (Mediterranean) anemia, with observations on the pathogenesis of the siderosis and fibrosis, Amer. J. Path. **30**:287, 1954.
23. Embil, J. A., Folkins, D. F., Haldane, E. V., and van Roogen, C. E.: Cytomegalic virus infection following extracorporeal circulation in children; a prospective study, Lancet **2**:1151, 1968.
24. Elmlinger, P. J., Huff, R. L., and Oda, J. M.: Depression of red cell iron turnover by transfusion, Proc. Soc. Exp. Biol. Med. **79**:16, 1952.
25. Epstein, R. B., Clift, R. A., and Thomas, E. D.: The effect of leukocyte transfusions on experimental bacteremia in the dog, Blood **34**:782, 1969.
26. Forum: The "anemia" of prematurity: should it be treated by transfusion? Quart. Rev. Pediat. **8**:1, 1953.
27. Gens, R. D.: Transfusion reactions due to leukocyte agglutinins, Pediatrics **27**:370, 1961.
28. Grove-Rasmussen, M., Lesses, M. F., and Anstall, H. B.: Transfusion therapy, New Eng. J. Med. **264**:1034, 1961.
29. Haber, J. M., Erlandson, M., Miles, W., and Rowe, A. W.: A method for crossmatching frozen red cells, Med. Lab., Jan., 1969, p. 28.
30. Kevy, S. V., Schmidt, P. S., McGinniss, M. H., and Workman, W. G.: Febrile nonhemolytic transfusion reactions and the limited role of leukoagglutinins in their etiology, Transfusion **2**:7, 1962.
31. Klinman, A.: No hepatitis after packed red cells? New Eng. J. Med. **279**:1290, 1968.
32. Krugman, S., and Giles, J. P.: Viral hepatitis; new light on an old disease, J.A.M.A. **212**:1019, 1970.
33. Leeksma, C. H. W., and Cohen, J. A.: Determination of the life of human blood platelets using labelled diisopropylfluorophosphate, Nature **175**:552, 1955.
34. McGovern, J. J.: Platelet transfusions in pediatrics, New Eng. J. Med. **256**:922, 1957.
35. Miller, G., McCoord, A. B., Joos, H. A., and Clausen, S. W.: Studies of serum electrolyte changes during exchange transfusion, Pediatrics **13**:412, 1954.
36. Mirick, G. S., Ward, R., and McCollum, R. W.: Modification of post-transfusion hepatitis by gamma globulin, New Eng. J. Med. **275**:59, 1965.
37. Mollison, P. L.: Blood transfusions in clinical medicine, ed. 3, Oxford, 1961, Blackwell Scientific Publications.
38. Mollison, P. L.: Blood transfusions in clinical medicine, ed. 4, Philadelphia, 1967, F. A. Davis Co., p. 145.
39. Murphy, S., and Gardner, F. H.: Platelet preservation; effect of storage temperature on maintenance of platelet-viability, deleterious effect of refrigerated storage, New Eng. J. Med. **280**:1094, 1969.
40. Newman, C. G. H.: Intraperitoneal transfusion of blood in a child with Cooley's anemia, Lancet **1**:230, 1959.
41. Penick, G. D., and Brinkhous, K. M.: Relative stability of plasma antihemophilic factor

(AHF) under different conditions of storage, Amer. J. Med Sci. 232:434, 1956.
42. Pickles, M. M.: Haemolytic disease of the newborn, Springfield, Ill., 1949, Charles C Thomas, Publisher.
43. Prince, A. M.: An antigen detected in the blood during the incubation period of serum hepatitis, Proc. Nat. Sci. 60:814, 1968.
44. Prince, A. M.: Relation of Australia and SH antigen, Lancet 2:462, 1968.
45. Richards, A. G.: Loss of blood group B antigen in chronic lymphocytic leukaemia, Lancet 2:178, 1962.
46. Robertson, O. H.: The effects of experimental plethora on blood production, J. Exp. Med. 26:221, 1917.
47. Rowe, A. W., Eyster, E., and Kellner, A.: Liquid nitrogen presentation of red blood cells for transfusion; a low glycerol-rapid freeze procedure, Cryobiology 5:119, 1968.
48. Schulman, I., Smith, C. H., Stern, G. S.: Studies on the anemia of prematurity, Amer. J. Dis. Child. 88:567, 1954.
49. Schwarzenberg, L., Mathé, G., Amiel, J. L., Cattan, A., Schneider, M., and Schlumberger, J. R.: Study of factors determining the usefulness and complications of leukocyte transfusions, Amer. J. Med. 43:206, 1967.
50. Smith, C. H., Schulman, I., Ando, R. E., and Stern, G.: Studies in Mediterranean (Cooley's) anemia. I. Clinical and hematologic aspects of splenectomy with special reference to fetal hemoglobin synthesis, Blood 10:582, 1955.
51. Smith, C. H., Schulman, I., Ando, R. E., and Stern, G. S.: Studies in Mediterranean (Cooley's) anemia. II. The suppression of hematopoiesis by transfusions, Blood 10:707, 1955.
52. Stefanini, M., and Dameshek, W.: Collection, preservation and transfusion of platelets; with special reference to the factors affecting the "survival rate" and the clinical effectiveness of transfused platelets, New Eng. J. Med. 248: 797, 1953.
53. Strumia, M. M.: The preservation of blood for transfusion, Blood 9:1105, 1954.
54. Waite, M. E., Colucci, D. D., and Glaser, J.: Blood transfusion by the intraperitoneal route, Amer. J. Dis. Child. 91:561, 1956.
55. Wiener, A. S.: Prevention of accidents in blood transfusions, J.A.M.A. 156:1301, 1954.

# 8 JAUNDICE—DIFFERENTIAL DIAGNOSIS IN THE NEONATAL PERIOD

The differential diagnosis of jaundice in the first weeks and months of life embraces a variety of conditions of a hemolytic and hepatic nature, some of which are specific and others ill defined. These conditions may be interrelated to the extent that they appear as a hemolytic process at the outset but eventually give the clinical picture of liver disease. Common to most of these conditions in the first days of life is accelerated red cell destruction, resulting in overproduction of bilirubin in amounts exceeding the excretory capacity of the liver for their disposal. On the other hand, jaundice may date from the newborn period on a purely hepatic basis without significant intensity until the second or third week of life. Here malformations of the bile ducts or an inflammatory process accounts for the jaundice uncomplicated by a hemolytic component.

Erythroblastosis plays a prominent role in the differential diagnosis of jaundice, both in the neonatal period when the disease is active and in the early months of life when it is an important factor in the pathogenesis of the inspissated bile syndrome. Since erythroblastosis will be dealt with fully in Chapters 9 and 10, in this discussion it will be referred to only in connection with syndromes from which it needs to be differentiated.

The pediatrician is confronted with making a diagnosis in infants with syndromes characterized by jaundice either during the first week of life (early neonatal period), as in those with erythroblastosis, or in the remainder of the neonatal period (second to fourth weeks of life), as in those with prolonged obstructive jaundice.

*Types of bilirubin.* Different types of bilirubin have been identified with each process on the basis of their reaction with van den Bergh's diazo reagent. The serum from patients with bilirubinemia resulting from red cell destruction produces a predominantly delayed or indirect reaction, whereas the serum from those with jaundice due to diseases of the liver and biliary system produces a direct (1-minute) reaction. Bilirubinuria is absent in patients with hemolytic anemia in whom there is a retention of *unconjugated* bilirubin (water-insoluble form) in the plasma, giving an *indirect* van den Bergh reaction. In patients with obstructive and hepatogenous jaundice in whom the plasma contains largely *conjugated* bilirubin (water-soluble form), giving a predominantly *direct* van den Bergh reaction, bilirubinuria is present.

Originally, van den Bergh developed a method for the estimation of bilirubin in serum by combining it in an alcoholic solution with freshly diazotized sulfanilic acid. Later, van den Bergh and Müller noted that by the omission of alcohol they could distinguish two types of reaction. Pigments from bile and serum from cases of obstructive jaundice developed a color in the absence of alcohol. This was called "direct" reaction. Normal serum and that of patients with hemolytic jaundice required alcohol for the development of color, and they were said to give an "indirect" reaction.[38]

*Enzymatic conversion of indirect to direct bilirubin.* Indirect bilirubin formed by the reticuloendothelial cells is transported in the plasma attached to proteins, mainly albumin.[151,152] Bilirubin excretion includes the following steps: (1) transfer of unconjugated bilirubin from the plasma across the cell membrane into the hepatic cells, (2) conjugation, (3) secretion of the conjugated pigment into the lumen of the biliary canaliculus, and (4) passage through the biliary tree and intestine.[108] In the process of conjugation the two carboxyl groups of bilirubin are esterified with glucuronic acid, forming an alkali-labile acyl diglucuronide.[107] The reaction is catalyzed by a microsomal enzyme, glucuronyl transferase, which is probably located in the smooth portion of the endoplasmic reticulum; the nucleotide uridine diphosphoglucuronic acid (UDPGA) serves as the donor.[11] In this reaction nonpolar, lipid-soluble unconjugated bilirubin is converted to a polar, water-soluble compound.[18,19] Free glucuronic acid, however, does not enter into the conjugation of indirect bilirubin. This conversion may be schematically represented as follows:

| Indirect bilirubin | Glucuronyl | Direct bilirubin |
|---|---|---|
| (Insoluble) | transferase | (Bilirubin- |
| + | $\longrightarrow$ | glucuronide |
| Glucuronic acid | | soluble) |

According to this concept, before birth the placenta and not the liver is responsible for removal of bilirubin from the fetal blood.[61] The infant, therefore, is not born jaundiced and only becomes so if the enzyme system responsible for the conjugation of bilirubin has not yet been fully developed. It may be assumed that the fall in pigment concentration during the first week of life depends upon a corresponding rise in glucuronyl transferase activity toward adult levels.[19]

Bilirubin forms two glucuronides: pigment I, believed to represent bilirubin monoglucuronide,[38] and pigment II, which represents bilirubin diglucuronide conjugated with two moles of glucuronic acid. Although solvent partition techniques have been described for their separation, more recent information suggests that the monoglucuronide is a complex of unconjugated bilirubin and bilirubin diglucuronide.[78] Bilirubin is not conjugated exclusively with glucuronide, but also with sulfate[98] and possibly with phosphate. In man, inducers or stimulators of glucuronyl transferase activity in newborn infants have not been so effective as they have been in newborn guinea pigs.[113] The glucuronide donor, uridine disphosphate glucuronic acid (UDPGA), is the unique substance in man through which the glucuronic acid is made available for the conjugation system. Aside from being demonstrable in hepatic parenchymal cells, glucuronyl transferase activity has been described in the kidney and gastrointestinal tracts.[54] The appearance of direct-reacting bilirubin in the plasma of hepatectomized dogs may be attributed to extrahepatic conjugation, possibly taking place in the kidney and gastrointestinal mucosa.[83]

The effect of this enzyme deficiency is manifested particularly in patients with erythroblastosis, as a result of which the newborn infant is exposed to high plasma concentrations of bilirubin. Excessive hyperbilirubinemia, occurring occasionally in the full-term and premature infant in connection with physiologic jaundice and unrelated to blood group incompatibility, is based on the same difficulty of converting indirect to direct bilirubin.[26] An unidentified substance in the plasma of the pregnant woman that inhibits the in vitro conversion of indirect bilirubin to direct bilirubin has been demonstrated by rat liver slices. This inhibitor may conceivably contribute to the development of hyperbilirubinemia in the newborn infant.[102]

A transient, familial form of neonatal hyperbilirubinemia has been described. In each of five women more than one deeply jaundiced infant was born for whom no available diagnosis seemed appropriate.[115] Postmortem examinations revealed that three infants had kernicterus. Sera from two infants and three pregnant mothers were three to four times as inhibitory to bilirubin conjugation by rat liver slices as the maximal inhibitory effect of sera from twenty normal pregnant women and their newborn infants. In this group there was no evidence of familial anemia, jaundice, diabetes, syphilis, erythroblastosis, or spherocytosis.

Conditions such as Gilbert's disease[62,69] familial nonhemolytic jaundice,[44] and the Crigler-Najjar syndrome,[42] in which the jaundice is due to the accumulation of unconjugated bilirubin, may now be explained as a failure of the liver to form conjugated bilirubin because of a deficiency of the specific enzyme transferase.

It has been observed[109] that unconjugated hyperbilirubinemia may be associated with a wide variety of disease states such as cardiac, hepatobiliary, and gastrointestinal disorders and infections. The retention is occasionally due to increased pigment production as a consequence of compensated hemolysis or ineffective hematopoiesis, but in most cases it appears to be related to a defect in the uptake, conjugation, or excretion of bilirubin by the liver. The fact that hyperbilirubinemia usually subsides following recovery establishes an etiologic relationship and demonstrates further that the underlying disease need not be one of the known hereditary or congenital entities.

It has been pointed out that, since the newborn infant's plasma bilirubin concentration begins to rise shortly after severance of the cord, it is a fair assumption that fetal blood is cleared of excess bilirubin by way of the placenta.[108] The transfer of unconjugated $^{14}C$ bilirubin across the placental barrier has been demonstrated in both guinea pigs[149] and monkeys.[105] The placenta resembles the intestinal mucosa,[106] in being freely permeable for the lipid-soluble conjugate. This mechanism undoubtedly accounts for the fact that during gestation the human fetus is protected against devel-

Table 8. Diagnostic features of the various types of neonatal jaundice*

| Diagnosis | Nature of van den Bergh reaction | Jaundice Appears | Jaundice Disappears | Peak bilirubin mg. % | Peak bilirubin Age in days | Bilirubin rate of accumulation mg. % per day | Remarks |
|---|---|---|---|---|---|---|---|
| 1. Physiologic jaundice | | | | | | | Usually relates to degree of maturity |
| Full-term | Indirect | 2–3 days | 4–5 days | 10–12 | 2–3 | < 5 | |
| Premature | Indirect | 3–4 days | 7–9 days | 15 | 6–8 | < 5 | |
| 2. Hyperbilirubinemia due to metabolic factors, etc. | | | | | | | Metabolic factors: hypoxia, respiratory distress, lack of carbohydrates, infants of diabetic mothers<br>Hormonal influences: cretinism, maternal hormones<br>Genetic factors: Crigler-Najjar syndrome, transient familial hyperbilirubinemia<br>Drugs: vitamin K, novobiocin |
| Full-term | Indirect | 2–3 days | Variable | 12 | First week | < 5 | |
| Premature | Indirect | 3–4 days | Variable | 15 | First week | < 5 | |
| 3. Hyperbilirubinemia of late onset | | | | | | | |
| (a) Some breast-fed infants | Indirect | 1–2 weeks | Variable 6 weeks | Unlimited | 2–6 weeks | Usually > 5 | (a) Relates to level of pregnanediol in breast milk; jaundice clears when patient is taken off breast feeding |
| (b) Pyloric stenosis | Usually indirect | Usually after 2 weeks | After pylorotomy | Unlimited | 2–6 weeks | Usually > 5 | (b) Carbohydrate starvation may contribute to jaundice; role of enterohepatic circulation of bilirubin not known |
| 4. Hemolytic states and enclosed hemorrhage | Indirect | May appear in first 24 hours | Variable | Unlimited | Variable | Usually > 5 | Erythroblastosis: Rh, ABO<br>Congenital hemolytic states: spherocytic, non-spherocytic, infantile pyknocytosis<br>Drugs: vitamin K₃<br>Enclosed hemorrhage: hematoma |
| 5. Mixed hemolytic and hepatoxic factors | Indirect and direct | May appear in first 24 hours | Variable | Unlimited | Variable | Usually > 5 | Infection: bacterial sepsis, pyelonephritis, hepatitis, toxoplasmosis, cytomegalic inclusion disease<br>Drugs: vitamin K₃ |
| 6. Hepatocellular damage | Indirect and direct | Usually 2–3 days | Variable | Unlimited | Variable | Variable: can be > 5 | Biliary atresia: galactosemia, hepatitis, and infection as for mixed hemolytic and hepatoxic factors |

*Modified from Brown, A. K.: Neonatal jaundice, Ped. Clin. N. Amer. 9:575, 1962.

oping hyperbilirubinemia, even when erythroblastosis occurs in utero.

Jaundice may occur as the result of two distinct but often associated derangements.[108] Overproduction of pigment, inadequate hepatic uptake, or failure of the conjugating mechanism may result in plasma retention of unconjugated bilirubin. "Regurgitation" into the plasma of bilirubin glucuronide is produced by functional cholestasis, disruption of the hepatic architecture, or extrahepatic biliary obstruction.

The following outline classifies the causes of jaundice in the early and late neonatal periods. The diagnostic features are presented in greater detail in Table 8.

I. Early neonatal period (first week)
  1. Physiologic jaundice: full-term and premature
  2. Erythroblastosis fetalis
  3. Hereditary spherocytosis
  4. Hereditary nonspherocytic hemolytic disease
  5. Hereditary elliptocytosis
  6. Heinz body anemia in the newborn infant
  7. Infections
      (a) Congenital syphilis
      (b) Sepsis
      (c) Toxoplasmosis
      (d) Cytomegalic inclusion disease
      (e) Urinary tract infection
      (f) Rubella
      (g) Herpes simplex
  8. Galactosemia
  9. Bleeding in enclosed spaces
      (a) Hematomas
      (b) Intraventricular hemorrhage
  10. Pyknocytosis
  11. Drug-induced hemolytic anemias
      (a) Enzyme deficiency—glucose-6-phosphate dehydrogenase
      (b) Vitamin K
      (c) Maternal ingestion of drugs—i.e., naphthalene, vitamin K
  12. Miscellaneous
      (a) Hypoxia in infants of diabetic mothers
      (b) Respiratory distress syndrome
      (c) Premature infants
      (d) Breast milk ingestion
      (e) Novobiocin

II. Later neonatal period (second to fourth weeks)
  1. Congenital atresia of the intrahepatic and extrahepatic ducts
  2. Neonatal hepatitis
  3. Biliary obstruction due to inspissation of bile (?)
  4. Familial nonhemolytic jaundice with kernicterus (Crigler-Najjar)
  5. Pyloric stenosis
  6. Cretinisim
  7. Miscellaneous
      (a) Gilbert's disease
      (b) Dubin-Johnson syndrome
      (c) Rotor-Schiff syndrome

## JAUNDICE IN EARLY NEONATAL PERIOD

*Physiologic jaundice (icterus neonatorum).* Jaundice appears commonly in newborn infants from the second to the fifth day of life. After reaching a maximum intensity between the second and third days, the jaundice begins to diminish, with bilirubin dropping to normal levels (0.25 to 0.75 mg. per 100 ml. of serum), generally between the first and second weeks of life. Immaturity of the liver, previously held responsible for the failure to excrete bilirubin resulting from normal or slightly accelerated red cell destruction,[177] now finds more precise definition in the delayed development of an enzyme system required for the conversion of indirect to direct bilirubin.

Mechanical fragility of the red cells in the first days of life indicates their increased susceptibility to hemolysis.[89] On the other hand, two studies relating to the transfusion of placental blood into another infant[131] or an adult[84] indicate that fetal red cells have only a somewhat shorter survival than those of the adult. Only the red cells produced during late fetal life survive for a shorter time than expected.[131] Using autotransfusion of red cells tagged with $^{51}$Cr as an index of hemolysis, it has been found[176] that differences in the rate of red cell destruction do not play an important role in the genesis of physiologic jaundice. No relation existed between erythrocyte survival on the one hand and peak bilirubin in the serum and duration of hyperbilirubinemia on the other.

The serum bilirubin of the full-term infant seldom exceeds 10 mg. per 100 ml. of serum at its height on the second and third days of life and usually reaches no more than 7 mg. per 100 ml. In the premature infant unaffected by erythroblastosis there is a tendency toward excessive bilirubinemia[86,136] as compared with the full-term infant. The bilirubin level follows that of the full-term infant in the first 2 days of life but then continues its rise to the fourth and sometimes fifth day before a decline occurs. The premature infant tends, therefore, to accumulate bilirubin beyond the 2-day period of the full-term baby. Peak levels in the premature infant average 12 mg.[86] and may exceed 20 mg. per 100 ml. of serum.[26] According to some authors, hyperbilirubinemia exists in the premature infant if a level of more than 10 to 15 mg. per 100 ml. occurs during the first week of life. Physiologic jaundice is present in infants with lower levels.[112]

Jaundice in the first 24 hours of life is never physiologic. In infants with erythroblastosis, in contrast to those with physiologic icterus, jaundice develops rapidly, with high bilirubin levels on the first day of life and maximum concentrations often reached in less than 2 days. In the absence of isoimmunization, excessive bilirubin levels in the full-term or premature infant develop more slowly and usually present initial problems of management beyond the first 48 hours of life.

The common denominator of all neonatal jaundice, however, is the limited capacity of the liver of the newborn infant for the conversion of bilirubin to the soluble pigment bilirubin glucuronide.[24] The principal source of bilirubin is the normal daily destruction of red cells, amounting to about 1% of total hemoglobin mass per day. Some hemoglobin is also derived from the degradation of hemoglobin derived from immature erythrocytes at the site of formation.[24]

The newborn monkey has an indirect reacting type of hyperbilirubinemia during the first 2 days of life. An analysis of the hepatic microsomal fraction glucuronyl transferase activity reveals a diminished activity during intrauterine life and in the early neonatal period.[116] In the guinea pig fetus it has been shown that enzymes responsible for the conjugation reaction are virtually absent and that levels found in the adult guinea pig are not reached until about the fifteenth day of life.[27]

One may also speculate that, if enzymes concerned with the excretion of bilirubin are not specific, then other substances which are detoxified by the process of conjugation in the liver (cortisone, chloramphenicol, salicylates, estrogens, aspirin, menthol, progesterone) may interfere by a process of competitive inhibition with excretion of bilirubin.[112]

Another aberration in bilirubin metabolism has been described in which the defect appears to be inability of the hepatic cell to excrete bilirubin glucuronide.[150] Persistence of this intrahepatic excretion block after the development of mature glucuronide synthesis[149] may explain the "inspissated bile syndrome"[82] (pp. 117 to 118).

*Hyperbilirubinemia of the newborn infant unrelated to isoimmunization.* Hyperbilirubinemia unrelated to erythroblastosis may reach a magnitude in the full-term and the premature infant sufficient to place the infant in jeopardy of brain damage. In a series of such infants, bilirubin levels (indirect-reacting) ranged from 12 mg. per 100 ml. on the first day of life to 20 mg./100 ml. and above (maximum 32 mg./100 ml.) during the ensuing week.[26] The peak level was reached earlier in the week in the full-term infant than in the premature infant. The degree of hyperbilirubinemia is regarded as an accentuation of the mechanism involved in the pathogenesis of physiologic jaundice. The premature infant particularly requires careful watching because of the tendency toward excessive bilirubinemia and subsequent kernicterus.

In a compilation of the mean concentrations of serum bilirubin of over 800 premature infants, Lucey and Driscoll[118] found that 12% of premature infants develop concentrations of serum bilirubin of more than 20 mg. per 100 ml.

In this group of patients with nonerythroblastotic hyperbilirubinemia there are conflicting views as to the critical levels for exchange transfusion or even for its routine use.[158] The low incidence of kernicterus in untreated premature infants (less than 1%) led one group of investigators to conclude that preventive treatment of kernicterus should be on an individual rather than a routine basis.[144] This was based on the fact that the existence of a critical peak concentration of plasma bilirubin in premature infants above which kernicterus could be expected to develop could not be demonstrated in their series. Nevertheless, levels of 20 mg./100 ml. and more of indirect bilirubin serve as well-established guideposts for orientation and management in this group as in that with erythroblastosis. The treatment of this type of hyperbilirubinemia will be discussed further in Chapter 10.

The normal newborn infant cannot conjugate bilirubin because of a relative deficiency in glucuronyl transferase activity as well as in the synthesis of uridine diphosphate glucuronic acid (UDPGA). A direct relation between lack of carbohydrate and of exaggeration and prolongation of physiologic jaundice is suggested by the frequency of hyperbilirubinemia in infants who do not have enough carbohydrate available for added demands. Such a situation presumably prevails in the respiratory distress syndrome, in infants of diabetic mothers,[168] and in premature infants who may be starved for the first 72 hours of life. Since glucose is the source of the glycogen from which the carbohydrate entering into the enzymic steps leading to the formation of uridine diphosphate glucuronic acid is derived, it is not difficult to imagine that deprivation of glucose in vivo has a detrimental effect on the developing glucuronide conjugating system.[25,188] In the children of diabetic mothers a lower bilirubin is noted by early feeding. The amelioration of the hyperbilirubinemia in this group of infants results from the effect of an early provision of water, glucose, and sodium chloride on bilirubin excretion by the liver.[92]

The administration of novobiocin to a group of newborn infants with staphylococcal infection was noted to result in a threefold increase of serum bilirubin levels.[166] Further studies based on experimental observations with novobiocin indicated that hyperbilirubinemia results from its direct inhibiting effect on the enzyme glucuronyl transferase,[75,82] preventing bilirubin conjugation with glucuronic acid.

*Phenobarbital therapy in neonatal jaundice.* Encouraged by the publications of Crigler and Gold[41] and Yaffé and his associates,[183] each describing a case of hyperbilirubinemia caused by Crigler-Najjar syndrome in a child in the first year of life in whom phenobarbital administration caused a decrease in serum bilirubin concentration, Maurer and his associates[125] treated twelve pregnant women with phenobarbital (30 to 120 mg. daily) for 2 weeks or longer prior to delivery. Concentrations of serum bilirubin in their offspring and in sixteen control babies were compared during the first 4 days of life. Premature babies and those sensitized by maternal-fetal Rh-Hr or A-B-O incompatibility were excluded. Serum bilirubin levels were significantly lower in babies of treated mothers. These data suggested that phenobarbital received during pregnancy may enhance hepatic metabolism and biliary excretion in the fetus and newborn infant. The data further suggested that the administration of phenobarbital for 2 weeks or longer before delivery altered the course of "physiological" hyperbilirubinemia in the neonatal period.

Trolle[173] also investigated the effect of this drug on decreasing the serum bilirubin concentration in infants during the first week of life. A large group of newborn babies of birth weight over 2,500 grams were treated in accordance with one of these programs: administration to the pregnant woman only, to the infant only, or to both. The treatment given the last group, 50 to 100 mg. phenobarbital (oral) given daily to the pregnant woman for at least 3 days before delivery, followed by 5 mg. intramuscularly to the newborn seven to ten times in all, proved most effective. The decrease in infants with 13 mg./100 ml. or more of bilirubin initially was 94%. The lowering of serum bilirubin concentration was attributed to the induction of the enzyme in liver microsomes by the phenobarbital.

Ramboer and his associates[143] found a daily dose of 60 mg. of phenobarbital given from the 32nd week of pregnancy effective in reducing the serum bilirubin concentration of the neonate. The mean plasma bilirubin in the babies of treated mothers was 4.4 mg./100 ml. on the third day of life as compared with 8.2 mg./100 ml. in babies of control mothers. In other series,[43,98,170,181] treatment of either normal or low-weight babies starting immediately after birth but without treatment of the mothers beforehand was less effective. In these infants and in those of Trolle[173] it should be emphasized that phenobarbital given to babies alone results in some reduction in bilirubin levels but less than if the mother had been previously treated.

In the Crigler-Najjar syndrome, severe jaundice occurs within hours after birth and is lifelong. This condition of chronic nonhemolytic unconjugated hyperbilirubinemia associated with defective glucuronide formation in vivo and markedly reduced hepatic glucuronyl transferase activity in vitro is of two types. Type I, in which hyperbilirubinemia is usually more severe (serum bilirubin, 20 to 45 mg. per 100 ml.) and kernicterus is frequent, is unaffected by prolonged phenobarbital administration. Patients with Type II disease generally have less severe hyperbilirubinemia (serum bilirubin, 8 to 22 mg. per 100 ml.) without kernicterus. The latter group of patients responds dramatically to treatment with phenobarbital. Jaundice recedes within 5 to 12 days and the level of unconjugated bilirubin declines to approximately 1.6 to 2.2 mg. per 100 ml. Upon cessation of phenobarbital administration, hyperbilirubinemia recurs in approximately 10 days.[41]

The paper by McMullin[127] regarding infants with Rh-Hr hemolytic disease brings the subject nearer home. McMullin did a controlled trial of phenobarbitone therapy in infants with Rh-Hr incompatibility. Treatment did not influence the requirement for a first exchange transfusion (which would have been carried out before treatment had become effective), but it significantly reduced the need for subsequent exchanges. Combined maternal and neonatal treatment might conceivably reduce even further the number of exchanges needed in this situation. Though the numbers are small, the results indicate that phenobarbitone is of benefit in the prophylaxis of Rh-Hr hemolytic disease. Phototherapy has not always been effective in lowering the serum bilirubin concentration in all low-birth-weight infants with physiologic or idiopathic jaundice.[139] In a group of eight infants (five with O-A incompatiblity, one Rh-Hr incompatibility, and two premature infants with idiopathic hyperbilirubinemia) bilirubin values did not fall as expected, and in two of the six exchange transfusions were needed. The observations emphasized the necessity of carefully monitoring the response to phototherapy in order to promptly initiate an exchange transfusion when indicated.

Phenobarbital causes a marked proliferation of the smooth-surfaced membranes of the endoplasmic reticulum in the liver cells. It is a known inducer of uridine diphosphate-glucuronyl transferase in animals.[31,32] Present evidence is inferential, and it is possible that phenobarbital has some other effect on bilirubin metabolism.[181]

Behrman and Fisher[15] emphasized the dangers of phenobarbital given to the mother during gestation and to the infant after delivery. The risks, however, of potential neonatal respiratory depression and hypotension after birth, of drug depression, and of untoward effects on neurobehavioral development introduce elements of caution in the administration of phenobarbital in the management of neonatal jaundice.

It has been postulated that the administration of phenobarbital stimulates the activity of other drug metabolizing enzymes in liver microsomes. It has been suggested, however, that such studies should proceed cautiously since phenobarbital is known to stimulate the activity of liver microsomal enzymes that metabolize steroid hormones and other normal body substrates. It is not known whether this effect, if it occurred in the human fetus or neonate, would be harmful.[125]

**Hyperbilirubinemia in breast-fed infants.** Newborn infants occasionally exhibit severe and prolonged unconjugated hyperbilirubinemia in the absence of erythroblastosis or prematurity. Jaundice in each infant is minimal during the first 5 days of life and is attributed to physiologic hyperbilirubinemia. Severe clinical jaundice is not apparent until the seventh to the tenth day, and in one series the bilirubin concentration reached levels of 14.7 to 24.5 mg./100 ml.[10] Breast milk obtained from the mothers of infants with this syndrome contains pregnane-3 (alpha), 20 (beta)-diol. Of particular interest is the demonstration that the excretion of pregnanediol in breast milk may cause severe and prolonged unconjugated hyperbilirubinemia in breast-fed infants.[9,10,134,164] This steroid, which competitively inhibits glucuronyl transferase activity in vitro, has been isolated from inhibitory but not from noninhibitory human milk. Approximately 75% of the infants nursed by these mothers will develop this syndrome. The mothers secrete this unusual isomer of pregnanediol in their urine during lactation and presumably have an inheritable defect in steroid metabolism that affects the course of hyperbilirubinemia in their neonates.[64] Kernicterus is said not to occur in this syndrome, because the high concentration of unconjugated bilirubin occurs at the end of the first week of life when the blood-brain barrier may be resistant to the passage of bilirubin.[63]

The elevation of indirect-reacting bilirubin has been attributed to interference with the normal conjugating mechanism by this substance in breast milk. It is not at all clear why high levels of this pregnanediol exist in the milk of certain mothers after childbirth. Of significance is the fact that both the milk and the crystallized product strongly inhibit the formation of o-aminophenol glucuronide and the direct-reacting bilirubin by rat, guinea pig, and rabbit liver homogenates and microsomes in vitro.[9] Indirect bilirubin levels above 20 mg./100 ml. are not infrequently observed. Hyperbilirubinemia occurs at 2 weeks of age and may persist from 2 to 6 weeks following birth and throughout the course of breast feeding.[134] Following replacement of human milk by cow's milk formula, the bilirubinemia clears rapidly. It had previously been shown[88] that serum from pregnant women, immediately postpartum women, and newborn infants possessed a similar inhibitor substance to the one described.

Although the syndrome of breast milk

jaundice may be suspected on the basis of the family history and the relation to jaundice to breast milk ingestion, definitive diagnosis requires the demonstration of inhibition of glucuronyl transferase by milk in vitro. Breast feeding may be resumed after the diagnosis is established. When the bilirubin level exceeds 20 mg./100 ml., interruption of nursing for 3 or 4 days usually results in a substantial reduction of hyperbilirubinemia.

*Transient familial neonatal hyperbilirubinemia (Lucey-Driscoll syndrome).*[118] In another group all infants of certain mothers develop severe nonhemolytic unconjugated hyperbilirubinemia within the first 4 days of life. These infants have a high risk of kernicterus unless exchange transfusion is carried out. During the last trimester of pregnancy serum from these mothers is found to contain a factor that markedly inhibits glucuronyl transferase activity in vitro. This unidentified factor increases in titer immediately before term and disappears rapidly after delivery from the maternal and infant serum. This factor disappears from the mothers' serum when they are not pregnant. The inhibitor is probably a progestational steroid, possibly of material origin. It is postulated that the inhibitor factor crosses the placenta and inhibits hepatic glucuronyl transferase in the neonate. This is superimposed on a normally occurring delayed development of the hepatic glucuronide conjugating systems, particularly glucuronyl transferase activity.

Lucey and Driscoll[118] had suggested that in some instances of extreme hyperbilirubinemia in the newborn period a genetic defect exists in the timing of maturation of the enzyme system responsible for conjugation of bilirubin. They noted that four mothers each gave birth to more than one infant in whom serum bilirubin levels of 12 to 65 mg. per 100 ml. developed in the neonatal period and that kernicterus followed in two of the infants.

After known causes of severe unconjugated hyperbilirubinemia have been eliminated in these infants, the final diagnosis rests upon the demonstration of increased inhibition of glucuronyl transferase activity by sera from both the mother and infant.[13]

*Phototherapy for hyperbilirubinemia.* Phototherapy as a method for reducing hyperbilirubinemia was first reported in 1958 by Cremer and co-workers.[40] A nurse had noted that babies exposed to sunlight did not become as jaundiced as infants away from the light. This form of treatment has recently been revived and numerous studies in various parts of the world have demonstrated that exposure to light could influence serum bilirubin levels. This treatment had not been widely used because of doubts as to its effectiveness and concern for the possible toxicity of the photochemical decomposition products of bilirubin. Experimental evidence indicates, however, that these products are nontoxic. A controlled study by Lucey and associates[114,119] has been carried out among 111 premature infants (fifty-three light-treated, fifty-eight controls) to test the effectiveness of artificial blue light in preventing hyperbilirubinemia of prematurity. They found that continuous phototherapy is effective in modifying hyperbilirubinemia of prematurity if used continuously between 12 and 144 hours of age. They were able to maintain bilirubin levels under 12 mg./100 ml. and it did not seem reasonable to expect to attribute any brain damage in this group to the effects of serum bilirubin. Broughton and co-workers[23] demonstrated that the products evolving from in vitro bilirubin illumination do not have any effects upon oxidative phosphorylation of liver and brain mitochondria.

Giunta and Roth[70] conducted a controlled study involving ninety-six babies weighing under 2,500 gm. by placing forty-seven completely exposed infants except for diapers under environmental lights averaging 90 footcandles and forty-nine fully clothed infants under lights averaging 10 footcandles. A significantly lower serum bilirubin occurred in the group with the greater intensity of light exposed from the second to the sixth day. No detectable toxic effects were noted during hospitalization of the exposed babies. Cool white lights were used and found to be effective.

Phototherapy has also been successfully employed in older infants to reduce serum bilirubin concentration. Two infants with congenital nonobstructive nonhemolytic jaundice have been reported, one receiving phototherapy at 19 months,[71] the other from earlier infancy when exchange transfusions had failed to stabilize the indirect bilirubin levels.[96] In each infant a presumptive diagnosis of Crigler-Najjar syndrome was made when a defect in ability to conjugate orally administered sodium salicylate was demonstrated. In both cases phototherapy was found effective in controlling the rise in bilirubin when there was no response to phenobarbital. Phototherapy given intermittently for several months on an average of 12 hours daily served to maintain the bilirubin at reasonable levels. Caution was urged in the use of phototherapy for prolonged periods because the biologic effects of chronic administration of light in the developing organism are unknown.[71]

Marked damage to the photoreceptors (rods and cones) of the retinae of newborn piglets exposed to blue fluorescent light has been reported by Sisson and associates[156a]; Kopelman and co-workers[98a] reported a syndrome of diarrhea, skin pigmentation, and red cell membrane damage occurring in newborn infants treated with phototherapy.

In a symposium on phototherapy for hyperbilirubinemia, Behrman and Hsia[16] pointed out that the possible untoward effects of phototherapy have not yet been determined. They emphasize that, while the treatment of term infants with light is rarely indicated, there were certain clinical situations in which they would use phototherapy to treat a jaundiced premature infant. Phototherapy is indicated for infants in whom the risks of hyperbilirubinemia are thought to outweigh the risks of phototherapy. They did not believe that phototherapy should be employed routinely in the premature nursery in an attempt to prevent elevations in the serum concentrations of bilirubin in all infants. They pointed out that some investigators have started therapy soon after birth, others have started at 12 to 72 hours. Therapy has been continued for varying periods of time, continuously or intermittently, through the sixth day of life. There is no good comparison available to judge the relative effectiveness and safety of blue, white, or daylight lamps in photo-oxidizing in the human infant. Blue light, however, was regarded as an effective source for rapidly lowering serum bilirubin levels, but daylight is also adequate and may be safer. It should be cautioned that, if an infant when first seen has sufficient indications for an exchange transfusion, the transfusion should not be delayed for a trial of phototherapy.

Porto and his associates[140] found that Caucasian and Negro infants had a similar response to phototherapy, suggesting that skin pigmentation does not interfere with the photo-oxidation of bilirubin in the newborn infant. These authors[141] also found that the photo-oxidation derivatives of bilirubin are not bound to albumin, or at least show less affinity to albumin than either bilirubin or salicylate.

**Relation of vitamin K to hyperbilirubinemia, kernicterus, and hemolytic anemia.** Large intramuscular doses of a vitamin K preparation (Synkavite) have been shown to increase the serum bilirubin levels in infants during the first week of life.[130] The most severe bilirubinemia, hence the risk of kernicterus, tends to occur in the premature infant, in whom elevated bilirubin levels are normally prone to exist.[21] Large dosages of vitamin K are also hepatotoxic, hemolytic, or both. The liberation of excessive amounts of bilirubin resulting from increased hemolysis in the newborn premature infant following excessive vitamin K dosage has been demonstrated.[4] Because of these possibilities it is unwise to exceed stated dosages for the prophylaxis and treatment of hemorrhagic disease of the newborn infant. There is ample evidence that a single dose of a water-soluble analogue equivalent to 1 mg. of synthetic vitamin K (menadione) is adequate to prevent hemorrhagic disease in the newborn infant. This would correspond to 3 mg. of menadione sodium diphosphate (Synkavite) vitamin K analogue.[48] At present, vitamin $K_1$ (phytonadione) is in common use. It is administered intramuscularly to the newborn infant, whether premature or full-term (Chapter 26), in the delivery room in a dosage not exceeding 1 mg. No untoward complications have been observed with this dosage.

It has been observed[117] that the parenteral administration of a large amount of a vitamin K analogue (Hykinone) to mothers during labor resulted in marked early hyperbilirubinemia in newborn premature infants which caused central nervous system involvement in several cases.

The hemolytic effects of vitamin K have been explained on the basis of an inherent glutathione instability exhibited by the red cells of newborn infants. Incubation of the red cells of newborn infants with vitamin K analogues results in a characteristic fall in glutathione content which accounts for their in vivo hemolysis.[185] This phenomenon corresponds with the susceptibility to hemolysis of selected persons who are sensitive to primaquine and naphthalene.

It has been found that the defect in glutathione stability in newborn infants is due to a lack of available glucose. This renders the red cells more susceptible to the hemolytic action of certain drugs leading to hyperbilirubinemia and kernicterus.[184] The precise mechanisms of hemolytic anemia and hyperbilirubinemia development after the parenteral administration of large doses of water-soluble vitamin K analogues have not, however, been clearly characterized. In addition to instability of glutathione caused by the lack of available glucose with resulting hemolysis, other causes of jaundice may be toxicity to hepatic cells and competition for conjugating enzymes.[112]

In a group of seventeen Greek infants, in whom jaundice was not due to blood group incompatibility, ten showed glucose-6-phosphate dehydrogenase deficiency.[49] In a group of Australian children of Mediterranean origin, hyperbilirubinemia was also related to deficiency of the enzyme.[76] On the island of Lesbos, 29 (4.6%) of 634 infants tested were found to show the enzyme deficiency. Hyperbilirubinemia of 16 mg. per 100 ml. or over was observed in 34% of glucose-6-phosphate-dehydrogenase deficient newborn males and in 9.1% of those with normal activity.[51] Jaundice in these cases may be sufficiently marked to warrant exchange transfusion and may cause kernicterus. It is not known why the erythrocytes of susceptible infants are particularly prone to spontaneous hemolysis, unless perhaps it is due to exposure to unidentified drugs or chemicals. The significantly higher incidence of severe neonatal jaundice among the enzyme-deficient newborn males cannot, as yet, be attributed to either exogenous or endogenous causes, but perhaps to the influence of a genetic factor.[50,59]

It is interesting to note that in institutions in this country the incidence of unexplained hyperbilirubinemia could not be attributed to the enzyme deficiency, either in Caucasians or in the Negro.[85] The activity of the enzyme was not significantly different from babies with hemolytic disease of the newborn infant due either to Rh-Hr or A-B-O incompatibility.

An association of the deficiency of G-6-PD and severe hyperbilirubinemia has been reported in Chinese, Malays, Greeks, Italians, African Negroes, Sephardic Jews, Indians, Bantus, and Thais.[28] Hyperbilirubinemia among G-6-PD deficient infants is a common and serious problem in Singapore, where seven of the seventy-two enzyme-deficient newborns studied either required exchange transfusions or developed neurologic sequelae of hyperbilirubinemia. Hyperbilirubinemia occurs in at least 8% of G-6-PD deficient infants in Singapore, while the incidence in non–G-6-PD deficient newborns probably is less than 0.3%.

The incidence of serious hyperbilirubinemia in G-6-PD-deficient infants appears to vary greatly among ethnic groups. Bilirubin values were found to exceed 20 mg./100 ml. in 38% of deficient Taiwanese infants, to exceed 15 mg./100 ml. in 27% of forty-four Hong Kong Chinese infants, and to exceed 16 mg./100 ml. in 34% of infants in Lesbos.[28]

In the Singapore cases the factors responsible for hyperbilirubinemia in the G-6-PD deficient infants are: the ethnic group predisposition, the slightly excessive hemolysis in G-6-PD deficient infants, and exposure to exogenous hemolytic agents.

In another series[58] it was found that G-6-PD deficiency of the Negro premature infant, unlike that of the Negro term infant, appears to be associated with an increased risk of hyperbilirubinemia. Bearing on this relationship is the fact that the premature infant, at any given bilirubin level, is more prone to develop kernicterus than is the term infant.

*Hereditary spherocytosis.* Hereditary spherocytosis is manifested occasionally in the newborn period,[120,162] at which time it may be confused with erythroblastosis. Microspherocytosis is present in patients with both hereditary spherocytosis and A-B-O (not Rh-Hr) erythroblastosis. In those with erythroblastosis the microspherocytosis lasts a few days, whereas it persists in those with hereditary spherocytosis. Incompatibility between the blood groups of the mother and fetus and, frequently, a positive direct and indirect Coombs test characterize erythroblastosis. In patients with hereditary spherocytosis the Coombs test is uniformly negative, a positive family history is common, and an increased erythrocyte fragility is noted in the blood of affected persons.

Exchange transfusions to prevent kernicterus are indicated for the treatment of patients with hyperbilirubinemia, as in those with erythroblastosis. It is as important to remove congenitally defective and readily destructible red cells from the blood of patients with hereditary spherocytosis as it is to remove sensitized cells from the blood of those with erythroblastosis.

*Hereditary nonspherocytic hemolytic disease.* Hereditary nonspherocytic hemolytic disease may also present itself at birth with the clinical picture of erythroblastosis[29] Absence of spherocytosis, normal osmotic fragility, and failure to respond to splenectomy rule out hereditary spherocytosis. A negative Coombs test and the absence of Rh incompatibility eliminate erythroblastosis, and persistence of the jaundice rules out A-B-O involvement.

*Elliptocytic (ovalocytic) hemolytic anemia.* Elliptocytic (ovalocytic) hemolytic anemia associated with jaundice on the second day of life has been reported, but anemia was not noted until the infant was 1 month of age.[110]

**Heinz body anemia in newborn infant.** Heinz body anemia in the newborn infant has been described as a hemolytic anemia occurring in premature infants.[65] These babies develop a nonobstructive jaundice in the first few days of life, usually between the first and fifth days. Anemia appears in the second to the third week as the jaundice fades. The Coombs test is negative. Examination of the blood before the development of the anemia shows a progressive increase in the number of Heinz bodies (9 to 45% of the red cells). Originally described in premature infants and newborns with congenital defects of the erythrocytes, Heinz body anemia has also been reported in full-term infants.[175]

Heinz bodies are refractible intracellular inclusions in the red cells which are readily seen in fresh wet preparations or in preparations with supravital dyes such as brilliant cresyl blue. They are composed of denatured globin and serve as an indication of a hemolytic process. The blood smear shows anisocytosis, target cells, irregularly shaped fragmenting cells, microspherocytes, and basophilic stippling.

The disease is self-limited, provided the child survives the original hemolytic episode. No evidence of exogenous toxic substances is found before, during, or after birth. High dosages of vitamin K (Synkavite) have been incriminated as a possible cause of Heinz body anemia since severe hemolytic anemia with some Heinz body formation can be produced experimentally in animals by administration of relatively large doses of Synkavite.[5] Another possibility is the existence of an inherent defect in red cells, rendering them susceptible to hemolysis analogous to primaquine sensitivity, in which Heinz bodies also occur.

**Acute hemolytic anemia related to naphthalene.** The ingestion of naphthalene (moth balls and flakes) has been described in children as a cause of severe illness with fever, nausea, diarrhea, and evidences of an acute hemolytic anemia. The initial cases were described in four Negro infants.[187] Fatal naphthalene intoxication, resulting from absorption through the skin from diapers stored in mothballs and crystals, has been reported in newborn infants.[148] Profound anemia, hemoglobinemia, normoblastemia, methemoglobinemia, leukocytosis, jaundice, cyanosis, spherocytosis, occasional Heinz bodies, and hemoglobinuria are noted. Whole blood or packed cells are essential in treatment.[37]

As is true of primaquine sensitivity, the susceptibility to naphthalene poisoning depends upon an intrinsic and genetically determined defect of the red cells which renders them especially susceptible to hemolysis (Chapter 15). The abnormality is in glutathione metabolism, which expresses itself in the older erythrocytes. As stated elsewhere, the basic biochemical defect is a deficiency of glucose-6-phosphate dehydrogenase. This enzyme is essential in maintaining glutathione in a reduced state which is necessary to protect intracellular hemoglobin from the toxic effects of a number of drugs. These defects were described in two newborn infants with hemolytic anemia who had been exposed to articles of clothing impregnated with moth balls.[46] In another case[186] naphthalene and its metabolites passed through the placenta to the newborn infant, producing jaundice and evidences of a hemolytic anemia. The mother who had ingested moth balls had a profound hemolytic anemia. An exchange transfusion in the infant was performed when the indirect bilirubin rose to nearly 20 mg. per 100 ml., from which point the course was uneventful.

**Infections in newborn infants.** Icterus associated with congenital syphilis, sepsis,[160] toxoplasmosis, rubella, disseminated herpes simplex infection, and cytomegalic inclusion disease may result from excessive blood destruction as well as from liver cell damage. Pneumonitis, congenital heart disease, meningitis, urinary tract infection, and intracranial hemorrhage are some of the pathologic states associated with hyperbilirubinemia. The elevation of both the direct and indirect serum bilirubin levels in patients with these conditions reflects excessive hemolysis of red cells as well as hepatocellular damage.[68]

In some institutions[154] urinary tract infection associated with sepsis has been a common cause of jaundice. Jaundice develops in these infants as a result of both hemolytic and toxic hepatitis. Laboratory findings include elevations of both direct and indirect reacting bilirubin fractions, together with elevation of blood urea nitrogen, acidosis, leukocytosis with predominance of granulocytes and immature forms, and thrombocytopenia.

***Cytomegalic inclusion disease.*** Cytomegalic inclusion disease which may appear at or shortly after birth should be suspected, especially in the premature infant, in the presence of jaundice, purpura, hepatosplenomegaly, chorioretinitis, and neurologic disturbances.[128] Other features include hemolytic anemia, thrombocytopenia, petechiae, hematuria, erythroblastemia, moderate leukocytosis, hyperbilirubinemia of the obstructive type with an elevated direct fraction, pneumonitis, and cerebral calcification. In one series,[178] acute hemorrhagic phenomena and thrombocytopenia developed at or shortly after birth in nine of seventeen infants. The bleeding tendency rapidly disappeared regardless of corticosteroid therapy or exchange transfusions. Enlargement of the liver and spleen was present in all infants, but varied in degree and duration. The direct-reacting bilirubin exceeded 50% of the total.

Cytomegalic inclusion disease is caused by a species-specific cytomegalovirus first isolated by Smith[159] from the salivary gland. Although the virus produces no recognizable illness in the mother, it may give rise to severe, frequently fatal, disease in the fetus and newborn. Patients with the disease who die soon after birth are usually premature and generally show evidence of hemolysis, hepatitis, and generalized disease.

The disease is characterized pathologically by an inclusion-containing giant cell appearing predominantly in the lining of the ducts of various organs such as the alveoli of the lungs, tubular epithelium of the kidney, and the brain. The diagnostic cytomegalic or owl-eyed cells with the large intracytoplasmic or intranuclear inclusion bodies are found in the sediment of urine kept under refrigeration[121] and in gastric washings.[156] Cytopathogenicity of this virus obtained from the mouth and urine for tissue cultures of human fibroblasts provides a means for study of the human infection with this virus.[159]

Congenital cytomegalic inclusion disease is caused by a human cytomegalic infection acquired in utero from a mother with inapparent infection.[129] The widespread nature of this disease is suggested by the frequency of occult infections with the agent in childhood and the prolonged period that the virus can be recovered from the urine. Cytomegalic virus has been cultured from the urine in children undergoing treatment for malignant disease of the hematopoietic and reticuloendothelial systems.[74] Cytomegalic inclusion disease is also a rare terminal complication of leukemia and lymphosarcoma in childhood.[72]

Zuelzer and his associates[189] have demonstrated recurrent lymphadenitis attributable to cytomegalic inclusion disease during periods of hemolysis. Lymphadenopathy in children was a prominent finding in the majority of cases and appeared to correspond to periods of rapid virus multiplication. The lymph nodes showed marked diffuse hyperplasia, loss of follicular structure, crowding of the reticulum with pleomorphic large and medium-sized lymphocytes, numerous plasma cells, varying degrees of infiltration with neutrophilic leukocytes of focal necrosis, as well as acute and chronic periadenitis.

***Congenital toxoplasmosis.*** Congenital toxoplasmosis is a rare cause of neonatal jaundice, but is probably more frequent than is suspected. This disease may be confused at the onset with erythroblastosis fetalis.[14] Congenital toxoplasmosis may be associated with deep jaundice, and in one infant in our experience, the serum bilirubin totaled 16 mg. per 100 ml., of which 13 mg. was of the indirect type.

The hemoglobin and red cell count may be normal or moderately or greatly reduced. A negative Coombs test and absence of intragroup incompatibility help to differentiate this condition from erythroblastosis. Spinal fluid changes consisting of a pleocytosis and increased protein content are frequently present in congenital toxoplasmosis. In the active disease the parasites have been demonstrated in smears of the spinal fluid. Chorioretinitis is found in almost all cases of toxoplasmosis and less frequently in cytomegalic inclusion disease. Nonspecific intracranial calcifications which may recede have been found in both conditions.

Congenital toxoplasmosis may appear in the first week of life and is manifested by fever, jaundice, lymphadenopathy, hepatosplenomegaly, a diffuse maculopapular rash, microphthalmia, chorioretinitis, seizures, hydrocephaly or microcephaly, intracranial calcification, anemia, and thrombocytopenia.[56,57] The picture is similar to that encountered in cytomegalic inclusion body disease. Thrombocytopenia occurs but is not as frequent as in cytomegalic inclusion body disease. Eosinophilia has been observed in 18% of patients with the generalized form of the disease. A specific diagnosis can be determined by demonstrating the organism or by serologic methods.[55] Serologic confirmation is most easily obtained by use of the Sabin-Feldman dye test performed on the sera from the mother and infant. A complement-fixation test is also available, but it is not as commonly done as the dye test.

*Chronic idiopathic jaundice (Dubin-Johnson type, Dubin-Sprinz disease).* Chronic idiopathic jaundice of Dubin-Johnson type[52,53,153,161] manifests itself as a form of chronic or intermittent jaundice of fluctuating intensity, with abdominal pain, fatigue, dark urine, and slight enlargement and tenderness of the liver. The direct bilirubin accounts for about 60% of the total serum bilirubin. The liver cell is apparently able to conjugate indirect bilirubin with glucuronic acid and convert it to direct bilirubin but cannot excrete it into the bile. The most striking finding in all cases is the presence of a coarsely granular brown pigment in a sharp centrolobular distribution in the parenchymal cells. A familial history of jaundice has been occasionally obtained in siblings.[94] This type of bilirubinemia in which the direct bilirubin fraction predominates is to be differentiated from Gilbert's disease,[62,69] familial non-hemolytic jaundice of Dameshek and Singer,[44] and the Crigler-Najjar syndrome[42] in which the indirect-reacting bilirubin is in excess. Although the Dubin-Johnson syndrome has been observed principally in adults, it has been recorded occasionally in infancy but not specifically in the early or late neonatal period.

We have encountered an infant, jaundiced from birth, with blood groups compatible with those of the mother who probably had a variant of this disease. The Coombs test was negative. In the first 2 weeks of life the total bilirubin ranged from 47 to 59 mg./100 ml., with a direct fraction of 33 to 40 mg. and an indirect fraction of 13 to 19 mg. Although the Coombs test was negative, the infant was given an exchange transfusion on the third day of life because of the mounting indirect fraction. The mother, her sister, and her two brothers have been chronically jaundiced but in good health. Their total bilirubin ranged from 6 to 13 mg./100 ml., of which the direct-reaching fraction ranged from 4 to 11 mg. and the indirect from 1.3 to 4.1 mg./100 ml. Liver biopsy in the mother, however, showed no pathognomonic pigmentation of the parenchymal cells as described in the Dubin-Johnson syndrome. The infant's jaundice and bilirubinemia receded over the period of several months.

A closely allied disease, but without pigment changes in the liver, is that described by Rotor.[147] This, too, is a familial type of non-hemolytic jaundice characterized by a direct van den Bergh reaction. The case described may fall into this category. The condition differs from that seen in patients with the Dubin-Johson syndrome in that the gallbladder is visualized after dye ingestion, in the absence of pigmentation in liver biopsy, and in the marked increase of conjugated as well as unconjugated bilirubin in the serum.[80]

## JAUNDICE IN LATER NEONATAL PERIOD

*Prolonged obstructive jaundice.* Several diseases of early infancy are characterized by evidence of biliary obstruction which finds its inception in the first weeks of life. Patients with diseases associated with biliary obstruction and those with absence of the bile ducts have been designated as members of a group with prolonged obstructive jaundice. Individual diagnosis is usually difficult, but complexities are resolved at times by scrupulous and continuous appraisal of clinical and laboratory findings.

This group of cases has been classified by Hsia and co-workers[91] into the following categories: biliary obstruction caused by inspissation of bile, either from hemolysis as occurs in erythroblastosis or of multiple etiologies and congenital atresia of the intrahepatic and extrahepatic ducts, including the common bile duct. Neonatal hepatitis has been included as one of the causative factors in the inspissated bile syndrome of nonerythroblastotic origin.

Prolonged obstructive jaundice is characterized by jaundice increasing after the first week of life but varying in its intensity after a maximum has been reached. Additional features are light stools, dark urine, elevation of both total and direct serum bilirubin levels, decreased urobilinogen in the urine and stool, and moderate to marked enlargement of the liver and spleen. Whereas the level of serum bilirubin remains relatively constant in infants with biliary atresia, it may fluctuate in those with the other groups of disease. Extensive erythropoiesis is found in the liver of patients with the inspissated bile syndrome due to erythroblastosis, but none is found in patients with the other syndromes. The liver flocculation tests for liver function are negative but may be transiently positive. No single laboratory test can be used for specific differentiation. Individualization is necessary, and the course in each patient must be followed clinically and with a combination of diagnostic laboratory tests.

Persistent obstructive jaundice in the first weeks or months of life is a common diagnostic problem.[101] About 60% of infants so affected have biliary atresia and 15% have the so-called inspissated bile syndrome associated with erythroblastosis fetalis. The remaining 25% have an entity known as neonatal hepatitis or giant-cell hepatitis. Among the cases in the latter group, sixteen cases of neonatal cholestasis have been recorded arising in seven sibships of the same family in southwest Norway.[1] The infants were jaundiced at or soon after birth, stools were pale, and urine was dark. There was a strong tendency to hemorrhage in early infancy. The initial period of jaundice lasted 1 to 6 years and was associated with severe itching, malabsorption, and later failure to thrive. These features resolved when the jaundice cleared. All patients had one or more subsequent periods of cholestasis. Seven children died in infancy, at least five as a result of hemorrhages, but no death from hemorrhage has occurred since vitamin K has been regularly used.

Laboratory examinations showed hyperbilirubinemia (conjugated bilirubin), increased transaminase, alkaline phosphatase, and hyperlipemia. After the end of the cholestatic period (1 to 6 years) the children began to regain normal stature so that adult height was normal. From prepuberty patients tended to develop edema of the legs for no known reason. Liver histology in this syndrome showed "giant hepatitis," but this did not progress to fibrosis. This syndrome was termed "hereditary, recurrent, intrahepatic cholestasis from birth."

This syndrome differs from related conditions in the following manner: victims have their first cholestatic period at birth, they develop their edema in prepuberty, liver biopsies show giant cells in addition to the cholestasis, the disease is clearly genetic, and the patients always have hyperlipemia in the cholestatic periods. As the bilirubin of the patients in this group is primarily of the conjugated form, they do not fit into the Crigler-Najjar syndrome or Gilbert's syndrome.

*Obstructive jaundice complicating erythroblastosis—inspissated bile syndrome.* The jaundice in most infants with erythroblastosis fetalis begins to subside by the fourth or fifth day and terminates by the end of 10 days. Occasionally, the jaundice persists, the stools become pale, and bile appears in the urine, the entire picture closely simulating congenital biliary atresia. The obstructive phenomenon may be of short or long duration. When prolonged, it acquires the clinical and pathologic characteristics of the inspissated bile syndrome although, qualitatively, the basic features are similar regardless of duration.

Obstructive jaundice may occur at the height of the hemolytic process in erythroblastosis or not until some weeks later. Occasionally, an evanescent phase of hemolytic jaundice occurs soon after birth, with a recurrence of the jaundice associated with biliary obstruction after a few weeks.[137] When obstruction appears in the first days of life, the total serum bilirubin becomes progressively elevated mainly due to the direct fraction and then recedes slowly to normal levels within a few weeks. When it persists at intermediate levels for prolonged periods, it is categorized as obstructive jaundice due to the inspissated bile syndrome.

It is relatively uncommon for newborn infants with erythroblastosis fetalis to exhibit an increase of conjugated (direct) serum bilirubin in cord blood or in blood samples taken during the first 24 hours of life. This phenomenon is regarded by some as not "obstructive"[77] or "regurgitative" but due to inadequacy of secretion of the hepatic parenchymal cell. The defect in secretion may be maturational, as is apparently the case with the inability of the immature hepatic cell to respond to a big load of unconjugated bilirubin. The mortality rate for infants showing increased conjugated bilirubin early (in the cord blood or within the first 24 hours of life) was 38% in one series, while it was zero for those in whom the increase appeared after the first 24 hours.[77]

Exchange transfusions have a negligible effect on the percentage of direct bilirubin and do not alter the progression of biliary obstruction.[163] This procedure should be carried out, however, if there is a significant elevation of indirect-reacting pigment which, in contrast to direct-reacting bilirubin, carries the hazard of cerebral damage. In the reported cases[163] the elevated direct serum bilirubin level decreased in most patients spontaneously in 18 hours to 6 days. It is of interest that the levels of direct bilirubin in the cord blood were higher than those in normal blood (approximately 1 mg. per 100 ml.).

In a newborn infant under our observation the cord blood bilirubin rose from a total of 17 to 48 mg., with 12 to 35 mg./100 ml. direct-reacting and

5 to 13 mg./100 ml. indirect-reacting pigment by the fourth day of life. The next day this value was lower and continued to decrease during the following week although normal blood levels were not achieved until the second month. In another infant, who was not seen until the fifth day of life, liver involvement was apparent when the total bilirubin on that day measured 43 mg./100 ml., of which 31 mg. was direct and 12 mg. indirect. On the seventh day the total bilirubin was 121 mg./100 ml., of which 83 mg. was the direct fraction and 38 mg. indirect. Jaundice then began to recede, and by the third week the total bilirubin measured 17 mg./100 ml., the direct fraction 14 mg., and indirect 3 mg. In the ninth week there was a total of 7 mg./100 ml., with 6 mg. indirect. Except for a slight transient elevation of thymol turbidity in the second month, there was no evidence of liver involvement. At 13 months of age, the infant was still normal without signs of nervous system involvement.

The degree of biliary obstruction is usually partial—rarely complete. Jaundice occurs between 3 weeks and 6 months of age, with an average duration of 7 to 8 weeks.[90] In cases of prolonged jaundice extending into the second month, there is a progressive increase of direct as well as indirect bilirubin. The precise reason for the inspissated bile syndrome complicating erythroblastosis is unknown, whether it be due to hepatocellular[163] damage incurred by the hemolytic disease or to the overload of pigment causing stasis and complete block. Multinucleated giant liver cells found in neonatal hepatitis have also been described in this condition. Recovery has been ascribed to cessation of the hemolytic process and enlargement of biliary ducts with increasing age.[90]

Although it has been advocated[22] to discard the term *inspissated bile syndrome*, there is a degree of usefulness to justify its retention. The term was originally used loosely to indicate an overloading of the liver cells with bile pigment either because of an increased supply or an inability to conjugate, or difficulties of eliminating the pigment into the bile canaliculi. Swelling of the liver cells loaded with bile pigment was assumed to have caused compression of the bile canaliculi.

In the strict sense, the inspissated bile syndrome implies a defect involving the excretory mechanism for conjugated bilirubin. The term may be applied to the persistence of this intrahepatic excretion block after the development of adequate glucuronide synthesis and the delayed appearance of conjugated bilirubin in infants with erythroblastosis fetalis.[108] In the intracellular bile canaliculi the bile casts, consisting of inspissated bile-protein complex, have been interpreted as the result rather than the cause of the jaundice.[188] Inspissated bile syndrome has a definite usefulness limited to the obstructive jaundice that may follow or develop during the course of erythroblastosis fetalis. Pathologically, it has no basis. The increasing jaundice in this condition involves the direct fraction and represents a defect or inadequacy in the secretion ability of the parenchymal cell of the liver.[77]

In differentiating the inspissated bile syndrome from other categories of obstructive jaundice, the history, clinical observation, and laboratory tests are helpful. Patients with the inspissated bile syndrome due to erythroblastosis demonstrate the following clinical and laboratory features: clinical evidence of erythroblastosis during the early acute phase, jaundice on the first day of life which persists longer than the first 3 weeks, an obstructive type of jaundice with marked elevation in both direct and indirect bilirubin levels, negative liver flocculation tests, and demonstration of maternal-fetal blood group incompatibilities.[90] Spontaneous recovery is the rule in patients with obstructive jaundice in this category.

*Atresia of bile ducts (congenital obliteration of bile ducts).* The diagnosis and management of prolonged obstructive jaundice in the early months of life have been beset with difficulties.[22] Except for the transitory inspissated bile syndrome due to erythroblastosis, the most common causes of persistent jaundice in the first 6 months of life are atresia of the extrahepatic ducts and neonatal hepatitis. Bile stasis (cholestasis) is associated with a variety of conditions such as hepatitis, prematurity, galactosemia, esophageal atresia, erythroblastosis fetalis, duodenal atresia, lower small intestinal obstruction, and infection with gram-negative organisms. In these conditions the conjugated bilirubin in the serum is elevated.[132] Biochemical dysfunction of liver cells, duct obstruction, and disturbances of hepatic blood flow are contributing causes of bile stasis.

Congenital atresia of the extrahepatic bile ducts represents about 75% of the cases of obstructive jaundice in the first 2 months of life. About two-thirds of the remaining cases are caused by neonatal hepatitis. The other one-third is made up of a variety of relatively rare disorders, such as galactosemia, cystic fibrosis of the pancreas, syphilis, inspissation of bile secondary to erythroblastosis fetalis, sepsis, and choledochal cyst.[67] Despite persistent and progressive jaundice, affected infants appear well nourished in the first 3 or 4 months of life. The stools are acholic, the urine is dark, and the level of bilirubin is fairly constant. The stools may, however, be slightly bile stained, even in severely jaundiced infants. In both atresia of the bile ducts and neonatal hepatitis the serum bilirubin is elevated and is equally divided between conjugated and unconjugated bilirubin. The serum bilirubin in atresia of the bile ducts does not rise steadily until death, but reaches a peak that may lie between 8 and 35 mg./100 ml. It has been estimated that, of about 20% of the patients amenable to surgical anastomosis, only 2 to 3% of the total with chronic obstructive jaundice due to atresia of the extrahepatic duct system have been treated successfully.[167] The remainder succumb in the immediate postoperative period or later to biliary cirrhosis.

Congenital atresia of the intrahepatic ducts may occur with or without an associated extrahepatic atresia. Diagnosis is possible only by biopsy. In general, the findings resemble those in patients in whom atresia of both intrahepatic and extrahepatic ducts occurred together; the course is more benign with a life-span of 3 to 5 years.[2] It has been demonstrated that the intrahepatic bile ducts are present in the early months of life and disappear coincident with prolonged disturbance in bilirubin elimination through the hepatic cells into the biliary canaliculi, giving histologic evidence of cholestasis.[78] Associated with atresia of the intrahepatic bile ducts there are often anomalies of the extrahepatic ducts. With advancing age generalized skin xanthomatosis appears and with this is associated marked elevation of the serum lipids. (In one of our patients the cholesterol reached 1,296 mg./100 ml. at 8 years of age.)

Alpert and co-workers[6] found that, of nineteen autopsied cases of 17-18 trisomy syndrome ten confirmed by cytogenetic studies, seven cases of neonatal hepatitis were found including two of biliary atresia. Liveborn infants had an early onset of icterus with elevated total and conjugated serum bilirubin concentrations. All had intrahepatic cholestasis and variable combinations of hepatocellular and portal tract involvement. The nature of the association between the chromosome aberrations and hepatobiliary disease is unclear. They suggested, among other speculations, that the chromosomal aberration and the hepatitis may have a common causation—a possibility that seems more consistent with observed facts.

It is possible that hepatobiliary lesions may represent a developmental error due to chromosomal aberration. Furthermore, the chromosomal aberration and the hepatitis may have a common causation such as a viral infection.[135]

*Neonatal hepatitis (giant cell hepatitis).* When jaundice persists in the neonatal period and the inspissated bile syndrome due to erythroblastosis and congenital obliteration of the bile ducts have been eliminated, neonatal hepatitis is next to be considered. Its etiology is controversial and diagnosis and treatment are poorly understood. No unequivocal evidence has been offered for its causation by the agents of homologous serum hepatitis or the virus of infectious hepatitis.[87]

The pathologic changes vary with the course of the disease, but the most prominent features have been the appearance in the liver of multinucleated giant cells,[39] with a feathery degeneration of the cytoplasm, and occasional areas of necrosis.[27] Later in the course, the lobular architecture is destroyed and the liver parenchyma is replaced by syncytial giant cells separated by fibrous tissue.[30] Plugging by inspissated bile in biliary canaliculi is of secondary importance.[79] This giant cell transformation has also been observed with intrahepatic and extrahepatic biliary obstruction.[97] Some giant cell transformation may be found with approximately one-third of the cases of biliary atresia.[30] Another theory is that neonatal hepatitis represents a developmental defect of liver cells, resulting in aplasia of the bile capillaries and malformation of the liver cells.[157] The relation of these morphologic changes to neonatal hepatitis is by no means settled. Factors such as small bile ducts, dehydration, and hepatic immaturity contribute to biliary stasis. The recovery of an inclusion cell virus from three infants with neonatal hepatitis[179] suggests such an etiology for a special group of cases of this disorder.

Giant cell hepatitis of infancy is, therefore, increasingly regarded as a disorder of unknown etiology characterized by the presence in the liver, chiefly of young infants, of varying numbers of multinucleated giant cells of hepatocellular origin and by the absence of any other demonstrable pathologic condition responsible for the jaundice. It is probably not due to a single cause but rather to numerous viral agents such as cytomegalic inclusion virus, Coxsackie virus, homologous serum and infectious hepatitis virus, and herpes simplex virus.

Transplacental viral transmission of neonatal hepatitis from a carrier mother to infant was first described by Stokes and associates.[165] Giant cell hepatitis of the newborn infant was also observed in connection with the case of a mother who, after an attack of infectious hepatitis, gave birth to two children who died with giant cell hepatitis.[7] The five children born before the attack were normal. On this basis, giant cell hepatitis of the newborn infant was construed as a form of hepatitis, either of the infectious or the serum type, that was transmitted from the mother to the infant. Despite evidence of this type, the hypothesis of transplacental transmission of giant cell hepatitis has failed to be substantiated, due to inconsistencies of clinical incidence and failure of experimental production.

The low birth weight in neonatal hepatitis suggests that the liver parenchyma may have been damaged before birth.[45] In some cases giant cell formation in the liver is associated with the deposition of hemosiderin in the giant cells. This form of perinatal hemochromatosis is ascribed to an inborn error of iron metabolism.[60] In two female premature siblings born 4 years apart, severe neonatal hepatitis with heavy deposits of hemosiderin was present. In one of the patients hemosiderosis of the myocardium, spleen, pancreatic acini, islets, and renal tubules was also found.[103]

The urine contains bile, and the stools are acholic, green, or yellow. The direct and total serum bilirubin levels are always elevated and show either a slowly falling or variable trend. As a rule, the serum bilirubin levels in patients with atresia are lower than in patients with hepatitis. The transaminase is usually greatly elevated and an anemia of hemolytic type may develop.

Patients in this category are often noted to be poorly nourished as compared with those in other categories who exhibit good health. About 60% of these infants recover without sequelae, some develop cirrhosis, and others die of surgical complications.[87]

In a recent report the clinical and pathologic features of three male siblings with histologically proved giant cell hepatitis, together with similar familial cases in the literature, have lent weight to the importance of genetic factors.[30] A recessive mode of inheritance has been suggested in this syndrome.[87]

Idiopathic cirrhosis[169] in the newborn infant has been separated from the syndrome of neonatal hepatitis. It has an acute onset, with severe gastrointestinal disturbances and failure to thrive. Jaundice is initially mild or absent. The disease, characterized by hepatosplenomegaly, early ascites, and anasarca, is always fatal, usually within the first 3 months. Neonatal hepatitis, on the other hand, is characterized by an insidious onset of obstructive jaundice in an otherwise normal infant. The most notable microscopic feature in idiopathic cirrhosis is extensive periportal fibrosis. Heavy collagen trabeculae connect portal areas, encompassing lobules and often involving central veins. Cells vary in size, many exhibiting vacuolizations, swelling, and irregular staining characteristics. Giant cell formation that characterizes neonatal hepatitis is a rare finding. In neonatal hepatitis full recovery is usual, but it is stated that one out of every three affected infants eventually develops chronic liver disease.[169] When neonatal hepatitis is fatal during the acute stage, death is precipitated by an added insult to the diseased liver, such as surgery, infection, or acute dyspnea.

*Byler's disease.* In six infants of eleven Amish families, persistent jaundice with intermittent exacerbations, hepatosplenomegaly, foul-smelling steatorrhea, and dwarfism were found, followed by death between 17 months and 8 years of age in four of the six involved.[36] These patients had elevation of both indirect and direct bilirubin, hypoprothrombinemia, elevated alkaline phosphatase, and normal serum cholesterol. At laparotomy three were found to have normal extrahepatic biliary systems. Intrahepatic cholestasis and intracellular vacuoles containing bile pigment were present. Since all eight parents of the affected children were descended from Jacob Beiler, born in 1799, and his wife Nancy Kauffman, this disorder supports an autosomal recessive inheritance.

**Management of prolonged obstructive jaundice.** A variety of laboratory procedures are employed in the diagnosis of persistent jaundice. These consist principally of examination of the stool and urine for bile pigments, van den Bergh's reaction, serum glutamic oxalacetic transaminase (SGOT) and glutamic pyruvic transaminase (SGPT) levels, lactic dehydrogenase, alkaline phosphatase, cephalin flocculation test, specific tests for cytomegalic inclusion disease and toxoplasmosis, Bromsulphalein and rose bengal dye excretion tests, and the hematologic studies.

Some regard the serum transaminase carried out serially as the best means of arriving at a diagnosis.[100] Values up to 800 units are reached in hepatic cirrhosis due to biliary atresia, with values above this figure in neonatal viral hepatitis. Thus, a steadily rising transaminase suggests hepatitis rather than biliary atresia. It has also been observed that infants with a clinical picture of biliary obstruction may show normal neonatal levels of transaminase activity (SGOT) during the first 2 to 3 weeks of life. In such cases congenital malformation of the biliary tract is strongly suspected and surgical exploration warranted.[99]

Rose bengal tagged with radioiodine ($^{131}$I) has been helpful in diagnosing biliary obstruction.[180] In the normal infant the dye, when injected intravenously, is cleared from the blood by the liver and is promptly conveyed to the intestine. In hepatitis the blood is cleared slowly of the dye and appears in the intestine later, but in normal amounts. In biliary atresia, the blood is cleared of activity more slowly and no activity reaches the intestine. If less than 5% of the administered radioactive substance appears in the stools, then complete obstruction is said to be present. With all this information, it is still frequently impossible to differentiate biliary atresia from neonatal hepatitis.

Although evaluation from clinical and laboratory sources may be helpful, exploratory laparotomy is sometimes undertaken when jaundice is unduly prolonged. The problem becomes increasingly perplexing from the second to the fourth months of life when the type of liver involvement is not discernible and the possibility, even though vague, of biliary atresia is entertained. One of the drawbacks to surgical intervention was the earlier finding that such a procedure in infants under 3 months of age with liver damage is attended with serious risk.[126]

Gellis and Hsia[68] have provided indications for surgical exploration that are eminently practical. Operation is indicated if there is a consistent absence of bile in the stools or duodenal secretions and of urobilinogen in the urine, if the initial bilirubin level is low and shows a slowly progressive increase with no variability in pattern, if the flocculation tests are negative, and if there is no blood group incompatibility to suggest erythroblastosis. Operation should be deferred longer if there is bile in the stools or duodenal secretions even in small amounts, if urobilinogen is present in the urine in normal dilutions, if the initial bilirubin level is high or has shown a tendency to fall or be highly variable with no definite upward trend, if the flocculation tests are positive, and if the blood group incompatibility suggesting erythroblastosis can be demonstrated.

By examining liver tissue in cases of biliary atresia, Christy and Boley[35] have found that a large amount of fibrosis was already present within the first 2 months after birth and that it tended to increase with age. Instead of extensive abdominal explorations which are hazardous, Swenson and Fisher[167] have described a limited exploratory operation with direct cholangiography, utilizing the gallbladder and outlining the extrahepatic duct system with Diodrast. A liver biopsy is made at the same time. Subsequent extensive exploration is undertaken if no hepatic or common duct is visualized. With this program an exploratory procedure and correction can be undertaken before the third month of life.

Punch biopsy of the liver provides useful and often definitive information. There is a growing tendency to pursue the program[155] of surgical exploration and liver biopsy, if the precise nature of the jaundice is not diagnosed between the fourth week and the end of the second month. In the event that the final diagnosis rests between neonatal hepatitis and biliary atresia, an open liver biopsy is undertaken, the gallbladder and its contents identified, and an operative cholangiogram carried out using radiopaque material. If a normal duct system is demonstrated, the abdomen is closed, otherwise a thorough exploration for extrahepatic ducts is carried out. Many variations of this plan are in current use. In patients with a patent extrahepatic duct, anastomosis to the jejunum is possible. If none is available, a satisfactory operation is not possible.[83]

In a study of fifty-seven cases of neonatal obstructive jaundice Bennett[17] emphasized foremost the need for conservative management of neonatal obstructive jaundice. He found that clinical data and most laboratory tests were of little use in distinguishing between biliary atresia and neonatal hepatitis.

Serial bilirubin determinations were useful, since falling levels over a period of weeks is strong evidence for hepatitis. In only 12% of cases of biliary atresia was a correctable lesion found, but exploration carried an excessively high incidence of postoperative morbidity and mortality. Bennett found early operation in neonatal hepatitis was hazardous and there was evidence to indicate that if the operation is delayed until 3 months of age, many patients would show evidence of resolution of their disease. With a serial fall in bilirubin, exploration becomes unnecessary. His argument against early operation (4 to 8 weeks of age) is that an increasing number of patients with neonatal hepatitis will be subjected to a relatively dangerous and poorly tolerated procedure. From these divergent points of view, it is clear that each patient with obstructive jaundice must be subjected to individualized assessment as to the urgency of surgical intervention.

Medical treatment with magnesium sulfate and other cholagogues to establish an increased flow of bile has been reported,[137,139a] but has thus far proved unsuccessful. Steroids given orally will occasionally lower the bilirubin level in patients without biliary atresia, but experience with their use is still limited.

Thaler and Gellis[170] found that infants with neonatal hepatitis surgically explored for the possibility of biliary atresia developed cirrhosis three times as frequently as infants not surgically explored. Clinical, laboratory, and histological data did not permit differentiation of these two categories of cases. The fecal excretion of rose bengal sodium [131]I accurately revealed the presence of complete biliary obstruction. The higher incidence in infants operated upon was not due to the greater severity of the disease process but was associated with trauma sustained at surgery or with general anesthesia.

Results of repair of biliary atresia are notoriously poor. Only 3 of 135 cases of congenital biliary atresia were successfully reported.

In another study[171] they showed slow progression of cirrhosis over a period of several months. Factors other than age play a role in the development of cirrhosis in biliary atresia and suggest that once biliary flow is reestablished even advanced cirrhotic changes may regress completely.

Thaler and Gellis[172] also found that about 20% of cases of neonatal hepatitis cannot be distinguished by clinical or laboratory means from cases of extrahepatic biliary atresia during the first 4 months of life. As far as the diagnostic management of infants with neonatal hepatitis is concerned, a wait of up to 4 months of age is suggested before exploratory laparotomy is undertaken. This approach carries the least danger for infants with neonatal hepatitis, without jeopardizing the possibility of complete recovery in the salvageable case of biliary atresia.

*Galactosemia.* Galactosemia is almost always accompanied by obstructive jaundice during the first week of life and persists for a variable length of time thereafter. In the absence of anemia, hepatomegaly and a positive reaction for sugar warrant an examination for galactosemia. (The tape test does not detect galactose in the urine.) The congenital inability to convert galactose to glycogen in the liver is corrected by feeding the infant a milk substitute.[47,95] Anemia may be a prominent feature and appears to be partly hemolytic. In one series it occurred in twelve of forty-eight cases.[91] The hemoglobin may drop suddenly without bleeding, followed by an increased reticulocyte count. Purpura also is occasionally noted. Whether the accumulation of galactose-1-phosphate in erythrocytes that characterizes galactosemia plays a role in the anemia is unknown.

*Congenital familial nonhemolytic jaundice with kernicterus (Crigler-Najjar syndrome).* Congenital familial nonhemolytic jaundice with kernicterus has been reported by Crigler and Najjar.[42] Six of eight infants in a single large family had jaundice with severe neurologic disease from the second day of life until death, which usually occurred within the first year of life. There was no incompatibility of blood groups or evidence of hemolytic disease. The indirect serum bilirubin level was constantly elevated, with minimal elevations in the direct fraction. The affected infants showed evidence of kernicterus between 2 weeks and 3 months of age.

The abnormality depends upon a genetic defect consisting of an inability of hepatic cells to metabolize and excrete bilirubin. There is evidence to show that the abnormally high levels of indirect bilirubin represent defective conjugation with glucuronic acid required for conversion to soluble direct bilirubin. These patients are deficient in the same bilirubin glucuronyl transferase enzyme that is slow to develop in the newborn infant.

Exceptions to the occurrence of kernicterus were seen in two of the children in this family who have had persistent jaundice from birth but who have shown no neurologic disability, at 2 and 5 years of age.[34] In another case of this disease, not in the same family, neurologic symptoms did not appear until the patient was 3 years of age[146] despite the persistence of jaundice from birth. An infant was reported,[123] the eleventh infant with typical features of the syndromes described by Crigler and Najjar,[42] in whom jaundice was noted at 2 days, but who did not have definite signs of kernicterus until the age of about 9 weeks.

Except for the development of kernicterus, this condition corresponds to a type of retention jaundice which may be readily confused with chronic hemolytic jaundice—i.e., *familial nonhemolytic jaundice*.[44] It represents a form of constitutional hepatocellular dysfunction resulting in an accumulation of indirect bilirubin.

Anemia, microcytosis, spherocytosis, reticulocytosis, increased fragility of the red cells, splenomegaly, and increased excretion of urobilinogen in the urine and stools which characterize hereditary spherocytosis are absent in this condition. Jaundice in this form of familial nonhemolytic jaundice usually appears soon after birth and persists throughout life. The concentration of bilirubin in the serum seldom exceeds 15 mg. per 100 ml., with a range of 12 to 15 mg./100 ml., and is practically all of the indirect type. In most instances the disease (familial nonhemolytic jaundice) is found in young adults and follows a benign clinical course without bilirubin encephalopathy. The Crigler-Najjar syndrome,[42] on the other hand, is associated with severe hyperbilirubinemia with 10 to 44 mg. of serum bilirubin per 100 ml., with the greater portion primarily of the indirect type and the prognosis is poor.

In another section (p. 109) two types of the Crigler-Najjar syndrome are differentiated: in one with marked hyperbilirubinemia, kernicterus is frequent and unaffected by prolonged phenobarbital administration. In another type hyperbilirubinemia is less severe, kernicterus is absent, and the jaundice responds dramatically to phenobarbital therapy.

A patient with familial nonhemolytic jaundice (Crigler-Najjar) has been reported[20] who had been normal apart from his jaundice for all his life. At 16 years of age, however, he developed neurological disabilities which progressed to his death 6 months later. The signs were similar to those of kernicterus seen in infants. Attempts to reduce the bilirubin level of the blood (fourteen exchanges, peritoneal dialysis, phenobarbital, and a course of cholestyramine) and to reverse the nervous system damage were unsuccessful.

*Familial nonhemolytic jaundice (Gilbert's disease).* Gilbert's disease is a syndrome of chronic unconjugated hyperbilirubinemia without overt signs of hemolysis, occurring in adolescents and adults. It is based on an autosomal dominant gene with incomplete penetrance.[8] It represents a deficiency due to a defective conversion of unconjugated bilirubin to bilirubin glucuronide whereas in the Crigler-Najjar syndrome there is a total absence of glucuronyl transferase.

In Gilbert's syndrome the bilirubin ranges from 1.1 to 6.2 mg./100 ml., and this increase is in the unconjugated glucuronide fraction. Powell and co-workers[142] described fifty-five cases of idiopathic benign unconjugated hyperbilirubinemia, diagnosis made on the basis of chronic unconjugated hyperbilirubinemia, with normal serum transaminase, normal alkaline phosphatase, normal hepatic histology, no evidence of overt hemolysis, and no other illness that might cause hyperbilirubinemia. The distribution of serum bilirubin concentration in relatives fell into two groups, one closely approximating the normal range and the other similar to the patients. No relative was detected with an elevated conjugated hyperbilirubinemia and no patient showed abnormal pigmentation in the liver.

Familial nonhemolytic jaundice should be differentiated from congenital familial nonhemolytic jaundice with kernicterus, from the Dubin-Johnson syndrome where the diagnosis is based on liver biopsy and negative family history, from hereditary spherocytosis by absence of spherocytes and hemolysis, and from jaundice due to liver disease by liver function tests. No treatment is required for patients suffering from Gilbert's disease.

*Jaundice and carotenemia.* Carotenemia, occasionally confused with jaundice, refers to a harmless yellowish discoloration of the skin which occurs in infants and young children due to increased lipochromes in the blood from ingestion of carrots, squash, spinach, egg yolk, and other sources of dietary pigment. The discoloration appears especially in the skin of the palms, soles, forehead, and nasolabial folds. In contrast to jaundice it is absent from the conjunctivae and buccal mucous membranes. The icterus index is elevated, but the van den Bergh reaction is negative.[33]

*Jaundice due to pyloric stenosis.* Jaundice has been described[12,124] with a marked increase in the indirect-reacting bilirubin in the serum of patients with pyloric stenosis due to posterior angulation of the pyloric tumor and extrinsic pressure on the common bile duct. Another more likely explanation for the elevation of indirect bilirubin is that the flow of blood through the portal venous system is compromised by increased intra-abdominal pressure. With diminished venous flow, unconjugated or indirect bilirubin bypasses the conjugating mechanism located in the parenchymal cells of the liver.[133] The underperfusion of the liver prolongs the hyperbilirubinemia. With operative treatment, jaundice disappears promptly. This combination assumes importance only because of the need for differentiation from other contemporaneous types of obstructive jaundice.

*Jaundice and hypothyroidism.* Prolonged physiologic jaundice has been encountered in connection with congenital cretinism. This association may lead to an early diagnosis and treatment of the hypothyroid condition that might otherwise not have been suspected.[3] A cretinous infant has been reported[122] who exhibited prolonged jaundice which subsided on thyroid replacement therapy. Accidental withdrawal of treatment led to a return of jaundice. The second drop in bilirubin on readministering thyroid served to document the close association of thyroid insufficiency and unconjugated hyperbilirubinemia.

Another case was reported[81] of a hypothyroid baby who presented with jaundice in the newborn period. In this case the unconjugated fraction reached 23.9 mg. per 100 ml. An exchange transfusion resulted in a fall in bilirubin. Thyroxine was later administered and normal development was achieved.

*Hematomas.* Mild jaundice occasionally follows absorption of bilirubin from hematomas in diverse locations, including those in intracranial and subdural sites. On the other hand, extensive hemorrhage into the tissues of the newborn infant may result in severe hyperbilirubinemia from the breakdown of hemoglobin in enclosed areas such as in the face, extremities, or in giant cephalhematoma.[104,145] Exchange transfusions may be required as in other cases in which indirect bilirubin rises to dangerous levels. Thrombocytopenia may accompany the sequestered blood accumulations.

Two types of cephalhematoma may be differentiated, the subperiostic and the subaponeurotic (subgaleal). In the subperiosteal type the periostium exerts a moderate degree of compression which tends to terminate bleeding. Reabsorption is slow so that there is no marked tendency to hyperbilirubinemia. Severe exsanguinating hemorrhages under the scalp are usually the second type, the subaponeurotic, often associated with a coagulation defect. Blood spreads along the fascial planes into the tissues of the neck, and substantial amounts of blood may be lost. The hemorrhage is reabsorbed quickly and the degree of hyperbilirubinemia reached may justify exchange transfusion. Both subperiosteal and subaponeurotic hemorrhages may occur together in the same infant.

*Miscellaneous.* In addition to cretinism and pyloric stenosis, prolonged "physiologic jaundice" may be due to other abnormalities such as congenital heart lesions and kidney disease.[66]

## REFERENCES

1. Aagenaes, Ø., Van de Hagen, C. B., and Rafsum, S.: Hereditary recurrent intrahepatic cholestasis from birth, Arch. Dis. Child. **43**:646, 1968.
2. Ahrens, E. H., Jr., Harris, R. C., and MacMahon, H. E.: Atresia of the intrahepatic bile ducts, Pediatrics **8**:628, 1951.
3. Akerren, Y.: Early diagnosis and early therapy in congenital cretinism, Arch. Dis. Child. **30**:254, 1955.
4. Allison, A. C.: Danger of vitamin K to newborn, Lancet **1**:669, 1955.
5. Allison, A. C.: Acute haemolytic anaemia with distortion and fragmentation of erythrocytes in children, Brit. J. Haemat. **3**:1, 1957.
6. Alpert, L. I., Strauss, L., and Hirschhorn, K.: Neonatal hepatitis and biliary atresia associated with 17-18 syndrome, New Eng. J. Med. **280**:16, 1969.
7. Alterman, K.: Neonatal hepatitis and its relation to viral hepatitis of mother; a review of the problem, Amer. J. Dis. Child. **105**:395, 1963.

8. Arias, I. M.: Chronic unconjugated hyperbilirubinemia without overt signs of hemolysis in adolescents and adults, J. Clin. Invest. 41:2233, 1962.
9. Arias, I. M., Gartner, L. M., Seifter, S., and Furman, M.: Neonatal unconjugated hyperbilirubinemia associated with breast-feeding and factor in milk that inhibits glucuronide formation in vitro, J. Clin. Invest. 42:913, 1963.
10. Arias, I. M., Gartner, L. M., Seifter, S., and Furman, M.: Prolonged neonatal unconjugated hyperbilirubinemia associated with breast feeding and a steroid, pregnane-3 (alpha) 20 (beta)-diol, in maternal milk that inhibits glucuronide formation in vitro, J. Clin. Invest. 43:2037, 1964.
11. Arias, I. M., and London, I. M.: Bilirubin glucuronide formation in vitro; demonstration of a defect in Gilbert's disease, Science 126:563, 1957.
12. Arias, I. M., Schorr, J. B., and Fraad, L. M.: Clinical conference; congenital hypertrophic pyloric stenosis with jaundice, Pediatrics 24:338, 1959.
13. Arias, I. M., Wolfson, S., Lucey, J. F., and McKay, R. J., Jr.: Transient familial neonatal hyperbilirubinemia, J. Clin. Invest. 44:1442, 1965.
14. Bain, A. D., Bowie, J. H., Flint, W. F., Beverly, J. K. A., and Beattie, C. P.: Congenital toxoplasmosis simulating haemolytic disease of the newborn, J. Obstet. Gynaec. Brit. Emp. 63:826, 1956.
15. Behrman, R. E., and Fisher, O. E.: Phenobarbital for neonatal jaundice, J. Pediat. 76:945, 1970.
16. Behrman, R. E., and Hsia, D. Y-Y.: Summary of Symposium on Phototherapy for Hyperbilirubinemia, J. Pediat. 75:718, 1969.
17. Bennett, D. E.: Problems in neonatal obstructive jaundice, Pediatrics 33:735, 1964.
18. Billing, B. H., and Lathe, G. H.: The excretion of bilirubin as an ester glucuronide, giving the direct van den Bergh reaction, Biochem. J. 63:6, 1956.
19. Billing, B. H., and Lathe, G. H.: Bilirubin metabolism in jaundice, Amer. J. Med. 24:111, 1958.
20. Blumenschein, S. D., Kallen, R. J., Storey, B., Natzschka, J. C., Odell, G. B., and Childs, B.: Familial nonhemolytic jaundice with late onset of neurological damage, Pediatrics 42:786, 1968.
21. Bound, J. P., and Telfer, T. P.: Effect of vitamin K dosage on plasma—bilirubin levels in premature infants, Lancet 1:720, 1956.
22. Brent, R. L.: Persistent jaundice of infancy, J. Pediat. 61:111, 1962.
23. Broughton, P. M., Rossiter, E. J., Warren, C. B., and Goulis, G.: Effect of blue light on hyperbilirubinemia, Arch. Dis. Child. 40:666, 1965.
24. Brown, A. K.: Neonatal jaundice, Ped. Clin. N. Amer. 9:575, 1962.
25. Brown, A. K.: Bilirubin metabolism with special reference to neonatal jaundice. In Levine, S. Z., editor: Advances in pediatrics, vol. 12, Chicago, 1962, Year Book Medical Publishers, Inc.
26. Brown, A. K., and Zuelzer, W. W.: Studies in hyperbilirubinemia; hyperbilirubinemia of the newborn unrelated to isoimmunization, Amer. J. Dis. Child. 93:263, 1957.
27. Brown, A. K., and Zuelzer, W. W.: Studies on the neonatal development of the glucuronide conjugating system, J. Clin. Invest. 37:332, 1958.
28. Brown, W. R., and Boon, W. H.: Hyperbilirubinemia in G-6-PD deficient Singapore infants, Pediatrics 41:1055, 1968.
29. Bruton, O. C., Crosby, W. H., and Motulsky, A. G.: Hereditary non-spherocytic hemolytic anemia presenting as hemolytic disease of the newborn infant, Pediatrics 13:41, 1954.
30. Cassady, G., Morrison, A. B., and Cohen, M. M.: Familial "giant-cell hepatitis" in infancy; clinical, pathologic and genetic studies on a large family, Amer. J. Dis. Child. 107:456, 1964.
31. Catz, C. S., and Yaffé, S. J.: Pharmacological modification of bilirubin conjugation in newborn, Amer. J. Dis. Child. 104:516, 1962.
32. Catz, C. S., and Yaffé, S. J.: Barbiturate enhancement of bilirubin conjugation and excretion in young and adult animals, Pediat. Res. 2:361, 1968.
33. Cecil, R. L., and Loeb, R. F., and others, editors: Textbook of medicine, ed. 9, Philadelphia, 1955, W. B. Saunders Co., p. 926.
34. Childs, B., and Najjar, V. A.: Familial non-hemolytic jaundice with kernicterus; a report of two cases without neurologic damage, Pediatrics 18:369, 1956.
35. Christy, R. A., and Boley, J. O.: The relation of hepatic fibrosis to concentration of bilirubin in the serum in congenital atresia of the biliary tract, Pediatrics 21:226, 1958.
36. Clayton, R. J., Iber, F. L., Ruebner, B., and McKusick, V. A.: Byler's disease; a fatal familial intrahepatic cholestasis in an Amish kindred, J. Pediat. 67:1025, 1965.
37. Cock, T. C.: Acute hemolytic anemia in the neonatal period, Amer. J. Dis. Child. 94:77, 1957.
38. Cole, P. G., and Lathe, G. H.: The separation of serum pigments giving the direct and indirect van den Bergh reaction, J. Clin. Path. 6:99, 1953.

39. Craig, J. M., and Landing, B. H.: Form of hepatitis in neonatal period simulating biliary atresia, Arch. Path. 54:321, 1954.
40. Cremer, R. J., Perryman, F. W., and Richards, D. H.: Influence of light on the hyperbilirubinemia of infants, Lancet 1:1094, 1958.
41. Crigler, J. F., and Gold, N. J.: Sodium phenobarbital-induced disease in serum bilirubin in an infant with congenital nonhemolytic jaundice and kernicterus, J. Clin. Invest. 45:998, 1966.
42. Crigler, J. F., and Najjar, V. A.: Congenital familial nonhemolytic jaundice with kernicterus; a new clinical entity, Pediatrics 10:169, 1952.
43. Cunningham, M. D., Mace, J. W., and Peters, E. R.: Clinical experience with phenobarbitone in icterus neonatorum, Lancet 1:550, 1969.
44. Dameshek, W., and Singer, K.: Familial nonhemolytic jaundice; constitutional hepatic dysfunction with indirect van den Bergh reaction, Arch. Intern. Med. 67:259, 1941.
45. Danks, D., and Bodian, M.: A genetic study of neonatal obstructive jaundice, Arch. Dis. Child. 38:378, 1963.
46. Dawson, J. P., Thayer, W. W., and Desforges, J. F.: Acute hemolytic anemia in the newborn infant due to naphthalene poisoning; report of two cases, with investigations into the mechanism of the disease, Blood 13:1113, 1958.
47. Dormell, G. N., and Lann, S. H.: Galactosemia; report of four cases, Pediatrics 7:503, 1951.
48. Doses of water-soluble vitamin K analogues in hemorrhagic disease of the newborn, J.A.M.A. 164:1331, 1957.
49. Doxiadis, S. A., Fessas, Ph., and Valaes, T.: Glucose-6-phosphate dehydrogenase deficiency; a new aetiological factor of severe neonatal jaundice, Lancet 1:297, 1961.
50. Doxiadis, S. A., and Valaes, T.: The clinical picture of glucose-6-phosphate dehydrogenase deficiency in early infancy, Arch. Dis. Child. 39:545, 1964.
51. Doxiadis, S. A., Valaes, T., Karaklis, A., and Stavrakakis, D.: Risk of severe jaundice in glucose-6-phosphate-dehydrogenase deficiency of the newborn, Lancet 2:1210, 1964.
52. Dubin, I. N.: Chronic idiopathic jaundice; a review of fifty cases, Amer. J. Med. 24:268, 1958.
53. Dubin, I. N., and Johnson, F. B.: Chronic idiopathic jaundice with unidentified pigment in liver cells; a new clinico-pathologic entity with a report of 12 cases, Medicine 33:155, 1954.
54. Dutton, G. J., and Stevenson, I. H.: Synthesis of glucuronide and the uridine diphosphate glucuronic acid in kidney cortex and gastric mucosa, Biochim. et Biophys. Acta 31:568, 1959.
55. Eichenwald, H. F.: The laboratory diagnosis of toxoplasmosis, Ann. N. Y. Acad. Sci. 64:207, 1956.
56. Eichenwald, H. F.: Toxoplasmosis; a study of 150 cases, Amer. J. Dis. Child. 94:411, 1957.
57. Eichenwald, H. F.: A study of congenital toxoplasmosis with particular emphasis on clinical manifestations, sequellae and therapy. In Siim, J. Chr., editor: Human toxoplasmosis, Copenhagen, 1960, Ejnar Munksgaard Forlag.
58. Esbaughpoor, E., Oski, F. A., and Williams, M.: The relationship of erythrocyte glucose-6-phosphate dehydrogenase deficiency to hyperbilirubinemia in Negro premature infants, J. Pediat. 70:595, 1967.
59. Fessas, Ph., Doxiadis, S. A., and Valaes, T.: Neonatal jaundice in glucose-6-phosphate-dehydrogenase deficient infants, Brit. J. Med. 2:1359, 1962.
60. Fienberg, R.: Perinatal idiopathic hemochromatosis; giant-cell hepatitis interpreted as an inborn error of metabolism, Amer. J. Clin. Path. 33:480, 1960.
61. Findlay, L., Higgins, G., and Stanier, W.: Icterus neonatorum; its incidence and cause, Arch. Dis. Child. 22:65, 1947.
62. Foulk, W. T., Butt, H. R., Owen, C. A., Jr., Whitcomb, F. F., Jr., and Mason, H. L.: Constitutional hepatic dysfunction (Gilbert's disease); its natural history and related syndromes, Medicine 38:25, 1959.
63. Gartner, L. M.: Jaundice in the newborn. In Barnett, H. L., editor: Pediatrics, ed. 14, New York, 1968, Appleton-Century-Crofts.
64. Gartner, L. M., and Arias, I. M.: Formation, transport, metabolism and excretion of bilirubin, New Eng. J. Med. 280:1339, 1969.
65. Gasser, C.: Die hämolytische Frühgeburtenanämie mit spontaner Innenkörperbildung, ein neues Syndrom, beobachtet an 14 Fällen, Helv. Paediat. Acta 8:491, 1953.
66. Gellis, S. S., editor: Year Book of Pediatrics, 1956-1957 Series, Chicago, 1956, Year Book Medical Publishers, Inc., p. 310.
67. Gellis, S. S.: Current problems in liver disease in infancy and childhood. In Progress in liver disease, New York, 1961, Grune & Stratton, Inc.
68. Gellis, S. S., and Hsia, D. Y-Y.: Jaundice in infancy, Ped. Clin. N. Amer. 2:449, 1955.
69. Gilbert, A., and Lereboullet, P.: La cholemie

simple familiale, Semaine Méd. **21**:241, 1901.
70. Giunta, F., and Rath, J.: Effect of environmental illumination in prevention of hyperbilirubinemia of prematurity, Pediatrics **44**:162, 1969.
71. Gorodischer, R., Levy, G., Krasner, I., and Yaffé, S. J.: Congenital nonobstructive nonhemolytic jaundice; effect of phototherapy, New Eng. J. Med. **282**:375, 1970.
72. Gottman, A. W., and Beatty, E. C., Jr.: Cytomegalic inclusion disease in children with leukemia or lymphosarcoma, Amer. J. Dis. Child. **104**:180, 1962.
73. Gregory, C. H.: Studies of conjugated bilirubin. III. Pigment I complex of conjugated and free bilirubin, J. Lab. Clin. Med. **61**:917, 1963.
74. Hanshaw, J. B., and Weller, T. H.: Urinary excretion of cytomegaloviruses by children with generalized neoplastic disease, J. Pediat. **58**:305, 1961.
75. Hargreaves, T., and Holton, J. B.: Jaundice of the newborn due to novobiocin, Lancet **1**:839, 1962.
76. Harley, J. D., and Robin, H.: Glucose-6-phosphate dehydrogenase deficiency: prenatal and post-natal implications, M. J. Australia **1**:198, 1963.
77. Harris, L. E., Farrell, F. J., Shorter, R. G., Banner, E. A., and Mathieson, D. R.: Conjugated serum bilirubin in erythroblastosis fetalis; analysis of 38 cases, Proc. Staff Meet. Mayo Clin. **37**:574, 1962.
78. Harris, R. C., and Anderson, D. H.: Intrahepatic bile duct atresia, Amer. J. Dis. Child. **100**:783, 1960.
79. Harris, R. C., Anderson, D. H., and Day, R. L.: Obstructive jaundice in infants with normal biliary tree, Pediatrics **13**:293, 1954.
80. Haverback, B. J., and Wirtschafter, S. K.: Familial nonhemolytic jaundice with normal liver histology and conjugated bilirubin, New Eng. J. Med. **262**:113, 1960.
81. Henchman, D. C., and McIntosh, A. J.: A Cretin with jaundice requiring exchange transfusion, Australian Paediat. J. **4**:203, 1968.
82. Hoffmann, H. N. II, Whitcomb, F. F., Jr., Butt, H. R., and Bollman, J. L.: Bile pigments of jaundice, J. Clin. Invest. **39**:132, 1960.
83. Holder, T. H.: Atresia of the extrahepatic bile duct, Amer. J. Surg. **107**:459, 1964.
84. Hollingsworth, J. W.: Life span of fetal erythrocytes, J. Lab. Clin. Med. **45**:469, 1955.
85. Hsia, D. Y-Y.: In Gellis, S. S., editor: Year Book of Pediatrics, 1961-1962 Series, Chicago, 1961, Year Book Medical Publishers, Inc., p. 297.
86. Hsia, D. Y-Y., Allen, F. H., Jr., Diamond, L. K., and Gellis, S. S.: Serum bilirubin levels in the newborn infant, J. Pediat. **42**:277, 1953.
87. Hsia, D. Y-Y., Boggs, J. D., Driscoll, S. G., and Gellis, S. S.: Prolonged obstructive jaundice in infancy, the genetic components in neonatal hepatitis, Amer. J. Dis. Child. **95**:485, 1958.
88. Hsia, D. Y-Y., Dowben, R. M., Shaw, R., and Grossman, A.: The inhibition of glucuronosyl transferase by progestational agents from pregnant serum, Amer. J. Dis. Child. **100**:599, 1960.
89. Hsia, D. Y-Y., Goldbloom, R. B., and Gellis, S. S.: Studies of the mechanical fragility of erythrocytes; relation to physiologic jaundice of the newborn infant, Pediatrics **13**:24, 1954.
90. Hsia, D. Y-Y., Patterson, P., Allen, F. H., Jr., Diamond, L. K., and Gellis, S. S.: Prolonged obstructive jaundice in infancy; general survey of 156 cases, Pediatrics **10**:243, 1952.
91. Hsia, D. Y-Y., and Walker, F. A.: Variability in the clinical manifestations of galactosemia, J. Pediat. **59**:872, 1961.
92. Hubbell, J. P., Jr., Drorbaugh, J. F., Rudolph, A. J., Auld, P. A. M., Cherry, R. B., and Smith, C. A.: "Early" versus "late" feeding of infants of diabetic mothers, New Eng. J. Med. **265**:835, 1961.
93. Isselbacher, K. J., and McCarthy, E. A.: Studies on bilirubin sulfate and other non-glucuronide conjugates of bilirubin, J. Clin. Invest. **38**:645, 1959.
94. John, G. G., and Knudtson, K. P.: Chronic idiopathic jaundice; two cases occurring in siblings, with histochemical studies, Amer. J. Med. **21**:128, 1956.
95. Johns, D.: Galactosemia; an unusual cause of neonatal jaundice, Amer. J. Dis. Child. **85**:575, 1953.
96. Karon, M., Imach, D., and Schwartz, A.: Effective phototherapy in congenital nonobstructive jaundice, New Eng. J. Med. **282**:377, 1970.
97. Kasai, M., Yakavac, W. C., and Koop, C. E.: Liver in congenital biliary atresia and neonatal hepatitis; a histopathologic study, Arch. Path. **74**:152, 1962.
98. Khanna, N. N., Stern, L., Levy, G., and Yaffé, S. J.: Effect of phenobarbital on neonatal hyperbilirubinemia, Program, 38th meeting Soc. for Ped. Res. 1968.
98a. Kopelman, A. E., Brown, R. S., and Odell, G. B.: The "bronze baby," a complication of phototherapy, American Pediatrics Society Program and Abstracts, 1971, p. 3.
99. Kove, S., Dische, R., and Wroblewski, F.:

Early diagnosis of biliary tract malformation in newborn infant by serum transaminase pattern, New York J. Med. **63**:3497, 1963.
100. Kove, S., Perry, R., and Wroblewski, F.: Diagnosis of neonatal jaundice by patterns of serum transaminase, Amer. J. Dis. Child. **100**:47, 1960.
101. Lancet Editorial: Neonatal hepatitis; a new syndrome? Lancet **1**:1011, 1969.
102. Lathe, G. H., and Walker, M.: The inhibitory effect of human pregnancy serum, neonatal serum, and steroids on the conjugation of bilirubin by rat liver slices, Biochem. J. **68**:6P, 1958.
103. Laurendeau, T., Hill, J. E., and Mannings, G. B.: Idiopathic neonatal hemochromatosis in siblings, Arch. Path. **72**:410, 1961.
104. Leonard, S., and Anthony, B.: Giant cephalhematoma of newborn, Amer. J. Dis. Child. **101**:170, 1961.
105. Lester, R., Behrman, R. E., and Lucey, J. F.: Transfer of bilirubin—$C^{14}$ across monkey placenta, Pediatrics **32**:416, 1963.
106. Lester, R., and Schmid, R.: Intestinal absorption of bile pigments. I. Enterohepatic circulation of bilirubin in rat, J. Clin. Invest. **42**:736, 1963.
107. Lester, R., and Schmid, R.: Intestinal absorption of bile pigments. II. Bilirubin absorption in man, New Eng. J. Med. **269**:178, 1963.
108. Lester, R., and Schmid, R.: Bilirubin metabolism, New Eng. J. Med. **270**:779, 1964.
109. Levine, R. A., and Klatsken, G.: Unconjugated hyperbilirubinemia in the absence of overt hemolysis, Amer. J. Med. **36**:541, 1964.
110. Lipton, E. L.: Elliptocytosis with hemolytic anemia; the effects of splenectomy, Pediatrics **15**:67, 1955.
111. Lokietz, H., Dowben, R. M., and Hsia, D. Y-Y: Studies on the effect of novobiocin on glucuronyl transferase, Pediatrics **32**:47, 1963.
112. Lucey, J. F.: Review article; hyperbilirubinemia of prematurity, Pediatrics **25**:690, 1960.
113. Lucey, J. F.: In May, C. D., editor: Prenatal pharmacology, report of the 41st Ross Conference on Pediatric Research, Columbus, Ohio, 1962, Ross Laboratories.
114. Lucey, J. F.: Phototherapy of jaundice, 1969; Birth Defects; Original Article Series, vol. VI, no. 2, Baltimore, 1970, The Williams & Wilkins Co., p. 63.
115. Lucey, J. F., Arias, I. M., and McKay, R. J., Jr.: Transient familial neonatal hyperbilirubinemia, Amer. J. Dis. Child. **100**:787, 1960.
116. Lucey, J. F., Behrman, R. E., and Warshow, A. L.: "Physiologic" jaundice in new born rhesus monkey, Amer. J. Dis. Child. **106**:350, 1963.
117. Lucey, J. F., and Dolan, R. G.: Injections of a vitamin K compound in mothers and hyperbilirubinemia in the newborn, Pediatrics **22**:605, 1958.
118. Lucey, J. F., and Driscoll, T. S.: Physiologic jaundice re-examined. In Sass-Kortsak, A., editor: Kernicterus, Toronto, 1961, University of Toronto Press, pp. 29-36.
119. Lucey, J. F., Ferreiro, M., and Hewitt, J.: Prevention of hyperbilirubinemia of prematurity by phototherapy, Pediatrics **41**:1047, 1968.
120. Macauley, D.: Acholuric jaundice in a newborn infant, Arch. Dis. Child. **26**:241, 1951.
121. Margileth, A. M.: The diagnosis and treatment of generalized cytomegalic inclusion disease of the newborn, Pediatrics **15**:270, 1955.
122. MacGillivray, M. H., Crawford, J. D., and Robey, J. S.: Congenital hypothyroidism and prolonged neonatal hyperbilirubinemia, Pediatrics **40**:283, 1967.
123. Martin, H. F., Black, O., and VanLeevwen, G.: Congenital nonhemolytic icterus; report of a case, Amer. J. Dis. Child. **107**:195, 1964.
124. Martin, J. W., and Siebenthal, B. L.: Jaundice due to hypertrophic pyloric stenosis, J. Pediat. **47**:95, 1955.
125. Maurer, H. M., Wolff, J. A., Finster, M., Poppers, P. J., Pantuck, K. E., Kuntzman, R., and Conney, A. H.: Reduction in concentration of total serum-bilirubin in offspring of women treated with phenobarbital during pregnancy, Lancet **2**:122, 1968.
126. McGovern, R.: Resident's meeting, section on pediatrics, New York Academy of Medicine, Dec. 13, 1951.
127. McMullen, G. P.: Phenobarbitone and neonatal jaundice, Lancet **11**:978, 1968.
128. Medearis, D. N., Jr.: Cytomegalic inclusion disease; an analysis of the clinical features based on the literature and six additional cases, Pediatrics **19**:467, 1957.
129. Medearis, D. N., Jr.; Observations concerning human cytomegalovirus infections and disease, Bull. Johns Hopkins Hosp. **114**:181, 1964.
130. Meyer, T. C., and Angus, J.: The effect of large doses of "Synkavit" in the newborn, Arch. Dis. Child. **31**:212, 1956.
131. Mollison, P. L.: Blood transfusion in clinical medicine, ed. 2, Oxford, 1956, Blackwell Scientific Publications, p. 130.
132. Nakai, H., and Landing, B.: Factors in the genesis of bile stasis in infancy, Pediatrics **27**:300, 1961.

133. Nakai, H., and Margaretta, W.: Protracted jaundice associated with hypertrophic pyloric stenosis, Pediatrics 29:198, 1962.
134. Newman, A. J., and Gross, S.: Hyperbilirubinemia in breast-fed infants, Pediatrics 32:995, 1963.
135. Nusbacher, J., Hirschhorn, K., and Cooper, L. Z.: Chromosomal abnormalities in congenital rubella, New Eng. J. Med. 276:1409, 1967.
136. Obrinsky, W., Allen, E. L., and Anderson, E. E.: Physiologic hyperbilirubinemia in premature infants, Amer. J. Dis. Child. 87:305, 1954.
137. O'Donohoe, N. V.: Obstructive jaundice in haemolytic disease of the newborn treated with magnesium sulphate, Arch. Dis. Child. 30:234, 1955.
138. Okcuoglu, A.: Erythrocyte glucose-6-phosphate dehydrogenase; a study of the enzyme activity in children, Amer. J. Dis Child. 107:116, 1964.
139. Patel, D. A., Pildes, R. S., and Behrman, R. E.: Failure of phototherapy to reduce serum bilirubin in newborn infants, J. Pediat. 77:1048, 1970.
139a. Patterson, P.: Study of the duodenal fluid in infants with jaundice, Amer. J. Dis. Child. 84:415, 1952.
140. Porto, S. O., Pildes, R. S., and Goodman, H.: Studies on the effect of phototherapy on neonatal hyperbilirubinemia among low-birth-weight infants. I. Skin color, J. Pediat. 75:1045, 1969.
141. Porto, S. O., Pildes, R. S., and Goodman, H.: Studies on the effect of phototherapy on neonatal hyperbilirubinemia among low-birth-weight infants. II. Protein binding capacity, J. Pediat. 75:1048, 1969.
142. Powell, L. H., Hemingway, E., Billing, B. H., and Sherlock, S.: Idiopathic unconjugated hyperbilirubinemia (Gilbert's disease), New Eng. J. Med. 277:1108, 1967.
143. Ramboer, C., Thompson, R. P. H., and Williams, R.: Controlled trials of phenobarbital therapy in neonatal jaundice, Lancet 1:966, 1968.
144. Rapmund, G., Bowman, J. M., and Harris, R. C.: Bilirubinemia in nonerythroblastotic premature infants, Amer. J. Dis. Child. 99:604, 1960.
145. Rausen, A. K., and Diamond, L. K.: "Enclosed" hemorrhage and neonatal jaundice, Amer. J. Dis. Child. 101:164, 1961.
146. Rosenthal, I. M., Zimmerman, H. J., and Hardy, N.: Congenital non-hemolytic jaundice with disease of the central nervous system, Pediatrics 18:378, 1956.
147. Rotor, A. B., Manahan, L., and Florentin, A.: Familial nonhemolytic jaundice with direct van den Bergh reaction, Acta Med. Philippines 5:37, 1948.
148. Schafer, W. B.: Acute hemolytic anemia related to napthalene, Pediatrics 7:172, 1951.
149. Schenker, S., Dawber, N. H., and Schmid, R.: Bilirubin metabolism in fetus, J. Clin. Invest. 43:32, 1964.
150. Schiff, L., Billing, B. H., and Oikawa, Y.: Familial nonhemolytic jaundice with conjugated bilirubin in the serum, New Eng. J. Med. 260:1315, 1959.
151. Schmid, R.: Jaundice and bilirubin metabolism, Arch. Intern. Med. 101:669, 1958.
152. Schmid, R., Axelrod, J., Hammaker, L., and Rosenthal, I. M.: Congenital defects in bilirubin metabolism, J. Clin. Invest. 36:927, 1957.
153. Schoenfield, L. J., McGill, D. B., Hunton, D. B., Foulk, W. T., and Butt, H. R.: Studies of chronic idiopathic jaundice (Dubin-Johnson syndrome). 1. Demonstration of hepatic excretory defect, Gastroenterology 44:101, 1963.
154. Seeler, R. A., and Hahn, K.: Jaundice in urinary tract infection in infancy, Amer. J. Dis. Child. 118:553, 1969.
155. Silverberg, M., Craig, J., and Gellis, S. S.: Problems in diagnosis of a biliary atresia; review and consideration of histologic criteria, Amer. J. Dis. Child. 99:574, 1960.
156. Silverman, W. A.: Cytomegalic inclusion disease, Pediatrics 21:682, 1958.
156a. Sisson, T. R. C., Glauser, S. C., Glauser, E. M., Tisman, W., and Kuwabara, T.: Retinal changes produced by phototherapy, J. Pediat. 77:22, 1970.
157. Smetana, H. F., and Johnson, F. B.: Neonatal jaundice with giant cell transformation of hepatic parenchyma, Amer. J. Path. 31:747, 1955.
158. Smith, C. H.: The magic of numbers—"20 milligrams of bilirubin," J. Pediat. 56:712, 1960.
159. Smith, M. G.: The salivary gland viruses of man and animals (cytomegalic inclusion disease), Prog. Med. Vir. 2:171, 1959.
160. Smith, R. T., Platou, E. S., and Good, R. A.: Septicemia of the newborn; current status of the problem, Pediatrics 17:549, 1956.
161. Sprinz, H., and Nelson, R. S.: Persistent nonhemolytic hyperbilirubinemia associated with lipochrome-like pigment in liver cells; report of four cases, Ann. Intern. Med. 41:952, 1954.
162. Stamey, C. C., and Diamond, L. K.: Congenital hemolytic anemia in the newborn; relationship to kernicterus, Amer. J. Dis. Child. 94:616, 1957.
163. Stempfel, R., Broman, B., Excardo, F. E., and Zetterstrom, R.: Obstructive jaundice

complicating hemolytic disease of the newborn, Pediatrics **17**:471, 1956.
164. Stiehm, E. R., and Ryan, J.: Breast milk jaundice; report of eight cases and effect of breast feeding on incidence and severity of unexplained hyperbilirubinemia, Amer. J. Dis. Child. **109**:212, 1965.
165. Stokes, J., Jr.: Wohlman, I. J., Blanchard, M. C., and Farquhar, J. D.: Viral hepatitis in the newborn; clinical features, epidemiology and pathology, Amer. J. Dis. Child. **82**:213, 1951.
166. Sutherland, J. M., and Keller, W. M.: Novobiocin and neonatal hyperbilirubinemia; an investigation of the relationship in an epidemic of neonatal hyperbilirubinemia, Amer. J. Dis. Child. **101**:447, 1961.
167. Swenson, O., and Fisher, J. H.: Surgical aspects of liver disease, Pediatrics **16**:135, 1955.
168. Taylor, P. M., Birchard, E. L., Bright, N. H., Wolfson, J. H., and Watson, D. W.: Hyperbilirubinemia in infants of diabetic mothers, Amer. J. Dis. Child. **98**:499, 1959.
169. Thaler, M. M.: Fetal neonatal cirrhosis; entity or end result? A comparative study of 24 cases, Pediatrics **33**:721, 1964.
170. Thaler, M. M., and Gellis, S. S.: Studies in neonatal hepatitis and biliary atresia. II. The effect of diagnostic laparotomy on long-term prognosis of neonatal hepatitis, Amer. J. Dis. Child. **116**:262, 1968.
171. Thaler, M. M., and Gellis, S. S.: Studies in neonatal hepatitis and biliary atresia. III. Progression and regression of cirrhosis in biliary atresia, Amer. J. Dis. Child. **116**:271, 1968.
172. Thaler, M. M., and Gellis, S. S.: Studies in neonatal hepatitis and biliary atresia. IV. Diagnosis, Amer. J. Dis. Child. **116**:280, 1968.
173. Trolle, D.: Decrease of total serum-bilirubin concentration in newborn infants after phenobarbital treatment, Lancet **2**:705, 1968.
174. Valaes, T., Petmezaki, S., and Doxiadis, S. A.: Effect on neonatal hyperbilirubinemia of phenobarbital during pregnancy or after birth; practical value of the treatment in a population with high risk of unexplained severe neonatal jaundice. In Bergsma, D., editor: Birth Defects, Original Article Series, Vol. VI, No. 2, Bilirubin metabolism in the newborn, Baltimore, 1970, The Williams & Wilkins Co., p. 46.
175. Varadi, S., and Hurworth, E.: Heinz-body anemia in the newborn, Brit. Med. J. **1**:315, 1957.
176. Vest, M. F., and Grieder, H. R.: Erythrocyte survival in the newborn infant as measured by chromium and its relation to the postnatal serum bilirubin level, J. Pediat. **59**:194, 1961.
177. Weech, A. A.: Genesis of physiologic hyperbilirubinemia. In Levine, S. Z., and others, editors: Advances in pediatrics, vol. 2, New York, 1947, Interscience Publishers, Inc., p. 346.
178. Weller, T. H., and Hanshaw, J. B.: Virologic and clinical observations on cytomegalic inclusion disease, New Eng. J. Med. **266**:1233, 1962.
179. Weller, T. H., Macauley, J. C., Craig, J. M., and Wirth, P.: Isolation of intranuclear inclusion producing agents from infants with illness resembling cytomegalic inclusion disease, Proc. Soc. Exp. Biol. Med. **94**:4, 1957.
180. White, W. E., Welsh, J. S., Darrow, D., and Holder, T. M.: Pediatric application of the radioiodine (I-131) rose bengal method in hepatic and biliary system disease, Pediatrics **32**:239, 1963.
181. Wilson, J. T.: Phenobarbital in the perinatal period, Pediatrics **43**:324, 1968.
182. Yaffé, S. J., Catz, C. S., Stern, L., and Levy G.: The use of phenobarbital in neonatal jaundice. In Bergsma, D., editor: Birth Defects, Original Article Series, Vol VI, No. 2, Bilirubin metabolism in the newborn, Baltimore, 1970, The Williams & Wilkins Co., p. 37.
183. Yaffé, S. J., Levy, G., Matsuzawa, T., and Baliah, T.: Enhancement of glucoronide-conjugated capacity in a hyperbilirubinemic infant due to apparent enzyme induction by phenobarbital, New Eng. J. Med. **275**:1461, 1966.
184. Zinkham, W. H.: An in vitro abnormality of glutathione metabolism in erythrocytes from normal newborns; mechanism and clinical significance, Pediatrics **23**:18, 1959.
185. Zinkham, W. H., and Childs, B.: Effect of vitamin K and napthalene metabolites on glutathione metabolism of erythrocytes from normal newborns and patients with naphthalene hemolytic anemia, Amer. J. Dis. Child. **94**:420, 1957.
186. Zinkham, W. H., and Childs, B.: A defect of glutathione metabolism in erythrocytes from patients with a naphthalene-induced hemolytic anemia, Pediatrics **22**:461, 1958.
187. Zuelzer, W. W., and Apt, L.: Acute hemolytic anemia due to naphthalene poisoning, J.A.M.A. **141**:185, 1949.
188. Zuelzer, W. W., and Brown, A. K.: Neonatal jaundice; review, Amer. J. Dis. Child. **101**:87, 1961.
189. Zuelzer, W. W., Stulling, C. S., Page, R. H., Teruya, J., and Brough, A. S.: Etiology and pathogenesis of acquired hemolytic anemia, Transfusion **6**:438, 1966.

# 9 ERYTHROBLASTOSIS FETALIS (HEMOLYTIC ANEMIA OF THE NEWBORN INFANT)—GENERAL CONSIDERATIONS

*Definition.* Erythroblastosis fetalis is a disease of the fetus and newborn infant, characterized by a hemolytic anemia due to incompatibility between the blood group of the mother and that of her offspring. The disease is designated as such because of the frequent appearance of nucleated red cells in the peripheral blood, resulting from their active proliferation in the liver, spleen, and bone marrow as a compensation for excessive hemolysis.

*Pathogenesis.* Isoimmunization results from the presence of an antigenic substance in the fetal red blood cell that is not present in the mother's red blood cells. Entrance of this antigenic factor into the maternal circulation either by direct transfusion or by transfer across the placenta from the fetal circulation results in the elaboration of a specific antibody by the mother. The transplacental transfer of red cells is facilitated by the existence in man of a single syncytial cell layer separating the villi containing fetal blood vessels and the maternal sinuses, by thinning out the expanding placental surfaces, and by small leaks in the placental barrier which permit leakage of fetal blood. The loss of fetal cells through the placenta into the maternal circulation and the reverse process have been well documented. Neonatal plethora in some cases has been ascribed to a maternal-fetal transfusion.[64] The identification of fetal red cells in the maternal blood has been described (p. 5). Radioactive tagged red cells,[77] elliptocytes,[43] and sickle cells[61] have been injected into the maternal circulation prior to delivery and later recovered from the fetal circulation. Wider experience with confirmatory techniques is necessary to determine to what extent neonatal polycythemia, not based on twin births, is dependent on the passage of red cells from mother to fetus.

Sensitization during pregnancies occurs classically when fetal Rh-positive blood enters the circulation of the Rh-negative mother. A similar mechanism is postulated with respect to the A-B-O groups in heterospecific pregnancies. Maternal antibodies cross the placenta, gaining access to the fetal circulation where they become attached to fetal red cells, resulting in their removal from the circulation and subsequent destruction. The various pathologic, clinical, and hematologic manifestations of erythroblastosis stem from the reaction of these antibodies with fetal red cells in utero and in the neonatal period. It has been estimated that only minute amounts of fetal blood (0.03 to 0.07 ml.) are required for immunization.[51]

Zipursky and co-workers[113] postulated that the mechanism of sensitization in pregnancy consists of a primary stimulus because of the transfer of 0.5 ml. of fetal blood. Antibodies usually appear only after "booster" stimuli of smaller transfusions of the order of 0.1 to 0.2 ml. of fetal blood in subsequent pregnancies. This hypothesis deserves support from the relative infrequency of Rh-Hr sensitization in the first pregnancy.

With aid of the acid elution technique, the blood for fetal cells was drawn within the first 24 hours postpartum from 1,190 Rh-negative women.[111] A scan count of 5 or more cells (representing approximately 0.1 ml. or more of fetal erythrocytes in the maternal circulation) was selected as indicative of a "large" transplacental hemorrhage. In the total group of 1,190 Rh-negative women, 5.1% had a scan count of 5 or more. High scan counts (5 cells or more) clearly occurred more often in the A-B-O compatible group (59 out of 948) than in the incompatible (2 out of 242). These studies indicated that fetal erythrocytes in quantities of 0.1 ml. or more are found in 5.1% of postpartum women and in highest frequency in A-B-O compatible pregnancies.

A mother sensitized by previous transfusions is likely to have an infant with erythroblastosis in her first pregnancy, whereas the firstborn of a mother immunized during pregnancy is usually free of the disease. In the latter situation anti-Rh antibodies cannot be detected in the maternal circulation until there is a subsequent pregnancy with an Rh-positive fetus. This means that a healthy child usually results from the first pregnancy and that subsequent children are often affected since later pregnancies provide an effective stimulus to an antibody-forming mechanism set in motion by the first pregnancy.

From a study of the interaction of Rh-negative daughters by their Rh-positive mothers, Taylor[98] concluded that, after three Rh-positive A-B-O compatible pregnancies, women with Rh-positive mothers are more likely to have children affected with erythroblastosis than are women with Rh-negative mothers. In some Rh-negative women an in utero exposure to blood of their Rh-positive mothers is equivalent to the sensitizing stimulation of an Rh-positive pregnancy. These data shed no light on the existence of a transitory immunologic tolerance at the time of birth of an Rh-negative infant to an Rh-positive woman. Rather, it indicates the reverse—that a pregnancy sensitization of some women who had Rh-positive mothers occurred, as shown by an increased incidence of erythroblastosis among their children. Immunologic tolerance was considered possible because maternal red cells cross the placenta to the fetus in at least some pregnancies.

**Clinical features.** The diverse symptomatology of erythroblastosis fetalis reflects variations in the degree of red cell destruction, blood production, and extramedullary hematopoiesis in the liver. In about 15 to 20% of Rh-positive infants of Rh-negative immunized mothers, clinical illness will be absent or hardly perceptible. The intensity of the hemolytic process is influenced largely, but not entirely, by the titer of maternal anti-Rh antibodies. A high titer (usually 1:64 and over) or a rising titer usually carries a serious import and is reflected in the severity of the anemia and degree of jaundice.

The clinical findings include jaundice, anemia, enlargement of the liver and spleen, and, in severe cases, petechiae, hemorrhages, and edema. The liver and spleen may be moderately enlarged at birth or may become palpable as the disease progresses in the first week of life. Formerly the disease was classified according to increasing severity: congenital anemia of the newborn infant, the mild form in which pallor becomes apparent as jaundice fades in the first week of life; icterus gravis neonatorum, in which the infant is more seriously affected with progressive anemia and jaundice, and hydrops fetalis (universal edema, generalized edema of the newborn infant), the stage in which the stillborn infant is often markedly edematous. Except for hydrops fetalis, the term *erythroblastosis* qualified by the degree of severity has supplanted the terminology of the first two categories. They represent each end of a continuous range of increasing severity with marked variation in the two salient features of the disease—i.e., anemia and jaundice.

The markedly hydropic infant, although usually stillborn and premature, may be born alive but seldom survives more than a few hours. The cause of the massive edema is not known but has been attributed to heart failure and hypoproteinemia. Mild edema is not necessarily fatal since survival is possible with active treatment. Placental excretion of bile pigments in utero supposedly accounts for the lack of jaundice in these infants.

In addition to the characteristic anatomic features of anasarca, serious effusion, anemia, hepatomegaly, and cardiomegaly, the hydropic infant with hemolytic disease also has an enlarged placenta which often weighs 1,500 gm. or more. The enlargement is mainly due to edema but also results from proliferation of villous trophoblasts and stroma. Some hydropic infants with hemolytic disease seem to have suffered retardation of intrauterine growth. Hyperplasia of the pancreatic islets occurs in most babies with hemolytic disease and hydrops. Similar hyperplasia has been observed in hydrops associated with alpha-thalassemia. Although the hydropic fetus or infant with hemolytic disease always has severe anemia, there does not seem to be a threshold of anemia, according to Driscoll,[26] at which hydrops is invariably found.

A number of conditions other than Rh disease have been associated with hydrops fetalis. The conditions in the following list should be considered in the absence of isoimmunization.[26]

Hematologic—feto-maternal hemorrhage, twin-to-twin transfusion (recipient twin usually affected), alpha-thalassemia

Infections—toxoplasmosis, cytomegalovirus, syphilis, congenital hepatitis

Renal—congenital nephrosis, renal vein thrombosis

Placental/maternal—diabetes mellitus, chorionic vein thrombosis, neuroblastomatosis, dysmaturity

Cardiopulmonary—pulmonary lymphangiectasis, cardiopulmonary lymphoplasia, cystic adenomatoid lung malformation

Congenital anomalies—achondroplasia, multiple anomalies, Turner's syndrome
Idiopathic

Phipps and associates[54] found that the presence of hydrops and a high aortic and central venous pressure were not necessarily indicative of heart failure, hypervolemia, or the need for phlebotomy. These patients have a normal blood volume and severe acidosis. For the anemia the hydropic babies initially had a small exchange transfusion with packed cells, keeping the blood volume constant. Following the small exchange of 75 to 100 cc., a larger exchange with whole blood is given.

The estimated mortality rate in infants with hydrops treated with a conventional exchange transfusion is about 90%. Since the infants with hydrops have normal blood volume and severe acidosis, they do not require phlebotomy; correction of the severe acidosis is necessary.

Of thirty-one infants with hydrops fetalis in northern Thailand, twenty-seven were found to be associated with Bart's hemoglobin. The incidence of Bart's hemoglobin (homozygous alpha-thalassemia) is shown to be 0.34% in this population.[99]

In the infant with erythroblastosis jaundice of the skin and sclerae is almost never present at birth but appears in the first hours of life. The amniotic fluid is often pale yellow or yellowish brown and the vernix normal or dark yellow. In the latter case the skin underlying the discolored vernix is usually not icteric.

**Detection of early jaundice of the newborn infant.** The need for the early detection of jaundice has been emphasized[3] in infants with erythroblastosis not caused by the Rh-Hr factor in whom jaundice is not anticipated, such as in those with immunization by A-B and rare blood factors. In the newborn infant jaundice is generally not apparent until the blood level reaches 4 to 6 mg. per 100 ml. The absence of clinically detectable jaundice at lower levels may be due to differences in capillary permeability in the newborn baby as compared with the adult or may be due to a diminished affinity to pigment in the skin of newborn infants.[44] To safeguard those in whom jaundice is not anticipated, it is suggested that all infants should be inspected frequently during the first 2 days of life.

According to Kramer,[50] in infants with progressive hyperbilirubinemia, the jaundice begins in the face and proceeds to the trunk, the extremities, and finally to the palms and soles. He postulated that albumin-bound indirect bilirubin maintains an equilibrium with tissue protein. This bilirubin is then transported to the elastin of collagen tissue by the tissue protein. This elastin-bound indirect bilirubin gives skin its yellow pigmentation. Kramer concludes that clinical jaundice does not appear in newborn infants until the serum indirect bilirubin reaches 4 mg./100 ml. concentration. In an infant whose serum indirect bilirubin is 18 mg./100 ml., the face and trunk will be orange yellow, while the hands and feet are a pale yellow. It is not until the serum bilirubin reaches 20 to 22 mg./100 ml. that the hands and feet will turn the same orange-yellow. At this point complete saturation of the entire subcutaneous tissue mass occurs and the central nervous system tissue, which is more resistant to staining by indirect bilirubin, begins to take up this toxic material with the well-known development of kernicterus.

The premature infant, on the other hand, often becomes totally yellow from head to foot with lower concentrations of serum indirect bilirubin. His smaller subcutaneous tissue mass is unable to bind much indirect bilirubin and therefore becomes more susceptible to kernicterus at lower serum indirect bilirubin levels.

This relationship existed in infants with unexplained icterus, with A-B-O hemolytic disease, and in certain infants with Rh-Hr hemolytic disease and appeared to depend on the rate of rise of serum bilirubin concentration. The more rapid progression of skin icterus in infants of low birth weight than in full-term infants is noteworthy.

**Kernicterus.** Brain damage (kernicterus) represents the most serious complication of erythroblastosis and is associated with high concentrations of indirect bilirubin from any cause. The extent of potential bilirubin accumulation that may be involved in erythroblastosis can be estimated. Each gram of hemoglobin constitutes a potential source of 35 mg. of bilirubin. For an infant weighing 3 kg. a decrease of 1 gm. of hemoglobin per 100 ml. of blood represents the destruction of 3 gm. of hemoglobin and the source of 105 mg. of bilirubin. A newborn infant, handicapped by immature liver enzyme systems, therefore may accumulate toxic amounts of bilirubin without evidence of marked anemia.

Kernicterus thus can be regarded as a bilirubin encephalopathy. Cerebral involvement should be suspected in an infant 36 hours or more after birth who feeds poorly, becomes lethargic, and develops muscular twitching or whose cry is sharp and high pitched. Alteration of the Moro reflex, displayed in response to jarring of the crib or a loud noise, from the normal embrace reflex of the arms with fists clenched in the affected infant is significant.[4] Opisthotonus and respiratory failure follow in the severe and fatal cases. Signs of nervous system involvement should be sought in severely affected full-term infants in whom jaundice reaches a peak intensity at thirty-six hours and in severely affected premature infants in whom jaundice reaches a peak intensity by the fifth or sixth day.

The toxicity in vivo bilirubin has been ascribed to the uncoupling of oxidative phosphorylation.[110] At certain concentrations bilirubin can almost completely inhibit phosphorylation by a partial inhibition of respiration, as demonstrated in isolated liver mitochondria of the rat. With a rise in indirect bilirubin, injury and death of nerve cells result from uncoupling of oxidative phosphorylation. Since the course and severity of kernicterus vary greatly from one patient to another, more than one factor must be involved. In some infants, for instance, kernicterus develops at a relatively low level of bilirubin, whereas other infants sustain higher levels without injury.[89]

The incomplete development of the blood-brain barrier has been suggested as contributory to the development of kernicterus.[96] This barrier is supposedly located in the capillaries of the central nervous system and is endowed with selective permeability. The permeability of the barrier tested for a number of aniline dyes, toxins, virus antibodies, and drugs[32] is greater in premature infants than in term infants. These observations may explain the susceptibility of the newborn subjects, in general, and premature infants, in particular, to the toxicity of bilirubin. The turnover of $^{32}P$ has also been found to be faster in the fetal and young animal than in the adult.[6] By the time the animal is several weeks old, the capillary wall gradually tightens and the blood-brain barrier resumes its protective wall.

That indirect bilirubin can pass the blood-brain barrier is confirmed by its presence in the spinal fluid in the first 4 days of life, varying to some extent with the degree of hyperbilirubinemia. In all cases, however, the concentration of bilirubin in the spinal fluid is only a fraction of that in the blood.[96]

Kernicterus has been established as a postnatal complication and is almost completely preventable. Although there is a variation in susceptibility, the likelihood of kernicterus in the infant with erythroblastosis when indirect bilirubin concentrations reach 20 mg./100 ml. and above has been well documented. Signs of neurologic damage appear 36 hours or more after birth.

Assiduous attention to maintaining serum bilirubin concentrations at levels below 20 mg./100 ml. by one or more exchange transfusions has led to a remarkable reduction in the incidence of kernicterus. Since kernicterus is correlated with the intensity of bilirubinemia, it is important to observe closely those infants who are severely affected clinically at birth and whose cord blood shows elevated bilirubin levels and lowered hemoglobin content. This is especially important in premature or immature infants and in male infants with a high maternal antibody titer since they have been shown to be especially susceptible.

Staining of the basal ganglia occurs not only in association with isoimmunization but with significant accumulation of indirect hyperbilirubinemia irrespective of the cause—e.g., with prematurity,[1,20,114] spherocytosis,[94] congenital familial nonhemolytic jaundice,[19] in newborn infants given large doses of vitamin K,[5,63] in premature infants given sulfisoxazole (Gantrisin) in the first 5 days of life,[42,92] and even in the newborn infant with severe physiologic jaundice. The use of sulfonamides and salicylates may be hazardous in the newborn infant with hyperbilirubinemia because of the ability of these substances to displace serum bilirubin from protein-binding sites on serum protein and therefore allow its diffusion to other body compartments.[78,79]

Attention has recently been focused on groups of small premature infants with nonhemolytic hyperbilirubinemia in whom death occured in the first days of life with only moderate elevations of indirect bilirubin.[2,34] In the group whose peak bilirubin was aproximately 9 to 15 mg./100 ml. of indirect bilirubin, kernicterus was complicated by high frequency of intracranial hemorrhage; in the second group with levels of 18.5 to 23 mg./100 ml. of indirect bilirubin, kernicterus was associated with skin hemorrhages. In the first group death occurred between the third and sixth days of life; in the second, definite or probable kernicterus occurred in five of seven small premature infants. In the latter, exchange transfusions were ineffective in preventing kernicterus. Possible factors responsible for an increased incidence of kernicterus at relatively low levels of serum bilirubin were hypoxia, acidosis, hypothermia, and low serum albumin. It is still uncertain if vigorous therapeutic measures should be applied, including exchange transfusion and/or administration of albumin intravenously to prevent bilirubin encephalopathy at relatively low bilirubin levels, or whether phototherapy should be employed to keep bilirubin from reaching elevated levels. Certainly the policy of carrying out exchange transfusions at a level of 20 mg./100 ml. is inadequate to prevent death or neurologic damage in the small premature infant.

In babies who develop kernicterus, the injury is produced by the bilirubin which penetrates the brain cells. It follows that tissue bilirubin should be of greater concern than serum bilirubin. The serum bilirubin is not always elevated, however, when the tissue bilirubin is excessive. There are several reasons for this discrepancy. Since indirect bilirubin exists in serum in combination with albumin, a reduced serum albumin (e.g., hypoproteinemia, prematurity) results in reduced binding sites for bilirubin and relatively increased unbound bilirubin to enter tissues.

Infants on sulfisoxazole (Gantrisin), which competes with bilirubin for binding sites on albumin, may therefore develop kernicterus even with low serum bilirubin levels.[92] Heme pigments, metabolic or respiratory acidosis, nonesterified fatty acids (e.g., fasting, hypoglycemia, following heparin therapy), and drugs such as sulfonamides and salicylates, given not only to the infants but to the mother prior to delivery, may displace bilirubin from albumin and result in brain damage, even though the serum bilirubin level remains under 20 mg. per 100 ml.[104]

Kernicterus identical with that seen in human beings occurs naturally in a strain of jaundiced rats.[40] Kernicterus and typical nervous system lesions have been experimentally produced in previously asphyxiated rhesus monkeys exposed to injections of indirect-reacting bilirubin.[57] Sustained concentrations of serum bilirubin of over 30 mg. per 100 ml. in these animals were associated with decreased concentrations of oxygen in the tissues. This effect may render the cells more susceptible to the inward diffusion of bilirubin and actually precede the intracellular action on oxygen uptake and phosphorylation.[7] The defect is the same in both species, i.e., a lack of the conjugating glucuronyl transferase enzyme in the liver. In the animals as on human beings the administration of sulfonamides results in a lowering of the serum bilirubin and intensification of nervous signs and nuclear staining.[49]

Here, too, the suggested explanation is that kernicterus results from the competition between bilirubin and the sulfonamides for binding sites on the serum albumin so that unbound bilirubin becomes available for damage to nerve tissue.

Since the red cells of the premature infant may be susceptible to hemolysis with the development of jaundice in the infant, drug therapy such as excessive doses of vitamin K and sulfonamides should be avoided unless a specific need exists.[35]

It has been estimated that approximately 5 to 15% of all live-born infants with erythroblastosis will develop kernicterus if untreated. About 70% of babies with kernicterus will succumb within 7 days of birth. Of the 30% that survive the acute stage of cerebral symptoms, neurologic sequelae are likely to develop at a later date. They constitute about 10% of all cases of cerebral palsy.[46] More specifically, a fatal outcome is to be expected when signs of cerebral involvement develop on the second day, and survival is more common when such signs appear on the fifth day.[37] In the group that survive, evidences of cerebral damage so frequently present consist of mild to severe spasticity, athetosis, auditory disturbances, and defects of ocular movements.[83]

Intense jaundice without signs of kernicterus may be followed by slight mental impairment amounting to a reduction of the intelligence quotient of about 12%.[38] High tone deafness is a common sequel of kernicterus and should be investigated in all affected infants despite the absence of other signs of damage to the nervous system.

Children who have recovered from hemolytic disease may show green pigmentation of the deciduous teeth. It is of interest that an acute enamel hypoplasia of the deciduous teeth has been observed in patients with kernicterus following erythroblastosis.[30]

Diamond[24] suggests that the concept of "immaturity" of the blood-brain barrier is not supported by recent experimental evidence with other compounds, and indeed a functional blood-brain barrier has been demonstrated even in the fetus. Although in normal plasma the unbound bilirubin fraction is minute, it may be increased in the presence of organic anions which compete with the pigment for common binding sites on albumin. Since the brain probably participates in this pigment shift, it would be expected that in jaundiced infants the potential danger of bilirubin encephalopathy would be lessened by increasing the pigment binding capacity of plasma. The administration of albumin can be expected[80] to increase the plasma volume 17 ml./gm. of albumin. This would necessitate an increase in donor blood employed for the exchange transfusion because of the expansion in the infant's blood caused by the albumin. Albumin is therefore not used in hemolytic disease where the primary purpose is to replace sensitized red cells.

*Pathology.* The pathologic changes in erythroblastosis reflect a number of factors: duration and intensity of the destruction of the red cells by maternal antibody in utero and in the first days of life, compensatory hematopoiesis, and effect of abnormal stresses upon the function and structure of immature tissues and organs.

In deeply jaundiced infants the entire brain may be pigmented. Staining is more intense, with a brighter yellow color in the basal ganglia and other nuclei in the brainstem and medulla in the kernicteric infants. Ganglion cells degenerate and disappear, leaving empty spaces.[56] The mechanism of these changes is unknown, but it may be related to inhibition by excessive bilirubin of oxygen uptake within the cells.[22]

The liver and spleen are invariably enlarged. Histologically, the most striking feature is widespread extramedullary hematopoiesis in these and other organs such as the pancreas, kidneys, adrenals, lymph nodes, thymus, and placenta. Because of the persistent destruction of red blood cells, there is a reversion to the embryonic type of blood formation. The bone marrow shows active hematopoiesis with a predominance of immature nucleated red blood cells. An enormous proliferation of normoblasts is particularly noticeable within the liver sinusoids, compressing and displacing the liver parenchymal cells and resulting in pronounced degenerative changes. Many of the hepatic cells are vacuolated and in some cases are replaced by coarsened reticulum. Severely damaged livers show evidence of intrahepatic biliary obstruction with masses of bile pigment in the small bile ducts and in biliary canaliculi. Hemosiderosis may be found in the spleen and liver. Hypertrophy and hyperplasia of the pancreatic islet cells are striking. Petechiae, even frank hemorrhages, may be observed in the lungs. The adrenals reveal lipid degeneration of most of the cortical cells.[56]

Two cases have been reported[97] of placental involvement by congenital metastasizing neuroblastoma. The tumors apparently were in the adrenal sympathetic plexus. Clinically both cases resembled erythroblastosis fetalis. The mother gave no evidence of metastatic disease. The severe edema together with the gross appearance of the placenta produced a clinical picture resembling isoimmunization.

Edema may be localized or severe and generalized as it is in infants with hydrops. In this condition, extensive edema (especially of the face), varying degrees of maceration, effusions into serous cavities, and marked enlargement of the spleen and, to a lesser degree, of the liver are conspicuous findings. The placenta in cases of hydrops is edematous, bulky, and friable. The occurrence of erythroblasts in the pulmonary capillaries is the most important single diagnostic sign to be found in the macerated fetus.[89]

*Maternal antibodies—prenatal testing.* All pregnant women are initially typed for A-B-O group and the **Rh**$_o$ factor. Whether or not the mother is immunized, prenatal testing is carried out initially at the first visit or in the first trimester of pregnancy and is repeated at 28 or 30 weeks. Where no immunization is then detected, tests should be repeated at 4-week intervals to the end of pregnancy. When antibodies are detected, frequency of testing should be increased to 2- or 1-week intervals.

When antibodies develop for the first time, they are usually not detectable until about the fourth month of pregnancy. They may increase as gestation proceeds. Although they are almost invariably detected by the thirty-fifth week, an unusual later development of antibodies may rarely result in a severly affected fetus. The absence of antibodies in the mother's serum at termination of the pregnancy indicates that the infant will not be affected by erythroblastosis due to the **Rh**$_o$ factor.[66] On the other hand, when antibodies are present at the beginning of pregnancy, even in weak concentration, the birth of an infant with erythroblastosis must be anticipated.

*Maternal anti-Rh$_o$ titer.* There is some general but not very close correlation between the type and concentration of antibodies and the clinical severity of the disease in the affected child. In general, the disease tends to be milder when the predominant anti-**Rh**$_o$ antibodies are of the saline agglutinating type rather than the immune or incomplete form.

By and large, higher titers of incomplete antibodies are associated with severe disease and a worse prognosis (1:32 to 1:64 and over). Exceptions to severe and fatal cases (stillbirths) with low titers and mild symptoms despite high titers have been noted.[107]

Because of the risk of kernicterus, a high maternal anti-$Rh_o$ titer (1:64 or higher) of incomplete antibodies previously had been regarded as a sufficient indication for exchange transfusion immediately after birth in the infant with erythroblastosis, regardless of the physical findings or hemoglobin level.[101] Currently the use of amniocentesis (p. 143) has modified the reliance on the anti-$Rh_o$ titer alone as a guide to immediate exchange transfusion.

A rising anti-$Rh_o$ titer in a first immunized pregnancy indicates that the fetus is $Rh_o$ positive. Antibody titers in subsequent pregnancies cannot be interpreted with the same degree of confidence. The antibodies derived from immunization with a previous Rh-positive fetus usually persist during a subsequent pregnancy even with an Rh-negative infant (heterozygous father) and have been stated to actually increase in titer.[59] This has been challenged by Wiener and co-workers,[106] who found that pregnancy with an Rh-negative fetus and the birth of an Rh-negative infant had no effect on the $Rh_o$-antibody titer of an Rh-negative woman sensitized to the $Rh_o$ factor. In this institution, two cases have been observed in which remarkable increases in antibody titer occurred during pregnancies when the mother was known to have been previously sensitized and when the infant was Rh negative. In one instance the titer increased from 1:4 to 1:128 and in the other, from undectable to 1:512.

In general, if the father is heterozygous and the antibody titer of a previously immunized mother is low and remains constant, the chances are fairly good that the infant will be Rh negative.

There is great variability in the titer of the sensitized mother following delivery. It generally falls somewhat or may continue to be high for prolonged periods.

*Effect of previous transfusions on the mother.* Transplacental immunization can be detected in pregnancy when there is a history of blood transfusions or fetal death. Transfusions of $Rh_o$-positive blood or intramuscular injections of $Rh_o$-positive blood increases an $Rh_o$-negative mother's susceptibility to immunization by an $Rh_o$-positive fetus. Repeated transfusions are especially potent agents in producing a high degree of sensitization, stillbirths, and hydrops.

Since the majority of blood currently given by transfusion has been tested for compatibility of the $Rh_o$ (D) factor, the incidence of $Rh_o$(D) sensitization by transfusion is decreasing. However, since compatibility with regard to other factors in the Rh-Hr system, such as **rh″** (**E**), **hr′(c)**, and **rh′(C)**, as well as factors outside this system, is not routinely determined, antibodies against these later factors have become more usual types found in women sensitized by transfusions given in more recent years. Proper identification of the antibody is necessary for protection of the mother, should she need blood, as well as for care of the infant.

In all instances in which sensitization is known or suspected to have resulted from transfusion, the husband's blood should be tested. Results may indicate that the infant cannot have blood of a type that can be affected by the maternal antibody and the concern with regard to erythroblastosis thus may be eliminated.

In addition, all women known to have been transfused should be investigated for presence of antibodies whether these women are $Rh_o$ negative (d/d) or $Rh_o$ (D) positive.

*Immunization in the Rh-positive mother and infant.* At times there is no obvious incompatibility between mother and child, both being $Rh_o$ positive; yet sensitization is indicated by neonatal hemolysis and a positive Coombs test. In the absence of A-B-O incompatibility, consideration must be given to immunization with **hr′(c)**, **rh″(E)**, **Kell** and other less frequent factors. In such cases the husband's blood also should be examined, regardless of his reaction to anti-$Rh_o$ (anti-**D**) serum, for his erythrocytes may possess a minor blood group antigen lacking in those of his wife.

*Heterozygous and homozygous status of the husband.* If the husband is Rh positive, it is important in management to determine whether he is homozygous or heterozygous for the $Rh_o$ factor. Although this may be reflected to some degree by the presence or absence of the $Rh_o$ factor in previous offspring, appropriate tests will determine this with greater accuracy. The use of anti-**rh′** (anti-**C**), anti-**rh″** (anti-**E**), anti-**hr′** (anti-**c**), and anti-**hr″**

(anti-**e**) provides a means of determining the husband's probable genotype. Since anti-**Hr₀** (anti-**d**) serum is unavailable, the diagnosis remains presumptive. In the heterozygous father the chances are 50% that the offspring will be Rh positive or Rh negative. For the homozygous father (for **Rh₀** [**D**]) it can be fairly safely predicted that all the children will be **Rh₀** positive.

*Different types of antibodies.* Antibodies react under varying physical conditions. Some agglutinate red cells suspended in saline solutions, whereas others will only coat them. Both forms are found in the blood of mothers sensitized to Rh-positive cells. The saline-active or "complete" antibodies agglutinate red cells containing the **Rh₀** factor; they do not cross the placenta and hence are not involved in the causation of erythroblastosis. The second type will fail to agglutinate Rh-positive cells when suspended in saline solution but will do so when these cells are suspended in colloid medium such as plasma, serum, or albumin. These antibodies are variously termed incomplete, univalent, hyperimmune, cryptagglutinoid, glutinin, immune, and albumin. Of these, incomplete and immune are most commonly used.

"Blocking" antibodies are a variety of "incomplete" agglutinins which fail to agglutinate test cells suspended in saline solution or in colloid media. They sensitize saline-suspended cells by coating their surface. The antibody (globulin) coating will be detected with the use of an antihuman globulin (Coombs) serum which agglutinates sensitized cells (direct Coombs test). Many affected Rh-positive (**Rh₀**[**D**]) infants appear to be Rh negative on typing, because the cells are heavily coated with incomplete antibodies. The most dependable test to determine the presence of such blocked or coated cells is the direct Coombs test.

Naturally occurring antibodies such as anti-**A** and anti-**B** isoagglutinins in persons with group O blood are those normally present throughout life which can be attributed to no known antigenic stimulus. Immune anti-**Rh₀** (anti-**D**) antibodies are of pathologic and diagnostic significance and originate as a response to a specific stimulus during pregnancy and to transfusion.

*Transmission of antibodies.* Only the incomplete or immune form of anti-**Rh₀** (anti-**D**) antibodies are capable of crossing the placenta, and this transmission can occur at any early stage of pregnancy. When the incomplete and complete forms are present together in maternal serum, only the incomplete form appears in the fetal serum.[12] While there is evidence that the milk of sensitized mothers may contain Rh-Hr antibody for 3 weeks after birth, the amount after the first 2 or 3 days is too small to produce harmful effects in nursing the erythroblastotic baby. Although antibody absorption takes place, the amount is insignificant.[10] Present practice has been to allow mothers to nurse their infants if they want to do so—certainly after the second day. Weaning infants with erythroblastosis because maternal milk contains antibodies is not justified.

The absence of erythroblastosis in certain infants demonstrating incompatibility with mothers with relatively high titers of Rh-Hr antibodies finds an explanation in structural differences among the Rh-Hr antibodies. By means of sensitive techniques for immune globulin analysis, it has been demonstrated that Rh-Hr agglutinins (saline, complete) are 19S macroglobulins in contrast to "blocking" antibodies (the immune, incomplete, and albumin type), which are 7S gamma globulins. With the realization that 19S antibodies essentially do not cross the placenta, the clinical correlation between affected infants and the type of Rh-Hr antibody synthesized is clarified.[86] In view of the fact that virtually all anti-**Rh** sera contain some 7S anti-**Rh** antibody, it is to be expected that Rh-positive infants born to mothers whose serum contains anti-**Rh** antibody will almost always have a positive antiglobulin test.[66]

*Coombs test (antiglobulin test).* The Coombs test is a sensitive method of demonstrating the presence of an antibody absorbed or bound to red cells. This test has come into common use since Coombs and associates[18] found that serum from rabbits immunized with human globulin agglutinated human erythrocytes coated with Rh-Hr antibodies. Experience has shown this to be an invaluable method of detecting incomplete Rh-Hr antibodies. The essential component of the Coombs serum is the antigamma globulin. There are two forms of the Coombs antihuman globulin test, the direct and the indirect.

*Direct Coombs test.* The direct test is used to detect antibodies fixed to infants' cells in vivo. Antiglobulin serum is added to a suspension of cells which has been washed three times with saline solution. After the mixture is centrifuged, it is observed for agglutination. Cells of the cord blood following delivery of an infant to an immunized woman are commonly used in the test to determine coating or sensitization while in utero. It is useful in confirmation of the typing of an infant presumably Rh negative. A positive Coombs test on such blood indicates that the red cells have been sensitized and that the infant is Rh positive. The earlier negative test was due to the blocking action of maternal antibody. A positive Coombs test establishes the diagnosis of erythroblastosis but is not in itself an indication for exchange transfusion.

The direct Coombs test on cord blood from babies with typical signs of erythroblastosis fetalis that had heretofore been negative may become positive after prior exposure of the red cells to fresh human serum. This suggests the possibility of converting a negative direct Coombs test of obviously affected babies to positive by the addition of complement prior to performing the traditional Coombs test.[88] This two-stage direct antiglobulin test was explored in A-B-O erythroblastosis, using serum A-B as a source of complement. Of nine clinical affected infants, seven showed strongly positive serologic reactions. None of the clinically affected incompatible infants showed a positive reaction.[15]

Clifford and co-workers[17] described the findings with antiglobulin testing of cord blood of 7,340 unselected newborn infants. In this study 100% of instances of hemolytic disease secondary to Rh-Hr system incompatibility and 93% of those with hemolytic disease related to A-B-O incompatibility were identified. The direct Coombs test on cord blood is suggested as a useful screening test, particularly when Rh-Hr or A-B-O grouping of the parents is either not known or so related to each other that a potential immunization may be apparent in the infant.

Except for erythroblastosis due to anti-**A** and anti-**B** antibodies when the reaction is often weak or negative, a weak reaction due to anti-**Rh** antibodies is usually associated with clinically mild forms of the disease.

Positive Coombs tests are obtained not only in patients with A-B-O and Rh-Hr erythroblastosis, but also in those with idiopathic acquired hemolytic anemia, acquired hemolytic anemias secondary to leukemia, lymphosarcoma, disseminated lupus erythematosus, and thrombotic thrombocytopenic purpura.

Two varieties of antibody have been encountered in the Coombs antiglobulin serum, one variety reacting as gamma globulin and the other as nongamma globulin. Antigamma globulin serum reacts best with cells coated with antibodies of the Rh-Hr system. Antinongamma globulin is specifically needed for reaction with such antibodies as anti-**H**, some anti-**Lewis**, and anti-**Kidd**. An ideal serum for routine use contains a combination of antigamma globulin and nonantigamma globulin reactivity.

*Indirect Coombs test.* The indirect test is used to demonstrate circulating antibodies which coat but do not agglutinate cells suspended in saline solution. In this in vitro test the serum in question is incubated with corresponding Rh-positive red cells of a compatible A-B-O group. Antiglobulin serum is added to the incubated red cell suspension that has been thoroughly washed. Readings for agglutination are made as in the direct test. If the patient's serum contains incomplete or immune anti-Rh antibodies, they coat the test red cells and agglutination follows on the addition of Coombs serum. The serum can be titrated by preliminary dilution with saline solution and made even more sensitive with the use of trypsinized test cells.

At present, potent antihuman globulin sera are readily available from several commercial sources. Falsely negative Coombs tests are therefore usually a result of technical errors rather than of inadequate reagents. The most common of these appear to be inadequate washing of the erythrocytes to be tested, inadequate drainage of wash solutions from around erythrocytes, and introduction of protein into the test system by placing a finger over the tube during mixing.

*Tests with trypsinized cells.* Saline-suspended red cells are so altered by preliminary exposure to a trypsin solution as to give direct readings with incomplete or immune antibodies.[71] This test does not replace the indirect Coombs test, for it fails to detect such rare antibodies as **Duffy**, **Kell**, and **Kidd** factors. The method, however, is widely used and constitutes a valuable adjunct to tests employed for the detection of circulating antibodies.

*Elution.* The specificity of the antibody causing damage to the infant's erythrocytes in erythroblastosis can also be demonstrated by elution tests.[41,62,105] This is a method of releasing antibody from red cells that had adsorbed it. The exact nature of the antibody involved may be determined through the use of the heat elution test on umbilical cord blood samples showing a positive Coombs test. Eluates are prepared from erythrocytes of umbilical cord blood by preliminary washing of the red blood cells in cold buffered saline solution and later subjecting the suspension to 56° C. The eluates are tested for hemagglutination against known A or B red blood cells or positive cells of Rh-Hr or other systems. The test is particularly valuable when sensitization to antigens in both the Rh-Hr and the A-B-O systems is possible.

Briefly the heat elution test is as follows: The blood clot obtained from the umbilical cord is agitated until sufficient erythrocytes are freed in the serum to make a heavy suspension. The red blood cells are removed by a pipette and separated from the serum by centrifuge. The cells are then washed three times in three to four volumes of cold saline solution. One milliliter of packed, washed erythrocytes is added to 1 ml. of fresh 0.85% saline solution and resuspended. This suspension is subjected to 56° C. in a water bath for 5 minutes. At the end of this period, the suspension is immediately centrifuged at 3,500 rpm for 3 minutes while the temperature of the tube is kept at 56° C. The supernatant fluid is transferred to a clean tube and spun again at 3,500 rpm to remove any remaining red cells. The supernatant eluate is then siphoned off and used to test for eluted antibodies. When antibodies are present, agglutination of known adult A or B red blood cells can be shown by mixing one drop of the eluate with one drop of 2% red blood cell suspensions.

If clumping fails to occur, a Coombs antiglobulin test is performed to see if nonagglutinating (cryptagglutinoid and agglutinoid) antibodies are present in the eluate. The A and B antibodies can be noted by their selective action on the corresponding group A and B blood cells used in the test panel of blood. The anti-A plus anti-B produce agglutination of both A and B test erythrocytes. A variation of this method has been described also eluting antibody from the infant's erythrocytes and testing with adult cells.[109]

*Frequency of blood group factors causing erythroblastosis.* Until recent years incompatibility with respect to the **Rh₀(D)** factor has accounted for the majority of cases of erythroblastosis. A lowered incidence, however, is being noted due to the fact that many parents who have had one or two children with erythroblastosis are limiting the size of their families.

Erythroblastosis due to A and B incompatibility is being recognized more widely since there is at present a greater alertness to its presence on the first day of life. The frequency of erythroblastosis involving the **A** and **B** factors has been estimated as 1% of all newborn infants as compared with 0.5% with the Rh factor (**Rh₀** or **D**).[100] Immunization with **A** is more frequently encountered than with **B**.

Rh-incompatible mating occurs in 13% of all marriages. Of incompatible matings about 50% of the Rh-positive fathers will be heterozygous so that one half of the offspring may be Rh negative and, hence, without disease.

Erythroblastosis due to the Rh factor in a population with about 15% Rh-negative persons occurs in 1 in 150 to 1 in 200 of all full-term pregnancies. The fact that only 1 in every 20 to 26 full-term incompatible pregnancies results in an infant with erythroblastosis emphasizes the inability of most Rh-negative mothers to produce Rh antibodies.[52] Even in Rh-negative persons sensitized by transfusions with Rh-positive blood, there are many (about 10%) who fail to develop antibodies even after a second transfusion or an incompatible pregnancy. It has been estimated that with properly spaced repeated transfusions of small amounts of Rh-positive blood more than 75% of Rh-negative persons can become immunized. Also the number of cases of erythroblastosis fetalis occurring in second-born infants of Rh-negative mothers depends upon the frequency with which fetal blood enters the maternal circulation during pregnancy.[108]

Anti-**Rh₀** (anti-**D**) antibodies often in combination with anti-**rh'** (anti-**C**) or anti-**rh''** (anti-**E**) antibodies account for most of the cases of erythroblastosis due to the Rh factor. Outside of the Rh factor and **A** and **B** factors that constitute the majority of cases, **hr'(c)**, **rh''(E)**, **Kell**, and a lesser number of blood factors outside of the Rh system mentioned previously (Chapter 6) account for the remaining 1 or 2% of erythroblastosis.

The frequency of erythroblastosis is directly proportional to the frequency of the Rh-negative persons in any given population. The incidence is less in Negroes in the United States, with about 5% Rh negative, and is exceedingly rare in Chinese, Japanese, and American Indians, among whom only 1% or less are Rh negative.[53]

In a Philadelphia hospital from 1946 to 1962, hemolytic diseases of the newborn infants due to $Rh_o(D)$ factor were found to have lower morbidity and mortality rates in Negro than in white infants.[70] Negro mothers were also less likely to produce stillbirths due to $Rh_o(D)$ sensitization. The prognosis for an affected baby is less in the Negro mother sensitized by transfusion prior to pregnancy than for the white mother so sensitized. Yet Negro and white mothers have shown an equal ability to produce anti-$Rh_o$ (anti-D) antibody. There seems to be no explanation for the milder disease in Negro babies in this series. A-B-O hemolytic disease has been shown of equal severity in Negro and white infants.

*Prognostic considerations and family patterns of severity.* The titer of maternal anti-Rh constitutes a primary factor in determining the prognosis in the fetus in utero. If the anti-Rh titer is less than 1:64, the chances are nearly 90% that the baby will be in good condition at birth.[4]

Certain predictions can also be made with respect to the disease in successive siblings. The disease tends to be milder in the first affected infant than in those that follow. However, serious exceptions to this rule have been noted to occur in a number of cases in which severe and fatal erythroblastosis has occurred in the first immunized pregnancy.[28] Such exceptions apparently may be detected by the development of high antibody titers in the maternal serum. Furthermore, a trend of increasing severity is not uniform in every family, and mild cases follow severe cases, even if the infant with the severe case had been stillborn. About 5 to 10% of first affected infants will be stillborn, and, of those born alive, 40% will not require treatment.[103] If the first sibling is mildly affected, then those that follow are likely to be mildly affected, and the chances of a subsequent stillbirth are relatively low (about 2%).[21] If a previous baby was stillborn on an Rh basis, there is about an 80% chance that the next baby, if spontaneously delivered, will also be stillborn.[21]

In another series it has been estimated[16] that after a woman has had one stillbirth due to erythroblastosis the chance for the next Rh-positive fetus to be a stillbirth is 75%; born alive but with extreme anemia, 15%; and born alive but with readily treatable disease, 10%. When a woman has had two stillbirths due to erythroblastosis, the chance for the next Rh-positive fetus to be a stillbirth is 90%; born alive but with extreme anemia, 8%; and born alive with readily treatable disease, 2%.

Greater prognostic accuracy can be obtained by referring to severity of the disease in the immediately preceding sibling. Thus, there is a tendency for very severely affected and stillborn infants to be followed by stillbirths and for moderately and severely involved infants to be followed by somewhat more severely affected infants.[66] Since a woman who has had one stillbirth on an Rh basis has about four chances in five of losing her next Rh-positive fetus,[66] it would seem reasonable to advise premature induction of labor if the husband is homozygous.

*Laboratory findings—blood.* The blood findings include abnormalities of red blood cells, hemoglobin, carboxyhemoglobin, reticulocytes, leukocytes, platelets, and bilirubin.

*Red blood cells.* The blood shows striking evidence of a hemolytic process with signs of active regeneration. The number of red cells, reticulocytes, and hemoglobin concentration depend upon the severity of the disease and the ability of hematopoietic tissues to compensate for the destruction of red cells.

The hemoglobin and red cells may be normal but usually are moderately to markedly reduced at birth. The red cell count ranges from less than 2 million to as high as 5.5 million per cubic millimeter. The most prominent feature in the blood smear is the large number of nucleated red cells in every stage of maturation. This normoblastic outpouring reflects the accelerated regenerative activity of the bone marrow and extramedullary tissues. The red cells are predominantly macrocytic with slight anisocytosis and poikilocytosis. Spherocytosis is not a feature of the blood smear in Rh erythroblastosis as it is in erythroblastosis due to A-B incompatibility.

Although the number of normoblasts in the blood of the normal newborn infant does not exceed 10 per 100 white blood cells in the first 2 days of life, in the severely affected infant it may rise to 5 or 10 nucleated red cells for every white blood cell. In mild cases it is not increased above the normal. In addition to erythroblastosis, normoblastemia also may occur in infants with congenital heart disease, in premature infants, in infants whose mothers have diabetes, in infants who have had fetal hemorrhage, and in those with anoxia.

*Hemoglobin.* The hemoglobin varies from

3 gm. per 100 ml. to normal values of 15 to 18 gm. Infants with marked anemia are critically ill with edema. Although the hemoglobin concentration is normally measured in blood, pricked from the heel, Mollison and Cutbush[68] have emphasized that it is obligatory to obtain the hemoglobin level from the cord blood. Where available, cord blood hemoglobin serves[67] as a more accurate index of the status of fetal blood and a more precise guide to treatment than the higher values obtained from venous blood and even the more elevated reading acquired from blood obtained by finger puncture. The reasons for these differences stem from the delayed tying of the umbilical cord, during which time the normal infant receives varying amounts of blood from the placenta so long as its cord is left intact, and the rapid shift of plasma from blood vessels soon after birth. Thus, Mollison and Cutbush cite an instance of a cord blood hemoglobin value of 12.8 gm./100 ml. with venous and capillary blood samples of 15.4 and 18 gm./100 ml., respectively. Such discrepancies are frequently responsible for confusion in determining the need for an exchange transfusion within the first 24 hours of life.

Capillary blood, on an average, has a hemoglobin level of 3.6% higher than blood from a venous source in the first few days of life; this discrepancy is generally thought to be due to venous stasis and hemoconcentration in the periphery. This discrepancy is dependent on the amount of acrocyanosis. Hence for accurate hemoglobin determination a venous source should be used or capillary blood drawn after the extremities have been warmed to get a sample more representative of venous blood.

The normal cord blood hemoglobin of 16.6 gm./100 ml. (16.55 ± 1.5) reported by Mollison and Cutbush[68] corresponds almost exactly with the values of 16.4 gm./100 ml. (16.4 ± 1.09) found in our laboratory. The value of 13.6 gm./100 ml., therefore, represents the lower level of normal for cord blood. These authors give values of 14.5 gm./100 ml. for venous blood and slightly over 15.4 gm./100 ml. for capillary blood as the low limit of normal on the first day of life, which should serve as a guide to management when cord blood determinations are not available. Thus, the range of normal hemoglobin values in newborn infants[68,69] may be stated as follows: cord blood, 13.6 to 19.6 gm. per 100 ml.; venous blood (first day), 14.5 to 22.5 gm. per 100 ml.; blood obtained by skin prick (first day), 15.4 to 22.8 gm. per 100 ml.

Severity of erythroblastosis has been classified on the basis of cord hemoglobin concentration: mild disease, 14 gm. per 100 ml. and above; moderately severe disease, 11 to 13.5 gm./100 ml.; and severe disease, less than 11 gm./100 ml.

In erythroblastosis the concentration of fetal hemoglobin is significantly lower than normal, whereas the concentration of adult hemoglobin is the same as in normal infants. There is no preferential destruction of fetal hemoglobin-containing erythrocytes in this disease; rather there is a preferential regeneration of adult hemoglobin in response to hemolysis. In infants born with normal hemoglobin levels, the capacity to synthesize adult hemoglobin in amounts greater than normal appears to be an important mechanism serving to prevent anemia.[91]

*Carboxyhemoglobin levels.* Carbon monoxide, a normal metabolic product of hemoglobin breakdown, is increased in infants with Rh incompatibility. Normal, term infants show a mean carboxyhemoglobin concentration of 0.42%. Infants with Rh incompatibility had elevations ranging from 2.6 to 11.9%.[82] The degree of carboxyhemoglobin elevation tended to parallel the severity of the anemia but not the serum bilirubin concentration. Infants with A-B-O incompatibility show moderate elevations. Infants with hyperbilirubinemia without anemia or blood group incompatibility have carboxyhemoglobin values within the normal range.[82]

*Reticulocytes.* The reticulocytes range above 6% (upper limit of normal) in the infant with mild erythroblastosis and reach 40 to 50% in those with severe disease. The reticulocyte count may also be increased when the cord blood hemoglobin is normal, indicating the ability of erythropoietic tissue to compensate adequately for the demands of hemolysis. A normal hemoglobin level, therefore, may be deceptive, and the need for repeated reticulocyte counts in such a case cannot be overemphasized as an index of underlying blood destruction. An infant with a normal hemoglobin level and an elevated reticulocyte percentage in the first 2 days of life may be in a precarious condition, for in many cases the hemoglobin is known to drop precipitously on the third day with the development of severe disease and the need for urgent treatment. The reticulocytes are of great value, therefore, in assessing the regenerative process since they are often found in increased numbers when nucleated red cells are within normal limits.[85]

*Leukocytes.* In infants with severe erythroblastosis the leukocytes vary from 15,000 to 30,000 per cubic millimeter. Higher counts have been recorded, but these include large numbers of nucleated red cells. Myelocytes are common. Erythrocytes that have undergone phagocytosis by monocytes or neutrophils are occasionally found in blood smears.

*Platelets.* The platelet count may be normal or diminished in infants with severe erythroblastosis. Thrombocytopenia may be sufficiently marked to cause petechiae and purpura. Usually the thrombocytopenia parallels the degree of the hemolytic process.[95]

PLATELET CHANGES FOLLOWING EXCHANGE TRANSFUSION. Desforges and O'Connell observed[23] low platelet levels several days after an exchange transfusion (as low as 50,000 per cubic millimeter and less in some cases), with a gradual rise beginning with the third day and restoration of normal values in about a week. Despite lowered values, there was no bleeding tendency. The persistence of thrombocytopenia beyond the third or fourth day after an exchange transfusion with bleeding prompts a search for some other causative process. Congenital thrombocytopenic purpura with a failure of megakaryocytes or a pyogenic infection should be considered in such instances.[25]

*Bilirubin.* Since kernicterus can be prevented in almost every case of erythroblastosis by keeping bilirubin levels below critical levels of 20 mg. per 100 ml., it is essential that bilirubin determinations be carried out from birth and frequently repeated during the first 4 or 5 days of life. It should be remembered that kernicterus may occur at lower levels of serum bilirubin under certain conditions (see p. 108). Micromethods are now available[47] that require only a small quantity of blood obtained from heel puncture.

The need for close scrutiny of laboratory methods used to determine bilirubin concentrations cannot be overemphasized. In comparing two hospitals with a great variation in the incidence of hyperbilirubinemia among premature infants, forty-four of 160 premature infants required exchange transfusions in one, as compared with four of 156 premature infants in the other hospital. Lucey and associates[58] found that the differences could not be explained by any of the usual factors known to affect neonatal hyperbilirubinemia. Investigation disclosed that the method of preparation of the bilirubin standard and standard curve created the difference in the incidence of hyperbilirubinemia. Correction and subsequent control of this variable resulted in a decrease in the incidence of hyperbilirubinemia in the hospital with the high incidence.

The cord blood bilirubin levels in most normal infants are under 3 mg. per 100 ml. The average is 2.2 mg. (range 1.5 to 3.2) on the second day for the full-term infant and approximately 11 mg. (range 0.0 to 27) on the third to fourth day in the premature infant. Usually, the bilirubin level begins to fall spontaneously between the second and third day in the full-term infant and on the fourth or fifth day in the premature baby. The fall is more gradual in the premature infant, and original cord values may not be reached until the tenth day or later. (For the significance of increased conjugated bilirubin, see discussion of obstructive jaundice complicating erythroblastosis, pp. 116 to 118.)

A knowledge of these normal values serves as a background for the fluctuations in the infant with erythroblastosis. The cord blood bilirubin level of 3.5 mg./100 ml. and above in the affected infant is not much higher than that of the normal infant because of the clearing of this pigment in utero, probably by the placenta. Of greater importance in management is the rate of rise of bilirubin as determined by periodic estimations. This ranges from 0.3 to 1 mg./100 ml. per hour, depending upon the severity of the disease, with the upper occurring in advanced disease. In some instances the rise is gradual over the first 2 days and accelerates on the third or fourth day.

Another technique has been described in which the plasma heme pigments measured spectroscopically also serve as a guide to the need for one or more exchange transfusions.[9] Bilirubin determinations, however, are universally used.

*Amniocentesis.* In recent years examination of the amniotic fluid by puncture through the abdominal wall has proved a valuable means of forecasting the severity of erythroblastosis fetalis.\* This method has proved useful in management of the sensitized woman who has had one affected infant requiring therapy and who,

---

\*See references 8, 11, 14, 29, 31, 48, 55, 60, 90, 93, and 102.

during the current pregnancy, has shown a significant rise in antibody titer to at least 1:32.[31] In a pregnancy in which a patient first becomes immunized, serial anti-Rh₀ (anti-**D**) titers are generally a good indication of fetal condition.[90] In subsequent pregnancies or in pregnancies in which the immunization is caused by a prior blood transfusion, the titer may not reflect what is going on and amniocentesis becomes valuable. Mothers previously sensitized to the Rh factor have given birth to Rh-negative infants, despite marked increases in antibody titer during pregnancy. The problem is also accentuated in the case of a husband who is probably or definitely heterozygous. Also in spite of a rising titer, delivery may yield an Rh-positive infant without any evidence of erythroblastosis who is subsequently exposed to the risk of prematurity.[36] Examination of the amniotic fluid could possibly prevent unnecessary deaths and unnecessary cesarean sections with delivery of unaffected children by affording a more realistic evaluation of erythroblastosis in utero than fluctuations in the titer. The introduction of transfusing the fetus in utero in the hope of gaining a few weeks of intrauterine gestation has intensified the interest in amniocentesis (p. 145.)

Transabdominal puncture is carried out in the region of the nape of the neck or the fetal small parts. To reduce the risk of opening fetal channels, the placenta may be localized by the use of radioactive albumin or chromated cells.[31] Blood-stained amniotic fluid cannot be used for accurate determination of the amount of bilirubinoid pigment but could be used to determine fetal blood group and Coombs test. Amniocentesis is timed on an individual basis. Some aspirate amniotic fluid initially at 32 weeks, repeating it at 1- to 2-week intervals, as necessary.[31] Others carry out two tests between 28 and 35 weeks. The second test is timed on the result of the first test which, in turn, is based on antibody levels, history, and suspicion. When the assessment of the fetal condition is regarded even more at risk, amniocentesis may be performed at 24 to 27 weeks, and when the technique is available, the severely affected infant may receive the benefit of intrauterine transfusion of packed cells by the intraperitoneal route.

Bilirubin appears in the fluid mainly as the indirect type when determined by the van den Bergh reaction. More commonly the combined pigments that represent various degradation products of hemoglobin, including bilirubin, are measured spectrophotometrically. The optical density is plotted against wavelength $(m\mu)$ and a continuous recording is obtained as the spectrophotometer scans the specimen from 800 to 300 $m\mu$.[31] The bile pigments degraded from hemoglobin absorb over the range between 400 and 500 $m\mu$, and when they are present in significant amounts, a bulge appears on the curve at 450 $m\mu$. The more pronounced the bulge the more severely affected is the fetus. The prognosis is progressively worse the earlier the pigments appear.[54]

An increase in optical density at 450 $m\mu$ indicates that bilirubinoid pigments are present. The height of the peak, corresponding to the concentration of pigment, gives information about the severity of the disease. The value of repeated analysis of the amniotic fluid from sensitized pregnant women lies in the ability to measure the progression of the disease. With worsening of the condition of the fetus, the peak reaches the top zone and warns that early delivery or transamniotic intraperitoneal transfusion is necessary. On the other hand, evidence that the fetus is not in danger permits the opportunity for greater fetal maturity and a better chance for postnatal survival.[45]

While labor is usually induced at approximately 37 weeks, when there is a rapidly rising and excessive titer (1:64), especially when there has been a previously affected erythroblastotic infant, induction has been carried out on the basis of amniocentesis as early as 32 weeks with a viable infant.[14]

Although most workers find amniocentesis a relatively safe procedure, attention has been drawn to the possibility that fetal erythrocytes may enter the maternal circulation if the placenta were damaged during amniocentesis.[112] Fetal hemorrhage may conceivably result, compromising the life of the fetus, and may also precipitate a rise in antibody titer in the mother. On the other hand, in a review of a large number of cases[29] no evidence was found that amniocentesis gave rise to changes in maternal antibody titer or increased the severity of hemolytic disease in the current or subsequent pregnancy. It is as yet impossible to state that the titer will be unaffected by aminocentesis. There are potential dangers in amniocentesis itself, in the premature induction of labor, and in the prematurity of the infant after birth.[60] The objective, of course, is a drop in the stillbirth rate, with a commensurate drop in neonatal death rate from premature induction.

Amniocentesis serves in selected cases as an important means of assessing the severity of erythroblastosis fetalis in those cases where fetal life is at risk.

Odell[81] has recently appraised the accuracy of diagnostic amniocentesis measurements, reviewing the shortcomings of spectrophotometric estimations of bile pigment concentrations. For instance, such factors as contamination of the amniotic fluid by oxyhemoglobin, tetracyclines, and meconium have been found to invalidate the spectrophotometric technique of assay. Various supplementary measurements have been suggested to provide greater accuracy. These include measurements in the amniotic fluid of nonhematin iron and erythropoietin, as well as sequential determinations of bilirubin-to-albumin and hemopexin-to-albumin ratios.

Müller-Eberhard and associates[72,74] had demonstrated that hemopexin, a beta glycoprotein, serves as a major transport protein of heme in extravascular fluids. Similar to haptoglobin, plasma hemopexin concentrations are reduced during hemolytic episodes in association with increased clearance of heme from the circulation. Müller-Eberhard and Bashors[73] reported that ratios of bilirubin to albumin in amniotic fluid above 0.10 were found in most patients receiving intrauterine transfusions, and that a ratio below 0.05 indicated patients needing no or one transfusion. A rising ratio of hemopexin to albumin usually suggested no or mild involvement; leveling and falling ratios were found when exchange or intrauterine transfusions were needed.

In the light of the information available from the more recent measurements, one can conclude that it "is no longer necessary to depend solely on the indirectly determined bile-pigment concentration of amniotic fluid in the management of intrauterine hemolytic disease."[81]

In a recent study Bowman and Pollock[11] state that, with the examination of amniotic fluid and spectrophotometry, their accuracy of prediction of severity of the disease in utero has risen to 96.8% in all isoimmunized pregnancies studied (252 Rh-negative isoimmunized pregnancies). This figure compares with 62% accuracy of prognosis in the period before amniotic fluid was examined. The ability to forecast the degree of disease in utero provides an indication for induction at or after 32 weeks' gestation. The survival of fifty-four infants was thus attributed to early delivery. They recommend amniocentesis (1) in all isoimmunized pregnancies with a history of preceding disease severe enough to require treatment or to cause stillbirth, no matter what the titer, (2) in all isoimmunized pregnancies with a preceding history of stillbirth, cause unknown, (3) in all first sensitized pregnancies in which the antibody titer exceeds 8 in albumin by 32 weeks' gestation, and (4) in all second and subsequent isoimmunized pregnancies in which the previous Rh-positive infant did not require treatment and in which the titer exceeds 8 in albumin. Bowman and Pollock point out that the amniotic fluid sample must be protected from light, since light (particularly daylight, but also artificial light to a lesser extent) rapidly decolorizes the bilirubin and the bilirubin-like pigments in the fluid which are responsible for the diagnostic 450 m$\mu$ optical density rise. Also, contamination with blood may make the fluid valueless since a spurious 450 m$\mu$ rise may develop. They found that the procedure carries no risk to the mother, but if the placenta is traversed, her antibody titer may rise and the severity of the disease in the fetus may be increased. They found amniocentesis was of proved value in calling attention to the fetus so severely affected that survival is possible only through intraperitoneal fetal transfusions.

***Examination of amniotic fluid for genetic defects.*** The realization that the amniotic fluid constantly bathes the developing fetus and fetal membranes and is in a dynamic equilibrium with both the intrauterine contents and the mother led to the concept that much useful information regarding fetal health and disease can be obtained by examination of the fluid.[34]

The finding that amniotic fluid contains living cells which may be cultured provides an opportunity for determining early in pregnancy the diagnosis of chromosome anomalies when the mother is already known to have a high risk of producing an abnormal child. Prenatal diagnosis through amniocentesis provides a more accurate basis for the prevention of births of children with serious genetic mental defects and fatal genetic diseases than counseling by the calculation of probability risks.[65]

The exact origin and fate of amniotic fluid remains unknown.[65] It is stated[65] that the term fetus swallows about 450 ml. of fluid and passes about 500 ml. of urine every 24 hours. At 14 weeks' gestation the amniotic fluid volume is between 98 and 116 ml. and at 16 weeks between 208 and 285 ml.[33] At 20 weeks the volume rises to 350 ml.[87] The amniotic fluid cells are of fetal origin and are derived mainly from fetal skin and amnion. It is maintained that some disorders evident in cultured skin fibroblasts could also be diagnosed in cultured amniotic fluid cells. The composition of amniotic fluid resembles that of extracellular fluid, but as pregnancy progresses extracellular fluids include products of deglutition, micturition, and defecation.

Nadler and Gerbie[76] recently reported 162 transabdominal amniocenteses performed between the thirteenth and eighteenth weeks of

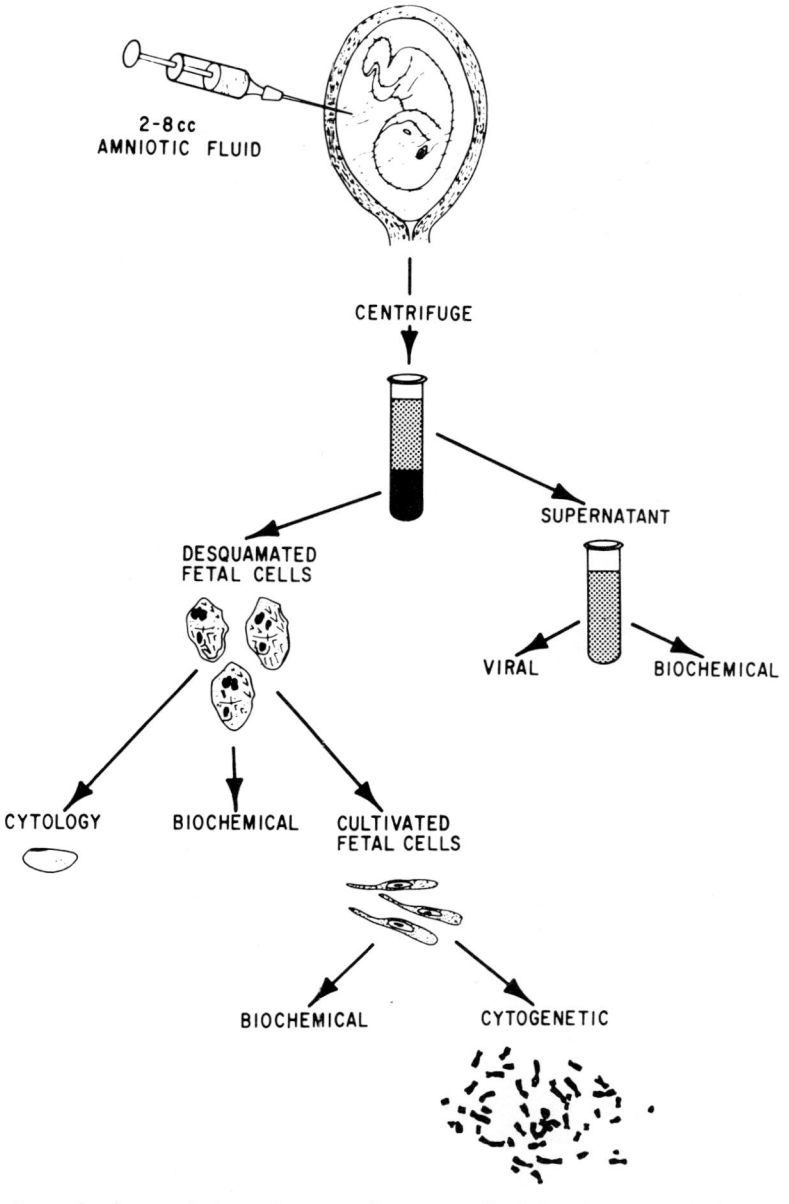

Fig. 11. General scheme of the utilization of amniotic fluid for the prenatal detection of genetic disorders. (From Nadler, H. L.: Prenatal detection of genetic defects, J. Pediat. 74:132-143, 1969.)

fetal gestation as part of the management of 155 "high risk pregnancies" where there was an appreciable risk that the child would be affected with a serious genetic disorder. They were able to culture successfully from amniotic fluid cells of fetuses with Down's syndrome, Pompe's disease, lysosomal acid phosphatase deficiency, and metachromatic leukodystrophy.

At present it would appear that the most suitable time to perform abdominal amniocentesis is at 16 weeks of gestation. The amniotic supernate is examined for amino acids, levels of 17-ketosteroids, and other less well-defined substances. It is also examined for desquamated amniotic fluid cells, for their cultivation, and for subsequent chromosome studies (Fig. 11). The familial metabolic disorders demonstrable in tissue culture include the following: Gaucher's disease, Niemann-Pick disease, Chediak-Higashi syndrome, Marfan's syndrome, orotic aciduria, and many others.[65,75] The list of metabolic errors detectable in cultivated amniotic cells is constantly increasing and includes galactosemia, cystathionuria, homocystinuria, Lesch-Nyhan syndrome, and the Hurler and Hunter syndromes.[76] Carter[13] postulated that a screening procedure by amniocentesis may come into common use for mothers over 40 years of age for the detection of chromosome anomalies, especially the G trisomy of Down's syndrome. He cites as an example the case of a mother who has a D/G translocation with a perhaps one in five chance of producing a live-born child with Down's syndrome; both parents requested a termination.[13]

Complications of this procedure have been reported in less than 1% of cases. In the adverse effects that have been reported, fetal mortality appears greater than maternal, with fetal deaths reported due to abruptio placentae, amnionitis, and fetal hemorrhage. The maternal mortality includes amnionitis, maternal hemorrhage, and peritonitis.

Several hereditary metabolic disorders are accompanied by changes in urinary composition.[27] Some of these disorders might therefore be detectable in utero by demonstrating changes in the composition of the amniotic fluid since fetal urine is known to contribute to the formation of amniotic fluid from at least the twelfth week of gestation. Twenty-seven amino acids and related compounds have been identified in human amniotic fluid. The concentrations of some substances remain more or less the same throughout pregnancy —e.g., cysteic acid, phosphoethanolamine, ethanolamine, and proline. In most cases concentration rises in the last months of pregnancy. The concentration of these substances might be useful in antenatal diagnosis. It seems likely that changes in the amino acid composition of amniotic fluid may prove diagnostic in such conditions as cystinuria, glycinuria, and Hartnup's disease. The untreated diagnosis of at least some genetic disorders associated with changes in urinary composition, by the biochemical analysis of amniotic fluid, therefore seems a distinct possibility.

## REFERENCES

1. Ackerman, B. D., Dyer, G. Y., and Leydorf, M. M.: Hyperbilirubinemia and kernicterus in small premature infants, Pediatrics 45:918, 1970.
2. Aidin, R., Corner, B., and Tovey, G.: Kernicterus and prematurity, Lancet 1:1153, 1950.
3. Allen, F. H., Jr.: Early jaundice in the newborn; aids to detection, New Eng. J. Med. 258:1302, 1958.
4. Allen F. H., Jr., and Diamond, L. K.: Erythroblastosis fetalis—including exchange transfusion technic, Boston, 1957, Little, Brown & Co.
5. Allison, A. C.: Danger of vitamin K to newborn, Lancet 1:669, 1955.
6. Bakay, L.: Studies on blood brain barrier with radioactive phosphorus. III. Embryonic development of the barrier, Arch. Neurol. Psychiat. 70:30, 1953.
7. Behrman, R. E., and Hibbard, E.: Bilirubin; acute effects in newborn rhesus monkeys, Science 144:545, 1964.
8. Bevis, D. C. A.: Blood pigments in haemolytic disease of the newborn, J. Obstet. Gynaec. Brit. Emp. 63:68, 1956.
9. Boggs, T. R., and Abelson, N. M.: An early and reliable guide in the prognosis and management of erythroblastosis, Amer. J. Dis. Child. 88:506, 1954.
10. Bowman, J. M.: Gastrointestinal absorption of isohemagglutinin, Amer. J. Dis. Child. 105:352, 1963.
11. Bowman, J. M., and Pollock, J. M.: Amniotic fluid spectrophotometry and early delivery in the management of erythroblastosis fetalis, Pediatrics 35:815, 1965.
12. Broman, B.: Incompatibility of blood, Acta Pediat. 36:585, 1948.
13. Carter, C.: Antenatal paediatrics by amniocentesis, Arch. Dis. Child. 47:157, 1970.
14. Cary, W.: Amniocentesis in haemolytic disease of the newborn, M. J. Australia 47:778, 1960.
15. Chan, A. C., Chung, F., and Keitel, H. G.:

ABO hemolytic disease serologic diagnosis with the two-stage direct antiglobulin test by means of fresh serum, J. Pediat. **61**:405, 1961.
16. Chown, B., and Bowman, W. D.: The place of early delivery in the prevention of foetal death from erythroblastosis, Ped. Clin. N. Amer. **5**:279, 1958.
17. Clifford, J. H., Mathews, P., Reiquam, C. W., and Palmer, H. D.: Screening for hemolytic disease of the newborn by cord blood Coombs' testing; analysis of a two-year experience, Clin. Pediat. **7**:465, 1968.
18. Coombs, R. R. A., Mourant, A. E., and Race, R. R.: A new test for the detection of weak and "incomplete" Rh agglutinins, Brit. J. Exper. Path. **26**:255, 1945.
19. Crigler, J. F., and Najjar, V. A.: Congenital familial nonhemolytic jaundice with kernicterus, Pediatrics **10**:169, 1952.
20. Crosse, V. M., Meyer, T. C., and Gerrard, J. W.: Kernicterus and prematurity, Arch. Dis. Child. **30**:501, 1955.
21. Davies, B. S., Gerrard, J., and Waterhouse, J. A. H.: The pattern of haemolytic disease of the newborn, Arch. Dis. Child. **28**:466, 1953.
22. Day, R. L.: Inhibition of brain respiration in vitro by bilirubin; reversal of inhibition by various means, Amer. J. Dis. Child. **88**:504, 1954.
23. Desforges, J. F., and O'Connell, L. G.: Hematologic observations of erythroblastosis fetalis, Blood **10**:802, 1955.
24. Diamond, I.: Kernicterus; revised concepts of pathogenesis and treatment, Pediatrics **38**:539, 1966.
25. Diamond, L. K.: Clinical pathological conference, J. Pediat. **50**:490, 1957.
26. Driscoll, S. G.: Hydrops fetalis, New Eng. J. Med. **275**:1432, 1966.
27. Emery, A. E. H., Burt, D., Nelson, M. M., and Scrimgeour, J. B.: Antenatal diagnosis and amino acid composition of amniotic fluid, Lancet **1**:1307, 1970.
28. Erlandson, M. E., and Haber, J. M.: Severe erythroblastosis fetalis in first immunized pregnancy, Amer. J. Obstet Gynec. **90**:779, 1964.
29. Fairweather, D. V. I., Murray, S., Parkin, D., and Walker, W.: Possible immunological implications of amniocentesis, Lancet **2**:1190, 1963.
30. Forrester, R. M., and Miller, J.: The dental changes associated with kernicterus, Arch. Dis. Child. **30**:224, 1955.
31. Freda, V. J., and Gorman, J. G.: Current concepts; antepartum management of Rh hemolytic disease, Bull. Sloane Hosp. Women **8**:147, 1962.
32. Friedman, V.: Blood-brain barrier, Physiol. Rev. **22**:125, 1942.
33. Fuchs, F.: Volume of amniotic fluid at various stages of pregnancy, Clin. Obstet. Gynec. **9**:449, 1966.
34. Fuchs, F.: Genetic information from amniotic fluid constituents, Clin. Obstet. Gynec. **9**:565, 1966.
35. Gellis, S. S., editor: Year book of pediatrics, 1957-1958 Series, Chicago, 1957, Year Book Medical Publishers, Inc., p. 17.
36. Gellis, S. S.: Year book of pediatrics, 1961-1962 Series, Chicago, 1961, Year Book Medical Publishers, Inc., p. 298.
37. Gerrard, J. W.: Kernicterus, Brain **75**:526, 1952.
38. Gerver, J. M., and Day, R.: Intelligence quotient of children who have recovered from erythroblastosis fetalis, J. Pediat. **36**:342, 1950.
39. Gitlin, D.: Some concepts of plasma protein metabolism A.D. 1956, Pediatrics **19**:657, 1957.
40. Gunn, C. K.: Hereditary acholuria jaundice in the rat, Canad. M.A.J. **50**:230, 1944.
41. Haberman, S., Krafft, C. J., Luecke, P. E., Jr., and Peach, R. O.: ABO isoimmunization; the use of the specific Coombs and heat elution tests in the detection of hemolytic disease, J. Pediat. **56**:471, 1960.
42. Harris, R. C., Lucey, J. F., and MacLean, J. R.: Kernicterus in premature infants associated with low concentrations of bilirubin in the plasma, Pediatrics **21**:875, 1958.
43. Hedenstedt, S., and Naeslund, J.: Investigations of the permeability of the placenta with the help of elliptocytes, Acta Med. Scandinav. (supp. 1) **170**:126, 1946.
44. Holman, G. H.: Studies on physiologic hyperbilirubinemia of Negro and white premature infants, Pediatrics **22**:1115, 1958.
45. Horger, E. O. III, and Hutchinson, D. L.: Diagnostic use of amniotic fluid, J. Pediat. **75**:503, 1969.
46. Hsia, D. Y-Y., Allen, F. H., Jr., Gellis, S. S., and Diamond, L. K.: Erythroblastosis fetalis; studies of serum bilirubin in relation to kernicterus, New Eng. J. Med. **247**:668, 1952.
47. Hsia, D. Y-Y, Hsia, H. H., Gofstein, R. M., Winter, A., and Gellis, S. S.: Determination of concentration of bilirubin in serum; rapid micro-method employing photoelectric colorimeter; rapid micro-method employing color standards, Pediatrics **18**:433, 1956.
48. Jennison, R. F., and Walker, A. H. C.: Amniocentesis, Lancet **2**:1387, 1963.
49. Johnson, L., Sarmiento, F., Blanc, W. A., and Day, R.: Kernicterus in rats with inherited deficiency of glucuronyl transferase, Amer. J. Dis. Child. **97**:591, 1959.

50. Kramer, L. I.: Advancement of dermal icterus in the jaundiced newborn, Amer. J. Dis. Child. 118:456, 1969.
51. Levine, P.: The mechanism of isoimmunization by the Rh factor of red blood cells, Arch. Path. 37:83, 1944.
52. Levine, P., Burnham, L., Katzin, E. M., and Vogel, P.: The role of isoimmunization in the pathogenesis of erythroblastosis fetalis, Amer. J. Obstet. Gynec. 42:925, 1941.
53. Levine, P., Vogel, P., and Rosenfield, R. E.: Hemolytic disease of the newborn. In Levine, S. Z., and others, editors: Advances in pediatrics, vol. 6, Chicago, 1953, Year Book Medical Publishers, Inc.
54. Lewis F., Schulman, H., and Hayashi, T. T.: Spectrophotometric analysis of amniotic fluid in erythroblastosis fetalis, J.A.M.A. 190:195, 1964.
55. Liley, A. W.: Liquor amnii analysis in the management of the pregnancy complicated by rhesus sensitization, Amer. J. Obstet. Gynec. 82:1359, 1961.
56. Lindsay, S.: Hemolytic disease of the newborn infant (erythroblastosis fetalis); a study of the pathologic lesions of twenty cases, J. Pediat. 37:582, 1950.
57. Lucey, J. F., Hibbard, E., Behrman, R. E., Gallardo, F. O., and Windle, W. F.: Kernicterus in asphyxiated newborn rhesus monkeys, Exp. Neurol. 9:43, 1964.
58. Lucey, J. F., Phillips, C. L., Utterback, J. G., and McKay, R. J., Jr.: A difference in the jaundice of hyperbilirubinemia among premature infants in two hospitals, Pediatrics 30:3, 1962.
59. Lucia, S. P., and Hunt, M. L.: A study of the occurrence of normal Rh-negative infants born to sensitized Rh-negative women, J. Pediat. 37:599, 1950.
60. MacKay, E. V., and Watson, D.: The diagnostic value of bilirubin levels in amniotic fluid in rhesus iso-immunized pregnancies, M. J. Australia 49:492, 1962.
61. Macris, N. T., Hellman, L. M., and Watson, R. J.: The transmission of transfused sickle-trait cells from mother to fetus, Amer. J. Obst. Gynec. 76:1214, 1958.
62. McElfresh, A. E., Kurkcuoglu, M., Vaughan, V. C., III, and Armbruster, R.: Elution of of anti-A and anti-B antibody from erythrocytes of incompatible newborn infants, J. Pediat. 56:39, 1960.
63. Meyer, T. C., and Angus, J.: The effect of large doses of "Synkavit" in the newborn, Arch. Dis. Child. 31:212, 1956.
64. Michael, A. F., Jr., and Mauer, A. M.: Maternal-fetal transfusion as a cause of plethora in the neonatal period, Pediatrics 28:458, 1961.
65. Milunsky, A., Littlefield, J. W., Kanfer, J. N., Kolodny, E. H., Shih, V. E., and Atkins, L.: Prenatal genetic diagnosis, New Eng. J. Med. 283:1370-1498, 1970.
66. Mollison, P. L.: Blood transfusion in clinical medicine, ed. 3, Oxford, 1961, Blackwell Scientific Publications.
67. Mollison, P. L.: Blood transfusion in clinical medicine, ed. 4, Philadelphia, 1967, F. A. Davis Co., p. 657.
68. Mollison, P. L., and Cutbush, M.: Haemolytic disease of the newborn; criteria of severity, Brit. Med. J. 1:123, 1949.
69. Mollison, P. L., and Cutbush, M.: A method of measuring the severity of a series of cases of hemolytic disease of the newborn, Blood 6:777, 1951.
70. Molthan, L.: Rh-D hemolytic disease in Negro and white infants; a comparison, J. Pediat. 62:474, 1963.
71. Morton, J. A., and Pickles, M. M.: Use of trypsin in the detection of incomplete anti-Rh antibodies, Nature 159:779, 1947.
72. Müller-Eberhard, U.: Hemopexin, New Eng. J. Med. 283:1090, 1970.
73. Müller-Eberhard, U., and Bashors, R.: Assessment of Rh disease by ratios of bilirubin to albumin and hemopexin to albumin in amniotic fluid, New Eng. J. Med. 282:1163, 1970.
74. Müller-Eberhard, U., Javid, J., Liem, H. H., Hanstein, A., and Hanna, M.: Plasma concentrations of hemopexin, haptoglobin and heme in patients with various hemolytic diseases, Blood 32:811, 1968.
75. Nadler, H. L.: Prenatal detection of genetic defects, J. Pediat. 74:132, 1969.
76. Nadler, H. L., and Gerbie, A. B.: Role of amniocentesis in the intrauterine detection of genetic disorders, New Eng. J. Med. 282:596, 1970.
77. Naeslund, J.: Studies on placental permeability with radioactive isotopes of phosphorus and iron, Acta Obst. et Gynec. Scandinav. 30:231, 1951.
78. Odell, G. B.: Studies in kernicterus. I. The protein binding of bilirubin, J. Clin. Invest. 38:823, 1959.
79. Odell, G. B.: The dissociation of bilirubin from albumin and its clinical implications, J. Pediat. 55:268, 1959.
80. Odell, G. B.: Comments on paper by Diamond, I.: Kernicterus; revised concepts of pathogenesis and treatment, Pediatrics 38:543, 1966.
81. Odell, G. B.: Evaluation of fetal hemolysis, New Eng. J. Med. 282:1204, 1970.
82. Oski, F. A., and Altman, A. A.: Carboxyhemoglobin levels in hemolytic disease of the newborn, J. Pediat. 61:709, 1962.

83. Perlstein, M.: Infantile cerebral palsy. In Levine, S. Z., and others, editors: Advances in pediatrics, vol. 7, Chicago, 1955, Year Book Medical Publishers, Inc., p. 209.
84. Phipps, R. H., Johnson, P., and Tooleg, W. H.: Circulatory changes in newborn with erythroblastosis with and without hydrops, Ped. Research 1:326, 1967.
85. Pickles, M. M.: Haemolytic disease of the newborn, Springfield, Ill., 1949, Charles C Thomas, Publisher.
86. Pinksy, L.: Genetic approaches to diseases of hypersensitivity, Amer. J. Med. Sci. 245:726, 1963.
87. Plentl, A. A.: Formation and circulation of amniotic fluid, Clin. Obstet. Gynec. 9:427, 1966.
88. Pollack, W., Reiss, A. M., and Reacy, M.: Observations on the direct Coombs' test on cord erythrocytes after the addition of complement, Vox Sang. 3:442, 1958.
89. Potter, E.: Diagnosis of erythroblastosis fetalis in the macerated fetus, Arch. Path. 41:223, 1946.
90. Queenan, J. T., and Adams, D. W.: Amniocentesis, Lancet 1:380, 1964.
91. Schulman, I., and Smith, C. H.: Fetal and adult hemoglobin in hemolytic disease of the newborn, Amer. J. Dis. Child. 87:167, 1954.
92. Silverman, W. A., Andersen, D. H., Blanc, W. A., and Crozier, D. N.: A difference in mortality rate and incidence of kernicterus among premature infants alloted to two prophylactic antibacterial regimens, Pediatrics 18:614, 1956.
93. Smith, C. H.: Crossing the chorion; amniocentesis, J. Pediat. 65:642, 1964.
94. Stamey, C. C., and Diamond, L. K.: Congenital hemolytic anemia in the newborn, Amer. J. Dis. Child. 94:616, 1957.
95. Stefanini, M., and Dameshek, W.: The hemorrhagic disorders, New York, 1955, Grune & Stratton, Inc.
96. Stempel, R., and Zetterström, R.: Concentration of bilirubin in cerebrospinal fluid in hemolytic disease of the newborn, Pediatrics 16:184, 1955.
97. Strauss, L., and Driscoll, S. G.: Congenital neuroblastoma involving the placenta; reports of two cases, Pediatrics 34:23, 1964.
98. Taylor, J. F.: Sensitization of Rh-negative daughters by their Rh-positive mothers, New Eng. J. Med. 276:547, 1967.
99. Thumasathit, B., Nondasuta, A., Silpisornkosol, S., Lousuebsakul, B., Unchalipongse, P., and Mangkornkanok, M.: Hydrops fetalis associated with Bart's hemoglobin in Northern Thailand, J. Pediat. 73:132, 1968.
100. Vaughan, V. C. III: Current status of hemolytic disease of the newborn, Postgrad. Med. 18:115, 1955.
101. Vaughan, V. C. III, Allen, F. H., Jr., and Diamond, L. K.: Erythroblastosis fetalis; further observations on kernicterus, Pediatrics 6:706, 1950.
102. Walker, A. H. C.: Liquor amnii studies in the prediction of haemolytic disease in the newborn, Brit. Med. J. 2:376, 1957.
103. Walker, W., and Murray, S.: Haemolytic disease of newborn as a family problem, Brit. Med. J. 1:187, 1956.
104. Waters, W. J., and Porter, E.: Indications for exchange transfusion based upon the role of albumin in the treatment of hemolytic disease of the newborn, Pediatrics 33:749, 1964.
105. Wheeler, W. E., and Scholl, M. L. L.: Determination of anti-Rh antibody in infants with erythroblastosis fetalis, Amer. J. Dis. Child. 74:274, 1947.
106. Wiener, A. S., Nappi, R., and Gordon, E. B.: Studies in Rh sensitization; methods; effect of Rh-negative pregnancies on Rh antibody titer, Blood 6:522, 1951.
107. Wiener, A. S., Nappi, R., and Gordon, E. B.: Studies on Rh sensitization, importance of the titer of Rh antibodies in the sensitized pregnant Rh-negative woman for prognosis, Amer. J. Obstet. Gynec. 63:6, 1952.
108. Wiener, A. S., and Wexler, I. B.: An Rh-Hr syllabus; the types and their application, ed. 2, New York, 1963, Grune & Stratton, Inc., p. 19.
109. Yunis, E., and Bridges, R.: The serologic diagnosis of ABO hemolytic disease of the newborn, Amer. J. Clin. Path. 41:1, 1964.
110. Zetterström, R., and Ernster, L.: Bilirubin, an uncoupler of oxidative phosphorylation in isolated mitochondria, Nature 178:1335, 1956.
111. Zipursky, A., and Israels, L. G.: The pathogenesis and prevention of Rh immunization, Canad. M. A. J. 97:1245, 1967.
112. Zipursky, A., Pollock, J., Chown, B., and Israels, L. G.: Transplacental foetal haemorrhage after placental injury during amniocentesis, Lancet 2:493, 1963.
113. Zipursky, A., Pollock, J., Neelands, P. J., Chown, B., and Israels, L. G.: The transplacental passage of fetal blood cells and the pathogenesis of Rh-immunization during pregnancy, Lancet 2:489, 1963.
114. Zuelzer, W. W., and Mudgett, R. T.: Kernicterus; etiology study based on an analysis of 55 cases, Pediatrics 6:452, 1950.

# 10 ERYTHROBLASTOSIS FETALIS (HEMOLYTIC ANEMIA OF THE NEWBORN INFANT)—TREATMENT

*Objectives of treatment.* The treatment of the infant with erythroblastosis fetalis has three major aims: (1) the prevention or control of cardiac failure, (2) the prevention or control of bilirubinemia in an effort to prevent the occurrence of kernicterus, and (3) the control of anemia (this is almost automatically associated with the first two aims). Severe anemia and its consequences appear to be primarily responsible for intrauterine and early neonatal deaths in erythroblastosis fetalis. Hemolysis, continuing after birth with even mild anemia, may be associated with increased amounts of bilirubin and other toxic products, which in turn may be injurious to tissues. It will be seen that, except in the infant with severe anemia and cardiac failure, treatment is primarily oriented toward keeping the blood bilirubin low rather than toward achieving a high hemoglobin level. It should be remembered that respiratory distress is the commonest cause of death. These babies are immature and attention should be paid to adequate ventilation.

To date the only effective therapy in controlling the aforementioned complications is exchange transfusion. In evaluating an infant for exchange transfusion, therefore, the physician must decide whether or not the disease state in the infant is severe enough to place him in danger of cardiac failure or subsequent hyperbilirubinemia of sufficient magnitude to cause kernicterus. Optimally, the decision concerning replacement transfusion should be made as soon as possible, since cardiac deaths often occur within the first few hours of life and since the prevention of bilirubinemia is much more efficient than the removal of the pigment once accumulation has been permitted to occur.

*Treatment.* The mainstay of treatment is the exchange transfusion, but its successful achievement depends upon many correlated items of procedure.

*Exchange transfusions*
*Rationale*: Exchange transfusions accomplish the removal of all but a small fraction of the infant's own "destroyable" and sensitized Rh-positive red cells and their replacement by an adequate concentration of normal nonsensitized Rh-negative cells. Unless the infant's red cells are replaced, they will continue to be destroyed by the maternal anti-Rh antibodies which persist in the circulation for 4 to 8 weeks after birth. With a two-volume exchange (twice the blood volume of the infant) 85 to 90% of the sensitized red cells are removed.

Although bilirubin is removed simultaneously with the red cells of the infant, by exchange of plasma, it frequently rebounds to approximately two-thirds of pretransfusion levels because of pigment sequestered in the extravascular reservoirs. It has been demonstrated that bilirubin accumulates in the plasma during exchange transfusion, even while it is being removed, and must therefore enter the circulation from the tissues.[18] Evidence from exchange transfusions is that about two-thirds of all bilirubin is extravascular.

There is suggestive evidence that the extravascular bilirubin pool is in two compartments: a "labile" part that is contiguous to, and in equilibration with, the plasma and can equilibrate during an exchange transfusion, and a "stable" fraction that is largely responsible for the rebound phenomenon.[128] The bilirubin withdrawn from tissue spaces is supplemented by that resulting from the breakdown of transfused red cells, especially if it has been stored for some time.[77] Bilirubin is most effectively removed by a slow exchange and with large volumes of blood. Anti-Rh antibodies are also inadequately removed by an exchange transfusion because of their wide distribution in extravascular spaces.

The rate of disappearance of haptoglobin from the infant's blood after exchange transfusion serves as an index of the rate of erythrocyte destruction in this period.[73] Plasma haptoglobin levels decrease in hemolytic states because the released hemoglobin is bound to haptoglobin, forming a molecule that is rapidly removed by the reticuloendothelial system. Based on this method, evidence of hemolysis, followed by a subsequent rise in bilirubin to a degree necessitating a second procedure, was found in fifteen of nineteen exchanges. Although many factors contribute to the bilirubin rebound, apparently a substantial segment is derived from hemolysis of donor blood, nonexchanged infant cells, and newly formed erythrocytes released from the bone marrow of the infant. Since newborn infants do not generally produce measurable amounts of haptoglobin during the first weeks of life, the rate of change in the level is from the donor-contributed exogenous source. A fall in the haptoglobin can only be influenced by the rate of removal of this substance.

In infants with Rh erythroblastosis the immediate objective is to replace the vulnerable Rh-positive cells, which are the sources of bilirubin, with the calculated amount of Rh-negative cells. The concurrent aim is the removal of pigment from the intravascular and extravascular fluid compartments. This procedure is usually accomplished expeditiously within 1 to 1½ hours. In the deeply jaundiced patient in whom correction of the anemia may not be so important as the removal of bilirubin, an interval of about 30 minutes to 1 hour may be permitted to elapse between each volume of the exchange. This delay will depend upon the condition of the infant and the general overall care in the treatment room.

The blood volume also can be adjusted by exchange transfusion, especially in infants with cardiorespiratory embarrassment. Infants with cord blood hemoglobin levels of 8 gm. per 100 ml. or less are often distressed at birth and can be shown to have elevated venous pressure and often cardiac failure.[92] One factor which may contribute to excessive blood volume and circulatory overload is the sudden passage of placental blood into the newborn infant at birth—hence the precaution of clamping the cord at the earliest moment. In this type of case every effort is made to reduce blood volume and venous pressure by establishing a deficit before beginning the exchange transfusion. The venous pressure is measured at intervals during the exchange, and appropriate deficits are created as necessary. Artifacts in venous pressure readings do occur. If the pressure is unusually high, the pulse and respiration will be increased. Therefore, these should be used together with venous pressure readings as criteria for the need to establish a deficit. The reduction in blood volume and correction of the anemia by an exchange transfusion at birth may be lifesaving in the severely anemic infant.

Recordings of venous pressure may be erroneously elevated in several situations.[43] A tight restraint over the lower thorax exerting pressure over the liver or the introduction of the catheter into a branch of the umbilical vein (a radicle of the portal system within the liver) rather than into the ductus venosus and inferior vena cava may result in unusually high recordings of pressure. If blood is continually removed to reduce the pressure, severe anemia may be induced. The misdirection of the catheter, which is usually associated with easy introduction but slow removal of blood, can be easily corrected by withdrawal and reintroduction.

*Indications*: The indications for exchange transfusion reside in the demonstration, by clinical and laboratory means, that the disease in the infant is, and may be expected to be, of sufficient severity to lead to the aforementioned complications. To a large extent the criteria for immediate exchange stem from clinical and laboratory evidence that a severe hemolytic process has been going on in utero. Thus clinical evidence of severe disease such as pallor, edema, poor respirations, and hepatosplenomegaly constitute indications for immediate exchange (jaundice at birth is practically never seen). Laboratory evidence of a severe prenatal hemolytic process includes the presence of anemia at birth (as determined by a low hemoglobin level in the cord blood), elevation of cord bilirubin (above 3 mg./100 ml.), and manifestations of marked attempts at blood regeneration (normoblastosis, reticulocytosis).

The baby threatened by cardiac failure always has severe anemia. On the other hand, an infant with good powers of regeneration in utero may be born with a nearly normal hemoglobin concentration and look clinically well but may still be in severe danger of subsequent hyperbilirubinemia. This is due to the fact that the hemolytic process will proceed unabated postnatally, but that the mechanism for excreting bilirubin will be inadequate. In utero, clearance of indirect reacting bilirubin is apparently carried out mainly by the placenta. Postnatally, however, bilirubin excretion is dependent upon the infant's liver function and the activation of a hepatic enzyme system which converts the insoluble indirect bilirubin to a water-soluble bilirubin diglucuronide (direct bilirubin) which may then be excreted. Development of efficient bilirubin excretion usually requires 3 to 4 days in a full-term baby and longer in a premature infant. It is essential, therefore, to detect early those infants with a severe hemolytic process and to prevent the occurrence of bilirubinemia by removing the Rh-positive antibody-coated cells and replacing them with Rh-negative cells.

In addition to the criteria described, there are reasons for close observation of certain infants who are particularly susceptible to kernicterus. These include premature infants, infants in a family with previous stillbirth and kernicterus, and infants born of mothers with very high antenatal titers.

It has been well established that the incidence of kernicterus may be reduced to extremely low levels if the indirect serum bilirubin is kept below 20 mg./100 ml. In the mature infant with erythroblastosis the likelihood of kernicterus has been estimated as about 1 in 10 for an indirect serum bilirubin of 20 to 25 mg./100 ml., about 1 in 5 for 25 to 30 mg./100 ml., and about 1 in 2 over 30 mg./100 ml.

The varying bilirubin levels obtained in the cord blood and the neonatal period from laboratory to laboratory and the significant differences in the number of exchange transfusions in the same areas (p. 143) led to the adoption of a uniform bilirubin standard. The recommendations include such items as absorptivity of the bilirubin, preparation and dilution of the standard, its preservation and calibration, and other items essential in performance of the test.[29]

In the small premature infant or in any premature infant whose condition is poor, it may be necessary to postpone the exchange transfusion because of the risk involved. The known susceptibility of such infants to kernicterus aggravates the problem. Under these circumstances careful observation is necessary, successive bilirubin determinations should be evaluated, and consultation with other physicians may be necessary before treatment is undertaken.

Before treatment is contemplated it is important to ascertain that the major portion of the bilirubin is of the indirect-reacting type. Whereas this pigment is associated with brain damage, increased concentration of direct bilirubin indicates obstruction or an inflammatory process in the biliary system. An exchange transfusion for a high direct-reacting bilirubin would be purposeless.

Indications for exchange transfusion may be summarized as follows:

*Indications for immediate exchange at birth*

Assuming that the direct Coombs test is positive, the indications for an immediate exchange are as follows:
1. Clinical signs of severe disease
   (a) Pallor
   (b) Hepatosplenomegaly
   (c) Poor respiration
   (d) Jaundice
   (e) Edema—with or without definitive signs of cardiac failure
2. Laboratory evidence of severe hemolytic disease
   (a) Cord hemoglobin of 14 gm./100 ml.* or below (less than 14.5 gm. venous blood or 15 gm. capillary blood)
   (b) Reticulocytosis over 6%
   (c) Normoblastosis greater than 10 per 100 white blood cells

   It should be remembered, however, that a low cord hemoglobin level may coexist with a low cord bilirubin level (below 3 mg./100 ml.); hence the greater importance of the former as a criterion for exchange at birth.

*Indications for initial exchange, late exchange, or repeated exchange*
1. Continued signs of cardiac failure or severe illness
2. Indirect bilirubin levels rising at greater than 0.5 mg./100 ml. per hour, reaching 7 mg. at 6 hours, 10 mg. at 12 hours, and approaching 20 mg./100 ml. at any time.

These indications may be restated as follows:

An exchange transfusion is performed at birth

---

*The cord hemoglobin level at which exchange transfusions are recommended varies for the full-term infant from below 11 gm./100 ml. to below 15.5 gm./100 ml. in different clinics. The level of 14 gm./100 ml. of hemoglobin is derived from the mean cord blood hemoglobin level obtained in a series of 133 normal infants in our clinic (16.4 ± 1.1 gm. per 100 ml.)

in an infant with a positive Coombs test who also presents one of the following abnormalities:
1. Clinical evidence of severe disease at birth with or without cardiac failure
2. Cord hemoglobin level of 14 gm./100 ml. and below
3. Cord bilirubin levels above 4 mg. per 100 ml.

A maternal titer of 1:64 or more as well as the results obtained by spectroscopic examination of the amniotic fluid should alert the pediatrician to the possible need for exchange transfusions. Wheeler and Ambuel[148] have pointed out that 80% of babies with a cord blood level above 4 mg. per 100 ml. eventually require an exchange transfusion, whereas only 20% of those with cord bilirubin below this level need treatment. These criteria for replacement transfusions are acceptable in most clinics, for severe disease is usually anticipated if the infant is untreated.

Odell and co-workers[101,102] have also included the level of serum protein as an indication for an exchange transfusion. A serum protein concentration below 5.5 gm. per 100 ml. is regarded as an indication, since additional bilirubin formation may not be reflected by a correlated rise in the serum bilirubin concentration in the presence of hypoproteinemia. Usually, the urgency of the condition does not permit time for this additional determination and reliance is placed on adequacy of the protein content of the donor blood.

It is important to evaluate the circumstances under which a positive Coombs test is found.[43] In the presence of a positive Coombs test and anemia, but with no significant reticulocytosis or normoblastosis, a normal cord bilirubin indicates that the anemia is due to some process other than hemolysis. Thus, an infant may have a positive Coombs test, but the anemia may stem from bleeding prior to or during delivery. Normoblastosis may result from anoxia from any cause prior to or following delivery.

If exchange transfusion is not performed at birth, the bilirubin level is determined every 4 to 6 hours during the first day and every 6 to 12 hours on the second and third days. Exchange transfusions are then given if bilirubin rises to 7 mg./100 ml. at 6 hours, and 10 mg./100 ml. or more in the first 12 hours, even if the hemoglobin level is above 15 gm./100 ml. (capillary blood). From one to four exchange transfusions may be required to keep the level of bilirubin below 20 mg. per 100 ml. In general, on the basis of indirect bilirubin levels, an exchange transfusion is given if the bilirubin reaches 10 mg./100 ml. at 24 hours, 14 mg./100 ml. at 48 hours, and 20 mg./100 ml. at any time. Brown[16] recommends levels of 8 to 10 mg. per 100 ml. at 8 hours, 10 to 12 mg./100 ml. at 16 hours, 12 to 15 mg./100 ml. at 24 hours, 18 to 20 mg./100 ml. at 48 hours, and 20 mg./100 ml. at any time.

It should be emphasized that after the initial cord blood hemoglobin level is determined subsequent hemoglobin levels serve no purpose in deciding on the need for exchange transfusions to prevent kernicterus. The later hemoglobin determinations merely indicate the need for correcting the anemia, which can be accomplished by small transfusions of packed cells. The bilirubin level, however, remains the only available index of the need for an exchange transfusion.[139]

It should also be stressed that the need for exchange transfusions in the first few days of life depends on the amount of unconjugated bilirubin rather than the total amount of bilirubin. Usually, within the first 48 hours most of the bilirubin is unconjugated and the total serum bilirubin serves as a satisfactory guide to the need for exchange transfusion. Later, infants with severe erythroblastosis may accumulate large amounts of conjugated bilirubin in their serum. To avoid unnecessary repetition of exchange transfusion, conjugated and unconjugated bilirubin should be determined separately.[90] High levels of conjugated bilirubin may lead to hypoprothrombinemia,[103] but do not contribute toward clinical kernicterus.

*Specific problems:* Specific problems relating to exchange transfusion include age at time of treatment, prematurity, and induction of labor.

AGE AT TIME OF TREATMENT. The late development of kernicterus can usually be avoided by early vigorous treatment when the trend of bilirubin levels is definitely upward during the first 24 to 48 hours. Following this policy, the problem of an initial transfusion beyond the second day of life is usually never pressing. Boggs,[9] for instance, has reported a cure in fifty-three of a group of fifty-six infants born to women who had had a previously affected infant, provided the infant was first seen before the age of 12 hours.

Individual problems arise, however, after the

first 72 to 96 hours, at which time the infant may be expected to begin excreting bilirubin momentarily. The question as to the age at which it is no longer beneficial to perform an exchange transfusion in the face of hyperbilirubinemia is most difficult to answer. No time limit in days can be set beyond which hyperbilirubinemia is no longer dangerous in the full-term infant, and in the premature infant it is even more difficult.

On the other hand, the need for an exchange transfusion is not readily assessed if the bilirubin level, which has risen slowly in the first days, reaches levels somewhat below 20 mg. per 100 ml. and if on the fourth day after birth the infant is vigorous, takes its feedings well, and shows no nervous system irritability. In such infants serial bilirubin levels must be observed through the first week of life, if necessary. High bilirubin levels cannot be ignored at any specific number of days following birth. Exchange transfusions are indicated in the infant at 7 days of age, for example, if the bilirubin is in excessive concentration.[4] Patients have even been described in whom the early signs of kernicterus have been reversed by one or more exchange transfusions. Except for the established bilirubin level of 20 mg. per 100 ml., there is no way of knowing at which of the lower levels a particular infant is in jeopardy of nervous system involvement. Infants with bilirubin levels greatly in excess of 20 mg./100 ml. have been known to be free of nervous system irritation, whereas some with much lower levels have had nervous system involvement. Since there is no uniform opinion at this juncture (i.e., in the older healthy infant with bilirubin levels fluctuating narrowly about 20 mg. per 100 ml.), the decision must ultimately be left to the clinical judgment of the attending physician who has full knowledge of both the hazard of hyperbilirubinemia and the potential risk of an exchange transfusion.

In contemplating exchange transfusion for hyperbilirubinemia, the direct reacting fraction of the serum bilirubin has been discounted in the causation of kernicterus. In other words, one does not exchange for direct bilirubin, regardless of the amount.[42]

PREMATURITY. In a premature infant in whom the maternal titer is high—i.e., reaching levels of 1:64—and in whom the cord blood bilirubin level is in the vicinity of 3 mg. per 100 ml. with hemoglobin levels of about 13 gm., it may be necessary to postpone exchange transfusion if the infant's condition would be jeopardized by the procedure. During the ensuing period, successive bilirubin determinations are made and evaluated before treatment is undertaken. This is not a simple matter, and no unequivocal measurement can be employed to fill all contingencies. The peculiar problems presented by the premature infant with erythroblastosis are similar to those in connection with exchange transfusion in physiologic hyperbilirubinemia of full-term and premature infants and are discussed further later in this chapter. Parents should be informed that an exchange transfusion carries a small but definite mortality per se on which are superimposed the handicaps of prematurity. Prematurity of 2 weeks or more constitutes a compelling indication for the prophylactic employment of exchange transfusions when the indications are otherwise equivocal.[139]

INDUCTION OF LABOR. In the infant with very severe disease the chances of survival diminish with the period of gestation. It has been estimated that a woman who has had one stillbirth caused by Rh erythroblastosis has about four chances in five of losing her next Rh-positive fetus if it remains in utero until term.[90] Most intrauterine deaths occur before the thirty-seventh week of gestation. Induction of labor, accordingly, has been recommended at or after 37 weeks of gestation in sensitized Rh-negative women when conditions are obstetrically favorable and the fetus is of good size and is viable.[3] Specifically, the indications are history of a severely affected infant, hydrops or stillborn baby, a homozygous father, a rising maternal antibody titer or one that has already reached 1:64, or amniocentesis results indicating a severely affected infant. Cesarean section is exceptionally advised if the mother's condition is unfavorable for induction of labor, usually after a trial of pitocin and ruptured membranes.[3] Based on a repetitive history of stillborn infants and a rising maternal titer, induction of labor has been recommended as early as 32 weeks in selected cases.[22] The present trend, however, is for early delivery for sensitized mothers in whom the prognosis for the infant seems good but at a time closer to term.[141]

Since the baby may be premature and may have already sustained the effects of blood destruction, exchange transfusion is prepared for in advance of delivery with a supply of type O Rh-negative blood at hand compatible with the mother's serum. The earlier fear of a high incidence of kernicterus in the slightly premature baby has now been dispelled by its known prevention with the use of multiple exchange transfusions.

Boggs[10] has presented evidence that interruption of carefully selected pregnancies has a role in the management of Rh sensitization. In high-risk pregnancies in which there has been a previous stillborn Rh-erythroblastotic infant or one who was live-born with hydrops, pregnancy is interrupted prior to 34 weeks. Of six such instances, two infants survived. Interference at 33 weeks' gestation or less offers little hope of success. On the other hand, after 33 weeks' gestation, there were only two neonatal deaths that could possibly have been attributed to the interruption of pregnancy. Both infants died from hyaline membrane disease. After 33 weeks' gestation, eleven of fourteen of the interrupted high-risk pregnancies resulted in surviving infants as compared to two of nine in the uninterrupted pregnancies. In intermediate and low-risk pregnancies the results were even more favorable. Boggs[10] advises the interruption of high-risk pregnancies believed to be associated with an Rh-positive fetus at 34 to 35 weeks, and of lower risk ones at 36 weeks and thereafter.

In a recent study it was emphasized that, contrary to the general impression, infants born of the first immunized pregnancy may (in rare instances) be affected severely enough to die in utero or in the early neonatal period. It was therefore suggested that a high titer (1:64) in the first immunized pregnancy is sufficient indication in itself for consideration of induction prior to term.[44]

*Whole blood versus sedimented red cells:* Although whole blood has been almost universally used in replacement, sedimented blood has its advocates.[90,123] The advantage of sedimented red cells is that the hemoglobin concentration is less likely to fall to levels requiring further transfusion. In this method, approximately 100 to 150 ml. of the supernatant ACD plasma layer is removed from a bag of previously stored Rh-negative blood.\*

Whole blood and packed red cells have been used in combination in a single procedure, with the latter employed for about one-third of the exchange transfusion.[114] The use of whole versus sedimented cells deserves further clinical and experimental evaluation because of increasing interest in the possible advantages of the latter. Sedimented red cells have already found a place in exchange transfusions in infants with profound anemia who are often in cardiac failure and show a high venous pressure.[147] In this case a one to one and one-half volume exchange is usually advisable because of the precarious state of the infant. Except for this emergency, whole blood is the preferred medium in exchange transfusions, especially in infants with elevated or rising bilirubin levels.[139]

In vitro and in vivo experiments have shown that sickle cell trait blood could be safely used for blood transfusion. A case has been reported,[143] however, of a premature infant with physiological jaundice who received an exchange transfusion of blood containing HbAS. Autopsy revealed generalized intravascular aggregation of sickled cells similar to that found in patients dying in sickle cell crisis.

For the present, whole blood is recommended in exchange transfusions, especially in infants with elevated and rising bilirubin levels.

*Use of concentrated serum albumin:* One of the primary objectives of exchange transfusions is the removal of maximal amounts of bilirubin already present in the plasma and that which enters the circulation from tissue depots during the exchange. An indirect advantage is that plasma protein, especially albumin, which serves as a vehicle for binding bilirubin, is supplied in larger quantity by whole blood than by restricted amounts present in sedimented blood. Transfusion with whole rather than sedimented blood receives strong support from the demonstration of the protective effect of albumin against the development of kernicterus.[15,98,99]

A protein-enriched exchange transfusion has been advocated as being more effective than whole blood exchange in removal of bilirubin because of the bilirubin binding of albumin.[99] In vitro, 2 moles of bilirubin interact with each mole of albumin, or 15 mg. of bilirubin are bound by 1 gm. of albumin at a pH of 7.4.[86] Albumin has been prescribed in several ways. It may be given intravenously as a 25% salt-poor albumin in amounts of 1 gm. per kilo-

---

\*From a mixture of 500 ml. of blood and 65 ml. of ACD (acid-citrate-dextrose) anticoagulant.

gram of body weight, 1 or 2 hours before the exchange transfusion.[101,102] Another method is to remove 50 ml. of plasma from a 500 ml. bag of donor blood and replace this with 50 ml. (12.5 gm.) of concentrated salt-poor human albumin. In some cases only 25 ml. (6.25 gm.) of albumin are added. The larger amounts of albumin raise the plasma albumin in the bag (normally averaging 3.8 gm. per 100 ml.) to 7 gm. per 100 ml. as compared with 5.5 gm. per 100 ml. when the smaller supplements are added.[144]

A method has been devised to determine the binding capacity of albumin using the dye phenolsulfonthalein (P.S.P.),[144] and hydroxybenzene azobenzoic acid (HBABA).[110] The capacity of serum to bind the dye has been related to the concentration of serum albumin and is inversely related to the concentration of bilirubin and other substances that are bound to albumin. A P.S.P.-binding capacity of over 100 $\mu$g per milliliter of serum or HBABA over 50% is considered adequate, and a capacity of less than 50 $\mu$g per milliliter of serum or HBABA value of less than 50% indicates the need for immediate treatment. According to Waters and Porter,[144] who developed the method, a serum bilirubin concentration of 20 mg. per 100 ml. or more was not considered alone as an indication for treatment, if the infant remained active and the binding capacity of serum was adequate. A P.S.P.-binding capacity of less than 50 $\mu$g per milliliter of serum or a low HBABA percentage saturation indicate that most or all of the sites for binding bilirubin to serum albumin are saturated either with bilirubin or competing substances. These tests show promise as valuable guides and with more extensive trial will undoubtedly determine, more precisely than the present criteria, the need for exchange and reexchange. Unless the P.S.P.-binding or HBABA-binding site test is employed, however, one does not know if the 20 mg. of bilirubin per 100 ml. is less threatening in the presence of a high plasma albumin than in the presence of a lower one.[21] Unless the reserve binding capacity of the serum albumin is known, it is still wise to keep the bilirubin level below 20 mg. per 100 ml.

*Estimation of the amount of blood to be used:* The infant's blood volume should be estimated on the basis of 85 ml. per kilogram of body weight. The total amount of blood to be used equals twice the calculated blood volume. The amount of blood actually exchanged by alternate withdrawal and introduction equals the total minus amount initially withdrawn. The remaining donor blood (equal to the amount withdrawn initially) may be carefully given as a terminal transfusion *only* if the venous pressure is normal.

*Example—3 kg. infant*
Blood volume: 255 ml.
Total blood ordered: 510 ml.
Initial withdrawal: 30 ml.
Exchange: 480 ml.

*Procedure:* Whenever possible, the exchange transfusion should be performed by catheterization of the umbilical vein. The operator must be prepared, however, to do a cutdown if necessary.

The necessary equipment should be completely assembled before the baby is exposed.

*Sterile pack* (also commercially available)
Plastic catheters (polyvinyl)
2 infant feeding tubes, sizes No. K31 and No. K32*
Sterile disposable plastic tubing (polyethylene), PE 190/S12 and PE 90/S12†
3 three-way stopcocks
15 cm. stainless steel rule
2 metal basins
1 cutdown set
1 transfusion set
12 syringes (10 ml.)
Plastic tubing (to fit the stopcocks)
Umbilical cord tape
Sterile drapes, dressing to include 1 circumcision sheet and 2 gowns
Sterile jar, 3 by 3 inches with Zephiran chloride solution
Sterile test tube with catgut with curved needle (plain 3-0)

*Unsterile equipment*
Operating board with facilities for heating, hot-water bottle, aquamatic K pad‡
Blood-warming apparatus§
Oxygen
Suction
Gravity pole
Waste bucket
2 Ace bandages (2-inch width)
1 circumcision board
Oscilloscope for monitoring baby's heart rate and ECG during procedure

―――――
*Pharmaseal Laboratories, Glendale, Calif.
†Intramedic, Clay-Adams, Inc., New York, N. Y.
‡Gorman-Rupp Industries, Inc., Belleville, Ohio.
§Hospital Instruments Co., Scotia, N. Y.

Also available should be heparin solution, 10% calcium gluconate solution, and specimen tubes for coagulated and uncoagulated blood. Blood for exchange transfusions should be as fresh as possible to avoid the risk of dangerous increases of potassium in the plasma and should be properly warmed before administration. The blood should never be placed in a water bath *above* 37° C. because of the danger of causing hemolysis.

The procedure for the exchange transfusion is as follows:

1. On a fairly large sterile field, all sterile equipment to be used should be laid out so that it will be within easy reach of the operator.
2. The tubing should be rinsed inside and out with saline solution and smoothed.
3. The three-way stopcocks are then fastened in tandem and attached to a 20 ml. syringe and to the catheter. The discharge tube is attached to the proximal stopcock so that removal of the syringe or emptying of the tube will not allow air to fall into the distal stopcock. The transfusion recipient set is attached to the distal stopcock.
4. One of the basins should be filled with sterile saline solution. The other should be filled with saline solution to which heparin solution has been added (1:300).
5. The syringes should all be rinsed with the heparin-saline mixture. The use of a commercially available kit obviates the need for multiple syringes and heparin-saline rinsing.
6. The baby should be completely immobilized on a Y board, leaving the abdomen exposed. The immobilization should allow for the provision of external heat, suction, and oxygen. The abdominal wall should be prepared by cleansing and draping as for a laparotomy.
7. When everything is ready, and after all equipment has been checked, the procedure should be started.
8. The umbilical cord should be cut squarely 1 cm. from the skin margin. The umbilical vein should be identified (it is the largest of the three vessels and at the 12 o'clock position). Any visible blood clots should be removed with forceps. One edge of the vein should be picked up with mosquito forceps. The catheter should then be inserted into the lumen of the vein, for a centimeter or so. Suction should be applied through the syringe and the catheter withdrawn so as to remove any deeper blood clots. After making certain that the catheter has been rinsed clear, it should be gently inserted into the vein until blood is obtained. If difficulty is encountered, slight caudal traction should be made on the vein and the catheter inserted and withdrawn until the proper channel has been found. It is advisable to restrict the insertion of the catheter to a length of 5 cm. from the skin surface. Its introduction through the umbilical vein to a distance of 8 to 9 cm. from the skin surface will place the tip of the catheter within the heart. When the catheter is in the right position, umbilical cord tape should be placed around the cord and catheter to provide an airtight seal. As previously stated, artifacts of venous pressure readings must be kept in mind and will be recognized if pulse and respirations are normal. In determining the venous pressure attention has been called to the possibility of a sudden increase in negative pressure in the thorax with sucking in of air through the open catheter. Under such circumstances occlusion of the catheter by some means may be lifesaving.[89]
9. The system should then be rinsed through with saline solution, the stopcocks disconnected from the catheter, and a venous pressure reading should be obtained by measuring the height of a column in the catheter against the steel rule placed just above the umbilicus or at the xyphoid process. (Normal venous pressure is 4 to 8 cm.)
10. The proper amount of blood should be withdrawn before any blood is administered. Specimens, both coagulated and uncoagulated, should be obtained for various determinations. For full-term infants with high hemoglobin values and without cardiac failure, 20 to 40 ml. of blood may be withdrawn be-

fore any blood is given. This deficit improves the efficiency of the exchange.

11. The infant should then be given 20 ml. of the donor blood. Thereafter, the exchange is continued with the alternate withdrawal and introduction of equal amounts of blood. For the average full-term baby 20 ml. increments are quite satisfactory. Volumes of 10 to 15 ml. are used in premature infants.
12. Throughout the procedure, care must be taken to keep syringes and tubing well rinsed to prevent clotting. If the infant struggles or cries, it may be an indication of an increased venous pressure. This should be checked before proceeding. A written record of the exact amount of blood introduced and withdrawn should be kept.
13. The infant should be given 1 ml. of 10% calcium gluconate solution after each 100 ml. of blood introduced. This should be diluted in saline solution and given over a period of several minutes, with careful auscultation or monitoring of heart sounds and rate during the administration.
14. When the required amount of blood has been exchanged, a final sample should be obtained for various determinations (Coombs test, total protein, hematocrit, hemoglobin, bilirubin, etc.).
15. The catheter should be withdrawn, the cord carefully tied, and a sterile dressing applied to the area. The cord is not kept moist even if a second exchange is contemplated for fear of later infection.
16. Sterile technique is mandatory throughout the procedure. In the case of infants taken directly from the delivery room to the exchange transfusion room, the deeper portion of the cord (area of transection after sterile preparation) may be assumed to be clean. Therefore, antibiotics should not be required. In infants housed in the nursery for periods of time prior to exchange transfusion, colonization of the cord stump will have occurred. However, since the organisms expected are amenable only to therapy by antibiotics too potentially toxic to be prescribed prophylactically, and since there is no evidence that prophylaxis with antibiotics prevents infection, antibiotics should be used only in cases in which additional clinical and laboratory indications exist.

Whether prophylaxis with standard antibiotics is effective for the type of infection to be encountered has been controversial.[147] Many workers prefer to treat infection due to specific organisms that have been isolated, despite the knowledge that blood culture following exchange frequently shows some growth.

In a study to determine the incidence of bacteremia in exchange transfusions, blood cultures were obtained from the umbilical vein catheter preexchange and postexchange of the last blood at the end of the procedure and a femoral vein blood culture taken immediately after the exchange transfusion.[06] Bacteria were isolated from 43% of the preexchange cultures, from 9% of the postexchange cultures, and from 10% of the femoral blood cultures. The organisms found in the blood cultures were in most instances the same as the flora of the umbilicus. There was no difference in the frequency of positive cultures in those receiving prophylactic antibodies before and/or after the exchange transfusion as compared with those receiving no antibiotics. It was concluded that routine prophylactic antibiotic therapy was not justified. Only in the event of suggestive clinical signs of infection should appropriate cultures be obtained and therapy instituted, whether it be before or after the exchange transfusion.

Extrahepatic portal vein obstruction and portal hypertension secondary to umbilical vein catheterization have been reported.[105] To avoid this complication, fluids should not be administered via an indwelling umbilical vein catheter. Catheters should not be left in the umbilical vein between exchange transfusions, and in the case of umbilical sepsis another site for catheterization should be sought.

The rapid movement of bilirubin into the plasma during or immediately following an exchange transfusion is known as the so-called "rebound phenomenon." To provide for this contingency the exchange transfusion is moderated to produce a slow continuous exchange.

*Saphenous vein method:* In the method described by Wiener and co-workers[151] the infant is bled from the radial artery while blood is introduced into the internal saphenous vein. Although this procedure constitutes an effective method of exchange transfusion, the intermittent substitution method utilizing the umbilical vein without the need for skin incision is the one in common use. If the umbilical vein is definitely unavailable, the femoral or saphenous vein is used instead.

*Heparinized blood:* Heparin instead of citrate has been employed as an anticoagulant for exchange transfusions[8,107,135] but not as yet on a widespread scale. Heparinized blood has many advantages: the blood is necessarily warm and not refrigerated since it is used within a short period after being drawn; it avoids citrate and potassium intoxication; calcium gluconate injections are unnecessary; and the blood is more concentrated with higher hemoglobin levels since dilution by acid-citrate-dextrose mixtures is avoided. The obvious disadvantages are that appropriate donors must be immediately available since heparinized blood keeps poorly and that there is the rare possibility of a coexisting bleeding tendency in the infant. Heparin is used in a dosage of 15 mg. per 500 ml. of blood. To avoid the danger of hemorrhage, 15 mg. of protamine sulfate solution is administered via the umbilical catheter at the end of the procedure.[107] This step is not always carried out.

Heparinized blood has been employed for exchange transfusion.[135] One of the objections to heparin is that it increases the plasma concentration of nonesterified fatty acids (NEFA). These acids have been shown in jaundiced rats to cause redistribution of the bilirubin, with a net diffusion away from the circulating plasma. The effect is apparently due to the competition of the unsaturated fatty acids for serum protein–binding sites. The fatty acids are bound by albumin and can interfere with the protein binding of bilirubin.[70] With heparinized blood the rebound of serum bilirubin followed as an index of the need for a second exchange transfusion may be artificially low due to the diminished ability of the circulating plasma to support bilirubin. More bilirubin is in the tissue and is not reflected by a correlated rise in the plasma concentration.[100,147] Despite this theoretic objection, the use of heparinized blood in 300 exchange transfusions in one institution during the past 10 years has been very satisfactory and has been regarded as superior to citrated blood.[147]

*Unexplained death:* Exchange transfusions are not without their dangers, and unexpected fatalities occur. It has been estimated that the frequency is about 1% of exchanges, but it is probably higher. In one series, in a 6-year period 351 exchange transfusions had been performed on 232 infants with 11 deaths.[146] The case mortality was 4.7% and the procedure mortality 3.1%. The mortality risk in premature infants was found to be no greater than that for the full-term infant. Cardiac arrest has been attributed to hyperkalemia, hypocalcemia, citrate toxicity, and acidosis. In any one case it is almost impossible to single out the causative factor. Cases of cardiac arrest during exchange transfusion have been reported which were successfully treated by thoracotomy and cardiac massage.[54,106]

Electrocardiographic monitoring during exchange transfusion is advisable. It may give warning of danger even when the heart rate is unchanged.[115] Bradycardia, heart rates outside of 100 to 160 per minute and the appearance of an abnormal complex are indications to stop the transfusion. These changes probably result from a combination of mechanical and biochemical factors and it is unwise to resume the transfusion until the electrocardiogram has returned to normal.[137]

Pierson and co-workers[109] noted that exchange transfusions have been performed using buffered and nonbuffered ACD blood. They pointed out that in low-risk infants receiving unbuffered blood severe acidosis may occasionally occur during transfusion. In infants with cardiorespiratory insufficiency in whom the mortality of exchange transfusion is increased, the use of buffered ACD blood would appear to lessen the risk. Acidosis during exchange transfusion was not observed in any of the twenty-six high-risk infants who were exchanged with buffered blood using THAM added to each unit of blood prior to exchange transfusion. Such maneuvers, particularly with THAM, appear to minimize citrate acidosis and subsequent alterations which are prone to occur, especially in infants exchanged with ACD blood. The benefits of such procedures are still under investigation.

Driscoll and Steinke,[41] and Hazeltine[58] have shown that insulin levels in the blood are elevated in infants with erythroblastosis fetalis and are comparable to levels observed in infants of diabetic mothers. This finding correlates with pancreatic hyperplasia that occurs in both diseases. If the diagnosis of hypoglycemia is established in these infants glucose should be administered intravenously until oral feedings are well taken.

Barrett and Oliver[7] observed hypoglycemia in five of sixteen (31%) of consecutively studied infants with moderate to severe erythroblastosis fetalis. Hyperinsulinemia was documented in each of four infants. They recommended that all infants with erythroblastosis should have measurements of blood glucose levels in the first hours of life and after exchange transfusion. If hypoglycemia develops in such an infant he should be treated with glucose intravenously. Hypoglycemia has not been thought to occur with increased frequency in the infant with erythroblastosis, even though hyperplasia of the islands of Langerhans is a well-recognized pathological finding in this condition. Hypoglycemia was defined as a blood glucose level less than 30 mg./100 ml. at term or 20 mg./100 ml. in preterm infancy.

Myocardial infarction has been reported[137] as occurring during an exchange transfusion; its thrombotic origin was demonstrated by postmortem coronary angiography and histological studies.

Another complication of exchange transfusion is the occurrence of colonic perforation and peritonitis.[20,30,53,83,104] Several hours or days after an exchange transfusion the infant has feeding problems and abdominal distension and passes blood by rectum. X-ray studies give evidence of pneumoperitoneum or intestinal obstruction. At laparotomy the colon is found to be perforated but the small intestine can also be involved with multiple perforations. The most common sites of perforation were the transverse and descending portions of the colon. In the etiology of this condition, it is possible that the catheter varies in position during exchange transfusion. The position of the umbilical venous catheter in the portal system may be crucial to the etiology of this condition. It is usually assumed that the catheter is in the inferior vena cava but it may in fact wander into the portal venous system or the right atrium.

*Miscellaneous treatment.* Some of the auxiliary measures of the past suggested for treatment of patients with erythroblastosis were ACTH and glucuronic acid; these have fallen into disuse. In current trial is phototherapy. Of historic interest was the use of glucuronic acid.

*Glucuronic acid:* The administration of glucuronic acid by oral and intravenous routes had been advocated as a means of converting the unconjugated bilirubin to the conjugated product which is excreted by the liver. Although lowering of indirect bilirubin has been reported by one group,[33,34] it has not been substantiated by others.[69] This approach bypasses the essential enzymatic nature of bilirubin glucuronide formation.[118] Uridine disphosphate-glucuronic acid is the source of the glucuronic acid of conjugated bilirubin and is transferred to bilirubin by an active enzyme system. Since free glucuronic acid does not enter into the sequence of reactions, the biochemical basis of this therapy is doubtful. Furthermore, it has been shown by animal experiments that kernicterus may develop despite a depression of serum bilirubin when glucuronic acid is given.[35,71] It has been suggested that this agent produces a redistribution of bilirubin from the blood to other body compartments with a potential increase in concentration in central nervous system tissue.[117] Claims for the efficacy of glucuronic acid were finally withdrawn when it was shown that the same effects on the concentration of bilirubin in the serum resulted from comparable amounts of glucose and saline solution given intravenously.[120]

PHOTOTHERAPY. In 1958 it was demonstrated that serum bilirubin concentration of newborn infants is reduced by exposure to light.

Broughton and co-workers[13] in 1965 treated a group of eleven infants with "physiological" jaundice, chosen by random selection, by irradiation with artificial blue light. The serum bilirubin concentration of the treated infants fell by an average of 2.9 mg./100 ml. during treatment; this was significantly greater than the change in bilirubin level in a similar untreated group of infants. Lucey and associates,[84] in a controlled study conducted on 111 low birth rate infants (53 light-treated, 58 controls), demonstrated that continuous phototherapy is effective in significantly modifying hyperbilirubinemia of prematurity if used continuously between 12 to 144 hours of age.

More extended remarks on phototherapy in the treatment of jaundice in the newborn are found in Chapter 8.

*Prevention.* Methods have been devised to prevent the formation or passage of anti-Rh antibodies in utero. Several will be described.

*Neutralization of antibodies with haptens.* Lipoid extracts of Rh-positive red cells (haptens)[19] have been prepared with the hope of neutralizing anti-Rh antibodies in the mother without, at the same time, stimulating fresh antibody production. Injections of this material have proved ineffective since immunization, once it has been established, appears permanent.

*Protection of mother with anti-Rh antibody.* The concept that Rh sensitization takes place by the transplacental passage of fetal red cells into the maternal circulation during labor and delivery led to methods for its prevention by administering Rh antibody to Rh-negative mothers[46,49] immediately following childbirth. The large numbers of fetal hemoglobin-containing red cells appearing in the maternal circulation within 72 hours of delivery could presumably be inactivated by the administration of anti-Rh (anti-D) sera.[46] The acid elution method for detecting fetal hemoglobin (p. 5) suggested that the passage of perhaps 1 to 5 ml. of fetal blood takes place during labor, due to trauma to the uteroplacental junction.[47] To test this hypothesis, Rh-negative volunteers were sensitized with Rh-positive blood and subsequently received anti-**Rh** (anti-**D**) serum. It was found that 60% of the Rh-positive red cells were eliminated within the first few hours and the cells not so destroyed, having been coated with anti-**Rh** (anti-**D**) serum, were likely to be removed from the circulation by the spleen. Another group of observers administered[51] a concentrated anti-Rh gamma$_2$-globulin (7S) preparation intramuscularly into unsensitized Rh-negative male volunteers 24 hours prior to each of several intravenous injections of Rh-positive blood. Three months after the last injection the positively acquired Rh antibodies were no longer in evidence and there was also no sign of active antibody production 6 months after the last injection of blood.

It was tempting to apply these results to the Rh-negative mother, hoping that a single injection of anti-Rh serum after the first sensitizing delivery could possibly prevent isoimmunization. The basic premise is that major Rh sensitization takes place at the time of delivery of the first unaffected pregnancy and not during the preceding months. Cohen and associates,[27] however, found that fetal erythrocytes entered the maternal blood in small quantities intermittently during pregnancy and that this was a physiologic event. Their studies indicated that fetal hemorrhage began well before the onset of labor and that labor, under ordinary conditions, was found to be of little or no significance with regard to the entry of fetal erythrocytes into the maternal circulation. Zipursky and co-workers[154] found that 15.8% of 1,019 blood specimens of 384 pregnant and postpartum women contained fetal red cells and that these were found in each trimester of pregnancy as well as in the postpartum period. Rh-negative patients become immunized to the Rh factor by exposure to Rh-positive erythrocytes. While fetal erythrocytes appear in the maternal circulation as early as 12 weeks of gestation, the major immunizing threat is generally believed to occur at the end of the third trimester and in the immediate postpartum period.[111]

The hypothesis that the anti-Rh antibody would destroy any Rh-positive cells (fetal erythrocytes) which enter the maternal circulation was first put to trial by Finn[45] in Rh-negative male volunteers. Later Woodrow and associates[153] demonstrated that injected Rh-positive fetal cells were rapidly cleared from the circulation of Rh-negative postmenopausal multiparas. It has now been abundantly shown that the injection of **Rh**$_o$(**D**) immune globulin (human) to an Rh-negative woman immediately after delivery of an Rh-positive infant is successful in preventing Rh-immunization.

*Prevention of the isoimmunization.*

MECHANISMS OF PROTECTION BY **Rh**$_o$ (**D**) IMMUNE GLOBULIN (RhoGAM). Several theories have been advanced to explain the mechanism by which immunization is prevented by the administration of **Rh**$_o$ (**D**) immune globulin to the negative woman.[24] One theory is that anti-Rh globulin coats and therefore blocks the Rh-positive antigen sites on the circulating fetal red cells from stimulating the antibody-forming cells of the maternal reticuloendothelial system. Expressed in another way, passively administered antibody causes the phagocytosis and destruction of antigen before it comes into contact with the antibody cells.[91] The second possibility is that the presence of excess passive antibody prevents the formation of immune antibody by a central "feedback" mechanism. This hypothesis is based on the concept of Smith,[127] who in 1909 demonstrated that mixtures of diphtheria toxin and antitoxin with antibody in excess did not immunize when injected.

The protective dose of anti-**Rh** gamma globulin to prevent antibody formation is a dose of 300 μg.[23,39,52] The anti-**Rh** gamma globulin is obtained from processing the plasma of naturally immunized women or of artificially immunized Rh-negative males. Since A-B-O incompatibility between the **Rh**$_o$ (**D**) negative mother and the **Rh**$_o$ (**D**) positive fetus offers only incomplete protection against Rh isoimmunization, the use of immune prophylaxis in these cases is also advisable. For RhoGAM, using a 2 ml. syringe, the total content of the vial is injected intramuscularly into the postpartum mother. Anti-**Rh** gamma globulin administration seems safe because gamma globulin disappears within a few months, but it is possible for mothers to become immunized to substances in the gamma globulin itself. Although a reaction is possible, the risk is small.

It can be concluded that a single dose of 300 μg of **Rh**$_o$ (**D**) immune globulin administered intramuscularly after each Rh-incompatible pregnancy is an effective prophylaxis against Rh immunization. This dosage is increased if the mother has had a large bleed from the fetus just before or during delivery.[53] This method has been shown to have the potential of almost entirely eliminating Rh immunization.

Furthermore, it has been suggested[50] that all Rh-negative nonimmunized women who have had an abortion at 2 months or beyond should receive Rh immune globulin whenever and wherever possible. It had been known that the 12% of Rh-negative women who have Rh-positive husbands develop Rh antibodies and that the average risk of immunization after abortion is about 3 to 4%. Freda and co-workers[50] determined that the risk varies considerably with the age of the fetus "virtually negligible at one month, definitely appreciable at 2 months (2 percent), and very substantial at 3 months and beyond ($\pm$ 9 percent)." It was therefore concluded that the risk of immunization in Rh-negative mothers who have an abortion is not negligible and that an appropriate dose of immune (anti-D) globulin should be given to such mothers who have an abortion at 2 months or beyond.

Zipursky and Israels,[54] among others, noted the frequency of fetal cells entering the maternal circulation and the possibility of primary immunization during the course of a first pregnancy. They considered this a reason for giving anti-D gamma globulin during pregnancy; this was done successfully in forty-seven cases. Despite this favorable experience, giving anti-D gamma globulin during pregnancy awaits further clinical trial.

While anti-D gamma globulin is effective in preventing Rh isoimmunization by pregnancy, it is unsuccessful in women who are already immunized against Rh antigen. Plasmapheresis has therefore been suggested in the latter as a means of reducing the amount of maternal anti-D antibody.

Intensive plasmapheresis of pregnant and nonpregnant women immunized to the Rh or Kell isoantigen was shown to lower the concentration of plasma proteins, including total IgG and individual antibodies.[25] In all, eight pregnant women were treated by plasmapheresis in addition to conventional therapy (intrauterine transfusions and in some cases exchange transfusions as well). Of these, five gave birth to live infants, of which four survived the early postnatal period. Studies showed that anti-D levels can be lowered, and it is possible that plasmapheresis may have contributed to the successful deliveries. What is needed, however, is "a comparison with a series of controls in which only conventional forms of treatment have been given."[25]

*Overall results of treatment of erythroblastosis fetalis.* With the reservations imposed by the uneven character of the severity of cases over the years, the drop in overall mortality and incidence of kernicterus has nevertheless been obvious. At The New York Hospital the improvement is reflected in the drop in mortality from 35.8% in the preexchange period (1932 to 1941) to 8.9% in the exchange transfusion period (1947 to 1955). The liberal use of exchange transfusions has resulted in a striking drop in the incidence of kernicterus from 25% of twenty-five infants with erythroblastosis in 1946, to a total absence of this complication in thirty-one infants in 1955. In a recent compilation at the same institution for the year 1962, a similar trend continues. Although the neonatal mortality was 7% due to erythroblastosis, the fetal mortality was much higher (21%) and emphasizes the need for early induction. No case of kernicterus occurred.

*Anemia in the previously treated infant.* One or more supplementary transfusions with packed cells (10 ml. per kilogram) are given before discharge from the hospital, to raise the hemoglobin to 10 to 12 gm./100 ml. Since anti-Rh antibody persists for at least 4 to 8 weeks following birth, weekly hemoglobin determinations are necessary during this period. Transfusions of packed cells are given in the clinic in the first 2 or 3 weeks following discharge from the hospital when the hemoglobin level falls below 7 gm./100 ml.

After this period, transfusions are usually unnecessary, particularly if a reticulocytosis appears, unless the 7 gm. concentration of hemoglobin is associated with illness. Transfusions above this level may suppress innate hemoglobin and red cell synthesis which is usually in progress between the sixth and eighth weeks of life. Hematinics are without value in the prevention or treatment of anemia at this time.

Hyman and Sturgeon[66] have shown that during the convalescent period of erythroblastosis fetalis there is often an increase in total hemoglobin despite a fall in hemoglobin levels. This discrepancy is explained on the basis of growth, since a simple calculation of blood volume will reveal that the infant is indeed regenerating hemoglobin which is not reflected in the reduced peripheral hemoglobin concentration.

In severe erythroblastosis, however, anemia may persist for several weeks following discharge from the hospital and is stated to exceed that which is expected from continuing hemolysis after successful replacement has been achieved or from an expanding blood volume due to growth of the infant. This form of anemia has been attributed to bone marrow hypoplasia as a complication of severe hemolytic anemia in the newborn infant,[38] from suppression of blood formation due to the known inhibitory effects of transfusion,[126] or from antibody specifically directed against the red cells in the fetus and extending into the neonatal period.[125]

Comprehensive bone marrow examinations, however, do not explain the continuing anemia following the acute hemolytic period on the basis of a decrease in the number of normoblasts in the bone marrow.[40,66] On the contrary, serial examinations indicate that the percentage of normoblasts in the bone marrow is increased in proportion to the anemia and that a true "normoblastopenic state" appears to be a rare occurrence.[40] The persistent anemia following the acute hemolytic stage of erythroblastosis probably represents a diminished reactivity of the bone marrow that may be more severe than is normally present.

On the other hand, bone marrow hypoplasia has been described with persistence of Rh antibody for a prolonged period after exchange transfusion. In one case[64] antibody was detected for between 11 and 14 weeks, causing a hemolytic and a hypoplastic anemia. At 4 weeks the bone marrow showed only 7% erythroid cells.[64,65]

A number of reasons may, therefore, be offered for the late anemia (after the first week) of infants with erythroblastosis.[64] These include persistence of antibody of a sufficient strength to destroy not only mature red cells, but also reticulocytes and normoblasts; an insensitivity to erythropoietin, even though abundantly produced by the erythroblastotic infant; sequestration of reticulocytes in the spleen, failure of the marrow to release reticulocytes, an abnormally short life-span of reticulocytes, and, finally, transient red cell hypoplasia. It has been emphasized that a high level of circulating hemoglobin at the end of exchange transfusion will protect the infant from the development of the late anemia in most cases.[96]

**Anemia in the previously untreated infant.** It is important to watch those babies closely after discharge who have not had previous exchange transfusions because their anemia was mild (10 to 11 gm. per 100 ml.) during the hospital stay. In an occasional case, a precipitious drop in the hemoglobin occurs in the second and third weeks of life. Death from severe and progressive anemia may result from excessive blood destruction, inadequate compensatory blood formation, and splenic trapping. Very careful observation and transfusions to maintain adequate hemoglobin levels are urgent in these infants.

*Rupture of the spleen.* Splenic rupture is a rare complication of erythroblastosis occurring regardless of therapy. Many factors have been incriminated: extramedullary hematopoiesis, increased phagocytosis, weakening of the supportive structures, and the tendency to hemorrhage.[108,124]

*Management of the infant with erythroblastosis.* When a sensitized mother enters the hospital for delivery of her baby, the pediatric service and the blood bank should be alerted immediately by the obstetric service. At the time of the delivery, a member of the pediatric staff should be in attendance. Observation should be made of the color of the vernix and of the amniotic fluid. They may be stained yellow in erythroblastosis fetalis. When the baby is delivered, the cord should be clamped immediately. This is done for several reasons. There is no advantage to the baby in a transfusion of antibody-coated red blood cells and circulating antibody. A great many of the more severely affected infants have an elevated venous pressure and would do better with a smaller blood volume. It is estimated that the child may receive up to 100 ml. of blood from the placenta.

It is of the greatest importance that the umbilical cord be cut so as to allow a segment at least 3 inches long between the umbilicus and the tie. Former precautions of keeping the cord moist have not been found necessary and may actually increase the chance of infection.

The child should be examined for manifestations of hemolytic disease: jaundice (rarely immediately at birth), pallor, hepatosplenomegaly, edema, and petechiae. At the same time, several blood specimens should be carefully collected from the placental portion of the cord.

A 5 to 10 ml. specimen of oxalated umbilical venous blood is examined for hemoglobin, A-B-O group, Rh-Hr type, and direct antiglobulin.* In the event of a positive Coombs test a serum bilirubin determination and a complete blood count, including reticulocytes and nor-

---

*At The New York Hospital 5 ml. of clotted blood is sent to the blood bank for routine typing and the Coombs test. The remainder of the blood specimen is saved for cross-matching. From 5 to 10 ml. of EDTA umbilical blood is set aside for determination of the serum bilirubin and the complete blood count, including reticulocytes.

moblasts, are carried out. When there is any suspicion of erythroblastosis and the Coombs test has been erroneously reported as negative, complete blood tests should nevertheless be carried out until the Coombs test is verified; this should be done without delay. When cord blood is not available, venous blood or blood obtained by pricking the heel can be used for the initial tests. The capillary blood may be more suitable for study of red and white cell morphology and reticulocytes.

After the preliminary studies have been performed, the subsequent course may be decided. It must first be determined, of course, whether or not the child is erythroblastotic.

Group-specific A-B-O Rh-negative blood is usually given. When a severely affected infant is anticipated, group O Rh-negative blood should be available before delivery. In any case the blood used should always be compatible with the mother's serum. The prospective donor's red blood cells also should be crossmatched with the serum of the infant's mother, and the compatibility should be confirmed by the indirect Coombs technique. The mother's serum not only contains much more anti-**Rh** antibody than the infant's serum, but may contain antibodies other than $Rh_o$ (**D**). It is only by such tests that other incompatibilities between mother's and infant's blood can be completely eliminated. Group O Rh-negative blood should be selected with low anti-**A** and anti-**B** titers.

The volume of blood used in exchange transfusion is best referred to in terms of multiples of the infant's own blood volume. Thus, for a child with an estimated blood volume of 250 ml., the commonly used 500 ml. replacement transfusion is a two-volume replacement. Such an exchange provides an 87% replacement of the blood, but the exchange of the red blood cells is dependent upon the hematocrit of the donor blood and upon the infant's initial hematocrit. The higher the donor hematocrit and the lower the infant's initial hematocrit, the higher the percentage of Rh-negative cells that will be present in the infant's circulation at the end of the transfusion.

For an exchange of 500 ml. of blood with the average hematocrit of 36%, the hematocrit of Rh-negative cells at the end of the transfusion (and this will be the infant's ultimate hematocrit when all of his own Rh-positive cells have been destroyed) will be 32%. The percentage of Rh-negative cells will range from 82% for an infant with an initial hematocrit of 50%, to 96% for an infant with an initial hematocrit of 10%. The size of the transfusion can also be determined according to the nomogram of Veall and Mollison,[142] which provides about 90% replacement with donor blood and a final total hematocrit of 50% in the infant.

Thrombocytopenia, occasionally encountered in erythroblastosis, can be further aggravated by the use of stored blood in which platelets are depleted.[119] To maintain some residuum of platelets, blood used for exchange should be relatively fresh, preferably under 24 hours old. In one child marked melena, which was attributed to severe thrombocytopenia, occurred after the fifth exchange transfusion. Treatment with platelet transfusions and prednisone (1 mg. per kilogram) was effective in establishing hemostasis.

*Treatment of the infant in cardiac failure.* In most cases the signs of congestive failure (pallor, dyspnea, restlessness, grunting respirations, cyanosis) will be found in severely anemic infants. Blood is withdrawn cautiously initially, the amounts depending upon the elevation of venous pressure and general condition of the infant. In infants with congestive failure usually 30 to 60 ml. are withdrawn; however, as much as one-third of the infant's blood volume may be withdrawn. Sedimented cells (150 ml. of supernatant ACD-plasma removed) are recommended for the anemic infant with heart failure. Replacement is carried out slowly, and less than the calculated amount is given—approximately one to one and one-half volumes of blood. Antibiotics should not be administered through the umbilical vein for fear of an adverse reaction through an effect directly on the cardiac musculature.

Administration of digitalis has usually been found unnecessary. Treatment of the anoxic, anemic, hypervolemic infant in cardiac failure is usually so urgent that there is little time for digitalization. The important thing is to relieve the excessive load on the heart by correcting the anemia and administering oxygen, decreasing the high venous pressure and blood volume by phlebotomy, and replacement by sedimented cells. Where it is felt that digitalization would contribute to the treatment of heart failure, Cedilanid, a rapidly acting cardiac glycoside, may be given intravenously in conjunction with the exchange. Most observers are not convinced that digitalization is of any value.

Varying degrees of endocardial fibroelastosis were found in twenty-six cases in a group of forty infants who died of erythroblastosis fetalis.[59] This condition was probably related to the long-sustained anemic anoxia and cardiac dilatation. The lesions are not visible to the naked eye and thus differ quantitatively from the striking lesions of idiopathic fibroelastosis.

*Intraperitoneal transfusion of the fetus.* The past history, husband's homozygosity for the Rh factor, and high antibody titers offer the means of selecting women for amniocentesis studies (pp. 143 to 145). Increased experience with amniocentesis and evaluation of pigment fluctuations by spectrophotometric examination permits the detection of very severe erythroblastosis in the fetus and a more accurate estimate of the prognosis of the degree of disease in the fetus. A dramatic technique of intraperitoneal transfusion was devised by Liley[80,81] for treatment of infants who would otherwise have been stillborn, hydropic, or hopelessly immature. In one instance[14] intraperitoneal transfusions of packed red cells were given as early as 26 weeks' gestation, followed by three others at 28, 30, and 32 weeks. The amount of blood given was 55, 80, 110, and 130 ml. of packed red cells, respectively. (Approximately 5 gm. of hemoglobin are transfused to raise the hemoglobin of the fetus 1 gm.) Group O Rh-negative blood is given compatible with the mother's serum. At the time of delivery (34 weeks' gestation) 85 to 90% of the baby's circulating red cells were adult Rh negative of the type which had been transfused.

While this technique salvages some infants, the overall mortality associated with this procedure was 70% in 238 fetuses receiving intrauterine transfusions in erythroblastosis fetalis.[116] The complications and risks associated with intrauterine fetal transfusions are numerous.[82] These include fetal trauma (hemothorax, hepatic and splenic lacerations, cardiac tamponade, insertion of dye into spinal cord, bowel and bladder perforation), maternal risks (premature labor, peritonitis, hepatitis, psychologic problems, bleeding), and neonatal disease (conjugated hyperbilirubinemia, hepatic damage, peritonitis, graft-versus-host reaction). The fetal mortality is related to fetal age at the time of the intrauterine transfusion and is between 90 and 100% when carried out before 25 weeks of gestation, between 50 and 80% between 25 and 30 weeks of gestation, and below 50% after 30 weeks of gestation. In the light of this high mortality and significant morbidity, careful assessment is required before this procedure is undertaken. Criteria for intrauterine transfusion vary from institution to institution, but the analysis of amniotic fluid remains the major indication— not a single value—but the rising trend of repeated values is the important criterion. Since the mortality from this procedure is so high before 30 weeks of gestation or when there is evidence of fetal hydrops, these two conditions should be regarded as contraindications in the light of our present knowledge. Fetal hydrops can be diagnosed from the amniogram (scalp and soft tissue edema, and abdominal protuberance due to ascites).

Forty-one infants (of forty-two discharged alive) who had intrauterine transfusions were followed up once, ranging in age from 6 months to 4½ years.[36] The forty-one infants represented the "end product" of 139 pregnancies during which the fetuses received one to four fetal transfusions. These infants averaged 34 weeks of gestation at birth. When the incidence of renal damage and other physical abnormalities and psychological scores were considered, a total of eleven infants (27%) had an abnormal outcome. The prognosis for these forty-one infants seemed less ideal than that expected of comparable infants not undergoing fetal transfusion.

Fong and associates[48] reported a series of 110 intrauterine transfusions performed on seventy-three fetuses selected primarily on the basis of serial amniotic fluid analysis. Eighteen (two hydropic and sixteen nonhydropic) of the seventy-three fetuses survived. The presence of excessive ascitic fluid at the time of paracentesis indicated that the intrauterine transfusion would be of questionable value. The survival rate of nonhydropic fetuses was better than 50% when slow blood infusion and the use of smaller blood volumes was initiated. One of the sixteen nonhydropic infants suffered severe respiratory depression after birth, which resulted in cerebral damage. No neurological, developmental, or immunological aberrations were observed in the remaining fifteen survivors after 4 years of follow-up. Elective delivery was planned generally for 35 to 36 weeks of gestational age. Transabdominal amniocentesis was performed on women with a previous history of hemolytic disease in their newborn infants or when the maternal indirect Coombs titer was greater than 1:8.

Another complication of intrauterine transfusion is the possibility of producing human runt disease by inducing a graft-versus-host reaction through the transplantation of donor white cells.[94]

Such a train of events occurred with an illness characterized by jaundice, aplastic anemia, and striking histiocytic reaction in the bone marrow in an 8-week-old infant who survived three intrauterine transfusions for Rh erythroblastosis fetalis. In spite of initial hematologic improvement, the infant's condition deteriorated to multiple infections and progressive weight loss, with death occurring at 13 weeks of age. The immune mechanisms of the young fetus may not be sufficiently mature to provide complete protection from a graft-versus-host reaction by lymphocytes of the donor blood (see Chapter 11, p. 201).

In other clinics amniocentesis is performed at 24 and 27 weeks so that infants who are severely affected may be supported by intraperitoneal transfusion of the fetus until the infant is 33 to 34 weeks, if possible. At birth, exchange transfusions are often necessary to keep the bilirubin within safe limits. Intraperitoneal transfusions are at present undergoing widespread trial.[60] The possibility of trauma, infection, fetal hemorrhage, and, perhaps, early exposure to x-rays are hazards to consider in the final decision before carrying out this procedure, even where amniotic pigment concentrations fall in the range of maximal risk. Despite these hazards, this method holds out hope of prolonging intrauterine life sufficiently to allow the delivery of a viable infant.

**Exchange transfusion in physiologic hyperbilirubinemia of the full-term and premature infant.** In exceptional cases the indirect-reacting bilirubin level in the normal full-term infant, and especially in the premature infant, reaches critical levels comparable to those in infants affected with Rh-Hr and A-B-O erythroblastosis. Neonatal jaundice not caused by blood group incompatibility is considerably more common in premature than in mature infants. Exposure to concentrations of bilirubin of 20 mg. per 100 ml. and above carries the same hazard of kernicterus, especially in the premature infant. It may be that the peculiar susceptibility of the premature infant to kernicterus is due to the greater permeability of bilirubin through the blood-cerebrospinal barrier in the premature infant than in the full-term infant,[95] or is associated with the lower serum albumin of premature infants. Jaundice can be controlled by exchange transfusions as it is in the infant with erythroblastosis. The exchange, however, must be carried out more slowly, and reexchange may be required since the objective is the removal of bilirubin from the circulation rather than the removal of sensitized cells, as in cases of erythroblastosis. The transfused blood should be of the same group and Rh subtype as that of the infant.

It is still too early to judge the efficacy of exchange transfusions in this group of infants because of limited experience. The problem is particularly trying in the premature infant whose physical condition does not warrant exposure to a prolonged technical procedure. Under these circumstances evaluation of serial bilirubin determinations provides the only means of controlling the situation. It may be necessary to defer treatment, even with a rising bilirubin, in the case of a small premature infant whose physical condition is precarious. In general one cannot as yet be too dogmatic as to the exact bilirubin level at which an exchange transfusion should be undertaken in these infants.[97] Clinical judgment in the individual case is needed, and in the group of premature and full-term infants a rigid yardstick cannot as yet be applied until a great deal more information is obtained.

It is of interest that, although available evidence has emphasized the susceptibility of premature infants with hyperbilirubinemia to kernicterus, Holman[61] pointed out the difficulties of assigning critical levels over which the nonimmunized premature infant requires treatment by exchange transfusion. For instance, in his series of fourteen such premature infants with bilirubin concentrations exceeding 18 mg. per 100 ml., there was no clinical evidence of kernicterus in the neonatal period. Undoubtedly, multiple factors play a role in determining the ultimate concentration of bilirubin or are actually involved in producing kernicterus. Prolonged follow-up is necessary to determine minor and major neurologic sequelae in this group of infants. The complexity of this subject is reflected in the comments on Holman's paper.[78] Crosse and colleagues[32] emphasize that replacement should be performed promptly in premature infants if the serum level of indirect bilirubin is over 18 mg. per 100 ml. or at a lower level if the bilirubin is rising rapidly. Meyer[88] cautions that there might even be justification for replacement transfusion with a rapidly rising bilirubin before levels of 18 and 20 mg./100 ml. are reached. Newns and Norron[97] would give transfusions to those infants with a serum bilirubin of 30 mg./100 ml. and below "if they become lethargic, irritable, difficult to feed, or if there is a rapid rise of serum bilirubin on the third or fourth day." After reviewing their cases of hyperbilirubinemia without blood group incompatibility, Mores and co-workers[93] claim that "prophylactic exchange transfusion in full-term infants is useless; in premature infants it is theoretically unfounded and its practical value has not been proved, not even by those performing it."

Jaundice due to Rh disease is generally considered to be potentially more serious than in neonatal idiopathic hyperbilirubinemia. The presence of an additional pigment, such as hematin, in the circulating blood of patients with hemolytic disease may be the complicating factor.[1] Hematin may in itself be toxic to nerve tissue or compete with bilirubin for protein-binding sites, displacing it from its combination with albumin.[36] In addition, infants with Rh disease are frequently premature and have respiratory distress syndrome, acidosis, and hypoproteinemia—all of which are predisposing factors in the development of kernicterus.

Killander and co-workers,[74] in a follow-up study of ninety-three full-term infants with hyperbilirubinemia not due to Rh hemolytic disease, of whom only forty-six patients were treated by exchange transfusion, could find no cases of kernicterus in either group between 2 and 2½ years of age. They suggested that exchange be withheld in these infants unless bilirubin levels exceeded 26 mg. per 100 ml. Shiller and Silverman[121] found no significant correlation between uncomplicated hyperbilirubinemia and neurologic deficits at 3 years of age among premature infants with peak serum bilirubin levels of 18 to 22 mg. per 100 ml. as compared with premature infants with lower peak levels of bilirubin. In a review of the sequelae of hyperbilirubinemia in infants of low birth weight, Hsia[62] concluded that kernicterus appears as an all-or-none phenomenon. Escape from gross neurologic damage in the neonatal period is likely to lead to motor and mental development similar to that of other infants of the same gestational length and birth weight. In a group of sixty-eight prematurely born children examined at 7 years of age, six, or 22%, of the twenty-seven children who had serum bilirubin concentrations above 20 mg. per 100 ml. had brain damage in the production of which hyperbilirubinemia may have been an important factor.[75] Presumably these six would have profited by exchange transfusions.

In a series of 204 infants with neonatal jaundice of undetermined origin, Jablonski[67] found no indication for exchanging full-term and larger premature infants with uncomplicated hyperbilirubinemia unless the bilirubin reached at least 25 mg./100 ml. The hazard of exchange transfusion was dramatically described by Trolle.[134] He estimated that, on the basis of a serum bilirubin of 20 mg./100 ml. as an indication for exchange transfusion, 2,140 term infants would have to be transfused to prevent one case of athetoid cerebral palsy, but twenty-one infants would probably die as a result of the procedure itself. In the case of premature infants, ninety-two would have to be exchanged to prevent athetosis in one, but four exchange deaths would result in the process. Based on these and other considerations, McKay[87] proposed bilirubin levels of 23 to 25 mg. per 100 ml. in premature infants and of 28 to 30 mg. per 100 ml. in term infants who were otherwise well as criteria for exchange transfusion in idiopathic hyperbilirubinemia. In sick infants and in premature babies exchange is advised for serum bilirubin levels of 18 to 22 mg. per 100 ml. and 20 to 24 mg. per 100 ml. in term infants. Such factors as asphyxia, prolonged cyanosis due to hyaline membrane disease or other causes, hypoglycemia, hypoproteinemia, and relative immaturity would call for exchange transfusions at the lower levels of bilirubin.[87]

In six small premature infants kernicterus occurred in the absence of hemolytic disease. Their gestational age ranged from 28 to 30 weeks. All six infants died within 12 hours of onset of symptoms. In four, bilirubin levels ranged from 17.1 to 18.8 mg. per 100 ml. On the basis of these findings, earlier exchange was recommended in small premature infants with a known antecedent history of asphyxia or respiratory difficulty.[131]

While the risk of treatment must be balanced against that of kernicterus, some workers are reluctant to recommend a level of serum bilirubin higher than 20 mg. per 100 ml. as a criterion for exchange transfusions.[36] To exceed this level requires an assessment of multiple factors, not the least of which is the experience and skill of the person doing the transfusion. Boggs[11] encountered no mortality in his own series of 506 exchange transfusions performed on 341 infants, approximately half of whom were premature infants. He elects to perform exchange transfusions on all premature babies with total serum bilirubin concentrations of 18 mg. per 100 ml. or more and on all full-term babies with 20 mg. per 100 ml. or more until such a time as a better means can be devised to prognosticate kernicterus on the basis of given serum bilirubin concentrations. In general, the trend seems to be to give exchange transfusions to affected infants with the reservation that critical levels cannot be stated categorically. (See Chapter 8 for additional comments on physiologic hyperbilirubinemia.)

*Exchange transfusions as a treatment of poisonings.* The removal of toxic substances from the blood and tissues of children in acute poisoning has been achieved by exchange transfusion. The procedure has been successfully used in children with a wide variety of poisonings, including barbiturates, boric acid,[12] methyl salicylate poisoning,[2,37] and ferrous sulfate poisoning.[5]

*A-B-O erythroblastosis.* In recent years incompatibility within the A-B-O blood group system has been established as a common cause of erythroblastosis. The failure to recognize A-B-O disease in the past was due to the fact that frequently it was so mild that it was commonly overlooked. From the 20 to 25% of heterospecific pregnancies in which fetal red cells possess an **A** or **B** factor not present in the mother's blood, a substantial number of cases of erythroblastosis develop. In approximately 95% of these infants the blood type of the mother has been group O; in the others, A or B. In recent years these appear to have outnumbered those due to the Rh factor. With few exceptions, the cases are confined to A or B offspring of group O mothers, with the A factor predominating.

The restriction of A-B-O erythroblastosis to 5% of incompatible matings is due to several mechanisms by which fetal erythrocytes are protected from the action of maternal antibodies. The most important probably relate to the neutralization or fixation of potentially harmful maternal antibody by specific A or B blood group substances located in fetal and placental tissues.[132,157]

The fact that most affected infants in A-B-O erythroblastosis are born to group O mothers in contrast to mothers belonging to group A or B is explained as follows. When stimulated by A or B antigens, group O individuals form 7S antibodies which traverse the placenta, while individuals who belong to group A or B synthesize the 19S variety, which are impermeable.[112,113] When the mother's serum contains a mixture of 19S and 7S isoagglutinins, the 7S component is readily transported across the placenta and the titer of 7S isoagglutinin is similar in mother and infant.[76] These molecules were found to occur in equilibrium on both sides of the placenta. Usually, the A-B-O isoagglutinins, having traversed the placenta, combine with extra-erythrocytic antigens. This combination exerts a protective effect as evidenced by the low frequency of erythroblastosis despite the common occurrence of diffusible agglutinins. Those cases in which the isoagglutinins escape combination, as tested by resistance to inhibition by specific soluble blood group substances, are candidates for severe erythroblastosis.

A case of A-B-O erythroblastosis has been reported[6] in which hemoglobinuria occured. Investigation of the maternal serum demonstrated the presence of a hemolytic antibody which was complement-dependent and was capable of destroying fetal B positive cells in vitro.

It has long been accepted that the development of isoantibodies in the rhesus system is much less frequent in rhesus negative-mothers who bear A-B-O incompatible children than in those in whom the fetus is A-B-O compatible. It has been assumed that this is because fetal cells leaking into the maternal circulation are rapidly destroyed by maternal isoantibodies in the A-B-O system, and therefore are eliminated from the maternal circulation before they can stimulate the production of rhesus isoantibodies. In the study by Cohen and colleagues,[28] 126 infants who developed Rh hemolytic disease despite A-B-O incompatibility with their mothers were compared with 366 cases of Rh hemolytic disease in A-B-O compatible infants. The incompatible group showed a milder disease with higher levels of hemoglobin, lower levels of bilirubin, no cases of hydrops, and fewer exchange transfusions. These data confirmed previous findings that Rh hemolytic disease was milder in the presence of A-B-O incompatibility. The sensitization caused by heterospecific pregnancy in 22% of the mothers analyzed showed low titer Rh antibody, which indicates only partial protection by heterospecific pregnancy. It is of interest that in 53 of the 126 infants both Rh and homologous isoantibody could be eluted from the erythrocytes and this group was considered to have combined Rh and A-B-O hemolytic disease. But in this group the characteristic hematologic finding in A-B-O hemolytic disease, namely, spherocytosis, was absent. This study demonstrated that the low levels of the maternal Rh antibody titer in the doubly sensitized group could not be the sole factor responsible for the mildness of the disease. The fact remains, however, that the fetus A-B-O incompatible with its mother will usually have very mild Rh hemolytic disease, requiring few exchange transfusions, especially if the erythrocytes are doubly sensitized.

*Clinical features.* In about 50% of cases the firstborn is usually affected, in contrast to Rh incompatibility in which the firstborn escapes unless the mother has been sensitized by previous transfusions. The occurrence of A-B erythroblastosis is therefore unanticipated unless a previous pregnancy has established the possibility of incompatibility from these blood factors.

An important distinguishing feature of A-B erythroblastosis is the development of jaundice within the first 24 hours of life—hence the designation "icterus precox."[57] Therefore, jaundice appearing before 24 hours of age almost invariably means erythroblastosis due to A or B factor. This must not be confused with physiologic jaundice which appears on the second or third day, when jaundice due to A-B incompatibility is frequently at its peak. In the severe type of A-B disease, the icterus increases in intensity from the first day and may be as pronounced as corresponding cases of Rh incompatibility. Anemia at birth is rare, and if it is present it is usually mild. Splenomegaly is slight to absent. Stillbirth and hydrops are exceedingly rare, and the prognosis for succeeding pregnancies is excellent. A tendency toward early recovery is characteristic. Hyperbilirubinemia can occur and, if untreated, results in kernicterus as in cases of Rh incompatibility. The occurrence in the firstborn has been attributed, among other causes, to diverse A and B antigen-like substances contained in material used for immunization procedures.

The usual immune response to the A and B antigens consists of macroglobulins that are unable to cross the placenta. In some cases gamma globulin antibodies are formed by the mother which are directed toward the A and B antigens and which do cross the placenta. In the fetus, A and B antigenic structures are present not only in erythrocytes but also in other tissues, such as the endothelial lining of blood vessels.[132] At this site these structures could effectively compete with fetal red cell antigens for those maternal A-B-O antibodies that cross the placenta.

*Laboratory findings—blood.* The hemoglobin level and red blood cell count are usually either normal or slightly reduced. In most infants hemoglobin levels usually range from 15 to 18 gm. per 100 ml. in the first days of life. There is seldom a substantial fall in the hemoglobin level during the course of the disease. Increased normoblasts are less common than in Rh disease. The white blood cell count is moderately elevated. It is of interest that infants with erythroblastosis due to anti-A antibody belong to subgroup $A_1$.[159]

The reticulocyte count is an essential test of special significance in A-B erythroblastosis. As in patients with Rh incompatibility, reticulocytosis indicates overactivity of the bone marrow to compensate for the destruction of red cells of a shortened life-span. A normal hemoglobin level and reticulocytosis (over 5 to 7%) indicate excessive blood destruction and are usually accompanied by rising bilirubin levels.

The most characteristic hematologic finding in A-B erythroblastosis is the presence of microspherocytosis as revealed by the blood smear. This feature is in contrast with the almost uniform macrocytosis present in Rh disease (Fig. 12). Spherocytosis is best observed in the first days of life. As would be expected, there is an associated increase in osmotic and mechanical fragility. Differentiation from hereditary spherocytosis is sometimes difficult. The absence of a positive Coombs test and the presence of the disease in other members of the family are important features in the diagnosis of hereditary spherocytosis.

SEROLOGIC FINDINGS. Without the use of refined methods, the Coombs test with infant's cells (direct antiglobulin test) is generally negative or weakly positive in A or B incompatibility. With specialized techniques, however, the Coombs test will be positive in as high as 90% of cases of A-B-O erythroblastosis. A strongly positive test is more likely to be observed in cord blood specimens than in blood samples from infants 24 to 48 hours of age. At The New York Hospital a record of the maternal major blood group is made available to the pediatrician during pregnancy. Blood typing and the Coombs tests are performed in cord specimens of all infants of group O mothers. If a positive Coombs test is found, a hemoglobin determination, reticulocyte count, and blood smear are carried out to look for nucleated red blood cells and spherocytes in an effort to establish the presence of active hemolytic disease in the infant.

Maternal serum in cases of A-B erythroblastosis contains natural saline-active antibodies anti-A and anti-B which are normally present in group O individuals. Only if the titer is excessively high

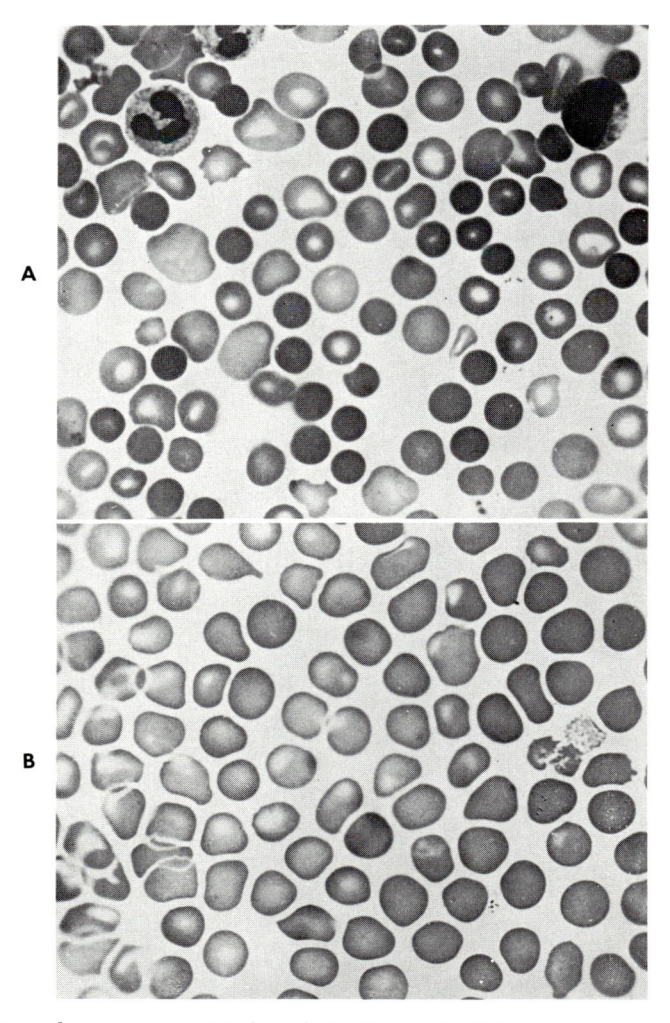

Fig. 12. **A,** Microspherocytosis in A-B hemolytic disease. **B,** Uniform macrocytosis in Rh hemolytic disease. (From Levine, P., Vogel, J. P., and Rosenfield, R. E.: Advances in pediatrics, vol. 6, Chicago, 1953, Year Book Medical Publishers, Inc.)

(over 1:1024 against A agglutinogens and 1:512 against B agglutinogens) may it help in diagnosis.[156]

Mothers of affected infants also possess hyperimmune or incomplete anti-**A** and anti-**B** antibodies which sensitize the red cells of the fetus. The presence of immune antibodies in the blood of the mother with affected children can be demonstrated by their failure to be neutralized with soluble A and B group substances. This is the basis of a test for the titration of anti-**A** and anti-**B** antibodies after partial neutralization of the naturally occurring antibodies.[52] Maternal serum containing these immune antibodies is capable of hemolyzing the infant's cells in vitro.[31] Added complement is sometimes necessary to demonstrate this property. The immune bodies reach their peak during the first 10 days postpartum and remain steady for the next 4 to 6 weeks. After that the majority diminish slowly in titer.[55]

Spontaneous agglutination of the infant's coated red cells, termed conglutination, can be demonstrated in A-B erythroblastosis. Conglutination refers to the tendency of thick suspensions of sensitized or coated red cells (with anti-**A**, anti-**B**, or **Rh**-immune antibodies) to clump spontaneously in protein media such as adult serum, plasma, and bovine albumin and in colloidal media such as gum acacia.[149] (For a discussion of elution tests to determine whether Rh or A-B-O sensitization is principally involved, see p. 139.)

One of the most reliable serologic methods for the diagnosis of A-B erythroblastosis is the demonstration of free antibody in the infant's plasma capable of agglutinating adult erythrocytes of the same blood group as the patient.[156] The presence of such homologous antibody is presumably derived from the transplacental passage of excess maternal antibody into the fetal circulation. In addition to these features the red blood cells of the affected infant clump spontaneously in plasma or colloid media.

Erythrocyte acetylcholinesterase activity is reduced in A-B-O hemolytic diseases of newborn infants.[72] The enzyme alteration is not present in all infants with A-B-O disease, nor in all erythrocytes of affected infants. In contrast, this enzyme is normal in Rh-Hr–hemolytic disease. The measurement of erythrocyte acetylcholinesterase activity is suggested as a simple colorimetric test to confirm the diagnosis of A-B-O disease of the newborn infant. Paroxysmal nocturnal hemoglobinuria is the only other disease in which there is a similar reduction in activity of this surface-located erythrocyte enzyme.

*Relation of A-B-O compatibility and Rh-Hr immunization.* It has been pointed out that erythroblastosis due to the Rh-Hr factor occurs more frequently when A-B-O compatibility exists between mother and child.[79] In one series[85] Rh-Hr compatibility between the mother and child was found to be present in 80% of an unselected obstetric population in contrast to 95% in a group of sensitized Rh-negative women who bore infants afflicted with hemolytic disease.

It has also been shown[129] that Rh-negative men in whom Rh-positive blood has been injected are six times more likely to develop anti-**Rh** antibody of the blood when A-B-O compatible than incompatible.

Wiener[150] ascribed the protective action of a heterospecific pregnancy on the basis of competition of antigens. Since both A and B are better antigens than Rh in man, the antigenicity of the weaker antigen may be suppressed. It seems more likely that the destruction of A and B cells leaves fewer red cells for Rh sensitization. However, exceptions have been reported in which erythroblastosis resulted from combined effects of Rh and hyperimmune anti-**A** antibodies found in the mother.[56] Neutralized group O Rh-negative blood is the recommended treatment.

Another explanation for the protection of A-B-O incompatibility against Rh-Hr sensitization is the "clonal competition for antigen."[130] If Rh-positive red cells of incompatible A-B-O group are injected into Rh-negative subjects, they are much less likely to stimulate the formation of antibody than Rh-positive cells of a compatible A-B-O group. In a study by Stern and associates,[130] 40% of the subjects who failed to form Rh-Hr antibodies after injection of A-B-O incompatible blood did form Rh-Hr antibodies after the subsequent injection of A-B-O compatible blood. The clonal competition for antigen has been postulated to explain this phenomenon—i.e., that the presence of large numbers of antibody-forming cells for one red cell may interfere with antibody response to another blood factor contained in the same red cell.

Differences in sites of visceral sequestration have been described for sensitized Rh-Hr and A-B-O red cells. Jandl and co-workers[98] have demonstrated preferential splenic sequestration of Rh-sensitized erythrocytes, while isoagglutination with hepatic trapping is the chief mechanism of destruction of transfused A-B-O incompatible red cells.

*Treatment.* It must be emphasized that the proper indication for exchange transfusion in infants with A-B-O erythroblastosis is the degree of bilirubinemia and not the anemia. The prevention of kernicterus due to hyperbilirubinemia, therefore, constitutes the major objective in management of A-B erythroblastosis as in Rh-Hr disease. Exchange transfusion is performed and repeated if necessary to keep the level of indirect serum bilirubin below 20 mg. per 100 ml. Although the majority of infants with A-B erythroblastosis are mildly affected and require no treatment, they nevertheless bear scrupulous watching. About 20 to 30% of infants with A and B incompatibility who develop icterus within the first 36 hours of life will need treatment. This compares with an estimated 80 to 90% of Rh-positive infants who were born to sensitized mothers and who require one or more exchanges.[139]

A level of 10 mg./100 ml. of bilirubin on the first day of life suggests the possibility of higher levels in the next few days, whereas the same level on the second or third day indicates a more benign course.[156] A reticulocytosis over 6% and a rapidly rising bilirubin level of more than 0.5 mg./100 ml. per hour constitute indications for treatment. All infants with A-B erythroblastosis should be closely observed during the first 2 days of life, with measurement of daily hemoglobin and frequent serum bilirubin levels. With increasing jaundice, bilirubin levels may be required every 6 to 8 hours. If the bilirubin exceeds 10 mg. per 100 ml. in the first 12 to 24 hours, an exchange transfusion is required. Deepening jaundice with a rise in bilirubin approaching levels of 20 mg./100 ml. on the second day of life also necessitates treatment.

Because jaundice is frequently mild and is overlooked in the first days of life, the pediatrician is often confronted with unexpected hyperbilirubinemia on the third or fourth day. To avoid this contingency, the A-B-O blood group and Rh-Hr typing of the mother and infant should be conspicuously placed on the chart and susceptible infants kept under scrutiny. Any infant who is jaundiced before 24 hours of age, who has an indirect serum bilirubin level exceeding 10 mg. per 100 ml. in the first 24 hours, and who is incompatible with the mother for A and B groups may be presumed to have erythroblastosis and should be treated.

The management of situations in which the bilirubin level approximates 20 mg./100 ml. on the third and fourth days of life when jaundice has gone unnoticed for the first 48 to 72 hours presents some difficulty. In these infants the rise in the concentration of bilirubin has probably been gradual. There is no unanimity of opinion regarding treatment in these circumstances. Exchange transfusion in this group has not always been considered necessary because of the gradual rise in the concentration of serum bilirubin which eventually did not greatly exceed 20 mg. per 100 ml.[122] So many borderline cases of A-B-O erythroblastosis are encountered, especially on the third and fourth day of life, that it is difficult to abide by hard and fast rules. It is hoped that adequately effective liver function will be established at 96 hours and that bilirubin levels will begin to drop. Unfortunately, this does not always occur. Many regard it safe to postpone treatment for an additional day in a full-term infant who is in good clinical condition and who is taking feedings well, if the bilirubin slightly exceeds 20 mg./100 ml. on the fourth day. As in cases of Rh-Hr erythroblastosis, the ultimate decision in each case must be left to the clinical judgment of the attending physician who is aware both of the sequelae of nervous system damage and of the potential hazard of an exchange transfusion.

In the anemic infant in whom the level of bilirubin is low or moderate and not rising, small transfusions of packed group O cells of compatible Rh type are given in the first days of life.

The blood used in all cases in the exchange transfusion should be fresh group O with low "a" and "b" isoagglutinins and appropriate Rh type. As in cases of Rh-Hr sensitization, reexchange may be necessary if hyperbilirubinemia persists, exceeds original levels, and shows evidence of rising to 20 mg./100 ml.

As for subsequent pregnancies, there is no fear of increasing severity as there is with Rh-Hr sensitization. On the other hand, since A-B incompatibilities occur in at least 20% of pregnancies, it is a good plan to be alert to the recurrence of the disease. However, there is no evidence that antibody titers caused by heterospecific pregnancies ordinarily persist or affect unfavorably the outcome of future pregnancies.[157]

*Differential diagnosis.* The following conditions must be excluded: physiologic jaundice, hereditary spherocytosis, congenital nonspherocytic hemolytic anemia, neonatal hepatitis, toxoplasmosis, cytomegalic inclusion disease, congenital syphilis, and bacterial sepsis in the newborn infant (Chapter 8). Jaundice should be controlled by exchange transfusion in patients with those conditions in which bilirubin of the indirect-reacting type is increased, before critical levels of hyperbilirubinemia appear and kernicterus threatens. These include jaundiced infants with hereditary spherocytosis and congenital nonspherocytic hemolytic anemia. The same consideration applies to newborn infants, especially premature ones in whom "physiologic" jaundice is intense and whose blood shows excessive bilirubin concentrations.[17] The differential diagnosis of jaundice in the neonatal period is given in greater detail in Chapter 8.

## REFERENCES

1. Abelson, N. M., and Boggs, T. R., Jr.: Plasma pigments in erythroblastosis fetalis. II. The level of heme pigment; an early guide to management of erythroblastosis fetalis, Pediatrics 17:461, 1956.
2. Adams, J. T., Bigler, J. A., and Green, O. C.: A case of methyl salicylate intoxication treated by exchange transfusion, J.A.M.A. 165:1563, 1957.
3. Allen, F. H. M., Jr.: Induction of labor in the management of erythroblastosis fetalis, Quart. Rev. Pediat. 12:1, 1957.

4. Allen, F. H., Jr., and Diamond, L. K.: Erythroblastosis fetalis—including exchange transfusion technic, Boston, 1957, Little, Brown and Co.
5. Amerman, E. E., Brescia, M. A., and Aftahi, F.: Ferrous sulfate poisoning, J. Pediat. 53:476, 1958.
6. Angella, J. J., Prieto, E. N., and Fogel, B. I.: Hemoglobinuria associated with hemolytic disease of the newborn infant, J. Pediat. 71:530, 1967.
7. Barrett, C. T., and Oliver, T. K., Jr.: Hypoglycemia and hyperinsulinism in infants with erythroblastosis fetalis, New Eng. J. Med. 278:1260, 1968.
8. Bentley, H. P., Ziegler, N. R., and Krivit, W.: The use of heparinized blood for exchange transfusion in infants, Amer. J. Dis. Child. 99:8, 1960.
9. Boggs, T. R., Jr.: Clinical experience with hemolytic disease of newborn infants, J.A.M.A. 165:9, 1957.
10. Boggs, T. R., Jr.: Survival rates in Rh sensitization; 140 interrupted versus 141 uninterrupted pregnancies, Pediatrics 33:758, 1964.
11. Boggs, T. R., Jr.: Comment on the pitfall of overuse of exchange transfusion for treating neonatal hyperbilirubinemia, Ped. Clin. N. Amer. 12:99, 1965.
12. Boggs, T. R., Jr., and Anrode, H. G.: Boric acid poisoning treated by exchange transfusion, Pediatrics 16:109, 1955.
13. Broughton, P. M. G., Rossiter, E. J. R., Warren, C. B. M., Goulis, G., and Lord, P. S.: Effect of blue light on hyperbilirubinemia, Arch. Dis. Child. 40:666, 1965.
14. Bowman, J. M., and Friesen, R. F.: Multiple intraperitoneal transfusions of the fetus for erythroblastosis fetalis, New Eng. J. Med. 271:703, 1964.
15. Bowen, W. R., Poter E., and Waters, W. J.: The protective action of albumin in bilirubin toxicity in newborn puppies, Amer. J. Dis. Child. 98:568, 1959.
16. Brown, A. K.: Bilirubin metabolism with special reference to neonatal jaundice. In Levine, S. Z., editor: Advances in pediatrics, vol. 12, Chicago, 1962, Year Book Medical Publishers, Inc., p. 121.
17. Brown, A. K., and Zuelzer, W. W.: Studies in hyperbilirubinemia; hyperbilirubinemia of the newborn unrelated to isoimmunization, Amer. J. Dis. Child. 93:263, 1957.
18. Brown, A. K., Zuelzer, W. W., and Robinson, A. R.: Studies in hyperbilirubinemia, clearance of bilirubin from plasma and extravascular space in newborn infants during exchange transfusion, Amer. J. Dis. Child. 93:274, 1957.
19. Carter, B. B.: Rh haptens; its preparation, assay and nature, J. Immunol. 61:79, 1949.
20. Castor, W. R.: Spontaneous perforation of bowel in newborn following exchange transfusion, Canad. M. A. J. 99:934, 1968.
21. Chown, B., and Bowman, J. M.: Hemolytic disease of newborn. In Gellis, S. S., and Kagan, B. M., editors: Current pediatric therapy, Philadelphia, 1964, W. B. Saunders Co.
22. Chown, B., and Bowman, W. D.: The place of early delivery in the prevention of foetal death from erythroblastosis, Ped. Clin. N. Amer. 5:279, 1958.
23. Clarke, C. A.: Prevention of Rh-haemolytic disease, Brit. Med. J. 2:417, 1967.
24. Clarke, C. A.: Prevention of rhesus-isoimmunization, Seminars in Hematology 6:201, 1969.
25. Clarke, C. A., Elson, C. J., Bradley, J., Donohoe, W. T. A., Lehane, D., and Hughes-Jones, N. C.: Intensive plasmapheresis as a therapeutic measure in rhesus-immunized women, Lancet 1:793, 1970.
26. Cochran, W., Stark, A., and Schulhoff, C.: Prognosis of live infants who had intrauterine transfusions, Ped. Res. 4:373, 1970.
27. Cohen, F. Zuelzer, W. W., Gustafson, D. C., and Evans, M. M.: Mechanisms of isoimmunization. I. The transplacental passage of fetal erythrocytes, Blood 23:621, 1964.
28. Cohen, F., Zuelzer, W. W., Hsu, T. H. J., and Teruya, J.: Rh hemolytic disease in ABO-incompatible offspring, Amer. J. Obstet. Gynec. 105:232, 1969.
29. Committee on Fetus and Newborn, American Academy of Pediatrics: Recommendations on a uniform bilirubin standard, Pediatrics 31:878, 1963.
30. Corkery, J. J., Dubowitz, V., Lister, J., and Moosa, A.: A colonic perforation after exchange transfusion, Brit. Med. J. 4:345, 1968.
31. Crawford, A., Cutbush, M., and Mollison, P. L.: Hemolytic disease of the newborn due to anti-A, Blood 8:620, 1953.
32. Crosse, V. M., Walles, G. P., and Walsh, A. M.: Replacement transfusion as a means of preventing kernicterus of prematurity, Arch. Dis. Child. 33:403, 1958.
33. Danoff, S., Boyer, A., and Holt, L. E., Jr.: The treatment of hyperbilirubinemia of the newborn with sodium glucuronate, Pediatrics 23:570, 1959.
34. Danoff, S., Grantz, C., Boyer, A., and Holt, L. E., Jr.: The conversion of indirect to di-

rect-reacting bilirubin in vivo, Science **127**:759, 1958.
35. Day, R. L.: Discussion on observations on the control of bilirubinemia, Amer. J. Dis. Child. **96**:440, 1958.
36. Day, R. L.: Physiologic jaundice—1961, Ped. Clin. N. Amer. **8**:539, 1961.
37. Diamond, E. F., and DeYoung, V. R.: Acute poisoning with oil of wintergreen treated by exchange transfusion, Amer. J. Dis. Child. **95**:309, 1958.
38. Diamond, L. K.: Discussion of current problems regarding the Rh factor, Blood Spec. Issue No. 2, The Rh factor, p. 180, 1948.
39. Diamond, L. K.: Protection against Rh sensitization and prevention of erythroblastosis fetalis, Pediatrics **41**:1, 1968.
40. Dillon, H. C., and Krivit, W.: Serial study of bone marrow in hemolytic disease of the new born (erythroblastosis fetalis), Pediatrics **23**:314, 1959.
41. Driscoll, S. G., and Steinke, I.: Pancreatic and insulin content in severe erythroblastosis fetalis, Pediatrics **39**:448, 1967.
42. Dunn, P. M.: Obstructive jaundice and haemolytic disease of the newborn, Arch. Dis. Child. **38**:54, 1963.
43. Erlandson, M. E.: Current status of exchange transfusion, J. Pediat. **63**:357, 1963.
44. Erlandson, M. E., and Haber, J. M.: Severe erythroblastosis in first immunized pregnancies, Amer. J. Obstet. Gynec. **90**:779, 1964.
45. Finn, R.: Erythroblastosis, Lancet **1**:526, 1960.
46. Finn, R., Clarke, C. A., Donohoe, W. T. A., McConnell, R. B., Heppard, P. M., Lehane, D., and Kulke, W.: Experimental studies on the prevention of Rh hemolytic disease, Brit. Med. J. **1**:1486, 1961.
47. Finn, R., Harper, D. T., Stallings, S. A., and Krevans, J. R.: Transplacental hemorrhage, Transfusion **3**:114, 1963.
48. Fong, S. W., Margolis, A. J., Westberg, J. A., and Johnson, P.: Intra-uterine transfusion; fetal outcome and complication, Pediatrics **45**:576, 1970.
49. Freda, V. J., and Gorman, J. G.: Antepartum management of Rh hemolytic disease, Bull. Sloane Hosp. Women **8**:147, 1962.
50. Freda, V. J., Gorman, J. G., Galen, R. S., and Treacy, N.: The threat of Rh immunization from abortion, Lancet **2**:147, 1970.
51. Freda, V. J., Gorman, J. G., and Pollack, W.: Successful prevention of experimental Rh sensitization in man with an anti-Rh gammaglobulin antibody preparation; a preliminary report, Transfusion **4**:26, 1964.
52. Freda, V. J., Gorman, J. G., and Pollack, W.: Rh factor; prevention of isoimmunization and clinical trial on mothers, Science **151**:828, 1966.
53. Friedman, A. B., Avellera, R. M., Lidsky, I., and Lubert, M.: Perforation of the colon after exchange transfusion in the newborn, New Eng. J. Med. **282**:796, 1970.
54. Glassford, G. H., and Motamedy, F. F.: Successful treatment of cardiac arrest during exchange transfusion, Amer. J. Dis. Child. **97**:616, 1959.
55. Gunson, H. H.: An evaluation of the immunohematological tests used in the diagnosis of A-B hemolytic disease, Amer. J. Dis. Child. **94**:123, 1957.
56. Gunson, H. H.: Combined Rh and AB hemolytic disease of the newborn, Amer. J. Clin. Path. **27**:35, 1957.
57. Halbrecht, I.: Role of hemagglutinins anti-A and anti-B in pathogenesis of jaundice of the newborn (icterus neonatorum precox), Amer. J. Dis. Child. **64**:248, 1944.
58. Hazeltine, F. G.: Hypoglycemia and Rh-erythroblastosis fetalis, Pediatrics **30**:696, 1967.
59. Hogg, G. R.: Cardiac lesions in hemolytic disease of the newborn, J. Pediat. **60**:352, 1962.
60. Holman, C. A., and Karnicki, J.: Intrauterine transfusion for haemolytic disease of the newborn, Brit. Med. J. **2**:594, 1964.
61. Holman, G. H.: Studies on physiologic hyperbilirubinemia of Negro and white premature infants, Pediatrics **22**:1115, 1958.
62. Hsia, D. Y-Y.: Bilirubin metabolism, Ped. Clin. N. Amer. **12**:713, 1965.
63. Hughes-Jones, N. C., and Mollison, P. L.: Failure of a relatively small dose of passively administered anti-Rh to suppress primary immunization of a relatively large dose of Rh-positive red cells, Brit. Med. J. **1**:150, 1968.
64. Hurdle, D. A. F., and Davis, J. A.: The 'late' anemia of hemolytic disease of the newborn, Brit. J. Haemat. **11**:247, 1965.
65. Hurdle, D. A. F., and Walker, A. G.: Bone marrow hypoplasia in the course of hemolytic disease of the newborn, Brit. Med. J. **1**:518, 1963.
66. Hyman, C. B., and Sturgeon, P.: Observations on the convalescent phase of erythroblastosis fetalis, Pediatrics **16**:15, 1955.
67. Jablonski, W. J.: Risks associated with exchange transfusions, New Eng. J. Med. **266**:155, 1962.
68. Jandl, J. H., Jones, A. R., and Castle, W. B.: The destruction of red cells by antibodies in man. I. Observations on the sequestration, analysis of red cells altered by immune mechanisms, J. Clin. Invest. **36**:1428, 1957.

69. Jeliu, G., Schmid, R., and Gellis, S.: Administration of glucuronic acids to icteric newborn infants, Pediatrics 23:92, 1959.
70. Johnson, L., Garcia, M. L., Figueroa, E., and Sarmeinto, F.: Kernicterus in rats lacking glucuronyl transferase. II. Factors which alter bilirubin concentration and frequency of kernicterus, Amer. J. Dis. Child. 101:322, 1961.
71. Johnson, L., Sarmiento, F., Blanc, W. A., and Day, R.: Kernicterus in rats with inherited deficiency of glucuronyl transferase, Amer. J. Dis. Child. 97:591, 1959.
72. Kaplan, E., Herz, F., and Hsu, K. S.: Erythrocyte acetylcholinesterase activity in ABO hemolytic disease of the newborn, Pediatrics 33:205, 1964.
73. Kauder, E., and Mauer, A. M.: Hemolysis as a contributing factor in the bilirubin rebound after exchange transfusion, J. Pediat. 60:163, 1962.
74. Killander, A., Michaëlsson, M., Müller-Eberhard, U., and Sjölin, S.: Hyperbilirubinemia in full-term newborn infants; a follow-up study, Acta Paediat. 52:481, 1963.
75. Koch, C. A.: Hyperbilirubinemia in premature infants; a follow-up study. II, J. Pediat. 65:1, 1964.
76. Kochwa, S., Rosenfield, R. E., Tallal, L., and Wasserman, L. R.: Isoagglutinins associated with erythroblastosis, J. Clin. Invest. 40:874, 1961.
77. Lathe, G. H.: Exchange transfusion as a means of removing bilirubin in haemolytic disease of the newborn, Brit. Med. J. 1:192, 1955.
78. Letters to the editor, Pediatrics 23:814, 1959.
79. Levine, P.: Serological factors as possible causes in spontaneous abortions, J. Hered. 34:71, 1943.
80. Liley, A. W.: Intrauterine transfusion of foetus in haemolytic disease, Brit. Med. J. 2:1107, 1963.
81. Liley, A. W.: The use of amniocentesis and fetal transfusion in erythroblastosis fetalis, Pediatrics 35:836, 1965.
82. Lucey, J. F.: Diagnosis and treatment of the fetus with erythroblastosis, Ped. Clin. N. Amer. 13:1117, 1966.
83. Lucey, J. F.: Colonic perforation after exchange transfusion, New Eng. J. Med. 280:724, 1969.
84. Lucey, J., Ferriro, M., and Hewitt, J.: Prevention of hyperbilirubinemia of prematurity, Pediatrics 41:1047, 1968.
85. Lucia, S. P., and Hunt, M. L.: The significance of ABO compatibility and its relationship to the intensity of Rh immunization, Blood 5:767, 1950.
86. Martin, N. H.: Preparation and properties of serum and plasma proteins: interaction with bilirubin, J. Amer. Chem. Soc. 71:1230, 1949.
87. McKay, R. J., Jr.: Current status of use of exchange transfusion in newborn infants, Pediatrics 33:763, 1964.
88. Meyer, T. C.: A study of serum bilirubin level in relation to kernicterus and prematurity, Arch. Dis. Child. 31:75, 1956.
89. Mintz, A. A., and Vallbana, C.: A hazard of exchange transfusion in newborn infants—negative pressure in the umbilical vein, Pediatrics 26:661, 1960.
90. Mollison, P. L.: Blood transfusion in clinical medicine, ed. 3, Oxford, 1961, Blackwell Scientific Publications.
91. Mollison, P. L.: Suppression of Rh-immunization by passively administered anti-Rh, Brit. J. Haemat. 14:1, 1968.
92. Mollison, P. L., and Cutbush, M.: Haemolytic disease of the newborn; criteria of severity, Brit. Med. J. 1:123, 1949.
93. Mores, A., Fargasova, I., and Minarikova, E.: The relation of hyperbilirubinemia in newborns without isoimmunization to kernicterus, Acta Paediat. 48:590, 1959.
94. Naiman, J. L., Punnett, H. H., Lischner, H. W., Destine, M. L., and Arey, J. B.: Possible graft-versus-host reaction after intrauterine transfusion for Rh erythroblastosis fetalis, New Eng. J. Med. 281:697, 1969.
95. Nasralla, M., Gawronska, E., and Hsia, D. Y-Y.: Studies on the relation between serum and spinal fluid bilirubin during early infancy, J. Clin. Invest. 37:1403, 1958.
96. Nelson, J. D., Richardson, J., and Shelton, S.: The significance of bacteremia with exchange transfusions, J. Pediat. 66:291, 1965.
97. Newns, G. H., and Norron, K. R.: Hyperbilirubinemia in prematurity, Lancet 2:1138, 1958.
98. Odell, G. B.: Studies in kernicterus. I. The protein binding of bilirubin, J. Clin. Invest. 38:823, 1959.
99. Odell, G. B.: The dissociation of bilirubin from albumin and its clinical implications, J. Pediat. 55:268, 1959.
100. Odell, G. B.: In Thompson, S. G., editor: Techniques of exchange transfusion, supplement No. 1 to reports of Ross Conferences on Pediatric Research, Columbus, Ohio, 1962, Ross Laboratories.
101. Odell, G. B., Bryan, W. B., and Richmond, M. D.: Exchange transfusion, Ped. Clin. N. Amer. 9:605, 1962.
102. Odell, G. B., and Cohen, S. N.: Albumin priming in the management of hyperbilirubinemia by exchange transfusions, Amer. J. Dis. Child. 102:699, 1961.
103. Oppé, T. E., and Oalaes, T.: Obstructive

jaundice and haemolytic disease of the newborn, Lancet 1:536, 1959.
104. Orme, R. L. E., and Eades, S. M.: Perforation of the bowel in newborn as a complication of exchange transfusion, Brit. Med. J. 4:349, 1968.
105. Oski, F. A., Allen, D. M., and Diamond, L. K.: Portal hypertension—a complication of umbilical vein catheterization, Pediatrics 31:297, 1963.
106. Pew, W. L.: Cardiac arrest during exchange transfusion, J. Pediat. 47:645, 1955.
107. Pew, W. L.: Exchange transfusion using heparinized blood, J. Pediat. 49:570, 1956.
108. Philipsborn, H. D., Traisman, H. S., and Greer, D., Jr.: Rupture of the spleen; a complication of erythrobyastosis fetalis, New Eng. J. Med. 252:159, 1955.
109. Pierson, W. E., Barrett, C. T., and Oliver, T. K., Jr.: The effect of buffered and nonbuffered acid blood on electrolyte and acid-base homeostasis during exchange transfusion, Pediatrics 41:802, 1968.
110. Porter, E. G., and Waters, W. J.: A rapid micromethod for measuring the reserve albumin binding capacity in serum from newborn infants with hyperbilirubinemia, J. Lab. Clin. Med. 67:660, 1966.
111. Queenan, J. J.: Modern management of the Rh problem, New York, 1967, Harper and Row, Publishers.
112. Rawson, A. J., and Abelson, N. M.: Studies of blood group antibodies. III. Observations on the physiochemical properties of isohemagglutinins and isohemolysins, J. Immunol. 85:636, 1960.
113. Rawson, A. J., and Abelson, N. M.: Studies of blood group antibodies. IV. Physiochemical difficulties between isoanti-A, B and isoanti-A or isoanti-B, J. Immunol. 85:640, 1960.
114. Robertson, S. E. S.: A study of the anemia following exchange transfusion in haemolytic disease of the newborn, M. J. Australia 43:250, 1956.
115. Robinson, A., and Barrie, H.: The electrocardiogram during exchange transfusion, Arch. Dis. Child. 38:334, 1963.
116. Ross Conference: Intrauterine transfusion and erythroblastosis fetalis, 53rd conference, Aspen, Colorado, March, 1966, p. 14.
117. Schmid, R.: Discussion on observations on the control of bilirubinemia, Amer. J. Dis. Child. 96:441, 1958.
118. Schmid, R.: Jaundice and bilirubin metabolism, Arch. Intern. Med. 101:669, 1958.
119. Schmidt, P. J., Peden, J. C., Bercher, G., and Baranovsky, A.: Extracorpuscular circulation, New Eng. J. Med. 265:1181, 1961.
120. Schwab, M., Perry, R., Boyer, A., Holt, L. E., Jr., Hallman, N., Backman, A., and Hjelt, L.: The influence of sodium glucuronate on hyperbilirubinemia of the newborn; further observations, Pediatrics 25:686, 1960.
121. Shiller, J. G., and Silverman, W. A.: "Uncomplicated" hyperbilirubinemia of prematurity, Amer. J. Dis. Child. 101:587, 1961.
122. Shumway, C. N., Miller, G., and Young, L. E.: Hemolytic disease of the newborn due to anti-A and anti-B, Pediatrics 15:54, 1955.
123. Sisson, T. R. C., Whalen, L. E., and Telek, A.: A comparison of the effects of whole blood and sedimented erythrocytes in exchange transfusion, Pediatrics 21:81, 1958.
124. Slotkowski, E. L., and Hand, A. M.: Rupture of spleen in erythroblastotic infant, Pediatrics 4:296, 1949.
125. Smith, C. H.: Chronic congenital aregenerative anemia (pure red-cell anemia) associated with iso-immunization by the blood group factor "A," Blood 4:697, 1949.
126. Smith, C. H., Schulman, I., Ando, R. E., and Stern, G.: Studies in Mediterranean (Cooley's) anemia; the suppression of hematopoiesis by transfusions, Blood 10:707, 1955.
127. Smith, T.: Active immunity produced by so-called balances in neutral mixtures of diphtheria toxin and antitoxin, J. Exp. Med. 2:241, 1909.
128. Sproul, A., and Smith, L.: The bilirubin equilibration during exchange transfusion in hemolytic disease of the newborn, J. Pediat. 65:12, 1964.
129. Stern, K., Davidsohn, I., and Masartis, L.: Experimental studies in Rh immunization, Amer. J. Clin. Path. 26:833, 1956.
130. Stern, K., Goodman, H. S., and Berger, M.: Experimental isoimmunization to hemoantigens in man, J. Immunol. 87:189, 1961.
131. Stern, L., and Denton, R. L.: Kernicterus in small premature infants, Pediatrics 35:483, 1965.
132. Szulman, A. E.: The histological distribution of blood group substances A and B in man, J. Exp. Med. 111:785, 1960.
133. Tovey, G. H.: A study of the protective factors in heterospecific blood group pregnancy and their role in the prevention of haemolytic disease of the newborn, J. Path. Bact. 57:295, 1945.
134. Trolle, D.: Discussion on the advisability of performing exchange transfusion in neonatal jaundice of unknown aetiology, Acta Paediat. 50:392, 1961.
135. Valentine, G. H.: Heparinized blood for exchange transfusions, Lancet 2:21, 1958.
136. Valentine, G. H.: Exchange transfusion by

continuous drip using heparinized blood, Lancet 1:10, 1962.
137. Van der Hauwaert, L. G., Loos, M. C., and Verhaeghe, L. K.: Myocardial infarction during exchange transfusions in a newborn infant, J. Pediat. 70:745, 1967.
138. Van Praagh, R.: Causes of death in infants with hemolytic disease of the newborn (erythroblastosis fetalis), Pediatrics 28:233, 1961.
139. Vaughan, V. C., III: Current status of hemolytic disease of the newborn, Postgrad. Med. 18:115, 1955.
140. Vaughan, V. C., III: Management of hemolytic disease of the newborn, J. Pediat. 54:586, 1959.
141. Vaughan, V. C., III: Early delivery for hemolytic disease of the newborn? J. Pediat. 56:713, 1960.
142. Veall, N., and Mollison, P. L.: The rate of red cell exchange in replacement transfusions, Lancet 2:792, 1950.
143. Verga, S., and Vathianathan, T.: Massive intravascular sickling after exchange transfusion with sickle cell trait blood, Transfusion 3:387, 1963.
144. Waters, W. J., and Porter, E. G.: Dye-binding capacity of serum albumin in hemolytic disease of the newborn, Amer. J. Dis. Child. 102:807, 1961.
145. Waters, W. J., and Porter, E.: Indications for exchange transfusion based upon the role of albumin in the treatment of hemolytic disease of the newborn, Pediatrics 33:749, 1964.
146. Weldon, V. V., and Odell, G. B.: Mortality risk of exchange transfusion, Pediatrics 41:797, 1968.
147. Wheeler, W. E.: Antibiotics. In Thompson, S. G., editor: Techniques of exchange transfusion, Supplement No. 1 to reports of Ross conferences on Pediatric Research, Columbus, Ohio, 1962, Ross Laboratories.
148. Wheeler, W. E., and Ambuel, J. P.: The efficient use of exchange transfusions in the treatment of erythroblastosis, Ped. Clin. N. Amer. 4:383, 1957.
149. Wiener, A. S.: Conglutination test for Rh sensitization, J. Lab. Clin. Med. 30:662, 1945.
150. Wiener, A. S.: Competition of antigens in isoimmunization by pregnancy, Proc. Soc. Exp. Biol. Med. 58:133, 1945.
151. Wiener, A. S., Wexler, I. B., and Brancato, G. J.: Treatment of erythroblastosis by exchange transfusions, J. Pediat. 45:546, 1954.
152. Witebsky, E.: Interrelationship between the Rh system and the A-B system, Blood, Spec. Issue No. 2, p. 66, 1948.
153. Woodrow, J. C., Clarke, C. A., Donohoe, W. T. A., Finn, R., McConnell, R. B., Sheppard, P. M., Lehane, D., Russell, S. H., Kulke, W., and Durkin, C. M.: Prevention of Rh-haemolytic disease: a third report, Brit. Med. J. 1:279, 1965.
154. Zipursky, A., and Israels, L. G.: The pathogenesis and prevention of Rh immunization, Canad. M. A. J. 97:1245, 1967.
155. Zipursky, A., Pollock, J., Neelands, P., Chown, B., and Israels, L. G.: The transplacental passage of foetal red blood-cells and the pathogenesis of Rh immunization during pregnancy, Lancet 2:489, 1963.
156. Zuelzer, W. W., and Cohen, F.: ABO hemolytic disease and heterospecific pregnancy, Ped. Clin. N. Amer. 4:405, 1957.
157. Zuelzer, W. W., and Kaplan, E.: ABO heterospecific pregnancy and hemolytic disease. I. Patterns of maternal A and B isoantibodies in unselected pregnancies, Amer. J. Dis. Child. 88:158, 1954.
158. Zuelzer, W. W., and Kaplan, E.: ABO heterospecific pregnancy and hemolytic disease; patterns of A and B isoantibodies in the cord blood of normal infants, Amer J. Dis. Child. 88:179, 1954.
159. Zuelzer, W. W., and Kaplan, E.: ABO heterospecific pregnancy and hemolytic disease; pathologic variants, Amer. J. Dis. Child. 88:319, 1954.

# 11 ANEMIAS—GENERAL CONSIDERATIONS

Anemia may be defined as a condition in which the concentration of hemaglobin or the number of red blood cells, either singly or in combination, are reduced below normal. The volume of packed red blood cells per 100 ml. of blood measured by the hematocrit undergoes a simultaneous but not always parallel reduction. The physiologic defect caused by the anemia is a decrease in the oxygen-carrying capacity of the blood and a reduction in the oxygen available to the tissues. Usually, anemia is said to exist when the hemoglobin content of the blood falls below normal.

A humoral regulatory mechanism which appears to be responsive to changes in the relation between oxygen supply and tissue requirements most probably exists as a homeostatic control over erythropoiesis.[35]

*Classification.* On an etiologic basis anemia results from an increased loss or destruction of red blood cells or a decreased rate of production. Blood loss is due to acute or chronic hemorrhage and excessive hemolysis from intracorpuscular defects or extracorpuscular factors. Impaired hemoglobin and red cell formation are due to a deficiency of substances required for their synthesis. Defects of the red cells may be congenital or acquired, but in either case their shortened life-span frequently results in anemia due to a failure of red cell production to keep pace with red cell destruction. Erythropoiesis also may be depressed by toxic, chemical, or physical agents, by space-occupying or infiltrative lesions of the bone marrow, or by unrecognized causes. It will be noted that the classifications may overlap. For example, anemia may result from a combination of excessive destruction of erythrocytes with intracorpuscular defects as occurs in patients with hereditary spherocytosis and the hereditary hemoglobinopathies with inadequate compensatory erythropoiesis. (For the hemolytic anemias, see Chapter 15; for the hereditary hemoglobinopathies, see Chapter 16.)

Following is a classification of the anemias based on etiology.

1. Blood loss—acute and chronic hemorrhage
2. Excessive blood destruction
    a. Intracorpuscular or intrinsic defects, usually hereditary
        (1) Hereditary spherocytosis, elliptocytosis, stomatocytosis
        (2) Hereditary hemoglobinopathies, sickle cell anemia, thalassemia
        (3) Hemolytic anemia due to enzyme deficiencies and hereditary nonspherocytic anemia
    b. Extracorpuscular factors
        (1) Factors due to antibodies and isoagglutinins
        (2) Symptomatic hemolytic anemias
        (3) Lederer's anemia, march hemoglobinuria, paroxysmal cold hemoglobinuria
        (4) Miscellaneous causes such as infections and chemical and physical agents—hypersplenism
3. Decreased or impaired production
    a. Deficiency of substances required for hemoglobin and red cell formation: iron, vitamin $B_{12}$, folic acid, ascorbic acid, protein
    b. Depression or inhibition of bone marrow
        (1) Infection, chemicals, physical agents, metabolic products
        (2) Idiopathic depression and aplasia with or without congenital anomalies
    c. Mechanical interference and replacement by abnormal cells: leukemia, Hodgkin's disease, malignancies
    d. Miscellaneous: infection, renal failure, hypothyroidism

*Orientation.* The anemias constitute the major segment of the blood disorders of infancy and childhood. Anemia is a syndrome of multiple etiology in which the origins are frequently difficult to discern for reasons inherent in the developmental processes of the pediatric period. Many of the anemias undoubtedly are conditioned by factors operative in fetal life dating from the critical first months of gestation when the primary blood cell elements are established. Others are influenced by the postnatal physiologic and anatomic changes that originate within and outside of the hematopoietic system. Still others represent inherited inborn errors of metabolism such as the primaquine-sensitive group of the hemolytic anemias. The conditioning factors influencing the blood picture in the neonatal period and early infancy are given in the following list.* Each of these items is discussed elsewhere in the text.

1. The results of maternal isoimmunization by fetal blood factors
2. Bleeding from the placental surface: abruptio placenta, placenta previa, and other complications of delivery
3. Fetal hemorrhage into maternal circulation
4. Anemia from congenital bleeding disorders: overt or obscure hemorrhage
5. Fluctuations in blood volume as related to early or late clamping of the cord
6. Substitution of adult for fetal hemoglobin
7. The aregenerative phase of erythropoiesis which characterizes the early months of life
8. The possibility that a blood dyscrasia may represent a congenital or developmental defect
9. The effects of prematurity
10. The effects of rapid body growth
11. Tendency for the hematopoietic system to react excessively to a stimulus; reactivation of extramedullary foci of hematopoiesis
12. Inadequate fetal stores of iron from maternal deficiency of this mineral
13. Hemolytic anemia from maternal transmission of ingested drugs or chemical compounds

*Diagnosis.* The problems of diagnosis in the infant and young child are complicated by the fact that the anemias tend to develop insidiously so that the complete hematologic picture with its specific criteria may be slow in emerging. Despite these apparent difficulties, it is possible with minimal laboratory equipment to arrive at a diagnosis by the judicious appraisal of data derived from a variety of sources such as the following.*

1. History and physical examination
2. Basic blood studies: complete blood count, reticulocytes, interpretation of blood smear
3. Comparison with normal range of blood values for each age period
4. Etiologic classification
   a. Blood loss
   b. Excessive blood destruction and hemolysis of extracorpuscular and intracorpuscular origin
   c. Bone marrow depression or infiltration
   d. Deficiency of building materials for hemoglobin or red cell formation
5. Reference to age periods of most frequent occurrence
6. Bone marrow examination
7. Roentgenographic examination
8. Study of hereditary factors
9. Therapeutic response to iron, folic acid, vitamin $B_{12}$, transfusion
10. Specialized laboratory procedures
    a. Essential
       (1) Stool guaiac test
       (2) Serum bilirubin
       (3) Blood urea nitrogen
       (4) Coombs test
       (5) Red cell fragility
       (6) Autohemolysis test
       (7) Hemoglobin electrophoresis
    b. Helpful
       (1) Gastric acidity
       (2) Stool urobilin
       (3) Serum iron and latent iron-binding capacity
       (4) Bone marrow iron
       (5) Radioisotopes in diagnosis
          (a) Radioactive chromium ($^{51}$Cr) determination of red cell lifespan, red cell mass, plasma volume, blood loss, amounts appearing in body sites (surface scanning), such as liver, spleen, and bone marrow
          (b) Radioiron ($^{59}$Fe) in determining plasma clearance rate, plasma iron transport rate, appearance rate in erythrocytes, amounts appearing in body sites such as liver and spleen

---

*Based in part on Smith, C. H.: Anemias in infancy and childhood; diagnostic and therapeutic considerations, Bull. N. Y. Acad. Med. 30:155, 1954.

*Modified from Smith, C. H.: Anemias in infancy and childhood; diagnostic and therapeutic considerations, Bull. N. Y. Acad. Med. 30:155, 1954.

(c) Radioactive $B_{12}$ urinary excretion test for $B_{12}$ absorption (Schilling test) in diagnosis of pernicious anemia

The large number of items included in the list illustrates the wide scope of available information and the simpler technical procedures upon which the diagnosis is based. However, an insight into the nature of the anemia actually requires that relatively few of these topics be probed. Under ordinary circumstances a thorough history, physical examination, and basic blood studies, in conjunction with a simple classification based on etiology, are usually sufficient to arrive at a correct diagnosis.

*History and physical examination.* Interrogation along broad lines of causation should include the following: any change of behavior pattern such as irritability, anorexia, inactivity, fatigability, onset of pallor, prematurity, rate of weight gain, quantity of milk ingested, and attitude toward solid food. Inquiry should also extend into a history of exacerbations of pallor and jaundice, hematemesis, loss of blood from the bowel, infection with animal parasites, allergy, ingestion of drugs or household products known to depress hematopoiesis or to cause hemolysis, exposure to radiation, frequency of respiratory infection, skeletal pain, joint swellings, renal disease, and purpura.

Physical examination should include scrutiny of such diverse features as pallor, jaundice, skin pigmentation, enlargement of lymph nodes, liver, and spleen, petechiae, and purpura. In iron-deficiency anemia, acute leukemia, and severe loss of blood, the skin has a waxy whiteness. Cardiac enlargement and signs of cardiac failure may be present. A loud systolic murmur best heard at the apex and less commonly over the pulmonic area is frequently regarded as being of organic origin before the underlying severe anemia is discovered. These murmurs are of hemic origin and usually disappear following transfusions. In patients with advanced Cooley's anemia the facies have a characteristic appearance. In this disease as well as in other conditions requiring multiple transfusions, such as aplastic anemia and pure red cell anemia, pallor is replaced by dark pigmentation and bronzing of the skin. In patients in whom hemosiderosis is present and at times coexists with hemochromatosis, sexual retardation is noted. Increasing jaundice from the first day of life differentiates erythroblastosis fetalis from its slower development in icterus neonatorum. Eye ground and nervous system changes are to be looked for in patients with sickle cell anemia. Leg ulcers occur rarely in sickle cell anemia in children.

Splenomegaly is most noticeable in infants with disorders attended by blood destruction such as erythroblastosis, hereditary spherocytosis, acquired hemolytic anemia, and severe Cooley's anemia. The spleen is occasionally enlarged in patients with iron-deficiency anemia and those with megoblastic anemia of infancy. It is not palpable in infants with aplastic, hypoplastic, or pure red cell anemia. It should also be remembered that a spleen palpable about 1 to 3 cm. below the costal margin is present in a substantial number of otherwise normal infants and children. The soft edge of the spleen in these children is in contrast with the hard edge found in patients with pathologic conditions. Enlargement of the liver is occasionally found in patients with congestive heart failure and in those with sudden severe anemia from any cause. It is often enlarged in patients with the hemolytic anemias, especially in those receiving frequent transfusions and who have developed hemosiderosis and hemochromatosis.

Except for the anemia associated with infection or with leukemia, lymphadenopathy is not a conspicuous feature of anemia. Enlarged cervical nodes frequently associated with a palpable spleen occur in the child with anemia due to repeated infections of the upper respiratory tract. The superficial lymph nodes may be slightly enlarged in patients with severe Cooley's anemia and sickle cell anemia but not in those with the other intrinsic anemias. A generalized lymphadenopathy in the presence of a refractory anemia and leukopenia should arouse suspicion of leukemia.

*Age incidence in relation to diagnosis.* When infection, which is responsible for the major number of anemias in the pediatric age group, is excluded as an etiologic factor, the remaining hematologic disorders can be grouped for orientation according to the age periods of their most frequent incidence: newborn, infancy, and childhood.

In the newborn infant the anemia is usually due to erythroblastosis fetalis. If this can be eliminated, blood loss is to be considered. Acute fetal blood loss during labor and delivery, frequently resulting in posthemorrhagic shock, may be due to fetal bleeding from the placenta, occult transplacental loss of fetal blood into the maternal circulation, or rupture of a normal or shortened umbilical cord.[31]

According to Oski and Naiman,[41] the differential diagnosis of anemia in the neonate includes cognizance of many conditions. A comprehensive examination of the family and maternal as well as obstetric history are important in diagnosis. Hereditary spherocytosis, thalassemia major, and sickle cell anemia in another sibling or parent can be determined by history or by a few simple hematologic methods. The basic laboratory studies in the initial examination should include hemoglobin and hematocrit determinations, reticulocyte count, examination of the peripheral blood smear, and the direct Coombs test of the infant's blood. The reticulocyte count provides important information since it is elevated with a hemolytic process or hemorrhage. If the reticulocyte count is decreased, aregenerative anemia or some infiltrative disease such as leukemia should be considered. Bone marrow examination is required to establish diagnosis of the latter. When reticulocytes are elevated and obstetric hemorrhage has been eliminated, a positive direct Coombs test will pinpoint those infants who have been immunized with Rh-Hr or A-B-O or minor blood factors. If the Coombs test is negative, other types of hemolytic disease as well as occult bleeding should be considered. Anemia of the newborn associated with hypochromic microcytes may stem from fetomaternal hemorrhage or twin-to-twin transfusion. A search for red cells in the mother's circulation containing fetal hemoglobin will reveal transplacental loss of fetal blood. Spherocytes, elliptocytes, and pyknocytes found in examination of the newborn blood smear provide important diagnostic information. Enzymatic defects such as pyruvate kinase deficiency and glucose-6-phosphate dehydrogenase deficiency may be found as causative factors in hemolytic anemia of the newborn. A number of infections may cause hemolytic anemia in this period such as cytomegalic inclusion disease, toxoplasmosis, congenital rubella, and congenital syphilis, and are usually accompanied by prominent hepatosplenomegaly, jaundice, and thrombocytopenic purpura. Other infections may also be responsible for anemia and jaundice; for these, blood and urine cultures may reveal the cause of an obscure hemolytic anemia during the first weeks of life.

Anemia due to iron deficiency occurs most commonly between 6 months and 2 years of age, especially in the rapidly growing infant, in the premature infant, and in any infant whose dietary iron is restricted. Iron-deficiency anemia also occurs during infancy due to chronic gastrointestinal bleeding from embryonic structural defects such as diverticula. Megaloblastic anemia of infancy occurs chiefly between the ages of 2 and 18 months. Pure red cell (aregenerative) anemia is usually apparent at the age of 2 to 3 months or later in the first year. When the infant is at approximately 6 months to 1 year of age, the clinical and hematologic features of severe Cooley's anemia, sickle cell anemia, and hereditary spherocytosis are sufficiently conspicuous to be diagnosed. They can be distinguished even earlier in suspected cases because of a familial background.

Aplastic anemia, hypoplastic anemia, and Fanconi's anemia syndrome (aplastic anemia combined with multiple congenital anomalies) usually manifest their complete clinical and hematologic features after 3 years of age. At about this time, too, Banti's disease and other disorders are encountered which are associated with splenomegaly and varying degrees of a hypersplenic blood picture such as that seen in Gaucher's disease. It must be emphasized that the onset of the blood disorders first recognized in older infants and young children precedes by a variable period the time when the distinguishing features are fully established and unequivocal.

*Normal blood values in infancy and childhood.* Because of developmental changes, anemias in infancy and childhood must necessarily be interpreted in the light of the contemporary hematologic framework within which they are encountered. The range of normal values for the respective age periods that serve as a basis for evaluating an anemia are summarized in Table 9. A knowledge of the values for hemoglobin and red cells at birth and in the early newborn period is essential for an awareness of an anemia due to erythroblastosis or blood loss.

For comparative purposes the average hemoglobin level on the first day of life may be regarded as 20 gm. per 100 ml. of blood, with values ranging from 18 to 22 gm./100 ml., and the red cell count as 5,500,000 per cubic millimeter, with a range from 5 to 6 million. During the first 2 years of life the normal hemoglobin content ranges from approximately 10 to 12.5 gm. per 100 ml. of blood, with an average value of 11 gm./100 ml., and between 5 and 10 years of age from 13 to 13.5 gm./100

**Table 9.** Normal blood values significant in diagnosis of anemias in infancy and childhood*

| | |
|---|---|
| Hemoglobin | |
|     First day | 20 gm./100 ml. (18 to 22 gm.) |
|     2 weeks | 17 gm./100 ml. |
|     First and second years | 11 gm./100 ml. (10 to 12.5 gm.) |
|     3 to 5 years | 12.5 to 13 gm./100 ml. |
|     5 to 10 years | 13 to 13.5 gm./100 ml. |
|     10 years | 14.5 gm./100 ml. |
| Red blood cells | |
|     First day | 5,500,000/cu. mm. (5 to 6 million) |
|     Second week | 5,000,000/cu. mm. |
|     Older infant and child | 4,000,000/cu. mm. lower limit of normal |
| Nucleated red cells | |
|     Average—3 to 10 per 100 white cells (birth to 4 days of life) | |
| Reticulocytes | |
|     0.5 to 1.5% (6% upper limit of normal—from birth to 4 days of life) | |
|     (Below 0.5% in aplastic and hypoplastic anemia; increased in hemolytic anemia; in deficiency anemia rise from low to high levels with treatment) | |
| Volume of packed red cells (hematocrit) | |
|     Infants 1 month to 2 years | 34% |
|     Children 2 years to 12 years | 36% |
|     Older children | 40% |
| Serum bilirubin | |
|     Newborn full-term infants | 2 to 8 mg./100 ml. |
|     Newborn premature infants | 1 to 15 mg./100 ml. |
|     (Values given for both full-term and premature newborn infants are the low values at birth rising to maximum during first week of life) | |
|     Normal infants and children | Under 1 mg./100 ml. |
|     (Hemolytic anemias—elevated total bilirubin predominantly indirect fraction) | |
| Fragility test | |
|     Normal range | 0.425 to 0.325% sodium chloride |
|     (Increased fragility in hereditary spherocytosis and in some cases of acute hemolytic anemia; decreased fragility in sickle cell anemia, thalassemia [major and minor], and in iron-deficiency anemia) | |

*From Smith, C. H.: Anemias in infancy and childhood; diagnostic and therapeutic considerations, Bull. N. Y. Acad. Med. **30**:155, 1954.

ml.; during puberty it rises gradually to the adult value of 14.5 gm. per 100 ml. A count of 4 million red cells per cubic millimeter of blood may be regarded as the lower limit of normal for the older infant and child. In normal newborn infants the number of nucleated red cells in the first few days of life ranges from 3 to 10 per 100 white blood cells.

*Volume of packed red cells (hematocrit).* In all anemias the measurement of the volume of packed red blood cells by the hematocrit constitutes an important and essential guide for diagnosis and therapy. This determination reflects the total mass of cells in a unit volume of blood and has proved to be of fundamental value in the study of all anemias in which considerable alterations occur in size, shape, and thickness of the red blood cells. It has the advantage of being reliable and least subject to error in quantitative interpretation. In patients with iron-deficiency anemia, for instance, the extremely low hematocrit reflects the state of anemia more accurately than does the moderate reduction or even normal value in the number of red blood cells. Also, in the asymptomatic person with the trait of thalassemia the volume of packed red cells frequently remains at the same level in spite of wide fluctuations in the number of red cells.

Because of the variations noted in available

studies, it is difficult to state the optimum packed cell volume for different age groups. As a working basis, a hematocrit of 34% may be regarded as the lower limit of normal in infants after the first month of life, 36% from 2 to 12 years of age, and 40% in older children.

*Reticulocyte count and stain.* The reticulocyte count reflects the state of activity of the bone marrow; hence this determination provides a useful guide in the diagnosis of both deficiency and hemolytic anemias and in gauging the response to treatment. Normally from 0.5 to 1.5% of the red blood cells are reticulated; levels below 0.5% represent inactive bone marrow. A persistent depression in the percentage of the reticulocytes in spite of treatment usually occurs in patients with aplastic and hypoplastic anemia. In those with anemia due to a deficiency, a reticulocyte response from previously low levels follows appropriate treatment. In patients with hemolytic anemias the values for reticulocytes are constantly elevated and the high levels that are maintained prior to and without treatment represent intensified bone marrow regeneration. In such cases the Coombs test will be positive in infants with erythroblastosis fetalis and acquired hemolytic anemia. A negative test prompts a search for the diagnosis among the hereditary hemoglobinopathies, primaquine-sensitive hemolytic anemias, nonspherocytic anemia, and hereditary spherocytosis.

*Reticulocyte stain*: A glass slide is cleaned and polished. Two or three drops of a saturated alcohol solution of brilliant cresyl blue are put near one end of the slide and allowed to dry. Heavy streaks of precipitated stain are removed by rubbing with lens paper.

A small drop of blood is placed in the center of the stained area and mixed with the stain by stirring with the edge of a second slide. When thorough mixing has occurred, the stained blood is smeared across the remainder of the slide. It is allowed to dry and then is counterstained with Wright's stain. The number of reticulocytes per 1,000 red blood cells should be enumerated to obtain an accurate count. The result is expressed as percentage—i.e., the number of reticulocytes per 100 red cells. In order to estimate effective erythropoiesis, the corrected or absolute erythrocyte count must be determined—i.e., the percent of reticulocytes times the erythrocyte count.

Other methods of carrying out reticulocyte counts prescribe incubating mixtures of blood and stain before preparing the slide. The method of Seip[46] utilizes a solution of brilliant cresyl blue 1% and sodium citrate 0.4% in normal saline as a stain. One or two drops of heel blood is mixed well with an equal amount of staining fluid in a hollow-ground, silicone-coated slide. The mixing is carried out by means of a small glass rod, which is also silicone-coated. The slide is placed in a moist chamber for 20 minutes. The stained slide is thereafter stirred very well with the glass rod so that an even suspension is attained. Thin smears are made on thoroughly cleaned slides.

Another method[7] is to mix two drops of blood and two drops of staining solution on a clean slide. The mixture is drawn into a capillary tube and expelled onto the slide, and the procedure is repeated several times. The slide is then placed in a moist chamber for 10 minutes. A small drop of the mixture is spread on a clean slide or cover slip. When the smears are air-dry, the reticulated red cells are counted. Another method is to allow the staining solution to stand for 10 minutes in a capillary pipette. In this method the staining solution is diluted in water. Both of these methods preclude the use of alcohol solution of the stain as in the rapid method first cited.

*Relationship between the red cell count, hemoglobin, and volume of packed red cells in absolute measurements.* Morphologically, the anemias may be classified according to the size of the red cell: normocytic, microcytic, and macrocytic. A hemoglobin concentration within normal limits is called normochromic; below normal, hypochromic. Hyperchromic anemias are nonexistent. The increase in hemoglobin in the macrocyte may run parallel with the size of the macrocyte but does not exceed it. Since the macrocyte is thicker than the normocyte, the central pallor is less marked in the macrocyte which appears dark when stained.[59]

The indices calculated from the red cell count, hemoglobin concentration, and volume of packed red cells offer important clinical clues to treatment.

*Color index:* The color index, formerly a widely used measurement, is obtained by dividing the hemoglobin value in grams per 100 ml. by the red cell count, both values being designated as a percentage of normal. It defines the hemoglobin content of the individual cells as compared with the content of a normal cell. A color index of approximately 1 is either normal or connotes a normocytic, normochromic anemia; an index of below 0.8 characterizes a hypochromic anemia; an index above 1 denotes macrocytosis, which is usually associated with hypochromia.

Although the color index is, in general, a valid expression of the relationship between hemoglobin saturation and cell size, exceptions occur. In infancy and early childhood, especially, the color index may be unreliable because of the normal fluctuations in hemoglobin and red cell counts which accompany growth.

$$\text{Color index} = \frac{\text{Hemoglobin (\% of normal [14.5 gm. per 100 ml.} = 100\%])}{\text{Red cells \% (5 million/mm.}^3 = 100\%)}$$

More precise and instructive information regarding cell size and hemoglobin concentration in the younger age groups is obtained by measuring the mean corpuscular volume (MCV) and the mean corpuscular hemoglobin concentration (MCHC).

*Price-Jones curve:* The Price-Jones curve is a graphic method of recording the diameters of red blood cells of various sizes from the stained blood smear.[42] In the majority of normal subjects the peak diameters are approximately 6.69 to 7.7$\mu$, which are taken as the upper and lower limits of normal.[56] The average mean diameter is given as 7.2$\mu$. The sizes of the red cells are noted on the abscissa and the number of cells (frequency) in each size group on the ordinate. The results are plotted in frequency curves. Figures or curves above or below the two peaks indicate macrocytosis and microcytosis, respectively. Anisocytosis is indicated by spreading of the base of the curve and flattening of the peak. The effects of treatment on macrocytosis in patients with pernicious anemia are particularly well demonstrated in the Price-Jones curve. Since measurement of the red cell diameters is a laborious procedure unless automatic electronic cell counters are used, the simpler measurement of the mean corpuscular volume is frequently substituted for it.

*Red cell indices:* The designation of the anemia according to size of the red cell and hemoglobin content serves to suggest specific blood disorders and their therapy.

MEAN CORPUSCULAR VOLUME (MCV). This represents the mean or average volume of a single red cell. The result is expressed in cubic microns.

$$\frac{\text{Hematocrit, \%} \times 10}{\text{Red blood cell count, millions/mm.}^3}$$

Example:
Red blood cell count   5 million
Hematocrit             45%
MCV                    $\frac{45 \times 10}{5} = 90\ \mu^3$

Normal range MCV = 80 to 94 $\mu^3$

A MCV of more than 94 $\mu^3$ indicates macrocytes; 80 to 94 $\mu^3$, normocytes; less than 80 $\mu^3$, microcytes. According to Guest and Brown,[26] the MCV in the newborn averages 113 $\pm$ 0.8 $\mu^3$, and at 1 week it averages 106 $\pm$ 6$\mu^3$. At 6 months it drops to 78 $\pm$ 0.7$\mu^3$, at 1 year 73 $\pm$ 1.1$\mu^3$, and at 14 years 81 $\pm$ 1.1$\mu^3$.

MEAN CORPUSCULAR HEMOGLOBIN (MCH). Mean corpuscular hemoglobin represents the average quantity (weight) of hemoglobin per individual red cell. Results are expressed in micromicrograms.

$$\frac{\text{Hemoglobin, gm./100 ml.} \times 10}{\text{Red blood cell count, millions/mm.}^3}$$

Normal range MCH = 27 to 32 $\mu\mu$g

A MCH with normal hemoglobin content is called normochromic; above normal, hyperchromic; below normal, hypochromic.

MEAN CORPUSCULAR HEMOGLOBIN CONCENTRATION (MCHC). This represents the average concentration of hemoglobin in the individual red cell as calculated from the amount of hemoglobin per 100 ml. of cells rather than of whole blood. The result is expressed as percentage.

$$\frac{\text{Hemoglobin, gm./100 ml.} \times 100}{\text{Hematocrit, \%}}$$

Normal range = 32 to 38%

Red cells with MCHC of less than 32% are hypochromic. At approximately 34% hemoglobin the normal erythrocyte contains a maximal number of hemoglobin molecules. Hyperchromia in reality describes an increased intensity of staining of the red cells. A cell with increased thickness, as is observed in patients with hereditary spherocytosis, gives the impression of hyperchromia (thickness above normal value of 2 m$\mu$). MCH and MCHC measure the weight and concentration of hemoglobin, respectively, in the average red cell.

The absolute values of the mean corpuscular hemoglobin concentration and the mean cell volume offer practical guides for diagnosis and therapy. The combination of microcytosis (MCV below 60 $\mu^3$) and hypochromia (MCHC of less than 32%) is indicative of iron deficiency. Characteristic is a blood smear with a predominance of hypochromic microcytes and pronounced central pallor. Thalassemia minor, which possesses red cell indices and red cell morphology similar to those of iron-deficiency anemia, is characterized by a familial and hereditary pattern and the presence of $A_2$ hemoglobin. On the basis of the blood smear alone, the two conditions are virtually inseparable. In patients with the less common macrocytic anemias with mean red cell volumes exceeding 94 $\mu^3$, restoration to normal values can be expected with vitamin $B_{12}$ and folic acid therapy. Macrocytes may be fully saturated with hemoglobin or the pigment may be diminished; in the latter case iron therapy is also indicated.

In patients with chronic infections and in those with systemic diseases such as nephritis, the red cells may be microcytic or normocytic with little or no decrease in the content of hemoglobin. Patients with these infections and diseases fail to respond permanently to antianemia therapy unless the primary cause is treated. Transfusions are symptomatically required for patients with these conditions as well as for those with the normochromic and normocytic anemias resulting from bone marrow depression. These include aplastic and hypoplastic anemias and leukemia, in which marrow cell displacement occurs. A normocytic normochromic anemia in a child for which no definite hematologic basis can be discovered necessitates comprehensive survey for an underlying pathologic condition.

*Bone marrow examination.* Aspiration of the bone marrow constitutes a useful laboratory aid in the diagnosis of blood disorders. The accessibility of the marrow, its responses to stimuli producing depression or hyperplasia, its availability for repeated examinations, and the comparative ease of identifying the cellular elements account for frequency with which aspiration is performed.[47] Disturbances of each of the principal blood elements are frequently reflected earlier or are more conspicuous in the bone marrow than in the peripheral blood. In patients with leukemia, for instance, the bone marrow may be extensively infiltrated with leukoblastic cells, whereas they appear in the peripheral blood in such scant numbers as to be overlooked. In patients with hypoplastic-aplastic anemias and in those with the hemolytic anemias, bone marrow studies permit quantitative estimation of the cell types involved. Bone marrow examination serves as a guide to therapy with antianemia agents and especially with the chemotherapeutic compounds in leukemia.

NORMAL VALUES. The figures in Table 10 represent the approximate range and average values of the cellular elements which one may expect to find in samples of the bone marrow obtained from normal infants and children. Certain modifications must be made in view of the changing pattern of the percentages of the component cells. The granulocytic series predominate in the first week or two of life. By 1 month the lymphocytes increase in number and often extend beyond the 25% level noted in Table 10 to reach levels of 50% during the first year. The presence of a lymphocytosis of this magnitude need not give rise to unnecessary concern, provided the cells are morphologically normal. Between 4 and 8 years of age, the granulocytes equal the lymphocytes numerically and eventually predominate, reaching adult values at about 12 years of age.

DIAGNOSTIC FEATURES IN THE BLOOD DISORDERS. The individual cellular constituents in the bone marrow are in such close proximity to each other that it is difficult for one element to be affected independently of the others. This total stimulation is best observed in patients

Table 10. Normal values of cellular elements in bone marrow in older infants and children

|  | Range (%) | Average (%) |
|---|---|---|
| Myeloblasts | 1 to 5 | 2 |
| Myelocytes (including promyelocytes) | 10 to 25 | 20 |
| Nonsegmented polymorphonuclear cells (including metamyelocytes) | 15 to 30 | 20 |
| Segmented polymorphonuclear cells | 5 to 30 | 25 |
| Lymphocytes | 5 to 25 | 13 |
| Nucleated red cells (principally normoblasts) | 15 to 30 | 20 |
| Megakaryocytes | 10 to 35 per mm.³ |  |
| Total nucleated cell count | 100,000 to 200,000 per mm.³ |  |

with the hemolytic anemias and most regularly in those with acute hemolytic anemia. In the latter, regeneration of the red blood cells is associated with an increase in the number of granulocytes and platelets. The reverse occurs in patients with aplastic anemia in whom values for the three types of blood cells are depressed simultaneously. However, other factors must operate in addition to anatomic proximity, since involvement of a single type of cell may occur. This is illustrated in persons with pure red cell anemia, in whom the production of red blood cells is inhibited without equal depression of the other cellular elements. Similarly, selective hyperplasia occurs in persons with iron-deficiency anemia and in those with chronic loss of blood in whom the normoblasts and their immediate precursors alone are primarily increased.

In patients with the hemolytic anemias (i.e., erythroblastosis fetalis, hereditary spherocytosis, acute acquired hemolytic anemia, sickle cell anemia, and thalassemia major) the bone marrow is hyperplastic, and there is an increased proliferation of normoblasts and, to a lesser extent, of erythroblasts. Granulopoiesis may be active, especially in persons with acquired hemolytic anemia. In patients with iron-deficiency anemia and in those with chronic hemorrhagic anemia, the bone marrow is similarly hyperplastic and values for normoblasts are greatly elevated, but granulopoiesis is normal. In patients with acute hemorrhage, however, the activity of the myeloid elements is also increased. The increase of the nucleated red cells in patients with these disease processes in excess of 50% of all nucleated elements in the marrow constitutes an important diagnostic feature (Table 11).

Aplastic anemia is associated with profound anemia, leukopenia, neutropenia, and thrombocytopenia. The bone marrow shows a progressive decrease in cellularity, and there is a sharp reduction in the myeloid elements, megakaryocytes, and nucleated red cells, with a relative increase in normal lymphocytes. Occasionally, acute lymphoblastic leukemia in the leukopenic stage may simulate aplastic anemia, and diagnosis is difficult without histologic examination of the bone marrow. Bone marrow aspiration in patients with leukemia will reveal a cellular bone marrow in which the normal nucleated elements are replaced by primitive cells of the lymphoid or myeloid series. With the progressive reduction in the number of platelets, hemorrhages occur in patients with aplastic anemia which may stimulate thrombocytopenic purpura. The bone marrow in persons with idiopathic thrombocytopenic purpura reveals a hyperplasia of immature

Table 11. Diagnostic features of the bone marrow in the common anemias of infancy and childhood[*]

| Type of anemia | Diagnostic features |
| --- | --- |
| Hemolytic group (erythroblastosis fetalis, hereditary spherocytosis, sickle cell anemia, thalassemia major, acquired hemolytic anemia) | Hyperplastic marrow with increase of nucleated red cells, chiefly normoblasts; granulopoiesis may also be active; occasionally during crises, marrow aplastic instead of hyperplastic |
| Iron-deficiency anemia | Hyperplastic marrow with increase in normoblasts; granulopoiesis unchanged |
| Hemorrhagic anemia | Hyperplastic marrow with increase in nucleated red cells, chiefly normoblasts; granulopoiesis active in acute hemorrhage and unchanged in slow and chronic loss of blood |
| Megaloblastic anemia of infancy | Pattern similar to pernicious anemia in relapse; megaloblastic type of erythropoiesis and changes in granulocytes resembling pernicious anemia |
| Aplastic anemia | Usually decreased cellularity to acellular; sharp reduction in myeloid elements, megakaryocytes, and normoblasts; increase in lymphocytes |
| Hypoplastic anemia | Hypoplastic marrow with pronounced depression affecting normoblasts mainly |
| Aregenerative (pure red cell) anemia | Normal marrow except for absence of nucleated red cells |

*From Smith, C. H.: Diagnosis of anemias in infancy and childhood, J.A.M.A. **134**:992, 1947.

megakaryocytes. In secondary thrombocytopenic purpura occurring in patients with leukemia and aplastic anemia, megakaryocytes are reduced in number or are entirely absent in the counting chamber and the bone marrow smears.

## FERROKINETICS AND ERYTHROKINETICS

*General considerations.* Anemia has been regarded as an imbalance between the number of red blood cells delivered to the circulation each day and the number of cells lost from the circulation.[16] Any decrease in the rate of entrance or any increase in the rate of removal without a corresponding increase of production leads ultimately to a lower level of circulating erythrocytes. Blood production and destruction may be estimated by six measurements: erythroid-myeloid ratio, plasma iron turnover, reticulocyte count, red cell utilization of radioiron, red cell life-span, and fecal urobilinogen. By combining ferrokinetic measurements (using $^{59}$Fe) with measurements of red cell survival (using $^{51}$Cr), important information can be obtained on the rate of blood formation and blood destruction. With the aid of $^{51}$Cr, blood volume can be measured and, based on this value, plasma iron turnover and red cell utilization can be determined.[3]

Radioactive sodium chromate ($^{51}$Cr) has a half-life of 27.8 days and is employed in measuring circulating red cell mass, plasma volume, red cell survival, sites of red cell destruction, and gastrointestinal bleeding. By reinjecting blood that had been mixed with $^{51}$Cr into the circulation of the patient, the lifespan of the red cell is measured in its natural environment. When injected into a normal recipient, an intrinsic defect of the red cell may be detected.

The sites of destruction of red cells with special reference to the role of the spleen and liver can be determined by in vivo surface counting, using a scintillation counter placed respectively over the heart, liver, and spleen. The fall in counts over the heart reflects the elimination of labeled red cells from the circulation. Theoretically, there should be a parallel fall in the counts over the liver and spleen as in the heart, unless hemolysis or sequestration of red cells is taking place within the organs. Thus, in hemolytic anemias a much greater radioactive count over the spleen as compared with the liver suggests benefits to be derived from splenectomy. When blood contains $^{51}$Cr-labeled red cells, fecal radioactivity is minimal unless bleeding has taken place somewhere along the course of the gastrointestinal tract. Radioactivity in stool specimens provides a reliable measure of the extent of blood loss.

$^{59}$Fe, the radioactive isotope of iron, has a relatively short half-life of 45 days and serves as a label for hemoglobin after its ingestion and injection. When injected into the blood in tracer quantities, it provides a label for the plasma iron pool and its rate of disappearance from the plasma can be measured. Its subsequent appearance in erythrocytes permits a measurement of the rate of hemoglobin synthesis and of the extent to which iron is utilized for this process. In normal subjects there is a rise in the counting rate over the marrow as the level of activity falls in the plasma. Counting rates over both the liver and the spleen are invariably a good deal lower than over the marrow at all stages in normal subjects. In hemolytic anemias the initial counting rates over the marrow rise rapidly and to a lesser extent than normal. This is associated with a rise in radioactivity over the spleen. In hypocellular marrows there is little initial uptake over the marrow, the major portion is eventually located in the liver and spleen, while very little appears in the red cell mass.[3] Available data suggests that hemolysis accompanied by a high rate of uptake by the spleen indicates a favorable outcome of splenectomy, whereas a relatively low rate of uptake prognosticates a lack of benefit.

The plasma iron turnover is calculated from the plasma iron concentration and the rate of disappearance of injected radioiron from the plasma. The plasma iron turnover is a measure of total erythroid activity, since in the normal individuals and in patients with increased erythropoiesis, over 70% of the iron passing through the plasma is directed to the marrow for hemoglobin synthesis.[16] The prolonged plasma clearance of $^{59}$Fe and delay of its reappearance in the circulating erythrocytes is a most reliable ferrokinetic index of erythropoietic depression. Plasma turnover rate (plasma half clearance time), the number of milligrams of iron entering and leaving the plasma per unit of time, is shortened in hemolytic conditions and iron-deficiency anemia.

The percentage of injected radioiron that

appears in the circulating red cells by 14 days, combined with the plasma iron turnover, also reflects the number of new red cells entering the circulation. This measurement is of special value at low levels of erythropoiesis but may be inaccurate in many hemolytic states when erythropoiesis is increased. Fecal urobilinogen, another measurement of red cell breakdown, estimates pyrrole pigment derived not only from circulating blood but also from the marrow cells.

*In the diagnosis of anemias.* As stated, measurements of iron kinetics (ferrokinetics) include estimates of the rates and sites of red cell formation and destruction, mean erythrocyte life-span, and plasma-storage iron exchange. Ferrokinetics also permit a quantitative estimate of erythropoietic activity (erythrokinetics). With the information provided by ferrokinetic determinations in conjunction with absolute reticulocyte counts, myeloid-erythroid ratio of the marrow, total red cell mass, and fecal urobilinogen, the kinetics of erythropoiesis can be estimated.

Definitive information can be obtained in normal conditions as well as in aberrations occurring in blood disorders. Plasma iron turnover normally approximates 0.6 mg. per 100 ml. of whole blood per day.[3] In a normal individual of 70 kg., 30 to 40 mg. of iron pass through the plasma in 24 hours. This means that the plasma iron pool of about 3 to 4 mg. turns over approximately twelve times each day. The plasma iron turnover is increased in the hemolytic anemias, polycythemia, iron-deficiency anemia, and infections. In subjects with hypocellular marrows (aplastic anemia) and in refractory anemias, the plasma iron turnover tends to fall within a normal range with a below-average red cell utilization. In leukemia, lymphoma, myelofibrosis, and myeloproliferative diseases, the plasma iron turnover varies from below to slightly above normal. In myelofibrosis rapid clearance is by far the more common finding.[51]

The fraction of red cells renewed per day is equal to the product of the percentage of red cell utilization and plasma iron turnover. The degree to which radioiron is utilized depends on the needs of the bone marrow and on the iron load being presented to the reticuloendothelial system at any one time. The major value of erythrokinetic measurement is in localizing the abnormality as due to a premarrow effect (lack of stimulation), to an abnormality in the marrow itself, or to an increased removal of red cells from the circulation.[3] On this basis, anemias have been differentiated into proliferative and nonproliferative types. Proliferative anemias are those in which an optimal increase results in total erythropoiesis in response to anemia. In these anemias the production rate is three to six times normal. Anything short of this is regarded as a nonproliferative state. Examples of nonproliferative anemias are those associated with endocrinopathies, renal disease, infection, and iron-deficiency anemia. Proliferative anemias are exemplified by those occurring in hemorrhage, with hemolysis, in conditions with a deficiency of an essential erythropoietic factor such as vitamin $B_{12}$, folic acid, and pyridoxine, and in some hereditary hemoglobinopathies such as thalassemia.[3]

*Effective and ineffective erythropoiesis.* From these measurements, degrees of erythropoiesis can be estimated. Total erythropoiesis is defined as the total red cell or hemoglobin production, regardless of whether the new cells ever circulate. Effective erythropoiesis designates that fraction of red cells which enters and remains in circulation long enough to be measured (about 1 day). Ineffective erythropoiesis refers to the portion of red cells not appearing in the circulation. It indicates the discrepancy between the total red cell or hemoglobin mass in the peripheral blood and red cell production in the bone marrow unexplained by hemolysis or hemorrhage.[29] In thalassemia, for instance, measurements of total erythropoiesis (plasma iron turnover and erythroid-myeloid ratio) are increased to six to ten times normal, while those measurements reflecting effective erythropoiesis (red cell utilization of radioiron and corrected reticulocyte count) are not increased above normal. Total hemoglobin breakdown as estimated by fecal urobilinogen is also much greater than can be accounted for on the basis of circulating red cell destruction measured by $^{51}Cr$ life-span. These discrepancies serve as examples of ineffective erythropoiesis, indicating that only a small portion of total marrow activity is effective.[16]

INVASION OF THE BONE MARROW BY FOREIGN CELLS. Abnormal elements characterizing a specific pathologic condition occasionally appear in the bone marrow. In younger age groups these consist most commonly of Gaucher and Niemann-Pick cells, the abnormal histiocytes of Letterer-Siwe disease (non-lipid reticuloendotheliosis), and metastatic neoplastic cells such as are found in patients with neuroblastoma and lymphosarcoma.

In an examination of the bone marrow smears obtained by aspiration in seventy-nine children with a variety of neoplasms,[15] tumor cells were found in twenty-one of thirty patients with neuroblastoma, in three of eighteen with embryonal rhabdomyosarcoma, in one of two with retinoblastoma, in two of six with osteogenic sarcoma, and in one of eight with Ewing's sarcoma. All children with recognizable bone marrow invasion died within 6 months. No tumor cells were found in aspiration of Wilms' tumor. The authors state that only two patients with neuroblastoma reported as having recovered with bony invasion did so spontaneously (see favorable results with cyclophosphamide, Chapter 24).[1,21]

NEUROBLASTOMA. Characteristic tumor cells are found with such great frequency in patients with metastatic neuroblastoma that bone marrow examination is essential when this disease is suspected. In one series of cases the abnormal cells were found in fifteen of thirty-one infants and children. Their presence is not dependent upon the existence of radio-visible bone lesions.[19] In patients with this condition ball-like masses or clusters of large immature cells form syncytial masses or pseudorosettes with a mosaic pattern.[30] The individual cells are large, with nuclei possessing an immature chromatin pattern which stain deep blue. The cytoplasm is scant, faintly basophilic, and without granules[19] Neuroblastoma may occasionally be confused with leukemia on bone marrow aspiration. The presence of discrete syncytium and scattered cells resembling stem cells are more likely to be diagnostic of neuroblastoma. In contrast to acute leukemia, neuroblastoma cells do not appear in the peripheral blood (Figs. 13 to 15).

Increased catecholamine production has been reported in children with neuroblastoma. Neuroblastoma, which originates from percursor cells of sympathetic nerve tissues or adrenal medulla, produces excessive quantities of dopa, dopamine, and norepinephrine. These are converted to two major terminal urinary metabolites—homovanillic acid (HVA) and vanillyl mandelic acid (VMA). An abnormally high concentration of urinary HVA and VMA has been found before treatment of neuroblastoma, ganglioneuroma, or ganglioneuroblastoma. Simultaneous measurement of urinary HVA and VMA excretion provides an effective method for the diagnosis of a majority of these tumors and for following the results of treatment.[22,57] In one child after removal of neuroblastoma, urinary excretion of catecholamines returned to normal.[54] The increased catecholamine excretion during the active disease is sometimes associated with diarrhea and hypertension. Although the mechanism of diarrhea is unclear, its prompt cessation after removal of the tumor implies some causative relationship.[43]

In a series of thirty-five tumor cases in children, the urinary excretion of vanillyl mandelic acid (VMA) ranged from 10 to above 80 $\mu$g/mg. creatinine, whereas it fell within the normal range (below 10 $\mu$g/mg. creatinine) in ganglioneuroma and other malignant tumors, most of them Wilms' tumors.[2] The VMA was raised in pheochromocytoma as well as in cases of neuroblastoma. The excretion of homovanillic acid (HVA) was increased in neuroblastoma but not in pheochromocytoma. The normal adult urinary VMA range in 0.1 to 9.0 mg./24 hrs. Neuroblastoma and its variant ganglioneuroblastoma is the second most common solid malignant tumor of infants and children; this frequency of occurrence is exceeded only by tumors of the central nervous system[32] and second only to leukemia as a childhood neoplasm.[14]

Neuroblastoma may occur in any anatomical site where neural crest tissue existed in the embryo so that the neoplasm may be present at any place along the sympathetic nerve chain, in any of the sympathetic groups, or in the adrenal gland. Only about half of the neuroblastomas arise in the adrenal gland. It is probably the only tumor which has the ability to undergo histologic change from a malignant sympathicoblastoma to a mild form, ganglioneuroma. Many of the neuroblastomas are secreting tumors and the physiological response to increased serum norepinephrine may be reflected clinically in diarrhea, hypertension, or failure to thrive. Metastasis and invasion occur early and are present in two-thirds of patients when first seen. Metastases characteristically go to the bones, retro-orbital tissue, liver, meninges, pleura, and sometimes regional lymph nodes.

Retrobulbar metastases are particularly common and cause exophthalmos and extensive

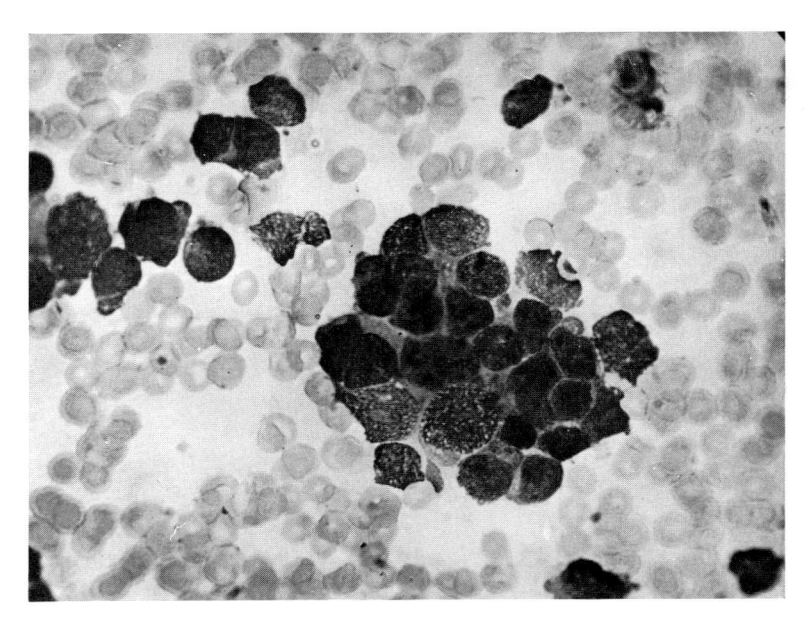

Fig. 13. Bone marrow smear in a case of neuroblastoma with splenomegaly and pancytopenia. Note tumor cells in ball-like clusters with scattering of cells resembling stem cells of leukemia in proximity. Diagnostic pseudorosettes are present in other portions of the smear. (×720.)

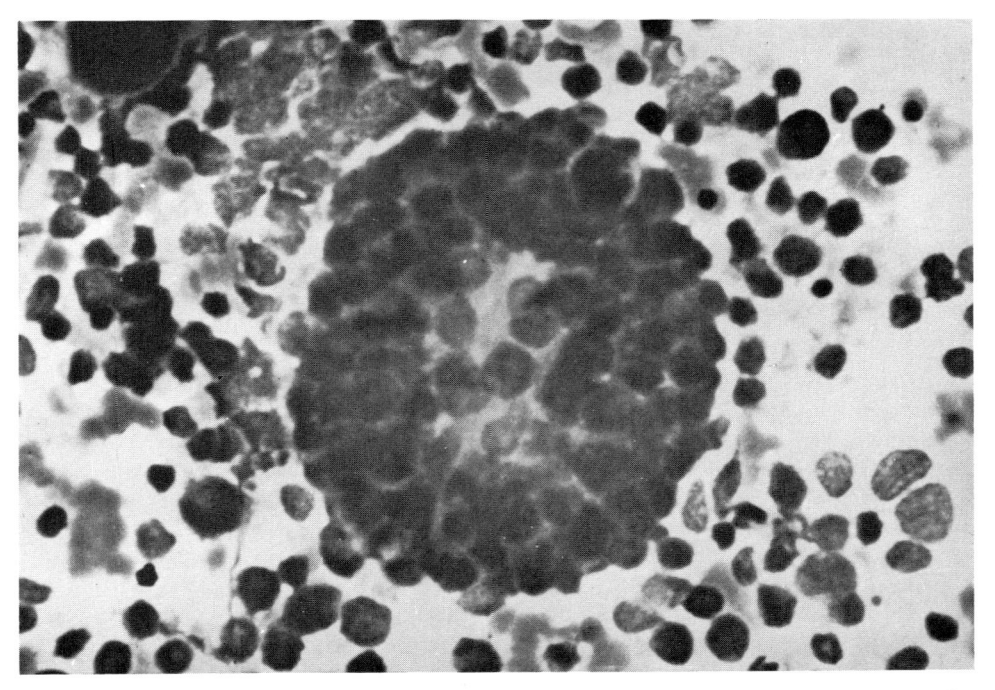

Fig. 14. Bone marrow smear in neuroblastoma in a 7-year-old child. Note the striking circular appearance of the rosette and the diffuse infiltration of neuroblastoma cells in the bone marrow. (Courtesy Dr. Philip Lanzkowsky, New York, N. Y.)

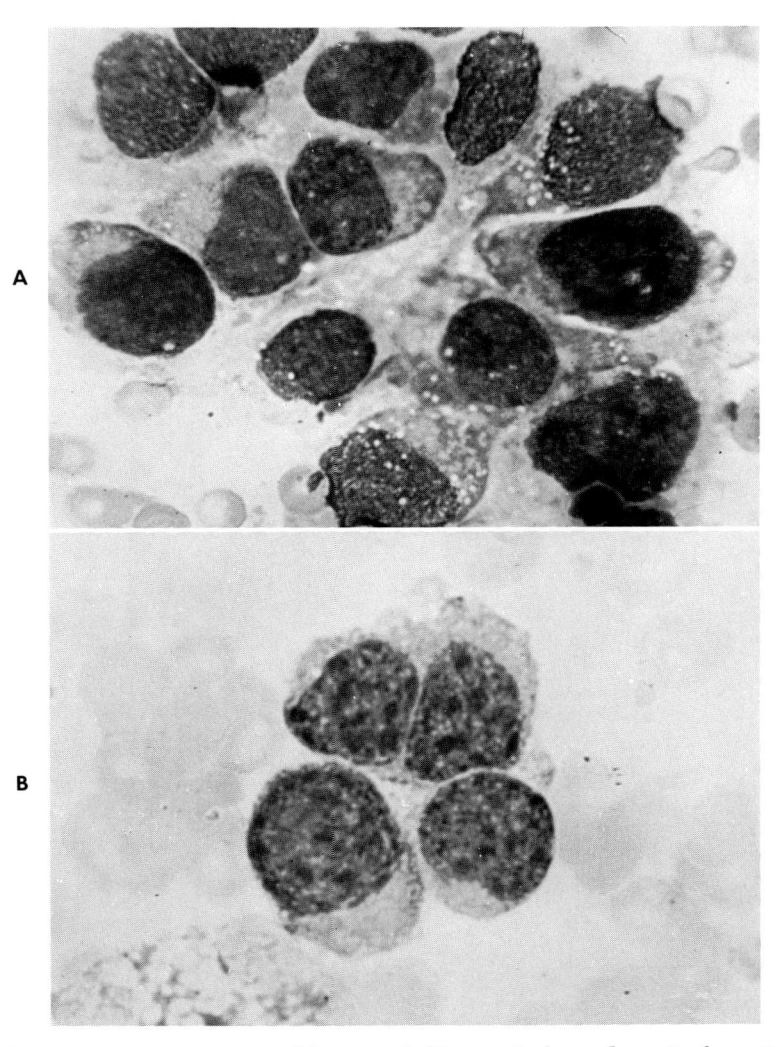

Fig. 15. Bone marrow smears in neuroblastoma. **A,** Note typical pseudorosette formation around a fibrillar network. **B,** Same formation as **A,** showing finer detail of individual cells in circular grouping (×1,200). (**A** courtesy Dr. Ralph L. Engle, Jr., New York, N. Y.)

destruction of the bony orbit. (Wilms' tumor, on the contrary, rarely metastasizes to bone but more commonly to lung.)

The diagnosis of neuroblastoma is based on the findings of bone marrow aspiration, skeletal survey (including the skull), intravenous pyelogram, lymphangiogram, chest x-ray, and inferior vena cavagram. Treatment consists of early surgical removal of resectable tumor, followed by x-ray therapy to the primary site and metastasis if present. As much tumor as can be removed should be resected, ligating the arterial blood supply where possible. Recent studies appear to indicate that there is a major immunologic factor in the spontaneous cure of neuroblastoma.

Complete excision of neuroblastoma results in highest survival rate. Partial excision even in the presence of metastases has occasionally produced cures, and in a small percentage of patients biopsy alone has been followed by long-term cures.[32]

Factors associated with improved prognosis include diagnosis under 1 year of age, mediastinal location, tumor maturation to ganglioneuroblastoma, and lack of dissemination.[14]

Some regard cyclophosphamide as the most effective single chemical agent, although antimetabolites and corticosteroids have also been used with beneficial results.[53] On the other hand, others state that chemotherapeutic regimens for neuroblastoma have not been notably successful. They state the total removal of the tumor followed by radiotherapy is associated with an excellent prognosis.[34]

A family has been reported in which the asymptomatic mother had abnormally high urinary excretion of dopamine, norepinephrine, and VMA. Four of her five offspring had neuroblastomas, and two of the affected siblings had other major diseases. These findings, together with other reports of familial neuroblastoma, are considered to suggest that this tumor may be inherited.[9]

Another patient in this hospital[37] represents one of the few recorded cases of a child with multiple skeletal metastasis and bone marrow infiltration secondary to disseminated neuroblastoma who survived 7 years and 6 months after the diagnosis without clinical, chemical, or radiographic evidence of disease.

In a study of twenty-seven cases of neuroblastoma[25] it was noted that the younger the patient at the time of diagnosis, the better the survival. In the 1950-1957 period, a cure rate of 36.7% was experienced by patients of all ages. During this period, those patients who were under 1 year of age were cured in 56% of the cases and those under 2 years, in 49%. In the same period, patients without metastases to bone, when first seen under 1 year of age, were cured in 70% of the cases and those under 2 years, in 65%.

Two cases of disseminated neuroblastoma, one occurring in a stillborn fetus and the other in a livebirth, have been reported[49] in which extensive placental involvement and hepatosplenomegaly mimicked erythroblastosis. Necropsy confirmed the diagnosis of metastasis to the placenta. These appear to be the first reported instances of placental metastasis of fetal neoplasms. Three years following delivery of the stillborn fetus in one of the cases, the mother gave no evidence of metastatic disease.

WILMS' TUMOR. Wilms' tumor accounts for about 6% of all renal malignant neoplasms. Approximately three-fourths of these tumors occur in children under the age of 4 years.

Infrequently bone marrow metastasis occurs in Wilms' tumor detected by bone marrow aspiration. In a report of a 2½-year-old boy with typical Wilms' tumor, routine bone marrow aspiration from the iliac crest showed tumor cells.[40] These cells resembled those associated with metastatic carcinoma and rhabdomyosarcoma and apparently different from neuroblastoma. Death of children with Wilms' tumor is invariably due to lung metastasis. Characteristically the lungs are the first sites involved and often the only site, although liver, brain, and rarely bony deposits are seen. Treatment comprises surgery, radiotherapy, and dactinomycin. Dactinomycin has a direct tumoricidal effect. A single course of dactinomycin consists of five successive daily doses of 15 $\mu$g per kilogram of body weight given intravenously. It may be given as a single course or as a part of maintenance dactinomycin therapy, given intermittently for 15 months in addition to postoperative radiotherapy.[61] Others claim that vincristine shares equal potency with dactinomycin in the treatment of Wilms' tumor.[50]

Hemihypertrophy[17] and aniridia[18] have been associated with Wilms' tumor.

TECHNIQUE OF BONE MARROW ASPIRATION. The sternal manubrium is rarely the optimal site for bone marrow aspiration in children. Other areas offer the advantages of being less dangerous, less painful, and less emotionally traumatic to the patient. Such sites are the lower thoracic or lumbar vertebral spinous processes, anterior iliac crest, posterior iliac crest, and tibia. In children older than 18 months to 2 years, the spinous processes are most useful. In younger children or infants selection of the iliac crest may expedite the procedure. It is probably wise to reserve use of the tibia for exceptional circumstances since fractures have resulted from such punctures at this site.

For children who are uneasy about bone marrow aspiration, the combination of the following drugs is administered approximately 1 hour before the precedure. Each of the drugs is given intramuscularly and in a separate syringe: demerol (Meperidine), 2 mg./kg.; phenergan (Promethazine) 1 mg./kg.; thorazine (Chlorpromazine) 1 mg./kg.

Skin preparation should include the use of pHisoHex as well as benzalkonium. Anesthesia is obtained by the use of 1% procaine solution. Following the intradermal injection of approximately 0.2 ml. of the procaine solution, a short time interval is necessary to allow adequate anesthetic effect to occur. If this step in observed, it is possible to ensure an almost painless procedure. The subcutaneous tissue is next infiltrated, with proper care being taken to avoid touching the periosteum. Another short interval of time will allow further specific injection of the periosteal layer without discomfort to the patient.

An 18-gauge, ¾- or 1-inch needle is used in the majority of children, although a smaller gauge may be employed for very young infants. Once the tip of the needle has been inserted through the periosteum, the needle is inserted with added pressure until it is firmly fixed within the bone. A sense of "give" is only occasionally felt as the needle enters the marrow cavity. The point of insertion should be in the midpoint of the spinous process or just 1 cm. below the lip of the ileum. The angle of insertion should be perpendicular to the spinous process or to the flat surface of the ileum. At all times the needle should be guarded at the skin's surface by the fingers of the operator's left hand to prevent it from slipping off the bony prominence while pressure is being exerted.

The stilette is then removed, and a 10 ml. syringe is attached to the needle. The actual aspiration of marrow contents is usually painful. It may be wise at this point to warn the patient that if pain occurs it will probably signify the end of the procedure. To minimize admixture with blood, only 0.1 to 0.2 ml. of marrow is withdrawn into the syringe. *Release the suction in the syringe.* This maneuver is necessary to avoid spreading the aspirate along the walls of the syringe when the needle is being removed from the bone. Remove the needle, still attached to the syringe, from the puncture site and expel the aspirate onto a glass slide. At this time speed is essential to avoid early coagulation and loss of cells, especially megakaryocytes.

A total nucleated cell count is made by diluting the fluid marrow in 3% acetic acid as for a peripheral white cell count. Cell types which may be particularly notable in the counting chamber include megakaryocytes and the large cells of Gaucher's and Niemann-Pick diseases.

Smears are made on glass slides which have been washed in 85% alcohol. Wright's stain is satisfactory for routine use.

Contraindications to bone marrow aspiration are hemophilia and related coagulation disorders. However, the bone marrow can be safely aspirated in thrombocytopenic purpura. Bone marrow fragments can be isolated from the aspirated sample and can be fixed and sectioned or be examined unstained for their fat content and hemosiderin granules. In patients with iron-deficiency hemosiderin is absent or present in only small amounts. It is thought by many that smears from these spicules offer a more accurate estimate of the cellular content and arrangement of the bone marrow than smears from the total aspirate. The differentiation between hyperplasia and hypoplasia of the bone marrow can be estimated by the total number of nucleated cells in the counting chamber or by inspection of the smear.

The posterior iliac crest as a preferential site for bone marrow biopsy has added another dimension to diagnostic morphology.[5] The aspiration smear does not invariably give a correct idea of the relative distribution of the cell types present. Architectural derangements of the marrow and especially significance of the "dry tap" are interpreted more accurately by biopsy taken from the posterior iliac crest. A generous plug of bone marrow can be obtained consistently and easily without recourse to a surgical procedure. The technique has been modified so that both aspiration and biopsy can be obtained during the same procedure. For biopsy use a Vim-Silverman needle, which consists of three parts: an outer needle 3 5/16 inches in length, an obturator, and cutting blades. With the cutting blades in position the overall length is 4½ inches. The biopsy needle is placed into the marrow cavity and the obturator is removed and replaced by the cutting blades. The marrow cavity is reached through the most medial and inferior part of the crest. Biopsy slides are the reliable indicator of marrow activity. Metastatic cells are most easily detected with a lower power objective. In general, metastatic cells are larger than normal hematopoietic elements. They tend to appear in groups or clusters and are usually found on the edges or ends of the smears.

Osteoblasts and osteoclasts may be confused with normal constituents of the bone marrow (Fig. 16). Osteoblasts superficially resemble plasma cells since both have a basophilic cytoplasm and an eccentric nucleus. The cells are oval, 25 to 50 $\mu$ in diameter, and each cell contains one to three nucleoli. Osteoclasts are giant cells about the size of a megakaryocyte, with which they may be confused. The diameter often exceeds 100 $\mu$. The cells contain several nucleoli scattered loosely over the whole cell. The nuclear chromatin is dense. Osteoblasts and osteoclasts are seen most frequently in fetal marrow.

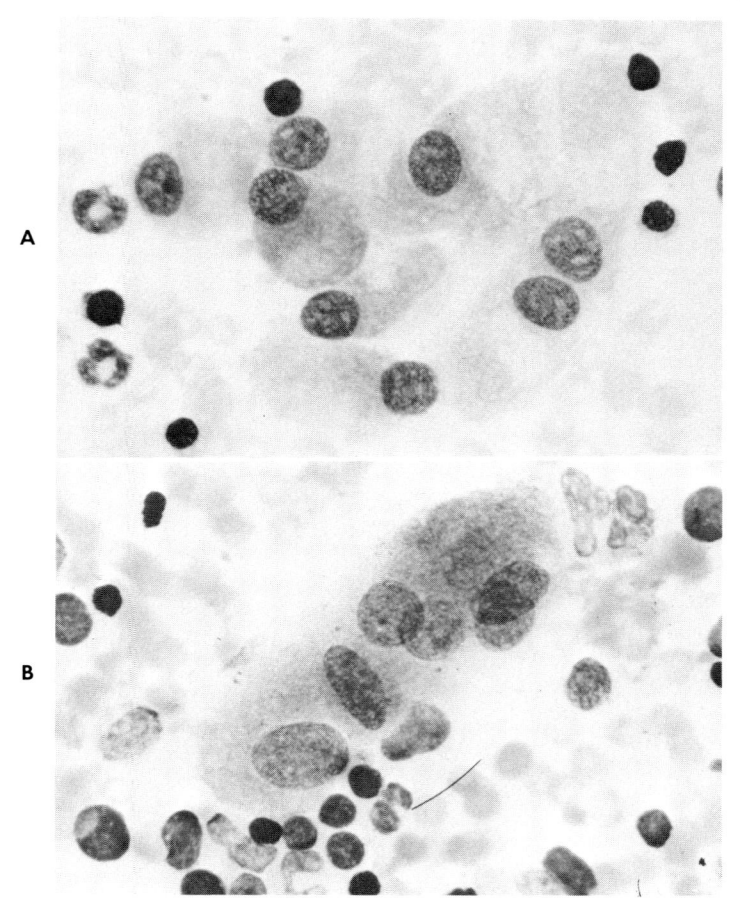

Fig. 16. **A,** Bone marrow aspirate with osteoblasts with eccentric, partially extruded nucleus. **B,** Bone marrow aspirate with multinuclear osteoclasts. (Courtesy Dr. Julius Rutsky, Royal Oak, Mich.)

*Myeloid:erythroid ratio.* The myeloid:erythroid ratio provides an index of depression or hyperactivity of the granulocytic elements as compared with nucleated red cells. In the newborn infant the M:E ratio rises from 2:1 on the first day of life to about 10:1 or 12:1 in the second week, indicative of granulocytic hyperplasia and a decline of erythrocyte production. Beyond infancy the M:E ratio is 2.5:1 to 3.5:1.[62]

*Roentgenographic examination.* The greater value of the roentgenogram in the diagnosis of blood dyscrasias in earlier life than in later childhood and adult life can be related to the developmental features of the bone marrow. The fact that all the bones are filled with red marrow is advantageous to the infant and young child in whom the demand for erythropoiesis is so active. Fat appears in substantial amounts in the long bones at about 7 years of age. Only with the appearance of nonfunctioning yellow marrow in the older child and its extension in the young adult is a potential reservoir available for the emergency formation of blood. In the absence of yellow marrow, the infant or young child faced with the need for excessive blood formation reactivates extramedullary fetal sites. In addition, the marrow hypertrophies and expands by absorption and atrophy of the bony trabeculae and the cortex. These changes are observed in the roentgenograms and are of value in diagnosis. More detailed discussions of the changes observed by roentgenography are described in connection with the specific blood disorders in this book and in the book by Caffey.[6]

Following is a list of the bone and joint manifestations of the blood disorders of infancy and childhood.

*Disorders affecting blood cells and bone marrow*
1. Red cells
   a. Aplastic anemia (Fanconi syndrome)
   b. Hereditary hemolytic anemias
      (1) Cooley's (thalassemia) anemia
      (2) Hereditary spherocytosis
      (3) Sickle cell anemia
2. White cells
   a. Leukemia
3. Bone marrow
   a. Marble-bone disease
   b. Myelofibrosis

*Coagulation disorders*
1. Classic hemophilia (antihemophilic globulin deficiency)
2. Christmas disease (plasma thromboplastin component deficiency)

*Hereditary hemolytic anemias (severe Cooley's anemia, sickle cell anemia, hereditary spherocytosis)*
   Common features:
1. Blood: increased hemolysis and blood production
2. Bone changes due to compensatory marrow hypertrophy
3. X-ray changes in skeleton, including skull and vertebrae
4. Bone changes most marked in severe Cooley's anemia and least in hereditary spherocytosis

*Cooley's anemia*
1. Skeletal changes confined to severe cases (rarely in thalassemia minor)
   a. Dilatation of marrow cavities
   b. Pressure atrophy of spongiosa and corticalis
      (1) Concave surfaces of metacarpals and long bones change to rectangular shape
      (2) Osteoporosis changing to sclerosis with age
      (3) Maturation and growth retarded
      (4) Pathologic fractures
2. Skull changes
   a. Widening of diploic space, "hair-on-end" appearance (also reported in patients with chronic iron-deficiency anemia)
   b. Swelling of zygomas
3. Vertebral changes; reticulated, occasionally compressed
4. In thalassemia intermedia, costal masses giving appearance of large bony masses in the thorax

*Sickle cell anemia*
1. Marrow hyperplasia less marked than in Cooley's anemia
2. Skull changes as in Cooley's anemia
3. Long bones in children, slight to no changes; in adults, fibrosis and thickening of cortex
4. Aseptic necrosis usually in femoral head, less common in humeral head
   a. Destructive and productive changes due to capillary thromboses and infarction
   b. Occurs in sickle cell anemia, sickle-heglobin C disease, and sickle cell-thalassemia disease
5. Tendency toward osteomyelitis in salmonella infection
6. Vertebrae—compression deformity

*Hereditary spherocytosis*
1. Skeletal and cranial change as in Cooley's anemia but infrequent and less marked; cranial changes more prominent than skeletal

*Fanconi syndrome*
1. Aplastic anemia in combination with congenital defects
   a. Affecting heart, skin, mentality, and genital development
   b. Skeletal—variable absence of thumb, calcaneal bones, radius; syndactylism

*Osteopetrosis (marble-bone disease, Albers-Schönberg disease)*
1. Cause—failure to resorb calcified cartilaginous matrix
2. Increased thickness and density of the cortical and spongy portions of the entire osseous system; bones brittle
3. X-ray—individual bones and skull opaque, heavy, and lacking in finer structure
4. Tendency toward fractures, slipping of epiphyses

*Leukemia*
1. Skeletal changes from encroachment upon functioning marrow by leukoblastic cells observed in metarcarpals, long bones, and pelvis
2. Destruction of spongiosa, erosion of cortex, lifting of periosteum
3. Osteoporosis, cystic rarefaction, moth-eaten appearance of long bones
4. Transverse zones of diminished density in metaphyses of long bones

*Hemophilia*
1. Skeletal lesions due to
   a. Bleeding directly into the bones

(1) Shafts and epiphyses
    (a) Rounded defects in spongiosa
    (b) Cystic areas of rarefaction
(2) Subchondral
    (a) Marginal bony defects at juxta-articular borders—flattening deformity of proximal epiphyses of femur (like coxa plana)
(3) Subperiosteal hematomas
    (a) Atrophy of underlying cortex
  b. Bleeding into joint spaces
    (1) Retained blood and clots
        (a) Inflammation, deformities and ankyloses, destruction of articular cartilage, thickened synovial membrane, connective tissue invasion into joints
        (b) Generalized rarefaction of epiphyses and shafts
    (2) Regional hyperemia and recurrent hemarthroses result in hypertrophy of adjacent epiphyses
  c. Hemarthroses—marked in both classic hemophilia (antihemophilic globulin deficiency) and in Christmas disease (plasma thromboplastin component deficiency)

*Hereditary factors as an aid in diagnosis.* The genetic aspects of disease are manifested in a variety of hematologic disorders, notably erythroblastosis fetalis, the hereditary hemoglobinopathies, the group of primaquine-sensitive hemolytic anemias, hereditary spherocytosis and elliptocytosis, and the coagulation defects. Specific genetic implications are discussed in connection with each entity elsewhere in the book. The discovery of hereditary factors depends upon the application of selected laboratory tests made not only on the affected patient, but also on his asymptomatic relatives for the signs of the trait. Tests in common use include examination of the blood smear for morphologic abnormalities, fragility tests, serologic techniques, starch and paper electrophoresis, exposure of red cells to specific chemical agents to determine their tendency toward hemolysis, coagulation studies, and a comprehensive investigation of the family for incidence of the disease. An analysis of the data provides insight into the genetic control of these disorders extending to their qualitative representation.

Thalassemia, sickle cell anemia, and hereditary spherocytosis may be cited as examples of familial diseases in which the hereditary trait may be recognized by suitable blood studies. Their hereditary nature is reflected in the relatively high incidence in members of the same family. The diagnosis of these diseases in a child with an obscure anemia of moderate severity often can be made earlier in its course and useless therapy avoided by detection of the trait in the parents and siblings. In the patient with thalassemia, for instance, the most important element in the diagnosis of the milder form with the simple means immediately available to the practitioner is the discovery of qualitatively similar alterations in the blood of other members of the same family. These persons are asymptomatic and have either mild anemia or no anemia. Regardless of the hemoglobin level, their blood shows hypochromic macrocytes, stippled erythrocytes, polycythemia, increased resistance of the red cells to hemolysis in hypotonic solutions of sodium chloride, and, less frequently, target or oval cells. The evidence is conclusive that in every family with a child having thalassemia major, requiring periodic transfusions, both parents reveal evidence of the disease. When this bilateral inheritance of the gene for thalassemia is nonexistent, a search is made by electrophoresis and sickle cell preparations for the presence of another abnormal hemoglobin in the seemingly unaffected parent.

*Diagnostic features of the blood smear.* Of all laboratory procedures, the most important for its diagnostic value, yet the simplest, is the examination of the blood smear. Although corroborative evidence from auxiliary sources may be required to establish a final diagnosis, the stained blood film constitutes a visual representation of the effect on morphology of the factors involved in the pathogenesis of a specific anemia. In describing the changes in the red blood cells, it should be pointed out that except for sickle cells, spherocytes, and leptocytes (the large pale, extremely thin, ridged erythrocytes with irregularly distributed hemoglobin observed in the blood of patients with thalassemia major), there are no specific red cells that are indicative of a particular disorder. Even the small, deeply stained spherocytes that characterize hereditary spherocytosis may also be observed in greater or lesser degree in patients with other conditions associated with hemolysis such as acquired hemolytic anemia, erythroblastosis due to sensitization by the A-B agglutinogens, and leukemia. Target cells, oval cells, hypochromic macrocytes and basophilic stippling, and hypochromic microcytes appear in varying percentage in certain stages of many anemias and therefore cannot be regarded as distinguishing features of a single disease. They are of

**Table 12.** Diagnostic features of the blood smear in the anemias of early infancy*

| Type of anemia | Diagnostic features |
| --- | --- |
| Erythroblastosis fetalis | Hyperchromic macrocytes; nucleated red blood cells |
| Hemorrhagic anemia | Acute blood loss: normochromic and normocytic red blood cells<br>Chronic blood loss: hypochromic microcytes |
| Iron-deficiency anemia | Hypochromic microcytes; marked central pallor of red blood cells; poikilocytes |
| Anemia of prematurity | Early—normocytic and normochromic red blood cells; later—hypochromic microcytes |
| Megaloblastic anemia of infancy | Unusually large macrocytes; microcytes; occasional nucleated red blood cells; abnormal neutrophils |

*From Smith, C. H.: Anemias in infancy and childhood; diagnostic and therapeutic considerations, Bull. N. Y. Acad. Med. **30**:155, 1954.

**Table 13.** Diagnostic features of the blood smear in the anemias of later infancy and childhood*

| Type of anemia | Diagnostic features |
| --- | --- |
| Anemia of infection | Normocytic and normochromic, occasionally microcytic and hypochromic red blood cells; with iron deficiency, hypochromic microcytes predominate |
| Aplastic, hypoplastic, and aregenerative (pure red cell) anemia | Normochromic and normocytic red blood cells |
| Acquired hemolytic anemia | Moderate spherocytosis; marked polychromasia; reticulocytosis |
| Congenital nonspherocytic hemolytic anemia (may appear at birth) | Normochromic and normocytic; reticulocytosis; occasionally macrocytosis, anisocytosis, and poikilocytosis |
| Hereditary spherocytosis (may appear at birth) | Spherocytes; polychromasia; reticulocytosis |
| Sickle cell anemia | Sickle cells; target cells; microcytes; occasional nucleated red cells; reticulocytosis |
| Thalassemia major (Cooley's anemia) | Very large thin hypochromic macrocytes; microcytes; nucleated red blood cells; marked poikilocytosis; anisocytosis; reticulocytosis |
| Thalassemia minor | Hypochromic macrocytes; microcytes; basophilic stippling; target and oval cells |

*From Smith, C. H.: Anemias in infancy and childhood; diagnostic and therapeutic considerations, Bull. N. Y. Acad. Med. **30**:155, 1954.

**Table 14.** Therapy of the common anemias of infancy and childhood

| Agent | Type of anemia |
| --- | --- |
| Iron | Iron-deficiency anemia, anemia of prematurity, chronic blood loss |
| Folic acid, vitamin $B_{12}$ (?) | Megaloblastic anemia of infancy |
| Transfusion | Exchange transfusions in erythroblastosis fetalis, blood loss—acute and chronic, chronic anemias, aplastic and hemolytic anemias, leukemia, hemorrhagic disease, coagulation defect, thrombocytopenia |
| Splenectomy | Hereditary spherocytosis, in selected cases of autoimmune hemolytic anemia, thalassemia major, sickle cell anemia, hypersplenism |
| Corticosteroids (including testosterone) | Autoimmune hemolytic anemia, aplastic anemia, pure red cell anemia |

diagnostic value only when they are considered in conjunction with pertinent information from other sources. The morphologic changes of the red cells in the most common anemias of infancy and childhood are summarized in Tables 12 and 13. Each of these disorders is described in greater detail elsewhere in the book.

*Principles of treatment.* The information gathered thus far has provided a sufficiently firm foundation with respect to pathogenesis to warrant a consideration of therapy. In Table 14 are listed the available agents in current use designed to correct an underlying deficiency or to ameliorate the disorder by accessory means when direct remedies are not available. The constant emphasis on the use of specific rather than indiscriminate mixtures of antianemia substances[58] applies with especial force to the pediatric age group. Iron salts given orally, preferably in the ferrous forms without the aid of supplementary minerals or vitamins, still constitute the most effective treatment of iron-deficiency anemia. Treatment with iron salts in patients with other conditions may not only be futile, but also potentially harmful. The anemias for which transfusions are indicated consist of two groups: those in which this measure constitutes a temporary expedient until spontaneous recovery sets in and those in which, in the absence of specific therapy, the need for restoration of optimum blood levels is continuous or urgent. The indications for splenectomy will be discussed in Chapter 25.

*Immunoallergic implications of blood disorders.* The clinical manifestations of many of the blood disorders are wholly or partially dependent upon immunoallergic reactions. The type of response resulting from the combination of an antigen with an antibody has its counterpart in the immunoallergic mechanisms underlying many of the blood disorders. Many of these are now classified under the heading of immunohematology and include the hemolytic anemias, granulocytopenia, and thrombocytopenia. The pathogenesis is based, to some extent, on antibodies to the respective formed blood elements, blood vessel hypersensitivity, incompatibility between blood elements of fetus and mother, transfusion reactions, and sensitivity induced by bacterial, chemical, and physical agents.[48] Hypersensitivity to drugs may result in hypoplastic or aplastic anemia in contrast to primaquine-sensitive hemolytic anemias, which are based on an inherited intrinsic defect of the red cells.

It is of interest to consider the extraordinary phenomenon by which antibodies that are capable of reacting with the patient's own red cells are elaborated. A similar situation occurs in those patients with thrombocytopenic purpura and agranulocytosis in whom antibodies are directed against the patient's platelets and polymorphonuclear cells. These disorders call attention to the remarkable tolerance developed from early fetal life by which the body in health avoids forming antibodies against its own tissues.[10] Such dire circumstances in which a living organism becomes capable of producing antibodies against its own body constituents was termed "horror autotoxicus" by Ehrlich.[60] The fundamental feature of autoimmune acquired hemolytic anemia and other disorders characterized by autoimmune antibodies to blood cell elements is the loss of this normally acquired tolerance with the development of antibodies to one's own cellular antigens.

Autoimmunization has, in recent years, embraced more than disorders of the red cells, platelets, and white cells. The theory of autoimmunity has also been extended to a number of pathologic states such as polyarteritis nodosa, systemic lupus erythematosus, Henoch-Schönlein syndrome, rheumatoid arthritis, myasthenia gravis, kidney and thyroid disease, multiple sclerosis, ulcerative colitis, and pernicious anemia.[12,38]

The concept of immunologic tolerance postulates that an antigen reaching the cells of the reticuloendothelial system during a critical period of fetal life may be accepted as "self" and, when subsequently reintroduced, may be tolerated without leading to the production of antibodies.[4] In autoimmune disease the normal safeguards by which the antibody-forming cells can distinguish between "self" and "not self" breaks down. Autoimmunity may be defined, therefore, as the development of abnormal immune antibodies (gamma globulins) within the patient's own body, with these antibodies having the capability of reacting against constituents of the patient's own cells or tissues. According to Dameshek,[11,12] the self-recognition mechanisms are at fault and this is due to the presence of groups or clones of abnormal immunocompetent cells that fail to recognize normal cell antigens and thus produce antibodies or autoantibodies against them.

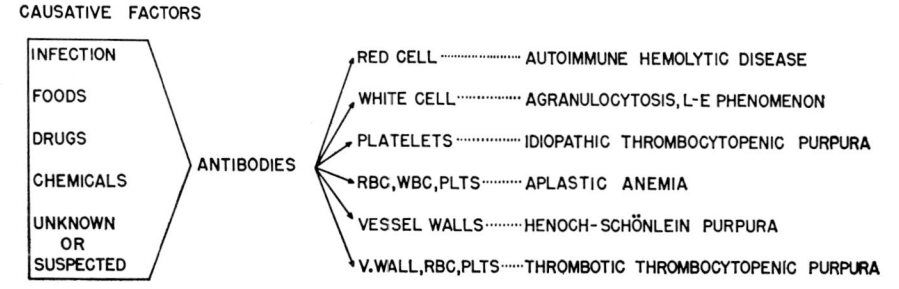

```
CAUSATIVE FACTORS
┌─────────────┐
│ INFECTION   │╲                    ╱ RED CELL ········· AUTOIMMUNE HEMOLYTIC DISEASE
│ FOODS       │ ╲                  ╱  WHITE CELL ······· AGRANULOCYTOSIS, L-E PHENOMENON
│ DRUGS       │  ANTIBODIES         ╱ PLATELETS ········ IDIOPATHIC THROMBOCYTOPENIC PURPURA
│ CHEMICALS   │  ╱                 ╲  RBC,WBC,PLTS······ APLASTIC ANEMIA
│ UNKNOWN     │ ╱                   ╲ VESSEL WALLS······ HENOCH-SCHÖNLEIN PURPURA
│ OR          │╱                     ╲V.WALL,RBC,PLTS··· THROMBOTIC THROMBOCYTOPENIC PURPURA
│ SUSPECTED   │
└─────────────┘
```

Fig. 17. Immunoallergic concept of blood disorders. (From Smith, C. H.: Allergic implications of blood disorders in infancy and childhood, Calif. Med. 86:366, 1957.)

The extent to which antitissue antibodies are produced and their significance in the pathogenesis of disease has been the subject of controversy. There remains very little doubt that allergic encephalomyelitis, experimental aspermatogenesis, and experimental thyroiditis result from autosensitization to the respective antigens. On the other hand, autoantibody formation cannot be considered as synonymous with autoimmune disease, intriguing as this hypothesis may be. Autoantibodies may be the result or by-product of tissue damage rather than the cause of the morbid process. In other words, the existence in the blood of one or more organ-specific antibodies is not necessarily evidence that it is a primary cause of disease in the organ against which it is immunologically directed. Indeed, circulating antiorgan antibodies may serve a protective role against extension of damage to the involved organ.[52] The problem has been, therefore, to distinguish between disease-producing and harmless antibodies. The truth probably lies between these extremes.[38]

Once the effects of the hypersensitive state are set in motion during the course of a blood disorder, therapeutic measures to slow their progress are often futile. Because it is not always possible to identify the potentially allergic child in whom these circumstances will occur, it is extremely important to weigh the advantages of the use of a drug before it is administered, especially when its side effects have not yet been thoroughly investigated.

Following is a list of blood disorders in infancy and childhood, in many of which the clinical and laboratory features lend themselves to an interpretation on an immunoallergic basis (also see Fig. 17).

*Disorders affecting blood cell and vascular elements*[*]

1. Red cells
    a. Acquired hemolytic anemia
        (1) Toxic products, drugs, favism
        (2) Antibodies against red cells
            (a) Erythroblastosis fetalis
            (b) Blood transfusion reactions
            (c) Associated with autoantibodies, primary autoimmune hemolytic anemia, secondary leukemia, Gaucher's disease
            (d) Pure red cell (chronic congenital aregenerative) anemia
2. White blood cells
    a. Agranulocytosis
        (1) Anticonvulsants
        (2) Antimicrobial agents
        (3) Antithyroid drugs
        (4) Sulfonamides
    b. Neonatal agranulocytosis
3. Platelets
    a. Thrombocytopenic purpura
        (1) Idiopathic
        (2) Congenital
        (3) Drug-induced: quinine, quinidine, sulfonamides, arsenicals
        (4) Eczema with purpura and otitis media
4. Red cells, white cells, and platelets
    a. Hypoplastic and aplastic anemia
        (1) Idiopathic
        (2) Drugs, chemicals, infection
5. Blood vessels
    a. Allergic purpura (Henoch-Schönlein syndrome)
    b. Idiopathic pulmonary hemosiderosis
    c. Polyarteritis nodosa and other collagen diseases

―――――――――
[*]From Smith, C. H.: Allergic implications of blood disorders in infancy and childhood, Calif. Med. 86:366, 1957.

d. Thrombotic thrombocytopenic purpura (vascular vessel wall in combination with platelets and red cells)

*Infections*
1. Infectious mononucleosis
2. Susceptibility following splenectomy

*Autoerythrocytic sensitization.* The symptoms in this condition are easy bruising with swelling, edema, and painful ecchymoses due to autosensitivity of patients to their own blood. Severe trauma with bruising characterizes the history. A stromal factor of red cells may be the responsible agent for the clinical manifestations and for the positive skin tests. Extremely painful reactions follow intradermal testing with red cells. This syndrome corresponds to the type of autosensitization noted in patients with lupus erythematosus, some forms of acquired hemolytic anemia, and thrombocytopenic purpura.[20] Suggestive evidence has been obtained that erythrocyte phosphatidyl serine may play a role in the initiation of the purpuric response in certain patients with autoerythrocyte purpuric disease.[24] In addition to sensitivity to phosphatidyl serine of the erythrocyte membrane, complex emotional problems may play a role in the pathogenesis of the purpuric lesions of this disease.[23]

Therapy for this disorder up to the present time has been unsatisfactory. Administration of corticosteroids, antihistamines, and antimalarials, and attempts at erythrocyte desensitization have been quite unsuccessful. In one group autoerythrocyte sensitization began after physical injury or surgery and in this group also the clinical features suggested a relationship between the patient's emotional problems and development of lesions.[44]

*DNA autosensitivity.* Autoerythrocytic hypersensitivity should be differentiated from DNA hypersensitivity. In the latter, the acute and painful ecchymoses are usually confined to the extremities. Several cases have been reported in adults,[8,33,45] and in one of these[8] the multiple painful bruises were scattered over the exposed areas of the body. Subsequently these hot, raised, reddened areas become ecchymotic and extremely painful and involved the extremities, trunk, and face. In the following typical case of a 14-year-old junior high school student,[36] the clinical picture was characterized as in other cases by painful, tender, ecchymoses of the extremities unrelated to trauma. Lesions identical both clinically and histologically with the spontaneous lesions were produced by the intradermal injection of calf thymus DNA and autologous lysed leukocytes. Treatment with chloroquine, primaquine, and hydroxychloroquine caused a dramatic clinical response, with rapid relief of pain and tenderness and with no further progression of the hemorrhages. Cessation of the drug allowed a return of symptoms and signs. It has been suggested[8] from clinical and theoretical considerations that DNA autosensitivity may be closely related to, or constitute a variant of, systemic lupus erythematosus.

*Graft-versus-host reaction (runt disease).* The graft-versus-host (GVH) reaction is not only of interest in transplantation immunology but is employed to explain the mechanism of various clinical syndromes. Runt disease is a peculiar wasting disease or syndrome resulting from an immunological disorder characterized by the formation of antibodies by the graft against the host. In this case antibody production is being stimulated by the antigens present in the host and not present in the graft. If a graft containing immunologically active cells is implanted into a host incapable of rejecting it either because of genetic constitution or because of other factors, disease results.

The term *immunocompetent cell* is commonly used to describe those cells which respond to antigen by producing antibody or by giving rise to cells which produce antibody.[13] The cell denotes its present status which, although not actually engaged in an immune response, is nevertheless fully qualified to initiate such a response when appropriately stimulated by antigen. In laboratory animals a graft becomes established, the host tissues become antigenic, and antibodies are produced by the graft which destroys the tissues of the host. Runt disease may be said to develop under the following circumstances: acceptance of the grafted tissues by the host animal, the presence of immunologically competent cells in the transplanted tissue, and an antigenic difference between the host and the graft.[13,55] Among the frequently observed features especially in neonatal runt disease are lymphadenopathy, splenomegaly, leukocytosis, skin lesions, diarrhea, wasting, and death. A hemolytic anemia and thrombocytopenia have been observed. Some of the small lymphocytes which lodge in the host's lymphoid tissue are responsible for initiating the disease. The host lymphohematopoietic tissues appear to bear the brunt of the graft-versus-host attack. Human counterparts of this syndrome have been described in infants with thymic alymphoplasia following transfusions with fresh whole blood and in adults with leukemia, Hodgkin's disease, and radiation sickness. In the animal it is characterized by retardation of growth, emaciation, dermatitis, alopecia, hepatosplenomegaly, lymphoid atrophy, diarrhea, and anemia.

Hathaway and colleagues[28] reported two cases of children with progressive vaccinia necrosum who had been given multiple transfusions and in whom erythrodermia, hepatomegaly, and a fatal aplastic anemia subsequently developed. One of the patients showed the features thymic alymphoplasia (Swiss-type agammaglobulinemia) and both had rudimentary thymuses. The clinical and pathological features were interpreted as manifestations of a graft-versus-host reaction and suggested the possibility that human runt disease had been produced by the transfusion of large numbers of viable leukocytes into patients who potentially were immunologically deficient. These workers also emphasized that the possibility of producing human runt disease might be much greater in infants receiving intrauterine transfusions of fresh blood containing leukocytes since some of the fetuses might be sufficiently immature to be tolerant to a hematopoietic graft. This caution was further defined by Naiman and co-workers,[39] who described the case of an 8-week-old infant who had received three intrauterine transfusions for Rh hemolytic disease. Two populations of lymphocytes were later found in the peripheral blood, one probably acquired from a donor. Multiple infections and progressive weight loss ensued, with death occurring at 13 months. Although lymphoid and thymic atrophy were evident at autopsy, these changes were considered to reflect atrophy (secondary to a graft-versus-host reaction) rather than primary immunologic disease. The authors state that this observation supported the recommendation of others that blood intended for transfusion in the fetus be first rendered free of viable lymphocytes.

The clinical and pathological findings in a 3½-month-old infant with hypogammaglobulinemia, lymphopenia, aplastic anemia, depletion of lymphoid tissue, and histiocytosis of spleen, lymph nodes, and bowel resembled most closely the findings of the graft-versus-host reaction or runt disease. The patient was treated with a bone marrow transplant without apparent benefit.[27]

# REFERENCES

1. Anderson, O. W.: Neuroblastoma with skeltal metastases and apparent recovery, Amer. J. Dis. Child. **83**:782, 1952.
2. Bettex, M., and Käser, H.: Diagnostic and prognostic value of the determination of urinary output of vanillyl-mandelic acid in tumours of sympathetic nervous system, Arch. Dis. Child. **37**:138, 1962.
3. Bothwell, T. H., and Finch, C. A.: Iron metabolism, Boston, 1962, Little, Brown & Co.
4. Burnet, E. M.: Enzyme, antigen and virus, London, 1956, Cambridge University Press.
5. Burney, S. W.: Bone marrow examination; technique and diagnostic value of a bone-marrow biopsy using a Silverman needle, J.A.M.A. **195**:171, 1966.
6. Caffey, J.: Pediatric x-ray diagnosis, Chicago, 1956, Year Book Medical Publishers, Inc.
7. Cartwright, G. E.: Diagnostic laboratory hematology, ed. 4, New York, 1968, Grune & Stratton, Inc., pp. 155-156.
8. Chandler, D., and Nalbandian, R. M.: DNA antisensitivity, Amer. J. Med. Sci. **251**:145, 1966.
9. Chatten. J., and Voorhess, M. L.: Familial neuroblastoma; report of a kindred with multiple disorders, including neuroblastoma in four siblings, New Eng. J. Med. **277**:1230, 1967.
10. Dacie, J. V.: Autoimmunization in respect of red cells, program of Sixth International Congress, International Society of Hematology, Boston, 1956, p. 488.
11. Dameshek, W.: Recent studies in autoimmunity, Acta haemat. **31**:187, 1964.
12. Dameshek, W.: Theories of autoimmunity. In Conceptual advances in immunology and oncology, New York, 1963, Harper & Row, Publishers.
13. Dameshek, W., Schwartz, R., and Oliner, H.: Current concepts of autoimmunization; an interpretive review, Blood **17**:775, 1961.
14. deLorimier, A. A., Bragg, K. V., and Linden, G.: Neuroblastoma in childhood, Amer. J. Dis. Child. **118**:441, 1969.
15. Delta, B. G., and Pinkel, D.: Bone marrow aspiration in children with malignant tumors, J. Pediat. **64**:542, 1964.
16 Finch, C. A., and Noyes, W. D.: Erythrokinetics in diagnosis of anemia, J.A.M.A. **175**:1163, 1961.

17. Fraumeni, J. F., Jr., Geiser, C. F., and Manning, M. D.: Wilms' tumor and congenital hemihypertrophy; report of five new cases and review of the literature, Pediatrics 40:886, 1967.
18. Fraumeni, J. F., Jr., and Glass, A. G.: Wilms' tumor and congenital aniridia, J.A.M.A. 206:825, 1968.
19. Gaffney, P. C., Hausman, C. F., and Fetterman, G. H.: Experience with smears of aspirates from bone marrow in the diagnosis of neuroblastoma, Amer. J. Clin. Path. 31:213, 1959.
20. Gardner, F. H., and Diamond, L. K.: Autoerythrocytic sensitization; a form of purpura producing painful bruising following auto sensitization to red blood cells in certain women, Blood 10:675, 1955.
21. Goldring, D.: Neuroblastoma sympatheticum with metastases; report of a case with apparent recovery, J. Pediat. 38:231, 1951.
22. Greenberg, R. E., and Gardner, L. I.: Catecholamine metabolism in a functional neural tumor, J. Clin. Invest. 39:1729, 1960.
23. Groch, G. S., Finch, S. C., Rogoway, W., and Fischer, D. S.: Studies in the pathogenesis of autoerythrocyte sensitization syndrome, Blood 28:19, 1966.
24. Groch, G. S., Rogoway, W., Fischer, D., and Finch, S. C.: Studies concerning the pathogenesis of autoerythrocyte purpura, Blood 22:814, 1963.
25. Gross, R. E., Farber, S., and Martin, L. W.: Neuroblastoma sympatheticum: a study and report of 217 cases, Pediatrics 23:1179, 1959.
26. Guest, G. M., and Brown, E. W.: Erythrocytes and hemoglobin of the blood in infancy and childhood. III. Factors in variability; statistical studies, Amer. J. Dis. Child. 93:486, 1957.
27. Hathaway, W. E., Brangle, R. W., Nelson, T. L., and Roeckel, I. E.: Aplastic anemia and alymphocytosis in an infant with hypogammaglobulinemia, J. Pediat. 68:713, 1966.
28. Hathaway, W. E., Githens, J. K., Blackburn, W. R., Fulginiti, V., and Kempe, C. H.: Aplastic anemia, histiocytosis and erythrodermia in immunologically deficient children; probable human runt disease, New Eng. J. Med. 273:953, 1965.
29. Haurani, F. I., and Tocantins, L. M.: Ineffective erythropoiesis, Amer. J. Med. 31:519, 1961.
30. Kato, K., and Wachter, H. E.: Adrenal sympathicoblastoma in children; with special reference to the biopsy of sternal marrow and of metastatic nodule in the skull, J. Pediat. 12:449, 1938.
31. Kirkman, H. N., and Riley, H. D.: Posthemorrhagic anemia and shock in the newborn; a review, Pediatrics 24:97, 1959.
32. Koop, C. E., and Hernandez, J. R.: Neuroblastoma; experience with 100 cases in children, Surgery 56:726, 1964.
33. Levin, M. B., and Pinkus, H.: Autosensitivity to desoxyribonucleic acid (DNA), New Eng. J. Med. 264:533, 1961.
34. Lingley, J. F., Sagerman, R. H., Santulli, T. V., and Wolff, J. A.: Neuroblastoma, management and survival, New Eng. J. Med. 277:1227, 1967.
35. Linman, J. W.: Physiologic and pathophysiologic effects of anemia, New Eng. J. Med. 279:812, 1968.
36. Little, A. S., and Bell, H. E.: Painful subcutaneous hemorrhages of the extremities with unusual reaction to injected deoxyribonucleic acid, Ann. Intern. Med. 60:886, 1964.
37. McGoldrick, K. E., and Lanzkowsky, P.: Prolonged survival in neuroblastoma with multiple skeletal metastases and bone marrow infiltration, Acta Paediat. Scand. 59:1, 1970.
38. Milgrom, F., and Witebsky, E.: Autoantibodies and autoimmune diseases, J.A.M.A. 181:707, 1962.
39. Naiman, J. L., Punnett, H. H., Lischner, H. W., Destine, M. L., and Arey, J. B.: Possible graft-versus-host reaction after intrauterine transfusion for Rh erythroblastosis fetalis, New Eng. J. Med. 281:697, 1969.
40. O'Neill, P., and Pinkel, D.: Wilms' tumor in bone marrow aspirate, J. Pediat. 72:396, 1968.
41. Oski, F. A., and Naiman, J. L.: Hematologic problems in the newborn, Philadelphia, 1966, W. B. Saunders Co., p. 59.
42. Price-Jones, C.: Red blood cell diameters, London, 1933, Oxford Medical Publications.
43. Rosenstein, B. J., and Engleman, K.: Diarrhea in a child with a catecholamine-secreting ganglioneuroma, J. Pediat. 63:23, 1963.
44. Ratnoff, O. D., and Agle, D. P.: Psychogenic purpura; a re-evaluation of the syndrome of autoerythrocytic sensitization, Medicine 47:475, 1968.
45. Schwartz, R. S., Lewis, F. B., and Dameshek, W.: Hemorrhagic cutaneous anaphylaxis due to autosensitization to deoxyribonucleic acid, New Eng. J. Med. 267:1105, 1962.
46. Seip, M.: The reticulocyte level and the erythrocyte production judged from reticulocyte studies, in newborn infants during the first week of life, Acta Paediat. 44:355, 1955.
47. Smith, C. H.: Bone marrow examination in blood disorders of infants and children, Med. Clin. N. Amer. 31:527, 1947.
48. Smith, C. H.: Allergic implications of blood disorders in infancy and childhood, Calif. Med. 86:366, 1957.
49. Strauss, L., and Driscoll, S. G.: Congenital

neuroblastoma involving the placenta; report of two cases, Pediatrics 34:23, 1964.
50. Sutow, W. W., and Sullivan, M. P.: Vincristine in primary treatment of Wilms' tumor, Texas Med. 61:794, 1965.
51. Szur, L., and Smith, M. D.: Red-cell production and destruction in myelosclerosis, Brit. J. Haemat. 7:147, 1961.
52. Thomas, L.: Circulating autoantibodies and human disease; with a note on primary atypical pneumonia, New Eng. J. Med. 270:1157, 1964.
53. Thurman, W. G., Fernbach, D. J., Sullivan, M. P., and the Writing Committee of the Pediatric Division of the Southwest Cancer Chemotherapy Study Group: Cyclophosphamide therapy in childhood neuroblastoma, New Eng. J. Med. 270:1336, 1964.
54. Voorhess, M. L., and Gardner, L. I.: The value of serial catecholamine determinations in children with neuroblastoma, Pediatrics 30:241, 1962.
55. Weiser, R. S., Myrvik, Q. N., and Pearsall, N. N.: Fundamentals of immunology, Philadelphia, 1969, Lea and Febiger.
56. Whitby, L. E. H., and Britton, C. J. C.: Disorders of the blood, ed. 8, New York, 1957, Grune & Stratton, Inc.
57. Williams, C. M., and Greer, M.: Homovanillic acid and vanilmandelic acid in diagnosis of neuroblastoma, J.A.M.A. 183:836, 1963.
58. Wintrobe, M. M.: Editorial: Shotgun antianemic therapy, Amer. J. Med. 15:142, 1953.
59. Wintrobe, M. M.: Clinical hematology, ed. 4, Philadelphia, 1956, Lea & Febiger.
60. Witebsky, E.: Ehrlich's side chain theory in the light of present immunology, Ann. N. Y. Acad. Sci. 59:168, 1954.
61. Wolff, J. A., Krivit, W., Newton, W. A., Jr., and D'Angio, G. J.: Single versus multiple dose dactinomycin therapy of Wilms' tumor, New Eng. J. Med. 279:290, 1968.
62. Wolman, I.: Laboratory applications in clinical pediatrics, New York, 1957, McGraw-Hill Book Co.

# 12 IRON-DEFICIENCY ANEMIA

Iron-deficiency anemia represents the most common nutritional deficiency in children and is especially prevalent in infancy. The unusual susceptibility of the infant is due to a variety of interrelated factors, inherent in this age period, which affect iron metabolism.

*Etiology.* Iron-deficiency anemia occurs most commonly between the ages of 6 and 24 months and reflects an inadequate supply or excessive demand for iron, or blood loss. These factors are interdependent and overlap. In the first 6 months the infant is dependent upon iron reserves acquired during fetal life. With the depletion of these stores the infant requires dietary iron to meet the demands of growth. The period before and after 6 months of age cannot be sharply circumscribed because of the individual variability of iron stores and the extent of growth. The major etiologic factors in iron deficiency in infancy and childhood are as follows.

1. Inadequate supply of iron
   a. Inadequate iron stores at birth
      (1) Low birth weight, premature, twin or multiple births
      (2) Severe iron deficiency in the mother
      (3) Fetal blood loss at or before delivery
         (a) Into maternal circulation
         (b) Retroplacental bleeding
   b. Inadequate intake—deficient dietary iron
2. Impaired absorption
   a. Chronic diarrhea
   b. Malabsorption syndrome
   c. Gastrointestinal abnormalities
3. Excessive demands for iron required for growth, especially prematurity and adolescence
4. Blood loss
   a. Acute or chronic hemorrhage—e.g., polypi, Meckel's diverticulum
   b. Parasite infestation—e.g., hookworm

In a series of 272 infants whose blood was found to contain less than 9 gm. of hemoglobin per 100 ml., Woodruff[223] found that the most common cause of hypochromic anemia was prematurity or a birth weight of less than 3 kg. The incidence of severe hypochromic anemia in infants weighing more than 4 kg. was extremely low. A first child was less likely to become anemic than were later siblings, single children were less likely than twins, and girls less likely than boys.[223] Guest and Brown[80] also found a significantly lower incidence of iron-deficiency anemia in firstborn infants than later-born infants.

Prenatal factors play an important role in influencing the iron content of the fetus. These include the length of gestation, uncommonly, maternal hemoglobin concentration, less frequently, occult or frank hemorrhage from the fetal surface of the placenta at or before delivery, and the transplacental passage of fetal blood into the maternal circulation—so-called fetomaternal transfusion.[32] Abnormal placental circulation in multiple births, especially in single-ovum twins, may result in the transfusion of one twin by another.[103] Such transfusions may explain the relatively frequent occurrence of hypochromic anemia in only one twin regardless of similar growth rates and diets.[223]

The only source of iron for the fetus is derived transplacentally from the maternal organism. To provide for increased needs incident to the rapid growth of the fetus in the last trimester of pregnancy, iron absorption in the mother is accelerated.[82,151]

The average adult has about 3 to 5 gm. of iron in his body, of which 2 to 3 gm. are found in the hemoglobin, 1 to 1.5 gm. in the body stores as ferritin and hemosiderin, and the rest in myoglobin, respiratory enzymes, and the plasma. Iron participates as iron-porphyrin complexes in reversible oxygenations as a key part of the respiratory pigments, hemoglobin, and myoglobin, as well as in oxidative enzyme systems such as the cytochromes, peroxidases, and catalases. In contrast, at birth the infant's supply is approximately 300 mg. provided by the mother; after birth, iron for the increasing needs of the growing body is derived from the diet.[27]

Although the iron transfer to the fetus is negligible during the first two trimesters of pregnancy, it rises in the third trimester to 4 mg. daily so that the total amount accumulated by the fetus at term approximates 300 mg.[153] Widdowson and Spray[216] found an average of 273 mg. of iron in six infants weighing more than 3,000 gm. They found that the iron concentration during fetal life was relatively constant, with an average value of 75 mg. per kilogram of body weight. Of this, the liver and spleen contained one-eighth of the total (34 mg.). The bulk of iron available to the infant at birth for eventual hemoglobin formation is that contained in the circulating hemoglobin. Josephs[97] estimated approximately 30 to 35 mg. in the liver. The amount of the nonhemoglobin iron fraction (myohemoglobin, cytochromes, and other respiratory enzymes) at birth has been variously estimated at 4 mg. per kilogram,[191] 6 mg. per kilogram,[185] and 7.5 mg. per kilogram.[97] The total hemoglobin mass may be computed by multiplying the blood volume of 85 ml. per kilogram (variation, 80 to 90 ml. per kilogram) by the hemoglobin concentration per 100 ml. of blood. Since each gram of hemoglobin contains 3.4 mg. of iron, the total hemoglobin value is multiplied by this figure to convert it to total body iron. With these values Sturgeon calculated[191] in a hypothetical infant weighing 4 kg., that 232 mg. of iron is present in circulating hemoglobin, 51 mg. in the liver and spleen, and 16 mg. as myoglobin and other parenchymal iron. In an infant weighing 3 kg. at birth, the figures accordingly would be 106 mg. in circulating hemoglobin, 11 mg. in stores, and 12 mg. in nonhemoglobin iron.

In an investigation[114] of 427 children 3 to 36 months of age attending forty New York City Department of Health Well Baby Clinics, 21.3% of 174 Negro children had hemoglobin levels of 10 gm./100 ml. or less, as compared with 11.4% of 158 Puerto Rican children and 2.4% of 82 Caucasian children.

While iron deficiency appears widespread in this group of young children of low socioeconomic backgrounds, in some of the reports which will be cited the incidence is strikingly lower in the preschool child.

Pearson and colleagues[149] in a survey of nearly 7,000 preschool children (4 to 6 years of age) from low socioeconomic backgrounds in five cities of the United States (New York City not included) found that the mean hematocrit was 36.32% ± 2.8%. Severe anemia was unusual and the incidence of significant anemia (hematocrit, 31%) showed considerable variation from city to city, ranging from 0.6 to 7.7% and was unaffected by iron supplementation. Of relevance was the observation that in Jacksonville, one of the cities investigated, where iron was routinely administered, the distribution of hematocrit was remarkably similar to that found in other cities where this was not done. The authors point out that not all anemic children necessarily suffer from nutritional deficiencies and where the incidence is in the order of only 1 to 2%, other etiologies such as thalassemia trait should be looked for.

In a later study the effects of a 5-week period of dietary and medicinal iron supplementation on hematocrit levels of 532 preschool children 4½ to 6½ years of age from low socioeconomic backgrounds were reported.[23] The initial mean hematocrit level of the entire group was 35.73% ± 2.5%. A hematocrit level less than 31% was found in only 1.5% of the children. Diet alone and diet plus 30 mg. of elemental iron per day were associated with significant increases in the mean hematocrit level. A strikingly greater increase in mean hematocrit was seen in the iron-supplemented group. The authors conclude that an increase in hematocrit or hemoglobin level following therapy may constitute a better indicator of the prevalence of nutritional anemia than a single measurement of such parameters as hemoglobin, hematocrit, or serum iron.

Contrasting findings are those of Owen and co-workers,[146] who studied 725 children 1 to 6 years of age of low economic background from fifteen states.

Premature, twin, and multiple births reduce the quantity of iron in the storage depots. These factors also tend to reduce the total amount of circulating hemoglobin and, therefore, the content of iron required for later hemoglobin synthesis. Less frequently, reduced stores result from hemorrhage due to loss of fetal blood into maternal circulation,[32] from placenta praevia, from abruptio placentae, and from injury to the cord during delivery.[215] Accidental bleeding from the cord following delivery reduces the initial iron stores in relation to the extent of hemorrhage. Early or late clamping of the cord is another important factor contributing to the iron endowment of the infant. Manual stripping of the cord can add as much as 75 ml. of whole blood or 40 mg. of iron to the storage depots.[191] It has been emphasized[211] that the technique of delayed ligation of the cord does not result in a significant increase in red cell volume unless the cord is initially stripped or milked.

Full-term infants born to nonanemic mothers receive sufficient iron during fetal life to meet their needs for at least the first 3 to 4 months of infancy.[222,223] With few exceptions infants born to mothers who have suffered iron depletion during pregnancy show normal hemoglobin concentrations at birth. The influence of an inadequate iron endowment does not become manifest until later in the first year. In markedly anemic mothers administration of iron before delivery of their babies prevents the development of anemia in the newborn infant.[182,188] Unless the anemia in the mother is marked (below 9 gm./100 ml.), iron deficiency usually does not occur in the infant.[225] Despite these facts, maternal iron depletion as indicated by severe anemia is not regarded as a common predisposing factor of iron deficiency in infants in the United States at the present time.[222] Administration of iron supplements to normal mothers overcomes the mild physiologic anemia of pregnancy but exerts little, if any, influence on the offspring's iron endowment at birth or iron nutrition in infancy.[111,192,193]

In another series[48] it was noted that the intramuscular injection of 1,000 mg. of iron-dextran or the daily administration of 78 mg. of elemental ferrous iron for 24 weeks to normal pregnant women resulted in higher hemoglobins and packed red cell volumes as compared with untreated women in the last trimester. Iron supplementation did not, however, affect the serum iron concentration of cord blood nor the hemoglobin levels of babies in the first year.

Iron-deficiency anemia in the full-term infant, which is noted at approximately 6 months of age, cannot be evaluated properly unless important hematologic events in the preceding period are considered. These two periods are not sharply circumscribed, but one merges with the other since both are affected by forces within and without the hematopoietic system. Of basic importance is the fact that the iron depots at birth, possessing variable amounts of this mineral (less in the premature and more in the full-term infant), are substantially increased by progressive accumulation of iron in the first months of life.[109] This major iron supplement is derived from the degradation of circulating hemoglobin mass with which the infant is born. Regardless of the amount, the initial iron tissue stores at birth cannot be underestimated for their value in hemoglobin synthesis.

A decrease in cytochrome C and myoglobin concentrations has been observed in young rats made anemic on a low iron diet.[44] They were most depleted in skeletal muscle which contains the major portion of these proteins. The results are in contrast with earlier observations that these enzymes were not affected by deprivation of iron.

An increased frequency of respiratory infections has been reported in infants with iron deficiency and reduced incidence of such infections in children receiving iron supplements.[6] These observations still await confirmation.

In 1959, Lanzkowsky[110] reported that iron therapy had cured a group of Cape Town children who suffered from pica. He described pica as "a perversion of appetite with persistent and purposeful ingestion of unsuitable substances, seemingly of no nutrient value." While it is true that pica is an important etiologic factor in lead poisoning, many children with pica apparently feel an instinctive need for iron to restore their hemoglobin levels. In this group treatment with iron was invariably followed by the rapid disappearance of pica. Another study[126] corroborating these findings emphasized that a permanent cure depends upon the maintenance of adequate hemoglobin levels.

In one series[11] it was found that the overall prevalence of pica was 22.8% of Negro children as compared with 14.8% of the white groups, with an overall prevalence of 18.5% for the two groups. In another group of children ranging in age from 1 to 6 years, Barltrop[11] found that 32.3% of Negro children had pica compared with 10% of white children. Prevalence of pica decreases with increasing age over this age range. Many of these cases were associated with iron deficiency.

Geophagia, the eating of earth or clay, has been observed frequently in children and adults in the southern and western portions of the United States. Also in New York City a group of non-pregnant patients were found to have iron deficiency and had ingested quantities of laundry starch.[150] Starch and clay ingestion varies from 250 to 1,300 gm./day and average hemoglobin was 6.2 gm./100 ml. Three patients who were followed received iron but despite correction of anemia continued to ingest clay or starch. It would seem that in adults iron deficiency was not the cause of the pica but that the latter contributed to the anemia. In children, however, there is a loss of pica with correction of the iron deficiency.[126]

Prasad and colleagues[152] described a syndrome occurring in males, natives of Iran, characterized by severe iron deficiency (hemoglobin levels ranging from 2.8 to 7.7 gm. per 100 ml.), hypogonadism, dwarfism, hepatosplenomegaly, and geophagia in nine of the patients. The age range was 14 to 21 years. Liver function tests were normal except for an elevated serum alkaline phosphatase.

Their diet consisted mostly of wheat and rice, with a little milk, and rarely meat, vegetables, and fruit. When these patients were properly treated with oral iron, the hemoglobin returned to normal and the liver and spleen diminished in size.

Iron lack has been associated with another perversion of appetite characterized by the ingestion of extraordinary amounts of ice—designated as "pagophagia." Coltman[36] reported a group of adult women with pagophagia who were iron deficient and consumed at least one ordinary tray of ice daily for a period in excess of 2 months. Iron administration in doses insufficient to correct the anemia or to replenish body stores promptly eliminated all craving for ice. The mechanism is related to iron lack but not specifically to iron-lack anemia.

It would seem that pica can be cured by the administration of iron, but a permanent cure is dependent on the maintenance of adequate hemoglobin levels. Pica has as its complications lead poisoning and ingestion of the ova of worms. Since available evidence indicates that pica is associated with iron-deficiency anemia and it is cured by iron administration, it seems possible that the widespread eradication of iron deficiency might eventually lead to a reduction in the incidence of pica and consequently lead poisoning.[113]

**Relation of physiologic anemia of the newborn infant to iron-deficiency anemia.** Following an inital week or 10 days of stable or mildly fluctuating blood levels, the hemoglobin and red cells drop, reaching a minimum at approximately 7 weeks of age in the premature infant and at 2 to 3 months in the full-term infant. This phase, designated as physiologic anemia of the newborn infant, is highly important in the iron economy of the infant since the iron liberated by red cell destruction is stored for later use in rebuilding hemoglobin. During this period the red cell count falls proportionately to hemoglobin so that a normochromic, normocytic anemia develops. It should be emphasized that the anemia at this stage is due to a depression of erythropoiesis and hemoglobin synthesis, during which red cells are destroyed at normal or at best slightly increased rates.[90]

The diminished hematopoiesis is explained by Gairdner and associates[62] as an adjustment to the changeover from the placenta to the lung as a source of oxygen. To maintain a normal postnatal oxyhemoglobin content of the blood, there is no need for elevated hemoglobin levels so that erythrogenesis and hemoglobin synthesis are retarded until such a time as the hemoglobin level drops from elevated blood levels at birth to approximately 11 to 12 gm. per 100 ml. Any decrease below this point induces increased hematopoietic activity, whereas elevations above this level will tend to decrease marrow activity. When the designated concentrations are reached in the full-term infant at 2 to 3 months of age, marrow erythroid activity is resumed[62] as reflected by reticulocytosis and the gradual rise in the circulating hemoglobin mass. A fundamental principle in the kinetics of iron metabolism is that once iron is introduced into the body it is used again and again. The amount excreted is small and is assumed to be less than 1 mg. daily.

At approximately 16 weeks of age in the full-term infant the total amount of circulating hemoglobin is restored to the initial birth values. A humoral erythropoietic stimulating factor, erythroprotein,[59] may also be involved in these fluctuations, functioning when anemia develops and being inactive at the high hemoglobin concentrations at birth.

With the resumption of active erythropoiesis, reticulocytes appear and the circulating mass expands. In both full-term and premature infants the amount of hemoglobin synthesized will be limited by the iron that has accumulated in the stores during the postnatal drop in hemoglobin. This, in turn, depends principally upon hemoglobin concentration and hemoglobin mass available at birth and supplemented by a variable component of pre-existing iron in the liver and spleen. Increase in weight and the blood volume obscures the improvement in the hemoglobin concentration during the period of recovery.

The supply of iron becomes strained with rapid growth so that the infant is exposed to an anemia based on the exhaustion of storage iron. Following the period of reutilization of iron and hemoglobin synthesis and increase in total hemoglobin mass, the supply of this mineral becomes depleted unless the stores are replenished by exogenous iron from an adequate diet. These demands are met in the average full-term infant. The failure to add foods containing significant quantities of iron leads to iron-deficiency anemia, especially if the demands are excessive. Iron-deficiency anemia, accordingly, is observed in clinical practice in infants who are growing rapidly and are fed almost exclusively on diets of milk and cereals with low iron content and present feeding difficulties.

Another feature of note in iron deficiency is the high incidence of unexplained occult blood loss.[89] Guaiac-positive stools are normally found without roentgenographic evidence of gastrointestinal lesions. This finding called attention to other interesting and associated functional and morphologic changes in the gastrointestinal tract. Iron-deficient infants frequently demonstrate a loss of plasma proteins in the gastric juice[217] and also a high incidence of precipitating antibodies to cow's milk in their sera.[217] Milk precipitins in such cases probably reflect an underlying pathologic process in which unaltered proteins cross the bowel into the bloodstream. Such a phenomenon had been described earlier in infants suffering from malnutrition and diarrhea.[7] In many respects the loss of plasma proteins in the lumen of the gastrointestinal canal corresponds to a protein-losing enteropathy.[106] In a group of fourteen infants and children with nutritional iron-deficiency anemia, a high incidence of abnormalities was found consisting of gastric achlorhydria, impaired absorption of xylose and vitamin A, and steatorrhea. Occult blood was found in the stools of six patients. Duodenal biopsies revealed varying degrees of chronic duodenitis and mucosal atrophy. Following treatment with oral iron, most of the abnormalities reverted to normal, indicating that a diffuse and reversible enteropathy exists in children as a result of iron deficiency.[143] These abnormalities are not seen in patients who are anemic from causes other than iron deficiency.

Guha and co-workers[81] studied a group of twenty-six children aged 4 to 12 years suffering from iron deficiency. More than two-thirds of the children showed evidence of altered gastrointestinal function and structure. Before treatment there was a varying degree of duodenal-jejunal mucosal atrophy. This consisted of partial villous atrophy and significant shortening of the villi, which were blunted and fused over wide areas. In a high proportion of cases there was occult blood in the stool and impaired absorption of fat and d-xylose. Following iron therapy the biochemical and biological changes in the small bowel disappeared. The severity of the intestinal changes was not directly correlated to the levels of hemoglobin or serum iron. These findings are comparable to the enteropathy due to iron deficiency in children aged less than 3 years previously reported.[143]

A method for quantitating the amount of blood lost in the feces by means of erythrocytes labeled with radioactive chromium has been described by Ebaugh and associates.[52] They also demonstrated that the sensitivity of the benzidine test could be increased by examining for hemoglobin in aqueous solutions rather than for hemoglobin present in the stools.

Iron deficiency, it would seem, through some as yet unknown mechanism provokes the leakage of plasma proteins in infants, leading to edema, poor growth, and decreased serum concentration of albumin, gamma globulin, transferrin, and ceruloplasmin.[106] In support of this hypothesis is the prompt disappearance of edema and hypoproteinemia after the administration of iron.

*Clinical features.* Infection, which plays a dominant role as an etiologic factor in anemia in infancy and childhood, frequently highlights an underlying state of iron deficiency. However, pallor, irritability, anorexia, and listlessness usually direct attention to severe grades of this disorder. A history of repeated upper respiratory difficulties is not uncommon.

In no condition is the sheetlike or waxy pallor so striking as in advanced iron-deficiency anemia. Except for pallor of the skin and mucous membranes and occasionally a slightly enlarged spleen, the patients present no significant physical abnormalities. As in patients with other severe anemias, a soft blowing apical systolic murmur is frequently heard, but the heart is not enlarged. The changes in the epithelial structures characterizing iron deficiency in adults, such as atrophic glossitis, dysphagia, and spoon-shaped or concave nails (koilonychia), do not occur in infants and are only rarely observed in older children. Because of gradual development of the anemia, signs of cardiac dysfunction are usually not encountered even in infants with severe grades of hemoglobin reduction.

*Laboratory data.* Important laboratory information is obtained from a study of the peripheral blood, bone marrow, and plasma of patients with iron-deficiency anemia.

*Blood.* The anemia of iron deficiency is characteristically hypochromic and microcytic in contrast to the normochromic, normocytic type of physiologic anemia in the postnatal period. Since iron deficiency primarily affects hemoglobin synthesis and red cell formation to a lesser degree, the red cell count may be normal, near normal, or moderately reduced. The hematocrit levels are lower than normal. The decreased hemoglobin content of the individual erythrocyte is the specific abnormality present in iron-deficiency anemia. The hemoglobin is reduced out of proportion to the red cell count. The red cell count varies, usually ranging from 3 to 5 million, with a hemoglobin level from 3 to 9 gm. per 100 ml. The following criteria of hypochromic anemia may be designated: hemoglobin concentrations below 9 gm. per 100 ml., a mean corpuscular hemoglobin (MCH) less than 27 $\mu\mu$g, a mean corpuscular hemoglobin concentration (MCHC) of less than 30%,[223] and a mean corpuscular volume (MCV) of less than 78$\mu^3$.[80]

The blood smear shows microcytes, poikilocytes, elliptical and elongated pencil forms, and target cells (Fig. 18). Many of the red cells are diminutive in size. A small number of normal-sized red cells and macrocytes are usually present, often with a normal hemoglobin content. The characteristic appearance of the blood smear is the presence of a majority of small red cells with marked central pallor with fine and poorly staining rims of hemoglobin. In severe iron deficiency, occasional stippled red cells and normoblasts may be present. Reticulocytes are normal or reduced, but in severe anemia a reticulocyte count of 3 to 4% is encountered. The fragility of the red cells may be normal or may show a moderate resistance to hemolysis in hypotonic solution of sodium chloride. The platelet count varies from thrombocytopenia to thrombocytosis. Although usually within a normal range, elevated platelet counts may accompany moderate anemia, and in some severely anemic individuals thrombocytopenia may be observed.[79] In one series the mean hemoglobin of the thrombocytopenic group (platelet counts of 170,000 per cubic millimeter) was 4 gm. per 100 ml. and for those with increased platelets (mean platelet count of 420,000 per cubic millimeter) it was 6 gm.

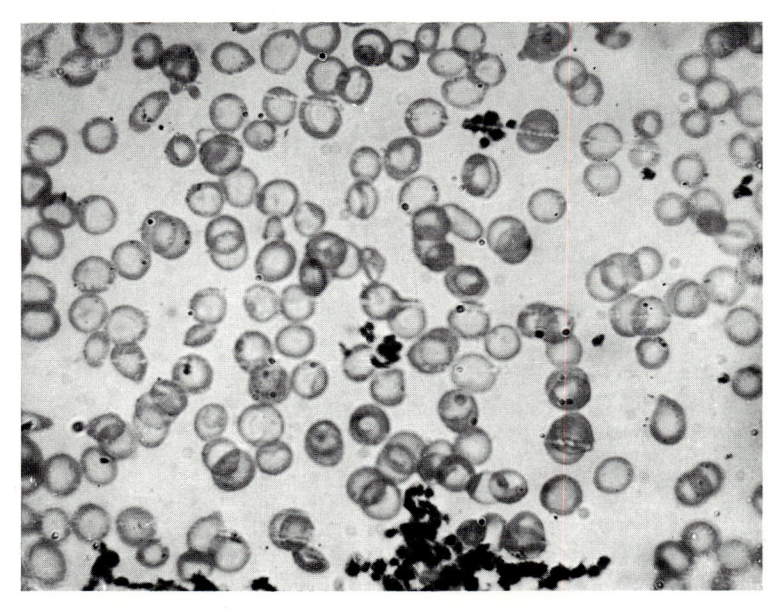

Fig. 18. Blood smear of an infant with iron-deficiency anemia. Note predominance of hypochromic microcytes, fairly uniform in size and shape, in which the outstanding feature is marked deficiency in hemoglobin indicated by central pallor. Note also large numbers of platelets (in lower portion of smear), sometimes found in this condition. (×840.)

per 100 ml. Platelets rose with iron therapy, although much more rapidly with parenteral iron administration. Thrombocytopenia may reflect a depletion of iron as iron enzymes, platelets being known to contain iron, or it may be due to associated folate deficiency or a transient thrombopoietin defect. The leukocytes are usually normal or slightly reduced.

A decreased red cell survival has been demonstrated in iron-deficiency anemia and has been ascribed to increased activity of the enzymes involved in the Embden-Meyerhof pathway and hexose-monophosphate shunt.[118] This increased metabolic activity declines during iron therapy and returns to normal within 3 months.

Normally, stock piles of porphyrin, iron, and globin become depleted as hemoglobinization of the red cell is completed. A deficiency or excess of these compounds may be found in abnormalities of heme synthesis. Thus, when the supply of iron to the marrow is restricted, iron granules within the normoblast disappear, protoporphyrin accumulates, and the total hemoglobin production is reduced, resulting in a hypochromic, microcytic red cell.

Following the administration of iron, a short intermediate phase of response is occasionally encountered in which the hemoglobin concentration is still very low, the platelets may be sharply reduced, and a marked leukocytosis is present. The latter constitutes a leukemoid reaction with large numbers of metamyelocytes, myelocytes, and normoblasts. At this time the bone marrow is hyperplastic. With recovery, platelet values may reach almost 1 million. Such extreme degrees of leukocytosis occur infrequently.

A normoblastic response to iron-deficiency anemia may occasionally become excessive. Also a leukoerythroblastosis has been reported[21,164] when parenteral iron (Imferon) is administered in severe iron deficiency. It has been suggested[21] that in a marrow avid for iron the rapid delivery of this substance from the iron-dextran combination produces a transient stimulus to granulocytopoiesis as well as erythropoiesis. Such a response should not be confused with leukemia, neoplasia, or a myeloproliferative process. These changes can occur as early as the third day after treatment with Imferon and can persist for about 10 days.

The occurrence of megaloblastoid changes consisting of increased lobe averages and hypersegmentation in a group of infants and children with iron-deficiency anemia was described by Vossough and associates.[203] They postulated that iron deficiency may produce a functional deficiency of folate or vitamin $B_{12}$ at the cellular level in the marrow. None, however, had decreased serum levels of vitamin $B_{12}$ and only two were considered to be folic acid deficient.

*Bone marrow.* The bone marrow shows erythroid hyperplasia with a predominance of polychromatophilic normoblasts often smaller than normal. The cytoplasm may be diminished to the extent that it forms a small rim around the nucleus. Granulopoiesis is normal. Megakaryocytes are normal in number and in appearance. They may be occasionally increased in patients with high platelet counts. Occasionally, when platelets are decreased, diminished numbers of megakaryocytes are associated with evidences of megaloblastic marrow.[79] Contributory evidence of diminished iron stores may be directly determined by bone marrow examination which reveals a decrease of iron granules in the normoblasts (sideroblasts)[35,98] and an almost complete absence of stainable iron or hemosiderin in marrow aspiration. This depletion of hemosiderin is contrasted with the increased quantities noted in infection and in hemolytic anemias.[93,187]

*Plasma.* The serum iron is reduced, varying from 10 to 60 µg per 100 ml. and averaging about 30 µg per 100 ml. (normal, approximately 120 µg). The latent iron-binding capacity of the serum is increased to approximately 450 µg per 100 ml. and above (normal, 250 µg). The saturation of serum iron (serum iron divided by serum iron plus latent iron-binding capacity) is reduced and averages 6%[183] (normal, 32%). A greatly reduced serum iron and a markedly elevated latent iron-binding capacity have not been found in any other condition than iron deficiency and are, therefore, of diagnostic value. With treatment the serum iron is increased, the latent iron-binding capacity undergoes a moderate contraction, and serum iron saturation increases. In addition to hypoferremia and reduced saturation of total serum iron, other chemical manifestations of iron deficiency include increased blood copper levels (hypercupremia) and increased free erythrocyte protoporphyrin.[190]

Of the many diagnostic features delineating the hematologic picture of an anemia due to a primary deficiency of iron, the simplest is the presence of microcytic hypochromic red cells that dominate the stained blood smear.

*Diagnosis.* The characteristic small, pale, red blood cells of iron-deficiency anemia in the stained smear, a history of an iron-deficient diet, and the marked pallor of the patient are usually sufficient to make the diagnosis in the infant over 6 months of age. The stool examination for unrecognized chronic blood loss is essential.

Hypochromic anemia is a descriptive term and is not synonymous with iron-deficiency anemia. There are other varieties of hypochromic anemia, such as thalassemia, pyridoxine deficiency, and sideroachrestic or refractory normoblastic anemia, in which there is an inability to synthesize hemoglobin in spite of a plentiful supply of iron (Fig. 19).

Early in iron therapy, short-lived macrocytes appear.[138] Under intense erythroid stimulation with iron therapy there is a shortening of the maturation interval with skipping of cell divisions. As recovery from the anemia progresses, the intensity of the erythroid stimulation decreases and more nearly normal cells are provided. The mechanism of the macrocytic response may be mediated by erythropoietin. Erythropoietin, which is demonstrated in cases of iron deficiency with hemoglobin levels below 5 gm., is not found at higher levels.[202] This inability to demonstrate erythropoietin at higher hemoglobin levels is probably due to utilization of erythropoietin by a functional competent stem cell compartment.[138]

Leventhal and Stohlman[116] have demonstrated that in iron-deficiency anemia the red cell size is related to the rate of maturation, which in turn is governed by the level of erythropoietin and the availability of precursors for hemoglobin such as iron. When high doses of iron were given macrocytes were produced, low doses produced an increased hemoglobin level but with increased production of microcytes, and intermediate doses resulted in the production of normocytes. In the presence of normal or excess iron stores the level of erythropoietin will govern the rate of maturation and hence the red cell size. With high erythropoietin output together with adequate precursors (iron-deficient group treated with high doses of iron) macrocytes are found.

Macdougall and co-workers[120] found decreased red cell survival in 24 of 38 children with nutritional iron-deficiency anemia. Decreased red cell survival appeared to be related to the severity of the anemia and the presence of a functioning spleen. Iron-deficient cells survived normally when transfused into a splenectomized recipient. A progressive increase in red cell hexokinase activity (without reticulocytosis) was noted in association with increasing severity of the anemia and decreasing red cell life-span. Red cell adenosine triphosphate concentration was normal or slightly decreased and showed marked instability on incubation. Iron-deficient cells that have increased metabolic requirements are more vulnerable to the adverse effects of the splenic environment situation that is exaggerated in the most severely anemic patients with the greatest increase in hexokinase activity. Moderate splenic enlargement was present in thirteen (34%) of the iron-de-

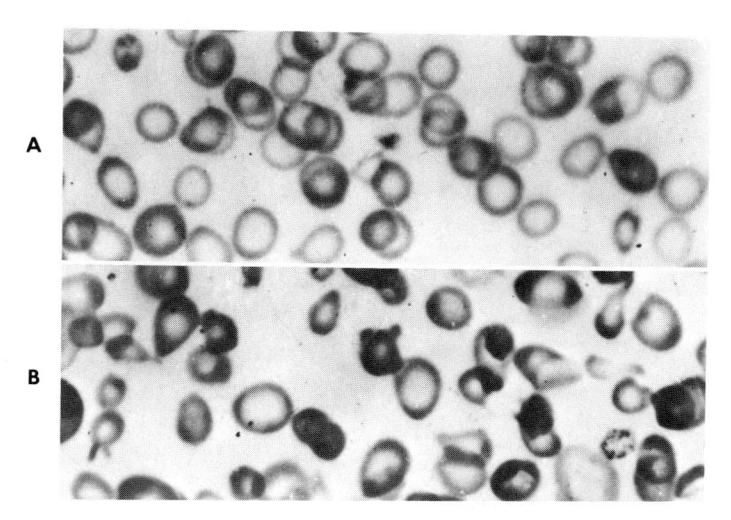

Fig. 19. Comparison of blood smears of iron-deficiency anemia and thalassemia major. A, Iron-deficiency anemia—note predominance of hypochromic microcytes of fairly uniform size and shape and central pallor. B, Thalassemia major, pre-splenectomy—note microcytes, hypochromic macrocytes, marked anisocytosis and poikilocytosis, normoblasts, and tear-drop cells.

ficient children studied, twelve of whom had decreased red cell survival. Overt bleeding was not noted in any of the iron-deficient children, although all had one or more stools positive for occult blood. Blood loss could not therefore be related to reduction in red cell survival.

Iron-deficiency anemia and milder forms of thalassemia are often indistinguishable. The red cells in both conditions show moderate stippling and target and oval forms, but the larger number of hypochromic macrocytes in the blood smear and the familial hereditary pattern are important diagnostic features of thalassemia minor. The blood smear of patients with mild thalassemia and of those with iron deficiency may both show, however, a more or less uniform hypochromic microcytic picture, and other diagnostic aids are necessary.

Confusion with the severe homozygous type of Cooley's anemia may occur only in the infant in the first year of life. The large, pale, extremely thin erythrocytes with irregularly distributed hemoglobin and scattered normoblasts interspersed among microcytes in the blood smear are in contrast with the more uniform microcytes of iron-deficiency anemia. Occasional hypochromic macrocytes are, however, also found in the latter. The significant splenomegaly and the presence of the trait in both parents and siblings further differentiates Cooley's anemia from iron-deficiency anemia.

Changes of the skull identical with the "hair-standing-on-end" appearance observed on the roentgenogram of patients with the chronic hemolytic anemias have been described in patients with chronic iron-deficiency anemia, especially in premature infants and

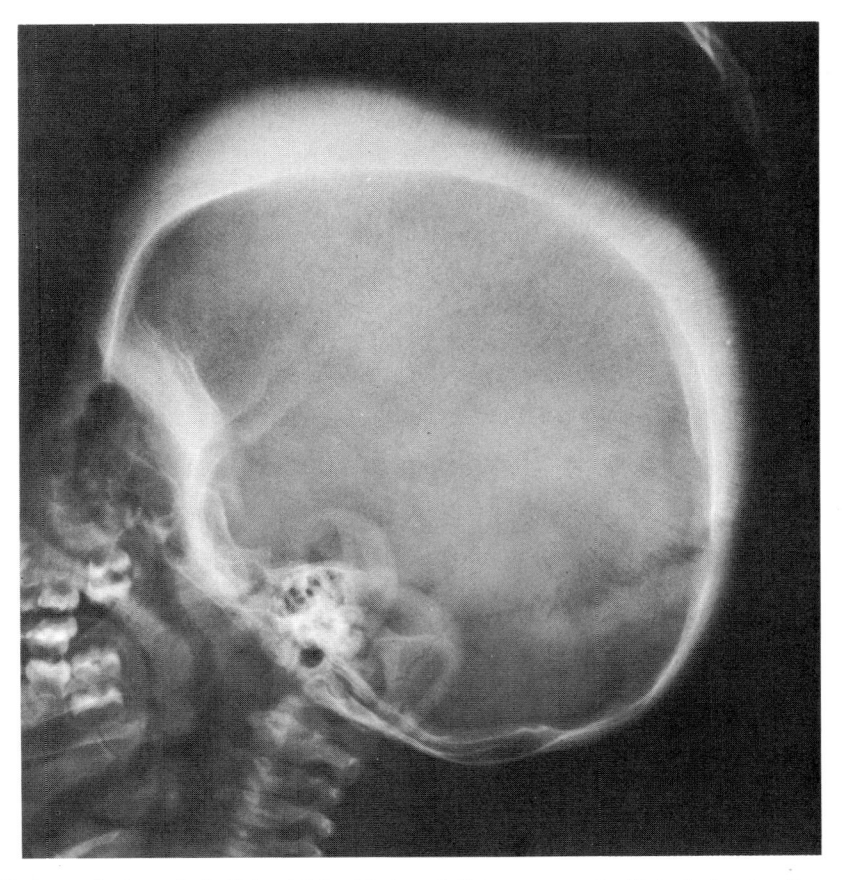

Fig. 20. Lateral view of skull in child with iron-deficiency anemia. Note hair—standing-on-end appearance. (From Lanzkowsky, P.: Radiological features of iron-deficiency anemia, Amer. J. Dis. Child. 116:16, 1968.)

twins.[2,25,56,112,177] These changes are associated with erythroid hyperplasia in the bone marrow. In contrast to changes observed in patients with Cooley's anemia, these changes are usually confined to the skull (Fig. 20).

***Treatment.*** Simple iron salts are effective in correcting iron-deficiency anemia. Nevertheless, successful management requires a thorough investigation of basic etiologic factors such as faulty diet, malabsorption due to chronic diarrhea, or blood loss due to a structural gastrointestinal defect such as polyps or Meckel's diverticulum. Most commonly, the history will reveal a dependence on foods notably poor in iron content such as milk, unfortified cereals, and other carbohydrate foods. Often this situation will have developed unwittingly from a failure of parents to understand the need for a well-balanced diet, particularly in the rapidly growing infant. Each of these factors can be eliminated by diagnostic and therapeutic procedures and the diet can be adjusted. Restriction of milk to one pint a day, the introduction of meat, vegetables, and fruit, and supplementation by an iron preparation will usually suffice to correct the anemia (Table 15).

Of importance in all infants, the full-term and especially the premature, is the insistence upon serial hemoglobin determinations from the second month, and at appropriate intervals thereafter, for the detection and control of the anemia. The necessity for this measurement stems from the variability in the hemoglobin mass at birth, from which iron is derived for later hemoglobin synthesis, and the individual needs for exogenous iron due to growth of tissues and expanding blood volume.

Iron-rich foods include the following: commercially prepared, dry, ready-to-serve infants' cereals (0.92 mg. of iron per tablespoon), green and yellow vegetables (0.05 mg. per tablespoon in spinach), green beans (0.28 mg. per tablespoon), and liver (0.56 mg. per tablespoon).

Josephs[98] gives the iron content of milk as follows: as it comes from the cow, it contains about 0.4 to 0.5 mg. of iron per liter. Commercial pasteurization increases the iron to 0.7 to 1 mg. per liter. Processed milk, whether powdered or condensed, may contain 1 to 2 mg. per liter. Breast milk contains 0.7 to 1 mg. per liter.

The recommended dietary intake of iron varies widely among individual infants depending on age, growth rate, stores, and other factors.

The Committee on Nutrition of the American Academy of Pediatrics formulated the needs for iron in infancy as follows:[37] they stated that the endowment of the newborn is proportional to the initial hemoglobin mass. This in turn depends upon the birth weight and initial hemoglobin level. The presence of low birth weight or decreased hemoglobin level in the first few days of life may identify infants with special iron requirements during the first months of life. The iron content of the circulating blood can be fairly accurately estimated from the red cell mass. More than three-quarters of the infant's iron endowment is in the red cell. On the basis of these fundamental assumptions, the Committee recommended an iron intake of 1 mg./kg./day to a maximum of 15 mg./day by age 3 months for normal, term infants. This amount can be easily provided by a diet that includes appropriate amounts of iron-supplemented foods such as infant cereals or milk formulas. Infants with low birth weight and others with reduced iron endowment by virtue of low initial hemoglobin values and who have experienced significant blood loss require as much as 2.0 mg. of iron per kilogram per day, beginning by 2 months of age. This amount is not ordinarily provided by the diet, even when iron-supplemented cereals are included. Attainment of these larger amounts requires the use of medicinal iron or iron-supplemented milk formula. The Committee further states, "Iron fortified milk or medicinal iron should be prescribed in order to assure an iron intake of at least 2 mg./kg./day for infants with reduced iron endowment."

When established iron-deficiency anemia is diagnosed, oral therapy with simple ferrous salts assures a satisfactory response. A total of 6 mg./kg./day of elemental iron in three divided doses between meals provides an adequate amount. This should be continued for a month or so after normal hemoglobin levels have been attained in order to assure replacement of iron stores.

**Table 15.** Iron content of infant foods

| Food | Iron (mg.) | Unit |
|---|---|---|
| Milk | 0.5 | Liter |
| Fruits (strained) | 0.2-0.4 | Ounce |
| Vegetables (strained) | | |
|     Yellow | 0.1-0.3 | Ounce |
|     Green | 0.3-0.4 | Ounce |
| Meats (strained) | | |
|     Beef, lamb, beef liver | 0.4-2.0 | Ounce |
|     Pork, liver, and bacon | 6.6 | Ounce |
| Cereal | 3-5 | Ounce |
| Eggs | 1.2 | Each |

Iron-enriched staples are to be used for feeding American infants between 3 and 18 months of age. At the present time iron-fortified cereals and milk formulas are the iron-supplemented foods most generally available. Cereal in the diet of American infants provides the most important source of iron since it is artificially fortified with reduced iron or iron-pyrophosphate during its processing. Such cereals contain 8.6 to 22 mg. of iron in each dry ounce. Limited amounts of eggs and meats supplied during the first year of life usually provide a small fraction of the total iron requirements.[37]

At a recent conference[100] on iron nutrition in infancy, the following recommendations were made:
1. All infants who are given artificial feeding should receive heat-processed, iron-fortified formula containing 10 to 15 mg. of elemental iron per reconstituted quart.
2. Such formula feedings be continued for the first year of life.
3. All milk formulas and milk-substitute formulas designed for infant feeding should contain adequate iron.
4. The use of iron-fortified cereals should be encouraged during infancy. Implicit in the public health approach to the problem is that steps must be taken to assure that all infants have access to such formulas and that education of the public and medical profession to the need for such an approach be instituted.

Others have claimed that a daily iron intake of 0.5 mg. per kilogram in food is adequate to maintain normal hemoglobin levels in most (full-term) infants.[12]

To achieve maximum improvement in hemoglobin concentration, Sturgeon[192] has suggested that the recommended daily allowance\* of 6 mg. of food iron through the first year and 10 mg. from 1 to 3 years of age be increased to intakes of 6 to 9 mg. daily at 3 months of age, to 8 to 12 mg. by 6 months, and to 10 to 15 mg. at 12 months. One egg yolk supplies approximately 1 mg. of iron, and peaches, the best source of iron among the fruits, provide 0.32 mg. per tablespoon.[156]

The average full-term infant requires a total of 8 mg. of iron daily from about 6 months of age and with optimal intake may derive this amount from dietary sources alone. The term infant with deficient body iron at birth may require this amount of iron as early as 3 months, and the premature infant at 2 months. In premature infants a total daily intake of about 2 mg. per kilogram should be assured by the third month, gradually decreasing to about 1 mg. per kilogram by the end of the first year.[169] While iron supplementation is indicated for all premature infants, a decided advantage is noted from the fourth month of life with negligible differences at 3 months.[160] Gorten and co-workers[73] have demonstrated, however, that premature infants absorb and utilize iron during the first 10 weeks of life. Examination of hemoglobin levels during the early periods reveal no substantial elevation of hemoglobin levels.

A significant number of premature infants demonstrate some laboratory evidence of a folate deficiency during the first 3 months of life.[180] The deficiency does not appear to be related either to the anemia or to morbidity of prematurity. The need for dietary folic acid supplementation is questionable at the present time.

*Iron therapy.* Treatment with a soluble iron salt, preferably ferrous iron, corrects the deficiency more promptly than the ingestion of foods rich in iron, although both should be given simultaneously. Ferrous iron permits significantly higher hemoglobin values in well children than does ferric iron of the same dosage.[144] Ingested iron is absorbed in the ferrous form largely from the duodenum. Ferrous sulfate is the preparation of choice in most infants because the metallic iron content is adequate and it is efficiently absorbed, inexpensive, and easily administered. Normal infants will absorb an average of 10 to 20% of orally administered ferrous sulfate in solution, and iron-deficient children absorb 5 to 10% more.[172]

Normal children absorb an average of about 10% of the naturally occurring iron in milk, eggs, chicken liver, and iron supplements added to commercially prepared infants' cereals.[171] Iron-deficient children absorb two to three times as much food iron as do normal children.[171] In normal adult subjects, on the contrary, approximately 5 to 15% absorption takes place from ferrous salt given in 100 mg. amounts.[50] With uncomplicated iron-deficiency anemia the absorption is increased to between 25 and 70%. With food iron, the percentage of absorption is 1 to 10%, which is increased to 20 to 30% in the iron-deficient subjects.[134] Reducing substances, especially ascorbic acid, enhanced the absorption of food iron.[134] With nearly 5 to 10% of iron in food assimilated by normal adults, the daily retention on a diet containing 12 to 15 mg. is approximately equivalent to the amount of iron lost from the body each day.[137] Charlton and Bothwell[30] state that the "present methods of food refining provide an average American diet with an iron concentration of about 6 mg./1000 calories. Normal males consuming a 2500 calorie diet would, therefore, obtain 15 mg. of iron per day of which between 0.5 and 1 mg. would be absorbed." They calculated that the range of absorption from a nor-

---
\*Based on data from Food and Nutrition Board of the National Research Council.

mal diet is a relatively small one, extending as it does from 0.5 in the iron replete individual to a maximum of little more than 3 mg. in the iron-deficient subject.

DOSAGE AND MODE OF ADMINISTRATION. Since the percentage of metallic iron content is a fraction of the entire compound, iron should be prescribed with this fact in mind. Such preparations are now available and are suitably designated according to iron content.

For infants, ferrous sulfate is available in concentrated solutions that can be given in drop dosage in which each drop contains a measured amount of elemental iron. The recommended oral dose is 1.5 to 2 mg. per kilogram of elemental iron given three times daily (4.5 to 6 mg. per kilogram per day).[224] The total dose of elemental iron recommended for an infant during the period of iron deficiency (6 to 24 months) ranges from 60 to 90 mg. Ideal treatment consists of the administration of such a soluble iron preparation in divided dosage, preferably between meals.

There are a large variety of iron salts, ferrous and ferric alike, available in solution form that produce a satisfactory hemoglobin response; the ferric solutions require a somewhat higher dosage. The pediatrician should have knowledge of several preparations with respect to details of administration and content of elemental iron since it is occasionally necessary to interchange them because of gastrointestinal irritation or anorexia produced by one or another preparation.

Theoretically milk has been regarded as being an unfavorable vehicle for iron, either because it combines with phosphates to form insoluble salts or because it shares with other foods of increased phosphorus content a basic difficulty in absorbing iron.[85] Phytates contained in cereals also make nonionized precipitates with iron. Despite these findings, iron salts in therapeutic doses added to milk have produced satisfactory hemoglobin responses in our experience and in that of others.[144] Furthermore, the iron in iron supplemented cereals now in common use in infant feeding is also well absorbed.[131]

Oral administration of iron usually results in the stool becoming a deep black color due to the increased content of iron sulfides. The absence of this change may serve as a clue to the irregular administration of the iron.[184] Ingestion of liquid iron preparations may produce a black staining of the teeth. Brushing the teeth after each administration is of value in reducing this untoward effect, although the staining is only temporary.

For older children, tablets of ferrous sulfate or ferrous gluconate are preferable to the concentrated liquid preparations used with infants. Gastric irritation, nausea, vomiting, and abdominal pain are less likely to occur if the tablets are taken with meals. Iron tablets are best taken three times daily at meal time. Tablets of ferrous sulfate (0.2 gm., 3 grains) or ferrous gluconate (0.3 gm., 5 grains) given three times daily provide a daily total of 100 to 200 mg. of elemental iron.

In the infant, as in the older child, full therapeutic doses of iron should be given for at least 6 to 8 weeks after the hemoglobin has been restored to normal levels. If oral therapy is withdrawn too soon, the iron stores will remain unreplenished[183] and anemia will eventually recur.

A simple test for the detection of iron in stools was described by Afifi and associates[1] and applied by Macdougall[119] to children with iron deficiency who failed to attain acceptable hemoglobin levels after 3 months of prescribed oral iron therapy. Macdougall[119] found uniformly positive stool tests within 48 hours of initiation of iron therapy. The test depends on the contact of one drop of 0.25% potassium ferricyanide with liquified stool specimen. In positive tests there is an immediate development of a blue crescent (ferrous cyanide) at the junction of this mixture. This test provides a rapid and effective means of determining the reliability of those responsible for administering iron medication to the children.

A basic difficulty in the treatment of iron-deficiency anemia is the standard set for the normal hemoglobin level at the end of the first year of life.[49] Although 11 to 12 gm. of hemoglobin per 100 ml. is a commonly accepted standard, at best this range is arbitrary since an infant with 10 gm. may be just as healthy. In the absence of information as to the differences between the normal, average, and optimal hemoglobin levels, and without ancillary data such as the serum iron for a particular infant, 11 to 12 gm. per 100 ml. may be regarded as an acceptable, normal value. The need for reaching for values above these by a variety of antianemia medications is sometimes questioned.

Between 3 and 18 months of age a hemoglobin of about 12 gm./100 ml. or a hematocrit of 36% may be considered optimal. Hemoglobin as low as 11 gm./100 ml. and hematocrit as low as 33% will fall within one or two standard deviations of these means and should be considered normal.

Trials of iron supplements in two at-risk groups (adolescent girls and adult women who had lately been iron deficient) revealed an effect on hemoglobin level of a supplement of 10 mg. of iron per day (as ferrous fumarate), but gave no clear evidence of an effect of a smaller supplement.[55] Elwood and associates[55] suggest that the long-term administration of tablets (of iron) is impractical and that if iron intake is to be supplemented iron should be added to a foodstuff. They pointed out, however, the problems involved in incorporating sufficient iron in a foodstuff.

*Iron-dextran for intramuscular use.* Parenteral iron therapy is indicated when patients fail to respond to adequate oral dosage, because of gastrointestinal irritation, gastrointestinal pathology, or, more rarely, refractoriness to oral therapy because of failure to absorb iron. The commonest causes of failure to respond to prescribed iron is unreliability of parental administration and an incorrect diagnosis where the anemia is due to causes other than iron deficiency. In such cases iron-dextran mixture for intamuscular use (Imferon) has proved a valuable adjunct to therapy. This preparation is well tolerated and provides 50 mg. of elemental iron in each milliliter. The total amount of iron needed to raise the hemoglobin level to normal and replenish stores is calculated as follows:

$$\frac{\text{Normal hemoglobin} - \text{Initial hemoglobin}}{100} \times \text{Blood volume (ml.)} \times 3.4 \times 1.5$$

1. Normal hemoglobin — 11 to 12 gm. in infants; 12.5 to 13.5 gm. in children; 14 to 15 gm. at puberty
2. Blood volume = 80 ml. per kilogram or 40 ml. per pound of body weight
3. 3.4 converts grams of hemoglobin into milligrams of iron
4. Factor 1.5 provides extra iron to replace depleted tissue stores

*Example:* Infant weighing 10 kg. with 5 gm of hemoglobin per 100 ml.
Blood volume = 80 ml. per kilogram × 10 kg. = 800 ml.
Hemoglobin deficit = 12 gm. (approximately normal for age) − 5 gm. = 7 gm. per 100 ml.
Total hemoglobin deficit = 7 gm. × $\frac{800}{100}$ = 56 gm.
Iron to restore hemoglobin to normal = 56 gm. × 3.4 mg. = 190 mg.
Iron to replenish stores = 50% of 190 mg. = 95 mg.
Total dose of iron to be injected = 190 + 95 = 285 mg. of iron

Iron-dextran has been administered to thirty-seven patients (presumably adults) with iron-deficiency anemia and to eight additional patients with acute gastrointestinal bleeding in doses up to 3,000 mg. intravenously, by a single injection.[121] No serious untoward results were observed. The indications were similar to those for the intramuscular route: an unwillingness to take oral iron, an inability to tolerate it well (e.g., ulcerative colitis, regional ileitis), difficulties in absorption of iron (e.g., sprue), and bleeding from gastrointestinal lesions nonamenable to surgical treatment (e.g., inoperable cancer, obscure blood loss). In a later report by Clay and colleagues,[34] 150 maternity patients were treated with intravenous Imferon by the total-dose Imferon technique. Mixed reactions occurred of which seven were severe and demanded emergency treatment. All those who suffered reactions were later safely delivered of healthy infants. This account was published in order to point out that, despite the reported safety of this method, such was not the experience of these investigators. Iron-dextran is, therefore, best administered intramuscularly. It is to be emphasized, however, that iron given orally is the treatment of choice in iron-deficiency anemia and iron-dextran given intramusclarly as the secondary route.

In experimental administration, intravenously, of iron to rabbits, hemosiderin formation never precedes ferritin formation.[179] For instance, iron from iron-dextran goes first to ferritin, and when ferritin concentration reaches a critical level, a process is started which results in a gradual cessation in the increase of ferritin and a reciprocal increase in the rate of hemosiderin production.

Intraperitoneal injection of iron-dextran is followed by the appearance of ferritin in the small intestine. Histologic studies indicate that iron is carried into the intestinal tissues by daipedesis of iron-laden phagocytes.[195]

The total dosage of iron-dextran according to age has also been estimated by Wallerstein and Hoag[207] as follows: 100 mg. for infants under 6 months of age; 200 mg. under 12 months of age; 300 mg. from 12 to 24 months of age; and 400 mg. over 24 months of age. Injections are given daily or, when this is impractical, at weekly intervals. In small infants the initial dosage is 50 mg. (1 ml.). With daily injections newly formed red cells well filled with hemoglobin are recognizable in blood smears within 48 hours after therapy. About the fifth day of treatment reticulocyte counts reach maximum values, which are probably initiated after 24 hours of therapy. In patients with severe anemia the hemoglobin level reaches 11 gm. per 100 ml. after 3 weeks and higher in patients with moderate anemia. The magnitude of the hemoglobin response varies, therefore, with the degree of anemia. If hemoglobin values do not rise at least 2 gm. in 3 weeks, other possible causes of anemia should be considered, and more iron should not be administered.

Injections into the upper outer quadrant of the gluteus muscle are given through skin which has been displaced laterally prior to the injection to prevent superficial staining. In rare cases local or generalized reactions, angioneurotic edema, and recurrent arthralgia occur.[176]

RESPONSE TO ORAL IRON THERAPY. The recovery is reflected by a reticulocyte response that reaches its maximum on the fifth to the tenth day after the institution of iron therapy. The magnitude of the response is related to the degree of anemia. Following the reticulocyte rise, the hemoglobin level, volume of packed cells (hematocrit), and red cell count increase. Following the peak of the reticulocyte rise, the hemoglobin rises at an average of 0.17 to 0.25 gm. per 100 ml. per day.[220] A substantial hemoglobin rise should be observed at approximately 3 weeks after beginning iron therapy. The failure to achieve a level of at least 11 gm. per 100 ml. in this period with adequate iron therapy indicates that the diagnosis of anemia on a purely nutritional basis is to be questioned and suggests the continuation of an infectious process, underlying renal abnormality, continued blood loss, or impaired absorption.

It is unwise to increase the dosage in refractory cases, for it is theoretically possible to induce hemosiderosis by indiscriminate administration of excessve amounts of parenteral iron. Iron given parenterally is stored, and a maximum daily excretion of only 1 mg. compels selectivity of patients and control of treatment by this route.

ADJUVANTS TO IRON THERAPY. Adjuvants to iron are unnecessary in the treatment of iron-deficiency anemia. It is unnecessary to add copper, molybdenum, cobalt supplements, vitamin $B_{12}$, or folic acid in treatment of iron-deficiency anemia. Since iron is absorbed in the ferrous form, the reduction of ferric salts to the bivalent form depends upon reducing mechanisms present in the small intestine. Moore and associates[136] demonstrated that the ingestion of vitamin C with ferric salts resulted in an increase in serum iron, probably by its reducing action. On the other hand, in a study of children of school age Schulze and Morgan,[173] employing soluble ferric pyrophosphate and small supplements of copper, found that the addition of ascorbic acid was unnecessary for the synthesis of hemoglobin.

Notwithstanding the diverse opinions with regard to ascorbic acid, Brise and Hallberg[24] found that ascorbic acid, when given in sufficient amounts, increased the absorption of ferrous iron and that the absorption-promoting effect increased with increasing amounts of ascorbic acid. The absorption-promoting effect of ascorbic acid is mainly due to its reducing action within the gastrointestinal tract, preventing or delaying formation of insoluble or less dissociated ferric compounds.

*Cobalt* has been advocated in the treatment of of anemia because of the known development of polycythemia when it is fed to experimental animals. Plasma from animals injected with cobaltous chloride rapidly develops a high titer of erythropoietin.[70] Cobalt is an essential element in vitamin $B_{12}$ (cyanocobalamin). Despite these considerations and reported beneficial results in the treatment of anemia associated with renal disease,[64] cobalt has been effective as a therapeutic agent in patients with iron-deficiency anemia, hypoplastic anemia, and other instances of bone marrow failure.[147] Of even greater concern is its possible toxicity in some patients, producing a goitrogenic effect in young infants,[104] hence the danger of recommending cobalt alone or cobalt with iron for clinical use.

*Copper* is normally found in the blood in both the plasma and the red corpuscles. Serum copper increases in pregnancy, infection, and iron deficiency. In adult males the concentration of copper in the serum is 105 $\mu$g per 100 ml. with the standard deviation of $\pm 16$.[107] In normal infants beyond 8 months of age the serum copper values are elevated. The range from 140 to 200 $\mu$g per 100 ml. is evidence of iron depletion during infancy.[101]

Experimental studies have shown that copper plays a role in the absorption and utilization of iron.[221] With serious depletion of copper not only is iron absorption impaired but also erythropoiesis is decreased and the defective erythrocytes that are produced have a shortened survival.[220]

In spite of the striking evidences of anemia in copper-deficient experimental animals, the usefulness of copper in the therapy of anemia in man has still to be demonstrated.[220] Copper is known to exist as an impurity in the therapeutic iron salts. It is of interest that processed baby foods such as strained beef liver and cereals and, to a lesser extent, fruits and vegetables possess the highest levels of copper. These foods are certainly sufficient to ensure the infant's daily requirement of copper of 0.05 mg. per kilogram of body weight per day.[92] The major portion of copper in the plasma is found in the $A_2$ globulin ceruloplasmin.

*Transfusions.* With the availability of suitable iron preparations for oral and parenteral administration, transfusions are left for the infant with a hemoglobin level of about 4 gm. per 100 ml. or less who is debilitated from an infection, especially when signs of cardiac dysfunction are present. In these instances packed red cells and not whole blood should be employed for a transfusion. With such severe grades of anemia, hospitalization is safer than ambulatory treatment.

Partial exchange transfusion has been recommended in the management of a severely anemic child under two circumstances.[154] One is in the case of a surgical emergency when a final hemoglobin of 9 to 10 gm. per 100 ml. should be attained to permit safe anesthesia. The other is when anemia is associated with congestive heart failure, in which case it is sufficient to raise the hemoglobin to 4 to 5 gm. per 100 ml. to correct the immediate anoxia. Rapid correction of the severe anemia (in the case cited, an infant with a hemoglobin of 1.8 gm. per 100 ml. presented with an intussusception) could not be carried out by simple transfusion without the risk of precipitating cardiac failure. Partial exchange transfusion was accomplished by the use of sedimented red cells with the alternate removal of the patient's anemic blood and administration of donor blood. To expedite attainment of the desired hemoglobin level at the end of the procedure, the exchange was completed by administering an excess of donor blood to the patient.

**Anemia of the premature infant.** The tendency of the premature infant to develop lower hemoglobin levels as compared with the full-term infant results from the impact of similar factors, which are exaggerated in the premature infant. The differences between the anemia of prematurity and the physiologic anemia of the full-term infant are quantitative. The premature infant is subject to two phases of anemia, one early and the other late. The early anemia is present at the end of the neonatal decline; the late anemia dates from that period in the first year when the iron stores are exhausted. In both the premature and full-term infant the initial period is one of declining hemoglobin levels due to the decreased rate of hemoglobin synthesis. Both subsequently undergo a stage of hemoglobin regeneration from reutilization of iron released from the destroyed red cells. The late anemia in the premature infant is one of iron deficiency, when exogenous iron is not in adequate supply to meet the demands of growth. Characteristic in the premature infant are the more accelerated drop and the lower levels of hemoglobin which are obtained in the postnatal period as compared with the steadier and more prolonged drop in the hemoglobin level in the full-term infant. In the premature infant, erythropoietic activity begins, therefore, at 5 to 7 weeks of age, which is earlier, by a month or more, than in the full-term infant.

The relatively lower initial hemoglobin mass at birth of the premature infant, the decreased synthesis of hemoglobin in the first weeks of life, and the very rapid growth and expansion of blood volume constitute the fundamental factors involved in the pathogenesis of the anemia. A decreased life-span in the erythrocytes of the premature infant has also been cited as a cause of the more exaggerated drop of the hemoglobin in the initial phase,[168,170] but more extensive data are needed with regard to this factor.

*Management.* The greater tendency of iron deficiency in the premature infant prompts a consideration of the most favorable time for iron supplementation. Most premature infants exhaust iron stores (derived from the hemoglobin mass at birth) by the fourth month of life.[168] Seip and Halvorsen[174] found little or no stainable iron in the bone marrow of the premature infant immediately after birth and a marked increase between 4 and 8 weeks of age. Iron stores decreased until finally no hemosiderosis could be demonstrated at 6 to 12 weeks of age. In the full-term infant, on the contrary, the bone marrow did not become hemosiderin-free until 16 to 20 weeks of age. It is questionable whether it is necessary to administer iron prophylactically to premature infants during the postnatal period of declining hemoglobin and red cell values when the bone marrow is nonreactive and when iron from degraded hemoglobin is being conserved. Available evidence indicates that iron administered soon after birth fails to retard the postnatal drop in hemoglobin but does reveal its effectiveness in infants with higher values from the third to the fourth month. Essentially, the same results are observed when iron is given by injection. When iron-dextran (Imferon) was given intramuscularly over a period of 2 to 4 days during the second or third week of life, a significant increase in hemoglobin was not observed until the infant was 3 months of age. The iron administered by this method accelerates the recovery of the early anemia and prevents the late (iron-deficiency) anemia.[53,83]

In a group of premature infants in whom the diet was supplemented in the early weeks with a formula containing 12 mg. of elemental iron per quart, accelerated recovery from early low hemoglobin concentration was noted.[72] These values were significantly higher than for infants not so fed. These studies demonstrate the ability of the infant to absorb and to utilize iron from fortified milk for hemoglobin synthesis. Early routine administration of elemental iron to all premature infants, without depending on the ingestion of a specified quantity of milk, will achieve the same results. It should be remembered that, in any case, iron therapy does not alter the initial physiologic drop in hemoglobin but hastens recovery from early low values when iron contained in the initial circulating hemoglobin mass reaches exhaustion.

For prophylaxis a daily dose of 15 mg. of elemental iron to be administered in a small quantity of milk is prescribed on discharge from the hospital. A dosage of 30 to 45 mg. of elemental iron given from 2 months should protect the majority of premature infants from iron-deficiency anemia and allow for iron storage. In instances in which iron deficiency already exists, the dosage is increased to 60 to 90 mg. daily. The iron is given in divided doses according to the principles outlined for iron-deficiency anemia in the full-term infant. In most premature infants iron should be continued for several months after the hemoglobin concentration has returned to normal to ensure adequate stores. Periodic hemoglobin determinations are required to assure the maintenance of normal blood values. Prophylaxis by means of parenteral iron (iron-dextran) may be advisable before discharge from the hospital, when it is anticipated that oral administration will be unreliable. The dosage in this case is 100 mg. of parenteral iron.

The management outlined for the premature infant also applies in cases of multiple births. In instances in which the hemoglobin level drops to 7 gm. per 100 ml. or less between 3 and 6 weeks of age, transfusions are required, especially when the infant is listless, eats poorly, and is not gaining weight. It should be mentioned, however, that besides the known complications of transfusions there is the possibility that repeated administration of blood may suppress inherent hematopoiesis at a time when the bone marrow may have become responsive.

*Iron transport—serum iron and iron-binding capacity.* Recent studies dealing with the metabolism of iron with respect to the phases of absorption, transport, and storage have provided another diagnostic tool in characterizing an anemia based on iron deficiency. Iron entering the plasma is derived from heme pigments, from body stores, and from gastrointestinal absorption. It is transported in the plasma in combination with a specific protein, a $beta_1$ globulin, variously designated as metal-combining globulin, siderophilin, or transferrin, the movement of which is responsible for the redistribution of iron in the body. This protein carries two iron atoms in the ferric state. In the process of iron turnover the transferrin delivers the metal to the liver, spleen, or bone marrow either for storage in a labile iron pool or for hemoglobin synthesis and erythropoiesis. Iron is stored both as ferritin and as hemosiderin, which are equally available for use in erythropoiesis. Ferritin is soluble and not visible in the tissues, whereas hemosiderin (a polymer of ferritin) is insoluble and is easily discerned as golden granules when unstained or as blue granules after staining with potassium ferrocyanide. The major portion of iron leaving the plasma is normally directed toward the bone marrow where it is used for hemoglobin synthesis.[18]

Several methods have been described by which iron enters immature erythrocytes in the bone marrow. Electron microscopy has demonstrated the passage of iron from ferritin and transferrin of central reticular cells (nurse cells) in erythroblastic islands to surrounding rows of erythroblasts.[14] In other words, the marrow reticulum cells contribute a significant fraction of the iron necessary for hemoglobinization of erythroid cells. Others[95,100] have shown that during the process of iron transfer, the iron-transferrin complex adheres to the surface of the reticulocyte. This attachment permits the active removal of the metal from the transferrin and its incorporation into the red cells. The displaced transferrin reenters the plasma, where in the course of its circulation more iron is acquired from storage sites, enabling it to repeat this cycle once more.

Normally, transferrin is about one third saturated, the bound fraction representing the segment linked to iron as serum iron. The unsaturated or latent capacity of this protein to combine with additional iron is subject to measurement. Serum iron is defined as the acid-soluble iron in the serum, the latent (unsaturated) iron-binding capacity is defined as that amount of additional iron capable of being bound by the unsaturated protein in serum. The total iron-binding capacity represents the sum of these two components. The percentage of saturation represents the percentage of iron-binding protein that is saturated with iron and is calculated by dividing the serum iron by the total iron-binding capacity. The total iron-binding capacity constitutes in effect an indirect estimate of the circulating iron-binding protein.

The normal metabolism of iron for hemoglobin synthesis requires a daily turnover of six to ten times the amount of serum iron so that the transport nature of the protein is clear. The single beta-globin found in almost all sera was designated as C, the faster moving variant observed in Caucasians was named type B, and the slower variant observed in Negroes was named type D.[13] There are at least seventeen transferrin variants, all separated by their mobilities in starch-gel electrophoresis. Transferrin C is by far the most frequent in all population studies.[186]

*Iron absorption.* Granick[74,75] has suggested that iron is absorbed by the mucosal cells of the duodenum in the ferrous form and stored there as ferritin. Upon entering the mucosal cells, the iron apparently is oxidized to the ferric form and, as ferric hydroxide, polymerizes and is attached in micelles or clusters to the colorless, iron-free protein apoferritin. It is this iron-containing form that is known as ferritin. The ferritin molecule consists of a central nucleus of high iron content surrounded by a shell of protein, somewhat spherical in shape.[140] The molecular weight of apoferritin is 465,000. A mucosal block against excessive absorption is said to occur when the available apoferritin is fully saturated with iron. In the presence of an anemia it has been postulated that the relative tissue anoxemia creates a greater reducing tendency in the intestinal mucosal cells. The conversion of the ferric iron present as a ferritin to circulating ferrous iron is thereby enhanced. This ferrous iron then rapidly attaches itself to the iron-binding protein transferrin, where it is converted to the ferric form. An additional amount of apoferritin is thus made available, and iron is once again absorbed through the intestinal mucosa.

According to this concept, control of iron absorption is mediated through the intestinal mucosa which can refuse or accept iron, depending upon the state of the stores. Evidence has been increasingly available that in patients with refractory anemia, pernicious anemia in relapse, hemolytic anemia, and hemochromatosis, the mucosal block does not prevent iron from being absorbed, in spite of adequate body iron stores.[4,50] Such data throw doubt upon ferritin and the mucosal cell as sole regulators of iron absorption and demonstrate that the mucosal block to iron absorption is only relatively complete.[31]

Mazur and associates[123,124] have shown that, when transferrin-bound iron is incubated with liver slices, adenosine triphosphate (ATP) and ascorbic acid mediate the transfer of iron to ferritin. ATP is thought to stimulate the oxidation of ascorbic acid in the presence of iron. This reaction reduces the plasma-bound ferric iron to the ferrous state, thus releasing iron from its protein bond and making it available for incorporation into ferritin. They have also demonstrated[76,125] the close relationship existing between purine and iron metabolism that is mediated through liver xanthine oxidase. They have shown that, with oxidation of hypoxanthine and xanthine to uric acid, ferric-ferritin is reduced to ferrous-ferritin, a step before the transport of iron from the liver. Xanthine oxidase acts as the oxidizing and reducing agent for these reactions. A case of xanthinuria and hemochromatosis has been reported[9] in an adult in which a postulated failure of xanthine oxidase to reduce ferric-ferritin to ferrous-ferritin existed. In this case assay of liver tissue revealed a marked decrease in xanthine oxidase activity.

Further support for the hypothesis that the release of iron from ferritin stores in the liver is mediated by the enzyme xanthine oxidase comes from studies in the experimental animal. The fact that the fetal and newborn rat is able to store iron from maternal serum is explained by the absence of hepatic xanthine oxidase and an associated high liver ferritin iron content. As soon after birth as hepatic xanthine oxidase activity increases, the liver ferritin iron content is simultaneously decreased.[122]

On the other hand, a xanthine-oxidase inhibitor, allopurinol, in three-dose schedules in normal subjects showed no effect on iron absorption.[46] This study also provided indirect evidence that the ferritin-oxidase system is not of major importance in the mucosal control of iron absorption. Allopurinol is a potent inhibitor of xanthine oxidase, the enzyme that catalyzes the oxidation of hypoxanthine to xanthine and xanthine to uric acid. Inhibition of xanthine oxidase might conceivably affect iron metabolism because the ferritin-xanthine oxidase system has been proposed as a mechanism for the mobilization of iron from the liver and intestinal mucosa. According to this hypothesis, reduction of ferric to ferrous ferritin is linked to the oxidation of xanthine by xanthine oxidase. This study does not, however, contribute information about the effect of the drug on the mobilization of iron from the liver.

In another study, oral and intravenous ferrokinetic studies were carried out in patients with gout or hyperuricemia to determine the effect of allopurinol on iron absorption.[22] Allopurinol had no measurable effect on iron metabolism.

The half-life of the iron-binding protein transferrin varies, probably from 8 to 10 days.[8] The iron-binding protein is probably a true carrier of iron, similar to the role of hemoglobin with respect to oxygen. With starch block electrophoresis it had been demonstrated that there were at least eight genetically controlled variants of human transferrins, differing in electrophoretic mobility.[197] Transferrin, thus, is not a single molecular entity but represents a species of protein. The eight transferrins represent allelomorphic genes at a single locus. These are all antigenically related and bind and deliver iron in equivalent fashion. Deficiency of transferrin has also been reported in a child who showed a hypochromic microcytic anemia and yet whose tissues had excessive iron deposits. This case was characterized by a decreased level of iron-binding protein in the parents and its absence in the child.[87]

That the duodenum is the most important site of gastrointestinal absorption of iron has been demonstrated by histochemical studies for guinea pigs, chemical analysis of tissues from guinea pigs, feeding studies in dogs, and with the use of everted duodenal pouches from rats. More distal intestinal segments (jejunum and ileum) do not appear to function as well with respect to iron absorption.[57] In one study, however, in dogs in which the duodenum had been removed, no significant decrease in iron absorption was observed.

Other intestinal areas must, therefore, also participate in this process.[51]

The erythropoietic labile pool receives a major portion (70 to 90%) of iron leaving plasma in a normal person, or 37 mg. a day. Approximately 23 mg. go into hemoglobin in erythrocytes and 14 mg. return to plasma. Iron from destroyed erythrocytes also approximates 23 mg. per day and reenters the labile pool.[57] Reticuloendothelial cells serve both to process iron from the heme moiety of nonviable erythrocytes by returning part to plasma transferrin and by retaining nearly half of the iron for at least 12 days. The degree of retention is not affected by the plasma iron but by the iron requirements of the erythroid marrow. The spleen releases its iron more rapidly to the plasma than does the liver.[145]

The main flow of iron normally takes place from plasma to marrow to erythrocytes and, following their destruction, back to the plasma. Other factors, such as intestinal absorption, storage exchange, and extracellular fluid exchange, play a smaller role, accounting for less than 10% of the daily amount going to the marrow. The extent of marrow uptake of iron correlates well in proportion to the degree of incorporation of $^{59}$Fe into newly formed red blood cells.[150] More iron goes to the bone marrow than the 20 to 25 mg. needed each day for hemoglobin synthesis. Normally, losses of iron from the body are small and range from 0.5 to 1 mg., mainly from the stool, urine, and sweat.[129]

The biochemical mechanisms that control iron absorption remain unknown.[135] Increasing evidence suggests than an active transfer system exists for transporting iron across the mucosal cells to the plasma and that this system is influenced to some extent both by the amount of iron in tissues and by the rate of erythropoiesis. The intestinal mucosa could still exert an important effect on iron metabolism, not through a ferritin-mediated mucosal block but by variations in the activity of the absorptive mechanism. To summarize, the quantity of iron absorbed from the gastrointestinal canal is influenced by several factors: the quantity ingested, the body iron content, the rate of erythropoiesis, and the presence or absence of anemia.[129] Anemia per se can have a marked effect on the absorption of iron that is independent of the effects of alterations in the rate of erythropoiesis and the body iron content.[130]

In refractory anemias associated with erythroid hyperplasia, absorption is increased as compared with subjects with comparable degrees of anemia but having erythroid hypoplasia. A combination of several factors probably have additive effects on absorption. Thus, a greater increase in iron absorption occurs in the presence of anemia and accelerated erythropoiesis then when either of these factors alone is present.[58] Similarly, absorption is much increased in those hemolytic processes associated with ineffective erythropoiesis (i.e., thalassemia major).[57] (For ferrokinetics and erythrokinetics, see Chapter 11.)

Intestinal absorption of iron is increased three to four times during the first days of exposure to high altitudes. During this period red cell precursors are markedly hyperactive. In contrast, iron absorption is decreased during descent from high altitudes coincidental with a depression of bone marrow activity. The stimulus for intestinal absorption of iron is related to the greater or smaller erythropoietic demand associated with changing red cell production.[157]

Except for local factors within the intestine (phosphates, phytates), the state of iron stores and the rate of erythropoiesis are major factors in the control of iron absorption.[19] Absorption is increased when the erythroid marrow is hyperactive (hemorrhage, hemolytic anemia) or when iron stores are depleted (iron deficiency). Contrariwise, absorption of iron is reduced when iron stores are increased and when erythropoiesis is depressed as in the plethora produced by transfusion.

Jacobs and co-workers[94] have shown that, in anemic subjects with reduced gastric acidity, iron absorption is significantly lower than in those with normal gastric acidity. In a study of sixteen normal subjects and twenty patients with iron-deficiency anemia, absorption in the latter group was significantly below normal levels. In spite of such studies, it has never been necessary to administer hydrochloric acid in iron-deficiency anemia in pediatric practice.

Crosby and co-workers[39,209] have demonstrated that the iron content of the epithelial cell is important in the regulation of its ability to absorb iron. The mechanism by which unneeded iron is rejected by the intestinal mucosa and of changes in iron-deficient subjects has recently been clarified with the use of autoradiographs of the small intestine. Conrad and Crosby[38] suggested that ferritin in mucosal cells not only impedes iron absorption but serves an excretory function as well. In normal iron-replete subjects the mucosal cells may contain a variable amount of iron supplied from the body stores. This deposit regulates, within limits, the quantity of iron that can enter the cell from the intestinal lumen. As the columnar epithelial cells of the duodenal villi are formed, they incorporate a portion of the intrinsic iron from the body's iron store. With iron excess these cells are saturated with intrinsic iron, thus preventing the cell from accepting dietary iron. Bound iron is subsequently lost when epithelial cells are sloughed at the end of the life cycle. In iron deficiency the receptor system is inactive or diminished so that early entry of dietary iron into the body is relatively uninhibited. Iron sequestered in the columnar epithelial cells of the duodenal villi serves, therefore, as a means to frustrate the absorption of iron when it is not needed. Sequestration occurs in the villous epithelium of the duodenum and jejunum. The iron is accepted by these absorptive cells, but not all of it is allowed to pass into the animal's body. A portion is retained, and when the villous cells are desquamated, the iron is lost in the intestine.[41] The intestinal iron content is, in turn, closely controlled by the plasma iron turnover. For instance, following blood loss, as marrow activity increases, the change in plasma iron turnover reduces the intestinal content of iron and absorption is increased.[209]

Bothwell[16] summarizes the factors involved in iron absorption according to the following principles: absorption is increased in iron deficiency anemia and also in nonanemic subjects with decreased iron stores. When iron stores are increased there is a corresponding reduction in absorption. It therefore appears as if the rate of iron absorption is modified in a way calculated to maintain optimal body stores. It is likely that wide variations in absorption which occur in each individual reflect differences in their storage iron status. A second factor influencing mucosal behavior is the rate of erythropoiesis. There is an increase in iron absorption when erythropoiesis is actively stimulated, while the opposite occurs when erythropoiesis is depressed. Clinically this occurs more commonly in thalassemia in which a large proportion of the marrow activity is ineffective in terms of the production of viable red cells. This is a plausible explanation for iron overload in some subjects with long-standing hemolytic anemias.

Iron transfer across the mucosal cell is part of an active metabolic process. In this process a portion of the iron taken up by the mucosal cells is rapidly delivered to the transferrin of plasma. Most of the remaining iron taken up by the mucosal cells is deposited as ferritin. When absorption is enhanced little or no ferritin is formed and iron entering the mucosal cells is rapidly delivered to the plasma. On the other hand, when absorption is depressed the iron is trapped in ferritin and is lost to the body when the mucosal cells exfoliate. It therefore appears as if deviation of iron into ferritin represents a mechanism for preventing excessive absorption from the gut. At the same time it should be stressed, according to Bothwell,[15] that the mechanism is operative only when doses of iron within the physiological range are fed, and it can be easily overwhelmed if larger doses of iron are administered. Thus iron stores and erythropoietic activity influence mucosal behavior.

Despite these definitive observations there is still conflicting evidence as to the role of transferrin in regulating iron absorption. Some have claimed that the level of transferrin saturation plays a major part in regulating iron absorption and that the amount of iron that leaves the mucosal cell and enters the blood appears to be regulated by the unbound iron-binding capacity of the transferrin.[29] Other observations are in conflict and have shown that the level of transferrin saturation is not important in regulating iron absorption from the gastrointestinal tract.[210] These results indicate that, despite complete saturation of transferrin, iron continues to be absorbed.

Intestinal malabsorption of $^{59}$Fe-labeled hemoglobin was measured in children with severe dietary iron deficiency and in iron-replete controls.[101] Absorption was impaired in all iron-deficient children and returned to normal after iron repletion. A decrease in iron-containing or iron-dependent enzymes in the mucosa of iron-deficient subjects may be responsible for a secondary malabsorption phenomenon. The relative malabsorption of iron tends to increase the severity of iron deficiency.

Summarizing these views of iron absorption, Granick[74,75] proposed ferritin-apoferritin as key elements in this process. Ferritin acts as a vehicle for iron absorption and a participant in "mucosal" block. Crosby and associates,[39,209] on the other hand, suggest that ferritin in villous epithelioid cells cannot be released and hence is lost from the body when the cell is sloughed.

**Gastroferrin.** The gastric juice of healthy people contains a high molecular weight iron-binding protein which has been designated as gastroferrin.[47] Normally there is sufficient gastric juice to bind the 15 mg. of iron present in a typical day's diet. This binding substance is not identical with plasma transferrin. The iron-binding protein provides a mechanism whereby dietary iron will remain in solution in the alkaline medium of the duodenum, the site of iron absorption. The relative absence of this substance in patients with hemochromatosis would suggest that it normally acts to inhibit iron absorption. Hence hemochromatosis may be regarded as an inborn error of metabolism in which there is a failure to produce the gastric iron-binding protein.

The concentration of this iron-binding protein, gastroferrin, is considerably reduced in iron-deficiency anemia due to blood loss.[117] When hemoglobin values are restored either by blood transfusion or by normal blood regeneration, gastroferrin levels return to normal. The results support the concept that gastroferrin production is concerned with the regulation of iron absorption in health: normal levels acting to inhibit the absorption of excessive amounts of iron present in the normal diet and reduced levels permitting enhanced absorption of iron in iron deficiency. Hence gastroferrin controls iron absorption by inhibiting its uptake from the lumen of the intestine.

***Iron-binding capacity of plasma in various clinical conditions.*** The level of serum iron reflects the balance between the iron absorbed, the iron utilized for hemoglobin synthesis, the iron released by red cell destruction, and the size of the storage depots. More simply stated, at any particular time, the serum iron concentration represents a precise equilibrium between the iron entering and leaving the circulation.

In persons with iron-deficiency anemia, the depleted stores are represented by a greatly reduced serum iron, a markedly expanded iron-binding capacity, and a very low percentage of saturation. An increase in the total iron-binding capacity may be interpreted as an added facility for transporting this metal and is, therefore, an indication for iron therapy to replenish stores. In patients with acute and chronic infection, the impairment of hemoglobin synthesis is accompanied by a disturbance in erythropoiesis and a diversion of iron to tissue stores.[158,219] Both the serum iron and the latent iron-binding capacity are significantly reduced, but the percentage of saturation is not decreased to the extent noted in patients with iron-deficiency anemia. In patients with disorders in which hemoglobin synthesis and marrow function are depressed as in those with untreated pernicious anemia, hypoplastic anemia, and aplastic anemia, the serum iron is greatly elevated, and the latent iron-binding capacity is reduced and often absent when multiple transfusions have been given. In persons with conditions of iron excess such as the hemolytic anemias, transfusion hemosiderosis, and hemochromatosis, the body iron is markedly increased as a result of the preponderance of red cell destruction over formation and in part from increased iron absorption. When the serum iron is markedly elevated, the latent iron-binding capacity is absent so that the saturation is 100%. As shown in Fig. 21 and Table 16, the examination of the individual patterns occasionally helps in the differentiation of the various anemias and provides an insight into the separate phases of iron metabolism.

Fig. 21 is based on the following average values for serum iron and latent iron-binding capacity, respectively, in micrograms per 100 ml.: for normal children, 122 and 246 µg; iron deficiency, 27 and 472 µg; Cooley's anemia and the hemolytic anemias, 203 and 0 µg. The column for chronic infection represents a typical case in a child, in this instance, with findings of 37 and 200 µg per 100 ml., respectively, and corresponds to the average adult figures given by Cartwright and Wintrobe[28] of 30 and 165 µg per 100 ml. It is of interest that the concentration of serum iron is higher in the morning and lower in the evening. This diurnal variation has been ascribed to the adrenal cortex and to variations in the autonomic nervous system.[20] A high degree of variability exists in adolescents, with respect to serum iron and iron-binding levels. Boys tend to have higher serum iron levels than girls, slightly lower unsaturated iron-binding capacities, and a greater percentage saturation of the circulating transferrins, as well as higher mean hemoglobin levels, hematocrit values, and mean corpuscular hemoglobin concentration.[175]

The sequence of iron depletion proceeds in the following stages: (1) the storage forms of iron (hemosiderin and ferritin) disappear and cannot be demonstrated in the bone marrow and other reticuloendothelial tissues; (2) the level of serum iron decreases and concomitantly the level of iron-binding capacity increases, resulting in decreased percentage of iron saturation. A serum iron saturation of less than 15% is indicative of iron depletion.

The values for serum iron and iron-binding capacity in normal infants and children at various ages are given in Table 17.[183] The iron values noted in the period from 5 to 8 days of age represent a persistence of the finding in

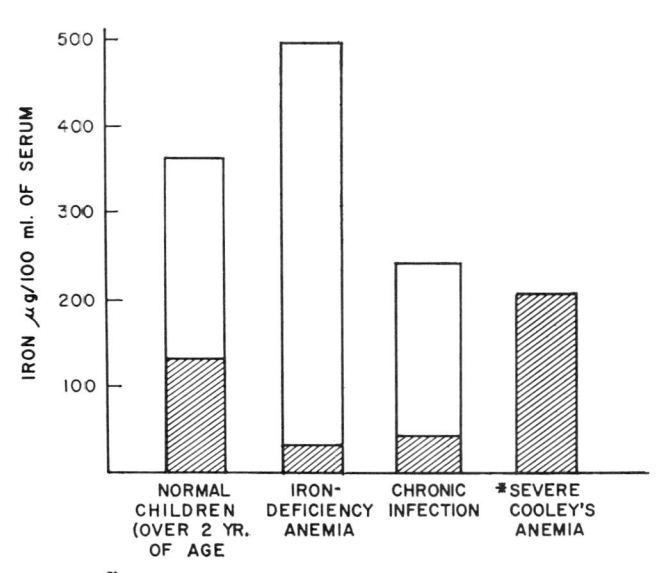

Fig. 21. Schematic representation of specific anemias. Shaded areas represent serum iron and clear areas latent iron-binding capacity. The total iron-binding capacity is the sum of these two fractions. The high serum iron and absent latent iron-binding capacity in patients with the hemolytic anemias are contrasted with the low serum iron and greatly expanded latent iron-binding capacity in those with iron-deficiency anemia.

**Table 16.** Serum iron and iron-binding capacity in various clinical conditions

| Decreased | Increased |
|---|---|
| *Serum iron* | |
| Iron deficiency | Hemolytic diseases |
| Acute and chronic infection | Hemosiderosis (transfusion) |
| Pregnancy | Hemochromatosis |
| Debilitating diseases (uremia, cancer, etc.) | Pernicious anemia (untreated) |
| | Cirrhosis |
| | Acute hepatitis |
| *Latent iron-binding capacity* | |
| Infection | Iron deficiency |
| Hemolytic disease | Pregnancy |
| Debilitating diseases | |
| Cirrhosis | |
| Hepatitis | |
| Pernicious anemia (untreated) | |
| Hemochromatosis ⎫ Absent | |
| Transfusion hemosiderosis ⎭ | |

**Table 17.** Normal values of serum iron and iron-binding capacity* (in micrograms per 100 ml. serum)

| | Serum iron | Latent iron-binding capacity | Total iron-binding capacity | Percentage saturation |
|---|---|---|---|---|
| Adults | 100 | 200 | 300 | 34 |
| Infants | | | | |
| 5-8 days | 148 | 114 | 262 | 65 |
| 1-2 years | 95 | 319 | 414 | 22 |
| Children | | | | |
| 2-6 years | 116 | 279 | 395 | 28 |
| 6-12 years | 127 | 213 | 340 | 38 |

*From Smith, C. H.: Anemias in infancy and childhood; diagnostic and therapeutic considerations, Bull. N. Y. Acad. Med. **30:**155, 1954.

cord blood—i.e., a higher serum iron and lower latent and total iron-binding capacities as compared to normal serum iron and higher latent and total iron-binding capacities in the mother. These findings represent the combined effects of transplacental iron transfer to build up fetal stores and an increased demand for iron in the mother so that she becomes relatively iron deficient. At about the end of the first month, erythropoietic function is gradually resumed, and the movement of stored iron in the direction of the bone marrow results in a low serum iron and high latent and total iron-binding capacities most marked at 2 years of age. This pattern, consistent with an iron-deficiency state despite the absence of anemia, indicates a continuous drain on storage depots.[191] As has been indicated, overt anemia, in which the serum iron shrinks further and the latent iron-binding capacity expands, occurs with rapid growth, dietary deficiency, and other causative factors. In general there is a direct correlation between the concentrations of serum iron and the state of iron storage.

Serum iron and iron-binding determinations may be employed as useful guides in gauging the adequacy and completeness of therapy in patients with iron-deficiency states. Iron administered orally or parenterally in patients with iron-deficiency anemia is utilized quantitatively for hemoglobin synthesis. If iron is administered parenterally only in amounts calculated to restore blood values to normal or if oral therapy is terminated as soon as normal levels are reached, the iron stores remain unreplenished. It is for this reason that iron therapy is continued for 1 or 2 months beyond the period when normal hemoglobin levels are achieved.

Brainton and Finch[10] differentiate between iron deficiency and iron-deficient erythropoiesis. Iron deficiency is regarded as a reduction in total body iron, best measured by the circulating hemoglobin and the hemosiderin within the reticuloendothelial cells of the marrow. Circulating red cells and reticuloendothelial cells represent about 95% of total body iron under normal conditions. Iron-deficient erythropoiesis is defined as a state of inadequacy of iron for optimal erythropoiesis in the developing red cell mass, resulting in a limitation of hemoglobin synthesis. This may occur as a result of depletion in total body iron or through inadequate supply of plasma iron, due either to a block in discharge of iron from the reticuloendothelial cell as occurs in infection or to an absence of circulating transferrin (protein deficiency or nephrosis when transferrin is lost). The relationship between iron supply and erythroid demand is estimated by comparing the serum iron level and percent saturation with percent sideroblasts in the marrow. Better correlation is found when percent saturation (ratio of the serum iron to total iron-binding capacity) is used as an expression of available iron supply. In iron-deficiency anemia, 16% or less saturation of plasma transferrin implies an inadequate supply of iron to the erythroid marrow and is associated in time with hypochromic microcytic anemia. In infection similar depression in transferrin saturation is observed. The best criterion of iron deficient erythropoiesis is the percent saturation of transferrin. The sideroblast count reflects not only iron supply, but also hemoglobin synthesis by the red cells. A discrepancy in sideroblast count from that predicted by the iron supply (percent saturation of transferrin) is a sensitive indication of a block in hemoglobin synthesis.

An interesting finding in a group of women with complaints of chronic fatigue, irritability, and neurasthenia was the observation that a number had hemoglobin levels of more than 12.0 gm. per 100 ml. and a saturation of less than 16% of total iron-binding capacity.[128] In other words, they were considered to be iron deficient without anemia.

**Hemosiderosis and hemochromatosis.** Hemosiderosis refers to excessive iron storage in various tissues of the body without associated tissue damage. Hemochromatosis is the term applied not only to a widespread increase in storage iron but also to resultant tissue damage.[60] The clinical and pathologic changes associated with excessive dietary intake of iron among Bantu suffering from malnutrition (cytosiderosis)[67] and with the deposition of iron due to multiple blood transfusions (transfusion hemosiderosis) may not always be distinguishable from those of classic hemochromatosis (bronze diabetes, pigment cirrhosis). The latter, a disease predominantly of middle-aged men, is characterized by cirrhosis of the liver, diabetes, skin pigmentation, hypogonadism, and congestive heart failure. The underlying defect in this disease is a disturbance in the normal mechanism of the intestinal mucosa for preventing unnecessary iron absorption, so that excessive quantities of iron are absorbed regardless of saturated body stores.[31] During the initial phase of excessive iron absorption, the plasma iron is elevated and the liver and reticuloendothelial tissues show an increased iron content. Eventually the liver becomes the chief site of iron storage.[60]

The widespread incidence of tissue siderosis in the adult Bantu population of South Africa is of great interest.[17] Judging from the findings in the liver and spleen, siderosis first becomes manifest in late adolescence and reaches its greatest degree in the forties. It has been related to an abnormally high absorption of iron from the intestine. Although maize and other foodstuffs consumed by the Bantu contain moderate amounts of iron, most of the ingested iron is derived from the iron utensils used in cooking and in the preparation of fermented beverages. It is, however, too difficult to overload animals with iron unless the phosphorus content of the diet is low.[85] In the Bantu (Kaffir) beer, the major source of iron, the phosphorus content is low. Other factors, such as the altered behavior of the bowel mucosa in association with a widespread metabolic defect induced by chronic malnutrition, may also account for the increased absorption of iron. There is a close relation between the iron concentration and histologic findings. With mild degrees of iron overload, iron is usually present only in the parenchymal cells of the liver. With increasing concentrations, iron appears in the Kupffer cells and in the portal tracts. Although the incidence of hepatic fibrosis and cirrhosis in the group is not high (15.6 and 1.4%, respectively), all subjects with iron concentrations above 2% dry weight showed portal fibrosis or cirrhosis. Splenic concentration of iron rises with the liver concentration and sometimes exceeds it.

The livers of thirteen Bantus with hemochromatosis were compared histologically with the livers of thirteen white subjects suffering from idiopathic hemochromatosis.[16] Clearcut differences were found in the cellular localization of iron deposits. In the livers from the Bantu subjects, most of the iron was located in the Kupffer cells and portal tract macrophages, with lesser amounts in the parenchyma. In contrast, the major deposits in subjects with idiopathic hemochromatosis were in the parenchymal cells and little iron was present in portal tract phagocytes. In addition, splenic concentrations of iron were far higher in the Bantu than in the subjects with idiopathic hemochromatosis.

Reports of hemochromatosis apparently resulting from orally administered iron medication are rare.[96] Such a typical case has been reported in an adult who over the period of 10 years had ingested over 1,000 gm. of elemental iron in iron medications together with an assortment of minerals and vitamins.

In patients with refractory anemias such as aplastic anemia, aregenerative anemia (pure red cell aplasia), and chronic hemolytic anemia, iron stores are increased by virtue of multiple transfusions (250 mg. in each 500 ml. of blood), greater iron absorption, and prolonged iron therapy.[208] Nutritional siderosis of the African Bantu and siderosis resulting from excessive parenteral iron therapy fall into the same category so that the complete histopathologic changes similar to classic hemochromatosis eventually develop.[68]

Whether or not hemosiderosis progresses to hemochromatosis is still being debated. Although extensive deposition of iron in tissues is a significant characteristic of hemochromatosis, this alone may not be the sole pathogenic factor in producing tissue changes.[102] In patients with Cooley's anemia, for instance, chronic anemia and tissue hypoxia may constitute the essential factors in the conversion of hemosiderosis to hemochromatosis.[54,91] Finch and Finch[60] state that there are no unique features in idiopathic hemochromatosis by which it can be distinguished pathologically from the terminal stage of other iron storage diseases, such as dietary or transfusion hemochromatosis. Those who are not convinced that excessive body iron is necessarily harmful point out the difficulties of producing the characteristic pattern of tissue damage of hemochromatosis in experimental animals by loading them with iron.[155] They claim that there is still no evidence that the accumulation of excessive iron is necessarily harmful nor that it produces the pathologic picture of idiopathic hemochromatosis. The fact remains, however, that many patients who receive multiple transfusions, as in thalassemia major, do develop an iron storage disease that clinically and pathologically is similar to idiopathic hemochromatosis.

*Diagnostic procedures.* Excessive body iron stores are indicated by an elevation of the plasma iron-binding protein and excessive hemosiderin deposits in the bone marrow. Actual diagnosis is only made by the demonstration of pigmentary cirrhosis of the liver.

Iron-containing macrophages present in various tissues in patients with iron-storage diseases have been demonstrated to pass from the intestinal villus into the intestinal lumen acting to transport iron as well as to store it. It was proposed by Yam and associates[226] that these cells may transport iron from one organ to another and thus might be present in the circulating blood. These were, therefore, sought in buffy coat preparations of venous blood in normal subjects and in patients with hemochromatosis and other iron-storage conditions such as transfusion siderosis. Circulating hemosiderin-containing cells were demonstrated in eight of the nine untreated patients with hemochromatosis and four of twenty with other iron-storage disorders. None were found in normal subjects. The discovery of such cells in the circulating blood suggests an iron-storage disease, although their absence does not exclude such a possibility. The iron-containing cells of patients with hemochromatosis differ from those of patients with transfusional siderosis. In hemochromatosis, the hemosiderin granules are few and small but in transfusion siderosis they are large and confluent. Further experience is needed before it can be known if the types and number of iron-containing leukocytes in the blood buffy coat is of reliable differentiated significance in the diagnosis of the iron-storage diseases.

Harker and co-workers[84] showed that desferrioxamine entered the liver parenchymal cells in which it finds excess storage iron. About two-thirds of the intracellularly formed ferrioxamine passes into the plasma to be excreted via the kidney and about one-third is excreted by way of the bile into the feces. Their data indicate that, when urinary chelate exceeds 4.0 mg., the patient has an excessive load of parenchymal iron. In patients with hemolytic anemia basal values of urinary iron excretion must be obtained, otherwise the high values associated with hemosiderinuria may be interpreted as representing increased stores. The test is ideal for screening and would be expected to reveal parenchymal iron overload before irreversible changes occur. It is now apparent than transferrin-bound iron is not vulnerable to chelate binding. There are now considerable data that indicate that chelate iron is quite independent of the rate of reticuloendothelial iron turnover. Thus chelate excretion does not appear to be related to red cell catabolism. It would appear that desferrioxamine enters the liver cells and there binds iron. In in vivo studies chelated iron is generally decreased in iron deficiency and is increased in patients with increased iron stores. It is possible to differentiate between the two storage sites—reticuloendothelial overload and parenchymal iron overload. The authors showed that patients with only reticuloendothelial iron overload and high plasma iron saturation do not excrete a significant amount of chelate iron. Although there was some correlation between total iron stores and chelate iron excretion, this relationship applied more specifically to liver parenchymal iron than to reticuloendothelial stores. Fecal iron losses with chelate (desferrioxamine) were about 40% of iron found in the urine. It is postulated that iron from both urinary and fecal excretion is derived from iron deposits within liver parenchymal cells.

*Treatment.* Mobilization of iron stores in idiopathic hematochromatosis has been successfully achieved by repeated phlebotomies.[40,60,141] In children having huge iron stores with refractory anemia, such as Cooley's anemia and pure red cell aplasia, the need for maintaining adequate hemoglobin levels precludes the use of this measure. The intravenous injection of chelating agents increases the urinary excretion of iron but until recently has been impractical in treatment of conditions in which massive iron overload exists.[77] Several newer chelating agents are undergoing trial, and one of these, desferrioxamine, has demonstrated its efficacy as a potent iron-binding substance. It is nontoxic and thus far has shown no side effects. It can be given intravenously by drip infusion or, preferably, by intramuscular injection. (For details of dosage, see Chapter 16.) Whether or not reversal of tissue damage will ensue, an important objective in hemochromatosis, awaits prolonged trial. The intravenous injection of chelating agents increases the urinary excretion of iron, but thus far has been impractical in treatment of conditions in which massive iron overload exists.[77] (For a discussion of recent chelating agents, see Chapter 16.)

*Transient dysproteinemia (copper deficiency in infants).* Several groups of infants have been described[108,194,200,201,227] who show pallor, edema, irritability associated with varying grades of hypochromic, microcytic anemia, hypoproteinemia, hypocupremia, and hypoferremia in the first year of life. Hypocupremia in these infants is contrasted with the usual increase in serum copper in those with iron-deficiency anemia. In one group these features were attributed to a primary abnormality in plasma protein marked by an increased rate of plasma protein degradation[201] without a compensatory rate of plasma protein synthesis. In other groups, patients were receiving cow's milk as their sole source of food intake.[108,194] It is probable that two clinical states with differing causes operate in these cases,[227] one with a primary plasma protein deficiency and the other with a nutritional deficiency due to an exclusive milk diet. Improved diet, the corrective effect of copper sulfate, and iron in various infants suggest that recovery occurs spontaneously and is unrelated to iron or copper therapy.[227]

Reviewing this syndrome, Schubert and Lahey[167] observed that iron-deficient infants cannot only be classified into those with and those without hypocupremia and hypoproteinemia, but that intermediate or transitional forms also exist. Hypoalbuminemia or hypocupremia and hypoalbuminemia occurred in infants with varying degrees of iron deficiency. The primary defect that they emphasized was one of iron deficiency, and with gradual development of moderately severe anemia a protein deficient state develops which in turn leads to dysproteinemia and copper deficiency. The role of copper in this syndrome may be incidental or of primary importance.

*Exudative enteropathy.* Hypoproteinemia has also been shown to result not only from excessive rates of protein destruction (hypercatabolic hypoproteinemia) or from a failure of protein synthesis, but also from the loss of plasma protein into the gastrointestinal tract. This process, termed *exudative enteropathy*,[71,198] can be tested by the intravenous injection of $^{131}$I-labeled polyvinylpyrrolidone—a plasma-protein substitute—which, gaining access to the lumen of the gastrointestinal tract, can be measured quantitatively by its radioactivity when excreted in the stool. $^{131}$I-labeled polyvinylpyrrolidone is excreted in the stools of normal subjects to the extent of 0 to 1.5% of the dose and up to 20% in those with exudative enteropathy. Lesions of the gastrointestinal tract may or may not exist. Hypoproteinemia, edema, and iron-deficiency anemia have been described in children with this syndrome. Anemia in these patients, in spite of the absence of gastrointestinal bleeding, is explained on the basis of nonhemoglobin iron lost in the stool.[199]

In addition to the use of [131]I-polyvinylpyrrolidone, intravenously administered albumin labeled with [51]Cr provides a means of demonstrating loss of protein into the gastrointestinal tract. It can also be used to determine the site of gastrointestinal protein loss.[204] Subjects without gastrointestinal disease excrete small amounts of the administered dose (0.06 to 0.63%), while those with enteric protein loss excrete 4.2 to 21% in the 4-day fecal excretion period.[107] The rapid disappearance from the blood of intravenously administered [131]I-albumin has also been demonstrated in patients in whom protein-losing enteropathy was proved by other techniques.[205]

Waldman and his associates[206] claim that this syndrome consisting of edema, anemia, hypoalbuminemia, eosinophilia, and growth retardation, is consistent with the concept of gastrointestinal allergy as a causative factor. They suggest that this syndrome may be attributable to an abnormal response of the gastrointestinal tract to certain dietary constituents, especially milk, and that this condition is distinct from gluten sensitive enteropathy. There was a distinct amelioration of the clinical symptoms and the disorders of protein metabolism in the three patients studied on an elimination diet. The presence of precipitating antibodies to milk in the serum, the clinical manifestations of allergy such as asthma, eczema, and persistent rhinitis, and the favorable response to the administration of corticosteroids were all regarded as consistent with allergy. The term *allergic gastroenteropathy* was suggested for this clinical syndrome.

According to another theory,[148] "protein losing enteropathy" should simply mean an increased leak of protein into the intestine. Like steatorrhea, it is a manifestation of many different diseases. Many patients with idiopathic hypoproteinemia and protein-losing enteropathy have a structural abnormality of the small bowel wall. This abnormality is characterized chiefly by dilatation of small lymphatics and has been termed *intestinal lymphangiectasia*. A child originally regarded as a case of idiopathic hypoproteinemia was shown later to have a protein-losing enteropathy, steatorrhea, and an abnormal small bowel histology with dilated lymphatic spaces and partial villous atrophy. If the anemia is moderately severe, whole blood is given.

Parfitt[148] found that three members of a sibship had neonatal edema due to hypoproteinemia. Two were shown to have an increased protein exudation and one had a structural abnormality of the small bowel.

In recent years the concept expressed by the terms *exudative enteropathy* and *protein-losing gastroenteropathy* has been extended to pathologic areas other than just the loss of plasma proteins exclusively into the gastrointestinal tract.[106] The loss of protein involving albumin predominantly may be the principal factor in the development of edema and hypoproteinemia. A variety of diverse disorders are now classified in the category of protein-losing enteropathy. The disorders include those in which the primary site of enteric involvement can be more or less designated and those in which precise localization has not been defined—e.g., agammaglobulinemia, nephrosis, and anorexia nervosa. Increasing evidence has demonstrated that many conditions heretofore ascribed to excess destruction of proteins are really loss from the body and the intestine.

Strober and co-workers[189] described four patients with protein-losing enteropathy, hypoalbuminemia, and lymphocytopenia secondary to tricuspid regurgitation and rheumatic heart disease. Following medical treatment in two patients, right atrial pressure declined and both protein loss and lymphocytopenia were ameliorated. It was suggested that patients with rheumatic tricuspid regurgitation and other patients with cardiac disease associated with protein-losing enteropathy have a secondary intestinal lymphangiectasia resulting from systemic venous and lymphatic hypertension. The lymphangiectasia leads to loss of protein-rich and lymphocyte-rich lymph into the gastrointestinal tract. The protein loss leads to hypoproteinemia, and lymphoctye loss presumably explains the immunologic deficiency. Hypoalbuminemia secondary to loss of serum protein into gastrointestinal tract is a rare accompaniment of cardiac disease. In several patients with constrictive pericarditis and associated protein-losing enteropathy, the lymphatics of the small bowel were markedly dilated. The venous hypotension causes an obstruction to normal lymph drainage, resulting in lymphatic hypertension as well as an increase in lymph production. Elevated central venous pressure is an important pathophysiologic mechanism in cardiac disease with protein-losing enteropathy. Thus tricuspid regurgitation appears to be a newly recognized cardiac cause of protein-losing enteropathy. As in patients with intestinal lymphangiectasia, the protein leak may be associated with lymphocytopenia and immunologic deficiency.

Wilson and colleagues[218] in another study showed that occasionally the ingestion of homogenized milk by infants may lead to a sufficient loss of intestinal blood to produce a hypochromic microcytic anemia. The substitution of a soybean diet or a heat-processed cow's milk diet will reduce fecal blood loss.

Copper is bound to an $alpha_2$-globulin, ceruloplasmin. Wilson's disease (cirrhosis of the liver, degeneration of the lenticular nucleus in the brain, and pigmentation of the cornea in the form of smoky-grown or grey-green ring) has been associated with a quantitative deficiency of the plasma ceruloplasmin. Almost all patients with Wilson's disease have less than 20 mg. of ceruloplasmin per ml. of serum, whereas normal people have from 20 to 35 mg. per 100 ml.[166] Wilson's disease is, therefore, an inborn error of metabolism in which ceruloplasmin synthesis is deficient.

*Acute iron intoxication.* The accidental ingestion of large doses of medicinal iron preparations, usually ferrous sulfate tablets, results in a fairly characteristic set of clinical features,[3,43,61,196] with a mortality of 50%.[33] Early symptoms include vomiting, diarrhea, dehydration, and the local effects due to the corrosive action of the metal on the stomach and other areas of the intestinal tract. Later evidences of severe and often irreversible cardiovascular collapse, shock, and coma may be associated with the marked increases in plasma iron. Postmortem examination reveals dilatation of the right heart, pulmonary congestion, hemorrhagic and necrotizing gastritis, cloudy swelling, and areas of hemorrhage in the lungs, brain, kidneys, and liver.

Treatment of iron poisoning is largely symptomatic, consisting of forced vomiting and prolonged and copious gastric lavage with sodium bicarbonate solution.[33] Sisson and Bronson[181] have advocated gastric lavage with 20% disodium phosphate dihydrate and intravenous administration of calcium disodium versenate. Blood volume and blood pressure are supported with solutions of glucose, saline, or appropriate electrolytes. Shock is treated with blood, plasma, and oxygen.

Desferrioxamine (Desferal), an iron-complexing agent employed in diseases associated with the pathologic iron deposition in tissues, is valuable in the treatment of acute iron poisoning in children. A combination of oral and intravenous desferrioxamine is the best form of therapy for acute iron poisoning. To counteract the toxic effect of excessive iron ingested, 5 to 12 gm. of this chelating agent dissolved in distilled water (10 ml. per 2 gm. of the drug) are immediately given by stomach tube[132,213] to neutralize the iron in the gastrointestinal tract. In addition, to counteract the toxic effect of the excessive iron absorbed, 500 to 2,000 mg. of desferrioxamine[132,213] is infused immediately.

Varying dosages of the drug are also currently given. Two cases of iron intoxication due to ferrous gluconate and ferrous sulfate ingestion in 14-month-old children were successfully treated with desferrioxamine.[88,165] The dosage of desferroxamine in one was 92 mg. per kilogram, given intravenously (800 mg. in 20 ml. of water) on three occasions at 12-hour intervals after an initial oral dose of 5 gm. (suspended in 200 ml. of isotonic saline solution given through a nasogastric tube). In the other case, 2 hours after ingestion of ten ferrous sulfate tablets (0.3 gm. tablet) 3,000 mg. of desferrioxamine dissolved in 200 ml. of isotonic saline solution was introduced through a gastric tube. Another 800 mg. of the same drug was given in a continuous intravenous drip for the first 24 hours. This was followed for the next 2 days by daily intramuscular injections of an additional 1,000 mg. in divided doses.

Additional studies in both animal experiments[212] and in the treatment of acute iron ingestion with desferrioxamine in children[127] have demonstrated the value of this drug. In the latter report of acute iron poisoning in twenty children, the stomach was initially emptied by vomiting induced by an emetic (15 ml. syrup of ipecac) followed by lavage with sodium bicarbonate solution. Five to 10 gm. of desferrioxamine is placed in the stomach before removing the lavage tube. Intravenous fluid therapy is initiated to correct acidosis and dehydration. If shock is present on admission, plasma or whole blood is given. Desferrioxamine is then given in the amount of 90 mg. per kg. body weight in 100 ml. of 5% aqueous dextran solution by intravenous drip over a period of 1 to 2 hours. A change of urine color to deep reddish brown indicates high urinary iron and additional desferrioxamine is administered continuously over the next 12 hours. Serial serum iron levels are used to determine the need for additional chelating therapy.

The removal of iron by exchange transfusion has been compared with that following administration of desferrioxamine in dogs with severe iron intoxication.[139] The mean removal of iron by exchange transfusion alone was thirty times greater than the mean urinary iron excretion following administration of desferrioxamine. Treatment of dogs with desferrioxamine did not improve the removal of iron by subsequent exchange transfusion.

It has been emphasized, however, that further studies are essential to establish criteria for determining the quantity of the drug needed to achieve maximum effectiveness and to prevent serious toxicity from the drug itself, notably marked hypotension noted in animal experiments.[214]

**Iron-deficiency anemia in patients with cyanotic congenital heart disease.** In most infants and children with cyanotic congenital heart disease, the bone marrow response to the persistent anoxic stimulus is polycythemia, in which the hemoglobin increase approaches the rise in the erythrocyte count. Occasionally the rise in hemoglobin does not keep pace with the erythrocytosis. Hemoglobin levels of 10 to 13 gm. per 100 ml., erythrocyte counts of 6 to 8 million, and hematocrit levels of 40%, accompanied by complaints of irritability, anorexia, and poor weight gain, have been observed in young patients.[142] Even hemoglobin levels of 16 to 18 gm. per 100 ml. may represent relative anemia in the presence of polycythemic blood levels. The administration of iron results in marked improvement in the clinical and hematologic status.[162] Iron therapy is stopped or decreased when the hematocrit level reaches 75%. Experience has shown that patients with appreciable arterial unsaturation function best with a hematocrit of 55 to 75%. Patients with values lower than these require iron medication.[142]

Although spread over a wide range, the mean platelet count in children with cyanotic congenital heart disease tends to be lower than normal.[78] Those patients with long-standing hypoxia and hemoglobin levels greater than 16.0 gm./100 ml. had the lowest platelet counts. The platelet values related directly to the mean oxygen saturation. Following correction of the cardiac defect, the platelet counts returned to normal.

**Refractory hypochromic anemia (sideroachrestic anemia, sideroblastic anemia, hypochromic iron-loading anemia).** Iron-loading anemia is characterized by the presence of a microcytic, hypochromic anemia in patients who have large iron stores, a high serum iron, and an ability to accumulate iron from the diet at a rapid rate.[42,86,163] The term *sideroachrestic anemia* has been applied to conditions characterized by the association of hypochromic anemia with excessive iron storage. Mollin[133] prefers the designation of *sideroblastic anemia* to the *sideroachrestic anemia* of Heilmeyer. The anemia is not due to blood loss or hemolysis. It is a hereditary hypochromic, hypersideremic anemia refractory to iron, transmitted through the female, affecting male members of a family.[26] The disease is attributed to a disturbance in heme biosynthesis so that anemia develops. Also featured is an accumulation of iron in the bone marrow and in other tissues, with large quantities present in erythroblasts and erythrocytes. While siderocytes and sideroblasts (erythrocytes and normoblasts, respectively, containing iron inclusions) may occur in moderate numbers in normal persons, in this group of refractory iron-loading anemias, these cells contain more iron than normal.[99] The number of sideroblasts is increased, but the iron granules are often strikingly coarse, arranged in a ring immediately around the nucleus of these cells. Patients are occasionally anemic in early childhood,[63] but the disease expresses itself fully in adult life. The blood picture shows anisocytosis, poikilocytosis, microcytosis, and hypochromia. Hepatosplenomegaly may be present. Serum iron is normal or increased, with almost complete saturation of the total iron-binding capacity. The plasma $^{59}$Fe clearance is often rapid. The blood picture resembles that of thalassemia, but fetal hemoglobin is absent and $A_2$ hemoglobin is not elevated. The number of sideroblasts is much greater than in thalassemia. Defective erythropoiesis involved in the pathogenesis of this anemia is attributed to abnormal intermediary metabolism of heme, probably an inability to utilize iron and porphyrin. In the cytoplasm of the erythroblasts the electron microscope reveals appreciable quantities of iron in the form of either ferritin molecules or iron-bearing micelles in the mitochondria.[14] Based on the response to phlebotomy, hypersideremic anemia has been explained as a failure to utilize iron.[42] Hemosiderosis and hemochromatosis are due to the excessive absorption of iron through the mucosal cells of the intestine and into the red cells. Treatment consists of transfusions since there is no response to iron and other hematopoietic agents.

One patient responded to the combined administration of pyridoxine and testosterone, though neither agent given alone was effective. The addition of oral crude liver extract caused further improvement.[65] In some cases improvement is produced by pyridoxine. For the excessive iron overload, chelating agents such as desferrioxamine are worthy of trial. Splenectomy may have a short-lived beneficial effect.[66]

In the differential diagnosis of hypochromic anemia a basic consideration is that an anemia with hypochromic red cells is generally attributable to impaired hemoglobin synthesis at one of several biochemical levels.[161] In iron-deficiency anemia the substrate iron is in poor supply. In hypochromic anemia, sometimes associated with infectious, inflammatory, or other debilitating disease, available iron stores are ineffectively used. The other hypochromic anemias are typically associated with excessive iron stores, often accompanied by iron loading of the mitochondria in red cell precursors. Staining of these cells for iron reveals the "ringed sideroblasts" characteristic of these diseases (i.e., refractory hypochromic anemia). The mitochondria are the sites in which protoporphyrin is chelated with iron by the enzyme heme synthetase. Iron loading suggests that the synthetase of the porphyrin moiety of heme is impaired. Defects in heme biosynthesis have been described in several forms of sideroblastic, hypochromic anemia: in thalassemia the primary defect is one of globin synthesis, but impaired heme production presumably secondary to the underlying abnormality may also be involved. Pyridoxine-responsive anemia appears to be due to depression of delta-aminolevulinic acid synthetase, the mitochondrial enzyme that limits the total rate of heme biosynthesis. The hypochromic anemia of chronic lead intoxication is associated with a number of metabolic abnormalities, including inhibition of several enzymes along the heme biosynthetic pathway. The basophilic material which contributed the stippling is the product of ribosomal agglutination.[161] In the course of the inhibited synthesis of heme two of its precursors, delta-aminolevulinic acid and coproporphyrin, are excreted in large quantity in the urine while there is an increase in free erythrocyte coproporphyrin.

In sideroblastic anemia the defect is in the terminal stage of heme synthesis,[160] that is, in the combination of iron and protoporphyrin to form heme. The erythrocyte porphyrin is high because of the block and the markedly reduced heme synthetase activity. Furthermore, deficient synthesis of heme, the product of the reaction, would explain the development of anemia, a hypochromic red cell population, and the reduction in the activity of erythrocyte catalase, a heme enzyme.

While in cases of hypersideremic anemia the marrow and hepatic reticulum cells are loaded with iron and sideroblasts are abundant, two siblings have been reported with a refractory, chronic, hypochromic, microcytic anemia, in which massive hepatic iron deposition was present but with absent stainable bone marrow iron stores.[178] In these cases iron infusion did not significantly increase bone marrow iron stores. The abnormality is probably a congenital lesion in which insufficient iron is delivered to the erythroid marrow rather than underutilization of iron and ineffective erythropoiesis.

A case of chronic hypochromic anemia has also been reported in a 15-year-old boy who was unresponsive to iron therapy. The serum iron was elevated and iron-binding capacity was completely saturated. Serum copper, pyridoxine, and vitamin $B_{12}$ concentrations were normal. Hypochromia, microcytosis, and a normoblastic marrow with a low iron content were present. The case was interpreted as a disturbance in hemoglobin synthesis, possibly related to impaired porphyrin metabolism.[63]

In a recent review of this syndrome, the term "sideroblastic anemia" has been applied to a large number of conditions characterized by a high serum iron,[133] a hyperplastic bone marrow with erythroblastic preponderance, and increased numbers of "ring form" sideroblasts. In these cells the iron granules are more or less concentrically situated about the nucleus. Dameshek[45] lists the current designations for this condition: primary refractory anemia, refractory anemia with hyperplastic marrow, refractory sex-linked hypochromic anemia with a high serum iron, chronic refractory anemia with sideroblastic bone marrow, sideroachrestic anemia, and refractory normoblastic anemia. He regards the first stage of the Di Guglielmo syndrome (a form of neoplasia of the bone marrow, especially of the red cell elements, i.e., erythremic myelosis), as often identical with what is variously known as sideroblastic or sideroachrestic anemia.

The acquired disorder is observed in either sex and usually in older patients. The acquired form is more often normocytic and normochromic or only slightly hypochromic. Lee and co-workers[115] described one such case in an adult with acquired sideroachrestic anemia and metastatic carcinoma of the prostate who possessed the characteristic features of sideroachrestic (sideroblastic) anemia: hypersideremia, abnormal ringed erythroblasts in the bone marrow, hypochromia of the erythrocytes, erythroid hyperplasia of the bone marrow, markedly reduced incorporation of radioiron into erythrocytes, and prominent siderosis of the bone marrow reticulum cells and liver parenchymal cells.

It was suggested that these were defects in the hemoglobin biosynthetic pathway: impaired incorporation of protoporphyrin into hemoglobin and defective delta-aminolevulinic acid synthesis. Pyridoxine had no effect on the former but partially corrected the latter.

In summarizing the sideroblastic anemias, Goldberg[69] regards them as a group of diseases of various etiologies, each with a final pathway of deranged hemesynthesis in the bone marrow. The sideroblastic anemias bear some resemblance to the hepatic porphyrias, which are also a group multifactorial in pathogenesis, each with a final pathway of deranged heme synthesis in the liver.

Pyridoxine-responsive anemia, which resembles sideroblastic anemia in that both manifest a hypochromic anemia, is accompanied by hyperferremia; these will be described on p. 460.

## REFERENCES

1. Afifi, A. M., Banwell, G. S., Bennison, R. J., Boothby, K., Griffiths, P. D., Huntsman, R. G., Jenkins, G. C., Lewin Smith, R. G., McIntosh, J., Qayum, O., Ross Russel, I., and Whittaker, J. N.: Simple test for ingested iron in hospital and domiciliary practice, Brit. Med. J. **1:**1021, 1966.
2. Aksoy, M., Camli, N., and Erdem, S.: Roentgenographic bone changes in chronic iron deficiency; a study of twelve patients, Blood **27:**677, 1966.
3. Aldrich, R. A.: Acute iron toxicity. In Wallerstein, R. O., and Mettier, S. R., editors: Iron in clinical medicine, Los Angeles, 1958, University of California Press.
4. Alper, T., and Savage, D. V.: Radioiron studies in a case of hemochromatosis, J. Lab. Clin. Med. **37:**665, 1951.
5. American Academy of Pediatrics, Committee on Nutrition: Trace elements in infant nutrition, Pediatrics **26:**715, 1960.
6. Andelman, M. B., and Sered, B. R.: Utilization of dietary iron by term infants, Amer. J. Dis. Child. **111:**45, 1966.
7. Anderson, A. F., and Schloss, O. M.: Allergy to cow's milk in infants with nutritional disorders, Amer. J. Dis. Child. **26:**451, 1923.
8. Awai, M., and Brown, E. B.: Studies on the metabolism of human transferrin, J. Lab. Clin. Med. **58:**797, 1961.
9. Ayvazian, J. H.: Xanthinuria and hemochromatosis, New Eng. J. Med. **270:**18, 1964.
10. Bainton, D. F., and Finch, C. A.: The diagnosis of iron deficiency anemia, Amer J. Med. **37:**62, 1964.
11. Barltrop, D.: The prevalence of pica, Amer. J. Dis. Child. **112:**116, 1966.
12. Beal, V. A., Meyers, A. J., and McCammon, R. W.: Iron intake, hemoglobin and physical growth during the first two years of life, Pediatrics **30:**518, 1963.
13. Bearn, A. G., and Parker, W. C.: Glycoproteins; their composition, structure and function, Amsterdam, 1966, Elsiever Publishing Company.
14. Bessis, M. C., and Breton-Gorius, J.: Iron metabolism in the bone marrow as seen by electron microscopy; a critical review, Blood **19:**635, 1962.
15. Bothwell, T. H.: The control of iron absorption, Brit. J. Haemat. **14:**453, 1968.
16. Bothwell, T. H., Abrahams, C., Bradlow, B. A., and Charlton, R. W.: Idiopathic Bantu hemochromatosis; comparative histological study, Arch. Path. **79:**163, 1963.
17. Bothwell, T. H., and Bradlow, B. A.: Siderosis in the Bantu; a combined histopathological and chemical study, Arch. Path. **70:**279, 1960.
18. Bothwell, T. H., Hurtado, A. V., Donohue, D. M., and Finch, C. A.: Erythrokinetics; the plasma iron turnover as a measure of erythropoiesis, Blood **12:**409, 1957.
19. Bothwell, T. H., Pirzio-Biroli, G., and Finch, C. A.: Iron absorption; factors influencing absorption, J. Lab. Clin. Med. **51:**24, 1958.
20. Bowie, J. W., Tauxe, W. N., Sjoberg, W. E., Jr., and Yamaguchi, M. Y.: Daily variation in the concentration of iron in serum, Amer. J. Clin. Path. **40:**491, 1963.
21. Bowman, H. S.: Hematopoietic responses to iron-dextran (studies in iron-deficiency anemia of infancy), Amer. J. Dis. Child. **99:**408, 1960.
22. Boyett, J. D., Vogler, W. R., Furtado, V. deP., and Schmidt, F. H.: Allopurinol and iron metabolism in man, Blood **32:**460, 1968.
23. Brigety, R. E., and Pearson, H. A.: Effect of dietary and iron supplementation on hematocrit levels of preschool children, J. Pediat. **76:**757, 1970.
24. Brise, H., and Hallberg, L.: Effect of ascorbic acid on iron absorption, Acta Med. Scand. (suppl. 376) **171:**51, 1962.
25. Britton, H. A., Canby, J. P., and Kohler, C. M.: Iron deficiency anemia producing evidence of marrow hyperplasia in the calvarium, Pediatrics **25:**621, 1960.
26. Byrd, R. B., and Cooper, T.: Hereditary iron-loading anemia with secondary hemachromatosis, Ann. Intern. Med. **55:**103, 1961.
27. Callender, S. T.: Iron absorption, Brit. M. Bull. **15:**5, 1959.
28. Cartwright, G. E., and Wintrobe, M. M.: The anemia of infection; a review. In Dock, W., and Snapper, I., editors: Advances in

internal medicine, vol. 5, Chicago, 1952, Year Book Medical Publishers, Inc., p. 165.
29. Charley, P. J., Sitt, C., Shore, E., and Saltzman, P.: Studies in regulation of intestinal iron absorption, J. Lab. Clin. Med. 61:397, 1963.
30. Charlton, R. W., and Bothwell, T. H.: Iron deficiency anemia, Seminars in Hematology 7:67, 1970.
31. Chodos, R. B., Ross, J. F., Apt, L., Pollycove, M., and Halkett, J. A. E.: The absorption of radioiron labelled foods and iron salts in normal and iron-deficient subjects and in idiopathic hemochromatosis, J. Clin. Invest. 36:314, 1957.
32. Chown, B.: The fetus can bleed, Amer. J. Obstet Gynec. 70:1298, 1955.
33. Clark, W. M., Jr., Jurow, S. S., Walford, R. L., and Warthen, R. O.: Ferrous sulfate poisoning, Amer. J. Dis. Child. 88:220, 1954.
34. Clay, B., Rosenberg, B., Sampson, N., and Samuels, S. I.: Reactions to total dose intravenous infusion of iron dextran (Imferon), Brit. Med. J. 1:29, 1965.
35. Coleman, D. H., Stevens, A. R., Jr., and Finch, C. A.: The treatment of iron deficiency anemia, Blood 10:567, 1955.
36. Coltman, C. A.: Pagophagia and iron lack, J.A.M.A. 207:513, 1969.
37. Committee on Nutrition: Iron balance and iron requirements in infancy, Pediatrics 43:134, 1969.
38. Conrad, M. E., Jr., and Crosby, W. H.: Intestinal mucosal mechanisms controlling iron absorption, Blood 22:406, 1963.
39. Conrad, M. E., Weintraub, L. R., and Crosby, W. H.: The role of the intestine in iron kinetics, J. Clin. Invest. 43:963, 1964.
40. Crosby, W. H.: Treatment of haemochromatosis by energetic phlebotomy; one patient's response to the letting of 55 litres of blood in 11 months, Brit. J. Haemat. 4:82, 1958.
41. Crosby, W. H.: The control of iron balance by intestinal mucosa, Blood 22:441, 1963.
42. Crosby, W. H., and Sheehy, T. W.: Hypochromic iron-loading anaemias; studies of iron and haemoglobin metabolism by means of vigorous phlebotomy, Brit. J. Haemat. 6:56, 1960.
43. Curtis, C. D., and Kosinski, A. A.: Fatal case of iron intoxication in a child, J.A.M.A. 156:1326, 1954.
44. Dallman, P. R., and Schwartz, H. C.: Distribution of cytochrome C and myoglobin in rats with dietary iron deficiency, Pediatrics 35:677, 1965.
45. Dameshek, W.: Sideroblastic anaemia; is this a malignancy? Brit. J. Haemat. 11:52, 1965.

46. Davis, P. S., and Deller, D. J.: Effect of a xanthine-oxidase inhibitor (Allopurinol) on radioiron absorption in man, Lancet 2:470, 1966.
47. Davis, P. S., Luke, C. G., and Deller, D. J.: Reduction of iron-binding protein in haemochromatosis; a previously unrecognized metabolic defect, Lancet 2:1431, 1966.
48. deLeeuw, N. K. M., Lowenstein, L., and Hsieh, Y-S.: Iron deficiency and hydremia in normal pregnancy, Medicine 45:291, 1966.
49. Diamond, L. K.: Iron intake, hemoglobin and growth, Letters to the Editor, Pediatrics 31:343, 1963.
50. Dubach, R. Callender, S. T. E., and Moore, C. V.: Studies in iron transportation and metabolism; absorption of radioactive iron in patients with fever and with anemias of varied etiolgy, Blood 3:526, 1948.
51. Duthie, H. L.: The relative importance of the duodenum in the intestinal absorption of iron, Brit. J. Haemat. 10:59, 1964.
52. Ebaugh, F. G., Clemens, T., Rodnan, G., and Peterson, R. E.: Quantitative measurement of gastrointestinal blood loss. I. The use of radioactive $Cr^{51}$ in patients with gastrointestinal hemorrhage, Amer. J. Med. 25:169, 1958.
53. Elliott, W. D.: The prevention of anaemia of prematurity, Arch. Dis. Child. 37:297, 1962.
54. Ellis, J. T., Schulman, I., and Smith, C. H.: Generalized siderosis with fibrosis of liver and pancreas in Cooley's (Mediterranean) anemia, Amer. J. Path. 30:287, 1954.
55. Elwood, P. C., Waters, W. E., and Greene, W. J. W.: Evaluation of iron supplements in prevention of iron-deficiency anaemia, Lancet 2:175, 1970.
56. Eng, L. L.: Chronic iron deficiency anaemia with bone changes resembling Cooley's anaemia, Acta Haemat. 19:263, 1958.
57. Erlandson, M. E.: Iron metabolism and iron deficiency anemia, Ped. Clin. N. Amer. 9:673, 1962.
58. Erlandson, M. E., Waldman, B., Stern, G., Hilgartner, M. W., Wehman, J., and Smith, C. H.: Studies on congenital hemolytic syndromes. IV. Gastrointestinal absorption of iron, Blood 19:359, 1962.
59. Erslev, A. J.: Humoral regulation of red cell production, Blood 8:349, 1953.
60. Finch, S. C., and Finch, C. A.: Idiopathic hemochromatosis, an iron storage disease; iron metabolism in hemochromatosis, Medicine 34:381, 1955.
61. Forbes, G.: Poisoning with a preparation of iron, copper and manganese, Brit. Med. J. 1:367, 1947.

62. Gairdner, D., Marks, J., and Roscoe, J. D.: Blood formation in infancy; normal erythropoiesis, Arch. Dis. Child. 27:214, 1952.
63. Garby, L., Sjolin, S., and Vallquist, B.: Chronic refractory hypochromic anaemia with disturbed haem-metabolism, Brit. J. Haemat. 3:55, 1957.
64. Gardner, F. H.: The use of cobaltous chloride in the anemia associated with chronic renal disease, J. Lab Clin. Med. 41:56, 1953.
65. Gardner, F. H., and Nathan, D. G.: Hypochromic anemia and hemochromatosis: response to combined testosterone, pyridoxine and liver extract therapy, Amer. J. Med. Sci. 243:447, 1962.
66. Gelpi, A. P., and Ende, N.: An hereditary anemia with hemochromatosis; studies of an unusual hemopathic syndrome resembling thalassemia, Amer. J. Med. 25:303, 1958.
67. Gillman, J., and Gillman, T.: Structure of the liver in pellagra, Arch. Path. 40:239, 1945.
68. Gillman, T., Lamont, N. Mc. E., Hathorn, M., and Canham, P. A. S.: Haemochromatosis, African nutritional siderosis, and experimental siderosis in animals, Lancet 2:173, 1957.
69. Goldberg, A.: Sideroblastic anaemia; a commentary, Brit. J. Haemat. 11:114, 1965.
70. Goldwasser, E., Jackson, L. O., Fried, W., and Plzak, L. F.: Studies on erythropoiesis; the effect of cobalt on the production of erythropoietin, Blood 13:55, 1958.
71. Gordon, R. S., Jr.: Exudative enteropathy, abnormal permeability of the gastrointestinal tract demonstrable with labelled polyvinylpyrrolidone, Lancet 1:325, 1959.
72. Gorten, M. K., and Cross, E. R.: Iron metabolism in premature infants. II. Prevention of iron deficiency, J. Pediat. 64:509, 1964.
73. Gorten, M. K., Hepner, R., and Workman, J. B.: Iron metabolism in premature infants. I. Absorption and utilization of iron as measured by isotope studies, J. Pediat. 63:1063, 1963.
74. Granick, S.: The chemistry and functioning of the mammalian erythrocyte, Blood 4:404, 1949.
75. Granick, S.: Iron metabolism and hemochromatosis, Bull. N. Y. Acad. Med. 25:403, 1949.
76. Green, S., and Mazur, A.: Relation of uric acid metabolism to releases of iron from hepatic ferritin, J. Biol. Chem. 227:653, 1957.
77. Greenwalt, T. J., and Ayers, V. E.: Calcium disodium EDTA in transfusion hemosiderosis, Amer. J. Clin. Path. 25:266, 1955.
78. Gross, S., Keefer, V., and Lieberman, J.: The platelets in cyanotic congenital heart disease, Pediatrics 42:652, 1968.
79. Gross, S., Keefer, V., and Newman, A. J.: Platelets in iron deficiency and response to therapy, Pediatrics 34:315, 1964.
80. Guest, G. M., and Brown, E. W.: Erythrocytes and hemoglobin of blood in infancy and childhood; factors in variability; statistical studies, Amer. J. Dis. Child. 93:486, 1957.
81. Guha, D. K., Walin, B. N. S., Tandon, B. N., Deo, M. G., and Ghai, O. P.: Small bowel changes in iron-deficiency anaemia of childhood, Arch. Dis. Child. 43:239, 1968.
82. Hahn, P. F., Carothers, E. L., Darby, W. J., Martin, M., Sheppard, C. W., Cannon, R. O., Beam, A. S., Densen, P. M., Peterson, J. C., and McClellan, G. S.: Iron metabolism in human pregnancy as studied with the radio-active isotope, $Fe^{59}$, Amer. J. Obstet. Gynec. 61:477, 1951.
83. Hammond, G. D., and Murphy, A.: The influence of exogenous iron on formation of hemoglobin in the premature infant, Pediatrics 25:362, 1960.
84. Harker, L. A., Funk, D. D., and Finch, C. A.: Evaluation of storage iron by chelates, Amer. J. Med. 45:105, 1968.
85. Hegsted, D. M., Finch, C. A., and Kinney, T. D.: The influence of diet on iron absorption; the interrelation of iron and phosphorus, J. Exp. Med. 90:147, 1949.
86. Heilmeyer, L.: Blut und Blutkrankheiten, Berlin, 1941, Springer-Verlag.
87. Heilmeyer, L., Keller, W., Vivell, O., Keideling, W., Betke, K., Wöhler, F., and Schultze, H. E.: Kongenitale Atransferrinämie bei einem sieben Jahre alten Kind, Deutsche med. Wchnschr. 86:1745, 1961.
88. Henderson, F., Vietti, T. J., and Brown, E. B.: Desferrioxamine in the treatment of acute toxic reaction to ferrous gluconate, J.A.M.A. 186:1139, 1963.
89. Hoag, M., Wallerstein, R., and Pollycove, M.: Occult blood loss in iron-deficiency anemia of infancy, Pediatrics 27:199, 1961.
90. Hollingsworth, J. W.: Life span of fetal erythrocytes, J. Lab. Clin. Med. 45:469, 1955.
91. Howell, J., and Wyatt, J. P.: Development of pigmentary cirrhosis in Cooley's anemia, Arch. Path. 55:423, 1953.
92. Hughes, A. A., Kelly, V. J., and Stewart, R. A.: The copper content of infant foods, Pediatrics 25:477, 1960.
93. Hutchinson, H. E.: The significance of stainable iron in sternal marrow sections; its application in the control of iron therapy, Blood 8:236, 1953.

94. Jacobs, A., Rhodes, J., Peters, D. K., Campbell, H., and Ealeins, J. D.: Gastric acidity and iron absorption, Brit. J. Haemat. 12: 728, 1966.
95. Jandl, J. H., Inman, J. K., Simmons, R. L., and Allen, D. W.: Transfer of iron from serum iron-binding protein to human reticulocytes, J. Clin. Invest. 38:161, 1959.
96. Johnson, B. F.: Hemochromatosis resulting from prolonged oral iron therapy, New Eng. J. Med. 278:1100, 1968.
97. Josephs, H. W.: Iron metabolism and the hypochromic anemia of infancy, Medicine 32:125, 1953.
98. Josephs, H. W.: Absorption of iron as a problem in human physiology, Blood 13:1, 1958.
99. Kaplan, E., Zuelzer, W. W., and Mouriquand, C.: The significance of visible iron in red cell precursors, Amer. J. Dis. Child. 86:462, 1953.
100. Katz, J. H., and Jandl, J. H.: The role of transferrin in the transport of iron into the developing red cell. In Gross, F., editor: Iron metabolism; an international symposium sponsored by Ciba, Berlin, 1964, Springer-Verlag.
101. Kimber, C., and Weintraub, L. R.: Malabsorption of iron secondary to iron deficiency, New Eng. J. Med. 279:453, 1968.
102. Kleckner, M. S., Jr., Kark, R. W., Baker, L. A., Chapman, A. Z., and Kaplan, E.: Clinical features, pathology and therapy of hemochromatosis, J.A.M.A. 157:1471, 1955.
103. Klingberg, W. G., Jones, B., Allen, W. M., and Dempsey, E.: Placental parabiotic circulation of single ovum human twins, Amer. J. Dis. Child. 90:519, 1955.
104. Kriss, J. P., Carnes, W. H., and Gross, R. T.: Hypothyroidism and thyroid hyperplasia in patients treated with cobalt, J.A.M.A. 157:117, 1955.
105. Kunkel, H. G., and Wallenius, G.: New hemoglobin in normal adult blood, Science 122:288, 1955.
106. Lahey, M. E.: Protein-losing enteropathy, Ped. Clin. N. Amer. 9:689, 1962.
107. Lahey, M. E., Gubler, C. J., Cartwright, G. E., and Wintrobe, M. M.: Studies on copper metabolism. VI. Blood copper in normal human subjects, J. Clin. Invest. 32:322, 1953.
108. Lahey, M. E., and Schubert, W. K.: New deficiency syndrome occurring in infancy, Amer. J. Dis. Child. 93:31, 1957.
109. Langley, F. A.: Haemopoiesis and siderosis in foetus and newborn, Arch. Dis. Child. 26:64, 1951.
110. Lanzkowsky, P.: Investigation into the treatment of pica, Arch. Dis. Child. 34:140, 1959.
111. Lanzkowsky, P.: The effect of intramuscular iron-dextran complex administered to women during pregnancy on their haematological values and on the haemoglobin levels of their infants, J. Obstet Gynaec. Brit. Emp. 68:52, 1961.
112. Lanzkowsky, P.: Radiological features of iron-deficiency anemia, Amer. J. Dis. Child. 116:16, 1968.
113. Lanzkowsky, P.: Iron supplementation of milk proposed to eliminate anemia, Pediat. News 9:1970.
114. Lanzkowsky, P., Nist, R. T., Bhardwaj, B., and Smith, C. H.: Prevalence of anemia in children in New York City, Program of American Pediatric Society, Inc., Atlantic City, New Jersey, May 1-4, 1968, page 49, 78th Annual Meeting.
115. Lee, G. R., Cartwright, G. E., and Wintrobe, M. M.: The response of free erythrocyte protoporphyrin to pyridoxine therapy in a patient with sideroachrestic (sideroblastic) anemia, Blood 27:557, 1966.
116. Leventhal, B., and Stohlman, F., Jr.: Regulation of erythropoiesis. XVII. The determinants of red cell size in iron-deficiency states, Pediatrics 37:62, 1966.
117. Luke, C. G., Davis, P. S., and Deller, D. J.: Changes in gastric iron-binding protein (Gastroferrin) during iron-deficiency anaemia, Lancet 1:926, 1967.
118. Macdougall, L. G.: Red cell metabolism in iron-deficiency anemia, J. Pediat. 72:30, 1968.
119. Macdougall, L. G.: A simple test for detection of iron in stools, J. Pediat. 76:764, 1970.
120. Macdougall, L. G., Judisch, J. M., and Mistry, S. P.: Red cell metabolism in iron deficiency anemia. II. The relationship between red cell survival and alterations in red cell metabolism, J. Pediat. 76:660, 1970.
121. Marchasin, S., and Wallerstein, R. O.: The treatment of iron deficiency anemia with intravenous iron dextran, Blood 23:354, 1964.
122. Mazur, A., and Carleton, A.: Hepatic xanthine oxidase and ferritin iron in the developing rat, Blood 26:317, 1965.
123. Mazur, A., Carleton, A., and Carlson, A.: Relation of oxidative metabolism to the incorporation of plasma iron into ferritin in vivo, J. Biol. Chem. 236:1109, 1961.
124. Mazur, A., Green, S., and Carleton, A.: Mechanism of plasma iron incorporation into hepatic ferritin, J. Biol. Chem. 235:595, 1960.
125. Mazur, A., Green, S., Saha, A., and Carleton, A.: Mechanism of release of ferritin iron in vivo by xanthine oxidase, J. Clin. Invest. 37:1809, 1958.

126. McDonald, R., and Marshall, S. R.: The value of iron therapy in pica, Pediatrics 34: 558, 1964.
127. McEmery, J. T., and Greengard, J.: Treatment of acute iron ingestion with deferoxamine in 20 children, J. Pediat. 68:773, 1966.
128. McFarlane, D. B., Pinkerton, P. H., Dagg, J. H., and Goldberg, A.: Incidence of iron deficiency with and without anaemia in women in general practice, Brit. J. Haemat. 13:790, 1967.
129. Mendel, G. A.: Studies on iron absorption. I. The relationships between the rate of erythropoiesis, hypoxia and iron absorption, Blood 18:727, 1961.
130. Mendel, G. A., Weiler, R. J., and Mangalik, A.: Studies on iron absorption. II. The absorption of iron in experimental anemias of diverse etiology, Blood 22:450, 1963.
131. Moe, P. J.: Iron requirements in infancy; longitudinal studies of iron requirements during the first year of life, Acta Paediat. (suppl. 150) 52:54, 1963.
132. Moeschlin, S., and Schnider, U.: Treatment of primary and secondary haemochromatosis and acute iron poisoning with a new, potent iron-eliminating agent (desferrioxamine B). In Gross, F., editor: Iron metabolism, Berlin, 1964, Springer-Verlag, p. 525.
133. Mollin, D. L.: A symposium on sideroblastic anaemia; introduction: sideroblasts and sideroblastic anaemia, Brit. J. Haemat. 11: 41, 1965.
134. Moore, C. V.: The importance of nutritional factors in the pathogenesis of iron-deficiency anemia, Amer. J. Clin. Nutr. 3:3, 1955.
135. Moore, C. V.: Iron metabolism and nutrition, The Harvey Lectures, Series No. 55, New York, 1961, Academic Press Inc., p. 67.
136. Moore, C. V., Arrowsmith, W. R., Welch, J., and Minnich, V.: Studies in iron transportation and metabolism; observations on the absorption of iron from the gastrointestinal tract, J. Clin. Invest. 18:553, 1939.
137. Moore, C. V., and Dubach, R.: Metabolism and requirements of iron in the human, J.A.M.A. 162:197, 1956.
138. Moores, R. R., Stohlman, F., Jr., and Brecher, G.: Humoral regulation of erythropoiesis. XI. The pattern of response to specific therapy in iron deficiency anemia, Blood 22:286, 1963.
139. Movassaghi, N., Purugganan, G. C., and Leikin, S.: Comparison of exchange transfusion and deferoxamine in the treatment of acute iron poisoning, J. Pediat. 75:604, 1969.
140. Muir, A. R.: The molecular structure of isolated and intracellular ferritin, Quart. J. Exper. 45:192, 1960.
141. Myerson, R. M., and Carroll, I. N.: Treatment of hemochromatosis by massive venesection; report of a case treated by removal of forty liters of blood in twenty-eight months, Arch. Intern. Med. 95:349, 1955.
142. Nadas, A. S.: Pediatric cardiology, Philadelphia, 1957, W. B. Saunders Co.
143. Naiman, J. L., Oski, F. A., Diamond, L. K., Vawter, G. F., and Shwachman, H.: The gastrointestinal effects of iron deficiency anemia, Pediatrics 33:83, 1964.
144. Niccum, W. L., Jackson, R. L., and Stearns, G.: Use of ferric and ferrous iron in the prevention of hypochromic anemia in infants, Amer. J. Dis. Child. 86:553, 1953.
145. Noyes, W. D., Bothwell, T. H., and Finch, C. A.: The role of the reticuloendothelial cell in iron metabolism, Brit. J. Haemat. 6: 43, 1960.
146. Owen, G. M., Nelson, C. E., and Garry, P. J.: Nurtritional status of preschool children; hemoglobin, hematocrit, and plasma iron values, J. Pediat. 76:261, 1970.
147. Panels in Therapy: The use of cobalt and cobalt-iron preparations in the therapy of anemia, Blood 10:852, 1955.
148. Parffit, A. M.: Familial hypoproteinemia with exudative enteropathy and intestinal lymphangiectasis, Arch. Dis. Child. 41:54, 1966.
149. Pearson, H. A., Abrams, I., Fernbach, D. J., Gyland, S. P., and Hahn, D. A.: Anemia in preschool children in the United States of America, Ped. Res. 1:169, 1967.
150. Pollycove, M.: Iron kinetics. In Wallerstein, R. O., and Mettier, S. R., editors: Iron in clinical medicine, Berkeley, Calif., 1958, University of California Press.
151. Pommerenke, W. T., Hahn, P. F., Bale, W. F., and Balfour, W. M.: Transmission of radio-active iron to the human fetus, Amer. J. Physiol. 137:164, 1942.
152. Prasad, A. S., Halsted, J. A., and Nadimi, M.: Syndrome of iron deficiency, hepatosplenomegaly, hypogonadism, dwarfism and geophagia, Amer. J. Med. 31:532, 1961.
153. Pribilla, W., Bothwell, T. H., and Finch, C. A.: Iron transport to the fetus in man. In Wallerstein, R. O., and Mettier, S. A., editors: Iron in clinical medicine, Los Angeles, 1958, University of California Press.
154. Purugganan, H. B., and Naiman, J. L.: Exchange transfusion in severe iron deficiency anemia prior to emergency surgery, J. Pediat. 69:804, 1966.
155. Rather, L. J.: Hemochromatosis and hemosiderosis; does iron overload cause diffuse

fibrosis of the liver? Amer. J. Med. **21**:857, 1956.
156. Report of committee on nutrition: On the feeding of solid foods to infants, Pediatrics **21**:685, 1958.
157. Reynafarje, C., and Ramos, J.: Influence of altitude changes in intestinal iron absorption, J. Lab. Clin. Med. **57**:848, 1961.
158. Robscheit-Robbins, F. S., and Whipple, G. H.: Infection and intoxication; their influence on hemoglobin production in experimental animals, J. Exp. Med. **63**:767, 1936.
159. Roselle, H. A.: Association of laundry starch and clay ingestion with anemia in New York City, Arch. Intern. Med. **125**:57, 1970.
160. Ross Conference: Iron Nutrition in Infancy, 62nd Conference on Pediatric Research, Ross Laboratories, Columbus, Ohio, 1970.
161. Rothstein, G., Lee, G. R., and Cartwright, G. E.: Sideroblastic anemia with dermal photosensitivity and increased erythrocyte protoporphyrin, New Eng. J. Med. **280**:587, 1969.
162. Rudolph, A. M., Nadas, A. S., and Borges, W. H.: Hematologic adjustments to cyanotic congenital heart disease, Pediatrics **11**:454, 1953.
163. Rundles, R. W., and Falls, H. F.: Hereditary (sex-linked) anemia, Amer. J. Med. Sci. **211**:641, 1946.
164. Samuels, L. D.: Leukemoid reaction to parenteral iron-dextran complex; a case report, J.A.M.A. **182**:1334, 1962.
165. Santos, A. S., and Pisciotta, A. V.: Acute iron intoxication, Amer. J. Dis. Child. **107**:424, 1964.
166. Scheinberg, I. H., and Sternlieb, I.: Wilson's disease and the concentration of caeruloplasmin in serum, Lancet **1**:1420, 1963.
167. Schubert, W. K., and Lahey, M. E.: Copper and protein depletion complicating hypoferric anemia of infancy, Pediatrics **24**:710, 1959.
168. Schulman, I.: Studies on the anemia of prematurity. In Wallerstein, R. O., and Mettier, S. A., editors: Iron in clinical medicine, Los Angeles, 1958, University of California Press.
169. Schulman, I.: Iron requirements in infancy, J.A.M.A. **175**:118, 1961.
170. Schulman, I., Smith, C. H., and Stern, G. S.: Studies on the anemia of prematurity, Amer. J. Dis. Child. **88**:567, 1954.
171. Schulz, J., and Smith, N. J.: A quantitative study of the absorption of food iron in infants and children, Amer. J. Dis. Child. **95**:109, 1958.
172. Schulz, J., and Smith, N. J.: Quantitative study of the absorption of iron salts in infants and children, Amer. J. Dis. Child. **95**:120, 1958.
173. Schulze, H. V., and Morgan, A. F.: Relation of ascorbic acid to effectiveness of iron therapy in children, Amer. J. Dis. Child. **71**:593, 1946.
174. Seip, M., and Halvorsen, S.: Erythrocyte production and iron stores in premature infants during the first months of life; the anemia of prematurity—etiology, pathogenesis, iron requirements, Acta Paediat. **45**:600, 1956.
175. Seltzer, C. C., Wenzel, B. J., and Mayer, J.: Serum iron and iron-binding capacity in adolescents. I. Standard values, Amer. J. Clin. Nutr. **13**:343, 1963.
176. Shafer, A. W., and Marlow, A. A.: Toxic reaction to intramuscular injection of iron, New Eng. J. Med. **260**:180, 1959.
177. Shahidi, N. T., and Diamond, L. K.: Skull changes in infants with chronic iron-deficiency anemia, New Eng. J. Med. **262**:137, 1960.
178. Shahidi, N. T., Nathan, D. G., and Diamond, L. K.: Iron deficiency anemia associated with an error of iron metabolism in two siblings, J. Clin. Invest. **43**:510, 1964.
179. Shoden, A., and Sturgeon, P.: Iron storage. III. The influence of rates of administration of iron on its distribution between ferritin and hemosiderin, Acta Haemat. **27**:33, 1962.
180. Shojania, A. M., and Gross, S.: Folic acid deficiency and prematurity, J. Pediat. **64**:323, 1964.
181. Sisson, T. R. C., and Bronson, W. R.: Studies in the treatment of acute iron poisoning, Amer. J. Dis. Child. **96**:463, 1958.
182. Sisson, T. R. C., and Lund, C. J.: Influence of maternal iron deficiency on the newborn, Amer. J. Clin. Nutr. **6**:376, 1958.
183. Smith, C. H., Schulman, I., and Morgenthau, J. E.: Iron metabolism in infants and children; serum iron and iron-binding protein; diagnostic and therapeutic implications. In Levine, S. Z., editor: Advances in pediatrics, vol. 5, Chicago, 1952, Year Book Medical Publishers, Inc., p. 195.
184. Smith, N. J.: Iron as a therapeutic agent in pediatric practice, J. Pediat. **53**:37, 1958.
185. Smith, N. J.: Considerations of iron metabolism in early infancy, J. Pediat. **54**:654, 1959.
186. Stanbury, J. B., Wyngaarden, J. B., and Frederickson, D. S.: The metabolic basis of inherited disease, ed. 2, New York, 1966, McGraw-Hill Book Co., pp. 1327-1329.
187. Stevens, A. R., Jr., Coleman, D. H., and Finch, C. A.: Iron metabolism: clinical eval-

uation of iron stores, Ann. Intern. Med. **38:** 199, 1953.
188. Strauss, M. B.: Anemia of infancy from maternal iron deficiency in pregnancy, J. Clin. Invest. **12:**345, 1933.
189. Strober, W., Cohen, L. S., Waldman, T. A., and Braunwald, E.: Tricuspid regurgitation; a newly recognized cause of protein-losing enteropathy, lymphocytopenia immunologic deficiency, Amer. J. Med. **44:**842, 1968.
190. Sturgeon, P.: Studies of iron requirement in infants and children; the influence on normal infants of oral iron in therapeutic doses, Pediatrics **17:**341, 1956.
191. Sturgeon, P.: Iron metabolism; a review, Pediatrics **18:**267, 1956.
192. Sturgeon, P.: Studies of iron requirements in infants and children. In Wallerstein, R. O., and Mettier, S. A., editors: Iron in clinical medicine, Los Angeles, 1958, University of California Press.
193. Sturgeon, P.: Studies of iron requirements in infants; influence of supplemental iron during normal pregnancy on mother and infant. B. The infant, Brit. J. Haemat. **5:**45, 1959.
194. Sturgeon, P., and Brubaker, C. A.: Copper deficiency in infants; a syndrome characterized by hypocupremia, iron deficiency anemia, and hypoproteinemia Amer. J. Dis. Child. **92:**254, 1956.
195. Thirayothin, P., and Crosby, W. H.: The distribution of iron injected intraperitoneally; evidence of serosal "absorption" by the small intestine, J. Clin. Invest. **41:**1206, 1962.
196. Thompson, J.: Two cases of ferrous sulfate poisoning, Brit. Med. J. **1:**640, 1947.
197. Turnbull, A., and Giblett, E. R.: Binding and transport of iron by transferrin variants, J. Lab. Clin. Med. **57:**450, 1961.
198. Ulstrom, R. A.: Exudative enteropathy, Pediatrics **24:**521, 1959.
199. Ulstrom, R. A., and Krivit, W.: Exudative enteropathy, hypoproteinemia, edema and iron-deficiency anemia, Amer. J. Dis. Child. **100:**509, 1960.
200. Ulstrom, R. A., Smith, N. J., and Heimlich, E. M.: Transient dysproteinemia in infants, a new syndrome; clinical studies, Amer. J. Dis. Child. **92:**219, 1956.
201. Ulstrom, R. A., Smith, N. J., Nakamura, K., and Heimlich, E.: Transient dysproteinemia in infants; studies on protein metabolism using amino acid isotopes, Amer. J. Dis. Child. **93:**536, 1957.
202. VanDyke, D. C., Layrisse, M., Laurence, J. H., Garcia, J. F., and Pollycove, M.: Relations between severity of anemia and erythropoietin titer in human beings, Blood **18:**187, 1961.
203. Vossough, P., Leikin, S., and Purugganan, G.: Evaluation of parameters of folic acid and vitamin $B_{12}$ deficiency in patients with iron deficiency anemia, Ped. Res. **2:**179, 1968.
204. Waldmann, T. A.: Gastrointestinal protein loss demonstrated by Cr-labelled albumin, Lancet **2:**121, 1961.
205. Waldmann, T. A., Steinfeld, J. L., Dutcher, T. F., Davidson, J. D., and Gordon, R. S.: The role of the gastrointestinal system in "idiopathic hypoproteinemia," Gastroenterology **41:**197, 1961.
206. Waldmann, T. A., Wochner, R. D., Laster, L., and Gordon, R. S., Jr.: Allergic gastroenteropathy; a case of excessive gastrointestinal blood loss, New Eng. J. Med. **276:**761, 1967.
207. Wallerstein, R. O., and Hoag, M. S.: Treatment with iron-dextran of iron-deficiency anemia in children, J.A.M.A. **164:**962, 1957.
208. Wallerstein, R. O., and Robbins, S. L.: Hemochromatosis after prolonged oral therapy in a patient with chronic hemolytic anemia, Amer. J. Med. **14:**256, 1953.
209. Weintraub, L. R., Conrad, M. E., Jr., and Crosby, W. H.: The significance of iron turnover in the control of iron absorption, Blood **24:**19, 1964.
210. Wheby, M. S., and Umpierre, G.: Effect of transferrin saturation on iron absorption in man, New Eng. J. Med. **271:**1391, 1964.
211. Whipple, G. H., Sisson, T. R. C., and Lund, C. J.: Delayed ligation of the umbilical cord, its influence on the blood volume of the newborn, Amer. J. Obstet. Gynec. **10:**603, 1957.
212. Whitten, C. F., Chen, Y-C., and Gibson, G. W.: Studies on acute iron poisoning. II. Further observations on desferrioxamine in the treatment of acute experimental ferrioxamine iron poisoning, Pediatrics **38:**102, 1966.
213. Whitten, C. F., Gibson, G., and Good, M.: Experiences with desferrioxamine in the treatment of acute iron poisoning, J. Pediat. **65:**1050, 1964.
214. Whitten, C. F., Gibson, G. W., Good, M. H., Goodwin, J. F., and Brough, A. J.: Studies in acute iron poisoning. I. Desferrioxamine in the treatment of acute iron poisoning: clinical observations, experimental studies and theoretical considerations, Pediatrics **36:**322, 1965.
215. Wickster, G. Z., and Christian, J. R.: Posthemorrhagic shock in the newborn premature, Ped. Clin. N. Amer. **1:**555, 1954.
216. Widdowson, E. M., and Spray, C. M.: Chemical development in utero, Arch. Dis. Child. **26:**205, 1951.

217. Wilson, J. F., Heiner, D. C., and Lahey, M. E.: Studies on iron metabolism. I. Evidence of gastrointestinal dysfunction in infants with iron deficiency anemia, J. Pediat. **60**:787, 1962.
218. Wilson, J. F., Heiner, D. C., and Lahey, M. E.: Studies on iron metabolism. IV. Milk-induced gastrointestinal bleeding in infants with hypochromic microcytic anemia, J.A.M.A. **189**:568, 1964.
219. Wintrobe, M. M.: Factors and mechanisms in the production of red corpuscles, The Harvey Lectures **45**:87, 1949-1950.
220. Wintrobe, M. M.: Clinical hematology, ed. 4, Philadelphia, 1956, Lea & Febiger.
221. Wintrobe, M. M., Cartwright, G. E., and Gubler, C. J.: Studies on the function and metabolism of copper, J. Nutrition **50**:395, 1953.
222. Woodruff, C. W.: Maternal factors in hypochromic anemia in infancy, J.A.M.A. **162**:659, 1956.
223. Woodruff, C. W.: Multiple causes of iron deficiency in infants, J.A.M.A. **167**:715, 1958.
224. Woodruff, C. W.: The utilization of iron administered orally, Pediatrics **27**:194, 1961.
225. Woodruff, C. W., and Bridgeforth, E. P.: Relationship between the hemogram of the infant and that of the mother during pregnancy, Pediatrics **12**:681, 1953.
226. Yam, L. T., Finkel, H. E., Weintraub, L. R., and Crosby, W. H.: Circulating iron-containing macrophages in hemochromatosis, New Eng. J. Med. **279**:512, 1968.
227. Zipursky, A., Dempsey, H., Markowitz, H., Cartwright, G., and Wintrobe, M. M.: Studies on copper metabolism; hypocupremia in infancy, Amer. J. Dis. Child. **96**:148, 1958.

# 13 MEGALOBLASTIC ANEMIA AND RELATED ANEMIAS

Megaloblastic anemias are characterized by the presence of megaloblasts in the marrow as well as evidence of macrocytosis in the peripheral blood and are usually but not invariably due to a deficiency of vitamin $B_{12}$ or folic acid. These two substances function as coenzymes in the synthesis of nucleoproteins, and in their absence specific clinical and hematologic abnormalities develop.

*Causes of megaloblastosis*

1. Vitamin $B_{12}$ deficiency
2. Folate deficiency
3. Thiamine responsive anemias
4. Hereditary orotic aciduria
5. Sideroblastic anemia (pyridoxine-responsive anemia)
6. Aplastic anemia—constitutional and acquired
7. DiGuglielmo's disease

**Vitamin $B_{12}$.** Vitamin $B_{12}$ is found principally in foods of animal origin, such as liver, kidney, and muscle, and, to a lesser extent, in eggs and milk. It is not usually present in higher plants but can be synthesized by certain bacteria, among them *Streptomyces griseus*. It occurs also as a by-product of streptomycin. In its pure form vitamin $B_{12}$ is a crystalline substance containing cobalt whose chemical name is cyanocobalamin. It functions as "extrinsic factor" in regard to erythropoiesis, and in the presence of the "intrinsic factor" of Castle secreted by gastric mucosa it is absorbed into the small intestine and passes into the bloodstream to the liver, where it is stored for use by the bone marrow and other tissues. The erythrocyte maturing factor (EMF) is probably identical with the extrinsic vitamin $B_{12}$ after its absorption. Vitamin $B_{12}$ exists in the serum, mainly in combined form as a heat-labile complex, with serum protein specifically in the alpha globulin fractions.[92] More specifically, a proportion of vitamin $B_{12}$ circulates in the plasma in a "free" or unbound state, probably loosely bound to the beta-globulins.[42] About 80 to 85% is carried in a bound form attached to a protein carrier, designated "erythroglobulin," and migrates as an alpha-globulin.[125]

While both $B_{12}$-bonding globulins may deliver the vitamin to reticulocytes and liver, Herbert's studies[48] suggest that the $B_{12}$-binding globulin is primarily a transport protein whereas the $B_{12}$-binding alpha-globulin functions primarily to conserve the vitamin. $B_{12}$-binding alpha-globulin has a greater affinity for $B_{12}$ and retains the vitamin more tenaciously than does the $B_{12}$-binding beta-globulin. He also found an elevated serum $B_{12}$ level and vitamin $B_{12}$-binding protein greatly elevated in chronic myelogenous leukemia and of value in diagnosing this condition.

In another terminology, the alpha 1 globulin binder has been designated as Transcobalamin I (TC I) and the beta globulin as Transcobalamin II (TC II).[40] The latter is the exogenous binder. In normal subjects, following absorption from the ileum or after parenteral injection of $B_{12}$, 85% of the vitamin is attached to TC II. It disappears from normal plasma so that less than 5% of the administered dose is present after 24 hours.[82] The endogenous binder, TC I, accounts for 90% of the $B_{12}$ in the serum of normal persons. An increase of TC I is found in all of the chronic myeloproliferative states, most striking in chronic leukemia.[40]

*Folic acid.* Folic acid, also a member of the vitamin B complex, is distributed in plant and animal tissues, chiefly in fresh leafy green vegetables such as spinach and cabbage and in liver, kidney, yeast, and mushrooms. Liver, beef, and fresh green vegetables are the common foods with a high folic acid content. Folic acid is readily absorbed from the gastrointestinal canal. In its synthesized form it is known as pteroylglutamic acid (PGA). For its metabolically active form it must be converted from its conjugated state to folinic acid (citrovorum factor) or to tetrahydrofolic acid.[39] The normal adult has a total body folic acid store of approximately 7.5 mg., with a daily requirement of 50 $\mu$g.[46] The major portion of folic acid (70%) is stored in the liver.[13]

Normal red cell folate measures 160 to 540 ng./ml. and serum folate 5 to 20 ng./ml. (vitamin $B_{12}$—normal 200 to 900 $\mu\mu$g/ml.).

Formiminoglutamic acid (FIGLU), a normal intermediate product of the metabolism of histidine, requires the active tetrahydrofolic acid for its further degradation to glutamic acid. When tetrahydrofolic acid is insufficient, formiminoglutamic acid accumulates and its excretion in the urine thus serves as a useful indicator of clinical folic acid deficiency.[71,112] Metabolic correction of the deficiency, following administration of folic acid, can be shown by the elimination of the increased urinary formiminoglutamic acid.

Histidine is normally metabolized to formiminoglutamic acid and then to glutamic acid through interaction with tetrahydrofolic acid. To increase the sensitivity of the test for FIGLU excretion when folic acid deficiency is suspected, loading doses of l-histidine are given orally to the patient. Normal subjects excrete less than 2 mg. per hour of FIGLU in the urine and usually a trace or none. In folic acid deficiency, excretion is greater than 3.5 mg. per hour, with especially high levels in idiopathic steatorrhea (30 to 80 mg.).[25]

FIGLU excretion, however, is occasionally increased in some patients with pernicious anemia whose serum levels of folic acid are not below normal, in some patients with iron-deficiency anemia, and in some cases of hereditary spherocytosis.[14] It has also been claimed that the large doses of histidine in the loading test may be unphysiologic and account for overlapping results noted in folic acid deficiency, vitamin $B_{12}$ deficiency, and other hematologic states.[44,49]

Urocanic acid is also a breakdown product of histidine to glutamic acid. When folic acid coenzyme is lacking, urocanic acid appears in the urine as does formiminoglutamic acid.[10]

Folic acid deficiency results principally from inadequate dietary intake, increased demand, antagonists to its utilization (such as occur in antileukemia therapy), and interference with intestinal absorption. Occasionally, ascorbic acid deficiency contributes to the causation of megaloblastic anemia by limiting the conversion of folic acid to its active form.

*Causes of folic acid deficiency*

1. Inadequate intake (dietary)
2. Defective absorption
    a. Specific folic acid
    b. Generalized malabsorption syndrome—i.e., celiac disease, idiopathic steatorrhea, congenital strictures, gastrointestinal resections, prolonged diarrhea
3. Increased requirements—i.e., rapid growth, hemolytic anemia, malignancies, chronic liver disease, infection
4. Presence of folic acid antagonists—i.e., methrotrexate, anti-epileptic drugs, pyrimethamine

In the body, folic acid exists in active forms that have coenzyme-like functions in cell metabolism in a number of reactions in which single carbon atoms are transferred to or built into intermediates.[4,42] Vitamin $B_{12}$ is also required in certain aspects of this metabolic process; it may be essential in methionine methyl neogenesis.[50] Herbert and Zalusky[50] have suggested that in vitamin $B_{12}$-deficient subjects "piled up" *Lactobacillus casei*-active folate activity ("probably $N^5$-methyl-tetrahydrofolic acid") tends to reduce the amount of folic acid available for other one-carbon unit transfers. Study of intermediary metabolism of the monocarbon pool and histidine in normal subjects and in patients with megaloblastic anemia can be utilized to differentiate between folic acid deficiency and vitamin $B_{12}$ as causative factors in pathogenesis of the anemia.[30]

The sequential pattern of developing folic acid deficiency was demonstrated in one adult[45] kept on a very low folic acid intake (5 $\mu$g daily). Low serum folic acid, the first evidence of the deficiency, appeared at 3 weeks, followed by the presence of hypersegmented neutrophils at 7 weeks, high urinary FIGLU (formiminoglutamic acid) excretion after histidine loading at 13 weeks, megaloblastic bone marrow changes at 19 weeks, and anemia at 19½ weeks.

Since folic acid is of fundamental importance in numerous metabolic processes and is intimately involved in DNA, RNA, and protein biosynthesis, it is to be expected that failure to absorb this substance would lead to serious consequences in growth and development. Such an event took place in a 19-year-old female in whom a clinical syndrome was observed characterized by specific malabsorption of folate from the gut with resultant megaloblastic anemia associated with mental retardation and cerebral calcification.[63]

The association of megaloblastic anemia with anticonvulsant therapy has been established in adults. Subnormal serum folic acid levels were found in 51% of epileptic children being treated with anticonvulsants.[83] Slight macrocytosis was found in 19%, all of whom had subnormal levels. Red cell indices and Arneth counts did not differ significantly from those found in a control group of children. Megaloblastic anemia was not seen in any patient. Values below 3 ng./ml. serum were regarded as deficient.

**Interrelationship of folic acid and vitamin $B_{12}$.** Folic acid is closely associated with vitamin $B_{12}$ in the synthesis of nucleic acids, acting as catalysts at different stages of this process.[88] There is evidence also that a balance exists between folic acid and vitamin $B_{12}$ and that a deficiency of one increases the requirement for the other.[95,126] Whereas a deficiency of either substance results in megaloblastic bone marrow and glossitis, the nervous system disturbance of pernicious anemia, for instance, is caused solely by vitamin $B_{12}$ deficiency. The prevention of neurologic symptoms requires vitamin $B_{12}$ therapy, and not folic acid. The deficiency of folic acid or vitamin $B_{12}$ not only results in the appearance of megaloblasts, but also affects other cells in the bone marrow. The constituents of nucleic acids (uracil, thymine, and thymidine) possess therapeutic activity in patients with megaloblastic anemia but not to the extent that folic acid and vitamin $B_{12}$ do.[88]

**Gastrointestinal absorption of folic acid and vitamin $B_{12}$.** According to Cooper and Castle,[23] the absorption of vitamin $B_{12}$ from food includes the following stages: release of the vitamin from its bound form in food, binding of the freed vitamin to the gastric intrinsic factor, adherence ("plastering") of the vitamin $B_{12}$ intrinsic factor complex in the ileal mucosa, splitting of the link between $B_{12}$ and intrinsic factor, either at or within the intestinal wall by a "releasing factor," and, finally, passage of vitamin $B_{12}$ into the bloodstream. The mechanism of intrinsic factor action in the intestine appears to be calcium-dependent. Vitamin $B_{12}$ is absorbed in the small intestine, mainly in the ileum, and both intrinsic factor and calcium ions are necessary for the absorption of physiologic amounts. Calcium chelating agents (EDTA) decrease and calcium lactate increases vitamin $B_{12}$ absorption. The ability to bind vitamin $B_{12}$ is one of the essential characteristics of intrinsic factor, and the most potent preparations of intrinsic factor have the highest binding capacity.[130]

In the absence of intrinsic factor none of the 2 to 10 $\mu$g of vitamin $B_{12}$ in the average daily North American diet can be absorbed. Vitamin $B_{12}$ deficiency develops over a period of 3 to 6 years, which is the time it takes for liver stores of vitamin $B_{12}$ to become nearly depleted. Inadequate ingestion of folic acid will lead to folic acid deficiency more quickly than inadequate ingestion of $B_{12}$. This is because tissue stores of folic acid will only remain normal for a little more than 1 month.[47]

Absorption studies in man, following resection of various segments of small intestine, suggest that the primary site of folic acid absorption is in the jejunum, whereas that of vitamin $B_{12}$ is in the ileum.[22] Megaloblastic anemia developed after massive resection of the small intestine in a newborn infant. Long-term therapy with vitamin $B_{12}$ was necessary to effect a cure.[26]

*Causes of vitamin $B_{12}$ deficiency*

1. Decreased intake (<1 $\mu$g daily, i.e., food fads, poverty or malnutrition)
2. Pernicious anemia (see table below)
3. Gastric mucosal disease—i.e., gastritis, corrosives, gastrectomy
4. Small intestine
   a. Generalized malabsorption—i.e., duodenal diverticulae, regional ileitis, strictures or stenosis of small bowel, intestinal resection, malignancy, lymphosarcoma
   b. Specific $B_{12}$ malabsorption—i.e., absent intestinal receptors, EDTA (chelates calcium)
5. Competition for vitamin $B_{12}$: blind loop syndrome, *Diphyllobothrium latum*

| Type | Juvenile | Adult | Adult and endocrinopathies |
|---|---|---|---|
| Intrinsic factor (I.F.) | Absent | Absent | Absent |
| Gastric histology | Normal | Atrophy | Atrophy |
| Acid secretion | Normal | Achlorhydria | Achlorhydria |
| I.F. and parietal cell antibodies | Absent | Present | Present |
| Family incidence | Present | Absent | Absent |
| Endocrinopathies | Absent | Absent | Hypothyroid Addison's disease Hypoparathyroidism |

As a unified concept, the megaloblastic anemias may be considered a single morphologic entity due to defective nucleoprotein synthesis from various causes.[50] The vast majority of patients with megaloblastic anemia have been found to have a deficiency of vitamin $B_{12}$, of folic acid, or of both vitamins. Herbert and Zalusky[50] have shown that folic acid activity piles up in human serum in the presence of vitamin $B_{12}$ deficiency. Vitamin $B_{12}$ is required for normal folic acid metabolism, and the apparent folic acid deficiency in many patients with vitamin $B_{12}$ deficiency may be due in large measure to secondarily deranged folic acid metabolism. Waters and Mollin[123] have also demonstrated that there is an accumulation of folic acid-like material in the serum of patients with pernicious anemia and that the level of this material falls rapidly after treatment with vitamin $B_{12}$.

Deficiencies of folic acid or vitamin $B_{12}$, or of both, account for at least 95% of all patients with megaloblastic anemia. The remainder, less than 5% includes patients who utilize these vitamins inadequately as in those with liver disease or orotic aciduria[53] or following therapy for leukemia with antipurines or antipyrimidines.[47]

Hereditary orotic aciduria associated with megaloblastic anemia unresponsive to vitamin $B_{12}$ and folic acid has been described in two children.[5,53] It is characterized by severe megaloblastic changes in the bone marrow, hypochromic macrocytes and microcytes, anisocytosis, poikilocytosis, multisegmented neutrophils and giant platelets in the peripheral blood, and the excretion of large amounts of orotic acid in the urine. These patients may be mentally retarded. The orotic acid cystalluria is due to a congenital defect in the pathway of synthesis of pyrimidine nucleotides. Hematologic remission is induced by the ingestion of adequate amounts of the pyrimidine nucleoside uridine. Investigation of parents and siblings indicate a heterozygous state without clinical abnormality and a minimal decrease in urinary orotic acid excretion. Orotic aciduria represents an inborn error of pyrimidine metabolism, in which there is a marked reduction in activity of two sequential enzymes in the major pathway of pyrimidine synthesis. The condition should be suspected in a child with a megaloblastic anemia with unexplained crystalluria or when mental retardation and anemia coexist.

The metabolic pathway of orotic acid is shown in the following diagram:

In another case the hemoglobin measured 7.7 gm./100 ml. at 2 months of age.[103] Treatment with iron produced no response. The bone marrow revealed erythroid hyperplasia and numerous megaloblastic erythroid precursors. The peripheral blood smear showed anisocytosis, poikilocytosis, hyperchromia, and hypersegmentation of granulocytes. Orotic acid crystalluria led to the diagnosis. With the administration of oral uridine (1.5 mg./kg.) a reticulocyte response appeared within 48 hours and a rise in hemoglobin followed. The mental development was normal at 2½ years. The enzymatic defect involves the two essential enzymes of normal pyrimidine synthesis, as shown in the diagram.

Investigation of the family revealed other heterozygous individuals. With the pedigrees of these families, an autosomal recessive mode of inheritance was demonstrated.

A urinary screening test for hereditary orotic aciduria has been described.[101] The test is based upon the conversion of orotic acid to barbituric acid by the action of saturated bromine water and subsequent reduction by ascorbic acid.

Available findings, according to some workers, indicate that a folic acid abnormality is basic to megaloblastic maturation, and this abnormality is secondary to vitamin $B_{12}$ deficiency. Unless an adequate amount of vitamin $B_{12}$ is available, folic acid and coenzymes cannot participate in their critical roles in nucleic acid synthesis and cell division. Others consider that vitamin $B_{12}$ is essential per se to prevent megaloblastic maturation[42] and that this vitamin rather than folic acid occupies a central role.

An 11-year-old Caucasian girl has been reported[102] with a megaloblastic anemia, refractory to folate and vitamin $B_{12}$, but responsive to treatment with thiamine. Withdrawal of supplemental vitamins resulted in a relapse within 3½ months. When the implicated vitamins were given sequentially, a reticulocytosis followed the administration of thiamine. Anemia again recurred 4 months after vitamin supplementation was discontinued. On this occasion the anemia was corrected by 20 mg. oral thiamine daily. The patient therefore appeared to have a thiamine-dependent megaloblastic anemia. Additional abnormalities included diabetes mellitus, aminoaciduria, and sensorineural deafness.

***Diagnosis of the megaloblastic anemias.*** The diagnosis of megaloblastic anemia is usually based on characteristic changes in the periph-

$$\text{Orotic acid} \xrightarrow[\text{Pyrophosphorylase}]{\text{Orotidylic}} \text{Orotidylic acid} \xrightarrow[\text{Decarboxylase}]{\text{Orotidylic}} \text{Uridylic acid} \longrightarrow \text{Nucleic acids}$$

$$\text{Uridine} \updownarrow \text{Uridylic acid}$$

eral blood and bone marrow: macrocytosis, oval red cells, pear-shaped poikilocytes, the presence in the peripheral blood of the polymorphonuclear neutrophils with hypersegmented nuclei, and megaloblasts and giant metamyelocytes in the marrow.[25] Confirmatory laboratory tests include the determination of vitamin $B_{12}$, folic acid, or both in the patient's serum and testing for the excretion of formiminoglutamic acid described previously.

Estimation of folic acid activity in serum is carried out by the microbiologic assay with *Lactobacillus casei* or with *Streptococcus faecalis*. *Lactobacillus casei* values of 7 to 15.9 $\mu\mu$g per milliliter are normal.[50] In normal subjects the serum level is also given as 5.9 to 21 $\mu\mu$g per milliliter (mean 9.9.)[122] For vitamin $B_{12}$ in serum, two microbiologic assays are available using *Euglena gracilis* and *Lactobacillus leichmanii*. With *Euglena gracilis* values of 200 to 900 $\mu\mu$g per milliliter are normally found. Besides microbiologic methods, tests are available for the determination of the capacity to absorb vitamin $B_{12}$: fecal excretion, urinary excretion (Shilling test), hepatic uptake, and plasma radioactivity determinations. Similarly, for folic acid, absorption and clearance tests (after oral or intravenous administration) and FIGLU determinations are available.[44]

The retention of small doses of parenteral folic acid in man provides good evidence of the state of the folic acid stores. Not only is a greater amount retained in patients with hematologic evidence of folic acid deficiency, but these doses, when given intravenously, are also cleared from the plasma to the tissue more rapidly than in control subjects.[12,13]

## MEGALOBLASTIC ANEMIA OF INFANCY

*Etiology.* Megaloblastic anemia of infancy is an acute anemia (rarely chronic), transitory in nature, due to a deficiency of folic acid. It is brought on by states in which reserves of folic acid are greatly diminished such as during periods of rapid growth, high nutritional demands, infection, and prolonged diarrhea.[77,134] Premature infants are especially susceptible.

The folic acid content of goat's milk is exceedingly low, 10.7 $\mu$g per liter as compared with whole cow's milk of 89.5 $\mu$g per liter, indicating the potential danger of megaloblastic anemia with excessive consumption of goat's milk.[86] Ascorbic acid and, to some extent, vitamin $B_{12}$ appear to play significant roles in the pathogenesis of this disease. The occasional case in which a response is obtained with large doses of vitamin $B_{12}$ is explained by the sparing action on folic acid.[71] Vitamin $B_{12}$ not only interacts with folic acid in the tissues as a coenzyme at different stages of nucleic acid synthesis, but also influences in some way the storage and intake of folic acid.[88] A disorder identical with that in the human being has been produced in monkeys fed a diet largely of powdered milk, notorious for its causative relationship to the disease in infants. Without additional ascorbic acid the animals develop scurvy and then megaloblastic anemia.[75] On the other hand, the severe deficiency of folic acid as a complication of scurvy in monkeys fed milk diets is probably due to nonspecific factors operating in scurvy.[75]

The participation of ascorbic acid in pathogenesis[76] is emphasized by the fact that the incidence of megaloblastic anemia has dropped precipitously since infant foods have been fortified with large amounts of this vitamin. This dramatic change applied particularly to powdered milk preparations that had been low in ascorbic acid. There is reason to believe that many cases reported as goat's milk anemia are indeed megaloblastic anemia of infancy.

Roberts and co-workers[99] studied the normal values for serum and red cell folate in seventy premature infants followed for the first 6 months of life. High levels of both serum and red cell folate were found in the infants at birth; the levels dropped rapidly until they reached low values at 3 months of age. At birth the mean serum folate was very high—the mean 18.7 ng./ml. (range 5.5-30.0). A marked fall in the mean value of the serum folate occurred in each 10-day period during the first 2 months of life; it then remained below 6 ng./ml. until 6 months of age. At 2 to 3 months the lowest values were reached, the mean being 1.9 ng./ml. Similarly, red cell folate dropped from a mean of 563 ng./ml. from 1 to 9 days to 140 ng./ml. at 3 to 4 months of age. These low levels were probably related to the low dietary folate intake, and the exhaustion of the high initial stores derived from the mother. There was probably an initial high intracellular level of folate at birth, which was gradually utilized with little or no replacement of folate for at least the first 3 months of life. Human colostrum contains a mean of 4.4 $\mu$g/liter of folate; mature milk more than 15 days postpartum, a mean of 16.5 µg/liter of folate. It is well known that the folate content of breast milk increases during the postpartum period. In fifty normal full-term infants the mean serum folate was 24.1 ng./ml. and mean red cell folate 460 ng./ml. It had previously been shown that in the healthy infant the level of whole blood "folic acid" was high at birth and dropped to a subnormal level by 8 weeks, and from then on to 1 year remained well below the adult norm.[74]

The normal adult levels of red cell folate have been considered to range between 160 and 640 ng./ml. of packed red cells. Others have given the upper normal value to be 530 ng./ml.[99]

*Clinical features.* The onset is insidious and usually makes its appearance between the ages of 2 and 17 months, with a mean age of 7 to 8 months.[71] Pallor, anorexia, irritability, failure to gain weight, persistent upper respiratory infections, intermittent fever, and diarrhea are common. Petechiae, mucous membrane hemorrhages, and ecchymoses, in conjunction with thrombocytopenia, are present in severely affected infants. The nutritional status is poor. The heart may be enlarged, and some degree of hepatomegaly is a common feature. Splenomegaly is unusual. There is no neurologic component as in patients with pernicious anemia. There may be transitory gastric achlorhydria, even after histamine administration and occasional hypoproteinemia.

*Laboratory findings.* Anemia is mild or severe. Hemoglobin levels below 5 gm. per 100 ml. are common.[133] The red blood cell count may be markedly reduced in occasional cases to less than 1 million per cubic millimeter. The blood smear shows anisocystosis, poikilocytosis, and either a normochromic or hypochromic anemia, and a moderate macrocytosis is noted. Except for leukocytosis with infections, leukopenia and neutropenia are common findings. The polymorphonuclear neutrophils are enlarged and hypersegmented. The platelets are reduced in number, often markedly so. In moderately or severely affected infants nucleated red cells appear in the peripheral blood. The bone marrow examination is diagnostic. The megaloblastic type of erythropoiesis corresponds to that of pernicious anemia (Figs. 22 and 23). The open structure of the nucleus, its finely divided chromatin, easily visible parachromatin, and basophilic cytoplasm characterize the megaloblasts.[115,133] Giant metamyelo-

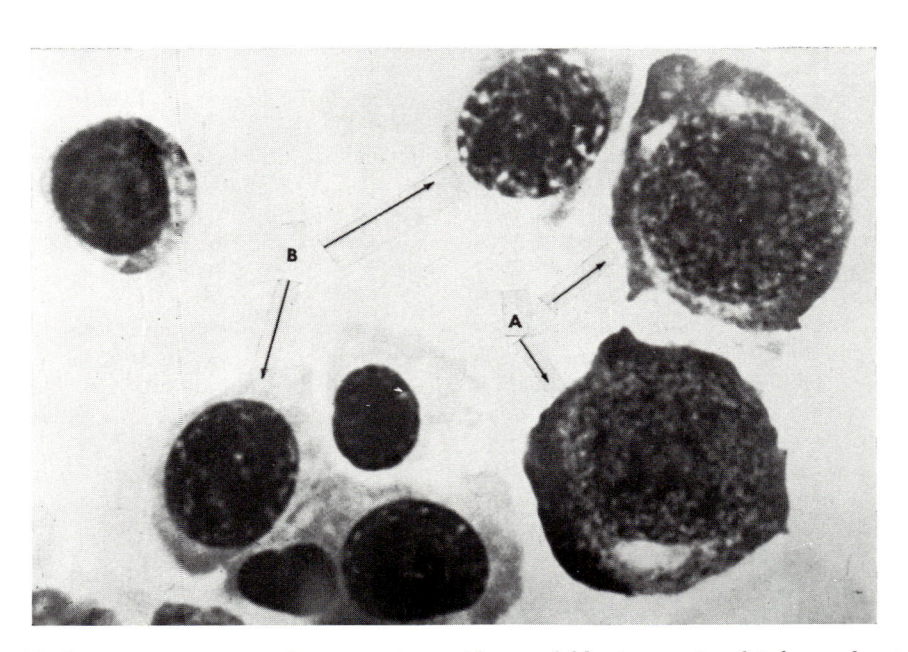

Fig. 22. Bone marrow smears from a patient with megaloblastic anemia of infancy showing megaloblastic erythroid precursors. Note the more typical megaloblastic chromatin structure in the early erythroblasts, **A**, and the less well-defined changes in the normoblasts, **B**. Cell at upper left is a small lymphocyte. (×900.) (From Luhby, L.: Megaloblastic anemia in infancy, J. Pediat. **54:**617, 1959.)

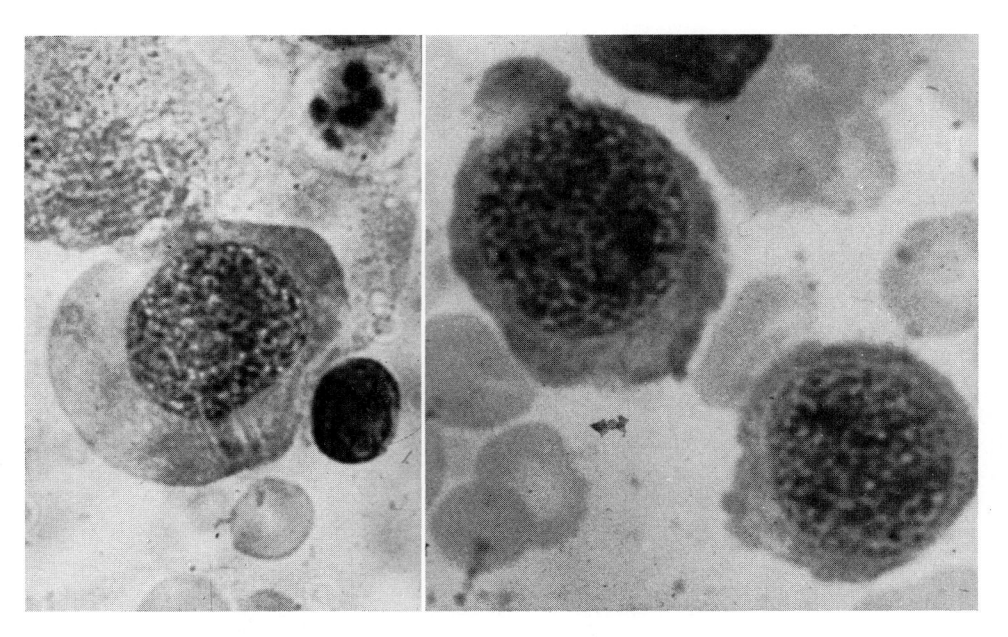

**Fig. 23.** Bone marrow smear from a 13-month-old child with severe megaloblastic anemia. Note three typical megaloblasts and in upper left a hypersegmented neutrophil. (Courtesy Dr. Philip Lanzkowsky, New York, N. Y.)

cytes and giant stab cells with distorted nuclei are pathognomonic of this disorder. Appearing at times in advance of megaloblasts, they are indications of the early stages of megaloblastic anemia. The variation in the number of megaloblasts, normoblasts, and abnormal metamyelocytes in different cases indicates that the deficiency may be partial and not always complete. Formiminoglutamic acid urinary excretion has been found useful as an indicator of folic acid deficiency.[71]

After the start of treatment for deficiency of vitamin $B_{12}$ or folate, it takes 1 to 4 months for hypersegmentation to disappear.

*Treatment.* The anemia responds readily and completely to oral administration of folic acid given daily in a dosage of 5 mg. over a period of 2 to 3 weeks, or until the blood and bone marrow picture returns to normal. A reticulocyte rise follows the administration of folic acid. Complete disappearance of the megaloblastic pattern is noted 2 days after the injection of folic acid.[133] Ascorbic acid should be given simultaneously in a dose of approximately 200 mg. if there is any suspicion of its deficiency. Some workers advocate a combination of folic acid and ascorbic acid from the outset as a routine procedure. In countries where malnutrition and poverty exist and megaloblastic anemia is prevalent, vitamin $B_{12}$ is also added.[69] An enriched diet containing folic acid and vitamin $B_{12}$ is essential. Antibiotic therapy is important, especially since infection plays such an important role in etiology. Transfusions are indicated when anemia is severe, but folic acid must be given at the same time. Where facilities are available, the precise deficiency should be determined so that appropriate therapy can be administered.

*Prognosis.* Complete recovery within a few weeks is expected following folic acid therapy. Although the administration of folic acid produces a permanent cure of megaloblastic anemia of infancy, juvenile pernicious anemia with a similar megaloblastic bone marrow is a lifelong disease requiring continuous therapy.

### JUVENILE PERNICIOUS ANEMIA

*Etiology.* Pernicious anemia in childhood is exceedingly rare.[6,84,90,96,104] Addisonian pernicious anemia is a megaloblastic anemia caused by a deficiency of vitamin $B_{12}$, which is based on a defective adsorption of the vitamin resulting from diminished or absent gastric secretion of intrinsic factor.[85] The essential abnormality in pernicious anemia is the failure of gastric secretion of an intrinsic factor needed for the ileal absorption of the extrinsic factor vitamin $B_{12}$. Continuous treatment is required to maintain the patient in a state of remission. Without vitamin $B_{12}$ normoblasts fail to mature and assume the cytologic features of the megaloblast. The absorption of substances other than vitamin $B_{12}$ is usually normal.[85] A familial tendency toward the disease has been noted.[96,114]

In its complete form juvenile pernicious anemia is characterized, as in the adult, by a macrocytic anemia, megaloblastic bone marrow, absence of intrinsic factor, atrophy of the papilla of the tongue and other features of recurrent glossitis, nervous system involvement, a specific response to parenteral injections of vitamin $B_{12}$, converting the bone marrow to a normoblastic pattern, and the need for continuous therapy to prevent relapses. Histamine refractory achlorhydria, one of the cardinal features of adult pernicious anemia, is an inconstant finding, however, in the juvenile form of the disease.

According to Castle,[9] pernicious anemia results from a vitamin $B_{12}$ deficiency associated with a lack of intrinsic factor of the normal human gastric secretion. "In the normal stomach the intrinsic factor is secreted by the parietal cells and avidly binds to itself the small amounts of vitamin $B_{12}$ found in most foods of animal origin and released during peptic digestion. Once so bound, the vitamin is then conveyed to the distal ileum where the intrinsic factor-vitamin $B_{12}$ complex is specifically adsorbed to the microvilli of the intestinal cell, and the vitamin is released to the cell interior and subsequently reaches the bloodstream."[9] Pernicious anemia in adults displays the characteristic defects of gastric secretion including volume, hydrochloric acid, pepsin, and intrinsic factor. In these patients the serum contains antibody directed against the intrinsic factor. The antibody becomes detectable at the stage in which the atrophic gastric mucosa no longer has sufficient antigen to absorb them. "Juvenile" pernicious anemia results from a congenital lack of intrinsic factor in an otherwise normal gastric secretion but is unassociated with anti-intrinsic factor antibodies.

By 1963, only twelve cases of pernicious anemia in childhood had been reported in which the diagnosis had been established beyond doubt. They had in common a deficiency of intrinsic factor in the gastric juice.[73] These children, in contrast to adults with pernicious anemia, usually had free hydrochloric acid in the gastric juice and a normal mucosa. In several instances temporary loss of acid secretion was observed during relapse of the anemia. Waters and Murphy[124] reported two additional cases of juvenile pernicious anemia and refer to another case of the anemia, probably present in a third brother who had died before their studies were initiated. Both parents and five other siblings absorbed subnormal or borderline amounts of a test dose of labeled vitamin $B_{12}$. It was concluded that both parents carried the gene for the deficient secretion of intrinsic factor as heterozygotes, and that the affected children were presumably homozygous for the gene, having inherited it from both parents. In several studies it was shown that relatives of patients with pernicious anemia have been reported to have a deficiency of intrinsic factor[7] and a defective vitamin $B_{12}$ absorption.[79] Typical juvenile pernicious anemia may result, therefore, from the homozygous inheritance of a gene responsible for the deficient secretion of intrinsic factor. The adult form is explained on the basis of an inherited heterozygous defect of intrinsic factor secretion, on which is superimposed an atrophic lesion of the mucosa.

A familial syndrome in children with megaloblastic anemia in whom there is selective malabsorption of vitamin $B_{12}$, an unexplained and persistent proteinuria, and an intrinsic factor activity present has been described.[38,51,54,113] Gastric achlorhydria is absent. The persistent proteinuria is of great interest. It is not orthostatic and is not corrected by vitamin $B_{12}$ therapy. There is no evidence of impairment in renal function. Patients with this familial megaloblastic anemia have pallor, weakness, anorexia, irritability, and fever. The onset of symptoms is from 5 to 6 months to 4 years of age. The bone marrow resembles that of pernicious anemia. The anemia responds to parenteral therapy with liver or vitamin $B_{12}$. Remissions as long as 14 to 15 months occasionally occur without treatment. With continued therapy patients appear to be in good health. This condition is probably due to intestinal malabsorption of vitamin $B_{12}$. The defect in vitamin $B_{12}$ absorption seems to be a specific one; no other abnormalities in intestinal absorptive function have been detected. X-ray examination of the stomach and small bowel have not disclosed any abnormalities. As in juvenile pernicious anemia, this megaloblastic anemia is also inherited in a simple, recessive genetic pattern.

Recent studies have focused attention upon autoimmune mechanisms in the etiology of pernicious anemia. Intrinsic factor antibodies have been demonstrated in a large percentage of known cases of adult pernicious anemia,[56,108,116] mainly those treated orally for some time and also in several untreated patients.[108] The presence of intrinsic factor antibodies was shown in 20 to 30% of patients with this disease.[56] The results of vitamin $B_{12}$ absorption tests utilizing human intrinsic factor and $^{60}CoB_{12}$ complex, mixed with normal and pernicious anemia sera, have demonstrated the inhibiting effect of some pernicious anemia sera. It has been estimated that the sera of approximately one-third of all individuals with pernicious anemia contain an antibody against human intrinsic factor.[94] Although there is apparently an abundance of evidence for autoimmunity in the etiology of pernicious anemia, its role in the pathogenesis of the disease is still unclear, since the antibody formed may be a secondary phenomenon. Intrinsic factor and parietal cell antibodies are usually absent in the juvenile form of the disease.

McIntyre and associates[78] extended the number of definitely proved cases of pernicious anemia in childhood to twenty-five and added an additional case of their own. In one group of nineteen patients, there was an early onset of a selective vitamin $B_{12}$ deficiency, lack of intrinsic factor with the preservation of normal acid secretion, and normal gastric mucosa histology. Antibodies to intrinsic factor were not found in the serum of these patients. In the second group of six patients, vitamin $B_{12}$ deficiency developed in later childhood. In this group deficient intrinsic factor secretion was present with gastric mucosa atrophy and histamine-fast achlorhydria. In four of these there was an associated endocrinopathy (hypoparathyroidism, hypothyroidism, or Addison's disease). In contrast to the first group, antibodies to gastric parietal cells or intrinsic factor were detected in sera of these patients. The authors suggest that the latter group of juvenile patients suffered from adult pernicious anemia, whereas the larger number of patients with intact acid secretion and histologically normal gastric mucosa were not genetically related to adult pernicious anemia.

A case of pernicious anemia has been reported in a 10-year-old girl with familial Addison's disease, idiopathic hypoparathyroidism, and moniliasis.[94] Pernicious anemia was diagnosed by the demonstration of a megaloblastic anemia, absence of intrinsic factor, and response to vitamin $B_{12}$ therapy. Several other cases of pernicious anemia associated with one or the other of these endocrinopathies have been previously reported. Unlike previous cases of pernicious anemia reported in children, this case presented achlorhydria and mild atrophic gastric mucosa. These findings do not contradict the belief that the gastric atrophy of adult pernicious anemia is secondary to chronic avitaminosis $B_{12}$. In this case antibody against human intrinsic factor was found.

A girl has been reported[29] now 11 years of age who has been shown to be suffering from pernicious anemia which first produced symptoms when she was under the age of 2. A congenitally determined defect in intrinsic factor synthesis was considered to be the likely cause, in contrast to the genetically determined disorder of the immunological mechanism which characterizes most of the cases of pernicious anemia in adults.

Although autoantibody to gastric parietal cells is found in up to 90% of all patients with pernicious anemia, this autoantibody is not considered characteristic of the disease.[35] Nevertheless, Goldberg and Fudenberg[35] believe that this antibody is found so frequently in pernicious anemia that its absence should make the clinician suspect another diagnosis. The antibody is known to occur in 5 to 8% of the random population between the ages of 30 and 60 years and in 14% of women over the age of 60. It has also been demonstrated that the administration of steroids to patients with pernicious anemia results in regeneration of atrophic gastric mucosa with subsequent production of intrinsic factor. With discontinuation of steroid therapy the disease state—atrophic gastric mucosa with absent intrinsic factor—recurs.[35]

*Clinical manifestations.* Many of the cases are detected during the first 2 years of life, whereas others become manifest during childhood until puberty. The onset is insidious, and pallor, apathy, fatigability, anorexia, and diarrhea are early symptoms. A beefy red, sore tongue, papillary atrophy, and other features of recurrent glossitis are common. Signs of subacute dorsolateral degeneration of the spinal cord occur infrequently.[96] Most common are neurologic signs, including ataxia, less often paresthesia of the hands and feet, inpaired vibratory perception, Babinski signs, and absence of tendon reflexes. Jaundice is absent, and there is no enlargement of the liver and spleen.

*Laboratory findings.* Macrocytes, many of

them oval, anisocytosis, poikilocytosis, polychromasia, and, occasionally, nucleated red cells characterize the blood smear and parallel the severity of the anemia. The hemoglobin ranges from 4 to 9 gm. per 100 ml., usually below 6 gm. The red blood cell count is comparatively lower than the hemoglobin level, varying from 1 to 2.5 million per cubic millimeter.

The anemia, being macrocytic, shows a high color index and an increase in the mean corpuscular volume (MCV) ranging from 110 to 140 $\mu^3$, which is well above the upper limit of normal of 92 $\mu^3$. The life-span of the red cells is moderately shortened.[24] The macrocyte, normally saturated with hemoglobin, takes a dark stain and conveys the impression of hyperchromia. Supersaturation is nonexistent. Leukopenia is common and may be marked, with the number of white cells ranging from 3,000 to 4,000 per cubic millimeter, and is caused by a depression of myeloid tissue in the bone marrow. Hypersegmentation of oversized polymorphonuclear leukocytes (macropolycytes) with bizarre-shaped lobes is common. The platelets are reduced in number. The leukopenia and thrombocytopenia are not so marked as to lead to susceptibility to infection or purpura.

The bone marrow is hyperplastic, with the nucleated red cells ranging up to 50% of the total cells. Of these the megaloblasts in different stages of maturation and hemoglobinization predominate. The typical megaloblast is larger and the cytoplasm more abundant than the normoblast of an equivalent stage of hemoglobinization. Their nuclear pattern is composed of strands more widely separated from each other than the comparable early normoblast. Mitotic figures are common. The abnormally large size of the polymorphonuclear cells and the metamyelocytes are characteristic features. The changes are particularly pronounced among the metamyelocytes, which are giant in size, possess a U shaped nucleus, and have a bulky, poorly granulated cytoplasm.

Ineffective erythropoiesis characterizes the anemia, i.e., erythroid cell death and phagocytosis within the marrow. More hemoglobin and red cell synthesis occurs in the marrow than can be accounted for in the peripheral blood.[87]

*Diagnosis.* Because of the rarity of pernicious anemia in children, it is important to eliminate other causes of megaloblastic anemia. A low serum vitamin $B_{12}$ suggests the diagnosis and it is confirmed by showing defective vitamin $B_{12}$ absorption using the Schilling test; vitamin $B_{12}$ absorption can be restored by the addition of intrinsic factor to the Schilling test. The difficulty in diagnosis has been the presence of free hydrochloric acid in the gastric contents and the inconsistency of histamine refractory achlorhydria in many of the reported cases.[104] Long-term follow-up is necessary to determine whether achlorhydria, essential for the diagnosis of the adult disease, will eventually develop. The presence of a megaloblastic bone marrow, the absence of intrinsic factor, a good reticulocyte response following the administration of vitamin $B_{12}$, and the continuous requirement of vitamin $B_{12}$ to maintain a remission of the disease constitute the basic diagnostic features.

A young man who was reported to have had pernicious anemia at the age of 13 months was found to be still suffering from vitamin $B_{12}$ deficiency at 18 years of age.[85] He secreted normal amounts of acid and pepsin in the gastric juice but was unable to absorb a test dose of radioactive vitamin $B_{12}$ unless this was given with a source of intrinsic factor. The gastric juice was deficient in intrinsic factor, but the gastric mucosal membrane was histologically normal. The patient's father suffered from typical addisonian pernicious anemia. It was suggested that vitamin $B_{12}$ deficiency itself could cause temporary gastric atrophy, which becomes permanent and complete if treatment is withheld too long. In another study[67] two children with pernicious anemia showed normal gastric function and structure. An inability to absorb vitamin $B_{12}$ from the gastrointestinal tract was demonstrated. The author postulated that the gastric manifestations of pernicious anemia are not an intrinsic part of the disease but are secondary to chronic deficiency of vitamin $B_{12}$.

Miller and co-workers[84] described three patients with juvenile pernicious anemia who were followed from infancy for long periods of time. They were characterized by the low levels of serum vitamin $B_{12}$, the early onset of megaloblastic anemia, absent intrinsic factor activity, but otherwise normal gastric secretions and normal gastric mucosal histology. The vitamin $B_{12}$ absorption was corrected by intrinsic factor but gastric-mucosa histology remained normal after 5, 11, and 29 years of the follow-up. Family studies in forty-three relatives demonstrated no increased incidence of intrinsic factor or parietal cell antibodies.

A 4-month-old infant has been described with megaloblastic anemia due to vitamin $B_{12}$ deficiency.[62] The anemia was attributed to insufficient vitamin $B_{12}$ in the mother, who was proved to have pernicious anemia. The infant was responsive to vitamin $B_{12}$ but not to folic acid. By 4 months the patient's stores of vitamin $B_{12}$ were sufficiently depleted to result in megaloblastic anemia.

McNicholl and Egan[80] reported three children, two of them siblings, who developed megaloblastic anemia around 1 year, showing a deficiency of intrinsic factor. They pointed out that growth retardation and acceleration appeared to be related to $B_{12}$ deficiency and treatment. The I.Q. of about 70 in each child may represent the effect of $B_{12}$ deficiency in cerebral growth. Cerebral damage may result from delay in recognition and lack of specific treatment with vitamin $B_{12}$.

A number of tests have been devised for the confirmation of the diagnosis of pernicious anemia.[33] The newer methods include biopsy of the gastric mucosa[131,132] to determine the presence of atrophic changes, estimation of serum vitamin $B_{12}$ level, and methods for determining the amount of radioactive vitamin $B_{12}$ absorbed from the intestine. The urinary excretion method of Schilling,[107] one of the simplest, consists of the oral administration of a small dose of radioactive vitamin $B_{12}$ followed by a flushing dose of 1 mg. of nonradioactive vitamin $B_{12}$ injected parenterally, immediately or within 2 hours. The nonreactive vitamin $B_{12}$ given parenterally serves to block the vitamin $B_{12}$-binding sites in the liver and plasma, thus causing the radioactive material to be flushed out.[111] Following the oral dose of radioactive vitamin $B_{12}$, substantial amounts of the vitamin are excreted in the urine of normal persons within 24 hours, as compared with minute amounts in patients with pernicious anemia. The normal urinary excretion is greater than 5% of the test dose. In pernicious anemia the excretion is 0 to 3% or from 3 to 30% if radioactive vitamin $B_{12}$ is given with intrinsic factor. In patients with pernicious anemia serum vitamin $B_{12}$ levels are low.

The need for accurate diagnosis of the type of megaloblastic anemia, so that appropriate treatment may be given, is emphasized in the report of a child with an onset of pernicious anemia in the first year of life.[89] At 18 months, a hypercellular marrow with megaloblastic erythropoiesis led to prolonged treatment with folic acid, with resulting hematologic remissions. When ataxia and coma developed at 32 months, vitamin $B_{12}$ therapy was instituted. Dramatic improvement resulted, except for partial deafness and mental retardation. The neurologic complications were probably the sequelae of prolonged vitamin $B_{12}$ deficiency, which was masked by the folic acid therapy. The administration of physiologic doses of folic acid (25 to 100 $\mu$g per day) has been suggested as both a diagnostic and therapeutic measure in cases of megaloblastic anemia in children. Such doses of folic acid will not be effective in pernicious anemia, while anemia secondary to folic acid deficiency will rapidly respond. An accurate diagnosis will be definitely established by vitamin $B_{12}$ absorption tests utilizing radioactive vitamin $B_{12}$ (Schilling test).

Cases of anemia associated with deficiency in vitamin $B_{12}$ and/or folate show distinct alterations in chromosome structure.[43] These consist of increased chromosome breakage, incomplete chromosome contraction, and centromere spreading. These abnormalities were not present after vitamin replacement. These cytogenic changes observed seem compatible with current concepts of megaloblastic cell division and with the role of folate and vitamin $B_{12}$ in DNA metabolism. All specimens examined were direct preparations of bone marrow.

**Course and prognosis.** With modern treatment, utilizing vitamin $B_{12}$ in adequate dosage, the outlook for reversal of the disorder is uniformly favorable, provided the patient does not have significant neurologic involvement when first seen. Complications arising from nervous system involvement do not respond to $B_{12}$ therapy.

**Treatment.** The response to vitamin $B_{12}$ is rapid and specific. The standard form of treatment consists of the parenteral injection of vitamin $B_{12}$. The dosage is to some degree an individual matter. In children a remission of the disease should be obtained with doses of 15 to 30 $\mu$g given every day or two for 2 to 4 weeks, followed by a maintenance dose of the same amount given every 2 to 4 weeks. Larger doses may be required. An alternate schedule is to give a large initial dose daily for five injections or every second or third day for 10 to 15 days, followed by one injection of 100 $\mu$g each month.[28] Liver extract may be given on the basis of its vitamin $B_{12}$ content.

The reticulocytes begin to increase on the third to fourth day, rise to a maximum on the sixth to eighth day, and fall gradually to normal about the twentieth day.[28] The height of the reticulocyte count is inversely proportional to the degree of anemia. Beginning bone marrow reversal from megaloblastic to normoblastic cells is obvious within 6 hours and is completely normoblastic in 72 hours.

Prompt hematologic responses are also obtained with the use of oral folic acid. Folic acid is, however, contraindicated since it has no effect upon neurologic manifestations and has been known to precipitate or accelerate their development. Indeed, megaloblastic anemia should never be treated before a serum folic acid or vitamin $B_{12}$ assay has determined the precise cause so that correct treatment can be administered. Iron is occasionally required when a generally inadequate diet has been given which is deficient in this mineral.

## NUTRITIONAL MEGALOBLASTIC ANEMIA

Nutritional megaloblastic anemia is a macrocytic anemia, occurring among underprivileged peoples in tropical and subtropical countries where malnutrition is prevalent due to poverty and dietary habits.[129] It results from an inadequate dietary intake, usually of folic acid and occasionally of vitamin $B_{12}$. The megaloblastic bone marrow, macrocytic anemia, and leukocytic changes respond to folic acid with or without vitamin $B_{12}$.[69] Correction of dietary defects is essential. Iron and transfusions are given as needed.

This type of anemia is to be differentiated from that occurring in kwashiorkor. The latter, originally described as a nutritional syndrome of African infants and children, is also prevalent in Central and South America,[109] India, China, and other countries and results from severe protein deficiency. The limiting nitrogenous factor in kwashiorkor is not one of the essential aminoacids, but nitrogen.[52] The intake of calories derived largely from starchy food is adequate. The anemia is usually normochromic and normocytic and, less commonly, macrocytic and microcytic.[36] Shortened red cell survival in young subjects with protein malnutrition (kwashiorkor and marasmus) appears to be due to both corpuscular and extracorpuscular factors.[65] Occasionally, it is aggravated by blood loss due to hookworm and malaria. The bone marrow is normoblastic or megaloblastic.[1,109] The anemia of kwashiorkor has also been found in association with aplastic crises (erythroblastopenia) in which giant proerythroblasts appeared in the marrow.[32,57,68,121] Patients with the normochromic, normocytic type of anemia respond to a well-balanced diet rich in protein but not in liver extract, folic acid, or vitamin $B_{12}$. Iron is occasionally effective. In those cases of kwashiorkor in which megaloblastic anemia of infancy is diagnosed, the bone marrow reverts to normal following the administration of folic acid.[120] The prothrombin is diminished in most cases and about 15% show purpura and thrombocytopenia.[81]

Nutritional megaloblastic anemia of pregnancy is also more common in underprivileged areas and is due to a chronic dietary deficiency. The prognosis for the mother and fetus has improved with the use of folic acid and vitamin $B_{12}$.[129] Riboflavin has also been recommended, especially in the recovery from crises of red cell aplasia.[32]

Megaloblastic anemia has been reported complicating the dietary treatment of phenylketonuria in infancy.[105] An infant in whom the diagnosis of phenylketonuria was made early in infancy was given a synthetic phenylalanine-restricted diet. Anemia was noted at 3 months, and at 6 months the bone marrow showed megaloblastic erythropoiesis. There was no response to vitamin $B_{12}$, and before folic acid could be administered, the infant's condition deteriorated and he died soon after. It was suggested that the marrow should be examined when infants are placed on such restricted diets and that folic acid should be given when necessary. Striking bone marrow vacuolizations of the erythroid series and, to a lesser extent, of other cellular elements were noted in a case of phenylketonuria on a restricted diet. The vacuolization disappeared with the addition of dietary phenylalanine.[110]

Kondi and associates[60] reported a group of cases of marasmus and kwashiorkor and found that, besides the low serum proteins on admission, there was a variety of complicating infections. Unless these were treated hematologic response was incomplete. Some anemias were either hypochromic or normochromic and were unrelated to the serum protein values. The blood findings in marasmus and kwashiorkor were indistinguishable, although the clinical picture was different. When hypoplasia or aplasia was diagnosed the cases were of two distinct types. One had an early onset and a short duration and was associated with giant proerythroblasts, neutrophilia, and infections responding without hematinics as the infection subsided.

Another type occurred late in recovery, was of longer duration, was unassociated with giant proerythroblasts or infections, but showed a lymphocytosis. These aplasias showed no folic acid deficiency. Some cases responded to riboflavin or prednisone but a small group of patients with anemia who were refractory to all other therapy eventually responded to pyridoxine. Megaloblastic anemia responding to folic acid was present in 17% of cases and these were associated with low serum folic acid and normal vitamin $B_{12}$ levels.

## MISCELLANEOUS MEGALOBLASTIC ANEMIAS

### Megaloblastic anemia with hemolytic anemias

Megaloblastic anemia is a rare complication of hemolytic anemia and has been reported in association with acquired hemolytic anemia, hereditary spherocytosis, thalassemia, sickle cell anemia, and paroxysmal nocturnal hemoglobinuria. The megaloblastic bone marrow is attributed to folic acid deficiency caused by the demands for this substance imposed by rapidly developing erythroid cells. The need for folic acid exceeds the dietary intake and results in tissue depletion.[16,59,128] Folic acid may be a limiting factor in the development of and recovery from the aplastic crisis of sickle cell anemia[91] and hereditary spherocytosis.[15] In each reported case pretreatment bone marrow demonstrated megaloblastic erythropoiesis.

Lindenbaum and Klipstein[70] summarized more than fifty cases of megaloblastic changes in patients with chronic hemolytic anemia reported in the literature. The administration of folic acid has been known to produce generalized bone pain in thalassemia major, either with a megaloblastic[100] or normoblastic marrow.[55,72] The onset of pain after folic acid therapy was related to expansion of an already fully occupied marrow cavity by an increase of the early erythrocyte forms. These early forms then matured and were released into the peripheral circulation.

Further reference to the development of megaloblastic bone marrow changes is cited in the course of discussing each of the hemolytic anemias in Chapters 15 and 16.

### Megaloblastic anemia with malignancies

The demands for folic acid in proliferating tissue of white cell origin may also account for megaloblastic anemia in patients with lymphosarcoma and chronic lymphocytic leukemia. The increased demands of rapidly growing neoplastic tissue for folic acid may be associated with a defect of this vitamin, due to malabsorption.[93]

### Megaloblastic anemia of pregnancy

It has been estimated that megaloblastic anemia occurs in 2.8% of all pregnancies.[17] The anemia responds to folic acid and its appearance in pregnancy may be prevented by giving folic acid supplements. This has suggested that the megaloblastic anemia in pregnancy is due either to a deficiency of folic acid or to interference with the utilization of this vitamin in pregnancy. Patients show an increased rate of clearance of folic acid from the plasma indicative of folic acid deficiency. This is a disease of late pregnancy and develops when the rate of fetal growth and therefore the fetal demand for folic acid is greatest. That megaloblastic anemia is eight times more frequent with twin pregnancies than with a single pregnancy supports this premise of the role of increased fetal demand.[17] Poor dietary intake or defective absorption of folic acid may contribute to the pathogenesis of this anemia. In one series,[18] eighteen out of 201 marrow specimens of affected pregnant women showed megaloblastic changes.

Megaloblastic anemia in pregnancy does not respond adequately to vitamin $B_{12}$ therapy but all patients respond completely to treatment with folic acid. The tendency is for the anemia to remit spontaneously after delivery.

### Megaloblastic anemia with hemochromatosis

The occurrence of a macrocytic anemia with a megaloblastic type of erythropoiesis has been observed in hemochromatosis. Its causation, as well as its formation and absorption, is related to the associated pigmentary cirrhosis hindering the storage of folic acid. In a patient with hemochromatosis with megaloblastic anemia there was a striking response to folic acid but not to vitamin $B_{12}$.[37]

### Megaloblastic anemia with fish tapeworm

The fish tapeworm (*Diphyllobothrium latum*) leads to megaloblastic anemia, indistinguishable from pernicious anemia. This type of anemia is caused by competition of the tapeworm with the host for the vitamin $B_{12}$ in the food in the intestinal tract necessary for the nutrition of the parasite.[119] Treatment depends upon expulsion of the parasite or the administration of vitamin $B_{12}$. On the other hand, patients with heavy hookworm infection develop a severe iron-deficiency anemia and lose about three times more blood than is provided in their bone marrow.[66]

## Megaloblastic anemia caused by anticonvulsant therapy

Extremely rare causes of megaloblastic anemia are the anticonvulsant agents phenytoin sodium (Dilantin)[106] and primidone (Mysoline).[34] The corrective effect of folic acid suggests that phenytoin and primidone may act as competitive inhibitors of some enzyme system normally involving folic acid.[34,127] A conditioning factor for the development of anticonvulsant megaloblastic anemia may be the presence in the patient of occult nutritional deficiency secondary to an inadequate diet, particularly of folic acid and to some extent of vitamin C.[31] Subnormal serum folic acid levels were observed in many patients receiving anticonvulsant drugs, especially Dilantin. In many of these patients slight or moderate macrocytosis was noted.[58]

In a study by Child and associates,[19] blood from 100 patients taking anticonvulsant drugs showed a high mean red cell volume (MCV) in 8%, low serum folate in 27%, and macrocytosis on a peripheral blood smear in 18%. These findings were not necessarily associated with an anemia. In another study,[98] megaloblastic changes in the bone marrow in patients on anticonvulsant drugs were not accompanied by anemia. Major blood dyscrasias are rare when minor blood abnormalities appear.

The folate clearance is abnormally fast in most patients with anemia but may be normal when there is a megaloblastic change with a relatively normal hemoglobin concentration.[11]

The administration of folic acid has been found to improve the mental state but to increase the frequency of seizures of chronic epileptic patients with folic acid deficiency due to anticonvulsant drug therapy.[97]

## MALABSORPTION SYNDROMES— SPRUE (TROPICAL), IDIOPATHIC STEATORRHEA (NONTROPICAL SPRUE), AND CELIAC DISEASE

Except for the common factor of impaired motility and absorption of the small intestine, there are no specific anatomic or pathologic changes in patients with sprue, idiopathic steatorrhea, or celiac disease. These diseases show a marked variation with regard to clinical features and causation.[33] Although the passage of stools containing an excess of fats (steatorrhea) is a characteristic feature of all of these diseases, patients also fail to absorb other nutrients. Thus, the body fails to absorb vitamins, minerals, proteins, carbohydrate, and such hematopoietic substances as folic acid, vitamin $B_{12}$, and iron. Diarrhea, weakness, and wasting are prominent symptoms.

Tropical sprue has a seasonal incidence and is limited largely to certain overcrowded and underdeveloped geographic areas in tropical and subtropical climates. It developes abruptly and runs a rapid course. Whether it is primarily or only secondarily a deficiency disease is not known.[27]

Idiopathic steatorrhea (nontropical sprue) is less common, occurs sporadically, has no seasonal or geographic incidence, and is usually a chronic and insidious disease.[20]

Celiac disease is included by some authors with nontropical sprue since it may persist into adult life. Celiac disease (Gee-Herter disease or gluten-induced enteropathy), a chronic disorder of infants and children, is characterized by diarrhea, wasting (especially noticeable in the flattened buttocks and groins), retardation of growth, and abdominal distention. The proteins (glutens) of wheat and rye are precipitating factors of the disorder, the gliadin fractions acting as toxic rather than allergic agents.[3,118]

In most cases of tropical sprue a macrocytic anemia indistinguishable from addisonian pernicious anemia is present and is associated with a megaloblastic bone marrow. Although a macrocytic anemia is commonly found in patients with nontropical sprue, it only occasionally presents the characteristics of pernicious anemia and may not be associated with megaloblastic bone marrow.[20] Glossitis is present in patients with tropical and nontropical sprue. Folic acid, vitamin $B_{12}$, and liver extract are specific therapeutic agents in the treatment of patients with tropical sprue with megaloblastic anemia. The deficiency pattern, including diarrhea, takes longer to reverse. Folic acid, vitamin $B_{12}$, and liver extract are also helpful in patients with nontropical sprue with megaloblastic anemia, although hematologic remission is not always complete and there is no demonstrable effect on the steatorrhea.[21] Hypochromic, microcytic anemia is by far more common than the macrocytic type in celiac disease. Iron administered orally or parenterally is given for the iron deficiency, and folic acid, liver extract, and vitamin $B_{12}$ are given for the macrocytic anemia.

The megaloblastic anemia associated with intestinal strictures, fistulas, and anastomoses is in some way dependent upon the invasion of the small intestine by organisms normally inhabiting the colon. In fistulas such as the ileocolic variety there is a direct contamination by organisms from the colon. In strictures and blind loops, stagnation predisposes to abnormal bacterial growth and absorption of toxic substances.[8,117] Most of the clinical and hematologic features are those of pernicious anemia or tropical sprue. Vitamin $B_{12}$ and especially folic acid have a beneficial effect on the anemia. Surgical correction of the intestinal disorder is often followed by relief of the anemia, but long-term parenteral vitamin $B_{12}$ administration may still be necessary. When intestinal stasis is a factor in the course of intestinal stricture and anastomosis, the impaired absorption of vitamin $B_{12}$ may be significantly improved by administration of the tetracycline group of antibiotics.[41]

Of the numerous tests for malabsorption, one of the simplest is the xylose excretion test.[64] It circumvents the need for stool collections. D-xylose in a dose of 0.3 gm./kg. with a maximum of 5 gm. dissolved in water to make a 5% solution is administered orally to fasting subjects. All urine excreted during the 5-hour period after ingestion is collected. In one group of children the mean percentage of recovery in younger infants (under 6 months) was 16.7%, from 6 months to 16 years from 25 to 38%, increasing with age, and in adults 36%.

In another group of children,[2] with an oral dose of 5 gm., values of 25% or more of the dose recovered indicated normal absorption in the upper gut and values below 15% indicated malabsorption.

## NORMOBLASTIC MACROCYTIC ANEMIAS

The normoblastic macrocytic anemias constitute a heterogenous group in which the bone marrow is normoblastic, but macrocytes appear in variable numbers in the peripheral blood interspersed among the red cells of a normocytic, normochromic anemia. These macrocytic anemias are secondary to aplastic anemia, lymphomas, and primary nonhematopoietic diseases such as hypothyroidism, scurvy, and liver disease.

### REFERENCES

1. Adams, E. B.: Anaemia in kwashiorkor, Brit. Med. J. 1:537, 1954.
2. Anderson, C. M.: Intestinal malabsorption in childhood, Arch. Dis. Child. 41:571, 1966.
3. Anderson, L. M., Frazer, A. C., French, I. M., Hawkins, C. F., Ross, C. A. C., and Sammons, H. G.: The influence of gluten and antibacterial agents on fat absorption in the sprue syndrome, Gastroenterologia 81:198, 1954.
4. Beck, W. S.: Metabolic functions of vitamin $B_{12}$, New Eng. J. Med. 266:708, 1962.
5. Becroft, D. M. O., and Phillips, L. I.: Hereditary orotic aciduria and megaloblastic anaemia; a second case, with response to uridine, Brit. J. Med. 1:547, 1965.
6. Benjamin, B.: Infantile form of pernicious (addisonian) anemia, Amer. J. Dis. Child. 75:143, 1948.
7. Callender, S. T., and Denborough, M. A.: A familial study of pernicious anaemia, Brit. J. Haemat. 3:88, 1957.
8. Cameron, D. G., Watson, G. M., and Witts, L. J.: The clinical association of macrocytic anemia with intestinal stricture and anastomosis, Blood 4:793, 1949.
9. Castle, W. B.: Current concepts of pernicious anemia, Amer. J. Med. 48:541, 1970.
10. Chanarin, I.: Urocanic acid and formiminoglutamic acid excretion in megaloblastic anaemia and other conditions; the effect of specific therapy, Brit. J. Haemat. 9:141, 1963.
11. Chanarin, I.: The megaloblastic anaemias, Philadelphia, 1969, F. A. Davis Co., p. 834.
12. Chanarin, I., Belcher, E. H., and Berry, V.: The utilization of tritium-labelled folic acid in megaloblastic anaemia, Brit. J. Haemat. 9:456, 1963.
13. Chanarin, I., and Bennett, M. C.: The plasma clearance of daily doses of folic acid in megaloblastic anaemia, Brit. J. Haemat. 8:95, 1962.
14. Chanarin, I., Bennett, M. C., and Berry, V.: Urinary excretion of histidine derivatives in megaloblastic anemia and other conditions and a comparison with the folic acid test, J. Clin. Path. 15:269, 1962.
15. Chanarin, I., Burman, D., and Bennett, M.: Familial aplastic crisis in hereditary spherocytosis; urocanic acid and FIGLU excretion studies in a case of megaloblastic anemia, Blood 20:33, 1962.
16. Chanarin, I., Dacie, J. V., and Mollin, D. L.:

Folic-acid deficiency in haemolytic anaemia, Brit. J. Haemat. 5:245, 1959.
17. Chanarin, I., MacGibbon, B. M., O'Sullivan, W. J., and Mollin, D. L.: Folic acid deficiency in pregnancy; the pathogenesis of megaloblastic anaemia in pregnancy, Lancet 2:634, 1959.
18. Chanarin, I., Rothman, D., Ward, A., and Perry, J.: Folate status requirement in pregnancy, Brit. J. Med. 2:390, 1968.
19. Child, J. A., Khattak, B. Z., and Knowles, J. P.: Macrocytosis in patients on anticonvulsant drugs, Brit. J. Haemat. 16:451, 1969.
20. Comfort, M. W., and Wallaeger, E. E.: Nontropical sprue; pathology, diagnosis and therapy, Arch. Intern. Med. 98:807, 1956.
21. Cooke, W. T., Frazer, A. C., Peeney, A. L. P., Sammons, H. G., and Thompson, M. D.: Anomalies of intestinal absorptions of fat; the haematology of idiopathic steatorrhea, Quart. J. Med. 17:9, 1948.
22. Cooper, B.: The absorption of folic acid and vitamin $B_{12}$ from the gastrointestinal tract, Blood 17:368, 1961.
23. Cooper, B. A., and Castle, W. B.: Sequential mechanisms in enhanced absorption of vitamin $B_{12}$ by intrinsic factor by rat, J. Clin. Invest. 39:199, 1960.
24. Dacie, J. V.: The haemolytic anaemias; congenital and acquired, New York, 1954, Grune & Stratton, Inc.
25. Dacie, J. V., and Lewis, S. M.: Practical haematology, ed. 3, New York, 1963, Grune & Stratton, Inc.
26. Dallman, P. R., and Diamond, L. K.: Vitamin $B_{12}$ deficiency associated with disease of the small intestine, J. Pediat. 57:689, 1960.
27. Dameshek, W., moderator: Panels in therapy; the treatment of spure, Blood 11:570, 1956.
28. DeGruchy, G. C.: Clinical haematology in medical practice, Springfield, Ill., 1958, Charles C Thomas, Publisher.
29. Dimson, S. B.: Juvenile pernicious anemia, Arch. Dis. Child. 41:216, 1966.
30. Fish, M. B., Pollycove, M., and Feichtmeir, T. V.: Differentiation between vitamin $B_{12}$-deficient and folic acid-deficient megaloblastic anemias with $C^{14}$-histidine, Blood 21:447, 1963.
31. Flexner, J. M., and Hartmann, R. C.: Megaloblastic anemia associated with anticonvulsant drugs, Amer. J. Med. 28:386, 1960.
32. Foy, H., Kondi, A., and MacDougall, L.: Pure red-cell aplasia in marasmus and kwashiorkor treated with riboflavine, Brit. J. Med. 1:937, 1961.
33. Girdwood, R. H.: The megaloblastic anaemias; their investigation and classification, Quart. J. Med. 25:87, 1956.

34. Girdwood, R. H., and Lenman, J. A. R.: Megaloblastic anaemia occurring during primidone therapy, Brit. Med. J. 1:146, 1956.
35. Goldberg, L. S., and Fudenberg, H. H.: The autoimmune aspects of pernicious anemia, Amer. J. Med. 48:489, 1969.
36. Gomez, F., Galvan, R. R., Cravioto, J., and Silvester, F.: Malnutrition in infancy and childhood, with special references to kwashiorkor. In Levine, S. Z., editor: Advances in pediatrics, Chicago, 1955, Year Book Medical Publishers, Inc.
37. Granville, N., and Dameshek, W.: Hemochromatosis with megaloblastic anemia responding to folic acid, New Eng. J. Med. 258:586, 1958.
38. Gräsbeck, R., Gordin, F., Kanero, I., and Kuhlbäck, B.: Selective vitamin $B_{12}$ malabsorption and proteinuria in young people; syndrome, Acta Med. Scand. 167:289, 1960.
39. Greenberg, G. R., and Jaenicke, L.: On the activation of the one-carbon unit for the biosynthesis of purine nucleotides. In Ciba Foundation Symposium: The chemistry and biology of purines, Boston, 1957, Little, Brown & Co., p. 204.
40. Hall, C. A.: Transport of vitamin $B_{12}$ in man, Brit. J. Haemat. 16:429, 1969.
41. Halsted, J. A., Lewis, P. M., and Gasster, M.: Absorption of radioactive vitamin $B_{12}$ in the syndrome of megaloblastic anemia associated with intestinal stricture or anastomosis, Amer. J. Med. 20:42, 1956.
42. Harris, J. W.: The red cell production, metabolism, destruction; normal and abnormal, published for The Commonwealth Fund, Cambridge, Mass., 1963, Harvard University Press.
43. Heath, C. W., Jr.: Cytogenetic observations in vitamin $B_{12}$ and folate deficiency, Blood 27:800, 1966.
44. Herbert, V.: The evaluation of assay methods in folic acid deficiency, Blood 17:368, 1961.
45. Herbert, V.: Experimental nutritional folate deficiency in man, Trans. Ass. Amer. Physicians 75:307, 1962.
46. Herbert, V.: Minimal daily adult folate requirement, Arch. Intern. Med. 110:649, 1962.
47. Herbert, V.: Current concepts in therapy; megaloblastic anemia, New Eng. J. Med. 268:201, 368, 1963.
48. Herbert, V.: Diagnostic and prognostic values of measurement of serum vitamin $B_{12}$-binding proteins, Blood 32:305, 1968.
49. Herbert, V., Baker, H., Frank, O., Pasher, I., Sobotka, H., and Wasserman, L. R.: The measurement of folic acid activity in serum;

a diagnostic aid in the differentiation of the megaloblastic anemias, Blood 15:223, 1960.
50. Herbert, V., and Zalusky, R.: Interrelationships of $B_{12}$ and folic acid metabolism: folic acid clearance studies, J. Clin. Invest. 4:1263, 1962.
51. Hippe, E.: Malabsorption of vitamin $B_{12}$; report of a case in a 1-year old boy; including studies of the absorption of $B_{12}$, Acta Paediat. Scand. 55:510, 1966.
52. Holt, L. E., Jr., Snyderman, S. E., Norton, P. M., Roitman, E., and Finch, J.: The plasma aminogram in kwashiorkor, Lancet 2:1345, 1963.
53. Huguley, C. M., Jr., Bain, J. A., Rivers, S. L., and Scoggins, R. B.: Refractory megaloblastic anemia associated with excretion of the orotic acid, Blood 14:615, 1959.
54. Imerslund, O.: Idiopathic chronic megaloblastic anemia in children, Acta Paediat., suppl. 119, p. 49, 1960.
55. Jandl, J. H., and Greenberg, M. S.: Bone marrow failure due to a relative nutritional deficiency in Cooley's hemolytic anemia; painful "erythropoietic crises" in response to folic acid, New Eng. J. Med. 260:461, 1959.
56. Jeffries, G. H., Hoskins, D. W., and Sleisinger, M. H.: Antibody to intrinsic factor in serum from patients with pernicious anemia, J. Clin. Invest. 41:1106, 1962.
57. Kho, L. K., Odang, O., Thajeb, S., and Markum, A. H.: Erythroblastopenia (pure red cell aplasia) in childhood in Djakarta, Blood 19:168, 1962.
58. Klipstein, F. A.: Subnormal serum folate and macrocytosis associated with anticonvulsant drug therapy, Blood 23:68, 1964.
59. Komninos, Z. D., Minogue, W. F., and Sarvajic-Dottor, J.: Folic acid deficiency in hereditary spherocytosis (failure of response to massive parenteral doses of cyanocobalamin), Arch. Intern. Med. 115:663, 1965.
60. Kondi, A., MacDougall, L., Foy, H., Mehta, S., and Mbaya, V.: Anaemias of marasmus and kwashiorkor in Kenya, Arch. Dis. Child. 38:267, 1963.
61. Koszewski, B. J.: Occurrence of megaloblastic erythropoiesis in patients with hemochromatosis, Blood 7:1182, 1952.
62. Lampkin, B. C., Shore, N. A., and Chadwick, D.: Megaloblastic anemia of infancy secondary to maternal pernicious anemia, New Eng. J. Med. 274:1168, 1966.
63. Lanzkowsky, P., Erlandson, M. E., and Bezan, A. J.: Isolated defect of folic acid absorption associated with mental retardation and cerebral calcification, Blood 34:452, 1969.
64. Lanzkowsky, P., Madenlioglu, M., Wilson, J. F., and Lahey, M. E.: D-Xylose test in healthy infants and children, New Eng. J. Med. 268:1441, 1963.
65. Lanzkowsky, P., McKenzie, D., Katz, S., Hoffenberg, R., Friedman, R., and Black, E.: Erythrocyte abnormality induced by protein malnutrition. II. 51-chromium labelled erythrocyte studies, Brit. J. Haemat. 13:639, 1967.
66. Layrisse, M., Paz, A., Blumenfeld, N., and Roche, M.: Hookworm anemia; iron metabolism and erythrokinetics, Blood 18:61, 1961.
67. Leikin, S. L.: Pernicious anemia in childhood, Pediatrics 25:91, 1960.
68. Lien-Keng, K.: Erythroblastopenia with giant pro-erythroblasts in kwashiorkor, Blood 12:171, 1957.
69. Lien-Keng, K., and Odang, O.: Megaloblastic anemia in infancy and childhood in Djakarta, Amer. J. Dis. Child. 97:209, 1959.
70. Lindenbaum, J., and Klipstein, F. A.: Folic acid deficiency in sickle-cell anemia, New Eng. J. Med. 269:875, 1963.
71. Luhby, A. L.: Megaloblastic anemia in infancy; clinical considerations and analysis, J. Pediat. 54:617, 1959.
72. Luhby, A. L., and Cooperman, J. M.: Folic-acid deficiency in thalassemia major, Lancet 2:490, 1961.
73. MacIver, J. E.: Megaloblastic anemia, Ped. Clin. N. Amer. 9:727, 1962.
74. Matoth, Y., Pinkas, A., Zamir, R., Mooallem, F., and Grossowicz, N.: Studies on folic acid in infancy. I. Blood levels of folic and folinic acid in healthy infants, Pediatrics 33:507, 1964.
75. May, C. D., Hamilton, A., and Stewart, C. T.: Experimental megaloblastic anemia and scurvy in the monkey; nature of the relation of ascorbic acid deficiency to the metabolism of folic acid compounds, J. Nutrition 49:121, 1953.
76. May, C. D., Nelson, E. N., Lowe, C. V., and Salmon, R. J.: Pathogenesis of megaloblastic anemia in infancy, Amer. J. Dis. Child. 80:191, 1950.
77. May, C. D., Stewart, C. T., Hamilton, A., and Salmon, R. J.: Infection as a cause of folic acid deficiency and megaloblastic anemia, Amer. J. Dis. Child. 84:718, 1952
78. McIntyre, O. R., Sullivan, L. W., Jeffries, G. H., and Silver, R. H.: Pernicious anemia in childhood, New Eng. J. Med. 272:981, 1965.
79. McIntyre, P. A., Hahn, R., Conley, C. L., and Glass, B.: Genetic factors in predisposition to pernicious anemia, Bull. Johns Hopkins Hosp. 104:309, 1959.
80. McNicholl, B., and Egan, B.: Congenital per-

nicious anemia: effects on growth, brain and absorption of $B_{12}$, Pediatrics 42:149, 1968.
81. Merskey, C., and Hansen, J. D. L.: Blood coagulation defects in kwashiorkor and infantile gastroenteritis, Brit. J. Haemat. 3:39, 1957.
82. Meyer, L. M., Osofsky, M., and Miller, I. F.: $Co^{57}$ vitamin $B_{12}$ clearance studies in pernicious anemia, Scand. J. Haemat. 4:301, 1967.
83. Miller, D. R.: Serum folate deficiency in children receiving anticonvulsant therapy, Pediatrics 41:630, 1968.
84. Miller, D. R., Bloom, G. E., Streiff, R. R., LoBuglio, A. F., and Diamond, L. K.: Juvenile "congenital" pernicious anemia, New Eng. J. Med. 275:978, 1966.
85. Mollin, D. L., Baker, S. J., and Doniach, D.: Addisonian pernicious anaemia without gastric atrophy in a young man, Brit. J. Haemat. 1:278, 1955.
86. Naiman, J. L., and Oski, F. A.: The folic acid content of milk; revised figures based on an improved assay method, Pediatrics 34:174, 1964.
87. Nathan, D. G., and Gardner, F. H.: Erythroid cell maturation and hemoglobin synthesis in megaloblastic anemia, J. Clin. Invest. 41:1086, 1962.
88. Nieweg, H. O., Faver, J. G., de Vries, J. A., and Stenfert Kroese, W. F.: Relationship of vitamin $B_{12}$ and folic acid in megaloblastic anemias, J. Lab. Clin. Med. 44:118, 1954.
89. Pearson, H. A., Vinson, R., and Smith, R. T.: Pernicious anemia with neurologic involvement in childhood, J. Pediat. 65:334, 1964.
90. Peterson, J. C., and Dunn, S. C.: Pernicious anemia in childhood, Amer. J. Dis. Child. 71:252, 1946.
91. Pierce, L. E., and Rath, C. E.: Evidence for folic acid deficiency in genesis of anemic sickle cell crisis, Blood 20:19, 1962.
92. Pitney, W. R., Beard, M. F., and van Loon, E. J.: Observations on the bound form of vitamin $B_{12}$ in human serum, J. Biol. Chem. 207:143, 1954.
93. Pitney, W. R., Joske, R. A., and Mackinnon, N. L.: Folic acid and other absorption tests in lymphosarcoma, chronic lymphocytic leukaemia, and some related conditions, J. Clin. Path. 13:440, 1960.
94. Quinto, M. G., Leikin, S. L., and Hung, W.: Pernicious anemia in a young girl associated with idiopathic hypoparathyroidism, familial Addison's disease, and moniliasis, J. Pediat. 64:241, 1964.
95. Reisner, E. H., Jr.: The nature and significance of megaloblastic blood formation, Blood 13:313, 1958.
96. Reisner, E. H., Jr., Wolff, J. A., McKay, R.
J., Jr., and Doyle, E. F.: Juvenile pernicious anemia, Pediatrics 8:88, 1951.
97. Reynolds, E. H.: Effects of folic acid on the mental state and fit-frequency of drug-treated epileptic patients, Lancet 1:1086, 1967.
98. Reynolds, E. H., Milner, G., Matthews, D. M., and Chanarin, I.: Anticonvulsant therapy, megaloblastic haemopoiesis and folic acid metabolism, Quart. J. Med. 35:521, 1966.
99. Roberts, P. M., Arrowsmith, D. E., Rau, S. M., and Monk-Jones, M. E.: Folate state of premature infants, Arch. Dis. Child. 44:637, 1969.
100. Robinson, M. G., and Watson, R. J.: Megaloblastic anemia complicating thalassemia major, Amer. J. Dis. Child. 105:275, 1963.
101. Rogers, L. E., and Porter, F. S.: Hereditary orotic aciduria. II. A urinary screening test, Pediatrics 42:423, 1968.
102. Rogers, L. E., Porter, S. F., and Sidbury, J. B., Jr.: Thiamine-responsive megaloblastic anemia, J. Pediat. 74:494, 1969.
103. Rogers, L. E., Warford, L. R., Patterson, R. B., and Porter, F. S.: Hereditary orotic aciduria. I. A new case with family studies, Pediatrics 42:415, 1968.
104. Rosensweig, L., and Bruton, O. C.: Pernicious anemia in an 8 year old girl, Pediatrics 6:269, 1950.
105. Royston, N. J. W., and Parry, T. E.: Megaloblastic anaemia complicating dietary treatment of phenylketonuria in infancy, Arch. Dis. Child. 37:430, 1962.
106. Ryan, G. M. S., and Forshaw, J. W. B.: Megaloblastic anaemia due to phenytoin sodium, Brit. Med. J. 2:242, 1955.
107. Schilling, R. F.: Intrinsic factor studies; the effect of gastric juice on the urinary excretion of radioactivity after the oral administration of radioactive vitamin $B_{12}$, J. Lab. Clin. Med. 42:860, 1953.
108. Schwartz, M.: Intrinsic factor antibody in serum of orally treated patients with pernicious anemia, Lancet 2:1263, 1960.
109. Schrimshaw, N. S., Behar, M., Perez, C., and Viteri, F.: Nutritional problems of children in Central America and Panama, Pediatrics 16:378, 1955.
110. Sherman, S. D., Greenfield, J. B., and Ingall, D.: Reversible bone-marrow vacuolizations in phenylketonuria, New Eng. J. Med. 270:810, 1964.
111. Silbertstein, E. B.: The Schilling test, J.A.M.A. 208:2325, 1969.
112. Spray, G. H., and Witts, L. J.: Excretion of formiminoglutamic acid as an index of folic acid deficiency, Lancet 2:702, 1959.
113. Spurling, C. L., Sacks, M. S., and Jiji, R.

M.: Juvenile pernicious anemia, New Eng. J. Med. 271:995, 1964.
114. Stamos, H. F.: Heredity in pernicious anemia, Amer. J. Med. Sci. 200:586, 1940.
115. Sunberg, R. D., Schaar, F., and May, C. D.: Experimental nutritional megaloblastic anemia; hematology, Blood 7:1143, 1952.
116. Taylor, K. B., Roitt, I. M., Doniach, D., Couchman, K. G., and Shapland, C.: Autoimmune phenomena in pernicious anaemia; gastric antibodies, Brit. Med. J. 2:1347, 1962.
117. Thompson, R. B., and Ungley, C. C.: Megaloblastic anemia associated with anatomic lesions in the small intestine, Blood 10:771, 1955.
118. Van de Kamer, J. H., Weijer, H. A., and Dickie, W. K.: Coeliac disease; an investigation into the injurious action on patients with coeliac disease, Acta Paediat. 42:223, 1953.
119. Von Bonsdorff, B., and Gordin, R.: Antianemic activity of dried fish tapeworm, Acta Med. Scand., suppl. 266, p. 283, 1952.
120. Walt, F., Holman, S., and Hendrickse, R. G.: Megaloblastic anemia of infancy in kwashiorkor and other diseases, Brit. Med. J. 1:1199, 1956.
121. Walt, F., Taylor, J. E. D., Magill, F. B., and Nestadt, A.: Erythroid hypoplasia in kwashiorkor, Brit. Med. J. 1:73, 1962.
122. Waters, A. H., and Mollin, D. L.: Studies on the folic acid activity of human serum, J. Clin. Path. 14:335, 1961.
123. Waters, A. H., and Mollin, D. L.: Observations on the metabolism of folic acid in pernicious anaemia, Brit. J. Haemat. 9:319, 1963.
124. Waters, A. H., and Murphy, M. E. B.: Familial juvenile pernicious anaemia; a study of hereditary basis of pernicious anaemia, Brit. J. Haemat. 9:1, 1963.
125. Weinstein, J. B., Weissman, S. M., and Watkin, D. M.: The plasma vitamin $B_{12}$ binding substance, J. Clin. Invest. 38:1904, 1959.
126. Welch, A. D., and Heinle, R. W.: Hematopoietic agents in macrocytic anemias, Pharmacol. Rev. 3:345, 1951.
127. Wickes, I. G.: Megaloblastic anaemia and anticonvulsants, Brit. Med. J. 2:1435, 1961.
128. Willoughby, M. L. N., Pears, M. Q., Sharp, A. A., and Shields, M. J.: Megaloblastic erythropoiesis in acquired hemolytic anemia, Blood 17:351, 1961.
129. Willis, L.: Pernicious anemia, nutritional macrocytic anemia and tropical sprue; a discussion, Blood 3:36, 1948.
130. Witts, L. J.: Some aspects of the pathology of anaemia. II. Investigation of Castle's hypothesis, Brit. Med. J. 2:404, 1961.
131. Wood, I. J.: Value of gastric biopsy in the study of chronic gastritis and pernicious anemia, Brit. Med. J. 2:283, 1951.
132. Wood, I. J., Doig, R. K., Motteram, R., Weiden, S., and Moore, A.: The relationship between the secretions of the gastric mucosa and its morphology as shown by biopsy specimens, Gastroenterology 12:949, 1949.
133. Zuelzer, W. W., and Ogden, F. H., Megaloblastic anemia of infancy, Amer. J. Dis. Child. 71:211, 1946.
134. Zuelzer, W. W., and Rutzky, J.: Megaloblastic anemia of infancy. In Levine, S. Z., editor: Advances in pediatrics, Chicago, 1953, Year Book Medical Publishers, Inc.

# 14 HYPOPLASTIC AND APLASTIC ANEMIAS

*General considerations.* The hypoplastic and aplastic anemias constitute a heterogenous group of anemias which include several well-defined entities and a larger number of still obscure hypoplastic states reflecting degrees of erythropoietic suppression. These anemias are not caused by excessive hemolysis, blood loss, nor in the majority of instances by space-occupying infiltrations of the bone marrow. The cardinal feature of this group of anemias is bone marrow hypofunction resulting from a failure of red cell production and hemoglobin synthesis to compensate for the normal rate of blood destruction. Erythropoiesis alone may be significantly decreased, or the defect may also extend to the granulocytes and platelets, resulting in a peripheral blood picture of pancytopenia. Bone marrow aspiration or biopsy reveals either the anticipated aplasia or a specimen varying from normal cellularity to hypercellularity, in which case depressed functional activity is postulated.[124] The difficulties of reconciling the state of the bone marrow with the peripheral blood picture and the resistance of the hypoplastic-aplastic group to all forms of antianemia therapy, except transfusion, have prompted their designation as refractory anemias.[18,123] Abnormalities in the metabolism of nucleic acids, particularly deoxyribonucleic acid, have been postulated as a cause of many refractory anemias in which peripheral pancytopenia is accompanied by a cellular hyperplastic bone marrow.[166]

It is also generally recognized that the mature human red blood cell depends primarily upon glycolysis for its energy-producing mechanisms. Maintenance of structural integrity and a normal life-span of the erythrocyte depends on the generation of this source of energy.[116,118] As yet, no effect upon a specific enzyme or enzyme system involving either process has been disclosed in the hypoplastic-aplastic anemias. There is only fragmentary evidence of any deficiency or impairment of enzymes or enzyme systems in these disorders comparable to a deficiency of glucose-6-phosphate dehydrogenase and of pyruvate kinase in the hemolytic anemias.

Interest in aplastic anemias has been intensified with the awareness of the potential depressive effect upon the bone marrow of newer agents to which the human organism is exposed. Especial attention has been focused upon the widespread use of the newly developed drugs among the antibiotics, tranquilizers, and anticonvulsants, together with chemicals in household use such as the insecticides, disinfectants, paints, and cleaning agents. The biologic effects of radioactive fallout from the fissioning or splitting of atoms of uranium and plutonium in the course of nuclear weapon testing are under serious scrutiny as bone marrow depressants. In the same category is the potential injury to blood-forming organs from diagnostic and therapeutic x-ray exposure.

The anemias are usually normochromic and normocytic, occasionally macrocytic with moderate anisocytosis, and are distinguished from other blood dyscrasias by a diminished number of reticulocytes and other evidences of inactive blood formation. The absence of enlargement of lymph nodes, liver, and spleen in patients with the major anemias of this group contributes a feature of diagnostic importance.

*Classification.* For purposes of simplification these anemias have been consolidated into two general categories—the hypoplastic and the aplastic anemias. Although overlapping obviously occurs, there are members of each group, nevertheless, which possess such well-defined characteristics as to constitute specific entities.

Aplastic anemia is characterized by a simultaneous depression of the three principal cellular elements in the bone marrow and a peripheral picture of profound anemia, leukopenia, neutropenia, and thrombocytopenia. It can be noted from the accompanying classification that aplastic anemia includes both primary (congenital, constitutional) and secondary forms, although the former are more prominent in infancy and childhood. Difficult to diagnose are the cases in which the clinical and blood pictures are consistent with a diagnosis of aplastic anemia yet the bone marrow in some cases has been cellular or even hyperplastic.

Hypoplastic anemia differs from aplastic anemia in that the formation of red cells is impaired, with lesser or no involvement of granulocytes and platelets. In recent years the term *hypoplastic anemia* has been applied rather loosely to intermediate or miscellaneous conditions. Reports of cases of hypoplastic anemia now range from conditions in which there is a failure of red cell production to those in which leukocytes and platelets are simultaneously depressed, but to a lesser degree than red cells. This tendency has been exaggerated by the knowledge that a transient anemia accompanied by a diminished reticulocyte count need not necessarily be correlated with a bone marrow deficient in erythroid tissue. To one of the members of this group, pure red cell anemia, a restrictive connotation should be applied. This is a chronic congenital aregenerative anemia which had been previously placed into a separate category,[152] but which is now classified with the hypoplastic anemias in contrast to the acquired forms of erythroblastopenia.

1. Hypoplastic anemia (major effect on erythropoiesis)
    a. Idiopathic—hypoplasia confined to erythropoiesis.
        (1) Congenital—pure red cell anemia (chronic congenital aregenerative anemia)
    b. Acquired—with varying degrees of erythrocytic hypoplasia
        (1) Anemias due to infections, drugs, chemicals, toxins, autoimmune and allergic states
        (2) Aplastic crisis in course of hemolytic syndromes, such as hereditary spherocytosis and sickle cell anemia
        (3) Anemia resulting from suppressive effect of multiple transfusions on erythropoiesis
        (4) Miscellaneous—moderate anemia with or without lesser involvement of granulocytes and platelets
2. Aplastic anemia (severe pancytopenia)
    a. Congenital or constitutional
        (1) With multiple congenital anomalies (Fanconi type)
        (2) Without associated anomalies
        (3) Nonfamilial and without associated anomalies, i.e., thrombocytopenia in newborn period progressing to pancytopenia
    b. Acquired—secondary
        (1) Anemia due to antimicrobial and other chemotherapeutic agents
        (2) Anemia due to industrial and household chemicals
        (3) Anemia due to irradiation
        (4) Miscellaneous causes—infections, endocrine factors, bone marrow invasion or replacement (myelophthisic anemias), hypersplenism
        (5) Idiopathic

## HYPOPLASTIC ANEMIAS
### Pure red cell anemia

*Definition.* Pure red cell anemia is also called chronic congenital aregenerative anemia, congenital hypoplastic anemia, congenital (erythroid) hypoplastic anemia, pure red cell aplasia, primary erythroid hypoplasia, erythrogenesis imperfecta, etc. The term *pure red cell anemia*[94] refers to a chronic, progressive anemia confined to a failure of erythropoiesis without an equivalent depression of the white blood cells or platelets.[32,83,168] The bone marrow is characterized by a complete or almost complete absence of cells of the erythroid series with normally proliferating cells of the granulocytic series and megakaryocytes. The failure of the bone marrow to provide adequate numbers of erythrocytes results in a persistent and progressive anemia with the need for long-term supportive transfusions. Pure red cell anemia has been observed at all ages, but it is particularly conspicuous as a congenital disease in early infancy and childhood.

*Pathogenesis.* The etiology is unknown, but several theories have been advanced to explain a condition in which only a single element of the bone marrow is affected. It is conceivable that the hematopoietic defect results from a noxious factor operating at critical periods of fetal development. Pure red cell anemia has been described in association with other developmental defects such as hypoplastic and cystic kidney,[152] as well as dwarfism, skeletal abnormalities, and webbed neck.[72] Complete[36] and temporary[52] pure red cell anemias have been reported in patients with autoimmune hemolytic disease. Pure red cell anemia may conceivably result from a similar mechanism—i.e., the action of such antibodies against the red cells in fetal life, producing prolonged and permanent depression of erythropoiesis.[151] Pure red cell anemia may be compared with other congenital anomalies caused by developmental defects.

Anthranilic acid, a metabolite formed in the breakdown of tryptophan, is excreted in relatively large quantities when a riboflavin-deficient animal is fed tryptophan. A similar defect in tryptophan metabolism has been reported in a number of patients with congenital pure red cell anemia.[9] The administration of riboflavin to these patients resulted in a decrease in the excretion of anthranilic acid but did not alter the hematologic status. The favorable response to corticosteroids in many cases of this disease suggested the possibility that this form of therapy stimulated an enzyme system, possibly tryptophan oxidase, comparable in this respect to the striking effect of cortisone on rat liver.[88] On the other hand, another group[155] found no excretion of large amounts of anthranilic acid in the urine in this disease on tryptophan loading, but found other abnormalities in several patients. These consisted of the excretion of 3-hydroxykynurenine, kynurenine, and xanthurenic acid in larger quantities than in any of the controls.

Pure red cell aplasia was observed in the course of galactoflavin-induced human riboflavin deficiency.[4] The anemia was normochromic and normocytic, in some instances hemoglobin levels fell as much as 9 gm. per 100 ml., and no changes were noted in the white cell and platelet counts. Serial marrow examinations revealed a gradual reduction in basophilic and polychromatophilic normoblasts. The administration of riboflavin resulted in a prolonged reticulocytosis, erythroid hyperplasia of the bone marrow, and correction of the anemia, despite continuation of riboflavin-deficient diet and galactoflavin administration. These studies are regarded as evidence of riboflavin requirement in human red blood cell formation.

A factor inhibiting erythropoiesis has been found in the plasma of two patients with red cell aplasia.[81] On this basis the inhibitory effect of plasma may be due to the presence of an antibody directed against the erythropoietic stimulating factor.

Others[90] have found in the plasma of an adult with red cell aplasia an antibody to erythroblast nuclei and another that inhibited heme synthesis. Treatment of the patient with cyclophosphamide results in disappearance of the inhibitors and a return of normal erythropoiesis.

*Clinical features.* Pure red cell anemia has an insidious onset with progressive pallor, anemia, irritability, listlessness, and anorexia, which are usually apparent at the age of 2 to 3 months or later in the first year. The infant appears healthy at birth, and general development proceeds normally. Exceptionally, the onset of the disease may be delayed; such a delay has been reported in a child 6 years old[60] and two brothers 17 years of age.[98] This occurrence in siblings has also been noted in other cases.[20]

Except for pallor, there is little to be observed at physical examination. The liver, spleen, and lymph nodes are not enlarged, jaundice is absent, and there are no manifestations of bleeding. In some patients a particular type of facies has been described,[22] consisting of tow-colored hair, snub nose, thick upper lips, rather wide-set eyes, and an intelligent expression.

The liver and spleen enlarge as transfusion hemosiderosis develops. Normal red cell survival, which is present when the spleen is not enlarged, is shortened as this organ becomes the site of increased red cell destruction. Long-standing administration of blood results in increased pigmentation of the skin. This is due to both iron deposition and excessive melanin formation.[93] Cardiac enlargement, multiple arrhythmias, and refractory heart failure are frequently inevitable consequences.

Pure red cell anemia also occurs as an acquired erythrocytic hypoplasia in adults without a proved common etiology.[141,162] Infection, allergy, red cell autoantibodies in hemolytic anemia, and chemical exposure have been incriminated.

A more constant finding is the coexistence of this disease with benign thymoma.[24,64,74,131] In one patient erythroblastic aplasia developed 4 years after removal of a symptomless thymic tumor.[63] It has been estimated that thymoma is present in approximately 50% of the reported cases of pure red cell anemia.[10,79] This association is not the experience, however, in pure red cell anemia in childhood where thymoma is infrequent.

The frequent occurrence of autoantibodies in diseases associated with abnormal proliferation of lymphoid tissue raises the possibility that antibodies directed against red cell precursors may be derived from thymic tumors.[10,64] According to Burnet,[21] the mutant cells, which give rise to forbidden clones involved in autoimmune disease, may have their origin in the thymus. The more pertinent observation is the recent recognition of the frequent association of thymic tumors with pure red cell anemia (erythroblastic aplasia[64]) and, in at least one report, with pancytopenic aplastic anemia.[12] It might be concluded from this association of thymic tumor and pure red cell anemia that the anemia is caused by an inhibitor of erythropoiesis originating in lymphoid tissue. The most challenging factor is that this association is not usually observed until late in adult life, notwithstanding definitive observations that humoral antibody production is impaired in a variety of animals thymectomized at birth.[11]

In a group of forty-three cases in adults (average age, 61 years) with benign thymoma, the incidence of red cell aplasia of the bone marrow was estimated at 5 to 10%. The incidence of thymoma in adults with erythroid aplasia was probably greater than 50%. The spindle cell type of thymoma predominated; all but one of the tumors was benign. Experimentally, it has not been possible to demonstrate a thymic principle which inhibits erythropoiesis. Thymectomy resulted in permanent remission in five cases of twenty-four and a temporary remission was obtained in two cases. The association of thymoma with agammaglobulinemia strengthened the evidence that aregenerative anemia may be related to some immunologic disorder.[128]

**Laboratory findings.** The outstanding feature is a chronic aregenerative and refractory anemia in which there is a striking absence from the marrow of the nucleated precursors of the red cells without a simultaneous depression of granulocytes, platelets, and their precursors. The anemia is normocytic and normochromic, with reticulocytes low in number or absent. Without supportive transfusions the hemoglobin falls to extremely low values. Fetal hemoglobin may be increased.

The number of platelets, white blood cells, and differential counts are normal. Marked leukopenia and moderate depression of platelets occur in rare instances in which the spleen enlarges and manifests a hypersplenic function. The bone marrow in such a patient shows normal myeloid activity and a normal number of megakaryocytes. In a 7½-year-old boy under observation, splenectomy resulted in a return of leukocytes and platelets to normal, but erythropoiesis remained hypoplastic. The serum iron level is elevated with complete saturation of the latent iron-binding capacity as a result of prolonged transfusion therapy.

In this condition, also, the bone marrow frequently contains varying numbers of primitive cells termed hematogones.[150,167] Although such cells usually are smaller than the ordinary lymphocytes, they resemble them closely in size and morphology. They possess a dense homogeneous matlike nucleus and a narrow rim of nongranular basophilic cytoplasm which are usually lacking in lymphocytes. These primordial cells possibly represent progenitors of the erythrocytic series. In one patient they were replaced by small numbers of normoblasts following the administration of cortisone.

In rare cases the cells in the marrow—erythrocytes, leukocytes, and myeloid elements—are heavily vacuolated. Their significance is unknown, but with steroid treatment the vacuoles disappear.

Initial diagnosis of pure red cell anemia is sometimes obscure if steroids have been given for any prolonged period. The bone marrow may show an erythropoietic hyperplasia and reticulocytes may be elevated. It will be necessary to eliminate all therapy so that an accurate diagnosis can be made.

**Pathologic findings.** The essential feature is widespread hemosiderosis, at times associated with evidence of hemochromatosis. In a 10-year-old patient who died of heart failure, postmortem examination revealed the typical syndrome of hemochromatosis, including diabetes mellitus and skin pigmentation. The heart was greatly enlarged, and many of the myocardial fibers contained iron pigment, scanty interstitial fibrosis, and occasionally necrosis of isolated fibers. In a 9-year-old child whose terminal illness was severe hepatitis, postmortem examination revealed massive liver necrosis and generalized hemosiderosis with fibrosis of the liver, pancreas, and thyroid. The myocardial fibers were hypertrophied, vacuolated, and contained moderate amounts of hemosiderin.

**Diagnosis.** In a typical congenital case the disease is fully established in early infancy. The need for frequent transfusions is soon found to be based on erythropoietic hypoplasia in the bone marrow. Occasionally, pure red cell anemia may follow erythroblastosis and be mistaken for the protracted depression of erythropoiesis which sometimes accompanies the latter disease. Pure red cell anemia can be differentiated from the hemolytic anemias, such as sickle cell disease, thalassemia major, and hereditary spherocytosis, by the lack of splenomegaly and the absence of icterus, reticulocytes, and morphologic abnormalities in the red cell.

There is as yet no unanimity as to the degree of erythroid hypoplasia, which the name of this anemia implies. Although the designation of pure red cell anemia relates to conditions in which the bone marrow is practically devoid of normoblasts (less than 2%), in some reports these elements, though reduced, are nevertheless present in moderate numbers. The myeloid-erythroid ratio which should be necessarily high in a typical case may be only moderately reduced in others. In one report[22] the disorder is referred to as "erythrogenesis imperfecta" in which several bone marrow examinations showed a variation between erythroid hypoplasia and hyperplasia. These cases, however, share the common feature of varying aplasia of erythropoiesis without involvement of leukocytes or platelets. The differentiation from aplastic anemia and the acquired erythroblastopenias will be discussed subsequently.

*Treatment.* Major therapy consists of transfusions, corticosteroids, and splenectomy.

*Transfusions.* Supportive transfusions to maintain the hemoglobin at levels compatible with freedom from symptoms constitute a basic need. The use of sedimented or packed cells is preferable to whole blood. As a guide to management we found that with few exceptions patients in this category of chronic anemia do not require transfusions until hemoglobin levels drop to 7 to 7.5 gm. per 100 ml., at which point clinical symptoms usually appear. These include anorexia, listlessness, apathy, and incipient signs of heart failure. It is apparent that hemosiderosis is to be expected following repeated transfusions. Another limitation of frequent transfusions is their potential depressant effect upon endogenous erythropoiesis and hemoglobin synthesis.[154]

*Corticosteroids.* In association with transfusions, adrenocortical hormones, prednisone, prednisolone, and similar synthetic substances are given primary consideration, since they represent a potent form of therapy.[5,31,51,113] Adrenocorticosteroids should be given early in treatment, since the response is less promising when hemosiderosis has resulted after prolonged transfusion therapy.[52] Depending upon the age of the patient, the steroid hormones (prednisone and prednisolone) are prescribed in a dosage of 1 to 2 mg. per kilogram of body weight, usually ranging from 15 to 60 mg. given in divided doses every 6 hours. The more common dosage is 30 mg. of prednisone daily, in divided doses. In the responsive patient evidence of bone marrow and blood remission should be manifested in 3 to 4 weeks. A favorable response is reflected in erythroid hyperplasia, reticulocytosis, and increased hemoglobin and red cell levels. If and when the patient responds, the dosage may be tapered to maintenance levels, the amount varying with the individual patient. Intermittent therapy is given to reduce the hazard of growth retardation. In this case, the dosage may be only 2.5 mg. of prednisone on two consecutive days a week, 2.5 mg. every other day, or 5 mg. once weekly. At times, 15 mg. in divided doses is needed. With a favorable response, reducing and stopping the drug entirely should be attempted periodically to determine the capacity of the patient to establish spontaneous erythropoietic function. Cobalt has been successfully employed in the treatment of pure red cell anemia.[169] The dangers, however, of using cobalt have been pointed out elsewhere (Chapter 12). Testosterone recommended for treatment of aplastic anemia is without value in pure red cell anemia.[32]

Any evidence of infection necessitates prompt search for its source and, if localized, appropriate antibiotic therapy should be administered. Despite the persistently low hemoglobin levels, these patients are not unduly susceptible to infection.

*Splenectomy.* Splenectomy, which is frequently recommended only as a last resort in the treatment of pure red cell anemia, has nevertheless proved effective on occasion both in reducing the number of transfusions and in restoring erythropoiesis.[22,36] When transfusions are required at increasingly frequent intervals to maintain a physiologically sufficient, although reduced, hemoglobin level, it is postulated that an extracorpuscular hemolytic component has developed which is presumably located in the spleen. Accelerated destruction can be confirmed by tagging normal donor red cells with radioactive chromium and noting their shortened survival.

In one of our patients with pure red cell anemia, marked enlargement of the spleen was present. This finding is contrary to an accepted criterion of the aplastic-hypoplastic group of anemias, i.e., the failure to palpate the spleen. In this patient, however, removal of the spleen resulted in extending the interval between transfusions, although depression of erythropoiesis persisted. Undoubtedly, in patients without enlargement, splenectomy is justified when a hemolytic factor for donor blood is demonstrated by techniques revealing a shortened survival of transfused normal erythrocytes. The presence of such a hemolytic factor would be clinically suspected when regularly spaced intervals for transfusions are suddenly shortened.

In patients whom no hemolytic component is apparent, splenectomy is considered on the basis that an abnormally functioning spleen may depress the erythropoietic function of bone marrow. This procedure is recommended when adrenocorticosteroids and transfusions have been given extensive trial and failed to achieve a remission. There is also less reluctance to remove the spleen when the bone marrow is not entirely devoid of erythroid elements in any stage of development. In any event the procedure may be justified on the basis of a splenic humoral factor which inhibits maturation of precursors, either visualized or potentially present in unidentified primordial cells such as hematogones. The fear that removal of the spleen deprives the patient of needed resources of erythropoietic tissue is not justified by results in patients with this disease. Although the majority of patients are not improved by splenectomy, the condition is not aggravated. Occasionally, splenectomy alone has a beneficial effect in restoring erythropoiesis. In other patients cortisone and other therapeutic agents have proved more effective after splenectomy. Increased experience may show that splenectomy will be efficacious in patients who respond initially to steroid therapy.[98]

In one reported series of pure red cell anemia,[31] the hazards of infection after splenectomy were demonstrated in three patients who died 3 months, 1½ years, and 4 years after splenectomy. Two died of pneumococcal sepsis and pneumonia and one of chickenpox, with complications including massive pericardial effusion and pneumonia.

*Prognosis.* Prior to corticosteroid therapy, the course of congenital pure red cell anemia was regarded as one of chronic and progressive anemia with a fatal outcome. It had been known, however, that in selected patients supportive transfusion therapy, corticosteroids, and splenectomy could maintain a concentration of hemoglobin compatible with health. It had also been observed that spontaneous recovery was possible.

In a recent long-term study of thirty patients with pure red cell anemia,[31] eighteen required regular transfusions for varying periods of time to maintain life. Six of the eighteen developed a spontaneous remission after periods ranging from 8 months to 13 years. Four of the six were alive at the last report,[31] two having died while in remission. Another patient had over 400 transfusions from 2 months to 14½ years of age, when a spontaneous remission occurred. At 16 years of age the patient was in surprisingly good clinical condition with a hemoglobin of 13 gm. per 100 ml. and a normal bone marrow. Of the thirty patients in this series, twenty-two had been given one or more trials of therapy with corticosteroids.[5] Twelve of the twenty-two developed a steroid-induced remission and three of these were well without medication at time of the report, having been treated for 11 months, 1 year, and 6 years. Seven of the patients were in remission on intermittent therapy and two patients have died. The only side effect of therapy was growth retardation. The final evaluation of corticosteroid therapy awaits long-term experience. In the meantime the prognosis must still be considered as extremely guarded.

Long-term transfusions, however, carry the hazards of hemosiderosis and hemochromatosis. Reported cases suggest that a more favorable response to steroid therapy could be expected in patients with moderate numbers of normoblasts in the bone marrow than in those in whom the normoblasts were practically depleted. In one of our patients, however, no response with corticosteroids was obtained, despite an initial finding of 5% normoblasts.

An important factor in evaluating therapy and in a consideration of prognosis is the possibility of spontaneous recovery. Such remissions occured in three of twelve patients cited by Diamond[30] and in others such as those reported by Palmen and Vahlquist.[111] Remission can occur at any period from early childhood to adolescence with stabilization at a lower hemoglobin level.

Death results from cardiac failure, hepatitis during the course of transfusions, and overwhelming infection and sepsis. In these terminal events the factor of hemosiderosis from excessive iron deposition resulting from transfusions and hemochromatosis may conceivably play an important complicating role.

### Acquired hypoplastic anemias

*Anemia due to infections, drugs, chemicals, toxins, and autoimmune and allergic states.* Under the heading of acute erythroblastopenias Gasser[50] described temporary aregenerative crises of 1 week's duration resulting in severe anemia in children as a result of toxic, infectious, or allergic causes. This acquired type of pure red cell anemia was noted in patients who had been given drugs such as amidopyrin, santonin, and barbiturates, in those with infections, including mumps, atypical pneumonia, bacterial sepsis due to meningococcus and staphylococcus, and those with autoimmune hemolytic disease.[52]

A case of acute transitory erythroid aplasia and vascular purpura has been reported in an otherwise hematologic normal child.[54] During the period of aplasia, bone marrow aspiration revealed an almost complete depletion of all erythroid elements and the presence of giant cells resembling proerythroblasts. On the eighth day reticulocytes appeared in the peripheral blood. In an adult an arrest of erythropoiesis followed an upper respiratory tract infection.[23] Megakaryocyte precursors resembling giant proerythroblasts appeared early, following the onset of the arrest.

*Aplastic crisis.* The aplastic crisis occurring in patients with a number of hemolytic conditions, notably hereditary spherocytosis, has been discussed elsewhere. Crises in these conditions are not hyperhemolytic as originally supposed, but are aplastic. The bone marrow shows a complete absence of erythropoiesis, the occasional presence of proerythroblasts, a shift to the left of the granulocytic series, and a decrease of megakaryocytes. The condition lasts only a few days and is followed by an erythroblastic hyperplasia in the bone marrow and a rise in reticulocytes and hemoglobin in the peripheral blood. The severity of the anemia is aggravated by the fact that the aplastic state occurs in patients with preexisting hemolytic disease in which the life-span of the red cell is already reduced.

The acute form of erythroblastopenia—the so-called aplastic crisis—was originally described by Owren[110] as a cause of the sudden, severe anemia in hereditary spherocytosis. He pointed out that crises in this disease, heretofore regarded as hyperhemolytic, were indeed aplastic. They represented a sudden disappearance of erythroblasts from the bone marrow and were associated with a reticulocytopenia in the peripheral blood. A variety of agents have been described as causes of aplastic crises[52]: drugs, insect bites, viral and bacterial infections, allergic episodes, and states of severe malnutrition (kwashiorkor).[48,87,171] Aplastic crises have been reported in hemolytic conditions other than hereditary spherocytosis, i.e., sickle cell anemia,[82,109] thalassemia major,[80] autoimmune hemolytic anemia,[36] and hereditary nonspherocytic hemolytic anemia.[70]

*Anemia resulting from suppressive effect of multiple transfusions on erythropoiesis.* The suppressive effect of multiple transfusions on erythropoiesis which has been demonstrated in connection with chronic hemolytic anemias[154] probably extends also to the refractory anemias in which transfusions are the mainstay of treatment.

*Miscellaneous.* The miscellaneous group of hypoplastic anemias is by far the most common. Persistent ill-defined anemias in children are often undiagnosed or are suspected of being an intermediate stage of idiopathic aplastic anemia. The normochromic and normocytic anemia that is found is at variance with the bone marrow, which is normal both with respect to total cellularity and in the content of erythroid elements. The anemia is moderately severe, resists treatment with iron and other hematinics, and may be corrected periodically by the administration of blood. Not until the basic difficulty, such as a specific hypersensitivity or the source of chronic upper respiratory infections, for instance, is eliminated or treated adequately will the hemoglobin level return to normal.

## APLASTIC ANEMIA (BONE MARROW FAILURE, REFRACTORY ANEMIA)

*Definition.* Aplastic anemia refers to a refractory anemia, characterized by severe anemia, leukopenia, and thrombocytopenia, and is usually associated with aplasia or hypoplasia of the bone marrow. Ehrlich is credited with the first description of the disease in a young adult in 1888.[35] The term *aplastic anemia* gained popularity as increasing numbers of cases with pancytopenia, often in the absence of a hypoplastic marrow, were reported.

*Etiology.* The search for a history of exposure to agents injurious to the hematopoietic system is often difficult to obtain in children, so that the majority of cases of aplastic anemia in younger age groups are eventually classified as idiopathic.

In a series of 334 patients with aplastic anemia Wolff[174] found 24.3% under the age of 15 years. Of the total number of patients, 57.2% gave no history of possible exposure to a toxic compound and were classified as having idiopathic anemia; 23.6% had been exposed to one or more antibacterials shortly before the onset of the disease; 9% had had an exposure to other types of possible toxic materials; and 10.2% gave a combined exposure history. In another series Scott and co-workers[139] found that seventeen of thirty-nine patients (thirteen below 20 years of age) could give no history of exposure to known or suspected marrow depressants and were therefore considered to have the idiopathic disease.

Aplastic anemia is classified as either idiopathic or secondary caused by a drug, chemical, or ionizing radiation. It is possible that patients who give no history of toxic exposure and are classified as having idiopathic anemia might well have been exposed to an unrecognized agent. In some patients an interval of several weeks may elapse following exposure to a toxic agent before clinical signs and symptoms appear. Even with a reliable history of exposure, the relationship between the toxic agent and bone marrow depressant may have been fortuitous. Idiopathic and secondary cases of aplastic anemia have similar clinical pictures, except that patients with the secondary type have a somewhat better prognosis.

### Congenital or constitutional aplastic anemia

Included among the cases of bone marrow failure of unknown etiology are two distinctive syndromes—one associated with congenital anomalies and the other without anomalies.

*Congenital aplastic anemia with multiple congenital anomalies (Fanconi type).* The best known group of congenital malformations in which anemia constitutes an outstanding symptom is represented by the Fanconi syndrome. This condition includes the rare association of pancytopenia, bone marrow hypoplasia, and a number of congenital anomalies, i.e., a patchy brown pigmentation of the skin due to a deposition of melanin, hypogenitalism, microcephaly, dwarfism, strabismus, ptosis of the eyelids, nystagmus, exaggerated deep tendon reflexes, mental retardation, anomalies of ears, deafness, and skeletal abnormalities. Anomalies of the thumb, radii, long bones, congenital dislocation of the hips, syndactyly, congenital heart disease, and kidney anomalies have been noted in various reports[28] (Fig. 24). Atrophy of the

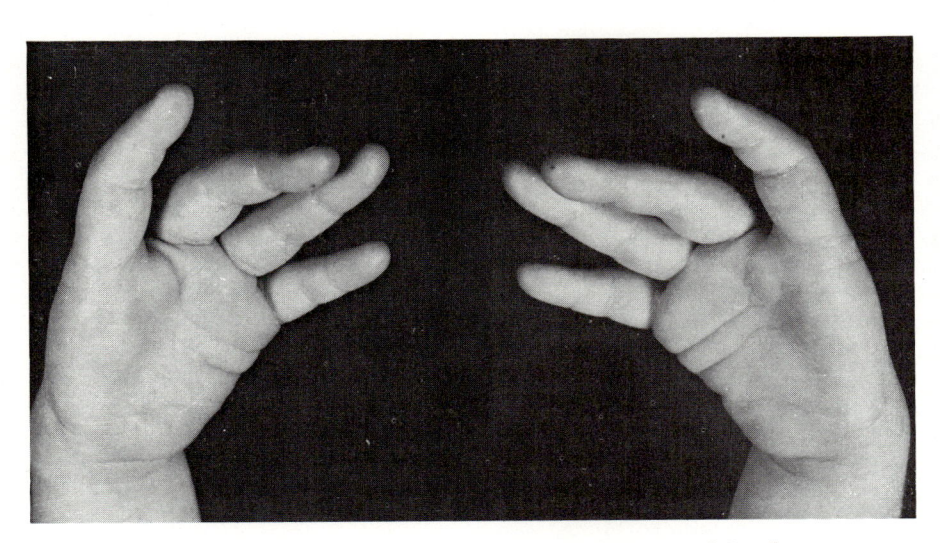

**Fig. 24.** Fanconi's syndrome, showing bilateral absence of thumbs.

spleen has been mentioned as an associated defect of development in this disease.[49] Originally, Fanconi[42] in 1927 reported cases occurring in three siblings. Sporadic as well as familial cases have been described. In most of the reported cases, hematologic abnormalities are initially detected between 4 and 12 years years of age. An earlier onset has been observed in one infant at 13 months of age, and in two brothers symptoms of a blood disorder appeared at the ages of 19 and 20 years, respectively.[127] The anemia is normocytic and slightly macrocytic, and leukopenia and thrombocytopenia coexist. As in the patients with aplastic anemia, the bone marrow content varies from acellular to hypercellular.

The asymptomatic period in a child with a skeletal defect before anemia becomes manifest has been unexplained. In an occasional patient studied during this period, the bone marrow surprisingly has revealed erythroid hyperplasia with megaloblastoid changes. During the period of anemia there also may be great variability in bone marrow response. Thus, in one 16-year-old girl anemia was associated with intense erythropoiesis, a rapid disappearance of radioactive iron from the plasma, and a low incorporation of iron in the red cells—events indicating marked hemolysis and compensatory erythropoiesis.[149]

The Fanconi syndrome appears to be transmitted by an autosomal recessive gene with variable penetrance.[71] Siblings of patients with the severe disease may possess congenital anomalies without blood changes.[49] Treatment consists of supportive transfusions, androgens, adrenocortical hormones, antibodies for infections, and splenectomy, in selected cases. The severe bleeding tendency associated with thrombocytopenia is difficult to control, and in one patient this was accomplished by splenectomy.[28] Patients with hypoplasia or maturation arrest have also been benefited by splenectomy.[120] Indications for splenectomy are the same as in other types of aplastic anemia. At the present time, splenectomy is reserved as a late therapeutic measure for patients with evidence of erythropoiesis in the bone marrow. Experience with testosterone therapy indicates that remissions are dependent on continued use of this hormone in contrast to acquired aplastic anemia, in which the drug can eventually be completely eliminated. As in acquired aplastic anemia, final assessment of testosterone therapy depends on long-term follow-up. (Details of hormone therapy appear in the section on acquired aplastic anemia.) Death usually results from hemorrhage into the brain or gastrointestinal tract.[28] Until the advent of hormone therapy, reported cases have had an almost uniformly fatal course. Exceptional cases have survived, probably due to the coexistence of congenital anomalies with minimal bone marrow depression.

In Fanconi's syndrome there have been many families with affected siblings and none with vertical transmission from parents to child. In a compiled series[43] consanguineous marriages were 20% of the total number, far in excess of the frequency of 0.5% in the general population. For rare recessive traits to manifest themselves there should be an increased prevalence of consanguinity between parents and affected individuals.

The demonstration of a high incidence of leukemia in the families of patients with Fanconi's syndrome is of interest. This coincidence may be due to chance or the influence of some hereditary fault.[49] In one series,[49] among forty-nine families in which Fanconi's syndrome was found, leukemia was reported four times, a rate of one in 12.2 cases, which is higher than the rate of familial leukemia (one in 450) or the rate in the overall population (60 per one million per year).

In addition to the wide variety of congenital anomalies characterizing Fanconi's anemia, associated specific chromosome abnormalities have also been observed in this condition.[17] In ten of the twelve patients of a series with this type of anemia chromosomal breaks, chromatid exchanges, and endoreduplication were noted in peripheral blood cultures and bone marrow examination. (These chromosomal aberrations are described in Chapter 22.) No correlation could be established between any of the congenital anomalies or the severity of the anemia and the chromosome disturbances. These findings were not related to therapy or other exogenous factors but rather to the basic pathologic process. This assortment of chromosome abnormalities was not found in a child with acquired aplastic anemia nor in a large group of patients with nonhematologic conditions. Chromosome breakage occurs in a variety of conditions in which radiation exposure occurs but the combination of aberrations of chromosome structure described in Fanconi's anemia serves to some extent as an excellent diagnostic criterion.

The increased incidence of leukemia found in Fanconi's anemia is of interest since similar chromosomal aberrations occur in both diseases. An increased incidence of leukemia has been observed in other disorders associated with similar cytogenetic abnormalities such as irradiation, benzene intoxication, patients with polycythemia vera treated with radioactive phosphorus, and Bloom's syndrome.[17] This relationship requires further study.

A family with two affected male children with Fanconi's anemia, one of whom developed acute myelomonocytic leukemia, has been reported.[33] Chromosome studies of the peripheral blood cultures of the patients revealed an increased frequency of chromosome and chromatid breaks, exchange figures, fragments, translocations, and gaps. Translocations produced by the abnormal recombinations of broken chromatids or chromosomes are the more important findings. Fibroblast cultures from both parents and one brother inoculated with simian virus 40, a known oncogenic agent, developed increased numbers of transformed colonies compared with normal control cultures similarly inoculated. Patients with Fanconi's anemia, Down's syndrome, and those treated with ionizing radiation demonstrate an apparent close relationship between chromosome abnormalities and an increased risk of malignancy.

Swift[159] compiled the death certificates and hospital records for clinically normal members of eight unrelated families in which there were one or more cases of Fanconi's anemia. In 102 deaths, a malignant neoplasm was the underlying cause of death in twenty-seven instances, a figure significantly greater than the unexpected value of 17.4. He concluded that the risk that a "Fanconi's anemia heterozygote will die from cancer or leukemia is between two and five times the normal risk."

Despite the absence of obvious anomalies, the kidney should be examined by intravenous pyelogram, since the only detectable abnormality in the Fanconi syndrome may reside in the urinary system.[25]

In the differential diagnosis other conditions are worthy of mention in which striking skeletal defects are present similar to those of Fanconi's aplastic anemia and which may be associated with hematologic changes.

A syndrome consisting of congenital hypoplastic anemia and triphalangeal thumbs has been described in two brothers.[1] The anemia appeared in early infancy, primarily affecting red cell precursors necessitating frequent transfusions. A congenital heart defect was present in one of the brothers.

Another disorder which possesses many of the features of the Fanconi syndrome is the combination of amegakaryocytic thrombocytopenia and various skeletal defects and is described in Chapter 27.

The Holt-Oram syndrome refers to a condition in which ventricular septal defects occur in conjunction with defective formation or absence of the radius and unassociated with hematologic abnormalities.

Holt and Oram[69] described a family in which the members of four generations were affected by both congenital heart disease and skeletal deformities. The most common heart lesion was an atrial septal defect and among the skeletal changes were webbing of the hand, supernumerary phalanx of the left thumb, absent terminal phalanx of the fifth finger, and absent radius.

In another series,[61] ventricular septal defects occurred in conjunction with defective formation or absence of the radius and sometimes absence of the thumb. Intermediate between the two syndromes is a third miscellaneous group of anomalies with some characteristics of both the Holt-Oram syndrome and ventriculoradial dysplasia, including severe pulmonary hypertension in some cases.

*Congenital hypoplastic anemia without associated anomalies.* Estren and Dameshek[41] have reported several siblings in each of two families who showed generalized hypoplasia of all elements of the bone marrow. Granulopoiesis and erythropoiesis were orderly and qualitatively normal, but quantitatively markedly diminished. Megakaryocytes were either virtually absent or decreased. All cases in the two families showed peripheral pancytopenia. In one of their patients showing severe anemia with an increased number of reticulocytes and thrombocytopenia, splenectomy resulted in moderate clinical and hematologic improvement.

## Acquired (secondary) aplastic anemia

Depressed blood formation may result from various forms of injury to the bone marrow. The clinical features are identical with those of primary aplastic anemia, but secondary anemia offers a better prognosis, especially if the condition is diagnosed early and the offending agent is eliminated.

*Anemia due to antimicrobial and other chemotherapeutic agents.* The offending drugs and chemicals are of two types: those which regularly produce bone marrow depression when given in sufficient dosage (such as the compounds used in the treatment of leukemia and malignant lymphomas) and substances which are occasional bone marrow depressants.[173] In the antileukemia group are nitrogen mustard, the folic acid antagonists, 6-mercaptopurine, busulfan (Myleran), and triethylenemelamine. Included in this category, also as depressants, are roentgen rays, radioactive phosphorus, radium, and products of atomic fission or atomic bomb explosions.

In the category of the occasional offenders are those drugs and chemicals which produce aplastic anemia with the initial dosage or in a subsequent course (Table 18). Tridione, Mesantoin,[125] and chloramphenicol are among the more common therapeutic agents which depress the bone marrow. Less common bone marrow depressants are sulfanilamide, sulfathiozole, and sulfapyridine, and, among the antibiotics, tetracyline, streptomycin, and penicillin. Atabrine, neoarsphenamine among the organic arsenicals, gold, and Butazolidin are also important etiologic agents but are of lesser importance in pediatric practice.

In the pathogenesis of aplastic anemia, chloramphenicol was probably the most frequent cause of aplastic anemia in the United States between 1949 and 1952.[96] A sharp decrease in the total number of cases followed 1952 when the hazard was pointed out and precautions were advised.[139] Because of a recent increase in the number of patients in whom chloramphenicol was associated with the development of aplastic anemia, the cautious use of this drug has been reemphasized.[121]

*Anemia due to industrial and household chemicals.* Benzol, benzene, and benzene derivatives, among the household and industrial chemicals, have a high priority among the marrow depressants because of their widespread

Table 18. Drugs associated with aplastic anemia*

|  | *All reports* | *Sole agent*† |
|---|---|---|
| Total reports of aplastic anemia in Registry (through December, 1963): 674 | | |
| Chloramphenicol (chloromycetin) | 299 | 157 |
| Sulfonamides (antibacterial)† | | |
| Sulfamethoxypyridazine (Kynex, Midicel) | 12 | 3 |
| Sulfisoxazole (Gantrisin) | 28 | 3 |
| Other | 118 | 18 |
| Sulfonamide derivatives (nonantibacterial)‡ | | |
| Acetazolamide (Diamox) | 10 | 3 |
| Chlorothiazide (Diuril) | 12 | 1 |
| Chlorpropamide (Diabinese) | 4 | 2 |
| Tolbutamide (Orinase) | 11 | 6 |
| Analgesics | | |
| Phenylbutazone (Butazolidin) | 34 | 16 |
| Anticonvulsants | | |
| Mephenytoin (Mesantoin) | 22 | 7 |
| Trimethadione (Tridione) | 5 | 2 |
| Benzene | 10 | 8 |
| Other organic solvents | 48 | 18 |
| Insecticides | | |
| Benzene hexachloride (Lindane) | 13 | 7 |
| Chlorophenothane (DDT) | 19 | 3 |
| Chlordane | 12 | 4 |
| Gold | 10 | 8 |

*From Erslev, A. J.: Drug-induced blood dyscrasias, J.A.M.A. **188**:531, 1964.
†Reports in which patient received listed drug either alone or with other, presumably innocent drugs.
‡Risk of aplastic anemia from most sulfonamide derivatives is slight, but as a group they are frequently associated with development of aplastic anemia.

use as solvents and in the manufacture of drugs, dyes, shellac, paint removers, and lacquers. Of importance also are DDT and other insectides which are especially injurious in concentrated exposure within enclosed and poorly ventilated areas.

*Anemia due to irradiation.* Roentgen rays and other forms of ionizing radiations are well-known physical agents which cause marrow depression. Radiations are of two kinds. The first are those which penetrate the body tissues, such as the roentgen rays (x-rays), gamma rays, and fast and slow neutrons. Gamma rays and neutrons are emitted from the explosion of atomic bombs and reach the blood-forming tissues rapidly. The second type are the alpha and beta particles which have a limited range of tissue penetration. They damage bone marrow directly when introduced into the body, as sometimes occurs in radium dial workers.[100]

Except when given in tremendous amounts, irradiation damages the precursors of the hematopoietic system rather than the formed elements in the peripheral blood.[91] The effect on the blood elements is related to their life-span (the leukocytes having the shortest and the red cells the longest life-span), the individual radiosensitivity of the precursors (the lymphocyte precursors being most sensitive), and the ability of hematopoietic tissue to regenerate (lymphatic tissue being most reactive). The leukocytes, therefore, show the first changes (i.e., a decrease in the number of lymphocytes being most noticeable), followed by a reduction in the number of platelets and red cells. Granulocytopenia and thrombocytopenia lead to infection and hemorrhage. Neutropenia is usually among the first manifestations of chronic overexposure. Individual susceptibility, dosage, and period of exposure account for the variation in blood alterations.

*Aplastic anemia following hepatitis.* Cases of pancytopenia and aplasia of the bone marrow following icteric hepatitis have been reported with increasing frequency in recent years. The outcome is usually fatal and the hepatic disorders appear to be of viral origin both clinically and pathologically.

Following several earlier reports,[89,99] Deller and colleagues[28a] in 1962 reported a 17-year-old boy in whom fatal pancytopenia developed during the early convalescent phase of acute viral hepatitis. An autoimmune mechanism was postulated to explain this complication on the basis of cross-reacting antibodies directed toward the cellular elements of the bone marrow.

Levy and associates[95] reported five patients 4 to 19 years of age in whom pancytopenia followed the onset of hepatitis by 1 to 7 weeks. In each case the hepatitis was improving when death occurred.

Schwarz and co-workers[138] reported three cases of aplastic anemia following hepatitis, two of whom responded with hematologic and clinical recovery after 2 to 3 weeks of prednisone and testosterone therapy.

In 1967 Rubin and his associates[133] reported that, in the preceding 10 years, sixteen cases of pancytopenia following hepatitis had been reported. With two exceptions, both middle-aged women, all the patients were young, ranging from 3½ to 22 years of age; most (twelve of sixteen) were males.

The interval between the onset of hepatitis and pancytopenia varied from an apparently simultaneous occurrence to 26 weeks. In almost all cases, pancytopenia developed after the hepatitis had subsided, and all but two patients died. Later, these same authors encountered six additional cases of hepatitis which were followed by aplastic anemia. Two patients had been treated with chloramphenicol 7 to 13 weeks before the onset of the hematological disorder.

Five cases are now on record in which children recovered from aplastic anemia following hepatitis.[133] The relationship between infectious hepatitis and the profound bone marrow depression is obscure. Some suggest that the pancytopenia may be due to invasion of the marrow by virus interfering with cellular proliferation, others that it is due to an autoimmune process.

Observations that the serum of patients with infectious hepatitis produces chromosomal abnormalities in cultured leukocytes from normal persons lend support to the hypothesis that chromosomal damage is involved in bone marrow hypoplasia.[37]

It has been suggested that some cases of idiopathic aplastic anemia in children may be a sequel to anicteric hepatitis.[133]

Treatment consists of adrenocortical steroids, blood transfusions, platelet transfusions, and antibiotics. Bone marrow transplantation was performed on a 12-year-old girl with this syndrome following cyclophosphamide as immunosuppressive therapy.[67] HLA-matched bone marrow from an uncle was given. A reticulocyte response appeared on the eighth to tenth day following transplantation. The white blood count rose slightly, and bone marrow aspiration revealed megakaryocytes and clusters of myeloid and erythroid cells, and XY pattern of chromosomes. Death followed evidences of consumption coagulopathy and graft-versus-host reaction.

Another case has been reported[178] of a boy aged 17 years who had been treated 7 weeks earlier for infectious hepatitis. He has hepatosplenomegaly and pancytopenia. The bone marrow showed total aplasia. A complete remission was achieved with corticosteroids, blood transfusions, and folic acid. The bone marrow reverted to normal granuloerythropoiesis, and the peripheral count was also returned to normal. He was symptom-free for 7 months and then was readmitted with bone marrow aplasia and pancytopenia. Despite vigorous treatment he expired in septic-hemorrhagic shock. At autopsy healed hepatitis with early fibrosis was found. The authors collected about forty case reports and all but seven of the patients ended fatally. In most cases the symptoms of pancytopenia appeared 2 to 6 months after the hepatitis.

*Miscellaneous causes.* Untreated pernicious anemia, overwhelming infections, and mechanical interference with erythropoiesis in the bone marrow may produce a blood picture of aplastic anemia. Anemias resulting from bone marrow invasion or replacement are the myelophthisic anemias due to bone marrow encroachment by foreign cells as occurs in patients with leukemia, lymphosarcoma, Hodgkin's disease, Niemann-Pick disease, Gaucher's disease, Letterer-Siwe disease, Albers-Schönberg disease (osteopetrosis), and myelofibrosis.

A case of fatal aplastic anemia has been reported in a 14-year-old boy due to airplane-glue sniffing.[117] Included with this case report were five other children with homozygous sickle cell disease who showed erythrocytic aplastic crises due to the same agent. Recovery was complete in the latter group after the offending agent was discontinued.

### Features common to congenital and acquired types of aplastic anemia

*Pathology.* The basic features of aplastic anemia are due to alterations of the bone marrow. It is probably best to restrict the term *aplastic anemia* to patients having hypocellular or acellular marrows associated with acute or chronic pancytopenia,[25] the important feature being the replacement of red marrow by fatty tissue.[39] During the course of the disease the bone marrow shows a progressive decrease in the total count so that the megakaryocytes eventually disappear, the myeloid elements and nucleated red cells are greatly reduced, and the lymphocytes predominate in the smears. Patients with normal or hyperplastic bone marrows with a peripheral blood picture of aplastic anemia have been diagnosed as having maturation arrest or bone marrow block. Quantitative variations in the total nucleated cell count and distribution of the blood elements may be due to the fact that areas of relatively acellular marrow alternate irregularly with areas of normal or increased cellularity. When aplastic, the normally red marrow appears yellow and fatty. The occasional increase in reticulocytes is due to patchy areas of active blood formation in the bone marrow. The liver, spleen, and lymph nodes are unaltered. Hemochromatosis may coexist with hemosiderosis due to iron deposition from multiple transfusions.[177] Infiltration with immature plasma cells may be so marked as to suggest myelomatosis.[105]

*Clinical features.* The onset is insidious, rarely abrupt, with anemia and cutaneous hemorrhages as early features. It is soon noted that the thrombocytopenia and purpura are insufficient to account for the degree of anemia. The clinical features are closely dependent upon the blood changes: anorexia, weakness, easy fatigue and dyspnea on exertion from anemia and loss of blood. Epistaxis, bleeding from the gums and gastrointestinal and renal tracts, menorrhagia, and retinal hemorrhage are prominent manifestations in later stages. Neutropenia is associated with sore throat and ulcerations of the mouth and pharynx. Fever due to secondary infections may be difficult to control with antibiotics. The spleen, liver, and lymph nodes are not enlarged.

A complicated relationship exists between hypoplasia of the marrow and paroxysmal nocturnal hemoglobinuria (PNH). Reports are now available of acute or chronic marrow failure in the course of PNH or of pancytopenia rather than hemolysis being the dominant sign. In some cases of PNH, marrow aspiration has shown definite hypocellularity where white blood counts and platelet counts have been low. In some the pancytopenia is transient.[26]

In a case reported by Dacie and Lewis,[26] the patient presented as one of aplastic anemia possibly drug-induced. A [51]Cr study showed excessive hemolysis and that radioactivity had accumulated in the spleen. Splenectomy was followed by alleviation of the hemolysis with eventual stabilization of the hemoglobin level. Seven months after splenectomy it was discovered that a small proportion (4%) of the erythrocytes reacted in vitro as if they were PNH erythrocytes. In another report,[119] four of six patients initially diagnosed as aplastic anemia subsequently manifested the hematologic failures of PNH (see Chapter 15).

Similar courses of aplastic anemia in identical twins exposed to chloramphenicol suggest that genetically determined predisposing factors were at work, according to Nagao and Mauer.[108] In one twin the onset lagged slightly behind and recovery occurred somewhat ahead of the other. Treatment in both infants consisted of packed red cell and platelet transfusions; no testosterone or corticosteroid therapy was given.

In tracing the course of the disease from an early phase to full recovery, it was observed in both twins that the earliest precursor cells (myeloblasts, promyelocytes, normoblasts, and basophilic normoblasts) were the first to disappear and also the first to reappear as recovery became evident. These observations were consistent with the concept that failure of delivery of differentiated forms from a damaged undifferentiated precursor cell line is the basic mechanism for the disease.

The possibility that patients who develop chloramphenicol-associated aplastic anemia may have a genetic defect which predisposes them to this disease has been postulated.[76] Others indicate that homozygosity may be necessary for a recessive gene to be related to the predisposition.[15] For identical twins, the operation of genetic factors are more in evidence.

Aplastic anemia has developed during pregnancy, frequently with a fatal outcome.[75,92] Occasionally remissions and even recovery may follow interruption of pregnancy. The infant may be stillborn or he may be unaffected at birth. It is not known whether pregnancy is a causal factor of the anemia. In one case pregnancy occurred while the patient was under treatment for aplastic anemia. Transfusions, which had been the mainstay of treatment, were increased during pregnancy. At delivery bleeding was excessive and large amounts of blood were required. The mother survived and a normal infant was delivered.

*Laboratory findings.* The red blood cell count fluctuates between 1.5 and 3 million per cubic millimeter; the hemoglobin drops proportionately. The reticulocytes number below 2% and are sometimes absent. The red cells are normochromic and normocytic, but macrocytes are often numerous. Poikilocytosis and red cell fragments may be prominent. The white cells tend to range between 1,500 and 4,000 per cubic millimeter, principally due to the lack of granulocytes. In a number of cases the cytoplasm of the neutrophils contains dark red-staining granules, coarser and larger than normal, regularly distributed through the cytoplasm, which are peroxidase positive.[97] In many cases the leukocyte alkaline phosphatase is high.[97] The platelets fall below 50,000 per cubic millimeter and frequently below 10,000 per cubic millimeter. Bone marrow aspiration discloses aplasia or hypoplasia. When aplastic, the normal red marrow appears yellow and fatty (Fig. 25). The sites for aspiration are the lower thoracic or lower lumbar spines, the anterior or posterior iliac crest, and the tibia in the first 2 years of life. If the hypocellular marrow is questioned, a more representative sample of bone marrow can be obtained with the Silverman needle.[114] The sample can then be fixed, blocked, sectioned, and stained. The value of obtaining an adequate sample and interpretation of the smear for the diagnosis of aplastic anemia cannot be overemphasized. Pancytopenia and a persistently cellular marrow suggest other diagnoses than aplastic anemia and are usually indicative of conditions associated with hypersplenism. On the other hand, variations in cellularity of the bone marrow may occur which range from total aplasia to apparent hyperplasia in adjacent areas or in specimens taken from different marrow sites.[3] While cases of pancytopenia with hyperplastic marrows have been reported in younger individuals,[62] they are infrequent, even when initially diagnosed.

Since the movement of iron is controlled by the formation and destruction of erythrocytes, it is to be expected that iron kinetics would be disturbed in states of bone marrow failure.[153] The extent of marrow uptake of iron correlates well in proportion to the degree of incorporation of [59]Fe into newly formed red blood cells. In aplastic anemia ferrokinetic

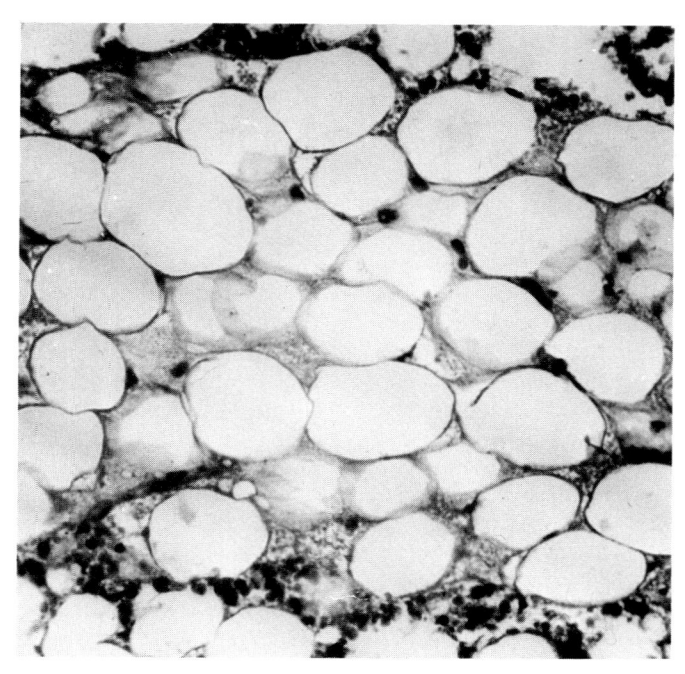

Fig. 25. Bone marrow biopsy from a 3½-year-old girl with idiopathic aplastic anemia, showing markedly hypocellular marrow with increased fat.

studies characteristically show a delayed clearance of isotope iron from plasma, decreased marrow uptake, and a reduction in the percentage incorporation of tagged iron into the red cells. The major portion of $^{59}$Fe given intravenously in aplastic anemia is diverted to the liver and a lesser amount to the spleen.

With the lack of iron utilization and its increased availability in the plasma, the serum iron is elevated and the iron-binding protein saturated. This observation has been employed to detect early drug-induced damage to blood. An increase in plasma iron content and in the saturation of iron-binding globulin have been found to precede the fall in hematocrit by an appreciable interval in erythropoietic depression induced by chloramphenicol and related drugs.[132] This measurement can thus serve as a reliable and sensitive index of early erythropoietic toxicity, permitting the discontinuance of a potentially noxious drug before changes become apparent in the peripheral blood.

There is still little doubt that in a large proportion of cases of aplastic anemia there is a hemolytic element. Red cell survival is frequently decreased, and surface counting over the spleen reveals red cell sequestration. On this basis it has been suggested that, if splenectomy is not contraindicated for other reasons, it may be beneficial in cases with excess hemolysis.[97]

*Erythropoietin in aplastic anemia.* The regulation of the production and maturation of red blood cells by humoral factors comes to an almost complete standstill in aplastic anemia (see Chapter 4 for full discussion of erythropoietin). That the plasma erythropoietin level is influenced by the functional state of the erythroid tissue of the marrow as well as the severity of the hypoxic stimulus is suggested by the high plasma values noted in refractory anemias and the relatively low values in most hemolytic disorders.[156] Erythropoietin is preferably utilized by a hyperplastic rather than an aplastic marrow. The plasma erythropoietin level is, therefore, related to the degree of erythroid activity of the bone marrow. In patients with an aplastic and hypoplastic bone marrow, erythropoietin is detectable when the hemoglobin concentration is as high as 10 gm. per 100 ml.[157] In patients with hemolytic anemias, erythropoietin activity can rarely be detected if the hemoglobin concentration is above 5 to 7 gm. per 100 ml.

In aplastic anemia, with the stem cell in a

refractory state, the uptake of erythropoietin is poor and the level of this factor, being unutilized, rises. The erythropoietin titer in patients with completely aplastic marrows is substantially greater than in patients with refractory anemia with cellular marrows. This concept is strengthened by observations that patients with chronic hypoplastic anemia (pure red cell anemia) in remission show no increased erythropoietin titer in their sera, whereas increased amounts are found in relapse when transfusions are needed.[59]

*Differential diagnosis.* True aplastic anemia with an acellular bone marrow and the typical picture of profound anemia, leukopenia, neutropenia, and thrombocytopenia is a rare occurrence in infancy and childhood. The marrow reveals progressive hypoplasia, although scattered areas of normal composition may be noted in samples from different sites. The anemia develops insidiously, so that diagnosis is difficult before pancytopenia is fully developed.

In differential diagnosis of aplastic anemia the following causes of pancytopenia are to be considered.

1. Leukemia with aleukemic blood picture
2. Aplastic anemia
3. Bone marrow infiltration or replacement
   a. Malignant lymphomas
      (1) Hodgkin's disease
      (2) Lymphosarcoma
      (3) Reticulum cell sarcoma
   b. Metastatic carcinoma
   c. Rare
      (1) Osteopetrosis (marble-bone disease)
      (2) Myelofibrosis, myelosclerosis
4. Hypersplenic syndromes
   a. Banti's disease
   b. Lymphomas
   c. Gaucher's disease
   d. Niemann-Pick disease
   e. Letterer-Siwe disease
   f. Splenic panhematopenia
   g. Disseminated lupus erythematosus
5. Miscellaneous
   a. Megaloblastic anemias
   b. Overwhelming infections

Hemorrhage based on thrombocytopenia or a blood picture of chronic anemia may constitute the dominant features until the deficiencies of the other cellular elements appear. As already mentioned, thrombocytopenic purpura, which may be considered early in the course of the disease, is associated with more than moderate anemia only as a result of blood loss. In the absence of overt hemorrhage, the anemia must, therefore, be explained on another basis.

Acute lymphoblastic leukemia in the leukopenic stage may stimulate aplastic anemia, but microscopic study of aspirated marrow usually reveals the precise nature of the illness. With an acellular marrow, the use of concentrated and volumetric bone marrow aspiration facilitates the differentiation between the two diseases.[158] A contracted or absent myeloid-erythroid (nucleated cell) layer and normal or increased percentage of fat in aplastic anemia are contrasted with leukopenia from other causes in which the fatty layer is absent and the myeloid-erythroid layer is variable.

Enlargement of the lymph nodes and spleen usually present in patients with acute leukemia is absent in those with aplastic anemia. In patients with splenic panhematopenia and secondary hypersplenism, the spleen is predominantly implicated in the pathogenesis of pancytopenia, and the bone marrow contains its full quota of each of the cellular elements. Myelofibrosis and neoplastic infiltration are also to be considered in the differential diagnosis.

*Management.* Comprehensive treatment consists of preventive measures, search for and elimination of the etiologic agent, transfusions and other supportive measures, stimulation of hematopoiesis, and a consideration of splenectomy.

*Preventive measures.* Because hypersensitivity is so variable and occurs so unexpectedly, a selection of a drug which is potentially myelotoxic requires some deliberation, and an attempt at supervision should be instituted if the drug is eventually to be used. These considerations apply particularly to patients with a history of allergic manifestations, such as eczema, urticaria, chronic rhinitis, hay fever, or asthma or who, in the past, have had skin rashes or constitutional reactions following exposure to a chemical or drug.

The extent to which precautionary measures are carried out depends, therefore, upon the known depressant effect of the drug, the benefits to be derived from its use, and the inherent nature of the patient with respect to hypersensitivity reactions. Myelotoxic drugs are difficult to control, because bone marrow hypoplasia can develop suddenly and because it is difficult to isolate the sensitive individual in whom treatment might be complicated by hematopoietic depression. Even with drugs such as Tridione, Mesantoin, Butazolidin, and chloramphenicol, which are known offenders, the incidence of toxicity is extremely low in comparison with the large number of patients so treated. The reported incidence of chloramphenicol, for instance, is estimated between 1 in 20,000 to 1 in 100,000 treated with this drug.[68] Nevertheless, a hemoglobin test, white blood cell count, and blood smear should be made periodically on patients receiving such drugs over prolonged periods and especially when treatment is intermittent. The exact intervals between these examinations cannot be specified. In the case of chloramphenicol weekly counts should be done initially and even more often when suspicious signs of toxicity appear. Fever, petechiae, purpura, epistaxis, oozing from the gums, mouth ulcerations, malaise, weakness, fatigue, and skin rashes are important signs of bone marrow depression. In the case of chloramphenicol, withdrawal of the drug at the stage of granulopenia and anemia usually results in complete hematopoietic recovery.[38,96] In the marrow, the signs of existing or impending bone marrow depression consist of a sudden shift to an immature level, the presence of promyelocytes and myelocytes, or marked reduction in the more mature elements and an increase in stem cells and lymphocytes.

In the prevention of drug-induced blood dyscrasias, early detection of bone marrow depression is important. Bone marrow toxicity may be reversed completely, if the drug is promptly withdrawn. Administration of chloramphenicol and drugs known to induce blood dyscrasias should always be preceeded by determination of the white blood cell count, hematocrit level, hemoglobin concentration, platelet count, and reticulocyte count. Of these, the reticulocyte count is the most sensitive indicator of a depression of red cell production.[40,103] In the case of chloramphenicol and other known offending agents, these tests should be determined at weekly intervals.

In a review comprising 408 cases of chloramphenicol administration, Best[14] found that in 10% of cases the development of a blood dyscrasia followed 4 days or less of therapy, in 50% of cases after 13 days or less, and in 10% after 150 days or more. In a few instances the drug was administered on only one occasion. The blood response developed in 10 days or less following the initial dose in 10% of cases, in 95 days or less in 50% of cases, and in 26 days or more in 10%. The overall mortality was approximately 50%; 10% of the patients in the entire series died within 2 weeks of the onset of the dyscrasia. In this series, the peak occurrence rate was noted at 3 to 7 years of age. Most patients develop manifestations of marrow depression after the drug has been stopped, often weeks or months later. For that reason monitoring blood counts during therapy would be of questionable value in preventing mortality[14] unless long-term blood studies are made.

Wallerstein and associates,[170] in a statewide staff study in California of the relation of chloramphenicol therapy and aplastic anemia, found that the ultimate risk of dying of aplastic anemia after ingestion of the drug was 1 in 36,118 with an average dose of 4.5 gm. per person; with average dose of 7.5 gm. per person the risk of death was 1 in 21,671. They found that dosage did not appear to play a part and that anemia might not appear until the second or third course of chloramphenicol. In five patients, aplastic anemia developed after a single dose of the drug.

Two types of toxicity have been described: a temporary erythroid depression and anemia, occasionally associated with thrombocytopenia and leukopenia, and severe pancytopenia with a usually irreversible aplastic marrow.[25] The hematopoietic reactions also range from mild reversible bone marrow depression to fatal aplastic anemia. The mechanism of bone marrow involvement has not been entirely elucidated, but there is evidence for depression of leukocyte respiration,[45] inhibition of nucleic acid synthesis by normal and leukemic cells,[175] and interference with heme synthesis.[165] Depression of erythropoiesis manifested by a drop in reticulocyte count is the first and most frequent warning of trouble, which is followed in order by suppression of thrombopoiesis and leukopoiesis.[103] A maturation arrest and vacuolization of the primitive red cell forms also occur principally around the periphery of the cells, occasionally in the nucleus. Vacuoles are also observed in the nucleus and cytoplasm of the granulocytic series. These morphologic changes disappear after chloramphenicol is withdrawn.[58,129,135] An acute erythroblastopenia without white blood cell and platelet depression has been observed with recovery following cessation of treatment.[19,53]

It is of interest that chloramphenicol rarely produced pancytopenia under 10 months of age. Apparently the "gray syndrome," a manifestation of chloramphenicol toxicity in newborn infants, is not associated with bone marrow damage. This age difference of marrow sensitivity is unexplained.[25]

The vacuoles in erythroid cell and myeloid cell cytoplasm, noted in the bone marrow in children treated with chloramphenicol, are morphologically identical with vacuolization observed in phenylalanine deficiency as well as in patients with erythremic myelosis and acute alcoholism. In a group of children treated with short courses of chloramphenicol for a variety of infections, the vacuoles disappeared in two patients[77] after treatment by mouth with 100 mg. L-phenylalanine per kilogram of body weight per day for 48 and 96 hours. Possibly the reversal of changes, associated with chloramphenicol administration by phenylalanine ingestion, suggests that chloramphenicol may act on the bone marrow by affecting phenylalanine metabolism.

In a study in adults[140] it was noted that bone marrow depression occurred regularly with plasma chloramphenicol levels of 25 $\mu$g per milliliter. Toxic plasma levels were regularly produced by daily doses of 50 mg. per kilogram of body weight. Doses of 25 to 30 mg. per kilogram per day produced adequate blood levels and were recommended for routine use. Progressive erythroid depression, a significant incidence of mild thrombocytopenia, and some evidence of disturbed granulocyte production occurred in patients given the larger dose for 2 weeks or more. These changes promptly disappeared after the drug was stopped. It was emphasized that in the individual case there should be a good clinical indication for the use of chloramphenicol in preference to other antibiotics. Hypoplasia of the bone marrow with pancytopenia has also been reported following the protracted use of chloramphenicol eyedrops.[130]

Recent investigations indicate that mammalian mitochondrial protein synthesis is sensitive to this drug. Chloramphenicol in concentrations within therapeutic range (10 $\mu$g/ml. to 50 $\mu$g/ml.) inhibits protein synthesis by rabbit and human bone marrow mitochondria without affecting mitochondrial respiration or oxidative phosphorylation.[101] Detailed electron microscopic study in bone marrow from patients receiving chloramphenical[176] indicated that the drug induces ultrastructural modification resulting in an increase in the density of the mitochrondrial matrix. Chloramphenicol produces a mitochondrial lesion which is directly related to the serum level of free chloramphenicol and is reversible. These observations do not, however, explain why the erythroid elevations are particularly vulnerable.

Chloramphenicol produces two types of toxic effect in bone marrow.[34] The first is a dose-related, reversible lesion occurring concurrently with chloramphenicol therapy and is characterized by a normally cellular marrow, maturation arrest, vacuolization in erythroid and myeloid cells, reticulocytopenia, and ferrokinetic changes reflecting a suppressed erythropoiesis. The second is a rare but serious complication characterized by a late clinical onset 3 to 6 weeks after the last drug dose resulting in bone marrow hypoplasia or aplasia, pancytopenia, and usually a fatal outcome from hemorrhage or infection. This second type shows a lack of dose-effect relationship. Apparently these two types of toxic effect are unrelated.

*Removal of the causative agent.* For obvious reasons recognition and elimination of the causative agent (such as a drug, chemical, insectide, or household chemical) are the first steps of treatment. Removal of the patient from further contact with the suspected toxic agent should be carried out immediately.

*Transfusion and other supportive measures.* Transfusions to combat anemia and provide platelets, adrenocortical hormones, and testosterone to stimulate hematopoiesis constitute the elements of treatment. Infections are usually brought under control with the liberal use of wide-spectrum antibodies. An environment free from infection is especially important in the early stages of the disease when remission with the newer therapeutic agents is awaited.

Thrombocytopenia almost invariably leads to excessive bleeding and is often responsible for a fatal outcome. Transfusion of fresh whole blood accomplishes the dual function of correcting anemia and supplying platelets. The administration, however, of platelet-rich plasma (obtained after sedimentation or centrifugation) and especially platelet concentrates is often lifesaving. Platelets are given in concentrated suspensions, one unit representing the amount removed from 500 ml. of whole blood. The sequential use of fresh whole blood followed by platelets is extremely useful and depends, of course, on the anemia. The value of transfusions as the sole treatment in producing permanent remissions in children falls far short of the notable success achieved in at least one series consisting principally of adults (eleven of forty-five patients).[78] The benefits of whole blood and fresh platelets, however, cannot be overestimated because they frequently sustain life until the belated effects of androgen-corticosteroid therapy become manifest.[13] Reliance is placed on adrenocortical steroids to control hemostasis. This is accomplished more by increasing capillary resistance than by elevating the number of platelets.[126] Epistaxis, an uncommon complication, may be controlled by packing with Surgicel or a similar preparation. When ineffective, the packing may be saturated with thrombin.

In one series,[57] patients with acute aplastic anemia became refractory to platelets obtained from random donors by a median of 8 weeks. Once a patient became refractory, the poor response to random donor platelets was not improved by splenectomy, corticoids, androgens, or any combinations of these. Platelets from family donors matched for histocompatibility antigens were given twice weekly for periods up to 77 weeks and continually provided excellent clinical responses. The therapeutic benefit from compatible platelet infusion was substantially greater than could be provided by a fivefold greater mass of incompatible platelets. Splenectomy or high-dose corticoid therapy improved the response to compatible platelets. When refractoriness to platelets is life-threatening, family members, particularly siblings, can be tried empirically as platelet donors.

Infections are often difficult to control, even with the liberal use of wide-spectrum antibiotics. Ampicillin, methicillin, and gentamicin are given until more specific information is obtained about the invading organism from blood cultures and examination of other accessible infected sites. In the event of marked neutropenia, antibodies are given if there are other clinical manifestations of active disease. The prophylactic use of antibiotics is hazardous because of possible bacterial resistance.

*Androgen-corticosteroid therapy.* The observation that androgenic hormones increased erythropoiesis to normal or polycythemic levels in patients with advanced breast cancer,[85,86] and that these hormones are a specific stimulus to erythroid activity, led to their use in aplastic anemia.[56,145,146] While the exact mechanism of erythropoietic action is still in question, testosterone has been effective in inducing a remission in a substantial number of acquired cases of aplastic anemia. Testosterone has been combined with corticosteroids and administered over prolonged periods. During the remission, the hemoglobin reaches normal levels, the number of reticulocytes increases, and the bone marrow is converted from a markedly hypocellular and fatty marrow to a hypercellular one with erythroid hyperplasia. In our experience and that of others, hemoglobin and red cell elevations may not occur until long intervals after therapy is instituted; usually not less than 3 months elapse and in many cases much longer. Awaiting a remission, patients must be kept free from infection and hemorrhage, and anemia must be promptly treated.

Until the advent of androgens, the corticosteroids were the principal hormones employed. In combination, the corticosteroids have an important place: to increase capillary resistance, decrease the rate of erythrocyte destruction, oppose the anabolic action of testosterone, and prevent increased bone maturation and premature closure of epiphyses.[145] In one of our cases in which corticosteroids were withdrawn because the patient was exposed to measles, testosterone was continued and the hemoglobin level dropped, and rose only when the steroids were later reintroduced.

Testosterone in the form of testosterone propionate or methyltestosterone is given preferably by the sublingual route in a daily dose of 1 or 2 mg. per kilogram of body weight. The dosage usually varies from a total of 30 mg. and should not exceed 50 mg. daily (in older children). Corticosteroids are given as prednisone (or substitutes in proportionate amounts) in a dosage of 10 or 15 mg. daily. These drugs are administered together in three divided doses. When testosterone cannot be given by the sublingual route, tablets of an appropriate oral compound are crushed and swallowed. In urgent conditions the drug is given parenterally, although hematomas form if patients are depleted of platelets. On occasion, methyltestosterone has been associated with mild jaundice, in which case testosterone propionate can be substituted, or this form can be given initially.

The evidence of maculinization, such as flushing of the skin, acne, deepening of the voice, hirsutism, and growth of pubic hair, are evidences of drug absorption. In our experience, except for the growth of pubic hair, all other evidences of androgen effect subside on withdrawal of the drug.

The most extensive experience has been with the sublingual administration of methyltestosterone. The other preparations listed below are still under trial and their dosages tentative. Caution is to be exercised particularly with preparations requiring intramuscular injections. A drug such as testosterone enanthate must be given in large dosages. The dosage suggested is 200 to 600 mg. weekly, usually divided in two or three injections over several months.[107] Another smaller dosage of the same preparation is suggested below. The clinical status of the patient may become so desperate, however, that recourse to parenteral preparations is necessary despite local bleeding complications.

1. Fluoxymestrone (Halotestin, Ultandren)—oral, (5 times as potent as methyltestosterone).
2. Methyltestosterone—sublingual (i.e., Metandren) or testosterone propionate—sublingual (i.e., Oreton). Dosage for either, 1 to 2 mg. per kilogram, usually 30 to 50 mg. daily in divided doses.
3. Testosterone enanthate in oil—intramuscularly, 4 mg. per kilogram once weekly.[144]
4. Testosterone cyclopentylpropionate (Depo-testosterone)—intramuscularly, dosage under trial.
5. Methandrostenolone (Dianabol)—oral, 0.25 to 0.5 mg. per kilogram.
6. Oxymetholone (Dihydrotestosterone)—oral, 2.0 to 6.5 mg. per kilogram.
7. Nandrolone decanoate—1 to 1.5 mg./kg./week intramuscularly for no less than 4 months.[27]

It is claimed[142] that smaller doses of methandrostenolone (Dianabol), 0.25 to 0.5 mg. per kilogram of body weight, will reduce the incidence of side effects produced by the high testosterone doses without diminishing its therapeutic effectiveness. This finding was confirmed in two children under our observation in whom methandrostenolone was substituted for methyltestosterone. Wider experience with this drug is necessary before it can be adequately compared with other testosterone compounds. Methandrostenolone, like other anabolic androgenic steroids, may also produce jaundice due to intrahepatic bile stasis.[84]

A synthetic derivative of testosterone, oxymetholone (2-hydroxymethylene-17 alpha-methyl-17β-hydroxy-3-androstanone) has also been found to be a potent bone marrow stimulant.[6,7,136,137] Mild virilization was the only side effect noted. In one series with oxymetholone given orally in a daily dosage of 2.0 to 6.5 mg./kg. body weight, significant improvement in peripheral blood appeared between the second and third months of treatment. Several of the children with acquired aplastic anemia have remained well without therapy for 18 to 24 months. Another patient with constitutional aplastic anemia had a good response to a second course of oxymetholone therapy but appeared to require continuous maintenance therapy.

As stated, the response to testosterone-corticosteroid therapy is usually not observed for 2 to 3 months and sometimes much later, or in many cases not at all. Reticulocytosis occurs but the peak is often missed and does not always herald an immediate rise in hemoglobin. When effective, the androgenic hormones potentiated by the corticosteroids increase erythroid activity, but return of granulocytes and platelets to normal levels is often delayed, particularly the latter. When the hemoglobin level reaches 12 to 14 gm. per 100 ml., androgen therapy is discontinued. Some prefer to continue corticosteroids for short periods, hoping to forestall a drop in hemoglobin and control bleeding.

While spontaneous remissions in aplastic anemia are known to occur in children, they are so rare that it is our procedure to initiate androgen-corticosteroid therapy with transfusions and other supportive therapy as soon as the diagnosis is made. Until more extensive experience is acquired, individual programs of treatment will be necessary with respect to dosage of hormones and the manner of withdrawal, once normal hemoglobin levels are established.

The response to androgen-corticosteroid therapy differs in the two groups of patients with aplastic anemia—the constitutional as compared with the acquired. The acquired type includes those exposed to myelotoxic agents and those with no history of ingestion of a toxic drug or exposure to a noxious agent—the so-called idiopathic aplastic anemia. The constitutional or congenital aplastic anemias include cases associated with congenital malformations such as found in Fanconi's syndrome, cases without demonstrable congenital defects but with pancytopenia in several members of the same family, and the recently described cases associated with pancreatic insufficiency and bone marrow dysfunction.[148] In favorable cases, patients with the acquired type recover without recourse to further therapy. Occasionally, a slight degree of hematologic relapse occurs, but spontaneous recovery is usual. In contrast, patients with the constitutional type of aplastic anemia require continuous testosterone therapy to maintain adequate hematopoiesis. In the recovered cases of either type, platelet response is much slower than in the attainment of normal hemoglobin and granulocyte levels. Patients showing evidences of mild bone marrow cellularity respond more favorably than those showing severe depression of the marrow.[29]

In one series[146] in which the acquired cases were predominantly due to chloramphenicol, nine of seventeen patients treated for periods ranging from 2½ to 15 months responded with a sustained remission. The remaining eight succumbed to hemorrhage or infection. In six of seven patients with constitutional aplastic anemia, there was a satisfactory rise in hemoglobin concentration and polymorphonuclear cells, but a slower platelet response. These patients were testosterone dependent since withdrawal of the drug produced a drop in blood values. In another group[29] of patients with acquired aplastic anemia, five demonstrated hematologic improvement within 1 to 6 months after the onset of therapy. A moderate degree of thrombocytopenia persisted in all patients.

Increased amounts of alkali-resistant hemoglobin have been found in patients with aplastic anemia (3 to 15%). While this level decreased steadily in most patients with acquired aplastic anemia in remission, it tended to fluctuate without dropping significantly in patients with the constitutional type of disease (Fanconi syndrome).[147] The level of fetal hemoglobin in acquired aplastic anemia may serve as an indicator of response to treatment.[16] Patients with severe aplasia have been found to have less total circulating fetal hemoglobin (hemoglobin gm./100 ml. × percent fetal hemoglobin) than those with milder forms of the disease. The majority of patients with acquired aplastic anemia who died had less than 400 mg./100 ml. of total fetal hemoglobin. On the other hand, the majority of those who are alive and doing well had more than 400 mg./100 ml. of fetal hemoglobin at the initial examination.

Patients with aplastic anemia show hypochromia of erythrocytes and an increase in free erythrocyte protoporphyrin during hematologic remission induced by testosterone therapy.[143] In the absence of iron deficiency, lead intoxication, and anemia of infection, in which the same findings are present, it is possible that testosterone enhances cellular maturation while incorporation of iron into hemoglobin in erythroid cells proceeds independently and at a slower rate.

Patients who apparently have recovered from acquired aplastic anemia may occasionally relapse after years of good health. One of our patients, a girl, was first observed in 1961 at 3 years of age, 1½ months after chloramphenicol therapy for asthmatic bronchitis. She responded with normal hemoglobin levels following androgen-corticosteroid therapy. By July, 1963, after all therapy was terminated, hemoglobin and white blood count levels had reached normal levels (hemoglobin, 13 gm./100 ml.; WBC, 8,500/cu. mm.). The platelets, however, remained at a subnormal value (50,000/cm.). After approximately 5½ years of remission, in 1969 the hemoglobin values dropped precipitously and oxymetholone and prednisone were administered. No etiologic factor, either drug or environmental, could be implicated. Investigations for paroxysmal nocturnal hemoglobinuria and occult malignancy were negative. The Coombs test was negative. With supportive blood and platelet transfusions another remission was obtained.

It would seem best until the platelets return to normal to follow patients with acquired aplastic anemia periodically during the period of remission.

Despite the emphasis on androgens in the treatment of acquired aplastic anemia, there are those who claim equally good results with supportive treatment alone. In the report by Heyn and her co-workers,[66] thirty-three children with acquired aplastic anemia were followed, fifteen of whom recovered and two still required transfusions. Sixteen (48.4%) died. All children received supportive care but no androgen treatment. Transfusions of either whole blood or packed cells were given to maintain a hemoglobin value of more than 6.0 gm./100 ml. or when the patient became symptomatic. Platelet transfusions were given to a few patients during major bleeding episodes. Antibiotics were used for specific pathogens when indicated. Potential etiologic agents were eliminated. The period for recovery in the survivors covered a wide span of time. Some children with markedly hypocellular marrow and extreme pancytopenia recovered completely in as little as 3 months, whereas others took 2 or 3 years to attain the same degree of recovery. Heyn and colleagues[66] claim that results with supportive treatment equaled the 50% responses with the use of androgens. Their conclusions are pertinent that "further observation on the natural course of the disease with reference to initial and sequential marrow and blood studies, causative agents, ancillary supportive care, and transfusion requirements might well benefit the future evaluation of modes of therapy."

*Splenectomy.* Bleeding in aplastic anemia, including the Fanconi type, is occasionally amenable to splenectomy. In two girls, 9 and 12 years of age, diminution of generalized bleeding and severe menorrhagia, respectively, resulted from splenectomy when all other available measures for controlling hemostasis failed. In a 15-year-old girl with the Fanconi type of aplastic anemia, splenectomy was performed because of severe thrombocytopenia and bleeding. At 20 years of age she was no longer anemic and the bleeding tendency had subsided but thrombocytopenia and leukopenia persisted.[28] The rationale for splenectomy has been reviewed in connection with pure red cell anemia. Recently this procedure has been recommended more freely in patients with unexplained refractory anemia, especially when any improvement in bone marrow function could be predicted. In one series, six of twelve patients with hypoplastic disease of the bone marrow,[65] in whom the indications for splenectomy were the presence of severe thrombocytopenic purpura, anemia, and granulocytopenia leading to increased susceptibility to infection, improved. Five of the twelve patients ranged in age from 2 to 9 years, and of these two showed hematologic improvement, but in only one was it sustained. In another series,[139] four of fifteen splenectomized patients have shown partial or complete recovery. It appears that splenectomy should be reserved not only for those patients in whom a hemolytic component can be demonstrated, but also for those in whom an inhibiting effect of an abnormal spleen on the marrow can be postulated. The criteria for patients with completely aplastic marrows still await formulation. In general, splenectomy is more likely to benefit the rare patient with pancytopenia in whom the bone marrow is hyperplastic with arrest of maturation. With the advent of hormonal treatment, it is possible that the need for splenectomy will be greatly reduced.

Flatow and Freireich[44] reported three patients with aplastic anemia treated with repeated platelet transfusions for periods of 11 to 14 months. Each of the patients became refractory to pooled platelet preparations from random donors, presumably as a result of antibody formation. Splenectomy was performed without complication in all three patients and resulted in improved response to platelet transfusion and longer posttransfusion survival of platelets. These authors suggest that splenectomy should be considered for patients with aplastic anemia who are refractory to platelet transfusions and are at risk from hemorrhage.

*Miscellaneous treatment.* The administration of iron is potentially harmful in patients with refractory anemias because of its increased absorption from the gastrointestinal tract, supplementing the already excessive iron stores within the tissues from transfusions. The use of cobalt has had many advocates, with sporadic reports of beneficial effects in pure red cell anemia and other refractory anemias. Cobalt has been shown to influence the production of the erythropoietic stimulating factor.[55] Its possible side effects, such as anorexia, nausea, and thyroid enlargement, preclude its widespread use except under controlled conditions.[112] Favorable results with cobalt, however, have been reported in several adults with the acquired erythrocytic hypoplasia.[46,141] In our experience the results with cobalt in congenital pure red cell anemia have been uniformly disappointing.

Each of the following vitamin B factors in suggested dosage has been given to patients with pure red cell anemia and other members of the hypoplastic-aplastic group of anemias: vitamin $B_{12}$, 1,000 µg intramuscularly three times weekly; riboflavin, 10 mg. three times daily; nicotinamide, 50 mg. daily; and folic acid, 5 mg. three times daily. In the doses mentioned, beneficial effects were obtained with riboflavin in the treatment of pure red cell anemia[47] and nicotinamide in hypoplastic anemia after the administration of chloramphenicol.[161] Although many of these substances are known to function in specific phases of erythropoiesis, their value in patients with refractory anemia is still debatable. Occasionally, they appear to stimulate red cell formation, particularly after splenectomy.

An ingenious treatment of aplastic anemia with phytohemagglutinin has been employed in a small series of adult cases.[73] This substance is an extract containing mucoproteins from the seeds of *Phaseolus vulgaris*, which in tissue culture causes human small lymphocytes to enlarge and undergo active mitotic division. The resemblance of these "phytohemagglutinin-altered" cells to hemocytoblasts and other primitive bone marrow cells prompted this treatment. The phytohemagglutinin is directed into the bloodstream by various devices. Although at best, partial remissions may have been achieved by this treatment; bone marrow stimulation was evident in increased cytoplasmic basophilia and granulation of lymphocytes and in persistent reticulocytosis.[73] A trial of phytohemagglutinin elsewhere gave disappointing results.[122]

*Marrow transplantation.* Efforts to suppress the immune spleen to permit marrow transplantation heretofore regarded as unsuccessful[172] have recently become more promising with the increased interest in the basic immunologic mechanisms involved in donor and recipient compatibility. It had been known[106,160] that a graft of isologous bone marrow (marrow from an identical twin) had a good chance of a successful outcome, provided the etiologic agent had been eliminated and an adequate number of viable cells transplanted. Sufficient cells can be obtained from the donor by aspiration from multiple sites along the iliac spines and crest. The report by Pillow and associates[115] in 1966 of recovery of an 18-year-old boy after a transplant from an identical twin brought to five the number of patients who at that time recovered following isogenic bone marrow infusion.

If an identical twin is not available, transplantation of allogenic marrow (from genetically dissimilar individuals) has met with limited success. In one series no differences were observed in the survival of twenty patients with aplastic anemia who received infusions of homologous marrow as compared with seventeen patients treated with other measures.[104] On the other hand, with the newer methods of preparing the recipient and often the donor, it is now possible to obtain successful grafts using allogeneic marrow.[102] In two patients with aplastic anemia, one due to chloramphenicol poisoning and the other to viral hepatitis, the graft was established. These patients had not received cytostatic drugs and all corticosteroid therapy had been withdrawn before giving antilymphocytic serum to the recipient.

If the host is immunologically competent, no allogeneic marrow is rejected by the host-versus-graft (HVG) reaction. On the other hand, if the graft contains immunologically competent cells, the graft will mount an immunologic attack against the host. If the host's immune mechanism is deficient because of impaired development or as a result of immunosuppressive agents, the graft produces the graft-versus-host (GVH) reaction, which may be fatal.

Various measures have been taken to suppress the recipient's immune response. Immunosuppression has been achieved by irradiation, by drugs such as cortisone, cyclophosphamide, azathioprine, methotrexate, and other antimetabolites, and by the use of antilymphocyte serum (ALS) or its purified fraction, antilymphocyte globulin (ALG).

An additional measure to ensure the success of the transplant (in this case, allogeneic marrow) is the use of donors who are in the same A-B-O blood group and who are also identical in the major histocompatibility locus in man, HL-A.[164] This common antigen is present in platelets, white blood cells, and tissue cells and is determined by lymphocyte typing. Experimental evidence indicates that leukocyte grouping is almost synonymous with tissue typing.[163] Originally a mixture of granulocytes and lymphocytes were used for leukocytic grouping. In current use are the lymphocytotoxic assays, tests with leukoagglutinins, and the mixed leukocyte culture technique (MLC).

Evidence that the induction of tumors by oncogenic viruses is favored by antilymphocytic serum is now available.[8,134] It is possible that long-term immunosuppression may allow the emergence of neoplastic cells because the normal immunologic control mechanism has been depressed.

*Course and prognosis.* Until the advent of androgen-corticosteroid therapy the outcome of idiopathic aplastic anemia in childhood was almost uniformly fatal. The favorable results with the newer therapy have already been detailed. Wider experience with testosterone therapy is needed, however, before results can be accurately assessed. When unresponsive to these agents and transfusions, the acute course of weeks and months is marked by intractable hemorrhage and infection. The prognosis is better in those cases in which the cause is known and in patients with cellular rather than acellular marrows. When a drug such as chloramphenicol is discontinued, hematologic improvement is gradual, the first sign of improvement being a decreased transfusion requirement, followed by a rise in the number of neutrophils and platelets. The platelets are the last of the blood elements to become normal in recovered patients.[139] Cerebral hemorrhage and septicemia are the common causes of death.

In a compilation of the results of combined

prednisone and testosterone treatment the prognosis for each of the types of aplastic anemia has been given as follows.[2] In the group of acquired aplastic anemia of seventy-nine cases, twenty-nine or 36% recovered or were responding; in the constitutional aplastic anemia of sixteen cases, thirteen or 81% responded. While patients with acquired aplastic anemia may continue for prolonged periods without medication, the children in the constitutional group are dependent on continuous steroid therapy.

## REFERENCES

1. Aase, J. M., and Smith, D. W.: Congenital anemia and triphalangeal thumbs; a new syndrome, J. Pediat. 74:471, 1969.
2. Abildgaard, C. F.: Hypoplastic and aplastic anemia. In Barnett, H. L., editor: Pediatrics, ed. 14, New York, 1968, Appleton-Century-Crofts, p. 1133.
3. Abt, A. F.: Aplastic anemias in childhood; report of a primary idiopathic refractory type, with splenectomy, in an eleven-year-old girl, Amer. J. Dis. Child. 78:516, 1949.
4. Alfrey, C. P., Jr., and Lane, M.: The anemia of human riboflavin deficiency, Blood 22:811, 1963.
5. Allen, D. M., and Diamond, L. K.: Congenital (erythroid) hypoplastic anemia; cortisone treated, Amer. J. Dis. Child. 102:416, 1961.
6. Allen, D. M., Fine, M. H., Necheles, T. F., and Dameshek, W.: Oxymetholone therapy in aplastic anemia, Blood 32:83, 1968.
7. Allen, D. M., and Necheles, T. F.: Oxymetholone therapy of aplastic anemia, Program and Abstracts, p. 56, American Pediatric Society, 79th Annual Meeting, 1969.
8. Allison, A. C., and Law, L. W.: Effects of antilymphocyte serum on virus oncogenesis, Proc. Soc. Exp. Biol. Med. 127:707, 1968.
9. Altman, K. I., and Miller, G.: A disturbance of tryptophan metabolism in congenital hypoplastic anemia, Nature 172:868, 1953.
10. Anderson, S. B., and Ladefoged, J.: Pure red cell anaemia and thymoma, Acta Haemat. 30:319, 1963.
11. Arnason, B. G., Janković, B. D., and Waksman, B. H.: A survey of the thymus and its relation to lymphocytes and immune reactions, Blood 20:617, 1962.
12. Barnes, R. D. S., and O'Gorman, P.: Two cases of aplastic anaemia associated with tumours of the thymus, J. Clin. Path. 15:264, 1962.
13. Bellanti, J. A., and Pinkel, D.: Idiopathic aplastic anemia treated with methyltestosterone and fresh platelets, J.A.M.A. 178:70, 1961.
14. Best, W. R.: Chloramphenicol-associated blood dyscrasias; a review of cases submitted to the American Medical Association Registry, J.A.M.A. 201:181, 1967.
15. Bithell, T. C., and Wintrobe, M. M.: Drug-induced aplastic anemia, Seminars Hemat. 4:194, 1967.
16. Bloom, G. E., and Diamond, L. K.: Prognostic value of fetal hemoglobin levels in acquired aplastic anemia, New Eng. J. Med. 278:304, 1968.
17. Bloom, G. E., Warner, S., Gerald, P. S., and Diamond, L. K.: Chromosome abnormalities in constitutional aplastic anemia, New Eng. J. Med. 274:8, 1966.
18. Bomford, R. R., and Rhoads, C. P.: Refractory anaemia, Quart. J. Med. 34:175, 1941.
19. Bridges, R. A., Dillon, H., and Good, R. A.: Acute erythroblastopenia due to chloramphenicol, Amer. J. Dis. Child. 96:508, 1958.
20. Burgert, E. O., Jr., Kennedy, R. L. J., and Pease, G. L.: Congenital hypoplastic anemia, Pediatrics 12:218, 1954.
21. Burnet, F. M.: The immunological significance of the thymus; an extension of the clonal selection theory of immunity, Australasian Ann. Med. 11:79, 1962.
22. Cathie, I. A. B.: Erythrogenesis imperfecta, Arch. Dis. Child. 25:313, 1950.
23. Chanarin, I., Barkhan, P., Peacock, M., and Stamp, T. C. B.: Acute arrest of erythropoiesis, Brit. J. Haemat. 10:43, 1964.
24. Clarkson, B., and Prockop, D. J.: Aregenerative anemia associated with benign thymoma, New Eng. J. Med. 259:253, 1958.
25. Clement, D. H.: Aplastic anemia, Ped. Clin. N. Amer. 9:703, 1962.
26. Dacie, J. V., and Lewis, S. M.: Paroxysmal nocturnal hemoglobinuria; variation in clinical severity and association with bone marrow hypoplasia, Brit. J. Haemat. 7:442, 1961.
27. Daiber, A., Herve, L., Con, I., and Donoso, A.: Treatment of aplastic anemia with nandrolone decanoate, Blood 36:748, 1970.
28. Dawson, J. P.: Congenital pancytopenia associated with multiple congenital anomalies (Fanconi type); review of the literature and report of a twenty-year-old female with a ten-year follow-up and apparently good response to splenectomy, Pediatrics 15:325, 1955.
28a. Deller, J. J., Cirksena, W. J., and Marcurelli, J.: Fatal pancytopenia with viral hepatitis, New Eng. J. Med. 266:297, 1962.
29. Desposito, F., Akatsaka, J., Thatcher, L. G., and Smith, N. J.: Bone marrow failure in pediatric patients. I. Cortisone and testosterone treatment, J. Pediat. 64:683, 1964.
30. Diamond, L. K.: Year book of pediatrics, 1954-1955 Series, Chicago, 1954, Year Book Medical Publishers, Inc., p. 308.

31. Diamond, L. K., Allen, D. M., and Magill, F. B.: Congenital (erythroid) hypoplastic anemia; A 25 year study, Amer. J. Dis. Child. **102**:403, 1961.
32. Diamond, L. K., and Blackfan, K. D.: Hypoplastic anemia, Amer. J. Dis. Child. **56**:464, 1938.
33. Dosik, H., Hsu, L. Y., Todaro, G. J., Lee, S. L., Hirschhorn, K., Selirio, E. S., and Alter, A. A.: Leukemia in Fanconi's anemia; cytogenic and tumor virus susceptibility studies, Blood **36**:341, 1970.
34. Editorial: Chloramphenicol-induced bone marrow suppression, J.A.M.A. **213**:1183, 1970.
35. Ehrlich, P.: Ueber einen Fall von Anämie mit Bemerkungen über regenerative Veränderungen des Knochenmarks, Charite Ann. **13**:300, 1888.
36. Eisenmann, G., and Dameshek, W.: Splenectomy for "pure red-cell" hypoplastic (aregenerative) anemia associated with autoimmune hemolytic disease, New Eng. J. Med. **251**:1044, 1954.
37. El-Alfi, O. S., Smith, P. M., and Biessle, J. J.: Chromosomal breaks in human leukocyte cultures induced by an agent in the plasma of infections, Hereditas **52**:1285, 1965.
38. Erslev, A.: Hematopoietic depression induced by chloromycetin, Blood **8**:170, 1953.
39. Erslev, A. J.: Drug-induced blood dyscrasias, J.A.M.A. **188**:531, 1964.
40. Erslev, A. J., and Wintrobe, M. M.: Detection and prevention of drug induced blood dyscrasias, J.A.M.A. **181**:134, 1962.
41. Estren, S., and Dameshek, W.: Familial hypoplastic anemia of childhood, Amer. J. Dis. Child. **73**:671, 1947.
42. Fanconi, G.: Familiäre infantile pernizosaartige Anämie (perniziöses Blutbild und Konstitution), Jahrb. Kindern. **117**:257, 1927.
43. Fanconi, G.: Die Hypothese einer Chromosomentranslokation zur Erklärung der Genetik der Familiären Konstitutionellen Panmyelopathic Typus Fanconi, Helv. Paediat. Acta **19**:29, 1964.
44. Flatow, F. A., and Freireich, E. J.: Effect of splenectomy on the response to platelet transfusions in three patients with aplastic anemia, New Eng. J. Med. **274**:242, 1966.
45. Follette, J. H., Shugarman, P. M., Reynolds, J., Valentine, W. N., and Lawrence, J. S.: The effect of chloramphenicol and other antibiotics on leukocyte respiration, Blood **11**:234, 1956.
46. Fountain, J. R., and Dales, M.: Pure red-cell aplasia successfully treated with cobalt, Lancet **1**:541, 1955.
47. Foy, H., and Kondi, A.: A case of true-red-cell aplastic anemia successfully treated with riboflavin, J. Path. Bact. **65**:559, 1953.
48. Foy, H., Kondi, A., and MacDougall, L.: Pure red-cell aplasia in marasmus and kwashiorkor treated with riboflavin, Brit. J. Med. **1**:937, 1961.
49. Garriga, S., and Crosby, W. H.: The incidence of leukemia in families of patients with hypoplasia of the marrow, Blood **14**:1008, 1959.
50. Gasser, C.: Akute Erythroblastopenie, 10 Fälle aplastischer Erythroblastenkrisen mit Riesenproerythroblasten bei allergisch-toxischen Zustandsbildern, Helv. Paediat. Acta **4**:107, 1949.
51. Gasser, C.: Aplastische Anämie (chronische Erythroblastophthise) und Cortison, Schweiz. med. Wchnschr. **81**:1241, 1951.
52. Gasser, C.: Aplasia of erythropoiesis, acute and chronic erythroblastopenias or pure (red cell) aplastic anemias in childhood, Ped. Clin. N. Amer. **4**:445, 1957.
53. Ghitis, J.: Acute benign erythroblastopenia possibly chloramphenicol induced, J. Pediat. **60**:566, 1962.
54. Ginsburg, S. M.: Acute erythroid aplasia (erythroblastopenia) and vascular purpura in an otherwise hematologically normal child, Ann. Intern. Med. **55**:317, 1961.
55. Goldwasser, E., Jacobson, L. O., Fried, W., and Plzak, L.: Mechanism of the erythropoietic effect of cobalt, Science **125**:1085, 1957.
56. Gordon, F. H., Nathan, D. G., Piomelli, S., and Cummins, J. F.: The erythrocythemic effects of androgen, Brit. J. Haemat. **14**:611, 1968.
57. Grumet, F. C., and Yankee, R. A.: Long-term platelet support of patients with aplastic anemia; effect of splenectomy and steroid therapy, Ann. Intern. Med. **73**:1, 1970.
58. Gussoff, B. D., Lee, S. L., and Lichtman, H. C.: Erythropoietic changes during therapy with chloramphenicol, Arch. Intern. Med. **109**:176, 1962.
59. Hammond, G. D., and Keighley, G.: The erythrocyte stimulating factor (ESF) in serum and urine in congenital hypoplastic anemia, Amer. J. Dis. Child. **100**:466, 1960.
60. Hansen, H. G.: Ueber die essentielle Erythroblastopenie, Acta Haemat. **6**:335, 1951.
61. Harris, L. C., and Osborne, W. P.: Congenital absence or hypoplasia of the radius with ventricular septal defect; ventricular-radial dysplasia, J. Pediat. **68**:265, 1966.
62. Hathaway, W. E., and Githens, J. H.: Pancytopenia with hyperplastic marrow, Amer. J. Dis. Child. **102**:389, 1961.
63. Havard, C. W. H., and Parish, A.: Thymic

tumor and erythroblastic aplasia, J.A.M.A. **179**:228, 1962.
64. Havard, C. W. H., and Scott, R. B.: Thymic tumour and erythroblastic aplasia; report of three cases and a review of the syndrome, Brit. J. Haemat. **6**:178, 1960.
65. Heaton, L. D., Crosby, W. H., and Cohen, A.: Splenectomy in the treatment of hypoplasia of the bone marrow with a report of twelve cases, Ann. Surg. **146**:637, 1957.
66. Heyn, R. M., Ertel, I. J., and Tubergen, D. G.: Course of acquired aplastic anemia in children treated with supportive care, J.A.M.A. **208**:1372, 1969.
67. Hilgartner, M. W., Lanzkowsky, P., Nachman, R. L., and Weksler, M. B.: Bone marrow transplantation for aplastic anemia following hepatitis. In press.
68. Hodgman, J. E.: Chloramphenical, Ped. Clin. N. Amer. **8**:1027, 1961.
69. Holt, M., and Oram, S.: Familial heart disease with skeletal malformations, Brit. Heart J. **22**:236, 1960.
70. Horsfall, W. R.: A case of congenital non-spherocytic haemolytic anaemia presenting with an aplastic crisis, M. J. Australia **2**:340, 1956.
71. Hsia, D. Y-Y.: Inborn errors of metabolism, Chicago, 1959, Year Book Medical Publishers, Inc., p. 221.
72. Hughes, D. W. O'G.: Hypoplastic anaemia in infancy and childhood; erythroid hypoplasia, Arch. Dis. Child. **36**:349, 1961.
73. Humble, J. G.: The treatment of aplastic anaemia with phytohaemagglutinin, Lancet **1**:1345, 1964.
74. Humphreys, G. H., II, and Southworth, H.: Aplastic anemia terminated by removal of mediastinal tumor, Amer. J. Med. Sci. **210**:501, 1945.
75. Hurwitt, E. S., and Field, L.: Aplastic anemia in pregnancy, Amer. J. Obstet. Gynec. **43**:42, 1942.
76. Ingall, D., and Sherman, J. D.: Chloramphenicol, Ped. Clin. N. Amer. **15**:57, 1968.
77. Ingall, D., Sherman, J. D., Cockburn, F., and Klein, R.: Amelioration by ingestion of phenylalanine of toxic effects of chloramphenicol on bone marrow, New Eng. J. Med. **272**:180, 1965.
78. Israels, M. C. G., and Wilkinson, J. F.: Idiopathic aplastic anaemia, Lancet **1**:63, 1961.
79. Jahsman, D. P., Monto, R. W., and Rebuck, J. W.: Erythroid hypoplastic anemia (erythroblastopenia) associated with benign thymoma, Amer. J. Clin. Path. **38**:152, 1962.
80. Jandl, J. H., and Greenberg, M. S.: Bone-marrow failure due to relative nutritional deficiency in Cooley's hemolytic anemia, New Eng. J. Med. **260**:461, 1959.

81. Jepson, J. H., and Lowenstein, L.: Inhibition of erythropoiesis by a factor present in the plasma of patients wtih erythroblastopenia, Blood **27**:425, 1966.
82. Jonnson, U., Roath, O. S., and Kirkpatrick, C. I. F.: Nutritional megaloblastic anemia associated with sickle cell states, Blood **15**:535, 1959.
83. Josephs, H. W.: Anaemia of infancy and early childhood, Medicine **15**:307, 1936.
84. Kaupp, H. A., and Preston, F. W.: Jaundice due to methandrostenolone therapy, J.A.M.A. **180**:411, 1962.
85. Kennedy, B. J., and Gilbertson, A. S.: Increased erythropoiesis induced by androgenic hormone therapy, New Eng. J. Med. **256**:719, 1957.
86. Kennedy, B. J., and Nathanson, I. T.: Effects of intensive sex steroid hormone therapy in advanced breast cancer, J.A.M.A. **152**:1135, 1953.
87. Kho, L. K., Odang, O., Thajeb, S., and Markum, A. H.: Erythroblastopenia (pure red cell aplasia) in childhood in Djakarta, Blood **19**:168, 1962.
88. Knox, W. E.: Two mechanisms which increase in vivo liver tryptophan peroxidase activity, Brit. J. Exp. Path. **32**:462, 1951.
89. Kosan, N.: Pancytopenie als Komplikation einer Hepatitis and Ursache einer Leberdystrophie, Medizinische Monatschrift **10**:794, 1956.
90. Krantz, S. B., and Kao, V.: Studies on red cell aplasia. II. Report of a second patient with an antibody to erythroblast nuclei and a remission after immunosuppressive therapy, Blood **34**:1, 1969.
91. Lawrence, J. S., Dowdy, A. H., and Valentine, W.: Effects of radiation on hematopoiesis, Radiology **51**:400, 1948.
92. Lennard-Jones, J. E., Hesse, deV., and Venn, R. J.: Aplastic anaemia during pregnancy, J. Obstet. Gynaec. Brit. Emp. **65**:92, 1958.
93. Lerner, A. B.: Melanin pigmentation, Amer. J. Med. **19**:902, 1955.
94. Lescher, F. G., and Hubble, D.: A correlation of certain blood diseases on the hypothesis of bone marrow deficiency or hypoplasia, Quart. J. Med. **1**:425, 1932.
95. Levy, R. N., Sawitsky, A., Florman, A. L., and Rubin, E.: Fatal aplastic anemia after hepatitis; report of five cases, New Eng. J. Med. **273**:1118, 1965.
96. Lewis, C. N., Putnam, L. E., Henricks, F. D., Kerlan, I., and Welch, H.: Chloramphenicol (Chloromycetin) in relation to blood dyscrasias with observations on other drugs; a special survey, Antibiot. Chemother. **2**:601, 1952.
97. Lewis, S. M.: Red-cell abnormalities and

hemolysis in aplastic anaemia, Brit. J. Haemat. **8**:322, 1962.
98. Loeb, V., Jr., Moore, C. V., and Dubach, R.: The physiologic evaluation and management of chronic bone marrow failure, Amer. J. Med. **15**:499, 1953.
99. Lorenz, E., and Quaisser, K.: Panmyelopathie nach Hepatitis Epidemica, Wien. Med. Wschr. **105**:19, 1955.
100. Martland, H. S.: Occupational poisoning in manufacture of luminous watch dials; general review of hazard caused by ingestion of luminous paint, with especial reference to the New Jersey cases, J.A.M.A. **92**:466, 1929.
101. Martelo, O. J., Manyan, D. R., and Smith, U. S.: Chloramphenicol and bone marrow mitochondria, J. Lab. Clin. Med. **74**:927, 1969.
102. Mathé, G., Amiel, J. L., Schwarzenberg, L., Choay, J., Trolard, P., Schneider, M., Hayatt, M., Schlumberger, J. R., and Jasmin, Cl.: Bone marrow graft in man after conditioning by antilymphocytic serum, Brit. Med. J. **2**:131, 1970.
103. McCurdy, P. R.: Chloramphenicol bone marrow toxicity, J.A.M.A. **176**:588, 1961.
104. McFarland, W., Granville, N., Schwartz, R., Oliner, H., Mirsa, D. K., and Dameshek, W.: Therapy of hypoplastic anemia with bone marrow transplantation, Arch. Intern. Med. **108**:91, 1961.
105. McKay, E.: Congenital hypoplastic anaemia; report of two cases, Arch. Dis. Child. **37**:663, 1962.
106. Mills, S. D., Kyle, R. A., Hallenbeck, G. A., Pease, G. L., and Cree, I. C.: Bone marrow transplant in an identical twin, J.A.M.A. **188**:1037, 1964.
107. Modell, W., editor: Drugs of choice, 1964-1965, St. Louis, 1965, The C. V. Mosby Co., p. 678.
108. Nagao, T., and Mauer, A. M.: Concordance for drug-induced aplastic anemia in identical twins, New Eng. J. Med. **281**:7, 1969.
109. Oliner, H. L., and Heller, P.: Megaloblastic erythropoiesis and acquired hemolysis in sickle-cell anemia, New Eng. J. Med. **261**:19, 1959.
110. Owren, P. A.: Congenital hemolytic jaundice; pathogenesis of "hemolytic crisis," Blood **3**:231, 1948.
111. Palmen, K., and Vahlquist, B.: Stationary hypoplastic anemia, Acta Haemat. **4**:273, 1950.
112. Panels in Therapy: The use of cobalt and cobalt-iron preparations in the therapy of anemia, Blood **10**:852, 1955.
113. Pearson, H. A., and Cone, T. E., Jr.: Congenital hypoplastic anemia, Pediatrics **19**:192, 1957.
114. Pearson, H. A., McFarland, W., and Cone, T. E., Jr.: Biopsy of bone marrow with the Silverman needle in children, Pediatrics **26**:310, 1960.
115. Pillow, R. P., Epstein, R. B., Buckner, C. D., Giblett, E. R., and Thomas, E. D.: Treatment of bone-marrow failure by isogeneic marrow infusion, New Eng. J. Med. **275**:94, 1966.
116. Ponder, E.: Present concepts of the structure of the mammalian red cell, Blood **9**:227, 1954.
117. Powars, D.: Aplastic anemia secondary to glue sniffing, New Eng. J. Med. **273**:700, 1965.
118. Prankerd, T. A. J.: The metabolism of the human erythrocyte; a review, Brit. J. Haemat. **1**:131, 1955.
119. Quagliana, J. M., Cartwright, G. E., and Wintrobe, M. M.: Paroxysmal nocturnal hemoglobinuria following drug induced aplastic anemia, Ann. Intern. Med. **61**:1045, 1964.
120. Reinhold, J. D. L., Neumark, E., Lightwood, R., and Carter, C. O.: Familial hypoplastic anemia with congenital abnormalities (Fanconi syndrome), Blood **7**:915, 1952.
121. Report of the Council on Drugs: Blood dyscrasias associated with chloramphenicol (Chloromycetin) therapy, J.A.M.A. **172**:2044, 1960.
122. Retief, F. P., Wasserman, H. P., and Hefmeyer, N. G.: Phytohemagglutinin in aplastic anaemia, Lancet **2**:1343, 1964.
123. Rhoads, C. P., and Barker, W. H.: Refractory anemia, J.A.M.A. **110**:794, 1938.
124. Rhoads, C. P., and Miller, D. K.: Histology of the bone marrow in aplastic anemia, Arch. Path. **26**:648, 1938.
125. Robins, M. M.: Aplastic anemia secondary to anticonvulsants, Amer. J. Dis. Child. **104**:614, 1962.
126. Robson, H. N., and Duthie, J. J. R.: Further observations on capillary resistance and adreno-cortical activity, Brit. Med. J. **1**:994, 1952.
127. Rohr, K.: Familial Panmyelophthisis: Fanconi syndrome in adults, Blood **4**:130, 1949.
128. Roland, A. S.: The syndrome of benign thymoma and primary aregenerative anemia; an analysis of forty-three cases, Amer. J. Med. Sci. **247**:719, 1964.
129. Rosenbach, L. M., Caviles, A. P., and Mitus, W. J.: Chloramphenicol toxicity; reversible vacuolization of erythroid cells, New Eng. J. Med. **263**:724, 1960.
130. Rosenthal, R. L., and Blackman, A.: Bone-marrow hypoplasia following use of chlor-

amphenicol eye drops, J.A.M.A. **191**:136, 1965.
131. Ross, J. F., Finch, S. C., Street, R. B., Jr., and Strieder, J. M.: Simultaneous occurrence of benign thymoma and refractory anemia, Blood **9**:935, 1954.
132. Rubin, D., Weisberger, A. S., and Clark, D. R.: Early detection of drug induced erythropoietic depression, J. Lab. Clin. Med. **56**:453, 1960.
133. Rubin, E., Gottlieb, C., and Vogel, P.: Syndrome of hepatitis and aplastic anemia, Amer. J. Med. **45**:88, 1968.
134. Russell, P. S., and Winn, H. J.: Transplantation, New Eng. J. Med. **282**:844, 1970.
135. Saidi, P., Wallerstein, R. O., and Aggeler, P. M.: Effect of chloramphenicol on erythropoiesis, J. Lab. Clin. Med. **57**:247, 1961.
136. Sanchez-Medal, L., Gomez-Leal, A., Duarte, L., and Rico, M. G.: Anabolic androgenic steroids in the treatment of aplastic anemia, Blood **34**:283, 1969.
137. Sanchez-Medal, L., Pizzuto, J., Torre-Lopez, E., and Derbey, R.: Effect of oxy-metholone in refractory anemias, Arch. Intern. Med. **113**:721, 1964.
138. Schwarz, E., Baehner, R. L., and Diamond, L. K.: Aplastic anemia following hepatitis, Pediatrics **37**:681, 1966.
139. Scott, J. L., Cartwright, G. E., and Wintrobe, M. M.: Acquired aplastic anemia; an analysis of thirty-nine cases and review of the pertinent literature, Medicine **38**:119, 1959.
140. Scott, J. L., Finegold, S. M., Belkin, A., and Lawrence, J. S.: A controlled double-blind study of the hematologic toxicity of chloramphenicol, New Eng. J. Med. **272**:1137, 1965.
141. Seaman, A. J., and Koler, R. D.: Acquired erythrocytic hypoplasia; a recovery during cobalt therapy; a report of two cases and a review of the literature, Acta Haemat. **9**:153, 1953.
142. Seip, M.: Aplastic anemia treated with anabolic steroids and corticosteroids, Acta Paediat. **50**:561, 1961.
143. Shahidi, N. T.: Morphologic and biochemical characteristics of erythrocytes in testosterone-induced remission in patients with acquired and constitutional aplastic anemia, J. Lab. Clin. Med. **62**:294, 1963.
144. Shahidi, N. T.: Aplastic and congenital hypoplastic anemias. In Gellis, S. S., and Kagan, B. M., editors: Current pediatric therapy, Philadelphia, 1964, W. B. Saunders Co., p. 255.
145. Shahidi, N. T., and Diamond, L. K.: Testosterone-induced remission in aplastic anemia, Amer. J. Dis. Child. **98**:293, 1959.
146. Shahidi, N. T., and Diamond, L. K.: Testosterone-induced remission in aplastic anemia of both acquired and congenital types; further observations in 24 cases, New Eng. J. Med. **264**:953, 1961.
147. Shahidi, N. T., Gerald, P. S., and Diamond, L. K.: Alkali-resistant hemoglobin in aplastic anemia of both acquired and congenital types, New Eng. J. Med. **266**:117, 1962.
148. Shwachman, H., Diamond, L. K., Oski, F. A., and Khaw, K. O.: Pancreatic insufficiency and bone marrow dysfunction, J. Pediat. **65**:645, 1964.
149. Sjölin, S., and Wranne, L.: Erythropoietic dysfunction in a case of Fanconi's anaemia, Acta Haemat. **28**:230, 1962.
150. Smith, C. H.: The anemias of early infancy, J. Pediat. **16**:375, 1940.
151. Smith, C. H.: Chronic congenital aregenerative anemia (pure red-cell anemia) associated with iso-immunization by the blood group factor "A," Blood **4**:697, 1949.
152. Smith, C. H.: Hypoplastic and aplastic anemias of infancy and childhood; with a consideration of the syndrome of nonhemolytic anemia of the newborn, J. Pediat. **43**:457, 1953.
153. Smith, C. H., Schulman, I., and Morgenthau, J. E.: Iron metabolism in infants and children; serum iron and iron-binding protein; diagnostic and therapeutic implications. In Levine, S. Z., editor: Advances in pediatrics, Chicago, 1952, Year Book Medical Publishers, Inc., p. 195.
154. Smith, C. H., Schulman, I., Ando, R. E., and Stern, G. S.: Studies in Mediterranean (Cooley's) anemia; the suppression of hematopoiesis by transfusion, Blood **10**:707, 1955.
155. Smith, N. J., Price, J. M., Brown, R. R., and Moon, R. L.: Urinary excretion of tryptophan metabolites by patients with congenital hypoplastic anemia, Amer. J. Dis. Child. **100**:752, 1960.
156. Stohlman, F., Jr.: Observations of physiology of erythropoietin and its role in regulation of red cell production, Ann. N. Y. Acad. Sci. **77**:710, 1959.
157. Stohlman, F., Jr.: Erythropoiesis, New Eng. J. Med. **267**:342, 392, 1962.
158. Sturgeon, P.: Idiopathic aplastic anemia in children; its early differentiation from aleukemic leukemia by bone marrow aspiration, Pediatrics **8**:216, 1951.
159. Swift, M. R.: Fanconi's anemia in the genetics of neoplasia, Nature **230**:370, 1971.
160. Thomas, E. D., Phillips, J. H., and Finch, C. A.: Recovery from marrow failure following isogenic marrow infusion, J.A.M.A. **188**:1041, 1964.
161. Todd, R. McL.: The treatment of hypoplas-

tic anaemia after chloramphenicol, Arch. Dis. Child. 29:575, 1954.
162. Tsai, S. Y., and Levin, W. C.: Chronic erythrocytic hypoplasia in adults; review of the literature and report of a case, Amer. J. Med. 22:322, 1957.
163. VanRood, J. J.: Leucocyte grouping and organ transplantation, Brit. J. Haemat. 16:211, 1964.
164. VanRood, J. J.: Tissue typing and organ transplantation, Lancet 1:1142, 1969.
165. Vas, M. R., Bain, B., and Lowenstein, L.: The effect of chloramphenicol on human bone marrow cultures, Blood 20:424, 1962.
166. Vilter, R. W., Jarrold, T., Will, J. J., Mueller, J. F., Friedman, B. I., and Hawkins, V. R.: Refractory anemia with hyperplastic bone marrow, Blood 15:1, 1960.
167. Vogel, P., and Bassen, F. A.: Sternal marrow of children in normal and in pathological states, Amer. J. Dis. Child. 57:245, 1939.
168. Vogel, P., Erf, L. A., and Rosenthal, N.: Hematological observations on bone marrow obtained by sternal puncture, Amer. J. Clin. Path. 7:436, 1937.
169. Voyce, M. A.: A case of pure red-cell aplasia successfully treated with cobalt, Brit. J. Haemat. 9:412, 1963.
170. Wallerstein, R. O., Condit, P. K., Kasper, C. N., Brown, J. W., and Morrison, F. R.: Statewide study of chloramphenicol therapy and fatal aplastic anemia, J.A.M.A. 208:2045, 1969.
171. Walt, F., Taylor, J. E. D., Magill, F. B., and Nestadt, A.: Erythroid hypoplasia in kwashiorkor, Brit. Med. J. 1:73, 1962.
172. Warren, S., and Dameshek, W., chairmen: Bone marrow transplantation conference, Spec. Sect. No. 2, Blood 13:296, 1958.
173. Wintrobe, M. M.: Clinical hematology, ed. 4, Philadelphia, 1956, Lea & Febiger.
174. Wolff, J. A.: Anemias caused by infections and toxins, idiopathic aplastic anemia caused by renal disease, Ped. Clin. N. Amer. 4:469, 1957.
175. Yunis, A. A., and Harrington, W. J.: Patterns of inhibition by chloramphenicol of nucleic acid synthesis in human bone marrow and leukemic cells, J. Lab. Clin. Med. 56:831, 1960.
176. Yunis, A. A., Smith, U. S., and Restrepo, A.: Reversible bone marrow suppression from chloramphenicol; a consequence of mitochondrial injury, Arch. Intern. Med. 126:272, 1970.
177. Zeltmacher, K., and Bevans, M.: Aplastic anemia and its association with hemochromatosis, Arch. Intern. Med. 75:395, 1945.
178. Zulik, R., and Bako, F.: Aplastic anemia and infectious hepatitis, Lancet 1:44, 1971.

# 15 THE HEMOLYTIC ANEMIAS

*Definition—general considerations of pathogenesis.* A hemolytic anemia may be defined as one due to excessive blood destruction. A large number of blood disorders of varied etiology and clinical and hematologic course are included in the group of hemolytic anemias which have in common the central feature of a red cell with a reduced life-span.

As has been pointed out, the presence or absence of anemia is dependent upon the ability of the bone marrow to respond to varying degrees of blood destruction. Abnormal degrees of hemolysis, therefore, need not result in anemia if the bone marrow is capable of regenerating adequate amounts of hemoglobin and red blood cells.[71] Bone marrow capacity has been estimated at six to eight times the normal so that when the average red cell survival is reduced to 15 to 20 days instead of the normal 120 days, the limit of compensation has reached its possible maximum. This situation represents a completely compensated hemolytic disease without apparent evidence of anemia. However, if the rate of destruction exceeds the ability of the body to increase the rate of red cell production, anemia will result. This is termed decompensated hemolytic disease. A new equilibrium is eventually reestablished when these forces are equalized at lower hemoglobin levels. The particular concentration of hemoglobin obtained is, therefore, determined both by the extent of the hemolytic defect present and by the particular capacity of the bone marrow to respond with an increase in the production of erythrocytes.

*Classification.* Hemolytic anemias may be classified as congenital (hereditary) and acquired—the former related to an intracorpuscular (intrinsic) abnormality and the latter related to an extracorpuscular (extrinsic) mechanism and due to the action of the external agents on structurally normal red cells. A combination of factors may be present in the same patient as in patients with Cooley's anemia in whom the abnormal cells have a shortened life-span within the circulation and transfused normal donor cells are destroyed by an extracorpuscular mechanism residing in the spleen (hypersplenism).

*Intracorpuscular or intrinsic abnormality*
1. Hereditary (congenital) hemolytic anemia
   a. Hereditary spherocytosis
   b. Thalassemia
   c. Sickle cell disease
   d. Hereditary hemoglobinopathies, including combinations of thalassemia and sickle cell disease
   e. Hereditary nonspherocytic hemolytic anemia
      (1) Enzymopathy
      (2) Unstable hemoglobin hemolytic anemia
   f. Hereditary elliptocytosis with hemolytic anemia
   g. Hemolytic anemia due to enzyme deficiency apparent after administration of drugs and other agents; primaquine naphthalene, fava bean (favism), etc.
   h. Hereditary stomatocytosis with hemolytic anemia
   i. Membrane lipid abnormalities with increased lecithin
2. Nonhereditary hemolytic anemia
   a. Paroxysmal nocturnal hemoglobinuria

*Extracorpuscular or extrinsic mechanism*
1. Acquired hemolytic anemia
   a. Due to antibodies
      (1) Autoimmune antibodies
         (a) Idiopathic acquired hemolytic anemias
      (2) Isoagglutinins
         (a) Erythroblastosis, mismatched transfusion (blood or plasma)
   b. Symptomatic hemolytic anemias
      (1) With Hodgkin's disease, lymphosarcoma, renal disease, lupus erythematosus, thrombotic thrombocytopenic purpura, etc.
   c. Paroxysmal cold hemoglobinuria
   d. Acute acquired hemolytic anemia (Lederer's anemia)

e. March hemoglobinuria
f. Miscellaneous causes
   (1) Infections
   (2) Chemical and physical agents
   (3) Vegetable substances
   (4) Drug sensitivity
   (5) Severe burns
   (6) Pyknocytosis; rarely acanthocytosis

It is reasonable to assume then that in any patient in whom the rate of destruction of erythrocytes is less than six to eight times the normal, no anemia need occur because of the inherent compensatory capacity of the bone marrow. An exception to this principle was noted in a series of pediatric patients with minimal clinical manifestations of hereditary spherocytosis in whom anemia was present in terms of a reduced total volume of red cells (red cell mass), despite a normal concentration of hemoglobin in the peripheral blood.[117] The capacity of the bone marrow was inadequate to compensate for rates of erythrocyte destruction of a magnitude less than six times the normal. The normal peripheral hemoglobin is explained by the contracted plasma component of the circulating blood. The studies of Crosby and Akeroyd,[72] therefore, need elaboration to determine the full range of the bone marrow's capacity under the stress of varying degrees of blood destruction.

**Principal features of increased hemolysis.** The varied clinical and hematologic manifestations of a hemolytic process stem from the release of products from red cell destruction and their disposal and the compensatory activity of the bone marrow. Many of these changes are observed in the urine, stool, and blood and are subject to quantitative measurement. The evidences of increased red cell destruction to be enumerated include anemia, structural abnormalities of the red cells, and increased pigment output.

*Hemoglobinemia and hemoglobinuria.* The concentration of hemoglobin normally found in the plasma is less than 5 mg. per 100 ml. and results from red cell destruction taking place within the cells of the reticuloendothelial tissues (amount usually less than 0.5 mg.). In the event of severe intravascular hemolysis, the concentration of plasma hemoglobin usually exceeds the renal threshold of 100 to 150 mg. per 100 ml. and the pigment appears in the urine.[69,73] Hemoglobinuria occurs with marked hemoglobinemia, when the rate of destruction is exceedingly rapid and severe, indicating that hemolysis is taking place in the circulating blood. Depending upon the amounts of pigment present, the urine is pink, red, brown, or almost black. Hemoglobinuria can be detected by benzidine and guaiac reactions. In patients with marked hemoglobinemia the plasma is red or brown. The absence of hemoglobinemia in patients with hemolytic disease indicates that extravascular hemolysis is principally involved. Hemoglobinemia is absent in patients with hereditary spherocytosis and hereditary nonspherocytic hemolytic anemia[69]; mild hemoglobinemia is present in those with sickle cell anemia and Cooley's anemia. Severe grades of hemoglobinemia occur in patients with acute acquired hemolytic anemia such as Lederer's anemia.

In patients with marked hemoglobinemia, iron-containing brownish granules of hemosiderin appear in the urine. Treating the urine with acidified potassium ferrocyanide reveals the presence of the Prussian blue hemosiderin.[69] The extent of hemosiderin excretion varies with the concentration of plasma hemoglobin. Hemosiderinuria is a characteristic finding in patients with nocturnal paroxysmal hemoglobinuria in whom hemoglobinemia is usually present.

*Haptoglobin in relation to hemoglobinemia.* When intravascular hemolysis occurs, the free hemoglobin in the plasma combines with a specific serum protein haptoglobin (Hp), comparable to the union of copper with ceruloplasmin and of iron with siderophilin or transferrin. Haptoglobin is an alpha$_2$ mucoprotein, 1 molecule of which is capable of binding 2 molecules of hemoglobin.[201] In adults the haptoglobins are present in amounts sufficient to bind up to 150 mg. of hemoglobin per 100 ml. of serum.[36] The haptoglobin-hemoglobin complex is removed from the plasma by the reticuloendothelial system where the hemoglobin is degraded into bilirubin.[246]

The large molecular weight of the hepatoglobin-hemoglobin complex (310,000) prevents its passage into the urine. Hemoglobinuria does not occur unless the amount of hemoglobin liberated intravascularly exceeds the binding power of the haptoglobin and the reabsorption capacity of the tubules. Unbound free hemoglobin is also oxidized into methemoglobin and methemalbumin, which are also eliminated into the urine. It has been demonstrated by starch gel electrophoresis that normal serum contains as many as twelve different haptoglobins.[60] These are genetically controlled,[332-334] and one or more may be present in the serum of a single person. The six more common haptoglobin variants are thought to result from the expression of three haptoglobins designated 1-1 and 2-2, both homozygotes, and 1-2, the heterozygote.[335] The pair of autosomal alleles expressed as Hp[1] and Hp[2] are responsible for the homozygotes Hp[1]/Hp[1], showing a single haptoglobin component and Hp[2]/Hp[2], with many components. The heterozygote Hp[1]/Hp[2] also shows several haptoglobin components. Hp[2m] is a modified Hp[2].[137] Congenital absence of haptoglobin, presumably on a genetic basis, apparently is not associated with unfavorable consequences,[225] and Hp[o] is designated as the responsible gene.

The concentration of haptoglobin is increased in patients with infections and malignancy and in those being given steroid therapy, and it is decreased or even absent in patients with increased hemolysis.[36,200] Liver disease may itself be associated with a diminished formation of haptoglobin, irrespective of rates of hemolysis. A reduced haptoglobin and, therefore, decreased hemoglobin binding may account for increased methemalbumin formation[200] and, in certain cases, for increased hemoglobinuria.

The three common variants of human haptoglobin (Hp) can be distinguished by starch gel electrophoresis (Fig. 26). All common Hp types have a strong affinity for hemoglobin.[175]

Haptoglobins cannot be demonstrated in cord blood or in the early neonatal period. They appear initially at the end of the first or second week of life.[4,17,328,354] In another study no evidence was found that this was due to their removal secondary to accelerated erythrocyte destruction during this period.[288]

Tuttle[355] has shown that hematin, which sometimes appears in normal cord blood, is bound to albumin as methemalbumin. Methemalbumin may appear as a constituent of cord serum in the normal newborn infant, although the concentration of this heme compound is extremely low and disappears from the circulation within the first day of life.

Contrary to other studies, the low haptoglobins in cord plasmas were interpreted not as a failure of production, but rather as the exhaustion of haptoglobin by the increased quantities of hemo-

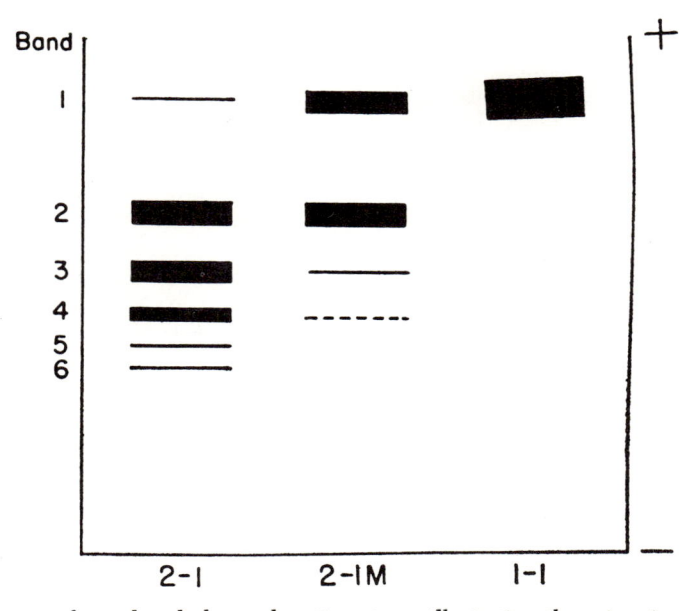

**Fig. 26.** Diagram of starch gel electrophoretic pattern illustrating the migration of the haptoglobin phenotypes Hp 2-1, Hp 2-1M, and Hp 1-1. (From Parker, W. C., and Bearn, A. G.: Control gene mutation as a possible explanation of certain haptoglobin phenotypes, Amer. J. Human Genet. 15:159, 1963. By permission of Grune & Stratton, Inc.)

globin released into the plasma during intravascular destruction of senescent erythrocytes.[5]

In still another study[305] the plasma of newborn infants who did not subsequently become icteric had a greater tendency to contain haptoglobins than those who did become icteric.

The term hypohaptoglobinemia rather than ahaptoglobinemia has been suggested for individuals with depressed levels of circulating haptoglobin. In one family an inherited deficiency of glucose-6-phosphate dehydrogenase and serum haptoglobin (hypohaptoglobinemia) were associated.[141] The concentration of serum of children suspected of ahaptoglobinemia will reveal exceptionally low but detectable quantities of haptoglobin.[373]

*Hemopexin.* Hemopexin, a $B_1$ globulin from human serum, forms with heme a red-colored complex which consists of one mole of hemopexin to one of heme.[159] Heme has a greater affinity for hemopexin than for albumin. Hemopexin serves as a major transport protein of heme. In states of excessive hemolysis part of the hemoglobin dissociates into its components of heme and globin. The heme complexes with both albumin (as methemalbumin) and with hemopexin, while globin as well as hemoglobin is bound by haptoglobin. Comparable to the behavior of haptoglobin, plasma hemopexin concentrations are reduced during hemolytic episodes.

The mean hemopexin level in adults is 77 mg./100 ml., with a range of 60 to 100 mg./100 ml. and the mean in the newborn is 18 mg. with a range of 6.5 to 25 mg./100 ml.[152] In hemolytic anemias the high plasma concentrations of heme are associated with low levels of hemopexin. Sears[317] found that the hemopexin level was not markedly depressed until the haptoglobin pool of plasma is depleted. Müller-Eberhard and co-workers[243] similarly encountered no instance in which the hemopexin concentration was diminished without a simultaneous reduction of haptoglobin level although the converse was frequently observed. Lundh and colleagues,[213] in a study of newborn premature and full-term infants, concluded that, due to the overlap in hemopexin concentration between children with and without grossly evident hemolysis, hemopexin determinations were of little value in appraising the degree of hemolysis in the newborn. These data confirmed previous observations that haptoglobin is absent or present in only small amounts in newborn infants, that haptoglobin acts as the first line of defense in hemolysis, and that hemopexin is affected only when the haptoglobin reaches the zero level and the plasma concentration of hemoglobin and of heme rises.

The correlation of measurements of hemopexin-to-albumin ratio in amniotic fluid with the severity of hemolytic disease in the fetus will be found in Chapter 7.

*Methemalbumin and methemalbuminemia.* Methemalbumin is formed in the plasma by the union of hematin with albumin when excessive amounts of hemoglobin are released in the course of severe red cell destruction.[126] Like haptoglobin, it serves as a means of transporting and neutralizing products of hemolysis, in this case hematin, in the bloodstream. When hemoglobinemia is intense, the spectroscopic picture of methemalbumin is distinct. In lesser amounts it can also be differentiated from methemoglobin and allied compounds by the effect of chemical reagents on their "a" bands. The large-sized molecule prevents its passage through the kidney and its presence in the urine.

Methemalbumin is now recognized as a reliable index of intravascular hemolysis of any etiology. It is of value, for instance, in detecting cases of suspected hemolytic transfusion reactions. Schumm's test is commonly employed to determine the presence of methemalbumin.[100] The serum or plasma is covered with a layer of ether. A one-tenth volume of saturated yellow ammonium sulphide is added. This results in the formation of a hemochromagen with an intense, narrow absorption band at 558 m$\mu$ that can be detected with a hand spectroscope.

In an 11-day-old infant with intracranial arteriovenous fistula causing heart failure and bilateral subdural hematomas, cyanosis was associated with methemalbuminemia.[253] Persistent hemorrhage from anastomosis between the carotid and jugular systems caused the formation of subdural hematomas. The rate of absorption exceeded the rate of removal of methemalbumin from the plasma, causing concentrations high enough to produce cyanosis. Drainage of the subdural spaces resulted in disappearance of methemalbuminemia and cyanosis.

*Hyperbilirubinemia and jaundice.* The extent of bilirubinemia depends upon the degree of hemolysis and the capacity of the liver to remove the pigment from the plasma and excrete it in the bile. In the infant in the first week of life the excretion of bile is retarded by the inability of the immature liver to conjugate indirect bilirubin because of enzyme deficiency. In the older patient the functional capacity of the liver may be impaired by the coexisting anemia. Usually, the liver is able to excrete increased amounts of bilirubin so that the degree of hyperbilirubinemia may not reflect the amount of blood destruction. In patients with hemolytic anemia the plasma bilirubin ranges from 1 to 3 mg. per 100 ml. and is occasionally normal so that the absence of jaundice does not necessarily eliminate a diagnosis of hemolytic anemia.

*Urobilinogen excretion.* The liver is able to excrete large amounts of bilirubin unless its function is impaired by severe anemia and anoxemia associated with the hemolytic process. Only small quantities of urobilinogen are excreted by the kidneys. Increased blood destruction is associated with excessive urobilinogen excretion in the feces and frequently in the urine. With the limitations already cited, elevated fecal urobilinogen may be considered as evidence of hemolytic disease, but the amount present in the urine is not a reliable measure of this process.

*Spherocytosis.* In addition to spherocytes which characterize the blood picture of hereditary spherocytosis, acquired types appear in hemolytic disease which are morphologically identical with the former. The presence of spherocytes may either indicate the production of intrinsically defective erythrocytes or reflect damage to normal cells by extrinsic factors. Spherocytes appear in patients with A-B-O erythroblastosis fetalis, hemolytic anemias due to drug sensitivity, and idiopathic acquired hemolytic anemia. In the latter, spherocytes are sometimes more numerous than in patients with hereditary spherocytosis. The acquired type of spherocyte represents a normal red cell whose surface has been damaged, causing irreversible contraction with an increase in osmotic and mechanical fragility. Spherocytes occur in so many hemolytic anemias of varied etiology that they are not diagnostic of any single one of them.

*Schistocytes.* Red cell fragments as well as shrunken and distorted red cells seldom seen in normal blood are present in appreciable numbers in patients with hemolytic disease. Red cell fragmentation has been described following severe burns[150] and exposure to chemicals.

Weed and Reed[370] described the formation of a tongue-like protrusion of the red cell in its passage through the capillary bed in general and the spleen in particular, and its ultimate sequestration from the red cell, producing irregularly shaped fragments of the red cell known as schistocytes. In a later paper Weed and his co-authors[369] suggested that a major role of adenosine triphosphate (ATP) in maintenance of red cell viability is related to preservation of red cell membrane deformability. They proposed that the changes seen in the physical properties of ATP-depleted erythrocytes represent ATP-calcium-dependent sol-gel changes occurring at the interface between the membrane and the cell interior, and that the sol-gel balance determines membrane deformability.

*Erythrophagocytosis.* Erythrocytes ingested by polymorphonuclear neutrophils and monocytes are rarely found in normal blood smears, but appear in those of patients with hemolytic anemias such as erythroblastosis, acquired hemolytic anemia, leukemia, chemical poisoning, and anemias associated with infections.

*Heinz bodies.* Heinz bodies are found in red cells damaged by toxic substances, giving the appearance of intracorpuscular particles and larger, rounder bodies. They represent oxidatively injured and denatured hemoglobin. A variety of drugs, such as phenylhydrazine, potassium chloride, naphthalene, primaquine, and related compounds, have been implicated in their formation. They are best observed in wet, unstained preparations, by supravital staining with methyl violet, or with the brilliant cresyl blue technique for reticulocyte staining.

*Folic acid deficiency.* The occurrence of megaloblastic anemia and folic acid deficiency in association with chronic hemolytic anemia has been the subject of an increasing number of reports. There is as yet no adequate explanation for the development of folic acid dependence in this type of anemia. Increased requirements consequent to accelerated erythropoiesis are the usual explanation. Serum folic acid determinations in twenty-four randomly selected patients with chronic hemolytic anemia (mainly sickle cell disease and hereditary spherocytosis) in the absence of any apparent aplastic crisis, infection, or diarrhea revealed that 54% of the patients showed some degree of folic acid deficiency.[323] The laboratory evidence of the deficiency, as shown by low serum folate levels in association with elevated urinary FIGLU (formiminoglutamic acid) excretion following histidine loading, was accompanied by hypersegmented neutrophils. (In the absence of folic acid, formiminoglutamic acid, an intermediate product of histidine metabolism, is not further metabolized to glutamic acid but appears in increased amounts in the urine, especially after an oral dose of histidine.) The existence of normoblastic bone marrows is explained by the fact that megaloblastic changes are late manifestations. Megaloblastic anemia, occurring in acquired hemolytic anemia, paroxysmal nocturnal hemoglobinuria, and the hereditary hemolytic anemias referred to in Chapter 13, is an extremely infrequent phenomenon.

Possibly the development of conditions with increased folic acid requirements such as pregnancy, infection, and diarrhea may precipitate unequivocal megaloblastic anemia. It is of interest that it is the unusual case of hemolytic anemia demonstrating a folic acid deficiency that shows a significant hematologic response with therapy. Following treatment with therapeutic doses of folic acid, FIGLU excretion may be converted to normal and serum folic acid increased, but the anemia is unresponsive.[270] Hypersegmented polynuclears may disappear and reticulocytes increase, but a rise in hemoglobin, or in the case of thalassemia a decrease in transfusion requirements, is infrequent. An aplastic crisis in association with folic acid deficiency has been reported in sickle cell anemia[276] and in hereditary spherocytosis.[49]

*Evidence of increased marrow activity.* In achieving equilibrium, red cell destruction is accompanied by graded increases of red cell production. The latter is marked by a compensatory hyperplasia of the bone marrow, resulting in proliferation of all types of nucleated red cells, ranging from the early proerythroblasts to the most mature normoblast. Also included in the blood picture of hemolysis are reticulocytosis, normoblastemia, macrocytosis, polychromatophilia, polymorphonuclear leukocytosis, and increased numbers of platelets.

*Reticulocytosis.* The appearance of nucleated red cells and reticulocytes in the blood smear indicates the premature delivery of red cells into the circulation. Reticulocytes usually range between 0.5 and 2% in the period beyond early infancy. They are increased in patients with hemolytic anemia and hereditary spherocytosis, and in those with acquired hemolytic anemia they may number approximately 20 to 50%. An increase of reticulocytes does not always serve as an accurate index of red cell production since bone marrow hyperplasia may be associated with only slight increases in reticulocytes, as frequently seen in patients with sickle cell anemia and severe Cooley's anemia. Reticulocytopenia has been noted during hemolytic (not aplastic) crisis in patients with acute immune hemolytic anemia. This is explained by the suppressive action of the autoimmune mechanism on the proliferating erythroid cells.[74] In the aplastic crisis reticulocytes disappear from the peripheral blood and nucleated cells from the bone marrow. Thrombocytopenia and leukopenia are accompanying features. The aplastic crisis is observed more frequently than the better known hemolytic crisis and is particularly common in patients with hereditary spherocytosis, sickle cell anemia, and Cooley's anemia.

A study of erythropoiesis during periods of phlebotomy-induced anemia of varying severity revealed that the percentage of reticulocytes varied not only in number but in their maturity.[162] As the hematocrit was lowered, large numbers of reticulocytes appeared and their relative reticulum content progressively increased. At the same time large numbers of polychromatophilic macroreticulocytes appeared in the circulation. Reticulocyte maturation was progressively prolonged as the severity of the anemia increased. Thus when the hematocrit was reduced to approximately 35% the maturation time of the circulating reticulocyte increased from 1.0 to between 1.5 and 1.7 days and with a hematocrit below 20% the maturation time rose to between 2.3 and 2.5 days. The prolonged survival of these "stress" or "shift" reticulocytes implies a need for correcting reticulocyte counts with variation in severity of an anemia.

*Normoblastemia.* The more anemic the patient and the higher the reticulocyte count, the more likely are normoblasts to appear in the peripheral blood. They are particularly noticeable in patients with erythroblastosis fetalis and severe autoimmune hemolytic anemia and after splenectomy in those with Cooley's anemia.

*Siderocytes.* Siderocytes are erythrocytes containing one or more granules of ferric iron which give a positive Prussian blue reaction for iron. They are increased in the peripheral blood of patients after splenectomy[70,196] as well as in patients with certain types of hemolytic anemia. These include erythroblastosis fetalis, hereditary spherocytosis, and autoimmune hemolytic anemia. Siderocytes appearing in the peripheral blood in patients with hemochromatosis reflect excessive red cell storage of iron.[128]

*Sideroblasts.* Sideroblasts are the precursors of siderocytes in the peripheral blood. Siderotic granules appear in the normoblasts of patients with normal bone marrow. They are diminished in patients with iron-deficiency states[184] and are exceptionally abundant in those with hemolytic disorders, severe Cooley's anemia, megaloblastic anemia, and lead poisoning.

*Macrocytosis.* An increased number of reticulocytes in the peripheral blood and macronormoblasts in the bone marrow account for a macrocytic blood picture in patients with hemolytic disease.

*Increased erythrocyte protoporphyrin and coproporphyrin.* The heme portion of hemoglobin is a ferrous protoporphyrin for whose synthesis porphyrin precursors and iron are required. The porphyrins are pigments whose structural unit consists of four pyrrole rings linked by four methene bridges. They differ depending upon the nature of the side chains attached to the eight free corners of the four pyrrole nuclei. Thus hemoglobin, myohemoglobin, cytochrome, and catalase represent porphyrin-protein compounds. Most porphyrins exist in the form of metal complexes (metalloporphyrin)—e.g., hemoglobin and chlorophyll, in which porphyrins are combined with iron and magnesium, respectively. Coproporphyrin, uroporphyrin, and protoporphyrin are the most common prophyrins occurring naturally. Two different isomer types (type I and type III) have been observed for uroporphyrin and coproporphyrin.

**The porphyrias.** Porphyrias refer to disorders of porphyrin metabolism associated with the increased formation and excretion of porphyrins. The term porphyrinuria applies to the excretion of porphyrins in excessive amounts in the urine and is not necessarily associated with the clinical syndromes of porphyria. Porphyrinuria occurs in a number of conditions such as liver disease, hemolytic anemia, and lead poisoning (see Chapter 17). The increased excretion of porphyrin may result from disordered synthesis of heme compounds other than hemoglobin.

The porphyrias are rare metabolic disorders in which abnormal amounts and kinds of porphyrins are excreted in the urine and feces.[219]

The two general groups of porphyrias are the erythropoietic and the hepatic types. In the former the central feature is the excessive production of porphyrins by the erythroid cells of the bone marrow. In the latter there is an excessive production of porphyrins and porphyrin precursors which takes place in the liver. Precise clarification of the porphyrias is still confused and awaits further documentation.

Specifically, porphyria is the designation applied to pathologic states produced by inherited errors of porphyrin metabolism in which the intermediates of porphyrin biosynthesis such as uroporphyrin, coproporphyrin, and porphobilinogen accumulate in the body and are excreted in excess in the urine.

Although coproporphyrin I and III might be found in many acquired disorders as well as in porphyria, increased excretion of uroporphyrin and porphobilinogen occurs, for all practical purposes, exclusively in the porphyrias.

The disease states resulting from disorders of porphyrin metabolism may be classified as follows (modified from Taddeini and Watson[348]):

1. Disorders of porphyrin synthesis in which excessive quantities of porphyrins are synthesized in the bone marrow
   a. Erythropoietic porphyria (erythropoietic uroporphyria)
   b. Erythropoietic protoporphyria
2. Disorders of porphyrin synthesis in the liver (excessive production of porphyrins and porphyrin precursors taking place in the liver)
   a. Porphyria hepatica
      (1) Intermittent acute
      (2) Cutanea tarda
      (3) Mixed types
3. Acquired toxic porphyria

Waldenström's classification[366] is as follows: congenital porphyria, porphyria cutanea tarda symptomatica, porphyria hereditaria (protocoproporphyria), and acute intermittent porphyria. Human erythrocytes contain free coproporphyrin (up to 2 $\mu$g per 100 ml. of red blood cells) as well as free protoporphyrin (normal, 15 to 60 $\mu$g per 100 ml. of red blood cells). In patients with iron-deficiency anemia and lead poisoning marked increases of protoporphyrin occur. Moderate increases are found in patients with hemolytic anemias and aregenerative anemias. In persons with hemolytic anemias there is a relatively greater increase in the erythrocyte coproporphyrins than in protoporphyrins.

Schmid[309] regards "the biosynthesis of heme as delicately synchronized, and regulated by a series of control mechanisms which prevent both the overproduction of the end product and significant accumulation of intermediates." Porphyria is regarded as a breakdown in these biologic control mechanisms resulting in the accumulation and excretion of metabolic intermediates (delta-aminolevulinic acid, porphobilinogen, porphyrinogens) or their oxidation products (porphyrins).

*Erythropoietic porphyrias (erythropoietic uroporphyrias).* Congenital porphyria[3,113] is a very rare metabolic disorder which is present at birth and is inherited as a mendelian recessive character.[56] In one series describing five cases in three generations of a family, a dominant type of inheritance was suggested.[146] The marked increase in the protoporphyrin and coproporphyrin in the red cells and the excessive amounts of porphyrins produced by the nuclei of the marrow normoblasts[216,310] led to the designation of this condition as erythropoietic protoporphyria.[310] Fluorescent microscopy of the bone marrow reveals intense red fluorescence of the normoblasts located chiefly in the nuclei. It is postulated that the nuclei of these cells form excessive amounts of porphyrin and release it into the plasma.[310] The basis for the disease is a constitutional disturbance in the biosynthesis of the heme of hemoglobin in the red cell precursors so that uroporphyrin, coproporphyrin, and porphobilinogen accumulate in the body.

The clinical features of congenital porphyria appear in infancy and childhood. It is characterized by sensitivity of the skin to sunlight, resulting in vesicles and bullae (hydroa aestivale), hirsutism, red urine, red or purplish brown staining of the teeth, an enlarged spleen, and a hemolytic anemia. Scarring occurs on the crusts of the vesiculobullous lesions and in other exposed areas.

The biochemical defect is ascribed to the inability to form uroporphyrin III from porphobilinogen with resultant accumulation of uroporphyrin I.[309] Uroporphyrin and coproporphyrin are the predominant porphyrins excreted. The continuous deposition of uroporphyrin in tissues, dentine, and the skeleton accounts for the hypersensitivity and pigmentation of bones and teeth. Its early appearance in infancy may be suspected by the child's diapers colored red by the urine. The color in fact ranges from pink to Burgundy red, and is attributable to the excretion of uroporphyrin I and coproporphyrin I.

*Erythropoietic protoporphyria.* This disorder was initially described by Magnus and his co-workers[216] who separated it from the classic erythropoietic porphyria. Erythropoietic protoporphyria is an inherited inborn error of porphyrin metabolism characterized clinically by excessive amounts of protoporphyrins and, at times, coproporphyrins in the erythrocytes and stool. The diagnosis of this disorder is confirmed by detecting excessive erythrocyte and fecal protoporphyrin levels.[292] Porphyrinuria does not occur. In the bone marrow fluroescent normoblasts containing excessive amounts of protoporphyrin and to a lesser extent coproporphyrin are observed.[56] Following exposure to sunlight burning, itching or prickling sensations develop and are followed by edema and erythema.

Magnus and associates[216] described a patient with light-sensitive urticaria whose urinary excretion of uroporphyrin, porphobilinogen, and delta-aminolevulinic acid were normal but the fecal protoporphyrin and coproporphyrin levels were elevated. The large variety of cutaneous lesions in this disease has led to the designation of polymorphic photodermatitis as an inconclusive designation for the abnormal responses to solar radiation.[76] In an 8-year-old girl with erythropoietic porphyria the free erythrocyte protoporphyrin ranged from 333 to 1,780 $\mu$g per 100 ml. of packed red cells.[153] In the same patient in vitro studies revealed a markedly abnormal photohemolysis within a period of 10 minutes, as compared with 10 to 12 hours in normal human red cells.

Congenital erythropoietic protoporphyria has been reported in two brothers, with attention drawn to the disease in one by the combination of photosensitivity, hemolytic anemia, and splenomegaly. The source of the large amount of porphyrin found in the liver was ascribed to excessive amounts of erythrocyte protoporphyrin.[280] The parents and close relatives in two cases were diagnosed as heterozygotes because of the increased uroporphyrin of their red cells.[160]

Reed and associates[292] conducted a genetic and clinical study of nine families, in which sixteen individuals were clinically affected and forty-three were carriers. A predominance of males in this study and in other studies was noted. Carriers were detected by increased fluorescing erythrocytes because fecal and erythrocyte protoporphyrin levels are often normal. The disorder is transmitted as an autosomal dominant with many carriers and few clinically involved individuals. In patients with lead poisoning there is no photosensitivity despite increased fluorescytes and blood protoporphyrin levels.

*Hepatic porphyria.* This disease is characterized by an excessive or abnormal formation of heme precursors in the liver. The acute intermittent type of hepatic porphyria occurs in young adults up to about 40 years of age. It is associated with periodic acute abdominal pain, severe colic, constipation, and vomiting, together with neurologic and emotional changes. Red urine may be voided during attacks.

While congenital erythropoietic porphyria, the metabolic defect, can be said to develop in red cells, in the hepatic type no such defect is found. Rather in the latter, the liver is the only organ containing large amounts of porphyrins and porphyrin precursors. Hepatic function is frequently impaired.[154]

Early during an attack the urine may be quite normal in color although porphobilinogen, which is itself colorless, may be present in high concentration. The characteristic finding in hepatic porphyria is the excretion in the urine of excessive amounts of the porphyrin precursors, delta-aminolevulinic acid and porphobilinogen. Several types of this entity have been described[56]: acute intermittent porphyria (Swedish type), porphyria variegata (South African type), porphyria cutanea tarda, and hereditary cutaneous porphyria.

In all types of porphyrias the excessive excretion of the porphyrins in the urine (and feces) permits recognition of the disease through urinalysis. In congenital porphyria, free uroporphyrin I constitutes the major product of the metabolic error and is therefore the abnormal pigment found in excess in blood and urine. The red color imparted to the urine by this product must be differentiated from that caused by other factors such as blood, hemoglobin, and myoglobin. Porphobilinogen is not found in the urine in congenital porphyria but does occur in hepatic porphyria. In the latter, the urine darkens on standing, turning to a Burgundy wine color due to the conversion of abnormal amounts of porphyrinogens and other heme precursors into porphyrins, porphobilins, and other unidentified pigments.

Treatment of the congenital photosensitive group (porphyrin erythropoietica) consists of shielding the patient against sunlight. Splenectomy, which is indicated with evidences of increased blood destruction, and splenomegaly often reduces the concentration of uroporphyrin and coproporphyrin in red cells, plasma, urine, and feces. The plasma porphyrins prior to splenectomy are probably derived from the destruction of circulating red cells containing these substances. Photosensitivity may be reduced or unaltered after splenectomy. Varadi[363] reported the case of a 6-month-old infant in whom splenectomy was followed by cure of the associated hemolytic anemia and thrombocytopenia. By diminishing the hyperactivity of the bone marrow the rate of porphyrin production was reduced and probably also the degree of photosensitivity. Treatment for other types of porphyria consists of symptomatic treatment. In the choice of drugs to relieve pain, barbiturates should be avoided since they may precipitate or aggravate attacks.

More specific therapy would aim at decreasing excessive production of porphyrins. The effect of purines and of corticosteroids has been of questionable value.[148] Polycythemia and anemia were induced in a patient with congenital erythropoietic porphyria as a possible means of altering erythropoiesis and its associated porphyrin production.[147] Throughout this study there was a constant relationship between porphyrin production and the utilization of iron by the marrow. Approximately 65% of the total porphyrin production at baseline was required for hemoglobin synthesis and 35% was excreted in excess. Maintenance of hematocrits at 50% and 60% for periods of 2 weeks decreased both erythropoiesis and porphyrin excretion to about half of their initial values. Conversely, with a hematocrit of 25% erythropoiesis and porphyrin production were increased to about twice the basal value. Examination of the marrow showed fluorescence in all late normoblasts.

During induced polycythemia, a shift in marrow erythroid population related to delayed enucleation was accompanied by retention of the reticulocyte pool and fluorescent cells within the marrow. During anemia, on the other hand, relatively more immature erythroid cells occurred and these were accompanied by a shift of the reticulocyte pool and fluorescent cells into the circulating blood.

Patients with erythropoietic protoporphyria with elevated levels of porphyrin in blood and stool and with severe photosensitivity on exposure of skin to both sunlight and artificial light were treated with an oral preparation of beta-carotene.[220] When the patients were carotenemic they reacted less intensely to artificial light. Beta-carotene appeared to counteract photosensitization in the skin of these patients. One of the patients was a 10-year-old girl. The itching, burning, and edema of the skin after brief exposure to the sun previously experienced were prevented by the oral administration of approximately 100,000 USP vitamin A units of beta-carotene per day.

*Additional tests for detecting abnormal hemolysis.* The vulnerability of the red cells to hemolysis may be determined by a few well-defined tests.

*Osmotic fragility test.* The resistance of the red corpuscles to varying dilutions of hypotonic sodium chloride solution constitutes an important laboratory procedure in the diagnosis of the anemias and is especially useful in the differentiation of the hemolytic group. The response of blood cells in the fragility test does not necessarily reflect their reaction within the circulating blood where conditions of isotonicity prevail. It constitutes, however, a useful gross index of the relative thickness of the major number of red cells in the sample of blood to be tested. If the red cell envelope is small in relation to its volume, as in the thick red cells of patients with hereditary spherocytosis, the resistance is decreased. Increased resistance to hemolysis is noted when the bulk of red blood cells possess relatively large surfaces in comparison with their substance, as occurs in the thin red cells of patients with thalassemia major and iron-deficiency anemia.

Increased fragility of the red cells in hypotonic solutions of sodium chloride, as compared with the fragility of normal blood occurs not only in persons with hereditary spherocytosis but occasionally in those with acute hemolytic anemia associated with infection and ingestion of drugs. Decreased fragility with complete hemolysis in solutions below 0.3% sodium chloride characterizes the blood of patients with sickle cell anemia, mild and severe forms of thalassemia, and iron deficiency.

METHODS. Osmotic resistance may be measured by placing small samples of blood in solutions of progressively diminishing concentrations of sodium chloride. After the solutions have been allowed to stand for a prescribed time, the points of minimal and maximal hemolysis are noted. Hemolysis normally begins in 0.42% solution and is complete in 0.33 to 0.30%.

An alternative and more precise method is the photoelectric determination of the degree of hemolysis in which the differences in the degree of hemolysis occurring in successive dilutions of hypotonic salt solution are plotted.[343]

The red cells in these solutions absorb water and grow progressively larger and more rounded until their membrane is stretched to the point of rupture when hemoglobin is liberated. Red cells already rounded, as those in patients with autoimmune acquired hemolytic anemia and hereditary spherocytosis, begin to hemolyze at more concentrated levels than normal. A thinner than normal red cell absorbs more water before rupture of the red cell membrane occurs.

It has been suggested that buffered sodium chloride solutions be employed in the determination of osmotic fragility.[48] A stock solution of buffered sodium chloride, osmotically equivalent to 10% sodium chloride, is prepared as follows: sodium chloride (NaCl), 180 gm.; dibasic sodium phosphate, 27.31 gm.; and monobasic sodium phosphate, 4.86 gm.; distilled water to make 2 liters. A 1% working solution is made from the 10% stock solution. The pH of this solution should be 7.4.

OSMOTIC FRAGILITY AFTER INCUBATION. The more rapid increase in the osmotic fragility of red cells after incubation for 24 hours at 37° C. is useful in detecting the asymptomatic subject with hereditary spherocytosis whose unincubated red cells show a normal fragility at room temperature. This method is especially applicable to the parent of a child with overt evidence of hereditary spherocyotsis in whom a hereditary pattern could not otherwise be elicited.[319]

*Screening fragility test using fingertip blood.* A screening test that has been shown to offer information of a decisive diagnostic character[350] employs blood from the finger and three dilutions of hypotonic solution of sodium chloride—0.37%, 0.35%, and 0.325%. The method as outlined here is not meant to replace the quantitative osmotic fragility test using venous blood,[47] which is more sensitive, but the use of finger blood provides a simple screening method. Since the blood from the finger is used, controls are readily available, and in normal persons the degree of hemolysis in the three tubes is as follows: with 0.375% solution of sodium chloride, 3+; with 0.35%, 3+ or 4+; and with 0.325%, 4+.

Two or three drops of blood from the finger, depending upon the severity of the anemia, are obtained by deep puncture and added to the three tubes, each containing 2 ml. of solution of the prescribed concentration of sodium chloride. After thorough mixing of the blood and solution, the tubes are allowed to stand at room temperature until sedimentation has occurred. The degree of hemolysis and the residue of unhemolyzed red cells are compared with the same factors in the blood of a normal control treated in the same manner. If any clotting occurs, the tube is centrifuged at low speed for a few minutes and the degree of hemolysis in the supernatant fluid is compared with that found in the corresponding tube of the control. Additional tubes with 0.45 and 0.425% of sodium chloride solution will detect the increased osmotic fragility of the blood from patients with hereditary spherocytosis. Complete hemolysis is found in all three tubes in hereditary spherocytosis and decreased hemolysis (increased resistance of the red cells), in thalassemia, sickle cell anemia, and other hemoglobinopathies.

*Autohemolysis test.* The hereditary hemolytic anemias comprise a large and miscellaneous number of diseases, among them the nonspherocytic congenital hemolytic anemias, which are due to specific enzyme deficiencies. This group of anemias is differentiated from congenital spherocytosis by the lack of spherocytes (prior to splenectomy), by normal osmotic fragility, and usually by failure to respond completely to splenectomy. Of the various red cell enzyme deficiencies grouped with congenital nonspherocytic hemolytic diseases, the most prevalent types are those associated with glucose-6-phosphate dehydrogenase deficiency and those associated with pyruvate kinase deficiency.

In 1954 Selwyn and Dacie[319] described the autohemolysis test which helped to screen the nonspherocytic congenital hemolytic anemias. The test for autohemolysis depends on the incubation of sterile defibrinated blood at 37° C. for 24 and 48 hours and the determination of the amount of spontaneous hemolysis which occurs. In comparison, the extent of hemolysis is determined when glucose or ATP is added to the blood. Normally minimal lysis occurs at the end of 48 hours (less than 5%) when incubated under sterile conditions. The addition of glucose or ATP in normal blood reduces the degree of autohemolysis only slightly (less than 1%).

In one of the standard methods[48] the patient's blood is collected in a sterile manner and defibrinated. Two milliliters of the sterile defibrinated blood are placed in sterile screw-capped vials. Glucose, 0.1 ml. solution (10 gm. in 0.85% saline to make 100 ml.), is added to one vial; 0.1 ml. of adenosine triphosphate solution (2.5 gm. in 0.85% saline to make 10 ml.) is added to another. One vial of the still defibrinated blood has no additive. All vials in duplicate are incubated at 37° C. and left undisturbed for 24 hours. After 24 hours the vials are rotated and then left to incubate for another 24-hour period. At 48 hours of incubation, the vials are again rotated and hematocrit plasma hemoglobins are determined on each vial. The amount of spontaneous hemolysis is estimated by measuring the amount of hemoglobin in the defibrinated supernatant layer or by changes in the volume of packed red blood cells as compared with the preincubation specimen.

The patterns of autohemolysis are noted in patients with congenital nonspherocytic hemolytic anemia. In the Type I pattern there is increased autohemolysis of the whole blood with partial correction by the addition of glucose or adenosine triphosphate. Type II pattern demonstrates greatly increased autohemolysis of whole blood but no correction by the addition of glucose and complete correction with adenosine triphosphate.

Type I autohemolysis has been observed in glucose-6-phosphate dehydrogenase deficiency, unstable hemoglobin hemolytic anemia, stomatocytosis, hexokinase deficiency, Heinz body anemias, and paroxysmal nocturnal hemoglobinuria. Type II is characteristic of pyruvate kinase deficiency. The third type of pattern is observed in hereditary spherocytosis and in triosephosphate isomerase deficiency; namely, correction almost to normal by the addition of glucose or adenosine triphosphate, rather than those of type I or type II nonspherocytic hemolytic anemia (Table 19).

It must be cautioned that exceptions to the above patterns have been found in individual cases.

In general, the rates of hemolysis parallel the degree of increased fragility before incubation.[78] Selwyn and Dacie[319] reported that spontaneous autohemolysis in patients with hereditary spherocytosis is not due to progressive swelling of the cells, but to a defective cell membrane which undergoes degenerative changes more rapidly than nor-

Table 19. Autohemolysis test (48 hours) in normal subjects and the three types of patterns observed in hemolytic anemia*

| Condition | Additive | | |
|---|---|---|---|
| | None | Glucose | ATP |
| | *Percent hemolysis* | | |
| Normal | 2.0 (0.2–4.0) | 0.3 (0.1–0.6) | 0.2 (0.1–0.8) |
| Type I | 9.0 (1–6) | 1.3 (0.5–4.0) | 1.0 (0.4–2.0) |
| Type II | 13.0 (8–44) | 15.0 (4–48) | 1.0 (0.2–2.0) |
| Hereditary spherocytosis | 16.0 (6–30) | 3.0 (0.2–14) | 3.0 (1–6) |

*From Cartwright, G. E.: Diagnostic laboratory hematology, ed. 4, New York, 1969, Grune & Stratton, Inc., p. 292.
Mean values and range (in parentheses) are listed.

mal. They also found that autohemolysis of the red cells of patients with hereditary spherocytosis was markedly retarded when appreciable amounts of glucose were added to the blood before incubation. Abnormally rapid autohemolysis had also been observed in patients with other types of spherocytosis and nonspherocytic hemolytic anemia.[384]

Selwyn and Dacie[319] demonstrated that the addition of glucose to whole normal blood did not prevent the increase in osmotic fragility during incubation, but did reduce the loss of potassium and the accumulation of sodium in erythrocytes which otherwise occurred. The normal red cell defends itself from osmotic lysis because its membrane is relatively impermeable to the free movement of cations. To prevent any gross leaks of sodium into the cell from surrounding plasma and potassium loss from the cell, an active energy-demanding "pump" operates in the cell to push sodium out and pull potassium in.[168,243] The pump activity balances the downhill leak of potassium out of the cell and the leakage of sodium into the cell. The energy necessary to provide this force is furnished by way of adenosine triphosphate (ATP), which is derived from glycolysis in the red cell. Ouabain inhibits the adenosine triphosphatase (ATPase), the cation pump, and thereby arrests cation transport.[281] The combination of deficient glucose consumption and accelerated breakdown of ATP, occurring in such red cell enzyme deficiencies as pyruvate kinase deficiency, deprives the cation pump of its energy source. Cation leaking is, therefore, ultimately unopposed and cell lysis follows.

The maintenance of osmotic fragility of erythrocytes during incubation in serum in autohemolysis tests is dependent on adequate energy production from glucose metabolism and the prevention of a decrease in the free cholesterol in the serum. The increase in osmotic fragility is also directly correlated with loss of erythrocyte cholesterol.[244]

Blood from newborn infants, both full-term and premature, appears to be more uniformly resistant to spontaneous autohemolysis in vitro than does blood from healthy adult controls.[303] Resistance to autohemolysis in the absence of glucose is uniformly greater than that noted in the red cells of healthy adults.

*Investigation of red cell survival in patients with hemolytic disorders.* The use of radioactive sodium chromate for labeling red cells provides a convenient method for estimating red cell survival. Since the isotope ($^{51}$Cr) remains attached to the erythrocyte for considerable periods of time, the life-span of the patient's red cells can be determined within his own circulation or in a normal recipient. By thus tagging the patient's red cells with $^{51}$Cr, it is possible not only to measure the rate of hemolysis but also to demonstrate the principal site at which this occurs. This is accomplished by reinjecting the patient's own $^{51}$Cr-labeled red cells and measuring the selective uptake of radioactivity over the heart, liver, and spleen. A shortened survival of labeled red cells in the circulation and a much greater radioactive count over the spleen as compared with the liver suggest that the patient would benefit from splenectomy.[166,173] Not only autogenous cells but also the shortened survival of normal donor cells in patients with the refractory hemolytic anemias such as severe Cooley's anemia may be accompanied by a progressive increase of radioactivity over the spleen. This finding incriminates the spleen as the site of excessive hemolysis for donor cells and serves as one of the criteria for splenectomy.

*Aplastic crisis in hemolytic anemia.* In the study of the course of hereditary spherocytosis, Owren[261] observed that the crisis which characterizes this disease was not associated with an increase in hemolysis but with a sudden cessation of erythropoiesis, reticulocytopenia, increased pallor rather than jaundice, a decreased concentration of serum bilirubin, and varying degrees of leukopenia and thrombocytopenia. Instead of an increased hyperplasia, the bone marrow was depressed, especially with respect to erythropoiesis. Spontaneous recovery was associated with the rapid regeneration of erythropoietic tissue, marked reticulocytosis, leukocytosis, and an increase in platelets. The crises are self-limited, lasting 1 to 2 weeks. Owren's conclusion that the crises in patients with hereditary spherocytosis are aplastic rather than hemolytic has been amply confirmed and observed in patients with other hemolytic anemias. There is no uniform causative factor for the crisis, although infection is regarded as the most common agent.

Aplastic crises have been described in children suffering from sickle cell anemia,[52,327] acquired hemolytic anemia,[101] and paroxysmal nocturnal hemoglobinuria.[68] Transient aplastic or hypoplastic states are occasionally observed in patients with severe Cooley's anemia during infection and often without a precipitating illness.[171] An infectious etiology explains the occurrence of aplastic crises within a brief period in several members of families with sickle cell anemia.[205] A transitory disappearance of normoblasts from the bone marrow has been described in allergic children as a result of infection due to sensitivity to a drug.[135]

It is obvious that the severity of the anemia during and following the aplastic crisis is correlated with the life-span of the red cells characterizing the anemia. The degree of anemia would be less marked in a person whose red cells had a normal life-span of 120 days as compared with the short life-span of the spherocyte or sickle cell. In the patient with sickle cell anemia an acute cessation of red cell production for a few days can result in a serious drop in hemoglobin and red cells. In a patient with infectious mononucleosis in whom the life-span of the red cell is normal, transitory erythroblastopenia was followed by minimal anemia.[52] Such minor degrees of anemia in previously nonanemic persons are readily remedied on the resumption of erythropoiesis.

Less commonly, a true hemolytic crisis is encountered in patients with sickle cell anemia as well as in those with the more common aplastic crisis. It is characterized by a severe pain in the back, abdomen, and extremities, with a significant drop in erythrocytes and hemoglobin level, and by an increase in serum bilirubin and reticulocytes. In this situation there is a dramatic fall in the circulating red cell volume accompanied by hyperplastic bone marrow.[315]

## CONGENITAL HEMOLYTIC SYNDROMES

The hereditary hemolytic syndromes, many of which exhibit an intrinsic abnormality of the red cell, hemoglobin, or both, include a large variety of disorders. They embrace hereditary spherocytosis, hereditary elliptocytosis, the nonspherocytic hemolytic anemias, Cooley's anemia, sickle cell anemia, the unstable hemoglobin hemolytic anemias, and many of the hereditary drug-induced hemolytic anemias. These erythrocytic abnormalities differ from each other morphologically and when this is not obvious they are distinguished by specific laboratory tests. The genetic patterns also serve as diagnostic aids. Paroxysmal nocturnal hemoglobinuria due to an inherent red blood cell defect is neither congenital nor hereditary. Sickle cell disease and thalassemia will be considered with the hereditary hemoglobinopathies in Chapter 16.

Many of the hemolytic aspects of the syndromes to be discussed are based on shortened survival of red cells in the circulation, due to innate defects which come to light when exposed to certain challenges. Hemolysis may be due to defects in the two factors which normally maintain the integrity of the red cell—its metabolic state and physical structure. The metabolic abnormalities include a deficiency on enzymes such as glucose-6-phosphate dehyrogenase, pyruvate kinase, and triosephosphate isomerase. The presence of certain stromal lipids also contributes to red cell survival. The hemolytic anemia of septicemia due to *Clostridium welchii* is thought to result from the action of lecithinase on red cell stroma. A number of lipids are included in the red cell membrane, one being cholesterol. The localization of cholesterol in definitive parts of the red cell plays an important role in maintaining its biconcave shape.[245]

*Hereditary spherocytosis (congenital hemolytic jaundice, congenital hemolytic anemia, spherocytic anemia, chronic acholuric jaundice, chronic familial jaundice)*

The designation hereditary spherocytosis emphasizes two important elements of the disease without excluding cases in which anemia and jaundice are absent. Hereditary spherocytosis is one of the chief congenital hemolytic syndromes that exhibits a hereditary abnormality of the red cell.

**Definition.** Hereditary spherocytosis is a genetically determined, chronic hemolytic disease characterized by spherocytes, increased osmotic fragility of the red cells, and, frequently, splenomegaly.

**Inheritance and race.** The disease is found chiefly among Caucasians and rarely among Negroes.[78,189] The prevalence of hereditary spherocytosis has been estimated at 220 per million with a mutation rate of $2.2 \times 10^{-5}$.[237] The defect is transmitted by either parent as a mendelian dominant so that males and females are equally affected. Discrepancies in the hereditary transmission which are difficult to explain are observed. In one series only 24% of the offspring of families with an affected parent showed spherocytosis, instead of the expected 50%.[382] Affected children have also been observed, both of whose parents possessed no clinical or hematologic evidence of this disease. Such exceptions are explained on the basis of doubtful paternity, mutation, or incomplete expressivity of the gene for hereditary spherocytosis. Occasionally, one of the apparently normal parents will reveal the red cell defect of spherocytosis by increased osmotic fragility or autohemolysis in excess of the normal after incubation of a blood sample at 37° C. for 24 to 48 hours.

**Etiology and pathogenesis.** The basic defect in patients with hereditary spherocytosis consists of the production of spherocytes which, because of their shape, are trapped in the spleen and are destroyed at a more rapid rate than normal. The pathogenesis of the abnormal shape of the spherocyte has been investigated with respect to its metabolic derangements and the effect of stasis within the spleen. The spheroidal configuration is not present in the corresponding nucleated red cells in the bone marrow but appears in the reticulocytes and is established thereafter.[382] Less often a definitive but slight reduction in size has been detected in the late normoblast.[92] Once having gained maturity in the circulation, the non-nucleated red cell is smaller and thicker than the corresponding normal red cell.

Extensive studies of various metabolic alterations in spherocytes have been under investigation.

Previous studies dealt with disturbances in carbohydrate metabolism in these cells and demonstrated slow regeneration of high-energy phosphate bonds.[283,319] With the aid of $^{32}P$ a defect in phosphorylation of adenosine triphosphate within the red cell has been observed with an increased uptake of the radioactive phosphorus into the pool of inorganic phosphorus. It was suggested that this defect contributed to the destruction of red cells in the spleen.[282] In later studies by Shafer[320] the phosphorylated carbohydrate intermediates of erythrocytes from normal adults and from five patients with hereditary spherocytosis were labeled in vitro with $^{32}P$ orthophosphate and then separated on columns of ion exchange resin. No qualitative or quantitative differences were found between normal erythrocytes and those of hereditary spherocytosis. The glycolytic mechanism of these abnormal erythrocytes was, therefore, open to further investigation.[395]

Recent studies suggest that an inherent increase in sodium permeability of the red cell membrane may be of importance in the pathogenesis of hereditary spherocytosis. Mention has already been made earlier in this chapter (p. 301) of the function of the red cell membrane in preventing the movement of sodium into the cell and of potassium loss from the cell. The bulk of the sodium-potassium ion interchange is under the direct control of several cation pumps which have been demonstrated to function in the membrane.[164] The metabolic alterations of the erythrocyte in hereditary spherocytosis have been explained in another manner. The cells have been found to possess a passive "leakiness" to sodium influx during incubation which is more than twice that of normal cells, while the potassium efflux remains similar to normal cells.[167] Under optimal conditions the cell can compensate for this sodium leak by increasing active transport from the cell via the sodium pump mechanism. As stated previously (p. 301 and p. 303), the sodium pump is largely ATP-dependent and the utilization of high energy phosphate is therefore increased in these cells. Similarly, anaerobic glycolysis on which the maintenance of ATP levels are dependent is also increased in these cells.[168] These observations indicate that hemolysis of red cells of hereditary spherocytosis is associated with overwork rather than a deficiency in energy metabolism.[168]

Entrapment and prolonged incubation in vitro reduce the supply of available glucose and render the cells incapable of preventing excessive sodium accumulation. They gain sodium and water and subsequently undergo osmotic hemolysis.[251] During metabolic stress, as is believed to occur in the spleen, sodium accumulates intracellularly, and irreversible changes in membrane permeability and ultimately hemolysis ensue. Splenectomy, by removing the source of conditioning, allows the cells to survive longer. Similarly the addition of glucose in in vitro incubation studies largely corrects the abnormal hemolysis.

It is now generally concluded that the lipid composition of the red cell is normal. The turnover of phospholipid, however, is increased, suggesting a possible connection between increased sodium pump activity and increased phospholipid turnover.[169] During incubation of hereditary spherocytosis cells in a glucose-containing medium, striking losses occur of both membrane cholesterol and phospholipid in proportion equal to those found in the intact membrane.[167] Entire units of cell membrane are lost during the incubation period and a budding type of cell fragmentation has been observed in spherocytosis.[291] With the loss of membrane lipid the microspherocyte is produced. Membrane lipid loss, phospholipid turnover, and microspherocytosis were viewed by Jacob and co-workers[167-169] as the direct result of the increased rate of active cation pumping that spherocytes maintain to counteract the influx of sodium. After splenectomy, lipid values previously decreased are restored to values obtained in normal subjects with spleens.[63]

The abnormalities of cation flux and phospholipid turnover represent secondary rather than primary abnormalities of the red cell membrane. Recent studies[169a] have suggested an instability of membrane proteins, but attempts to detect abnormalities in the pattern of membrane protein electrophoresis have yielded inconsistent results.[387a]

It is generally accepted that the globular shape of the red cells accelerates their removal from the circulation and their sequestration in the splenic pulp where they undergo lysis. This process is not dependent upon specific abnormalities of the patient's spleen, since it takes place as readily in the spleen of normal persons as in that of those suffering from diseases other than spherocytosis. The abnormal thickness of spherical cells does not permit them to escape readily from the pulp into the venous sinuses.[387] The stagnation of spherocytes in the spleen is apparent in the engorgement of the pulp with red cells, but the venous sinuses are, for the most part, inconspicuous and contain few red cells.[382] Increasing evidence has confirmed the hypothesis that many of the erythrocytes, having been trapped in the spleen, undergo lysis and others are so conditioned that they are incapable of prolonged survival in the circulation after release from the spleen.[115,387] Additional evidence that the spherocytes are primarily involved in the pathogenesis is the fact that removal of the spleen relieves the anemia, but the red cell defect as manifested by spheroidicity, increased autohemolysis, excessive permeability to sodium, increased osmotic and mechanical fragility, and hypermetabolism remains unaltered.

With phlebotomy, iron-deficiency anemia was produced in two patients with hereditary spherocytosis so that the red cells became hypochromic, smaller, thinner, and lost their spheroidal character. Although fragility tests were improved, the life-span in the circulation was not altered until after splenectomy, indicating that the shape of red cells per se in hereditary spherocytosis was not responsible for their premature destruction.[72]

Experimentally induced spherocytes show a marked shift of oxygen dissociation to the left. In contrast, in splenectomized animals, in which red cells thinner than normal appear, the curve is shifted to the right. The oxygen-carrying capacity of spherocytic erythrocytes, its alteration after splenectomy, and the possible role of 2-3 diphosphoglycerate in red cell pathophysiology in this condition are under intensive investigation.[206]

***Clinical features.*** The clinical manifestations are extremely variable, particularly with regard to the time of onset and intensity of symptoms. In individual patients and among members of the same family they vary widely at different times in the course of the disease. Jaundice, symptoms referable to anemia, and splenomegaly constitute the most common clinical features of the disease. In some infants hereditary spherocytosis may be evident at birth, whereas in others symptoms may not appear until late in adult life.

Jaundice is unusual in infancy and childhood except during the newborn period, when it may simulate erythroblastosis with the same susceptibility to kernicterus in the event of hyperbilirubinemia. In the older child, an icteric tint, which becomes more pronounced in the young adult and affected parent, is noticeable. Jaundice is accompanied by a highly pigmented urine and stool. The spleen is nearly always enlarged. In the young infant it may be palpable or may not be felt at all. Pallor with or without anemia and a sallow complexion are common. Lassitude, fatigability, anorexia, fever, and abdominal pain may call attention to the disease. Crises are ushered in by fever, extreme pallor, shortness of breath, nausea, vomiting, and extreme weakness. They are now known to be aplastic rather than hemolytic, as formerly assumed, and are associated with cessation of blood formation. Crises may occur in several members of the same family almost simultaneously.

Gallstones occur commonly in older persons, with an incidence as high as 85% of cases;[385] they are uncommon in young children but have been reported in a child 3 years old.[133] They usually increase in frequency after the age of 10 years.[14] Gallstone colic or biliary obstruction may constitute the first indication of existing hereditary spherocytosis. A history of cholelithiasis in a parent justifies examination for spherocytosis in the offspring who is pale, easily fatigued, and without appetite. The presence of gallstones in patients with hereditary spherocytosis depends upon the activity and duration of the hemolytic process.

Gallstones are of the pigment variety, resulting from increased concentration of bilirubin in the bile. Their presence leads to cholecystitis or cholangitis, which may be followed by formation of stones of the mixed type containing bile pigment and cholesterol. Mixed stones are radiopaque, pigment stones are not.[82]

Leg ulcers occur infrequently and are extremely rare in childhood. Their causation is not so readily explained as in patients with sickle cell anemia. Cardiac murmurs, especially in young children, may be so intense as to simulate congenital heart disease and eventually lead to recognition of the underlying disease. Their elimination by transfusion confirms a hemic origin. Roentgenologic changes are similar to those occurring in patients with other congenital hemolytic syndromes, but less in degree and incidence. They most commonly consist of thickening and striation of the frontal and parietal bones of the skull.[61]

Bony masses consisting of hemopoietic tissue are found in this condition as in thalassemia major. They represent heterotopic bone marrow and are usually situated in the thorax as slowly growing paraspinal mediastinal masses. The tumor produces no symptoms and is a manifestation of compensatory, extramedullary hematopoiesis.[64]

These masses may be erroneously diagnosed as malignant thoracic neoplasms.[151] They originate as extensions from the marrow or from embryonic rests or lymph nodes. Whether surgical excision is ever necessary is questionable.[64] While usually found in the thorax, the bony masses may appear lateral to the bodies of the dorsal vertebrae.[156]

Barry and associates[13] reported five cases of hemochromatosis secondary to hereditary spherocytosis. Only one had multiple blood transfusions and none were known to have had significant oral iron therapy. Massive iron overload was proved by venisection in two of the patients who are alive and well 7 and 5 years after presenting in heart failure. In one case heterotopic extramedullary hematopoietic masses were found characteristically situated in the thoracic paravertebral gutter where they masqueraded as pseudotumors. A persistently high serum iron with largely saturated total iron binding capacity was present. Failure to undertake effective prophylactic or definitive treatment of the iron overload by multiple venisections may result in progression to cirrhosis and ultimately hepatocellular failure. The experience with these cases reinforces current views that, once congenital spherocytosis has been diagnosed in the adult, splenectomy to prevent the occasional development of secondary hemochromatosis and the emergence of some of the other complications should not be delayed.

In another patient—a 29-year-old woman with hereditary spherocytosis who had a splenectomy 5½ years previously—hemochromatosis was present. There was no history of heavy and prolonged iron intake. The essential features were increasing skin pigmentation which had been reversed by phlebotomies, and massive iron deposition in hepatic, parenchymal, and reticuloendothelial cells associated with portal cirrhosis.

*Growth.* Among patients with hereditary spherocytosis who exhibit little in the way of symptoms but have a reduced volume of erythrocytes, growth has been normal. There was no deviation from the normal growth curve in any patient during the period of the expected preadolescent acceleration of growth. It is during this period that patients with other chronic anemias, such as thalassemia major, receiving transfusion therapy fail to keep pace with rates of growth observed in normal children. Thus adults with hereditary spherocytosis who are relatively asymptomatic except during periods of crisis are of normal height. In contrast to these patients, children who are moderately or severely anemic and require repeated transfusions show impairment in both growth and weight. In such patients it is undoubtedly wise to advise splenectomy at much earlier periods.

*Laboratory data.* The increased rate of red cell destruction produces anemia, hyperbilirubinuria, an elevated icterus index, increased fecal and urinary urobilinogen, and elevated serum iron concentration. The increased rate of red cell regeneration leads to reticulocytosis. The blood picture is characterized by anemia, spherocytosis, increased osmotic fragility, and an elevated serum bilirubin. The Coombs test is negative, and an abnormal hemoglobin is absent. The hemoglobin level may be normal but usually ranges from 7 to 11 gm. per 100 ml., and the red blood cell count ranges from 2.5 to 4.5 million per cubic millimeter. During a crisis the hemoglobin may fall to 3 to 4 gm. and the red cell count to 1.5 to 2 million. The reticulocytes range from 5 to 20%.

The spherocytes appear as small, bright, deeply stained cells that lack central pallor. Their decreased diameter and increased thickness contribute to the rounded appearance. Normoblasts may appear in the peripheral blood. Poikilocytosis is rare. Large polychromatophilic cells are common and appear in the blood smear in conjunction with normal and spherical cells. Spherocytes may be few in number or constitute the bulk of cells. Except in the mildest cases the osmotic fragility is increased. When this is uncertain, fragility is accelerated by prior incubation of the blood for 24 hours at 37° C. Mechanical fragility is increased. The autohemolysis test reveals greater than normal lysis of the red cells during sterile incubation at 37° C. for 48 hours. The addition of glucose causes marked inhibition of autohemolysis.[319,384] The leukocytes are usually normal in number or may be slightly increased. The platelets are normal. Bilirubinemia varies between 1 and 4 mg. per 100 ml. but often lies within the normal range despite other signs of active hemolysis.[78]

A normal or slightly lowered hemoglobin concentration may coexist with active hemolytic disease. An abnormally small total red cell volume may be present in such cases and, in combination with a rapid rate of red cell production, results in a partially compensated hemolytic anemia.[117] Whether or not anemia exists depends upon the ability of red cell production to compensate for the increased destruction of cells. The failure of the plasma volume to expand accounts for the apparently normal hemoglobin level in the peripheral blood. As yet there is no known explanation for the lack of expansion of the plasma volume in patients with this disease or for the greater than normal expansion in patients with sickle cell anemia.

Since hereditary spherocytosis is characterized by a chronic and persistent hemolytic process, one would expect episodes of exagerated hemolysis to occur. In contrast to an anticipated increase in hemolysis, the crisis in hereditary spherocytosis is now known to be aplastic. Instead of a hyperplastic bone marrow that is ordinarily present in this disease, an acute aplasia of erythroid tissue supervenes and is associated with reticulocytopenia, anemia, leukopenia, and thrombocytopenia. The serum bilirubin decreases and jaundice gives way to pallor.

A variant of hereditary spherocytosis has been described[374] in a 58-year-old white man in which red cell survival studies indicated splenic conditioning of nearly all the circulating red cells. Clinical features also suggested a severe form of the disease with anemia, splenomegaly, a history of leg ulcers, and retardation of growth in childhood. Autohemolysis was atypical for hereditary spherocytosis in that the increased hemolysis of incubated blood was not corrected by glucose supplementation, although after splenectomy the autohemolysis reverted to a normal pattern. Transfusion of the patient's red cell to a normal compatible recipient resulted in their removal by the spleen with a half-time (T½) of 12½ minutes equivalent to complete removal of these cells during a single passage through the spleen. After the patient's spleen had been removed, however, his red cells survived in a normal recipent with a T½ of 90 minutes. The difference in survival time demonstrates that splenic conditioning had a damaging effect on the in vivo survival of the patient's cells.

*Hereditary spherocytosis in the newborn period.* Hereditary spherocytosis may be manifest at birth.[215,322,338] The blood smear in the neonatal period shows both macrocytic cells from fetal life and spherocytes. The latter become increasingly numerous in the weeks following birth (Fig. 27). Excessive jaundice due to the accumulation of unconjugated bilirubin leads to confusion with erythroblastosis. The differentiation from cases of erythroblastosis due to A and B blood groups which are also characterized by spherocytosis may be difficult. The persistence of spherocytes and a negative Coombs test in patients with hereditary spherocytosis separate the two conditions. At any rate exchange transfusions are required in patients with hereditary spherocytosis in the event of hyperbilirubinuria since the same susceptibility to nervous system damage exists as in patients with erythroblastosis.

It is noteworthy that in patients with hereditary spherocytosis several supportive transfusions may be required during the first 3 weeks of life because of severe anemia. Thereafter, patients attain a steady state in which the anemia is minimal and symptoms are few.[116]

**Diagnosis.** The important diagnostic features of hereditary spherocytosis stem from the intrinsic red cell anomaly. As has already been indicated, the morphology of the red cells accounts for the increased osmotic fragility, reticulocytosis, jaundice, and splenomegaly. Spherocytosis and increased osmotic fragility are not exclusive features of spherocytosis and may be present in patients with other hemolytic disorders. A positive family history and one in which relatives manifest these hematologic features contribute to the diagnosis. Incubation of blood samples at 37° C. for 24 hours increases osmotic fragility in the asymptomatic and affected relative or the patient with the mild or latent disease. Diagnosis may be difficult in the child without a positive family history or in one who is initially observed in an aplastic crisis.

It should be emphasized that the absence of jaundice and absence of anemia are inadequate criteria for the diagnosis of a latent case or a spherocytic trait. Jaundice and bilirubinemia are largely dependent upon the excretory capacity of the liver since hemoglobin and red cell levels depend not only upon the rate of hemolysis, but also upon the capacity for regeneration. Thus, determination of fecal urobilinogen excretion may provide evidence of a marked hemolytic disorder in the absence of jaundice or hyperbilirubinemia. The reticu-

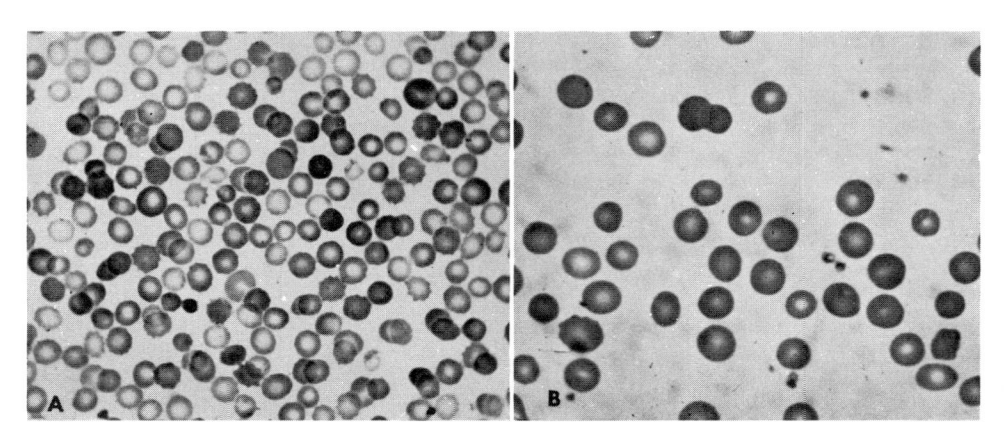

Fig. 27. Blood smear of a patient with hereditary spherocytosis. **A,** Low-power view showing dark staining of abnormally thick spherocytes. (×250.) **B,** Slightly increased magnification of **A.**

locyte count may reveal accelerated red cell regeneration in the absence of anemia. This determination is especially important in patients in whom the failure of the plasma volume to expand in the face of a diminished red cell mass results in a normal or slightly lowered hemoglobin level in the peripheral blood.

Autoimmune acquired hemolytic anemia usually shows marked spherocytosis, but the positive Coombs test and negative family history differentiate it from hereditary spherocytosis. In patients with hereditary nonspherocytic anemia, spherocytes are absent and osmotic fragility is normal.

*Treatment.* Splenectomy is followed by a complete and permanent relief from all signs and symptoms of the disease. Except for the asymptomatic patient in whom red cell destruction is well compensated, the operation is recommended once the diagnosis is established. Even in the mildly affected person without anemia or jaundice, splenectomy is advisable for the relief of a chronic hemolytic condition and proneness to crises and gallstone formation. Because of evidence that splenectomy in early childhood may cause increased susceptibility to infection,[331] it has been suggested that the operation be postponed until the patient is at least 5 years of age. Also, at this age gallstones tend to be formed.[386] Occasionally, an earlier operation at approximately 2 years of age is necessary when anorexia and fatigability seriously interfere with the health of the child. By pooling data from reported sources from 1934 to 1957 of the evidence of infection following splenectomy for hereditary spherocytosis in the first year of life, Burman[38] found that ten of forty-eight patients developed an infection and that four died. It would seem that splenectomy in the first year of life is definitely hazardous. The optimal age for the operation still awaits the results of more extended experience. Children require close supervision for several years postoperatively so that immediate and energetic treatment can be instituted in the event of sudden and severe illness. Since serious infections occur most frequently in the first 2 years after splenectomy, oral therapy with antibiotics (usually penicillin, 200,000 units once daily) has been prescribed as a continuous prophylactic measure during this period.

Spherocytosis as well as increased osmotic fragility of the red corpuscles persist after splenectomy. A sharp rise in platelets and leukocytes follows postoperatively. The reticulocyte count drops to normal but is occasionally slightly elevated, hemolysis ceases, and the bilirubin level falls significantly. The life-span of the red cells, previously shortened, becomes approximately but not quite normal after splenectomy. Despite the persistence of spherocytosis after splenectomy in hereditary spherocytosis, it has usually been assumed that the red cell life-span returns completely to normal. A study of splenectomized patients 2 to 27 years postoperatively showed a red cell survival of 96 days (range 78 to 118 days), significantly less than the 123± 14 days in normal individuals.[50] Despite the subsequent disappearance of anemia, reticulocytosis, and hyperbilirubinemia, the red cell life-span does not return to normal.

Blood transfusion is required in the early months of life until the hemoglobin stabilizes and for treatment of a crisis with severe anemia.

*Congenital hemolytic anemia with stomatocytes.* A variant of congenital hemolytic anemia has been described showing stomatocytes (Chapter 5), increased osmotic fragility and autohemolysis, storage instability greater at 5° C. than at 37° C., decreased concentration of reduced glutathione despite normal glucose-6-phosphate dehydrogenase and glutathione reductase. An 18½-year-old male with these abnormalities had severe hemolytic anemia, jaundice, and splenomegaly. Splenectomy resulted in improvement of the anemia but did not cure the hematologic disorder.[231]

Stomatocytes have also been observed in several instances in which the primary red cell defect was an extraordinary permeability to sodium and potassium. Zarkowsky and colleagues[389] reported a child with a hemolytic anemia of unknown cause in whom the sodium concentration in the patient's red cells ranged from 91 to 108 and the potassium from 35 to 47 mEq. per liter of cells as compared with normal values of 10 and 95 mEq. per liter, respectively. His anemia and hemolysis rate was greatly impaired but not cured by splenectomy. The vastly increased rate of active cation transport placed extraordinary metabolic demands on the patient's cells. The red cells were large, and numerous stomatocytes were seen in stained preparations. This increase in red cell membrane permeability of both sodium and potassium differs from the erythrocytes of hereditary spherocytosis in which the rate of entry of labeled sodium is greater than into normal cells but in which potassium loss is not increased.[168] In contrast, the erythrocytes in some cases of pyruvate kinase deficiency show an increased potassium leak but without clearcut evidence of excessive sodium leak.[250] Oski and co-workers[258] reported a young boy, his father, and his grandfather whose erythrocytes were found to have markedly reduced potassium and elevated sodium concentrations. The disease clinically mimics hereditary spherocytosis in its mode of inheritance and its association with increased red cell osmotic fragility in affected members. It differs in the absence of spherocytes in the peripheral blood and in red cell cation content. Mild anemia and macrocytosis were present in each of the affected subjects. In the propositus and his father approximately 20% of the cells had slitlike areas of central pallor ("stomatocytes") (Fig. 28). In the grandfather only 2% of cells had this unusual appearance. Autohemolysis was increased in all three patients and was reduced by glucose and ATP.

A mild chronic hemolytic anemia has been reported in an adult male characterized by the remarkable absence of all Rh-Hr factors, in other words, $Rh_{null}$.[342] The mild normocytic normochromic anemia was associated with persistent reticulocytosis. The red cell morphology showed minor but distinct aberrations. The area of the central pallor was slitlike rather than circular, corresponding to the morphology of stomatocytes. Microscopic hyperchromic spherocytosis involving a small number of cells was also present.

Ducrov and Kimber[112] found that stomatocytes were a relatively common finding in the peripheral blood in members of the Greek and Italian communities in South Australia. In this group there was a high incidence of recurrent abdominal pain, nausea, vomiting, low-grade pyrexia, and splenomegaly. Anemia was a common finding and there was a mild to moderate elevation of the reticulocyte count. A slight reduction in red cell survival was established in all cases. Osmotic fragility was normal in all cases. Bone marrow examination revealed normoblastic hyperplasia in three cases. In one the marrow was normal. It is not clear from this study whether the defect is acquired or inherited.

A new variant of congenital hemolytic anemia associated with stomatocytosis, reticulocytosis, decreased osmotic fragility, type I autohemolysis, shortened erythrocyte survival, three-fold increased intracellular sodium and slightly decreased intracellular potassium content was documented in three siblings of consanguineous parents. Active sodium efflux was eight to ten times greater than normal but potassium influx was normal. The syndrome differs from others associated with stomatocytosis in that the cells lose a disproportionate amount of potassium and become dehydrated. A membrane abnormality was proposed, but the exact nature of the defect is unknown.[229]

## Sporadic congenital spherocytosis associated with congenital hypoplastic thrombocytopenia and malformations

A syndrome characterized by congenital malformations (such as absent radii, cyanotic

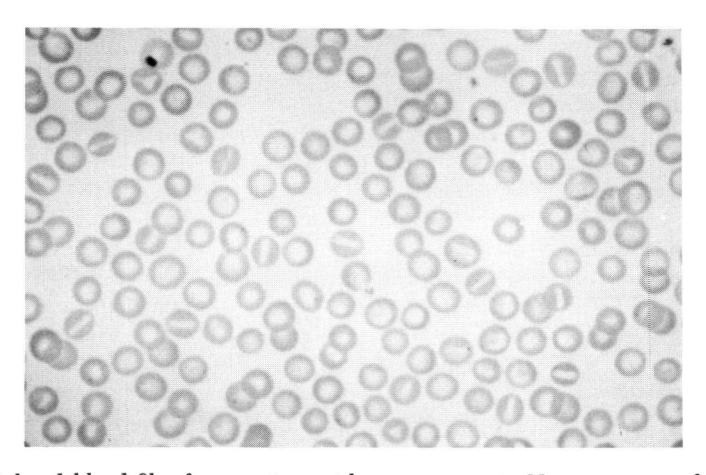

Fig. 28. Peripheral blood film from patient with stomatocytosis. Note presence of erythrocytes with slit-like rather than circular area of central pallor. (Courtesy Dr. Frank A. Oski, Philadelphia, Pa.)

heart disease, and bilateral hydronephrosis), thrombocytopenia, hypoplasia of megakaryocytes, and a sporadic form of spherocytic anemia has been described in infants.[390] The spleen may be transiently enlarged and petechiae may be present in early infancy. A follow-up into childhood is not yet available in these patients. Except for the presence of spherocytes, the combination of depleted megakaryocytes and platelets dating from the neonatal period resembles congenital hypoplastic thrombocytopenia. In many respects the clinical and hematologic features constitute a variant of Fanconi's syndrome to the extent that a severe anemia coexists with congenital abnormalities.

### Hereditary nonspherocytic hemolytic anemia (atypical familial hemolytic anemia, congenital nonspherocytic anemia)

Hereditary nonspherocytic hemolytic anemia applies to a form of chronic hemolytic anemia, frequently familial and genetically transmitted as either an autosomal recessive or x-chromosome-linked trait, in which the red cells possess an intrinsic defect usually without a manifest morphologic anomaly. In the latter respect it differs from hereditary spherocytosis, sickle cell anemia, and thalassemia in which an intrinsic defect coexists with a distinctive cellular malformation. Osmotic and mechanical resistance of red cells is normal, and the life-span of the red cells is shortened (12 to 17 days[239]). An abnormal type of hemoglobin has not been demonstrated. In contrast to hereditary spherocytosis, there is not only normal red cell fragility, but usually a failure to respond to splenectomy as well. The anemia varies in intensity from mild to severe, requiring transfusions. The red cells are normocytic but show a tendency toward macrocytosis, and occasionally ovalocytes are present.[183] The hematologic picture includes erythroid hyperplasia of the bone marrow, reticulocytosis, normoblasts in the peripheral blood, hyperbilirubinemia, and punctate basophilia of the erythrocytes.[127,194] Fecal urobilinogen is increased. The Coombs test is negative. Autohemolysis and osmotic fragility after incubation at 37° C. for 24 hours showed a slight increase over the normal. Clinical features include mild jaundice, slight to moderate enlargement of the liver and spleen, and, in rare instances, facial configuration of the mongoloid type. Thickening of the cranial bones and a hair-on-end appearance between the tables similar to that observed in patients with Cooley's anemia and sickle cell anemia have been reported.[183,252] A familial incidence is well documented,[65,183,329] but, as in patients with hereditary spherocytosis, it cannot always be demonstrated in the asymptomatic siblings or parent. Sickle cell anemia, Cooley's anemia, and hereditary spherocytosis are readily differentiated by clinical and hematologic criteria.

The metabolic aberrations which constitute the basis of the congenital nonspherocytic hemolytic anemias are best explained by a knowledge of the enzymes that function at important stages of the metabolic pathways; such knowledge serves as a frame of reference for deviations from the normal.

In Chapter 4 it was stated that the erythrocyte is a metabolically active cell and that glucose provides the energy for its various metabolic activities. The red cell must preserve its biconcave shape, maintain sodium and potassium gradients across its membrane, reduce methemoglobin formed by the oxidation of hemoglobin, and maintain enzymes in an active state.[20] After phosphorylation to glucose-6-phosphate in the hexokinase reaction, metabolism of the red cell transverses two main pathways. The predominant Emdben-Meyerhof pathway provides approximately 90% of all glucose metabolized anaerobically producing two moles of lactate for each mole of glucose metabolized. This pathway provides energy in the form of ATP and reduces NADP (TPN) to NADPH (TPNH) for methemoglobin reduction, mediated by methemoglobin reductase. The other route of red cell metabolism is the hexose monophosphate oxidate shunt. In this pathway no ATP is formed but NADP is reduced to NADPH. Normally, only 5 to 10% of glucose-6-phosphate is metabolized by this pathway. This route, which is outside of the strictly glycolic pathway, provides the NADPH which, linked to glutathione reductase, maintains glutathione (GSH) in its reduced form.

Increasing evidence indicates that hereditary nonspherocytic hemolytic anemia is not a single entity and that not all patients with this disease suffer from the same disorder. The disorders are similar with respect to a shortened red cell survival, normal osmotic fragility, failure to respond to splenectomy, and, often, development of hyperbilirubinuria and anemia shortly after birth. At least two distinct types have been separated in the basis of the extent of increased osmotic fragility and autohemolysis (with or without added glucose) after 24 hours of incubation at 37° C.[78] In patients with one of these types the greatly increased osmotic fragility and the failure of glucose to diminish autohemolysis, as occurs in patients with normal blood, suggest a metabolic defect[78] (type II). In patients with another type the red blood cells were found to possess the properties of cells sensitive to primaquine—i.e., a reduced glutathione content, a markedly abnormal glutathione stability test, and an extreme reduction of glucose-6-phosphate dehydrogenase (type I). In patients with this type the morphology of the red cells is normal and the degree of anemia mild, except during infections. The defect is present in other members of the family and in several generations. In both, the autohemolysis is correctable by provision of optimal amounts of adenosine triphosphate (ATP).

From these observations types I and II of nonspherocytic hemolytic anemia emerged. Patients with type I exhibited normal autohemolysis which could be decreased by the addition of glucose, but the decrease is not as great as in normal blood. Furthermore, in this type with glucose-6-phosphate dehydrogenase deficiency, adenosine triphosphate content (ATP) of the red cell is not reduced. In type II, on the other hand, there is markedly increased autohemolysis not corrected by the addition of glucose. De Gruchy and associates[104] showed also that adenosine triphosphate (ATP), an essential element in the glycolytic cycle in the red cell, when added in vitro to the red cells of type II cases, diminished the rapid rate of autohemolysis which glucose failed to do. This suggested that the failure to synthesize ATP might be responsible for the red cell's impaired life-span.

Tanaka and associates[350] later discovered a deficiency of the glycolytic enzyme pyruvate kinase (PK) in patients conforming to the type II pattern, which was confirmed by later reports.[31,35,257] In a series of twelve cases, all with red cell pyruvate kinase deficiency, Grimes and colleagues[143] found no correlation between the enzyme level and the apparent severity of the hemolytic anemia. All their patients had pyruvate kinase levels between 10 and 40% of the mean normal value. The levels of adenosine triphosphate and total diphosphopyridine nucleotide (oxidized plus reduced) in red cells were found to be low, while the 2,3-diphosphoglycerate concentration was high. All the cases studied conformed to the type II classification in that added glucose did not reduce the amount of in vitro hemolysis.

In a number of the families it appeared that this enzymatic disorder was inherited as a mendelian recessive. In one family the pyruvate kinase activity of both parents of the propositus was lower than normal; about half the normal was present in the heterozygotes. In the patients themselves the enzyme activity was almost absent.

As the reported cases of hereditary hemolytic anemia have multiplied, available techniques have been able to identify the specific enzymopathy. As enzyme assays are more widely emphasized the list of deficiencies will grow. These disorders have been classified by Valentine[356] as follows:

A. The hexose monophosphate-shunt enzyme deficiencies
 1. Glucose-6-phosphate dehydrogenase
 2. 6-Phosphogluconate dehydrogenase
B. Nonglycolytic-enzyme deficiencies
 1. Glutathione reductase
 2. Adenosine triphosphatase
 3. Glutathione peroxidase
 4. Glutathione synthetase
C. Glycolytic-enzyme deficiencies
 1. Pyruvate kinase
 2. Triosephosphate isomerase
 3. Hexokinase
 4. Glucosephosphate isomerase
 5. Phosphoglycerate kinase
 6. Diphosphoglyceromutase

The two most common of the enzymopathies are glucose-6-phosphate dehydrogenase deficiency and pyruvate kinase deficiency.

*Glucose-6-phosphate dehydrogenase deficiency (G-6-PD deficiency).* With the clearer definition of enzyme deficiencies, Dacie[84] suggested that the classification of nonspherocytic hemolytic anemias might be revised, discarding type I and type II classifications and substituting the designation according to the basic defect. Type I would include those patients with a deficiency of the enzyme glucose-6-phosphate dehydrogenase[254,321,394] and other disorders discussed in the tests for autohemolysis described previously (p. 300).

G-6-PD is the enzyme which Carson and his associates[41] had demonstrated to be the underlying defect associated with the development of hemolysis following administration of drugs such as primaquine. Primaquine-sensitive cells have a diminished content of glutathione (GSH), and when such cells are incubated with acetylphenylhydrazine their glutathione rapidly disappeared, while glutathione from normal cells is unaffected. With the disappearance of reduced glutathione, Heinz bodies are precipitated within the red cell. The mechanism of drug-induced hemolysis in G-6-PD deficiency is thought to reside in the inability of affected cells to generate the necessary NADPH to maintain glutathione in its reduced form.

Investigation of primaquine sensitivity brought to light the intrinsic defects in red cells rendering them susceptible to hemolysis. These abnormalities are apparently harmless unless red cells are exposed to primaquine and other drugs commonly used in medicine.[18] It was shown that an antimalarial drug, primaquine, induced intravascular hemolysis in about 10% of American Negroes but rarely in Caucasians.[22] After approximately 50% of the original cells are hemolyzed, the younger population of red cells is resistant to further hemolysis and the anemia is thus self-limited.[107]

G-6-PD deficiency is a very widespread disorder, affecting perhaps 100 million individuals in the world.[43] Perhaps as many as 30% of the cases of chronic nonspherocytic hemolytic anemia are associated with a form of G-6-PD deficiency.

The gene for G-6-PD is located on the X chromosome. Studies of families reveal that transmission occurs from mother to son but not from father to son.[20] Females who are heterozygous for G-6-PD deficiency are often found to have levels of activity in their blood intermediate between those of fully affected males and normal subjects. Some women, however, who are shown to be heterozygotes have normal red cell G-6-PD activity, while others have as severe a degree of deficiency as hemizygotes.[21] (See p. 321 for further details of genetic transmission.)

Clinically G-6-PD deficient individuals may develop hemolytic anemia during the course of an infection or following the administration of small doses of drugs in patients with diabetic acidosis, pneumococcal pneumonia, hepatitis, streptococcal pharyngitis, chronic renal failure, malaria,[356] ingestion of fava beans, or in the neonatal state. Under such circumstances there is marked shortening of red cell life-span, with all the clinical signs of hemolytic anemia.[20] G-6-PD deficiency in the Caucasian as well as in the Oriental is more severe than that in the Negro. In the hemizygous male subject the enzymatic assay of red cell activity of G-6-PD ranges from 0 to approximately 15%, with blood from fully expressed Caucasians and Orientals being generally from 0 to 8% and from Negroes, 3 to 15%. Similar ranges of activity are also found in fully expressed homozygous female subjects.[43] G-6-PD deficiency is readily demonstrable in the leukocytes of affected Caucasians but is much less evident in Negroes.

It is generally believed that the leukocyte enzyme is identical to the erythrocyte enzyme.[25] When the enzyme activity of the red cell is low, leukocyte activity yields equivalent results.

Ramot and associates[287] reported a marked reduction in the mean value of the glucose-6-phosphate dehydrogenase activity of the leukocytes (white blood cell, glucose-6-phosphate dehydrogenase [WBC G-6-PD]) of persons with the erythrocyte defect in Israel. Later, it was reported by Marks and Gross[217] that, while Negro males with a severe RBC G-6-PD defect had WBC G-6-PD in the low normal range, similarly affected Caucasian males had subnormal G-6-PD in their leukocytes. In a study of a Greek family[304] in which classic RBC G-6-PD deficiency was found, there was a WBC G-6-PD defect strongly dominant in all affected members, regardless of sex. In two persons in this family with a high RBC G-6-PD, there was a similar WBC G-6-PD defect. In a family of Spanish ancestry four members had a severe WBC G-6-PD deficiency despite a high RBC G-6-PD. In American Negroes the results also were variable, that is, a WBC G-6-PD defect was found with low or normal (not elevated) RBC G-6-PD.

While the relatively mild form of this defect is found in American Negro males, the more severe form occurs in Sephardic Jews, Sardinians, Arabs, Greeks, and many other Southern European, Middle Eastern, and Oriental population groups.[19] It is of interest that no subjects with a glutathione deficiency and G-6-PD deficiency have been found among Ashkenazi Jews.[346,347] The incidence is also low among subjects of Chinese and Japanese descent.[215] Furthermore, individuals with the more severe type of defect develop hemolytic anemia in response to certain drugs that do not appear to cause hemolysis in American Negroes in the dose ordinarily used.

In Negroes with G-6-PD deficiency the hemolytic process affects only the older red cells with the lowest enzyme content, thus limiting the hemolytic episode. In Caucasians and Orientals it appears that the whole red cell population is susceptible to destruction, resulting in a more severe disorder than in the Negro.

Considerable biochemical heterogeneity exists in the glucose-6-phosphate dehydrogenase of G-6-PD deficient patients with congenital hemolytic disease. In this respect, glucose-6-phosphate dehydrogenase deficiency has been analagous to the hemoglobinopathies. The mutations which affect the glucose-6-phosphate dehydrogenase molecule correspond to the numerous mutations which affect the structure of the hemoglobin molecule. Beutler and associates[25] outlined the methods of separating the abnormal types of G-6-PD deficiency from the point of view of the activity of the enzyme toward its substrates, glucose-6-phosphate and TPN. A small number of patients inherit a G-6-PD which is so biologically ineffective that their red cell life-span is shortened even in the absence of stress.

Many variants of G-6-PD exist, some associated with decreased enzyme activity in the mature erythrocyte, others merely showing alteration in electrophoretic mobility. Of approximately fifty G-6-PD variants, twelve have been associated with nonspherocytic congenital hemolytic disease. In these the activity of G-6-PD ranged from 0 to 20% as compared with the normal of 100%.[20]

An example of such a variant was demonstrated in an 11-year-old boy who first experienced a hemolytic episode at the age of 8 years. The red cells contained a level of G-6-PD activity approximating 10 to 25% of the normal. This enzyme represented a new variant named G-6-PD Alhambra.[26]

While the vast majority of G-6-PD deficient subjects have erythrocytes with a normal or nearly normal life-span in the absence of stress, there are patients who demonstrate the clinical picture of nonspherocytic congenital hemolytic anemia in the absence of exposure to a situation of stress. Their G-6-PD enzyme activity is markedly decreased or the enzyme has poor stability in vivo.[20]

The knowledge of the self-limited nature of hemolysis in the G-6-PD deficient Negro obviates needless transfusions. Splenectomy is not generally useful in congenital nonspherocytic hemolytic anemia due to G-6-PD deficiency.

In the case of other variants with severe hemolytic anemia transfusions are required.[21]

*G-6-PD deficiency in infancy.* Doxiadis and co-workers[110] have shown that in one-third of the Greek full-term infants with severe neonatal jaundice, isoimmunization could be excluded. A deficiency of glucose-6-phosphate dehydrogenase in many of these infants may have been the causative factor in jaundice and kernicterus. A similar relationship has been reported in newborns in Singapore and China.[110]

It is noteworthy that, while such an increase has been observed in Greece,[110] it could not be documented in Israel.[345] It is of interest that the G-6-PD variant most prevalent in these regions is the same, G-6-PD Mediterranean.[20] Environmental factors may play a role in this type of hemolytic anemia of the newborn. A dye mixture used to sterilize the umbilical cord or the routine administration of Vitamin K derivatives have been suggested as etiologic agents. In most cases, however, no definite exogenous agent has been determined beyond the suggestion of normal enzymatic immaturity of the newborn erythrocyte.[20]

In Negro term infants no increased incidence of jaundice has been observed in G-6-PD deficient groups. In Negro premature infants, G-6-PD deficiency has been found to be associated with an increased incidence of hyperbilirubinemia and a greater frequency of exchange transfusions.[212]

**Pyruvate kinase (PK) deficiency.** The erythrocytes conforming to the type II category of Selwyn and Dacie[319] are those previously mentioned in which the addition of glucose to the incubating blood fails completely or almost completely to reduce the rate of hemolysis. This type of congenital nonspherocytic hemolytic anemia is a homogenous group confined to patients with a deficiency of the enzyme pyruvate kinase and represents an inborn error involving the main pathway of glycolysis. Such are the cases first described by Valentine and his associates in 1961 and 1962[350,360] of a deficiency of the enzyme pyruvate kinase which in the red cells of certain patients was associated with a form of congenital nonspherocytic hemolytic anemia, the type II referred to. Since these reports, about a hundred documented cases of hemolytic anemia due to a similar hereditary deficiency of this enzyme have been described.[356]

In hemolytic anemia due to glucose-6-phosphate dehydrogenase deficiency the defect involves the hexosemonophosphate shunt. Another differential feature is therefore that in the pyruvate kinase deficiency there is impairment of synthesis of ATP, as contrasted with type I, in which glucose-6-phosphate dehydrogenase deficiency produces no fall in ATP. As was previously stated, De Gruchy and colleagues[104] had noted that supplementation of whole blood with ATP would prevent autohemolysis in the type II disorder even when glucose was ineffective. The conversion of phosphoenol pyruvate to pyruvate, the step located just above the terminal lactate dehydrogenase, is not completed for the lack of the enzyme pyruvate kinase. The failure to produce ATP interferes with the transport of sodium and potassium and shortens the erythrocyte life-span. As a result also of the deficiency of pyruvate kinase, abnormal accumulations of phosphoenol pyruvate, trioses, and particularly 2,3-diphosphoglycerate result. The very high content of 2,3-diphosphoglycerate first reported by Motulsky and co-workers[240] and confirmed by Robinson and associates[296a] is the metabolic hallmark of PK deficiency. It appears thus far that, except for G-6-PD deficiency, this is the commonest heritable disorder of the enzyme deficiency group.[356]

An autosomal recessive inheritance has been found in all adequately studied kindreds. Both sexes are affected. Although the heterozygous subjects are clinically normal, great variation exists in the severity of the disease in homozygotes.[187] The spleen is enlarged, and bone changes simulating those in other hemolytic anemias have been described. The clinical manifestations which appear in the newborn may be marked by hyperbilirubinemia and may require exchange transfusion. Anemia in the affected patients may be severe, moderate, or minimal. The spectrum of severity thus ranges from severe neonatal anemia with kernicterus at one extreme to a fully compensated hemolytic process in adults at the other. Reticulocytes are often markedly increased after splenectomy, although they are not unusually high before splenectomy.[187] The reticulocyte count continues to rise gradually with age, as the extremely high reticulocyte counts observed after splenectomy are found mainly in adults splenectomized in childhood.[187] Most patients exhibit macrocytosis, the red cells tend to lose potassium in vitro, and the affected cells may show spicule formation of the red cell membrane resembling acanthocytes.[250] The membrane defect is sufficiently gross so that the liver rather than the spleen is the primary site of destruction of the affected cells. As a consequence, hemolysis persists after splenectomy.[187] Removal of the spleen may be accompanied by significant improvement, at times decreasing transfusion requirements.[248] Although splenectomy has not been curative in most cases of pyruvate kinase deficiency, improvement has been noted in patients so treated. On the basis of their findings, Nathan and colleagues[248] recommend splenectomy in the management of severe hemolytic anemia due to pyruvate kinase deficiency. Removal of the spleen appears to improve the survival of the younger erythrocytes.

In a child with severe congenital nonspherocytic hemolytic anemia associated with a deficiency of erythrocytic pyruvate kinase, the red cells presented spicules on their surface. These were not unlike the cells found in acanthocytosis, but differed from the latter in having normal serum beta lipoprotein.[183] Lysis of red cells and the resulting anemia may have been due to the leakage of potassium out of the cells at an accelerated rate.[177] The combination of deficient glucose consumption and breakdown of ATP regeneration resulting from the demands for an increased inward pumping action were probably contributory factors to the death of the patient's cells.

The leukocyte pyruvate kinase activity is normal.[350,360]

In the patients reported by Bowman and Procopio,[31] the disease occurred in five severly affected children in whom the syndrome appeared in the fourth generation of Amish kindred and was transmitted as a mendelian autosomal recessive trait. Siblings in whom the disease was unrecognized died in infancy. Erythrocyte enzyme assays disclosed intra-erythrocyte pyruvate kinase deficiency in homozygotes and intermediate levels of enzyme in heterozygotes. The survival of red cells was shortened both in the circulation of normal subjects and in the homozygous anemic infants. Splenectomy halted the transfusion requirements of these patients. Atypical cases of heritable hemolytic anemia have been noted[265] that conform clinically and biochemically to anemias of the pyruvate kinase (PK) deficient type except for the presence of apparently adequate quantities of erythrocyte-PK activity by the usual assay procedure. Four such anomalous cases are reported occurring in two unrelated families. Autohemolysis was modestly increased, partially corrected by glucose and better corrected by adenosine triphosphate.

*6-Phosphogluconate dehydrogenase (6-PGD) deficiency.* Moderate reductions of this enzyme have been found with[268] and without[314] associated hemolytic anemia.

*Glutathione reductase (GSSG-R) deficiency.* In 1959 Deforges reported studies of a patient with sulfoxone-induced hemolytic anemia whose red cell G-6-PD activity was glutathione reductase activity of only 60% of normal and who later was found to have a that of a normal control.[108] One of the early cases reported was one of hemolysis during the administration of quinine and isopentaquine.[41,46] Originally reported as due to G-6-PD deficiency, this enzyme was later found to be normal but possessed between 50 and 60% of GSSG-R activity. Another patient, when treated for a urinary tract infection with Gantrisin, developed hemolysis and was also found to have a low GSSG-R activity only 38% of normal.[44] Additional cases have been reported from various parts of the world in one family after the ingestion of poisonous mushrooms.[43] An electrophoretically fast red cell GSSG-R with increased activity and an autosomal mode of inheritance has been found in a Negro outpatient population.[43]

*Glutathione (GSH) deficiency.* A marked diminution of the content of both reduced and oxidized glutathione in red cells was first described by Oort and associates in 1961.[255] Glutathione deficiency is associated with a mild nonspherocytic hemolytic anemia.[284] Glutathione deficiency appears to be transmitted as an autosomal recessive. Stomatocytes were observed in the case of an 18½-year-old male who also showed decreased concentration of reduced glutathione and a severe hemolytic anemia.[231] Splenectomy resulted in improvement of the anemia but did not cure the hematologic disease. It seems likely that glutathione deficiency is due to an incapacity of the red cell to synthesize glutathione.[20] The life-span of the glutathione deficient erythrocytes is markedly shortened.[284]

*Triosephosphate isomerase (TPI) deficiency.* In family members with hemolytic anemia resembling that of pyruvate kinase deficiency, a separate deficiency has been demonstrated, that of triosephosphate isomerase involved in the process of anaerobic glycolysis. The autohemolysis test resembles that seen in hereditary spherocytosis, namely, the marked hemolysis is well corrected by glucose and adenosine triphosphate.

In a 13-month-old girl of French-Negro ancestry a marked deficiency of a glycolytic enzyme, triosephosphate isomerase, was present in both the erythrocytes and leukocytes with the clinical findings of chronic hereditary hemolytic anemia.[311] Transmission was by an autosomal-recessive mode of inheritance and the symptom-free heterozygotes manifested an intermediate enzyme deficiency.

An atypical severe and progressive neurologic deficit involving peripheral nerves and cerebral nervous tissue has been noted in a small number of affected children who have survived the first few months of life.[356]

Among the slightly macrocytic erythrocytes are a number of densely contracted red cells with a contour similar to acanthocytes, as well as small numbers of nucleated red cells. Sickle cell trait and G-6-PD deficiency has been reported in the same kindreds with coexisting triosephosphate isomerase deficiency.[359]

*Adenosine triphosphatase (ATPase) deficiency.* Adenosine triphosphatase (ATPase) is a sodium-potassium magnesium dependent ouabain inhibitable ATPase generally considered to play a central role in the active transport of sodium and potassium across cell membranes.[356] Chronic, apparently inherited hemolytic anemia has been reported in patients in whom ATPase levels in the red cell fell below normal values.[155]

*Hexokinase (HK) deficiency.* Another inherited erythrocyte enzyme abnormality is a deficiency of erythrocyte hexokinase.[358] A patient first examined at birth had a bilirubin of 13.0 mg./100 ml. and had an exchange transfusion. Anemia persisted, as well as mild jaundice. With splenectomy, transfusions were eliminated but mild anemia persisted. The erythrocytes of this patient with congenital hemolytic anemia were shown to have a specific deficiency of the glycolytic enzyme hexokinase. The leukocytes and platelets had normal enzyme activity. Family studies suggested an autosomal-recessive mode of inheritance.

*Glucosephosphate isomerase (GPI) deficiency.* A Caucasian male of French and Irish descent showed hemoglobin values ranging between 4.7 and 6.8 gm./100 ml. of whole blood in the first 7 months of life. This congenital hemolytic anemia was due to a deficiency in another glycolytic enzyme, glucosephosphate isomerase (GPI), the catalyst specific for the second step of the Embden-Meyerhof glycolytic pathway.[15] The leukocytes are also involved. Family studies were consistent with an autosomal recessive mode of inheritance with the asymptomatic heterozygotes demonstrating an intermediate enzyme deficiency and the symptomatic homozygote, the propositus, demonstrating a marked enzyme deficiency. In a 13-year-old girl[268] first noted to be anemic at 3 months of age, transfusions were required every 1 to 3 months thereafter until splenectomy at the age of 13 months. No transfusions were required after 5½ years of age. Over the past 2 years hemoglobin has varied between 6.7 and 7.8 gm. per 100 ml., with 53 to 73% reticulocytes and 2 to 7 nucleated erythrocytes per 100 leukocytes. In three other children similarly affected, splenectomy was followed by objective improvement. As with many PK-deficient hemolytic anemias, splenectomy in all four cases of GPI deficiency has been followed by clinical improvement with diminution of transfusion requirements although with continuation of hemolysis and reticulocytosis.

*Phosphoglycerate kinase (PGK) deficiency.* A hereditary hemolytic anemia associated with a deficiency in the activity of phosphoglycerate kinase, a glycolytic enzyme in erythrocytes and leukocytes, had been reported in an adult Caucasian female[193] and in a large Chinese kindred.[357] In the latter group the propositus, a 12-year-old Chinese boy, was admitted for an anemia at 3 years of age. PGK activity in the assay had been less than 5% of normal. The data were consistent with the hypothesis of a deficiency that is X-chromosome linked.

*2,3-Diphosphoglycerate mutase (2,3-DPGM) deficiency.* A deficiency of this enzyme has been reported as a cause of congenital nonspherocytic hemolytic anemia.[30]

*Hereditary nonspherocytic hemolytic anemia with an altered phospholipid composition of the erythrocytes.* A hemolytic disorder with mild hyperbilirubinemia and reticulocytosis of 6 to 15% was documented in eight members of a large family from the Dominican Republic and was presumed to be present in eight other members.[170] Analysis of phospholipids revealed a distinct increase in phosphatidyl choline (lecithin) in erythrocytes of affected members of the family but not in the cells of unaffected relatives. The clinical picture presented by affected members of the family was that of a fairly well-compensated hemolytic disorder. The increase in autohemolysis corrected nearly to normal by the addition of glucose was characteristic of the hereditary nonspherocytic hemolytic disease classified under type I of Dacie.

There are cases of congenital and hereditary nonspherocytic hemolytic disease that cannot be strictly classified with the groups just discussed. In some of these an abnormal hemoglobin has been demonstrated which, because of an amino acid substitution, is less stable than normal hemoglobin. While these hemoglobinopathies present a picture of nonspherocytic hemolytic anemia, they are not due to deficiencies of glycolytic enzymes or defects in the hexosemonophosphate shunt; a feature common to all of these is the presence of Heinz bodies in the red cells (see Chapter 16). Hemoglobin Zürich was the first of the unstable hemoglobins to be so characterized. Drug-induced hemolytic anemia has been noted with hemoglobin Zürich[131,132] with the same drugs that cause hemolysis of glucose-6-phosphate dehydrogenase deficient red cells.

*Summary.* Hereditary nonspherocytic hemolytic anemia should be considered in patients who present the clinical picture of erythroblastosis at birth without the characteristic laboratory findings of the latter disease.[37] Hyperbilirubinemia of the indirect type in the first days of life necessitates exchange transfusion, as in erythroblastosis, before critical levels are reached. It is characteristic, however, of hereditary nonspherocytic anemia that chronic anemia persists following discharge of the patient from the hospital. The diagnosis is often made by exclusion from a heterogeneous variety of intrinsic blood disorders.

Frequent transfusions to maintain hemoglobin levels of approximately 7 gm. per 100 ml. constitute the only reliable form of therapy. Excessive blood requirements may lead to an extracorpuscular hemolytic defect,[194] in which case splenectomy is beneficial although the basic hemolytic process remains unaltered. The congestion with spherocytes which is characteristic of the spleen of the patient with hereditary spherocytosis is strikingly lacking in the splenic pulp of the patient with non-spherocytic anemia, although hemosiderin deposits are abundant. The value of splenectomy was pointed out in several of the congenital hemolytic syndromes, notably in pyruvate kinase (PK) deficiency and in glucosephosphate isomerase (GPI) deficiency.

### Hereditary elliptocytosis with hemolytic anemia

Hereditary elliptocytosis is an uncommon hereditary anomaly characterized by the presence of large numbers of oval and elliptical cells in the peripheral blood and is usually discovered on routine examination.[111] It is transmitted as an autosomal dominant; either sex may be equally affected. Elliptocytes are usually found in one parent, but, despite this unilateral inheritance, about 12% of the offspring bearing the trait[272] show evidences of a hemolytic anemia. In only a few reported cases have both parents been affected and in these the offspring gave evidence of a severe hemolytic anemia.[210,285,381] At birth elliptical red cells are few in number and do not appear in significant numbers until the third to fourth month of life, although jaundice and anemia may be present in the first month.[161,381] The nucleated precursors of the elliptical cells in the marrow are round, with the abnormal cells making their initial appearance in the reticulocyte stage or later. No abnormal hemoglobin has been detected in the cells of patients with hereditary elliptocytosis. The gene determining elliptocytosis is located in the same chromosome as that carrying the genes for the Rh blood groups.[140] There is no sickling in wet preparations.

Variable expression of a single dominant gene is the basis for the spectrum of clinical severity of the elliptocytic syndrome. In one family[178] where it was possible to trace fifty individuals with elliptocytosis, pedigree studies indicated strongly that affected members of the family were the descendants of a common ancestor. A high incidence (over 57%) of signs and symptoms of hemolysis was found among the affected individuals at one time or another.

While elliptocytes made up 80 to 90% or more of the blood picture, the degree of hemolysis varied from otherwise normal hematologic values to severe hemolytic anemia with markedly abnormal red cell morphology. The variation in gene expressivity is therefore considerable. Pearson[271] reported two pedigrees of elliptocytosis. In one family, double heterozygosity for the genes for G-6-PD deficiency and elliptocytosis did not result in hemolytic anemia. In the second family, a woman with benign elliptocytic trait had children with hemolytic elliptocytosis by two normal unrelated fathers. The findings in this family and other recent reports make variable expression of a single dominant gene the best explanation for the spectrum of severity of the hemolytic manifestations associated with elliptocytosis.

***Clinical and blood findings.*** The characteristic cells are oval, elliptical, sausage shaped, elongated, and rod shaped[129] and together constitute over 50% of the red cell population. Osmotic resistance is normal, except in patients with overt hemolytic anemia, in whom it is decreased. The condition is usually benign without symptoms or signs of anemia, notwithstanding the presence of elliptical cells in the blood (Fig. 29). In the patient with the severe hemolytic form, the peripheral blood shows ovalocytes, elliptocytes, microspherocytes, distorted microcytes, and fragmented forms. Small numbers of oval cells (1 to 15%) may appear in the blood of normal persons.[129] There is limited evidence that in subjects without overt hemolysis, the red cell life-span may be either normal or slightly shortened. With overt hemolysis, all grades of shortening may be encountered.[82] Typical aplastic crises may occur with pallor, severe anemia, sharp decrease in reticulocytes, bone marrow showing an increase in early forms, and lack of more mature nucleated elements. Oval cells are found in increased numbers in conditions other than hereditary elliptocytosis. Such are conditions in which anisocytosis and poikilocytosis are prominent, as in patients with iron-deficiency anemia, mild and severe Cooley's anemia, macrocytic anemia, and severe anemia associated with leukemia and cancer.[242]

It has been suggested that at least 25% of the red cells in the stained blood film should be oval, elliptical, or rod shaped before the diagnosis of elliptocytosis is made.[11]

In the uncommon hemolytic cases two grades of severity are observed, one with hemolysis without anemia and the other with hemolytic disease and anemia.[242] In both types, splenomegaly, hematologic evidences of hemolysis, and bone marrow regeneration make their appearance, and the life-span of the red cells, usually normal, is shortened.[221,242] While the spleen has been reported to be enlarged in most patients with hereditary elliptocytosis

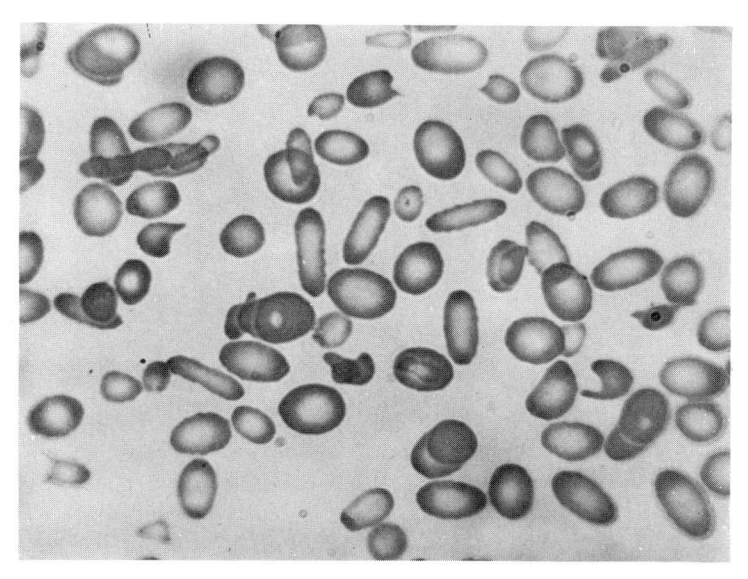

Fig. 29. Photomicrograph of blood smear of patient with hereditary ovalocytosis. Note larger number of elliptical, oval, and elongated cells. (×1200.)

and hemolytic anemia, in one series none of the six affected individuals showed splenomegaly.[371] Splenectomy was almost uniformly effective in relieving the hemolysis. In three generations of another family, seven members showed evidences of the disease, with uncompensated hemolysis in six. A remission was produced in the five patients subjected to splenectomy.[77] In one case megaloblastic anemia occurred in two pregnancies. The blood smear showed marked elliptocytosis, and it is possible that the patient may have had folic acid deficiency.

Three cases of hereditary elliptocytosis have been reported with hemolysis and hyperbilirubinemia in the newborn period requiring exchange transfusion.[7] The presenting morphologic picture was not diagnostic of elliptocytosis but of pyknocytosis. It was only later that the diagnostic picture of elliptocytosis appeared.

De Gruchy and co-workers[103] divide the cases of hereditary elliptocytosis into three groups. The first includes those without overt hemolysis in which the osmotic fragility (both of fresh and incubated blood), mechanical fragility, and autohemolysis are normal. The second includes those with overt hemolysis and no microspherocytosis. Here the osmotic fragility of fresh blood is normal, that of incubated blood is usually but not invariably increased, the mechanical fragility is usually increased, and the autohemolysis is increased. Finally, there are the cases with overt hemolysis and microspherocytosis in which the osmotic fragility of both fresh and incubated blood is increased, the mechanical fragility is usually but not invariably increased, and the autohemolysis is increased. When microspherocytes are present, as well as elliptocytes, signs of overt hemolysis are usually present.[103] De Gruchy and associates also suggested that the metabolic defect is a major factor in the premature destruction of cells in subjects with hemolysis. It seems probable that in hereditary elliptocytosis, as in hereditary spherocytosis, passage through the spleen stresses the red cell, bringing to light the metabolic defect, which in the absence of the spleen remains clinically latent. In their experience when microspherocytes as well as elliptocytes are present, signs of overt hemolysis are usually present. Considerable evidence now suggests that in hereditary elliptocytosis with hemolysis red cell destruction occurs mainly in the spleen and that splenectomy results in clinical remission. A low level of reduced glutathione and a deficiency of glucose-6-phosphate dehydrogenase have been found in association with elliptocytosis.[262]

In a genetic analysis, mutants at the elliptocytosis locus, which is linked to rhesus, tend to produce hemolysis less often or less severely than those at the locus or loci not linked to rhesus.[11]

Two New Guinea families with hereditary elliptocytosis have been reported.[285] All four patients demonstrated elliptocytes in blood films and the two fathers also had deficiency of red cell glucose-6-phosphate dehydrogenase activity. The parents of one family showed normal red cell survival, while there was evidence of increased red cell destruction in the parents of the other family. One child in each family had severe hemolytic anemia, and it is suggested that these were possibly homozygous for elliptocytosis. Splenectomy was performed in one case and resulted in clinical and hematologic improvement.

Diagnosis is made by the presence of elliptical cells in the patient, in a parent, and in other members of the family. Thalassemia minor, in which elliptical cells are also commonly seen, may be confused with elliptocytosis.[180] Elliptocytosis has been reported in association with other types of disease, among them the sickle trait.[124]

*Treatment.* Patients who are asymptomatic or give evidence of compensated hemolytic disease require no treatment. In addition to supportive treatment by transfusions, splenectomy has benefited most patients with severe uncompensated anemia.[27,210,242] Although red cell destruction is reduced, the characteristic oval and rod-shaped elliptical cells persist.

### Hemolytic anemia due to enzyme deficiency following administration of drugs and other agents

Beutler[19] summarizes the drug-induced blood dyscrasias as follows: the drugs most frequently associated with hemolytic anemia of this type are naphthalene, nitrofurantoin, salicylazosulfapyridine (Azulfidine), sulfamethoxypyridazine (Kynex, Midicel), aminosalicylic acid, and sodium sulfoxone (Diasone sodium). Most of these drugs can produce hemolysis of normal red blood cells when they are administered in doses larger than normal or when they are given to patients with impaired renal function.[19]

Favism, which occurs almost exclusively in enzyme-deficient subjects, is a hemolytic anemia caused by eating broad beans *(Vicia faba)* or from inhaling the pollen of the bean flower. In most, if not all, cases there is a low glutathione level in the red cells due to a deficiency of glucose-6-phosphate dehydrogenase enzyme. Not all persons with the enzyme defect are susceptible to the effects of eating broad beans. It has been demonstrated that the serum from normal persons as well as the serum from some patients with the enzyme deficiency can prevent normal red cells from becoming sensitized by an extract of beans. The serum from patients with favism does not possess this protective property.[302] Most, if not all, patients with favism are also susceptible to the hemolytic effect of primaquine.[18]

All individuals susceptible to favism probably have erythrocytes deficient in glucose-6-phosphate dehydrogenase. However, repeated exposure to fava beans does not provoke hemolysis in most enzyme-deficient individuals, and most patients who develop favism have previously been exposed to the bean without ill effects.[157] Confirmation of the hypothesis that enzyme deficiency is a necessary but not sufficient factor in favism comes from the experimental demonstration that the enzyme-deficient siblings of patients with favism did not manifest the disease when injected with a large dose of the fava bean extract.[142] There are different types of glucose-6-phosphate dehydrogenase deficiency, one of which predisposes the host to favism. This may explain why favism does not occur in all Negroes who have the enzyme deficiency.[188]

It is of interest that the fava bean appears to be a rich source of the amino acid L-DOPA, the drug used in the treatment of parkinsonism. Beutler[21] also points out that dopaquinone, the oxidation product of L-DOPA, has the capacity to destroy glutathione (GSH) in the lens, the metabolism of which has much in common with that of the red cell.

The clinical features of favism are reviewed in a later section of this chapter. Drug-induced hemolytic anemia may result from antibodies which, in the presence of the drug, agglutinate red cells. Among these are penicillin, quinine, quinidine, and acetophenetidin (Phenacetin).

Caucasian patients with erythrocyte glucose-6-phosphate dehydrogenase deficiency also have a deficiency in erythrocyte acid phosphomonoesterase, in contrast to Negroes in whom a deficiency of the latter enzyme is not present.[260]

The following agents are reported to induce hemolytic anemia in subjects with glucose-6-phosphate dehydrogenase deficiency*:

*Antimalarials*
1. Primaquine
2. Pamaquine
3. Pentaquine
4. Plasmoquine

---

*From Gross, R. T.: Bull. N. Y. Acad. Med. (Ser. 2) 39:90, 1963.

*Sulfonamides*
1. Sulfanilamide
2. Sulfapyridine
3. Sulfisoxasole (Gantrisin)
4. Salicylazosulfapyridine (Azulfidine)
5. Sulfamethoxypyridazine (Kynex, Midicel)
6. Sulfacetamide (Sulamyd)

*Nitrofurans*
1. Nitrofurantoin (Furadantin)
2. Furazolidone (Furoxone)
3. Furaltadone (Altafur)

*Antipyretics and analgesics*
1. Acetylsalicylic acid
2. Acetanilid
3. Acetophenetidin (Phenacetin)
4. Antipyrine
5. Aminopyrine (Pyramidon)
6. p-Aminosalicylic acid

*Others*
1. Sulfoxone
2. Naphthalene
3. Methylene blue
4. (?) Vitamin K
5. Phenylhydrazine
6. Acetylphenylhydrazine
7. Probenecid
8. Fava bean

*Infections*
1. Viral respiratory infections
2. Infectious hepatitis
3. Infectious mononucleosis
4. Bacterial pneumonias and septicemias

Increasing evidence emphasizes the importance of glutathione in maintaining red cell integrity and in allowing activation of enzyme systems through its reducing or protecting action.[102] The characteristics of the primaquine-sensitive erythrocytes are a decreased content of reduced glutathione, marked fall of glutathione after incubation of whole blood with acetylphenylhydrazine (glutathione stability test), and a deficiency of glucose-6-phosphate dehydrogenase. Both in vivo and in vitro exposure of the red cell to a drug of the primaquine type causes a further fall in the already decreased glutathione content.[23]

Glutathione exists in a reduced form (GSH) and an oxidized form (GSSG). The interconversion of these two is catalyzed by an enzyme, glutathione reductase, which requires reduced triphosphopyridine nucleotide (TPNH) for the reduction of glutathione. One of the principal sources of the required TPNH (which serves as a coenzyme) is the oxidation of glucose-6-phosphate to 6-phosphogluconic acid (successive intermediates in the direct oxidation of glucose) which is catalyzed by an enzyme glucose-6-phosphate dehydrogenase. It is this enzyme which is deficient in the red cells of persons sensitive to primaquine.[42] When this source of TPNH is unavailable because of enzymatic deficiency, the red cell is unable to maintain its glutathione in the reduced state.

Several relatively simple screening methods of detecting red cell glucose-6-phosphate dehydrogenase are available. Among these is a dye-decolorization technique,[241] a spot test,[125] and a methemoglobin test.[351] The later is based on observations that the rate of methemoglobin reduction by sensitive erythrocytes in the presence of methylene blue is markedly slower than normal. Modifications of this test can be employed to detect all individuals having the defect of sufficient severity to render them susceptible to hemolysis of clinical significance—i.e., fully expressed males and females and approximately 30 to 50% of heterozygous females. A simple colorimetric test is also available for the determination of reduced glutathione.[341] The normal glucose-6-phosphate dehydrogenase is 1.5 to 3 units per gm Hgb.

The glucose-6-phosphate dehydrogenase is in highest concentration in the younger cells of both sensitive and nonsensitive populations and is actually higher in the very young cells of the sensitive population than in the oldest cells of the nonsensitive population. The young cells of the sensitive population therefore, are resistant to hemolysis since they have enough enzyme to generate sufficient TPNH to keep the glutathione reduced. The defect in glutathione metabolism expresses itself in the older erythrocytes.

The red blood cells of susceptible persons who have a low glutathione level show an increased tendency to form Heinz bodies. The Heinz bodies are visible manifestations of oxidative damage to either hemoglobin and/or the stroma of the sensitive cells.[18] The chemical relationships between the drug and the oxidation of glutathione and between the oxidation state of the glutathione and hemolysis are not clear.

Utilizing radioactive labeling techniques ($^{32}$DFP and $^{51}$Cr), it has been demonstrated that red cells deficient in glucose-6-phosphate dehydrogenase die prematurely in vivo, even when not stressed by the presence of drugs.[33] Such studies indicate that this enzyme, or the pentose phosphate pathway of which it is a part, plays an important role in maintaining the red cell through a normal life-span. Catalase activity is only 60% of the normal in primaquine-sensitive cells.[352]

Similar mechanisms account for hemolytic anemia from exposure to fava beans,[344] naphthalene,[392] and vitamin K analogues.[391,392] Cells sensitive to primaquine have also been shown to be unusually susceptible to hemolysis by certain aniline derivatives, including sulfanilamide, phenacetin, Promizole, and acetanilid.[106] The fact that erythrocytes of sensitive persons are more susceptible to the in vitro Heinz body–forming action than are cells of nonsensitive persons serves as a valuable means of predicting primaquine sensitivity.[22]

A high proportion of asymptomatic parents and siblings of the affected person with a history of favism or hemolytic anemia due to drugs have a low glutathione content in their red cells[344] and a deficiency of glucose-6-phosphate dehydrogenase.[145] In a survey of randomly selected Negroes the incidence of persons sensitive to primaquine based on the glutathione stability test was found to be about 14% among males and 2% among females.[55] Among relatives of "reactors," males also predominated. The defects are apparently transmitted by a sex-linked gene with incomplete dominance.

The defect in glucose-6-phosphate dehydrogenase activity in erythrocytes is inherited as a sex-linked characteristic, with incomplete dominance in the heterozygous female. The defect is, therefore, transmitted by a gene of partial dominance carried on the X chromosome. Male hemizygotes ($\bar{X}Y$) and female homozygotes ($\bar{X}\bar{X}$) are invariably more severely affected than female heterozygotes ($\bar{X}X$) who manifest partial expression of the trait.[351] Apparent male-to-male transmission is rare. The usual picture is one of an intermediate female who produces reactive sons or intermediate daughters.[54] The mutant gene usually occurs in the more darkly pigmented racial ethnic groups and may reach a frequency of 50% in some populations. The geographic distribution is broad in tropical and semitropical areas and tends to parallel the occurrence of *Plasmodium falciparum* malaria against which it may have a biologic advantage.

Individuals with the electrophoretic variant A (fast) of G-6-PD have significantly lower parasite counts than those with the B (slow) variant of the enzyme. In a recently reported study,[20a] there was no evidence that enzyme-deficient males have greater resistance against malaria than normals.

Three patients were reported[505] who developed severe hemolytic anemia as a complication of acute viral hepatitis who offered evidence that the anemia was caused by destruction of G-6-PD deficient red cells. The hemolytic syndrome was characterized by a rapid decline in hemoglobin concentration accompanied by leukocytosis, reticulocytosis, and marked hyperbilirubinemia.

The defect in glutathione metabolism has been thoroughly investigated in relation to naphthalene-induced hemolytic anemia in infants and children.[102,392] Only a small percentage of children who have ingested naphthalene moth balls develop a hemolytic anemia and these are most often Negroes. Abnormal numbers of Heinz bodies also appear in the cells after incubation. The hemolytic effect is attributed not to naphthalene itself but to its derivatives. Transplacental passage of these compounds was noted in one case[392] in which both the mother and the newborn infant showed evidence of a hemolytic anemia after the mother ingested moth balls (Fig. 30).

A similar mechanism (glutathione instability) has been postulated for hemolysis occasionally encountered in newborn infants who are given excessive amounts of vitamin K at birth.[391]

From the group of diseases classified as hereditary nonspherocytic hemolytic anemia, one variety has also been found to possess the properties of primaquine-sensitive erythrocytes. These cells show a reduced glutathione content, markedly abnormal glutathione stability, and an extreme reduction of glucose-6-phosphate dehydrogenase. In this group similar defects also appeared in the families of these patients.[321,394] That a familial defect is not always in evidence was noted in a patient with congenital nonspherocytic hemolytic anemia, in whom the disease manifested itself in the absence of Gantrisin but was accentuated by the ingestion of this drug.[254]

### Nonhereditary hemolytic anemia— paroxysmal nocturnal hemoglobinuria (PNH, Marchiafava-Micheli syndrome)

Paroxysmal nocturnal hemoglobinuria, an uncommon type of chronic hemolytic anemia with an insidious onset, is characterized by attacks of hemoglobinuria occurring mainly at night. It is neither congenital nor hereditary. The attacks of hemoglobinuria are marked by the passage of dark urine, occurring during sleep regardless of the time of day. The disease occurs most commonly in adult life (usually

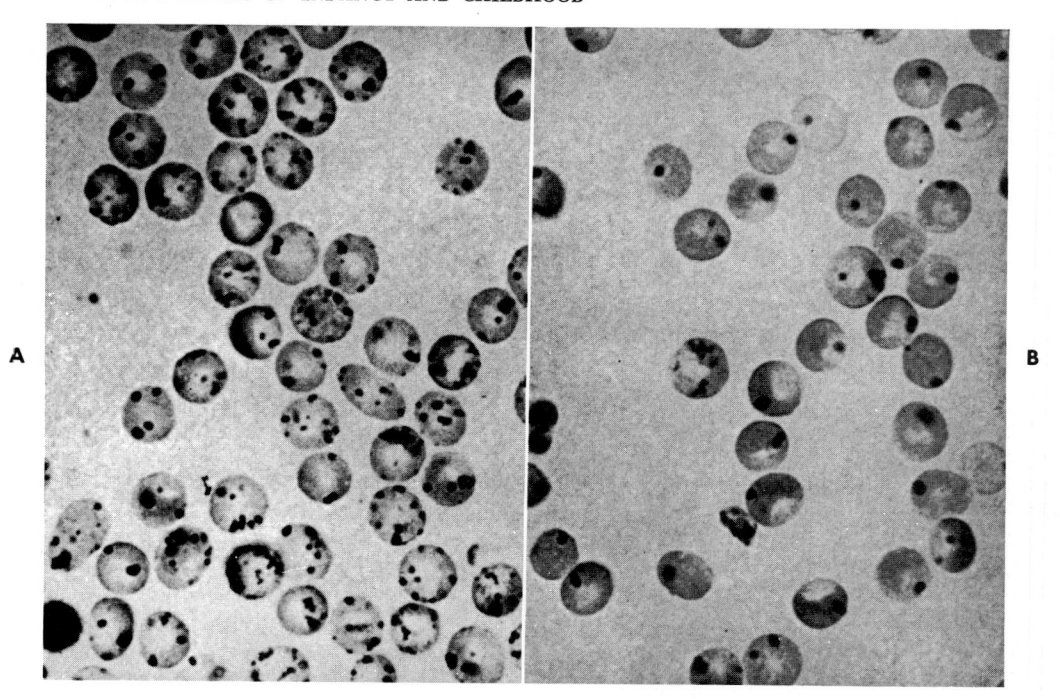

Fig. 30. Heinz body formation in sensitive, **A**, and nonsensitive, **B**, erythrocytes after incubation with 100 mg.% acetylphenylhydrazine solution for 4 hours (standard test procedure). Wet preparations stained with crystal violet. (×1300.) (From Beutler, E., Dern, R. J., and Alving, A. S.: Hemolytic effect of primaquine; in vitro test for sensitivity of erythrocytes to primaquine, J. Lab. Clin. Med. 45:40, 1955.)

the third decade), but a few cases have been described in children.[222,277] It is due to an inherent red blood cell defect, which makes the cells susceptible to hemolytic factors present in both the serum and plasma of normal persons and of the patient. These factors include complement, thrombin,[67] and properdin.[28] Properdin is a natural heat-labile serum protein which, in association with magnesium and complement, is involved in the destruction of bacteria and viruses.[278] The exact mode of action of these factors in hemolysis is complex and not yet established. The coagulation system also appears to be involved in some way in the precipitation of a hemolytic crisis. The red cells show a shortened survival when injected into normal subjects. Markedly reduced erythrocyte acetylcholinesterase activity which is localized to the stroma has been demonstrated in patients with this disease. This impairment possibly diminishes the integrity of the red cell.[6] A similar reduction in acetylcholinesterase activity is found in A-B-O hemolytic disease of the newborn.[182]

It has also been firmly established that the red cells of the PNH patient are exquisitely sensitive to lysis by complement.[86,300] The PNH erythrocytes appear to differ from normal cells in the availability of membrane sites for attachment of complement. The blood of patients with PNH have in effect two populations of erythrocytes—one, the "sensitive" population, is much more susceptible to lysis by complement than normal cells, while the other, the "insensitive" population, is more clearly normal in its susceptibility to lysis by complement but is usually not entirely normal.[195] These studies have also shown that the red cells of patients with PNH consist of a mosaic of distinct cell populations which differ in their content of acetylcholinesterase as well as in their sensitivity to complement lysis. The cells in the population most sensitive to complement lysis appear to have no acetylcholinesterase activity, whereas the cells in the population relatively insensitive to lysis have a somewhat reduced acetylcholinesterase activity. These cells, however, are somewhat more sensitive to complement than normal cells.

Bone marrow failure has been observed occasionally to occur during the course of this disorder. It has been well authenticated that PNH frequently develops on the basis of marrow hypoplasia and irrespective of whether the latter was of genetic, idiopathic, or drug-induced origin.[85] Many of the patients (approximately one-quarter) were originally diagnosed as having a drug-induced aplastic anemia in which red cell abnormality of paroxysmal nocturnal hemoglobinuria eventually developed.[89] There is, without a doubt, a complicated relationship between hypoplasia of the marrow and paroxysmal nocturnal hemoglobinuria. There are many reports of acute or chronic bone marrow failure occurring in the course of the disease or of pancytopenia rather than hemolysis being the dominant sign. In these patients with aplastic anemia an abnormality of the erythrocytes characterized by positive acid serum and thrombin tests are observed at some time during their illness.[286] It must not be supposed, however, that the paroxysmal nocturnal hemoglobinuria defect is a common phenomenon in aplastic anemia of either the congenital or acquired varieties.

A 7-year-old girl who presented initially with a typical picture of aplastic anemia eventually recovered after prolonged medical treatment and splenectomy.[299] She later developed the clinical and laboratory features of paroxysmal nocturnal hemoglobinuria. The deficiency in acetylcholinesterase activity was not limited to the erythrocytes but also was noted in the leukocytes.

Lewis and Dacie[209] described seven patients who suffered from the aplastic anemia–paroxysmal nocturnal hemoglobinuria syndrome. All had been diagnosed at first as having aplastic anemia. In discussing the relationship of these two diseases the authors postulated that the link between the diseases is the development of an abnormal clone of hemopoietic cells in a regenerating previously aplastic marrow. Survival studies in PNH showed increased rate of red cell destruction. The interrelationship between aplastic anemia and PNH varies from patient to patient. Some have signs of moderate or severe hemolysis but also evidence of chronic marrow hypoplasia and pancytopenia; others have one or more episodes of marrow failure of relatively short duration and finally there are others who appear to be suffering from typical aplastic anemia throughout their illness and in whom PNH is only a laboratory phenomenon.

There is much to indicate that PNH is not simply a peculiar hemolytic anemia but rather a disorder of the entire bone marrow.[94] Mature red cells are produced showing a variety of abnormalities: ready destruction within the circulation via complement, unusual reactivity with such antibodies as anti-I (cold hemagglutination), increased sensitivity to minor reductions in pH, reduced acetylcholinesterase activity. Pancytopenia is also present. The end result of such a myeloproliferative disorder may well be acute leukemia, myelosclerosis with myeloid metaplasia, polycythemia vera, and the DiGuglielmo syndrome. Cases of paroxysmal nocturnal hemoglobinuria have been reported which have terminated in acute myeloblastic leukemia.[165,176,186]

When the erythrocytes of paroxysmal nocturnal hemoglobinuria (PNH) are exposed to hydrogen peroxide they lyse excessively and form greater than normal quantities of lipid peroxide when compared to red cells of normal subjects and patients with most types of hematologic diseases.[226]

A patient (a 20-year-old male) with confirmed paroxysmal nocturnal hemoglobinuria was seen in an aplastic megaloblastic crisis.[267] The bone marrow initially was not hypoplastic for erythroid cells but showed maturation arrest at the megaloblastic level. Increased hemolysis was also evident. Classic helmet cells and schistocytes, most unusual findings in this disease, were found in the peripheral blood in the initial crisis. Folic acid and steroids were of value in treatment during crisis apparently by different mechanisms.

A rare disorder even in adults, paroxysmal nocturnal hemoglobinuria (PNH) had by 1967 been reported in only six children under 12 years of age and in an additional five adolescents under age 20. Two children in these groups[228] were: the first, a boy, presented at 7½ years of age with aplastic anemia; the second, a 15-year-old girl, was admitted initially with a Coombs positive hemolytic anemia, leukopenia, and thrombocytopenia. In the first case 5 years later the evidences of paroxysmal nocturnal hemoglobinuria were present. The second case had a course complicated by multiple thromboses requiring intravenous heparin therapy (approximately 100 units/kg. every 6 hours). In both patients the presence of chronic hemolysis, hemoglobinuria, hemosiderinuria, anhaptoglobinemia, positive acid hemolysis tests, erythroid hyperplasia in the bone marrow, with peripheral leukopenia, and thrombocytopenia, intermittent hemoglobinuria, decreased leukocyte alkaline phosphatase, and erythrocyte acetylcholinesterase activity was unequivocally consistent with a diagnosis of PNH. It is thought that the appearance of PNH after aplastic anemias may represent a somatic mutation of the hematopoietic tissue to the production of intrinsically abnormal cells.

Studies to date reveal no chromosomal abnormalities in paroxysmal nocturnal hemoglobinuria. Chromosome 21 shows no deletion or other abnormalities in this disease, despite the deficiency in both acetylcholinesterase and leukocyte alkaline phosphatase.[24]

Paroxysmal nocturnal hemoglobinuria has been described in association with sickle cell disease. One patient also had glucose-6-phosphate dehydrogenase deficiency.[274] It may be that latent paroxysmal nocturnal hemoglobinuria may be more common than generally believed and that its full expression may be dependent on coexistent hemoglobinopathies or erythrocyte enzyme deficiencies.

The patients are persistently anemic and slightly icteric and show a slight to moderate enlargement of the liver and spleen. They are fatigued, complain of headaches and abdominal and lumbar pain, and are febrile during a hemolytic crisis. Hemoglobinuria, hemoglobinemia, and hemosiderinuria which characterize the disease are evidence of intravascular hemolysis.

The blood picture reveals an anemia of varying severity with moderate reticulocytosis (10 to 20%), polychromasia, and macrocytosis. There is a tendency toward neutropenic leukopenia and thrombocytopenia. The leukocyte content of alkaline phosphatase is decreased below normal.[24,349] Lewis and Dacie[208] have found the neutrophil alkaline phosphatase is often very low or absent in the severe disease; in less serious cases it has been found to be normal or even above the upper limit of normal. Spherocytes are not present, and osmotic fragility is not increased. The bone marrow is hypercellular, indicative of increased regeneration, and rarely aregenerative. The serum bilirubin does not exceed 3 mg. per 100 ml. A tendency toward thrombosis in the systemic (including cerebral) and portal circulations accounts for varied symptomatology. The increased rate of hemolysis produced by lowering the pH of the blood has suggested that the mechanism of the disease is related to an accumulation of acid metabolites during sleep, inducing hemoglobinuria. Acute or chronic bone marrow failure rather than hemolysis has been observed.[90] Bone marrow aspiration reveals definite hypocellularity during such episodes.

In the differential diagnosis, the lack of a history of cold-precipitating hemolysis eliminates paroxysmal cold hemoglobinuria. Acute acquired hemolytic anemia (Lederer's anemia) in which hemoglobinuria is also present occurs commonly in children and is unaccompanied by pancytopenia or a congenital defect of the red cells.

The course is chronic, of varying severity, with occasional exacerbations often precipitated by infections. Death from anemia, thrombosis, and infection may occur. Prolonged survival, as well as spontaneous cures, has been reported. In one patient with moderately severe disease, hemoglobinuria ceased after 13 years and 7 years later recovery was complete.[90]

Some patients with PNH survive for many years. Three such patients have been reported with survivals of 43, 29, and 27 years.[51] Their histories and those of fourteen other patients who survived for more than 20 years suggest that prolonged survival is not necessarily related to amelioration of the disease. In spite of an apparent remission of the disease, laboratory abnormalities persist for many years.

Because of the wide variation in this disease, ranging from mild and refractory anemia to the classic case with marked hemoglobinuria, the concept has been put forward that paroxysmal nocturnal hemoglobinuria may represent a syndrome.[16] The basic findings of erythrocyte acetylcholinesterase deficiency, neutrophil alkaline phosphatase deficiency, and increased acid hemolysis constitute the features of a single disorder, although the clinical and laboratory findings show striking differences from case to case.

The diagnosis is confirmed by the Ham acid-serum test.[149] In a positive test the patient's cells undergo hemolysis in acidified normal serum at 37° C. Additional lysis of patient's cells can be achieved by addition of thrombin to the test.[66] A test based on the sensitivity of the red cells to high titer cold agglutinins shows a positive correlation with the acid-serum test.[82,91] The fact that they do not run exactly parallel may reflect a diversity of pathologic changes in different individuals and the effect of multiple causal mechanisms.

Another simplified diagnostic test for PNH is based on the observation that erythrocytes from such subjects are hemolyzed when incubated with autologous or isologous compatible normal serum or plasma in low ionic strength sucrose solutions.[158] The mechanism of this reaction remains to be established but appears to be related to the observation that normal cells as well as erythrocytes from PNH patients become loaded with complement components when incubated with serum diluted in sucrose solutions.

The "sugar-water" test is carried out for screening purposes as follows: one level tablespoon of commercial granulated sugar (sucrose) is dissolved in 3½ ounces (103 ml.) of distilled water or, alternately, 9 to 10 ml. of dry sugar in 100 ml. of distilled water. The pH of freshly prepared sugar-water was approximately 7.4. One volume of oxalated, citrated, or defibrinated whole blood is added to 9 volumes of sugar solution. The mixture is incubated at 37° C. for 30 minutes and centrifugated, and the supernatant is observed for hemolysis.

Sucrose hemolysis is greater than in the acid hemolysis test and frequently of the same order of magnitude as in the thrombin test. To date hemolysis of erythrocytes has been specific for PNH. No hemolysis has been observed in normal blood specimens and in a variety of non-PNH blood disorders. Blood collected in EDTA and in heparin should not be used. Also, 5% dextrose should not be substituted for sucrose.

There is no specific treatment. Splenectomy is disappointing, rarely beneficial, and potentially hazardous. Transfusion is the most beneficial form of treatment. Because of the possible hemolytic effect of plasma factors in the patient's erythrocytes, washed red cell suspensions have been employed with good results.

## ACQUIRED HEMOLYTIC ANEMIAS

The acquired hemolytic anemias embrace a group of heterogeneous disorders of varying etiology whose pathogenesis is dependent on an extracorpuscular mechanism rather than on an intrinsic defect of the red cell. They are classified as immune or nonimmune, depending upon whether or not an immune mechanism can be demonstrated. The immune group comprises those conditions in which antibodies contribute to the pathogenesis. They include autoimmune hemolytic anemia, erythroblastosis fetalis, transfusion reactions, and paroxysmal cold hemoglobinuria.

The nonimmune acquired hemolytic anemias appear after treatment with drugs such as quinine, phenylhydrazine and acetylphenlyhydrazine, sulfonamides, and arsenical compounds, after poisoning caused by chemicals such as naphthalene, benzene, and nitrobenzene, and after exposure to physical agents such as extreme heat or cold. They may follow infection by bacteria, bacterial products, viruses, and parasites. The action of these agents is characterized by direct destruction of erythrocytes or inhibition of immature forms in the bone marrow. Obviously, treatment necessitates elimination of the offending drug, chemical, or toxic agent.

Recent investigations have shown that such agents as sulfonamides, naphthalene, primaquine, and vegetable poisons (for example, fava bean) owe their action to a familial and intrinsic defect in the red cell which renders it susceptible to destruction. It is to be expected that other anemias in this group will eventually disclose the same relationship. In the case of favism,[224] as described in an earlier section of this chapter, ingestion of even small amounts of fava bean or inhalation of the pollen from the blossom of the plant produces in sensitive persons, especially children, a sudden acute attack of hemolysis accompanied by jaundice and often hemoglobinuria. The episode usually lasts less than a week and responds to transfusions. Favism occurs especially in Sicily, Calabria, Sardinia, and in countries about the Mediterranean. Sporadic cases have occurred in the United States and even England.[34] When due to pollen inhalation, the hemolytic episode may begin within a matter of minutes. After bean ingestion there is usually a lag period of 5 to 24 hours. The fresh and uncooked beans are thought to be more dangerous than those that have been dried or cooked. The presence of abnormal factors in the circulating blood or those adsorbed to the red cells has been of variable significance.

Hemoglobinuria occurs in severely burned patients with evidences of fragmented red cells, spherocytes, and increased susceptibility to osmotic and mechanical fragility.[150] The red cells with a shortened life-span appear to be destroyed intravascularly.

Hemolytic anemia and thrombocytopenia are present early in infants with congenital syphilis, often before the "classic" signs of syphilis develop. The anemia of congenital syphilis resembles that of erythroblastosis in many respects. Peripheral blood smears reveal normocytic, normochromic erythrocytes, (including macrocytes) with increased polychromasia and many nucleated erythrocytes. Reticulocytes are elevated. Penicillin therapy does not affect the anemia but platelet counts return to normal. Jaundice is frequent and is characterized by elevation of direct and indirect bilirubin.[372]

In newborn infants with congenital rubella a transient thrombocytopenic purpura, sparse numbers of megakaryocytes in the bone marrow, and evidence of a partially compensated hemolytic disease have been noted.[62,289,290] The latter was represented by fragmented cells, burr cells, teardrop forms, microspherocytes and target cells, transient anemia, normoblastemia, reticulocytosis, and erythroid hyperplasia of the bone marrow in the immediate neonatal period. Thrombocytopenia subsides in 1 month, whereas the bizarre morphology of the red cells and the reticulocytosis may persist for 3 months.

Malarial infection produces anemia by toxic inhibition of the marrow and actual parasitization of the red cells by the protozoa. The fulminating hemoglobinuria and severe associated clinical symptoms which occur in the condition known as blackwater fever occur in the majority of patients in the course of infection by *Plasmodium falciparum.*

The malarial organisms actually produce erythrocyte destruction through their presence in the erythrocytes. As the malarial parasites go through their cycle of development and invade and hemolyze new corpuscles, more anemia and deeper jaundice are produced. Methemalbuminemia, indirect hyperbilirubinemia, and hemoglobinuria appear. The anemia is of sudden onset and is severe; hemoglobin drops to low values. Constitutional symptoms are marked. In some cases death may occur from anemia and vascular collapse or renal failure. The attack is often precipitated by the ingestion of quinine. An autoimmune mechanism has been suggested as a causative factor.

Similar clinical and hematologic features occur in children in a form of acute acquired hemolytic anemia (Lederer's anemia, p. 336). The short, stormy course may simulate blackwater fever, but treatment with transfusions and adrenocortical steroids is usually effective.

Infection by organisms such as *Clostridium welchii* and *Bartonella bacilliformis* (in one of its clinical forms) is characterized by severe hemolytic anemia (Oroya fever). In this infection, which occurs in inhabitants of the central zones of Peru, Colombia, and Ecuador, numerous organisms invade the bloodstream, and stained smears reveal as many as 90% of the erythrocytes to be heavily invaded.[293]

A case of unsuspected toxoplasmosis in an adult with retroperitoneal fibrosis, profound anemia, hepatosplenomegaly, and marked erythroid hyperplasia of the bone marrow has been reported.[181] The identification of the organism as *Toxoplasma gondii* was made by electron microscopic recognition of its ultrastructural features.

In children and young people Wilson's disease may be combined with hemolysis.[214,223] The red cell half-life is shortened during the hemolytic crisis. During the acute hemolytic episodes large amounts of copper are excreted into the urine. The sudden release of copper from the tissues into the blood is associated with hemolysis of the red cells.[214,223]

Arsenic poisoning may be occasionally associated with a hemolytic anemia, leukopenia, and thrombocytopenia.[197] Bone marrow aspiration shows depressed or disturbed erythropoiesis. Hematologic abnormalities disappear within 2 or 3 weeks after cessation of arsenic ingestion.

Acute hemolytic anemia following the bite of unidentified insects was reported in two patients, one a child of 4 years. Severe hemoglobinuria, anemia, hyperbilirubinemia, and spherocytes were present. The clinical picture resembled the syndrome of necrotic arachnidism. Exchange transfusion has also been of value.[247] In another case the bite of a spider of a definitive species also produced severe hemolytic anemia.[233]

The immune acquired hemolytic anemias reveal antibodies in the blood which are detected by the Coombs (antiglobulin) test. These antibodies are globulins which are elaborated by the patient through some unknown mechanism and lead to premature destruction of the red cells—hence the designation of autoimmune antibodies. In patients with the hemolytic anemias caused by the agents enumerated previously, antibodies are only irregularly found. In persons with autoimmune hemolytic anemia, however, these antibodies play a dominant role in pathogenesis and constitute one of its major features.

Wallerstein and Aggeler[367] have recently reviewed the acute hemolytic anemias that occur in association with infections such as virus pneumonia, herpes simplex, infectious hepatitis, Newcastle disease, typhoid fever, malaria, bartonellosis, and infections with *Clostridium welchii,* hemolytic *Streptococcus,* and *Haemophilus influenzae.* In addition to being drug induced, acute hemolytic anemias also occur during the course of lymphosarcoma, Hodgkin's disease, infectious mononucleosis, acute glomerulonephritis, chronic ulcerative colitis, hemolytic-uremic syndrome, systemic lupus erythematosus, paroxysmal nocturnal hemoglobinuria, and thrombotic thrombocytopenic purpura. This type of anemia is characterized by bone marrow erythroid hyperplasia, the frequent presence of spherocytosis, Heinz bodies, methemalbuminemia, hemoglobinuria, and the absence of haptoglobins. The Coombs test was usually negative. The signs, symptoms, and laboratory findings depend to some extent on the stage of illness. Chills, high temperature, abdominal pain, and vomiting were initial symptoms. In the clinical management of these patients it was found important to prevent shock and acute tubular necrosis by transfusion and proper attention to fluid and electrolyte balance. Corticosteroids were seldom required. The prognosis for complete recovery was good in patients who had no serious underlying disease.[367]

The drug-induced acquired hemolytic anemias have been classified as follows[388]: (1) Immunologic—in which the drug induces serologically definitive changes in the susceptible individual that may or may not require the continuing presence of the offending agent for diagnosis. These drugs include acetophenetidin, alpha-methyldopa, chlorpromazine, penicillin, pyramidon, sulfonamides, quinidine, and quinine. (2) Metabolic—the genetically determined abnormalities in red cell metabolism described previously. The exposure to oxidant drugs (listed previously) results in Heinz body formation. Individuals whose erythrocytes are deficient in glucose-6-phosphate dehydrogenase have an inborn proclivity to hemolyze upon exposure to certain drugs or upon ingestion of fava beans. Next to blood group incompatibility, this metabolic error is the most common potential mechanism for hemolytic disease in man. (3) Hemoglobin instability—in which the amino acid substitutions have been localized to the region of heme. Such substitutions diminish the binding of heme by the affected globin chain. All these hemoglobinopathies (i.e., Hb Zürich and Hb Köln) are characterized by the presence of Heinz bodies in fresh and incubated blood and by increased thermolability of the hemoglobin. Drugs implicated in causing hemolytic anemia in this latter group include primaquine, sulfisomidines, sulfisoxazole, sulfaproxiline, and sulfamerazine.

Except for penicillin, alpha-methyldopa, and cephalothin, which will be discussed separately, the drug-induced immune hemolytic anemias cause a hemolytic anemia with these characteristics: the hemolysis is usually acute and intravascular, manifesting hemoglobinemia and hemoglobinuria; the dosage of the offending drug is low and there is usually a history of prior ingestion. The Coombs test is frequently negative, and the sera of affected patients will not react with normal cells unless the drug is also present.[388]

Several explanations have been offered for the formation of antibodies and the development of hemolysis. In one of these, antibody production is initiated from the drug becoming antigenic after combining with a soluble macromolecule.[227,324,388] On later exposure to the drug, the drug-antidrug complexes passively absorb the red cell which is regarded an "innocent bystander."[93] Either this complex or the initiation of the complement-fixation sequence damages the red cell. According to another hypothesis, the red cells act as a carrier for the drug in initiating antibody formation.[1] Readministration of the drug prompts specific interaction between antibody and the drug-carrier (red cell) antigen.

With penicillin administration, the hemolytic anemia is probably related to the presence of circulating antipenicillin antibody.[275] In many of the reported cases a positive direct Coombs test appeared. The direct Coombs test becomes weaker after cessation of the drug and gradually reverts to negative. Brisk hemolysis may occur and may persist for several weeks after cessation of penicillin administration.

The association of the positive Coombs test and hemolytic anemia with the antihypertensive drug alpha-methyldopa was first reported in 1966.[46,211,378,379] The severity of the anemia varies and is unrelated to the total dose of methyldopa. The Coombs reaction was entirely of the IgG type, the "warm antibody type." Fortunately the anemia responds rapidly to the withdrawal of the methyldopa. Incidence of a positive Coombs reaction rose with increasing the dose of the drug. The antibody can be easily eluted from patient's cells.[211,378,379] Of 572 patients on this medication, 20% showed a positive test but only two had overt hemolytic anemia. In another case, eluted antibodies were found to be related to the Rh complex.[10] The autoantibody population consisting of $\delta\beta$ globulins with both light and heavy chain subclasses was judged to be most compatible with a response of basically normal lymphoid tissue to some antigenic alteration brought about by alpha-methyldopa or a derivative.

In the majority of patients (forty-one of fifty-five cases) receiving antibiotic cephalothin at one hospital, a positive direct Coombs test developed, leading to difficulty in cross-matching.[236] This occurred especially in azotemic patients. Normal serum produced a positive Coombs test when incubated with cephalothin-coated cells. The median dose of drug was 4 gm. for patients with a positive Coombs test. The drug has the peculiar property of attaching itself or reacting with globulin, either plasma globulin on the surface of the red cell or cell membrane globulin. This causes a direct globulin reaction with Coombs serum. This drug, however, is unknown to cause hemolytic anemia.

## Autoimmune hemolytic anemia (chronic idiopathic autoimmune hemolytic disease, chronic acquired hemolytic anemia)

Autoimmune hemolytic anemia is characterized by the presence of demonstrable abnormal antibodies in the blood which are produced by the body and are directed against its own red cells. In this phenomenon an important factor is the coating of erythrocytes with an antibody of unknown nature, which renders the cells more susceptible than normal cells to erythrophagocytosis by the reticuloendothelial system. The causation may be unknown and hence be idiopathic or symptomatic of an underlying disorder. The latter disorders include chronic leukemia (mainly chronic lymphocytic leukemia), the lymphomas (Hodgkin's disease, follicular lymphoblastoma, reticulum cell sarcoma, and lymphosarcoma), disseminated lupus erythematosus and other collagen diseases (scleroderma, polyarteritis nodosa, dermatomyositis), neoplasms, and liver disease. Autoimmune hemolytic anemia also occurs with virus pneumonia in the second or third week of illness and after the onset of infectious mononucleosis. Recent studies have shown that 80% of patients with autoimmune hemolytic anemia were of the secondary or symptomatic type; the remainder were primary or idiopathic.[307]

*Clinical features.* Autoimmune hemolytic anemia occurs at all ages and has been reported in infants of 6 weeks,[294] 2½ months,[199] and 5 months of age.[78] The disease is usually chronic with an insidious onset and is prone to exacerbations of severe hemolytic anemia. In children, pallor, lethargy, fatigue, anorexia, and low-grade fever are common. Mild to moderate jaundice is present in about 75% of the patients. The spleen is usually palpable and varies in size; when it is greatly enlarged, an underlying disease should be suspected. Moderate enlargement of the liver is frequent, and lymphadenopathy is absent. Purpura is indicative of a secondary condition. Hemoglobinuria is unusual and is an occasional accompaniment of a hemolytic episode.

A type of autoimmune hemolytic anemia has been described in which a depression of red cells and reticulocytes in the peripheral blood is associated with a temporary disappearance of erythroblasts from the bone marrow.[114,136] This is explained by antibodies acting peripherally on erythrocytes and reticulocytes and in the bone marrow on the erythroblasts.

The rarity of autoimmune hemolytic anemia in early infancy has been construed as confirmation of the infant's limited ability to produce antibodies. However, the ability of the newborn infant to form antibodies has undergone critical reappraisal. With strong stimuli there is evidence that better responses may be produced.[294] In an infant with autoimmune hemolytic anemia reported by Ritz and Haber,[294] it seems that good antigenic capacity existed before the age of 6 weeks. A 7S agglutinin was demonstrated to be quite distinct from any antibody present in the mother. In this infant the bone marrow was almost devoid of erythroid precursors at a time when the Coombs test was strongly positive. Such aplasia has been interpreted as caused by bone marrow suppression, by viral infection, or by the antibody itself. The infant did not respond to relatively large doses of prednisone initially, but subsequently improved with ACTH therapy. He was maintained on prednisone and at 17 months was well without medication. The spleen was not enlarged at any time in the clinical course.

*Blood findings.* The blood picture varies with the extent of the anemia and the degree of bone marrow compensation. The hemoglobin usually ranges between 10 and 11 gm. per 100 ml. but may drop to levels of 3 to 5 gm. per 100 ml. in an acute attack. The blood smear shows a persistent reticulocytosis (up to 60% in severe hemolytic episodes), polychromatophilia, microspherocytosis, anisocytosis, and often a tendency toward macrocytosis. Spherocytosis is marked in the active phase and is less noticeable when the disease is quiescent. Normoblasts appear in small numbers. Erythrophagocytosis by monocytes and sometimes by neutrophils may be seen in the blood smear and in greater numbers from the buffy coat of incubated venous blood.[393] The polymorphonuclear leukocyte count varies during chronic periods and may be greatly elevated during an exacerbation. In one of our patients the total leukocyte count rose to 94,300 per cubic millimeter. The platelet count is usually normal but may be depressed. Thrombocytopenia has been interpreted as part of the immune antibody mechanism in which the red cells are intensely involved.[118,120] Simultaneous occurrence of thrombocytopenia and autoimmune hemolytic anemia is well recognized and is referred to as the Evans syndrome. Dausset and Colombani,[99] in a review of eighty-three "idiopathic" warm antibody cases, encountered thrombocytopenic purpura in eleven (13.2%) patients. In three instances the purpura had preceded the hemolytic anemia, in five it developed spontaneously, and in three the purpura developed after the hemolytic anemia. The serious nature of this association has been emphasized in many papers.[75,83]

Osmotic fragility and autohemolysis are both increased and parallel the degree of spherocytosis. The bone marrow is hyperplastic. An aplastic crisis indicated by reticulocytopenia, leukopenia, and erythrocytic aplasia of the bone marrow is rare. In an infant with a strongly positive direct and indirect antiglobulin test the bone marrow was hypoplastic for 7 weeks.[294] The major fraction of increased hemolysis occurs in normal extravascular sites with the formation of excessive amounts of bilirubin. With unimpaired liver function the bilirubin level is not greatly elevated and usually ranges from 1 to 4 mg./100 ml. in quiescent periods.

Rarely, acquired hemolytic anemia may be associated with a megaloblastic marrow and a macrocytic blood picture. A depletion of vitamin $B_{12}$ and/or folic acid may have been induced by the excessive erythroid turnover since the administration of either factor converts the marrow to a normoblastic state.[375]

*Serologic findings.* Three different autoantibodies affect the red cells in autoimmune hemolytic anemia: autoagglutinins, autohemolysins, and incomplete antibodies, permitting agglutination by antiglobin serum (Coombs test). The blood of patients with autoimmune hemolytic anemia commonly undergoes rapid spontaneous autoagglutination after withdrawal from the body, resulting in clumping of the red cells, so that blood counts are difficult. The autoantibodies may be nonspecific and therefore act as panagglutinins and panhemolysins. They react with normal erythrocytes in addition to the patient's own cells regardless of blood group or type. In some cases (about 30%) the sera react specifically and usually with well-recognized blood group antigens within the Rh system.[88]

The antibodies may be absorbed on the surface of the red cells, in which case they are detected by the direct Coombs antiglobulin test or are free in the serum. Their presence in serum may be demonstrated by the indirect Coombs technique in which normal red cells are initially exposed to the patient's serum before testing with the Coombs antiglobulin reagent. In neither case does the intensity of the Coombs test bear any relationship to the severity of the disease. The warm antibody can be eluted from the red cells and will then combine with most normal cells.[119]

An autoantibody refers to the production by an individual against an antigen that he himself possesses. Isoantibody refers to antibody production by an individual after introduction of antigen from another member of the same species.

For many years it has been known that the red cells of patients with autoimmune hemolytic disease may be coated or sensitized with gamma globulin, accounting for the positive Coombs test. More recently, however, it has been recognized that there are other cases in which the red cells have not been agglutinable by an antigamma globulin rabbit serum, but rather by an antiserum to whole human serum. Such an antiwhole serum can be exhastively absorbed with gamma globulin and still agglutinate these cells. Cells undergoing this latter type of agglutination are cells coated with a nongamma globulin. Some patients' red cells are agglutinated by both antigamma and antinongamma globulin sera and have, therefore, been said to be coated simultaneously by gamma and nongamma globulins. It has been suspected that the nongamma coating may be attributed to attachment of complement portein to the cells.[202]

Two types of antiglobulin reactions have been enumerated in patients with acquired hemolytic disease: those due to coating of the patient's red cells with autologous globulins, and those due to coating with autologous complement protein.[364] In two-thirds of the cases of idiopathic acquired hemolytic disease (hemolytic disease without any recognized underlying disorder), sensitization with globulins occurred. In the remaining third, the red cells exhibited complement sensitization. In patients with hemolytic disease accompanying systemic lupus erythematosus or other connective tissue diseases, the frequency of complement sensitization was much greater.

Two types of autoantibodies can be distinguished by their behavior in vitro: a warm type, active at 37° C. (the more common in the idiopathic autoimmune disease)[89] and the clinically infrequent cold type, active at temperatures of 4° C. High titer cold agglutinins are potentially hemolytic.[79] Both types give positive direct antiglobulin (Coombs) reactions.[81] Autoagglutination by cold antibodies is abolished at 37° C. Anemia, reticulocytosis, and spherocytosis are not as conspicuous as in the patient with the hemolytic anemia with warm agglutinins. Hemolytic anemia associated with high titer cold hemagglutinins are principally found in patients with virus pneumonia. In older persons they are also active in the development of a rare form of chronic hemolytic anemia with hemoglobinuria, high titer cold hemagglutinins, and Raynaud's phenomenon.[57,339] Cold antibodies are also involved in the pathogenesis of paroxysmal cold hemoglobinuria. The Donath-Landsteiner test which is diagnostic of this disorder requires cold for the union of antibodies with the red blood cells and warmth together with complement for eventual lysis. The titer of cold agglutinins is low in comparison with the elevated titer of agglutinins in patients with viral pneumonia.

Patients with acquired hemolytic anemia and negative Coombs tests have been described in whom IgG antibodies on the red cell surface have been identified by a sensitive complement-fixing antibody consumption technique.[138a] Thus immunohemolytic anemia may occur with concentrations of red cell autoantibodies below that necessary to produce agglutination by antihuman globulin (Coombs) serum.

Cold agglutinins are usually macroglobulin antibodies which agglutinate red cells strongly at reduced temperature and which usually cause little or no agglutination at body temperature. They are present in high titer in the serum of patients who have hemolytic anemia and cyanosis and other peripheral vasomotor phenomena of the extremities on exposure to cold.

It has been pointed out[201] that cold agglutinins will agglutinate all human red cells at 0° C. Those cold agglutinins which agglutinate normal adult red cells (adult "I" cells) more strongly than the cells of rare adults (adult "i" cells) or of newborn infants (cord "i" cells) are said to have specificity for the "I" antigen. Those antibodies which agglutinate adult "i" cells or cord "i" cells more strongly than adult "I" cells are said to have specificity for the "i" antigen. The studies of Rosse and Sherwood suggest that the difference between adult red cells and cord (or adult "i") red cells with regard to the fixation of cold agglutinin antibody is due in large part to a difference in the "affinity" of the antibody and the antigen on the red cell surface rather than to a major difference in the number of antigen sites.[201] These studies also suggest that the content of "I" antigen in adult "I" cells is not so different from cord "i" or adult"i" cells as the nomenclature would indicate.

Cold agglutinins can usually be demonstrtaed in cord blood but only if present in the mother's blood.[235] In general, autoimmune hemolytic anemia due to cold antibodies is fairly infrequent (7.7% in one series).[99] Clinically, it is characterized by the rarity of splenomegaly, the chance of cold paroxysmal hemoglobinuria and of Raynaud's syndrome, and, serologically, by the presence of a cold acid hemolysin along with an increased titer of cold agglutinins.[99] Complement is diminished or absent.

In all cases with cold antibodies, exposure to low temperature has to be carefully avoided. Steroids appear to be of less benefit than in the warm antibody type of disease. Cold antibodies probably do not exist in a demonstrably incomplete form. Agglutination by antiglobulin serum of red cells exposed to these antibodies is due to an interaction between the antiglobulin serum and sub-hemolytic amounts of adsorbed complement rather than between the antiglobulin serum and antibody. The reaction with antiglobulin serum is due to adsorption of complement on to the red cells, and it is, therefore, not inhibited by the addition of gamma globulin to the antiglobulin serum.[87]

Study of the autoantibodies of acquired hemolytic anemia has demonstrated that the warm types of antibodies are 7S gamma globulin and that the cold antibodies are 19S macroglobulins.[83]

A powerful antibody found in the serum of certain patients suffering from cold antibody hemolytic anemia has been designated as anti-I and its antigen as I. Fetal red cells and those of newborn infants contain mostly the i antigen and correspondingly less I, the latter becoming fully developed after about 18 months of life. (See Chapter 6 for a more complete discussion of this subject.)

In autoimmune hemolytic anemia antibodies have been known to develop against stored red cells. They were associated with false positive serologic reactions for syphilis. Stored cell antibodies may be rapidly identified by replacing the stored reacting cells with fresh cells from the same donor. Antigen may arise during storage by the action of intracellular enzymes reacting with a basic substance present in all red cells.[177]

Cryoglobulins, proteins that precipitate in the cold and redissolve on heating to 37° C., have been demonstrated in the serum of patients with autoimmune hemolytic anemia.[59]

**Pathogenesis.** It is of interest that the body in health avoids forming antibodies against its own tissues, a tolerance developed from early fetal life.[80] Such dire circumstances in which a living organism becomes capable of producing antibodies against its own body components has been termed "horror autotoxicus" by Ehrlich.[377] This situation apparently exists in autoimmune hemolytic anemia with the loss of normally acquired tolerance and the development of antibodies to the patient's own red cells.[377]

The situation in which abnormal autoantibodies are produced against the patient's own red cells in acquired hemolytic anemia and platelets in thrombocytopenic purpura has been explained by Burnet[39] to result from a breakdown of immunologic homeostasis. According to this concept, a physiologic state is established in fetal life in which immunologic tolerance for all normal body constituents develops. When the inhibitors controlling immunologic homeostasis disappears because of infections or environmental factors such as ionizing radiation or through mutation, immunologic competent cells, previously sequestered, emerge in the form of "forbidden clones." These emerging cells are capable of producing abnormal antibodies against the patient's own normal tissue and blood cells. Immune tolerance, usually present, is disrupted and an antibody is produced against some tissue of the patient, in this instance the red cell.[39]

The simultaneous attacks on the different blood elements in the same destructive process was emphasized by Evans and co-workers,[118,120] who observed that acquired hemolytic anemia with sensitization of the red cells is often accompanied by thrombocytopenia. Primary thrombocytopenia in turn frequently coexists with red cell sensitization with or without hemolytic anemia.

The formation of autoantibodies has also been ascribed to other mechanisms[79]: an alteration of patient's erythrocytes, making them foreign to his own antibody-forming mechanism and thus permitting the development of anti-red cell antibodies or the formation of abnormal proteins by the patient with an abnormal reaction on the part of his antibody-forming tissue. False positive Wassermann and Kahn tests sometimes found in patients with this disease fit in with the latter hypothesis.[79]

Zuelzer and associates[397] have drawn attention to the possible etiologic relationship of chronic acquired hemolytic anemia of autoimmune type to viral infection, most commonly the cytomegalovirus. In the young, lymphadenopathy was a prominent finding in the majority of cases and appeared to correspond to periods of rapid virus multiplication. In a later communication,[396] long-term studies of autoimmune hemolytic anemia in twenty-eight children were presented. These patients were separated into three groups: the first were patients of low age, acute onset with early full recovery, and normal immunoglobulins; a second showed a wide age range, acute onset, chronic course, occasional purpura, eventual recovery, and abnormal immunoglobulins. Dysgammaglobulinemia persisted long after cessation of hemolysis and lymphadenopathy of minor degree was often present. The third group had an indeterminate onset, frequency of growth failure, purpura, neutropenia, massive lymphadenopathy, and waning in parallel with hemolytic episodes, various illnesses and complications, high mortality, indefinite duration, and abnormal immunoglobulins, mostly IgA deficiencies. Splenectomy in this group was followed by cessation or decrease of hemolysis in half the patients, but the general condition did not improve. Neutropenia when present was unaffected. Chromosomal abnormalities were common in all groups but were not of a specific character. In these three categories the assumption that occult virus is essential for the development of autoimmune hemolytic anemia is based on the large number of cases in which at least one virus, the cytomegalovirus, could be incriminated on histopathologic or virologic grounds. It is noteworthy that five of the twenty-eight cases were under 1 year, ranging from 10 weeks to 5 months of age, but these are not always associated with a positive Coombs test at the onset.

*Destruction of sensitized red cells.* The spleen, liver,[174] and other portions of the reticulendothelial system contribute, by as yet unknown mechanisms, to the destruction of red cells coated by antibodies. Much evidence has isolated the spleen as the important organ in which sensitized red cells are filtered from the circulation, trapped and sequestered, phagocytosed, and lysed.[230,383] Spherical red cells are particularly susceptible to lysis.

Red cells coated with warm antibodies are sequestered in the spleen and antiagglutinin action seldom occurs. Red cells coated with cold antibodies are sequestered in the liver, bind complement at subnormal temperatures, agglutinate at a normal or near normal temperature, and may lyse spontaneously in the intravascular compartments.[238]

*Diagnosis.* For the diagnosis of autoimmune hemolytic anemia the following criteria have been specified[307]: a direct positive globulin test, suggestive evidence that the globulin which coats the red cell is an antibody produced by the host, and the coating antibody must be presumed to be responsible for damage and consequent shortened survival of the red cell.

The diagnostic features of autoimmune acquired hemolytic anemia consist of anemia, reticulocytosis, jaundice, splenomegaly, and elevated serum bilirubin with a positive Coombs test. A positive Coombs test in patients with acquired hemolytic anemia in contrast to the negative test in those with hereditary spherocytosis is helpful in differentiating the two conditions, since spherocytosis and reticulocytosis occur in both. In all patients with hemolytic anemia with a positive Coombs test, search should be made for one of the underlying diseases previously enumerated.

*Treatment.* Steroid hormones, blood transfusions, and splenectomy constitute the basis of treatment. Cytotoxic drugs to suppress immune responses are being carefully scrutinized.

*Adrenocortical steroids.* Cases of autoimmune acquired hemolytic anemia and often symptomatic cases usually respond favorably to hormonal therapy. Permanency of improvement with these agents has not yet been thoroughly ascertained. The steroid hormones either alone or combined with splenectomy represent the treatment of choice. As with other blood disorders in which steroid hormones are used, dosage must be individualized.

Prednisone or prednisone-like compounds are most commonly given initially in a total daily dosage of 2 mg. per kilogram of body weight divided in three or four doses. When the response of the patient and the severity of the disease are ascertained, the dosage may be adjusted accordingly. In favorable cases the dose is reduced within a week. This is marked by a fall in the reticulocyte count, a rise in the number of red blood cells and hemoglobin, and a reduction in the number of transfusions and their elimination. Once a remission is obtained, the steroid hormone is gradually reduced to a maintenance dose which, in our experience, is approximately 15 mg. daily. With relapse the initial dose is restored. In spite of improvement, a positive Coombs test may persist and should prompt an alertness to recurrences of the hemolytic state. If prednisone or a substitute fails to achieve a remission, ACTH should be tried before or after splenectomy. In summary, steroid hormones in adequate dosage represent a remarkably effective form of therapy, especially in the initial control of this disorder.[95] It has been estimated that from 70 to 80% of the patients with warm antibodies respond to steroid treatment.[139] As already stated, this response is less striking in patients with cold antibodies.

Cytotoxic agents capable of suppressing immune responses have been employed in the treatment of autoimmune hemolytic anemia and other conditions suspected of being immunologic in nature. The mechanism by which these agents exert their effects in blocking the production of antibodies against erythrocytes and other tissue elements is still unclear. Dameshek[97] has suggested that antimetabolites check the proliferation of abnormal antibody forming cells, presumably located in the lymphoid and reticuloendothelial tissues. 6-Mercaptopurine has been shown not to inhibit in vitro antigen-antibody union.[96] It remains to be determined whether beneficial results stem from a direct local effect on mononuclear cells in general, or on a small fraction of cells capable of participating in inflammatory reactions, or by an indirect effect in suppressing antibodies.[105]

Following the demonstration that 6-mercaptopurine (6-MP, Purinethol) could suppress immune responses in the experimental animal, this agent was used in human autoimmune disease. The same dosage as in leukemia, 2.5 mg. per kilogram, was employed.[313] Its use in a small series of patients produced beneficial results in a substantial percentage.[312]

Remissions have been obtained in systemic lupus erythematosus and other collagen diseases (dermatomyositis, neurodermatitis, scleroderma) with the use of another purine antagonist, 6-thioguanine.[105]

The immunosuppressive drug azathioprine (Imuran) has been successfully used in autoimmune hemolytic anemia in three infants—two at 3 and 4 months of age, respectively, and another at the age of 2 years.[163] One case was complicated with a rare hemoglobinopathy which may have been coincidental. Corticosteroid treatment in large doses was partially and temporarily effective in controlling the disease. Immunosuppressive therapy (azathioprine [Imuran], 2 to 5 mg./kg./day) produced a complete cure in one case and a marked decrease in steroid dosage in the other two cases. The authors caution that, before starting immunosuppressive treatment, a course of primary immunization (in infants) or a booster injection (in older children) with the normal antigens should be given to take advantage of the child's own antibody-forming capacity as much as possible.

It has been emphasized that these drugs are toxic, and routine use of antimetabolites cannot be recommended. Only when splenectomy and steroid therapy have failed in autoimmune hemolytic disease should 6-mercaptopurine be administered. The use of this and other chemical agents such as triethylenemelamine, chlorambucil, cyclophosphamide,[353] and 6-thioguanine in autoimmune disease await further assessment.

*Transfusions.* Blood transfusions are given when the hemoglobin level drops below 7 to 8 gm. per 100 ml. and are repeated in accordance with the demands of the patient to maintain normal activity without discomfort. Transfusions represent supportive therapy but do not alter the hemolytic process. Although of temporary value, they play an important role in tiding the patient over a severe hemolytic episode. In the severe case the transfused cells are rapidly destroyed, and the hemoglobin rise is not maintained. The extrinsic mechanism in this disease (the autoimmune antibodies) destroys not only the patient's cells but also transfused normal cells.

The presence of autoantibodies frequently interferes with the typing and cross-matching of blood. In these cases the least incompatible blood is utilized pending the effect of steroid hormones. Careful cross-matching, slow administration of blood, and alertness to reactions are essential. Occasionally, it is not feasible to maintain a hemoglobin at optimal levels, and the patient is required to make appropriate adjustments until other modes of therapy are introduced. Replacement transfusion was successfully employed in a patient with severe hemolysis with dramatic, although temporary, response. The purpose of this procedure was to remove large amounts of antibody and antibody-coated red cells.[32]

*Splenectomy.* Prior to the advent of ACTH and corticosteroid therapy, great reliance was placed on splenectomy for treatment. Results were unpredictable, however, and the recovery rate when splenectomy was done as an initial procedure was estimated as approximately 50% in patients with autoimmune hemolytic anemia. Permanency in the favorable case was extremely uncertain. Since autoantibodies are produced in large measure by the spleen, removal of this organ would be expected to result in a sharp decrease in their concentration. The variable effect of splenectomy, however, indicates that the spleen may not be the sole source of antibody.

At present, splenectomy is reserved for patients in whom steroid therapy alone is inadequate, especially when excessively large doses of prednisone are required to control the hemolysis without inducing serious metabolic side effects. Following splenectomy, the resumption of steroid hormones is usually necessary. At present, steroid therapy represents the treatment of choice and splenectomy should be reserved for those patients who fail to respond to hormone therapy.[53]

That splenectomy has a prejudicial effect on the course of lupus erythematosus when acquired hemolytic anemia complicates this disease has been challenged. On the contrary, splenectomy has been advised in the event that steroids do not satisfactorily control the hemolytic anemia.[306]

There are, however, no well-defined criteria on which to base the decision for splenectomy. In children the interference with growth by adrenocortical steroids and the other complications of hypercorticism, not the least of which are the embarrassing disfigurements, compel a consideration of splenectomy. The diminution in antibody titer and, in some cases, the disappearance of the positive Coombs' test following splenectomy suggest that the spleen acts both as a site of antibody production and destruction of sensitized cells. By some, extreme spherocytosis serves as an indication of successful splenectomy. In vivo studies with red cells labeled with $^{51}$Cr using a surface counting technique will aid in selection of the case with major blame on the spleen. If not entirely successful, it is sometimes possible to control the anemia with smaller doses of hormone than were required before splenectomy.

*Thymectomy.* On the basis that the thymus was the primary source of autoantibody-producing clones of cells,[40] this organ was removed in two infants with severe autoimmune hemolytic anemia.[185,376] In one infant in whom severe hemolytic anemia dated from 2½ months of age, thymectomy was performed 4 months later. The other was an infant whose hemolytic process started at 10 months of age and in whom the thymus was removed 2 months later. In both infants the hemolytic process could not be controlled by transfusion, corticosteroids, or splenectomy. At the last report, 6 and 7 months postoperatively, transfusions were no longer required in either patient, and in the second case negative direct and indirect Coombs tests were recorded. While spontaneous remissions are known to occur in this condition, the complete recovery after thymectomy is still intriguing. At this writing this measure is certainly not advocated, except in desperation, and then not until corticosteroid therapy has been thoroughly exhausted and the spleen removed. While splenectomy avowedly removes the main organ of destruction of antibody-coated red cells,[83] thymectomy supposedly eliminates the main organ of autoantibody production.[40] It may be that thymectomy in the infant with autoimmune hemolytic anemia responds favorably because the operation is performed at an age when the thymus has not yet involuted and may, therefore, still be functional. The normal thymus is known to exert its greatest immunologic function in the neonatal period, while later the other lymphoid organs progressively take over that function.[185]

*Prognosis.* The outlook in autoimmune acquired hemolytic anemia has greatly improved with the advent of steroid therapy. A complete and sustained remission rate of approximately 80% has been obtained with the use of corticosteroids or corticosteroids plus splenectomy.[234] Severe anemia, reticulocytopenia, thrombocytopenia, and leukopenia are associated with a high mortality rate.[75] The varied forms and combinations of therapy, however, still await a longer experience for ultimate evaluation. The effects of therapy are difficult to measure because of the uncertain course, remissions, exacerbations, tendency toward spontaneous recovery, and relatively recent introduction of immunosuppressive therapy. Fatalities have occurred in a relatively small number of children.[198,232]

In one series,[307] a mortality of 40 to 45% was to be anticipated for patients with a diagnosis of idiopathic or primary autoimmune hemolytic anemia. If death occurs it happens within 2 years of diagnosis. In this series 20% could be expected to be "cured." An indeterminate percentage of the remaining 35% could be expected to develop or manifest underlying lymphomatous or hypersensitivity state disease. Patients who have symptomatic or secondary autoimmune hemolytic anemia have a mortality rate based upon the underlying primary disease. Autoimmune hemolytic disease secondary to bacterial or viral infection rarely results in death. The multisystem aspects of this disorder are demonstrated by the increased frequency in the presence of serum antibodies directed not only against red cells and platelets but against white cells, thyroid, and deoxyribonucleic acid. The antibody related to production of the hemolytic anemia is usually of the incomplete warm type and in some way related to red cell Rh-Hr antigen. When viewed in its broadest aspects, autoimmune hemolytic anemia represents a manifestation of generalized altered immune response.[307]

### Paroxysmal cold hemoglobinuria

In paroxysmal cold hemoglobinuria, a rare syndrome, sudden attacks of intravascular hemolysis and hemoglobinuria are precipitated by exposure to cold. The disorder is due to the presence of an autohemolysin in the patient's blood which is biphasic, uniting with the red cells at a low temperature and destroying them in the presence of complement upon subsequent warming to body temperature. The antibody was discovered in 1904 by Donath and Landsteiner.[109] The Donath-Landsteiner test demonstrates this sequence of events by bringing together cells and serum in the cold and warming the suspension to allow complement to produce hemolysis. The direct antiglobulin (Coombs) test is positive at the height of a hemolytic episode and negative when the patient is symptom free.[78] The Donath-Landsteiner antibody causes agglutination as well as hemolysis.[78]

The clinical and hematologic picture is that which characterizes acute hemolytic anemia, especially when hemolysis is intravascular: fever, a shaking chill, headache, pain in the abdomen and back, and the passage of dark bloody urine. In addition to severe anemia and other features of hemolysis during the paroxysm, leukopenia and erythrophagocytosis appear,[179] the latter serving to remove damaged erythrocytes. Paroxysmal cold hemoglobinuria occurs usually in patients with syphilis, especially congenital syphilis. Occasionally, there is no clinical evidence of syphilitic infection, and a positive Wassermann or Kahn test is interpreted as being false. Treatment is directed toward the syphilitic infection when required and toward the avoidance of chilling. Transfusion of fresh whole blood is potentially harmful, because this might result in adding complement to the patient's blood and thus provoke hemolysis of his own and the transfused cells.[362]

A quite distinct type of IgG autoantibody is the Donath-Landsteiner antibody of paroxysmal cold hemoglobinuria. This antibody reacts with "$P_1$" and "$P_2$" cells irrespective of the other antigens present, but fails to react with "p" and "$P^K$" cells.[380] (The P blood group system is composed of two alleles, "$P_1$" and "$P_2$", plus the rare amorph "p" and the rarer "$P^K$"). This specificity within the P blood group system is of little practical importance since the patients seldom require transfusion. It is unlikely that the antibody will cause difficulties in cross-matching the blood. The reason for this unexpected specificity is unknown.

## Dysproteinemias

The dysproteinemias represent a group of disorders characterized by an abnormality of the plasma proteins. They include cryoglobulinemias, hyperglobulinemias, and macroglobulinemias (Waldenström's syndrome). They have in common hemorrhagic manifestations. Although these conditions do not occur in the pediatric age group, one of these, cryoglobulinemia, may be mentioned here because of its association with hemolytic anemia.

The macroglobulinemia of Waldenström[263,296] is characterized by the presence of macroglobulins in abnormal concentrations in the plasma, often accompanied by a hemorrhagic diathesis, hepatosplenomegaly, lymphadenopathy, lethargy, and recurrent infections chiefly in people over 50 years of age. The bone marrow, spleen, lymph nodes, and liver are infiltrated by lymphocytoid reticulum cells which are probably responsible for the production of the macroglobulins.[29] It may be a primary disease or secondary to multiple myeloma, cirrhosis, nephrosis, cancer, or congenital syphilis. The coating of the platelets by macroglobulins may account in some measure for the purpura in this condition.[2] The anemia of macroglobulinemia is attributed to inadequate red cell synthesis, iron deficiency, and decreased red cell survival.[58]

*Cryoglobulinemia.* Cryoglobulinemia refers to the presence in the serum of an abnormal globulin (cryoglobulin) which precipitates spontaneously in the cold and redissolves on subsequent warming.[12,206,207] Cryoglobulinemia is usually secondary to another disorder such as multiple myeloma, leukemia, or malignant lymphomas. It is associated with purpura and Raynaud's phenomenon, occurring after exposure to cold. Acute hemolytic anemia and high titer cold agglutinins have also been described.[59]

*Cryofibrinogenemia.* In this cryopathy chilling of heparinized plasma (4° C.) results in precipitation of a gelatinous, flocculent material that redissolves upon warming to 37° C.[295] Cryofibrinogenemia has been known to occur in the course of leukemia, multiple myeloma, fibrosarcoma and other neoplasms, with acute rheumatic fever and ulcerative colitis. Primary idiopathic cryofibrinogenemia, without an underlying disorder, is associated with cold sensitivity purpura, occlusive vascular phenomena, gangrene of the fingertips, ischemic necrosis of the toes and the nose, and, at times, hemorrhagic conjunctivitis and retinal vein thrombosis.[171] The severity of clinical symptoms cannot be correlated with the quantity of the cryofibrinogen.[171] A limited experience has shown some benefit from ascorbic acid, penicillin, streptokinase-streptodornase, and anticoagulants.

Four infants with respiratory infections[297] demonstrated a transient cryopathy resulting from cryofibrinogenemia. Three of the four had severe bilateral tender indurated swelling of the extremities without evidence of cyanosis. The fourth child had cold cyanotic swelling of his feet. Significant amounts of cryofibrinogen (but no cryoglobulin) were found in their plasma and disappeared when the respiratory infection cleared. Three of the four cases of cryofibrinogenemia occurred during the winter months and the fourth after 12 hours in a cold oxygen tent. The exact nature of this abnormal plasma protein is unknown.

## Acute acquired hemolytic anemia (Lederer's anemia)

Sporadic cases of acute hemolytic anemia, often referred to as Lederer's anemia,[203,204] occur most commonly in children. The condition is characterized by an acute onset, short duration, and spontaneous recovery. Hemoglobinuria, jaundice, vomiting, prostration, restlessness, elevation of temperature, leukocytosis, and marked anemia are predominant features. Splenomegaly is inconsistent. Azotemia, oliguria, and anuria may be present, but death from renal failure is rare. The infrequency with which antibodies and a positive antiglobulin (Coombs) test are found is probably explained by the rapid course. The peripheral blood picture is one of a regenerative anemia with polychromatophilia, reticulocytosis, spherocytes, normoblasts, and erythrophagocytosis. Marked polynuclear leukocytosis (66,000 per cubic millimeter in one of our patients) with numerous metamyelocytes and myelocytes is indicative of increased bone marrow activity. In its subacute and milder form the disease may be difficult to differentiate from the autoimmune hemolytic disease with respect to the blood picture and serologic findings.[98,232,298] The acute hemolytic episode may continue in a milder form which is indistinguishable from the autoimmune disease. When tested at appropriate times antibodies can be demonstrated in as many as 50% of patients.[89] In a case of an 8-year-old boy with this disease the globulin coating the red cells was of the nongamma globulin variety, corresponding to complement.

Despite the usual self-limited course, transfusions are required to maintain adequate hemoglobin levels. In the early stages when differentiation from an exacerbation of the chronic autoimmune disease has not yet been established, adrenocortical steroids are usually given. Regardless of the precise diagnosis, these agents are of great value at the onset of the acute fulminating disease when the anemia is severe and the patient is in a state of severe collapse.

The term Lederer's anemia should be applied to this type of hemolytic anemia in children with a short, stormy course. Lederer's anemia cannot strictly be applied to the acute hemolytic anemias that occur at any age period in association with a variety of conditions, including malignant disease, chronic ulcerative colitis, systemic lupus erythematosus, hemolytic-uremic syndrome, infectious mononucleosis, thrombotic thrombocytopenic purpura, and other blood disorders.[367]

*Idiopathic paroxysmal myoglobinuria.* Hemoglobinuria must be distinguished from myoglobinuria. Idiopathic paroxysmal myoglobinuria is a rare disease of unknown etiology in which myoglobin is liberated from the muscle and appears in the urine. Necrosis of skeletal muscle fibers results in the liberation of intracellular constituents, including myoglobin, into the bloodstream. If the mass of destroyed muscle is large and the process occurs rapidly, the concentration of myoglobin in the plasma may exceed the renal threshold and the pigment appears in the urine.[190]

Myoglobinuria can result from crushing injuries of muscle or can be idiopathic and unassociated with any specific or discernible cause. Episodic myoglobinuria may occur with Type VII glycogen storage disease in which a severe deficiency of phosphofructokinase in skeletal muscle has been demonstrated.[352a] Severe muscle pain, especially in the calves, thighs, and back, spasm, weakness, or complete paralysis may result with the excretion of burgundy-colored urine.[269,318,336]

Myoglobin, having one-fourth of the molecular weight of hemoglobin, passes readily through the glomerular membrane. The disease is prone to recur and to be precipitated by exercise. In many cases the attack of myoglobinuria is precipitated by infection, while in others a history of muscular exertion precedes the illness.[191] Myoglobin and hemoglobin give a positive benzidine reaction. Increased creatine from the release of phosphocreatine by damaged muscle cells is excreted in the urine.[8] Peculiar bands that stain like heme groups appear in the electrophoretic pattern of the urine but cannot be identified.[192] The absence of erythrocytes in the urine, the differences in the absorption bands observed by spectroscopic examination of the urinary pigment, and a negative test for porphyrin establish the diagnosis of myoglobinuria. Treatment is supportive.

Respiratory distress due to muscle weakness, hyperkalemia associated with cellular breakdown, and acute renal failure are the most important complications threatening life. Renal failure is treated by fluid restriction, dialysis if needed, and other methods of restoring kidney function.[8] The mortality rate is 30%,[318] with death caused by acute renal failure or respiratory paralysis. In the majority of cases, the patients become free of muscular symptoms and dark urine during the first week after onset. Long-term care is directed to avoidance of exertion and to prevention of infection.[192]

Myoglobin isolated from the muscle of two patients with childhood muscular dystrophy and one with dermatomyositis and another with idiopathic myoglobinuria were characterized by a marked decrease in myoglobin A (normal adult myoglobin) with a predominance of fetal myoglobin.[273]

### March hemoglobinuria

March hemoglobinuria is a rare and benign abnormality occurring in otherwise healthy young men in whom strenuous physical exertion carried out in the erect position is followed by the passage of dark urine.[138] Hemoglobinuria is secondary to hemoglobinemia; jaundice, anemia, and reticulocytosis are absent. The condition has been observed in soldiers after marching, in marathan runners, and in college athletes. The patient recovers spontaneously within a few months. Attacks recur in the same person after brisk exercise. The mechanism of hemoglobinuria is still unknown. Chilling of an extremity fails to produce the condition. A closely allied syndrome termed "exercise myohemoglobinuria" has been described in which painful swollen muscle groups and the excretion of dark urine after excessive exercise were the essential complaints.[337]

### Intravascular hemolysis following open heart surgery

Sayed and associates[308] described as a severe intravascular hemolytic anemia which developed in a patient in whom a ventricular septal defect was repaired with the use of Teflon felt. Hemolysis was attributed to mechanical conditions in the heart, presumably produced by a regurgitant jet of blood being driven against the bare Teflon felt or by tur-

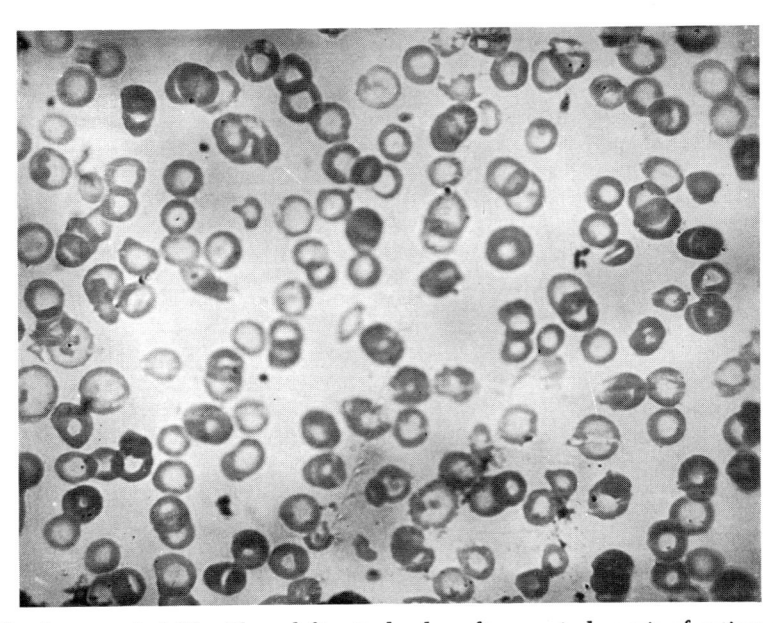

Fig. 31. Blood smear of child with a cleft mitral valve after surgical repair of ostium primum. Note hypochromia, poikiloanisocytosis, and fragmented red cells resulting from intravascular destruction. (×840.)

bulence of the blood flow. When the bare area of Teflon was covered by endocardium, hemolysis ceased and recovery set in (Fig. 31).

In another report of children with atrial[365] and atrioventricular septal defects[326] complicated by a cleft mitral valve, a similar hemolytic anemia developed in relation to a patch of Teflon felt used in repair. A precautionary covering of the patch with endothelium prevented red cell destruction. The hemolytic anemia was associated with a negative Coombs test, fever, petechiae, a shortened red cell lifespan, reduced serum haptoglobin, reticulocytosis, erythroid hyperplasia of the marrow, methemalbuminemia, hemoglobinemia, hemoglobinuria, and splenomegaly. The red cells showed bizarre poikilocytes consistent with red cell fragmentation. The low serum iron and elevated total iron-binding capacity and hypochromia reflected a superimposed iron-deficiency anemia. In other words, mechanical factors within the heart are capable of producing severe intravascular hemolytic anemia, accompanied by a persistent loss of hemoglobin and hemosiderin in the urine leading to an iron-deficiency state. As contrasted with the normal degradation of hemoglobin in the reticuloendothelial system, in intravascular hemolysis hemoglobin is released directly into the plasma when it is excreted by the kidneys. Evidence of iron depletion as an accompaniment of long-standing hemolysis is unusual since chronic hemolytic anemia is generally associated with elevated levels of serum iron and the presence of stainable iron in the tissues. If the dietary intake of iron does not keep pace with the amount of iron lost in the urine, an iron-deficient state ensues. (This syndrome of intravascular hemolysis has also been termed the Waring Blendor syndrome.[325])

Severe intravascular hemolysis has also been observed following aortic valve replacement with a Starr-Edwards prosthesis. It was attributed to mechanical damage to the red blood cells caused by turbulence or contact between the cells and the presence of a rigid prosthesis in the circulation.[218,340] With the same type of prosthesis for aortic valve surgery seven cases of acquired hemolytic anemia were reported.[279] Six of the seven patients had positive antiglobulin tests. The erythrocyte-coating material was identified as an erythrocyte antibody, and steroid therapy helped correct the hemolysis in four of the cases in which it was employed. It was postulated that the erythrocyte-surface antigenic state was modified through turbulent blood flow, with the development of a cross-reacting erythrocyte antibody. The febrile postcardiotomy lymphocytic splenomegaly syndrome[316] was also present in four of the seven cases in which hemolytic anemia developed (Chapter 21).

Twelve patients with symptomatic aortic valve disease and twelve patients with aortic ball valve prostheses were studied for evidence of traumatic hemolysis.[122] Low or absent haptoglobins suggesting an accelerated rate of red cell destruction were found in three of the twelve patients with diseased valves and in eleven of the twelve patients with ball valve prostheses. Two patients with diseased valves and three with ball valve prostheses had hemosiderinuria. It was concluded that mechanical hemolysis can result in iron-deficiency anemia in patients with aortic valve disease as well as in those with prosthetic aortic ball valves. Hemolysis occurred by random destruction of cells of all ages rather than as a consequence of cell aging in such patients.

In a patient with an aortic ball valve prosthesis who had traumatic hemolysis, hemoglobinuria and iron deficiency secondary to ball variance has been reported.[121] Hemolysis and urinary iron loss decreased when activity was restricted. The hemolysis also subsided following replacement of the swollen ball component (poppet).

Red cell osmotic fragility after incubation was increased in seventeen of thirty-five patients with aortic ball valve prostheses.[123] Osmotic fragility was increased in most but not all patients with significant intravascular hemolysis. In this study it was also noted that hemosiderinuria occurs more frequently with Starr-Edwards ball valve prostheses than with MacGovern valves, suggesting that red cell damage and chronic intravascular hemolysis are more severe with the former type of valve. In traumatic hemolysis, fragmentation is accompanied by the loss of a piece of membrane. Massive damage presumably leads to the production of cell fragments, which are rapidly removed from the circulation.

**REFERENCES**

1. Ackroyd, J. F., and Rook, A. J.: Allergic drug reactions. In Gell, P. G. H., and Coombs, R. R. A., editors: Clinical aspects of immunology, ed. 2, Edinburgh, 1968, Blackwell Scientific Publications, p. 693.
2. Adelson, E., Rheingold, J. J., and Crosby, W. H.: The platelet as a sponge; a review, Blood 17:767, 1961.
3. Aldrich, R. A., Hawkinson, V., Grinstein, M.,

and Watson, C. J.: Photosensitive or congenital porphyria with hemolytic anemia; clinical and fundamental studies before and after splenectomy, Blood 6:685, 1951.
4. Allison, A. A., and ap Rees, W.: The binding of haemoglobin by plasma proteins (haptoglobins); its bearing on the "renal threshold" for haemoglobin and the aetiology of haemoglobinuria, Brit. Med. J. 2:1137, 1957.
5. Anderson, R. L., and Chaplin, H., Jr.: Plasma hemoglobin concentration in umbilical cord blood, Amer. J. Dis. Child. 105:19, 1963.
6. Auditore, J. V., and Hartmann, R. C.: Paroxysmal nocturnal hemoglobinuria. II. Erythrocyte acetylcholinesterase defect, Amer. J. Med. 27:401, 1959.
7. Austin, R. F., and Desforges, J. F.: Hereditary elliptocytosis; an unusual presentation of hemolysis in the newborn associated with transient morphologic abnormalities, Pediatrics 44:196, 1969.
8. Baile, M. D.: Primary paroxysmal myoglobinuria; report of a case and review of the literature, New Eng. J. Med. 271:186, 1964.
9. Baird, R. L., Weiss, D., Ferguson, A., French, J., and Scott, R.: Studies in sickle cell anemia. XXI Clinico-pathological aspects of neurological manifestations, Pediatrics 34:92, 1964.
10. Bakemeier, R. F., and Leddy, J. P.: Erythrocyte autoantibody associated with alpha-methyldopa; heterogeneity of structure and specificity, Blood 32:1, 1968.
11. Bannerman, R. M., and Renwick, J. H.: The hereditary elliptocytoses; clinical and linkage data, Ann. Human Genet. 26:23, 1962.
12. Barr, D. P., Reader, G. G., and Wheeler, C. H.: Cryoglobulinemia, Ann. Intern. Med. 32:6, 1950.
13. Barry, M., Scheuer, P. J., Sherlock, S., Ross, C. F., and Williams, R.: Hereditary spherocytosis with secondary haemochromatosis, Lancet 2:481, 1968.
14. Bates, G. C., and Brown, C. H.: Incidence of gall bladder disease in chronic hemolytic anemia (spherocytosis), Gastroenterology 21:104, 1952.
15. Baughan, M. A., Valentine, W. N., Paglia, D. E., Ways, P. O., Simon, E. R., and De Marsh, Q. B.: Hereditary hemolytic anemia associated with glucosephosphate isomerase (GPI) deficiency—a new enzyme defect of human erythrocytes, Blood 30:850, 1967.
16. Beal, R. W., Kronenberg, H., and Firkin, B. G.: The syndrome of paroxysmal nocturnal hemoglobinuria, Amer. J. Med. 37:899, 1964.
17. Bergstrand, C. G., Czar, B., and Tarokosk, P. H.: Serum haptoglobin in infancy, J. Lab. Clin. Invest. 13:576, 1961.
18. Beutler, E.: The hemolytic effect of primaquine and related compounds; a review, Blood 14:103, 1959.
19. Beutler, E.: Drug-induced blood dyscrasias, III. Hemolytic anemia, J.A.M.A. 189:143, 1964.
20. Beutler, E.: Drug-induced hemolytic anemia, Pharm. Rev. 21:73, 1969.
21. Beutler, E.: Glucose-6-phosphate dehydrogenase deficiency, Brit. J. Haemat. 18:117, 1970.
22. Beutler, E., Dern, R. J., and Alving, A. S.: The hemolytic effect of primaquine; a study of primaquine-sensitive erythrocytes, J. Lab. Clin. Med. 44:177, 1954.
23. Beutler, E., Dern, R. J., and Alving, A. S.: The hemolytic effect of primaquine; an in vitro test for sensitivity of erythrocytes to primaquine, J. Lab. Clin. Med. 45:40, 1955.
24. Beutler, E., Goldenburg, E. W., Ohno, S., and Yettra, M.: Chromosome-21 and paroxysmal nocturnal hemoglobinuria, Blood 24:160, 1964.
25. Beutler, E., Mathai, C. K., and Smith, J. E.: Biochemical variants of glucose-6-phosphate dehydrogenase giving rise to congenital nonspherocytic hemolytic disease, Blood 31:131, 1968.
26. Beutler, E., and Rosen, R.: Nonspherocytic congenital hemolytic anemia due to a new G-6-PD variant; G-6-PD Alhambra, Pediatrics 45:230, 1970.
26a. Bienzle, U., Lucas, A. O., Ayeni, O., and Luzzatto, L.: Glucose-6-phosphate dehydrogenase and malaria, Lancet 1:107, 1972.
27. Blackburn, E. K., Jordan, A., Lytle, W. J., Swan, H. T., and Tudhope, G. R.: Hereditary elliptocytic haemolytic anaemia, J. Clin. Path. 11:316, 1958.
28. Blaisdell, R. K., Priest, R. E., and Beutler, E.: Paroxysmal nocturnal hemoglobinuria; a case report with a negative Ham presumptive test associated with serum properdin deficiency, Blood 13:1074, 1958.
29. Bouroncle, B. A., Datta, P., and Frajola, W. J.: Waldenström's macroglobulinemia, J.A.M.A. 189:729, 1964.
30. Bowdler, A. J., and Prankerd, T. A. J.: Studies in congenital non-spherocytic haemolytic anaemia with specific enzyme defects, Acta Haemat. 31:65, 1964.
31. Bowman, H. A., and Procopio, F.: Hereditary non-spherocytic hemolytic anemia of pyruvate-kinase deficient type, Ann. Intern. Med. 58:567, 1963.
32. Bowman, J. W.: Acquired hemolytic anemia, use of replacement transfusion in a case, Amer. J. Dis. Child. 89:226, 1955.
33. Brewer, G. J., Tarlov, A. R., and Keller, R. W.: The hemolytic effect of primaquine.

XII. Shortened erythrocyte life span in primaquine-sensitive male Negroes in the absence of drug administration, J. Lab. Clin. Med. 58:217, 1961.
34. Brodribb, H. S., and Woprssam, A. R. H.: Favism in an Englishwoman, Brit. Med. J. 1:1367, 1961.
35. Brunetti, P., Puxeddu, A., Nenci, G., and Migliorini, E.: Congenital nonspheroytic haemolytic anaemia due to pyruvate-kinase deficiency, Acta Haemat. 30:88, 1963.
36. Brus, I., and Lewis, S. M.: The haptoglobin content of serum in haemolytic anaemia, Brit. J. Haemat. 5:348, 1959.
37. Bruton, O. C., Crosby, W. H., and Motulsky, A. G.: Hereditary nonspherocytic hemolytic anemia presenting as hemolytic disease of the newborn infant, Pediatrics 13:41, 1954.
38. Burman, D.: Congenital spherocytosis in infancy, Arch. Dis. Child. 33:335, 1958.
39. Burnet, F. M.: The new approach to immunology, New Eng. J. Med. 264:24, 1961.
40. Burnet, F. M., and Mackay, I. R.: Lymphoepithelial structures and autoimmune disease, Lancet 2:1030, 1962.
41. Carson, P. E., Biswer, G. J., and Ickes, C. E.: Decreased glutathione reductase with susceptibility to hemolysis, J. Lab. Clin. Med. 58:840, 1961.
42. Carson, P. E., Flanagan, C. L., Ickes, C. E., and Alving, A. S.: Enzymatic deficiency in primaquine-sensitive erythrocytes, Science 124:484, 1956.
43. Carson, P. E., and Frischer, H.: Glucose-6-phosphate dehydrogenase deficiency and related disorders of the pentose phosphate pathway, Amer. J. Med. 41:744, 1966.
44. Carson, P. E., Okita, G. T., Frischer, H., Hirasa, J., Long, W. K., and Brewer, G. J.: Patterns of hemolytic susceptibility and metabolism. In Proceedings of the 9th Congress of the European Society of Haematologists, Lisbon, 1963, New York, 1963, S. Karger.
45. Carson, P. E., and Torlov, A. R.: Biochemistry of hemolysis, Ann. Rev. Med. 13:105, 1962.
46. Carstairs, K. C., Breckenridge, A., Dolery, P. T., and Worlledge, S. M.: Incidence of a positive direct Coombs test in patients on A-methyldopa, Lancet 2:133, 1966.
47. Cartwright, G. E.: Diagnostic laboratory hematology, ed. 3, New York, 1963, Grune & Stratton, Inc.
48. Cartwright, G. E.: Diagnostic laboratory hematology, ed. 4, New York, 1968, Grune & Stratton, Inc., pp. 291-292.
49. Chanarin, I., Burman, D., and Bennett, M. C.: Familial aplastic crisis in hereditary spherocytosis; urocanic acid and FIGLU excretion studies in a case of megaloblastic anemia, Blood 20:33, 1962.
50. Chapman, R. G.: Red cell life-span after splenectomy in hereditary spherocytosis, J. Clin. Invest. 47:2263, 1968.
51. Charache, S.: Prolonged survival in paroxysmal nocturnal hemoglobinuria, Blood 33:877, 1969.
52. Chernoff, A. I., and Josephson, A. M.: Acute erythroblastopenia in sickle-cell anemia and infectious mononucleosis, Amer. J. Dis. Child. 82:310, 1951.
53. Chertkow, G., and Dacie, J. V.: Results of splenectomy in auto-immune haemolytic anaemia, Brit. J. Haemat. 2:237, 1956.
54. Childs, B., and Zinkham, W.: The genetics of primaquine sensitivity of the erythrocytes. In Wolstenholme, G. E. W., and O'Connor, C. M., editors: Biochemistry of human genetics, Boston, 1959, Little, Brown & Co.
55. Childs, B., Zinkham, W. H., Browne, E. A., Kimbro, E. L., and Torbert, J. V.: A genetic study of a defect in glutathione metabolism of the erythrocyte, Bull. Johns Hopkins Hosp. 102:21, 1958.
56. Chisolm, J. J., Jr.: Symposium on porphyrins. Part II. Pediatric aspects of the porphyrias, J. Pediat. 64:159, 1964.
57. Christenson, W. N., and Dacie, J. V.: Electrophoresis of acquired haemolytic anaemia serum; abnormal gamma$_1$ peak composed of cold antibody protein, Transactions of Sixth Congress of the European Society of Haematology, Copenhagen, 1957.
58. Cline, M. J., Solomon, A., Berlin, N. I., and Fahey, J. L.: Anemia in macroglobulinemia, Amer. J. Med. 34:213, 1963.
59. Conn, H. O.: Acute hemolytic anemia, cryoglobulinemia and cold agglutination; report of a case, New Eng. J. Med. 253:1011, 1955.
60. Connell, G. E., Dixon, G. H., and Smithies, O.: Subdivision of the three common haptoglobin types based on hidden differences, Nature 193:505, 1962.
61. Cooper, E. L.: Familial acholuric jaundice associated with bone changes, Ann. Intern. Med. 15:858, 1941.
62. Cooper, L. Z., Green, R. H., Krugman, S., Giles, S. P., and Mirick, G. S.: Neonatal thrombocytopenic purpura and other manifestations of rubella contracted in utero, Amer. J. Dis. Child. 110:416, 1965.
63. Cooper, R. A., and Jandl, J. H.: The role of membrane lipids in the survival of red cells in hereditary spherocytosis, J. Clin. Invest. 48:736, 1969.
64. Coventry, W. D., and LaBree, R. H.: Heterotopia of bone marrow simulating mediastinal tumor; a manifestation of chronic he-

molytic anemia in adults, Ann. Intern. Med. 53:1042, 1960.
65. Crosby, W. H.: Hereditary non-spherocytic hemolytic anemia, Blood 5:233, 1950.
66. Crosby, W. H.: Paroxysmal nocturnal hemoglobinuria; a specific test for the disease based on the ability of thrombin to activate the hemolytic factor, Blood 5:843, 1950.
67. Crosby, W. H.: Paroxysmal nocturnal hemoglobinuria; plasma factors of the hemolytic system, Blood 8:444, 1953.
68. Crosby, W. H.: Paroxysmal nocturnal hemoglobinuria; relation to the clinical manifestations underlying pathogenic mechanisms, Blood 8:769, 1953.
69. Crosby, W. H.: The hemolytic states, Bull. N. Y. Acad. Med. 30:27, 1954.
70. Crosby, W. H.: Siderocytes and the spleen, Blood 12:165, 1957.
71. Crosby, W. H., and Akeroyd, J. H.: The limit of hemoglobin synthesis in hereditary hemolytic anemia; its relation to the excretion of bile pigment, Amer. J. Med. 13:273, 1952.
72. Crosby, W. H., and Conrad, W. E.: Hereditary spherocytosis; observations on hemolytic mechanisms and iron metabolism, Blood 15:652, 1960.
73. Crosby, W. H., and Dameshek, W.: The significance of hemoglobinemia and associated hemosiderinuria, with particular reference of various types of hemolytic anemia, J. Lab. Clin. Med. 38:829, 1951.
74. Crosby, W. H., and Rappaport, H.: Reticulocytopenia in autoimmune hemolytic anemia, Blood 11:929, 1956.
75. Crosby, W. H., and Rappaport, H.: Autoimmune hemolytic anemia; analysis of hematologic observations with particular reference to their prognostic value; a survey of 57 cases, Blood 12:42, 1957.
76. Curwen, W. L., and Pathak, M. A.: Abnormal porphyrin metabolism and polymorphic photodermatitis, New Eng. J. Med. 271:385, 1964.
77. Cutting, H. O., McHugh, W. J., Conrad, F. G., and Marlow, A. A.: Autosomal dominant hemolytic anemia characterized by ovalocytosis; a family study of seven involved members, Amer. J. Med. 39:21, 1965.
78. Dacie, J. V.: The haemolytic anaemias; congenital and acquired, New York, 1954, Grune & Stratton, Inc.
79. Dacie, J. V.: The autoimmune haemolytic anaemias, Amer. J. Med. 18:810, 1955.
80. Dacie, J. V.: Autoimmunization in respect of red cells, Program of Sixth International Congress of Hematology, Boston, 1956, p. 488.
81. Dacie, J. V.: Acquired hemolytic anaemias, Brit. M. Bull. 15:67, 1959.
82. Dacie, J. V.: The haemolytic anaemias congenital and acquired. Part I. The congenital anaemias, ed. 2, New York, 1960, Grune & Stratton, Inc.
83. Dacie, J. V.: The haemolytic anaemias congenital and acquired. Part II. The auto-immune haemolytic anaemias, ed. 2, New York, 1962, Grune & Stratton, Inc.
84. Dacie, J. V.: The hereditary nonspherocytic haemolytic anaemias, Acta Haemat. 31:177, 1964.
85. Dacie, J. V.: The haemolytic anaemias—paroxysmal nocturnal haemoglobinuria, haemolytic disease of the newborn, ed. 2, London, 1968, Churchill.
86. Dacie, J. V.: Paroxysmal nocturnal haemoglobinuria; an acquired disorder of the red cell membrane, XII Congress International Society of Hematology, Papers of the Plenary Session, 1968, p. 102.
87. Dacie, J. V., Crookston, J. H., and Christenson, W. N.: "Incomplete" cold antibodies; role of complement in sensitization to antiglobulin serum by potentially haemolytic antibodies, Brit. J. Haemat. 3:77, 1957.
88. Dacie, J. V., and Cutbush, M.: Specificity of auto-antibodies in acquired haemolytic anaemia, J. Clin. Path. 7:18, 1954.
89. Dacie, J. V., and de Gruchy, G. C.: Autoantibodies in acquired haemolytic anaemia, J. Clin. Path. 4:253, 1951.
90. Dacie, J. V., and Lewis, S. M.: Paroxysmal nocturnal haemoglobinuria; variation in clinical severity and association with bone-marrow hypoplasia, Brit. J. Haemat. 7:442, 1961.
91. Dacie, J. V., Lewis, S. M., and Tills, D.: Comparative sensitivity of the erythrocytes in paroxysmal nocturnal haemoglobinuria to haemolysis by acidified normal serum and by high-titre cold antibody, Brit. J. Haemat. 6:362, 1960.
92. Dameshek, W.: Hemolytic anemia; direct and indirect indications, pathogenetic mechanisms and classifications; seminars on the hemolytic anemias, Amer. J. Med. 18:315, 1955.
93. Dameshek, W.: Autoimmunity; theoretical aspects, Ann. N. Y. Acad. Sci. 124:6, 1965.
94. Dameshek, W.: Foreword and a proposal for considering paroxysmal nocturnal hemoglobinuria (PNH) as a "candidate" for myeloproliferative disorder, Blood 33:263, 1969.
95. Dameshek, W., and Komninos, Z. D.: The present status of treatment of autoimmune hemolytic anemia with ACTH and cortisone, Blood 11:648, 1956.

96. Dameshek, W., and Schwartz, R.: Treatment of certain "auto-immune" diseases with antimetabolites; a preliminary report, Trans. Ass. Amer. Physicians 73:113, 1960.
97. Dameshek, W., Schwartz, R., and Oliner, H.: Current concepts in autoimmunizations: an interpretive review, Blood 17:775, 1961.
98. Dameshek, W., and Schwartz, S. O.: Acute hemolytic anemia (acquired hemolytic icterus, acute type), Medicine 19:231, 1940.
99. Dausset, J., and Colombani, J.: The serology and the progress of 120 cases of autoimmune hemolytic anemia, Blood 14:1280, 1959.
100. Davidsohn, I., and Stern, K.: Diagnosis of hemolytic transfusion reactions, Amer. J. Clin. Path. 25:381, 1955.
101. Davis, L. J., Kennedy, A. C., Baikie, A. G., and Brown, A.: Haemolytic anaemias of various types treated with ACTH and cortisone, Glasgow M. J. 33:263, 1952.
102. Dawson, J. P., Thayer, W. W., and Desforges, J. F.: Acute hemolytic anemia in the newborn infant due to naphthalene poisoning; report of two cases, with investigations into the mechanism of the disease, Blood 13:1113, 1958.
103. De Gruchy, G. C., Loder, P. B., and Hennessy, I. V.: Haemolysis and glycolytic metobolism in hereditary elliptocytosis, Brit. J. Haemat. 8:168, 1962.
104. De Gruchy, G. C., Santamaria, J. N., Parsons, I. C., and Crawford, H.: Nonspherocytic congenital hemolytic anemia, Blood 16:1371, 1960.
105. Demis, J. D., Brown, C. S., and Crosby, W. H.: Thioguanine in the treatment of certain autoimmune, immunologic and related diseases, Amer. J. Med. 37:195, 1964.
106. Dern, R. J., Beutler, E., and Alving, A. S.: The hemolytic effect of primaquine; the natural course of hemolytic anemia and the mechanism of its self-limited character, J. Lab. Clin. Med. 44:171, 1954.
107. Dern, R. J., Beutler, E., and Alving, A. S.: The hemolytic effect of primaquine; primaquine sensitivity as a manifestation of multiple drug sensitivity, J. Lab. Clin. Med. 45:30, 1955.
108. Desforges, J. F., Thayer, W. W., and Dawson, J. P.: Hemolytic anemia induced by sulfoxone therapy, with investigations into the mechanisms of its production, Amer. J. Med. 27:132, 1959.
109. Donath, J., and Landsteiner, K.: Ueber paroxysmale Hämoglobinurie, Münch. med. Wschr. 51:1590, 1904.
110. Doxiadis, S. A., Fessas, P. H., and Valaes, T.: Glucose-6-phosphate dehydrogenase deficiency; a new aetiological factor of severe neonatal jaundice, Lancet 1:297, 1961.
111. Dresbach, M.: Elliptical human red corpuscles, Science 19:469, 1904.
112. Ducrov, W., and Kimber, R. J.: Stomatocytes, haemolytic anaemia and abdominal pain in Mediterranean migrants; some examples of a new syndrome, Med. J. Aust. 2:1087, 1969.
113. Dunsky, I., Smith, F., and Gibson, S.: Porphyria and porphyrinuria; report of a case; review of porphyrin metabolism with a study of congenital porphyria, Amer. J. Dis. Child. 74:305, 1947.
114. Eisenmann, G., and Dameshek, W.: Splenectomy for "pure red-cell" hypoplastic (aregenerative) anemia associated with autoimmune hemolytic disease, New Eng. J. Med. 251:1044, 1954.
115. Emerson, C. P., Jr., Shen, S. C., Ham, T. H., Fleming, E. M., and Castle, W. B.: Studies on the destruction of red blood cells; quantitative methods for determining the osmotic and mechanical fragility of red cells in the peripheral blood and splenic pulp; the mechanism of increased hemolysis in hereditary spherocytosis as related to the functions of the spleen, Arch. Intern. Med. 97:1, 1956.
116. Erlandson, M. E., and Hilgartner, M.: Hemolytic disease in the neonatal period and early infancy, J. Pediat. 54:566, 1959.
117. Erlandson, M. E., Schulman, I., and Smith, C. H.: Studes on congenital hemolytic syndromes; rates of destruction and production of erythrocytes in hereditary spherocytosis, Pediatrics 23:462, 1959.
118. Evans, R. S., and Duane, R. T.: Acquired hemolytic anemia; the relation of erythrocyte antibody production to activity of the disease; the significance of thrombocytopenia and leucopenia, Blood 4:1196, 1949.
119. Evans, R. S., Duane, R. T., and Behrend, T. V.: Demonstration of antibodies in acquired hemolytic anemia with anti-human globulin serum, Proc. Soc. Exp. Biol. Med. 64:372, 1947.
120. Evans, R. S., Takahashi, K., Duane, R. T., Payne, R., and Liu, C.: Primary thrombocytopenic purpura and acquired hemolytic anemia; evidence for a common etiology, Arch. Intern. Med. 87:48, 1951.
121. Eyster, E.: Traumatic hemolysis with hemoglobinuria due to ball variance, Blood 33:391, 1969.
122. Eyster, E., Mayer, K., and McKenzie, S.: Traumatic hemolysis with iron deficiency anemia in patients with aortic valve lesions, Ann. Intern. Med. 68:995, 1968.
123. Eyster, E., Rothchild, J., and Mychaljiro, O.: Red cell osmotic fragility after aortic valve replacement. In press.

124. Fadem, R. S.: Ovalocytosis associated with the sickle cell trait, Blood 4:505, 1949.
125. Fairbanks, V. F., and Beutler, E.: Simple method for detection of erythrocyte glucose-6-phosphate dehydrogenase deficiency (G-6-PD spot test), Blood 20:591, 1962.
126. Fairley, N. H.: Methaemalbumin, Quart. J. Med. 10:95, 1941.
127. Feinberg, A. W., and Watson, J.: Nonspherocytic chronic hemolytic anemia with basophilic stippling; report of a case in a Negro, Blood 6:357, 1951.
128. Finch, S. C., and Finch, C. A.: Idiopathic hemochromatosis, an iron storage disease; iron metabolism in hemochromatosis, Medicine 34:381, 1955.
129. Florman, A. L., and Wintrobe, M. M.: Human elliptical red corpuscles, Bull. Johns Hopkins Hosp. 63:209, 1938.
130. Fornaini, G., Bianchini, E., Leoncini, G., and Fantoni, A.: Metabolic aspects of red cells in congenital nonspherocytic haemolytic anaemia, Brit. J. Haemat. 10:23, 1964.
131. Frick, P. G., Hitzig, W. H., and Betke, K.: Hemoglobin Zürich. I. A new hemoglobin anomaly associated with acute hemolytic episodes with inclusion bodies after sulfonamide therapy, Blood 20:261, 1962.
132. Frick, P. G., Hitzig, W. H., and Stauffer, U.: Das Hämoglobin-Zürich-Syndrome, Schweiz. med. Wchnschr. 91:1203, 1961.
133. Gairdner, D.: Association of gallstones with acholuric jaundice in childhood, Arch. Dis. Child. 14:109, 1939.
134. Gardner, F. H., and Diamond, L. K.: Autoerythrocytic sensitization; form of purpura producing painful bruising following autosensitization to red blood cells in certain women, Blood 10:675, 1955.
135. Gasser, C.: Akute Erythroblastopenie, 10 Fälle aplastischer Erythroblastenkrisen mit Riesenproerythroblasten bei allergisch-toxischen Zustandsbildern, Helvet. Paediat. Acta 4:107, 1949.
136. Gasser, C.: Aplasia of erythropoiesis; acute and chronic erythroblastopenias or pure (red cell) aplastic anaemias in childhood, Ped. Clin. N. Amer. 4:445, 1957.
137. Giblett, E. R., and Steinberg, A. G.: The inheritance of serum haptoglobin types in American Negroes; evidence for a third allele Hp[2m], Amer. J. Human Genet. 12:160, 1960.
138. Gilligan, D. R., and Blumgart, H. L.: March hemoglobinuria; studies of clinical characteristics, blood metabolism and mechanism, with observations on three new cases, and a review of the literature, Medicine 20:341, 1941.
138a. Gilliland, B. C., Baxter, E., and Evans, R. S.: Red-cell antibodies in acquired hemolytic anemia with negative antiglobulin serum tests, New Eng. J. Med. 285:252, 1971.
139. Githens, J. H., and Hathaway, W. E.: Autoimmune hemolytic anemia and the syndrome of hemolytic anemia, thrombocytopenia and nephropathy, Ped. Clin. N. Amer. 9:619, 1962.
140. Goodall, H. E., Hendry, D. W. W., Lawler, S. D., and Stephen, S. A.: Data on linkage in man; elliptocytosis and blood groups, Ann. Eugenics 17:267, 1953.
141. Gottlieb, A., Wisch, N., and Ross, J.: Familial hypohaptoglobinemia; a genetically determined trait segregating from glucose-6-phosphate dehydrogenase deficiency, Blood 21:129, 1963.
142. Greenberg, M. S., and Wong, H.: Studies with destruction of glutathione, J. Lab. Clin. Med. 57:733, 1961.
143. Grimes, A. J., Meisler, A., and Dacie, J. V.: Hereditary non-spherocytic haemolytic anaemia; a study of red-cell carbohydrate metabolism in twelve cases of pyruvate kinase deficiency, Brit. J. Haemat. 10:403, 1964.
144. Gross, R. T.: Clinical applications of some recent studies of erythrocyte enzymes, Bull. N. Y. Acad. Med. 39:90, 1963.
145. Gross, R. T., Marks, P. A., Hurwitz, R. E., Beasley, J., and Sui, M.: Studies in the hereditary enzymatic defect in certain drug induced anemias, Amer. J. Dis. Child. 96:436, 1958.
146. Haeger-Aronson, B.: Erythropoietic protoporphyria; a new type of inborn error of metabolism, Amer. J. Med. 35:450, 1963.
147. Haining, R. G., Cowger, M. L., Labbe, R. F., and Finch, C. A.: Congenital erythropoietic porphyria. II. The effects of induced polycythemia, Blood 36:297, 1970.
148. Haining, R. G., Cowger, M. L., Shortleff, D. B., and Labbe, R. F.: Congenital erythropoietic porphyria. I. Case report; special studies and therapy, Amer. J. Med. 45:624, 1968.
149. Ham, T. H., editor: A syllabus of laboratory examination in clinical diagnosis, Cambridge, Mass., 1950, Harvard University Press.
150. Ham, T. H., Shen, S. C., Fleming, E. M., and Castle, W. B.: Studies on the destruction of red blood cells—thermal injury: action of heat in causing increased spheroidicity, osmotic and mechanical fragilities and hemolysis of erythrocytes; observations on the mechanisms of destruction of such erythrocytes in dogs and in a patient with a fatal thermal burn, Blood 3:373, 1948.
151. Hanford, R. B., Schneider, G. F., and Mac-

Carthy, J. D.: Massive thoracic extramedullary hemopoiesis, New Eng. J. Med. 263:120, 1960.
152. Hanstein, A., and Müller-Eberhard, U.: Concentration of serum hemopexin in healthy children and adults and those with a variety of hematological disorders, J. Lab. Clin. Med. 71:232, 1968.
153. Harber, L. C., Fleischer, A. S., and Baer, R. L.: Erythropoietic protoporphyria and photohemolysis, J.A.M.A. 189:191, 1964.
154. Hargreaves, T.: Inherited enzyme defects; a review, J. Clin. Path. 16:293, 1963.
155. Harrald, B., Hanel, K. H., Squires, R., and Traft-Jensen, J.: Adenosine-triphosphotase deficiency in patients with non-spherocytic haemolytic anaemia, Lancet 2:18, 1964.
156. Hartfall, S. J., and Stewart, M. J.: Massive paravertebral heterotopia of bone marrow in a case of acholuric jaundice, J. Path. Bact. 37:455, 1933.
157. Hartigak, J. D., and Garnett, T. J.: Favism; report of a case, J.A.M.A. 171:299, 1961.
158. Hartman, R. C., and Jenkins, D. E.: The "sugar-water" test for paroxysmal nocturnal hemoglobinuria, New Eng. J. Med. 275:155, 1966.
159. Heide, K., Haupt, H., Störiko, K., and Schultze, H. E.: On the heme-binding capacity of hemopexin, Clin. Chimica Acta 10:460, 1964.
160. Heilmeyer, L.: The erythropoietic porphyrias, Acta Haemat. 31:137, 1964.
161. Helz, M. K., and Meuten, M. L.: Elliptocytosis, a report of two cases, J. Lab. Clin. Med. 29:185, 1944.
162. Hillman, R. S.: Characteristics of marrow production and reticulocyte maturation in normal man in response to anemia, J. Clin. Invest. 48:443, 1969.
163. Hitzig, W. H., and Massimo, L.: Treatment of autoimmune hemolytic anemia in children with azathioprine (Imuran), Blood 28:840, 1966.
164. Hoffman, J. F.: The red cell membrane and the transport of sodium and potassium, Amer. J. Med. 41:666, 1966.
165. Holden, D., and Lichtman, H.: Paroxysmal nocturnal hemoglobinuria with acute leukemia, Blood 33:283, 1969.
166. Hughes Jones, N. C., and Szur, L.: Determination of the sites of red-cell destruction using $^{51}$Cr-labelled cells, Brit. J. Haemat. 3:320, 1957.
167. Jacob, H. S.: Abnormalities in the physiology of the erythrocyte membrane in hereditary spherocytosis, Amer. J. Med. 41:734, 1966.
168. Jacob, H. S., and Jandl, J. H.: Increased cell membrane permeability in the pathogenesis of hereditary spherocytosis, J. Clin. Invest. 43:1704, 1964.
169. Jacob, H. S., and Karnovsky, M. L.: Concomitant increase of membrane phosphotide metabolism and sodium transport in hereditary spherocytosis (HS), J. Clin. Invest. 44:1062, 1965.
169a. Jacob, H. S., Ruby, A., Overland, E. S., and Mazia, O.: A protein abnormality in red cell membranes of hereditary spherocytosis, J. Clin. Invest. 50:1800, 1971.
170. Jaffé, E. R., and Gottfried, E. L.: Hereditary nonspherocytic hemolytic disease associated with an altered phospholipid composition of erythrocytes, J. Clin. Invest. 47:1375, 1968.
171. Jager, B. V.: Cryofibrinogenemia, New Eng. J. Med. 266:579, 1962.
172. Jandl, J. H., and Greenberg, M. S.: Bone marrow failure due to nutritional deficiency in Cooley's hemolytic anemia; painful "erythropoietic crises" in response to folic acid, New Eng. J. Med. 260:461, 1959.
173. Jandl, J. H., Greenberg, M. S., Yonemoto, R. H., and Castle, W. B.: Clinical determination of the sites of red cell sequestration in hemolytic anemias, J. Clin. Invest. 35:842, 1956.
174. Jandl, J. H., Jones, A. R., and Castle, W. B.: The destruction of red cells by antibodies in man; observations on the sequestration and lysis of red cells altered by immune mechanisms, J. Clin. Invest. 36:1428, 1957.
175. Javid, J., and Yingling, W.: Immunogenetics of human haptoglobins. I. The antigenic structure of normal Hp phenotypes, J. Clin. Invest. 47:2290, 1968.
176. Jenkins, D. E., Jr., and Hartmann, R. C.: Paroxysmal nocturnal hemoglobinuria terminating in acute myeloblastic leukemia, Blood 33:274, 1969.
177. Jenkins, W. J., and Marsh, W. L.: Autoimmune haemolytic anaemia; three cases with antibodies specifically active against stored red cells, Lancet 2:16, 1961.
178. Jensson, O., Jonasson, T. H., and Olafsson, O.: Hereditary elliptocytosis in Iceland, Brit. J. Haemat. 13:844, 1967.
179. Jordan, W. S., Jr., Prouty, R. L., Heinle, R. W., and Dingle, J. H.: The mechanism of hemolysis in paroxysmal cold hemoglobinuria; erythrophagocytosis and leukopenia, Blood 7:387, 1952.
180. Josephs, H. W., and Avery, M. E.: Hereditary elliptocytosis associated with increased hemolysis, Pediatrics 16:741, 1955.
181. Kalderon, A. E., Kikawa, Y., and Bernstein, J.: Chronic toxoplasmosis associated with

severe hemolytic anemia, Arch. Intern. Med. 114:95, 1964.
182. Kaplan, E., Herz, F., and Hsu, K. S.: Erythrocyte acetylcholinesterase activity in ABO hemolytic disease of the newborn, Pediatrics 33:205, 1964.
183. Kaplan, E., and Zuelzer, W. W.: Familial non-spherocytic hemolytic anemia, Blood 5:811, 1950.
184. Kaplan, E., Zuelzer, W. W., and Mouriquand, C.: Sideroblasts; a study of stainable nonhemoglobin iron in marrow normoblasts, Blood 9:203, 1954.
185. Karaklis, A. Valaes, T., Pantelakis, S. N., and Doxiadis, S. A.: Thymectomy in an infant with autoimmune haemolytic anaemia, Lancet 2:778, 1964.
186. Kaufmann, R. W., Schechter, G. P., and McFarland, W.: Paroxysmal nocturnal hemoglobinuria terminating in acute granulocytic leukemia, Blood 33:287, 1969.
187. Keitt, A. S., and Bennett, D. C.: Pyruvate kinase deficiency and related disorders of red cell glycolysis, Amer. J. Med. 41:762, 1966.
188. Kirkman, H. N., and Riley, H. D., Jr.: Nonspherocytic hemolytic anemia; studies on a family with a qualitative defect in glucose-6-phosphate dehydrogenase, Amer. J. Dis. Child. 102:313, 1961.
189. Kline, A. H., and Holman, G. H.: Hereditary spherocytosis in the Negro, Amer. J. Dis. Child. 94:609, 1957.
190. Kontos, H. A., Harley, E. L., Wasserman, A. J., Kelly, J. J., III, and Magee, J. H.: Exertional idiopathic paroxysmal myoglobinuria; evidence for defect in skeletal muscle metabolism, Amer. J. Med. 35:283, 1963.
191. Korein, J., Coddon, D. R., and Mowrey, F. H.: Clinical syndrome of paroxysmal paralytic myoglobinuria; report of 2 cases and analytical review of the literature, Neurology 9:767, 1959.
192. Kossman, R. J., Camp, W. A., and Engle, R. L., Jr.: Idiopathic recurrent rhabdomyolysis and myoglobinuria; case report with diagnostic recommendations and demonstration of unusual heme compounds in urine, Amer. J. Med. 34:554, 1963.
193. Krauss, A. P., Langston, M. F., Jr., and Lynch B. L.: Red cell phosphoglycerate kinase deficiency; a new cause of nonspherocytic hemolytic anemia, Biochem. Biophys. Res. Commun. 30:173, 1968.
194. Krivit, W., Smith, R. T., Marvin, J. F., Read, R., and Good, R. A.: Congenital nonspherocytic hemolytic anemia; two non-familial cases with red cell survival studies, J. Pediat. 49:245, 1956.

195. Kunstling, T. R., and Rosse, W. F.: Erythrocyte acetylcholinesterase deficiency in paroxysmal nocturnal hemoglobinuria (PNH); a comparison of the complement sensitive and insensitive populations, Blood 33:607, 1969.
196. Kurth, D., Deiss, A., and Cartwright, G. E.: Circulating siderocytes in human subjects, Blood 34:754, 1969.
197. Kyle, R. A., and Pease, G. L.: Hematologic aspects of arsenic intoxication, New Eng. J. Med. 273:18, 1965.
198. Larson, A.: Chronic idiopathic autoimmune hemolytic disease in children, Acta Pediat. 46:144, 1957.
199. Laski, B., Wake, E. J., Bain, H. W., and Gunson, H. H.: Autohemolytic anemia in young infants, J. Pediat. 59:42, 1961.
200. Lathem, W., and Jensen, W. N.: Plasma hemoglobin-binding capacity in sickle cell disease, Blood 14:1047, 1959.
201. Laurell, C. B., and Nyman, M.: Studies on the serum haptoglobin level in hemoglobinemia and its influence on renal excretion of hemoglobin, Blood 12:493, 1957.
202. Leddy, J. P., Hill, R. W., Swisher, S. N., and Vaughan, J. H.: Observations on the immunochemical nature of red cell autosensitization. In Grabar, P., and Miescher, P. A., editors: Immunopathology, Third International Symposium, Basel, Switzerland, 1963, Benno Schwabe & Co.
203. Lederer, M.: Form of acute hemolytic anemia—probably of infectious origin, Amer. J. Med. Sci. 170:500, 1925.
204. Lederer, M.: Three additional cases of acute hemolytic anemia, Amer. J. Med. Sci. 179:228, 1930.
205. Leikin, S. L.: The aplastic crisis of sickle-cell disease; occurrence in several members of families within a short period of time, Amer. J. Dis. Child. 93:128, 1957.
206. Lerner, A. B., Barnum, C. P., and Watson, C. J.: Studies of cryoglobulins; spontaneous precipitation of protein from serum at 5° C. in various disease states, Amer. J. Med. Sci. 214:416, 1947.
207. Lerner, A. B., and Watson, C. J.: Studies of cryoglobulins; unusual purpura associated with presence of high concentration of cryoglobulin (cold precipitable serum globulin), Amer. J. Med. Sci. 214:410, 1947.
208. Lewis, S. M., and Dacie, J. V.: Neutrophil (leucocyte) alkaline phosphatase in paroxysmal nocturnal haemoglobinuria, Brit. J. Haemat. 11:549, 1965.
209. Lewis, S. M., and Dacie, J. V.: The aplastic anaemia—paroxysmal nocturnal anaemia haemoglobinuria syndrome, Brit. J. Haemat. 13:236, 1967.

210. Lipton, E. L.: Elliptocytosis with hemolytic anemia; the effects of splenectomy, Pediatrics 15:67, 1955.
211. LoBuglio, A. F., and Jandl, J. H.: The nature of the alpha-methyldopa red cell-antibody, New Eng. J. Med. 276:650, 1967.
212. Lubin, B. H., and Oski, F. A.: Observations of screening procedures for red cell glucose-6-phosphate dehydrogenase deficiency in the newborn infant, J. Pediat. 70:788, 1967.
213. Lundh, B., Oski, F. A., and Gardner, F. H.: Plasma hemopexin and haptoglobin in hemolytic diseases of the newborn, Acta Paediat. Scand. 59:121, 1970.
214. Lyle, W. H.: Hemolytic anemia in Wilson's disease, New Eng. J. Med. 276:475, 1967.
215. Macauley, D.: Acholuric jaundice in a newborn infant, Arch. Dis. Child. 26:241, 1951.
216. Magnus, I. A., Jarrett, A., Prankerd, T. A. J., and Rimington, G.: Erythropoietic protoporphyria; a new porphyria syndrome with solar urticaria due to protoporphyrin anaemia, Lancet 2:448, 1961.
217. Marks, P. A., and Gross, R. T.: Erythrocyte glucose-6-phosphate dehydrogenase deficiency; evidence of differences between Negroes and Caucasians with respect to this genetically determined trait, J. Clin. Invest. 38:2253, 1959.
218. Marsh, G. W.: Intravascular haemolytic anaemia after aortic-valve replacement, Lancet 2:986, 1964.
219. Martin, W. J., and Heck, F. J.: The porphyrins and porphyria; a review of eighty-one cases, Amer. J. Med. 20:239, 1956.
220. Mathews-Roth, M. M., Pathak, M. A., Fitzpatrick, T. B., Harber, L. C., and Kass, E. H.: Beta-carotene as a photoprotective agent in erythropoietic photoporphyrin, New Eng. J. Med. 282:1231, 1970.
221. McBryde, R. R., Hewlett, J. S., and Weisman, R., Jr.: Elliptocytosis; a study of erythrocyte survival using radioactive chromium ($Cr^{51}$), Amer. J. Med. Sci. 232:259, 1956.
222. McDougal, R. A., Shively, J. A., and Palmer, C.: Paroxysmal nocturnal hemoglobinuria in a Negro child, Amer. J. Dis. Child. 97:92, 1959.
223. McIntyre, N., Clink, H. M., Levi, A. J., Cumings, J. N., and Sherlock, S.: Hemolytic anemia in Wilson's disease, New Eng. J. Med. 276:439, 1967.
224. McPhee, W. R.: Acquired hemolytic anemia caused by ingestion of fava beans, Amer. J. Clin. Path. 26:1287, 1956.
225. Mehta, S. R., and Jensen, W. N.: Haptoglobins in haemoglobinopathy; a genetic and clinical study, Brit. J. Haemat. 6:250, 1960.
226. Mengel, C. S., Kann, H. E., and Meriwether, W. D.: Studies of paroxysmal nocturnal hemoglobinuria erythrocytes; increased lysis and lipid peroxide formation by hydrogen peroxide, J. Clin. Invest. 46:1715, 1967.
227. Miescher, P., and Straessle, R.: Experimentelle studien über den Mechanismus der Thrombocyten-Schädigung durch Antigen-Antikörperreaktion, Vox Sang. 1:83, 1956.
228. Miller, D. R., Baehner, R. L., and Diamond, L. K.: Paroxysmal nocturnal hemoglobinuria in childhood and adolescence, Pediatrics 39:675, 1967.
229. Miller, D. R., Rickles, F. R., Lichtman, M. A., LaCelle, P. L., and Weed, R. I.: A new variant of hereditary stomatocytosis, Blood 36:839, 1970.
230. Miller, G., Shumway, C. N., Jr., and Young, L. E.: Auto-immune hemolytic anemia, Ped. Clin. N. Amer. 4:429, 1957.
231. Miller, G., Townes, P. L., and MacWhinney, J. B.: A new congenital hemolytic anemia with deformed erythrocytes (?"stomatocytes") and remarkable susceptibility of erythrocytes to cold hemolysis in vitro. I. Clinical and hematologic studies, Pediatrics 35:906, 1965.
232. Millichap, J. G.: Acute idiopathic haemolytic anaemia, Arch. Dis. Child. 27:222, 1952.
233. Minton, S. A., and Olson, C.: A case of spider bite with severe hemolytic reaction, Pediatrics 33:283, 1964.
234. Modell, W.: Drugs of choice 1964-1965, St. Louis, 1965, The C. V. Mosby Co., p. 679.
235. Mollison, P. L.: Blood transfusion in clinical medicine, ed. 3, Oxford, 1961, Blackwell Scientific Publications.
236. Molthan, L., Reidenberg, M. M., and Eichman, M. F.: Positive direct Coombs tests to cephalothin, New Eng. J. Med. 277:123, 1967.
237. Morton, N. E., MacKinney, A. A., Kosower, N., Schilling, R. F., and Gray, M. P.: Genetics of spherocytosis, Amer. J. Human Genet. 14:170, 1962.
238. Moskowitz, R. M.: Autoimmune hemolytic anemia in a patient with a deficiency of red cell glucose-6-phosphate dehydrogenase activity, Johns Hopkins Med. J. 126:139, 1970.
239. Motulsky, A. G., Crosby, W. H., and Rappaport, H.: Hereditary nonspherocytic hemolytic disease; a study of a singular familial hemolytic syndrome, Blood 9:749, 1954.
240. Motulsky, A. G., Gabrio, B. W., Burkhardt, J., and Finch, C. A.: Erythrocyte carbohydrate metabolism in hereditary hemolytic anemia, Amer. J. Med. 19:291, 1955.
241. Motulsky, A. G., Kraut, J. M., Theime, W.

T., and Musto, D. F.: Biochemical genetics of glucose-6-phosphate dehydrogenase deficiency, Clin. Res. **7**:89, 1959.
242. Motulsky, A. G., Singer, K., Crosby, W. H., and Smith, V.: The life span of the elliptocyte; hereditary elliptocytosis and its relationship to other familial hemolytic diseases, Blood **9**:57, 1954.
243. Müller-Eberhard, U., Liem, H. H., Hanstein, A., and Hanna, M.: Plasma concentrations of hemopexin, haptoglobin and heme in patients with various hemolytic diseases, Blood **32**:811, 1968.
244. Murphy, J. R.: Erythrocyte metabolism. III. The relationship of energy metabolism and serum factors to the osmotic fragility following incubation, J. Lab. Clin. Med. **60**:32, 1962.
245. Murphy, J. R.: Role of cholesterol in determining shape of erythrocytes, Blood **24**:838, 1964.
246. Murray, R. K., Connell, G. E., and Pert, J. H.: The role of haptoglobin in the clearance and distribution of extracorpuscular hemoglobin, Blood **17**:45, 1961.
247. Nance, W. E.: Necrotic arachnidism, Amer. J. Med. **31**:801, 1961.
248. Nathan, D. G., Oski, F. A., Miller, D. R., and Gardner, F. H.: Life span and organ sequestration of red cells in pyruvate kinase deficiency, New Eng. J. Med. **278**:73, 1968.
249. Nathan, D. G., Oski, F. A., Sidel, V. W., and Diamond, L. K.: Extreme hemolysis and red-cell distortion in erythrocyte pyruvate kinase deficiency. II. Measurements of erythrocyte glucose consumption, potassium and adenosine triphosphate stability, New Eng. J. Med. **272**:118, 1965.
250. Nathan, D. G., Oski, F. A., Sidel, V. W., Gardner, F. H., and Diamond, L. K.: Studies of erythrocyte spicule formation in haemolytic anaemia, Brit. J. Haemat. **12**:385, 1966.
251. Neerhout, P. C.: Disorders of red cell membrane; A review of biochemical and physiologic alterations of erythrocyte membranes which may lead to morphologic changes and shortened red cell survival, Clin. Pediat. **7**:451, 1968.
252. Nelson, M. G.: Atypical congenital haemolytic anaemia, Arch. Dis. Child. **29**:457, 1954.
253. Newcomb, R., Liebman, J., Collins, W., and Shojania, A. M.: Cyanosis caused by methemalbuminemia, Amer. J. Dis. Child. **106**:507, 1963.
254. Newton, W. A., Jr., and Bass, J. C.: Glutathione-sensitive chronic nonspherocytic hemolytic anemia, Amer. J. Dis. Child. **96**:501, 1958.
255. Oort, M., Loos, J. A., and Prins, H. K.: Hereditary absence of reduced glutathione in the erythrocytes—a new clinical and biochemical entity? Vox Sang. **6**:370, 1961.
256. Origenes, M. L., Jr., Need, D. J., and Hartmann, J. R.: Treatment of the malignant lymphomas in children, Ped. Clin. N. Amer. **9**:769, 1962.
257. Oski, F. A., and Diamond, L. K.: Erythrocyte pyruvate kinase deficiency resulting in congenital nonspherocytic hemolytic anemia, New Eng. J. Med. **269**:763, 1963.
258. Oski, F. A., Naiman, J. L., Blum, S. F., Zarkowsky, H. S., Whaun, J., Shohet, S. B., Gren, A., and Nathan, D. G.: Congenital hemolytic anemia with high-sodium, low-potassium red cells, studies of three generations of a family with a new variant, New Eng. J. Med. **280**:909, 1969.
259. Oski, F. A., Nathan, D. G., Sidel, V. W., and Diamond, L. K.: Extreme hemolysis and red-cell distortion in erythrocyte pyruvate kinase deficiency. I. Morphology, erythrokinetics and family enzyme studies, New Eng. J. Med. **270**:1023, 1964.
260. Oski, F. A., Shahidi, N. T., and Diamond, L. K.: Erythrocyte acid phosphomonoesterase and glucose-6-phosphate dehydrogenase deficiency in Caucasians, Science **139**:403, 1963.
261. Owren, P. A.: Congenital hemolytic anemia; pathogenesis of the "hemolytic crisis," Blood **3**:231, 1948.
262. Ozer, L., and Mills, G. C.: Elliptocytosis with haemolytic anaemia, Brit. J. Haemat. **10**:468, 1964.
263. Pachter, M. R., Johnson, S. A., Neblett, R. T., and Truant, J. P.: Bleeding, platelets and macroglobulinemia, Amer. J. Clin. Path. **31**:467, 1959.
264. Paglia, D. E., Holland, P., Baughan, M. A., and Valentine, W. N.: Occurrence of defective hexosephosphate isomerization in human erythrocytes and leukocytes, New Eng. J. Med. **280**:66, 1969.
265. Paglia, D. E., Valentine, W. N., Baughan, M. A., Miller, D. R., Reed, C. F., and McIntyre, O. R.: An inherited molecular lesion of erythrocyte pyruvate kinase; identification of a kinetically aberrant isozyme associated with premature hemolysis, J. Clin. Invest. **47**:1929, 1968.
266. Palek, J., Mircevová, L., and Brabec, V.: 2,3-Diphosphoglycerate metabolism in hereditary spherocytosis, Brit. J. Haemat. **17**:59, 1969.
267. Parlic, G. J., and Bouroncle, B. A.: Megaloblastic crisis in paroxysmal nocturnal hemoglobinuria, New Eng. J. Med. **273**:789, 1965.
268. Parr, C. W., and Fitch, L. I.: Hereditary partial deficiency of human erythrocyte phos-

phogluconate dehydrogenase, Biochem. J. **93**:280, 1964.
269. Pearson, C. M., Beck, W. S., and Bland, W. H.: Idiopathic paroxysmal myoglobinuria, Arch. Intern. Med. **99**:376, 1957.
270. Pearson, H. A.: Megaloblastic crisis of sickle cell anemia, coincidence or fact. In Society for Pediatric Research Program Abstracts, 33rd Annual Meeting, Atlantic City, N. J., May, 1963.
271. Pearson, H. A.: The genetic basis of hereditary elliptocytosis with hemolysis, Blood **32**: 972, 1968.
272. Penfold, J. B., and Lipscomb, J. M.: Elliptocytosis in man associated with hereditary haemorrhagic telangiectasia, Quart. J. Med. **12**:157, 1943.
273. Perkoff, G. T.: Studies of human myoglobin in several diseases of muscle, New Eng. J. Med. **270**:263, 1964.
274. Perrine, R. P., and Gelpi, A. P.: The sickle cell paroxysmal nocturnal hemoglobinuria syndromes, Amer. J. Med. **37**:659, 1964.
275. Petz, L. D., and Fudenberg, H. H.: Coombs-positive hemolytic anemia caused by penicillin administration, New Eng. J. Med. **274**: 171, 1966.
276. Pierce, L. E., and Rath, C. E.: Evidence for folic acid deficiency in genesis of anemic sickle cell crisis, Blood **20**:19, 1962.
277. Pierce, P. P., and Aldrich, C. A.: Chronic hemolytic anemia with paroxysmal nocturnal hemoglobinuria (Marchiafava-Micheli syndrome); report of a case with marked thrombocytopenia in a five-year-old child, J. Pediat. **22**:30, 1943.
278. Pillemer, L., Blum, L., Lepow, I. H., Ross, O. A., Todd, E. W., and Wardlaw, A. C.: The properdin system and immunity; demonstration and isolation of a new serum protein, properdin, and its role in immune phenomena, Science **120**:279, 1954.
279. Pirofsky, B., Sutherland, D. W., Starr, A., and Griswold, H. E.: Hemolytic anemia complicating aortic-valve surgery, New Eng. J. Med. **272**:235, 1965.
280. Porter, F. S., and Lowe, B. A.: Congenital erythropoietic protoporphyria. I. Case reports, clinical studies and porphyrin analyses in two brothers, Blood **22**:521, 1963.
281. Post, R. L., Merritt, C. R., Kinsolving, C. R., and Albright, C. D.: Membrane adenosine triphosphatase as a participant in the active transport of sodium and potassium in the human erythrocyte, J. Biol. Chem. **235**:1796, 1960.
282. Prankerd, T. A. J.: Studies on the pathogenesis of haemolysis in hereditary spherocytosis, Quart. J. Med. **29**:199, 1960.
283. Prankerd, T. A. J., Altman, K. L., and Young, L. E.: Abnormalities of carbohydrate metabolism of red cells in hereditary spherocytosis, J. Clin. Invest. **34**:1268, 1955.
284. Prins, H. K., Oort, M., Loos, J. A., Zürcher, C., and Beckers, T.: Congenital nonspherocytic hemolytic anemia, associated with glutathione deficiency of the erythrocytes, Blood **27**:145, 1966.
285. Pryor, D. S., and Pitney, W. R.: Hereditary elliptocytosis; a report of two families from New Guinea, Brit. J. Haemat. **13**:126, 1967.
286. Quagliana, J. M., Cartwright, G. E., and Wintrobe, M. M.: Paroxysmal nocturnal hemoglobinuria following drug-induced aplastic anemia, Ann. Intern. Med. **61**:1045, 1964.
287. Ramot, B., Fisher, S., Szeinberg, A., Adam, A., Sheba, C., and Gafni, D.: A study of subjects with erythrocyte glucose-6-phosphate dehydrogenase deficiency. II. Investigation of leukocyte enzymes, J. Clin. Invest. **38**: 2234, 1959.
288. Rausen, A. R., Gerald, P. S., and Diamond, L. K.: Haptoglobin patterns in cord blood serums, Nature **191**:717, 1961.
289. Rausen, A. R., London, R. D., Mizrahi, A., and Cooper, L. Z.: Generalized bone changes and thrombocytopenic purpura in association with intrauterine rubella, Pediatrics **36**: 264, 1965.
290. Rausen, A. R., Richter, P., Tallal, L., and Cooper, L. Z.: Hematologic effects of intrauterine rubella, J.A.M.A. **199**:75, 1967.
291. Reed, C. F., and Swisher, S. N.: Erythrocyte lipid loss in hereditary spherocytosis, J. Clin. Invest. **45**:477, 1966.
292. Reed, W. B., Wuepper, K. D., Epstein, J. H., Redeker, A., Simonson, R. J., and McKusick, V. A.: Erythropoietic protoporphyria; a clinical and genetic study, J.A.M.A. **214**:1069, 1970.
293. Ricketts, W. E.: Bartonella bacilliformis anemia (Oroya fever); study of 30 cases, Blood **3**:1025, 1948.
294. Ritz, N. D., and Haber, A.: Auto-immune hemolytic anemia in a 6-week-old child, J. Pediat. **61**:904, 1962.
295. Ritzmann, S. E., and Levin, W. C.: Cryopathies; a review classification; diagnostic and therapeutic considerations, Arch. Intern. Med. **107**:754, 1961.
296. Ritzmann, S. E., Thurm, R. H., Truax, W. E., and Levin, W. C.: The syndrome of macroglobulinemia; review of the literature and a report of two cases of macrocryogelglobulinemia, Arch. Intern. Med. **105**:939, 1960.
296a. Robinson, M. A., Loder, P. B., and de Gruchy, G. C.: Red-cell metabolism in nonspherocytic congenital haemolytic anaemia, Brit. J. Haemat. **7**:327, 1961.
297. Robinson, M. G., Proiano, G., Cohen, H., and

Fundi, M.: Acute transient cryofibrinogenemia in infants, J. Pediat. **69**:35, 1966.

298. Rose, B. S., and Mabarro, S. N.: Four cases of acute acquired haemolytic anaemia in childhood treated with ACTH, Arch. Dis. Child. **28**:87, 1953.

299. Ross, J. D., and Rosenbaum, E.: Paroxysmal nocturnal hemoglobinuria presenting as aplastic anemia in a child; case report with evidence of deficient leukocyte acetylcholinesterase activity, Amer. J. Med. **37**:130, 1964.

300. Rosse, W. F., and Dacie, J. V.: Immune lysis of normal human and paroxysmal nocturnal hemoglobinuria (PNH) red blood cells. I. The sensitivity of PNH red cells to lysis by complement and specific antibody, J. Clin. Invest. **45**:736, 1966.

301. Rosse, W. F., and Sherwood, J. B.: Cold-reacting antibodies; differences in the reaction of anti-I antibodies with adult and cord red blood cells, Blood **36**:28, 1968.

302. Roth, K. L., and Frumin, A. M.: Studies on the hemolytic principle of the fava bean, J. Lab. Clin. Med. **56**:695, 1960.

303. Rudolph, N., and Gross, R. T.: Studies of in-vitro autohemolysis in blood from newborn infants, Brit. J. Haemat. **12**:351, 1966.

304. Sabine, J. E., Jung, E. D., Fish, M. B., Pestaner, L. C., and Rankin, R. E.: Observations on the inheritance of glucose-6-phosphate dehydrogenase deficiency in erythrocytes and in leucocytes, Brit. J. Haemat. **9**:164, 1963.

305. Salen, G., Goldstein, F., Havrani, F., and Wirts, C. W.: Acute hemolytic anemia complicating viral hepatitis in patients with glucose-6-phosphate dehydrogenase deficiency, Ann. Intern. Med. **65**:1210, 1966.

306. Sarles, H. E., and Levin, W. C.: The role of splenectomy in the management of acquired autoimmune hemolytic anemia complicating systemic lupus erythematosus, Amer. J. Med. **26**:547, 1959.

307. Sawitsky, A., and Ozaeta, P. B., Jr.: Disease-associated autoimmune hemolytic anemia, Bull. N. Y. Acad. Med. **46**:411, 1970.

308. Sayed, H. M., Dacie, J. V., Handley, D. A., Lewis, S. M., and Cleland, W. P.: Haemolytic anaemia of mechanical origin after open heart surgery, Thorax **16**:356, 1961.

309. Schmid, R.: The porphyrias. In Stanbury, J. B., Wyngaarden, S. B., and Fredrickson, D. S., editors: Metabolic basis of inherited disease, ed. 2, New York, 1966, McGraw-Hill Book Co., pp. 813-870.

310. Schmid, R., Schwartz, S., and Sundberg, R. D.: Erythropoietic (congenital) porphyria; a rare abnormality of the normoblasts, Blood **10**:416, 1955.

311. Schneider, A. S., Valentine, W. N., Hattori, M., and Heins, H. L., Jr.: Hereditary hemolytic anemia with triosephosphate isomerase deficiency, New Eng. J. Med. **272**:229, 1965.

312. Schwartz, R., and Dameshek, W.: The treatment of autoimmune hemolytic anemia with 6-mercaptopurine and thioguanine, Blood **19**:483, 1962.

313. Schwartz, R., Eisner, A., and Dameshek, W.: The effect of 6-mercaptopurine on primary and secondary immune responses, J. Clin. Invest. **38**:1394, 1959.

314. Scialom, C., Najean, Y., and Bernard, J.: Anémie Hémolytique Congénitale nonsphérocytaire avec déficit incomplet en 6-phosphogluconique-deshydrogenase, Nouv. Rev. Franc. Hemat. **6**:452, 1966.

315. Scott, R. B.: In Gellis, S. S., editor: Yearbook of Pediatrics, 1957-1958, Chicago, 1958, Year Book Medical Publishers, Inc., p. 294.

316. Seaman, A. J., and Starr, A.: Febrile postcardiotomy lymphocytic splenomegaly: a new entity, Ann. Surg. **156**:956, 1962.

317. Sears, D. A.: Plasma heme-binding in patients with hemolytic disorders, J. Lab. Clin. Med. **71**:484, 1968.

318. Segar, W. E.: Idiopathic paroxysmal myoglobinuria, Pediatrics **23**:12, 1959.

319. Selwyn, J. G., and Dacie, J. V.: Autohemolysis and other changes resulting from the incubation in vitro of red cells from patients with congenital hemolytic anemia, Blood **9**:414, 1954.

320. Shafer, W. A.: The phosphorylated carbohydrate intermediates from erythrocytes in hereditary spherocytosis, Blood **23**:417, 1964.

321. Shahidi, N. T., and Diamond, L. K.: Enzyme deficiency in erythrocytes in congenital nonspherocytic hemolytic anemia, Pediatrics **24**:245, 1959.

322. Shapiro, C. M., Josephson, A. M., Rozengvaig, S., and Kauffman, A.: Hereditary spherocytosis in the neonatal period, J. Pediat. **50**:308, 1957.

323. Shojania, A. M., and Gross, S.: Hemolytic anemias and folic acid deficiency in children, Amer. J. Dis. Child. **108**:53, 1964.

324. Shulman, N. R.: A mechanism of cell destruction in individuals sensitized to foreign antigens and its implications in autoimmunity, Ann. Intern. Med. **60**:506, 1965.

325. Sigler, A. T., Forman, E. N., Zinkham, W. H., Neill, C. A., and Bahnson, H. T.: The Waring Blendor syndrome, Amer. J. Dis. Child. **104**:470, 1962.

326. Sigler, A. T., Forman, E. N., Zinkham, W. H., and Neill, C. A.: Severe intravascular hemolysis following surgical repair of en-

docardial cushion defects, Amer. J. Med. **35:** 467, 1963.
327. Singer, K., Motulsky, A. G., and Wile, S. A.: Aplastic crisis in sickle cell anemia, J. Lab. Clin. Med. **35:**721, 1950.
328. Sklavurw-Zurukzoglu, S., and Malaka, K.: Serum haptoglobins in childhood, Lancet **2:**722, 1961.
329. Smiley, R. K., Dempsey, H., Villeneuve, P., and Campbell, J. S.: Atypical familial hemolytic anemia, Blood **11:**324, 1956.
330. Smith, C. H.: Diagnosis of anemias in infancy and childhood, J.A.M.A. **134:**991, 1947.
331. Smith, C. H., Erlandson, M. E., Schulman, I., and Stern, G.: Hazard of severe infections in splenectomized infants and children, Amer. J. Med. **22:**390, 1957.
332. Smithies, O.: Zone electrophoresis in starch gels; group variations in the serum proteins of normal human adults, Biochem. J. **61:** 629, 1955.
333. Smithies, O.: An improved procedure for starch-gel electrophoresis; further variations in the serum proteins of normal individuals, Biochem. J. **71:**585, 1959.
334. Smithies, O., and Walker, N. F.: Genetic control of some serum proteins in normal humans, Nature **176:**1265, 1955.
335. Smithies, O., and Walker, N. F.: Notation for serum protein groups and the genes controlling their inheritance, Nature **178:**694, 1956.
336. Spaet, T. H., Rosenthal, M. C., and Dameshek, W.: Idiopathic myoglobinuria in man; report of a case, Blood **9:**881, 1954.
337. Stahl, W. C.: March hemoglobinuria; report of five cases in students at Ohio State University, J.A.M.A. **164:**13, 1957.
338. Stamey, C. C., and Diamond, L. K.: Congenital hemolytic anemia in the newborn; relationship to kernicterus, Amer. J. Dis. Child. **94:**616, 1957.
339. Stats, D., Wasserman, L. R., and Rosenthal, N.: Hemolytic anemia with hemoglobinuria, Amer. J. Clin. Path. **18:**757, 1948.
340. Stevenson, T. D., and Baker, H. J.: Haemolytic anaemia following insertion of Starr-Edwards valve prosthesis, Lancet **2:**982, 1964.
341. Stevenson, T. D., McDonald, B. L., and Rosten, S.: Colorimetric method for determination of erythrocyte glutathione, J. Lab. Clin. Med. **56:**157, 1960.
342. Sturgeon, P.: Hematological observations in the anemia associated with blood type $Rh_{null}$, Blood **36:**319, 1970.
343. Suess, J., Limentani, D., Dameshek, W., and Doloff, M. J.: A quantitative method for the determination and charting of the erythrocyte hypotonic fragility, Blood **3:**1290, 1948.
344. Szeinberg, A., Asher, Y., and Sheba, C.: Studies on glutathione stability in erythrocytes of cases with past history of favism or sulfa-drug-induced hemolysis, Blood **13:**348, 1958.
345. Szeinberg, A., Oliver, M., Schmidt, R., Adam, A., and Sheba, C.: Glucose-6-phosphate dehydrogenase deficiency and haemolytic disease of the newborn in Israel, Arch. Dis. Child. **38:**23, 1963.
346. Szeinberg, A., and Sheba, C.: Hemolytic trait in Oriental Jews connected with an hereditary enzymatic abnormality of erythrocytes, Israel M. J. **17:**158, 1958.
347. Szeinberg, A., Sheba, C., and Adam, A.: Selective occurrence of glutathione instability in red corpuscles of the various Jewish tribes, Blood **13:**1043, 1963.
348. Taddeini, L., and Watson, C. J.: The clinical porphyrias, Seminars Hemat. **5:**335, 1968.
349. Tanaka, K. R., Valentine, W. N., and Fredricks, R. E.: Studies on leukocytic and erythrocyte enzymes in paroxysmal nocturnal hemoglobinuria, Clin. Res. **8:**132, 1960.
350. Tanaka, K. R., Valentine, W. N., and Miwa, S.: Pyruvate kinase (PK) deficiency hereditary nonspherocytic hemolytic anaemia, Blood **19:**267, 1962.
351. Tarlov, A. R., Brewer, G. J., Carson, P. E., and Alving, A. S.: Primaquine sensitivity glucose-6-phosphate dehydrogenase deficiency; an inborn error of metabolism of medical and biological significance, Arch. Intern. Med. **109:**209, 1962.
352. Tarlov, A. R., and Kellermeyer, R. W.: The hemolytic effect of primaquine. XI. Decreased catalase activity in primaquine-sensitive erythrocytes, J. Lab. Clin. Med. **58:**204, 1961.
352a. Tarui, S., Okuno, G., Ikura, Y., Tanaka, T., Suda, M., and Nishikawa, M.: Phosphofructokinase deficiency in skeletal muscle; a new type of glycogenosis, Biochem. Biophys. Res. Commun. **19:**517, 1965.
353. Taylor, L.: Idiopathic autoimmune hemolytic anemia; response of a patient to repeated courses of alkylating agents, Amer. J. Med. **35:**130, 1963.
354. Tuttle, A. H.: Demonstration of hemoglobin-reactive substance in human serum, Science **121:**701, 1955.
355. Tuttle, A. H.: Serum pigment studies in newborn infants, I. Erythroblastosis fetalis, Amer. J. Dis. Child. **89:**544, 1955.
356. Valentine, W. N.: Hereditary hemolytic anemias associated with specific erythrocyte enzymopathies, Calif. Med. **108:**280, 1968.
357. Valentine, W. N., Hsieh, H. S., Paglia, D. E., Anderson, H. M., Baughan, M. A., Jaffé, E.

R., and Garson, O. M.: Hereditary hemolytic anemia associated with phosphoglycerate kinase deficiency in erythrocytes and leukocytes, New Eng. J. Med. **280**:528, 1969.
358. Valentine, W. N., Oski, F. A., Paglia, D. E., Baughan, M. A., Schneider, A. S., and Naiman, J. L.: Hereditary hemolytic anemia with hexokinase deficiency; role of hexokinase in erythrocyte aging, New Eng. J. Med. **276**:1, 1967.
359. Valentine, W. N., Schneider, A. S., Baughan, M. A., Paglia, D. E., and Heins, H. L., Jr.: Hereditary hemolytic anemia with triosephosphate isomerase deficiency; studies in kindreds with co-existent sickle cell trait and erythrocyte glucose-6-phosphate dehydrogenase deficiency, Amer. J. Med. **41**:27, 1966.
360. Valentine, W. N., Tanaka, K. R., and Miwa, S.: A specific erythrocyte glycolytic enzyme defect (pyruvate kinase) in three subjects with congenital nonspherocytic anemia, Trans. Ass. Amer. Physicians **74**:100, 1961.
361. Valtis, D. S., and Baikie, A. G.: The influence of red-cell thickness on the oxygen dissociation curve of blood, Brit. J. Haemat. **1**:146, 1955.
362. Van Loghem, J. J., Jr., Mendes de Leon, D. E.: Frenkel-Tietz, H., and van der Hart, M.: Two different serologic mechanisms of paroxysmal cold hemoglobinuria, illustrated by three cases, Blood **7**:1196, 1952.
363. Varadi, S.: Haematological aspects in a case of erythropoietic porphyria, Brit. J. Haemat. **4**:270, 1958.
364. Vaughan, J. M., Barnett, E. V., and Leddy, J. P.: Autosensitivity diseases; immunologic and pathogenetic concepts in lupus erythematosus, rheumatoid arthritis and hemolytic anemia, New Eng. J. Med. **275**:1986, 1966.
365. Verdon, T. A., Jr., Forrester, R. H., and Crosby, W. H.: Hemolytic anemia after open-heart repair of ostium-primum defects, New Eng. J. Med. **269**:444, 1963.
366. Waldenström, J.: The porphyrias as inborn errors of metabolism, Amer. J. Med. **22**:758, 1957.
367. Wallerstein, R. O., and Aggeler, P. M.: Acute hemolytic anemia, Amer. J. Med. **37**:92, 1964.
368. Watson, D., and Porter, R.: On haemoglobin degradation in the newborn, Acta Haemat. **29**:37, 1963.
369. Weed, R. I., La Celle, P. L., and Merrill, S. W.: Metabolic dependence of red cell deformability, J. Clin. Invest. **48**:795, 1969.
370. Weed, R. I., and Reed, C. F.: Membrane alterations leading to red cell destructions, Amer. J. Med. **41**:681, 1966.
371. Weiss, I. H.: Hereditary elliptocytosis with hemolytic anemia; report of six cases, Amer. J. Med. **35**:455, 1963.
372. Whitaker, J. A., Sartain, P., and Shaheedy, M.: Hematological aspects of congenital syphilis, J. Pediat. **66**:629, 1965.
373. Whitten, C. F.: Studies in serum haptoglobins, Amer. J. Dis. Child. **102**:480, 1961.
374. Wiley, J. S., and Firkin, B. G.: An unusual variant of hereditary spherocytosis, Amer. J. Med. **48**:63, 1970.
375. Willoughby, M. L. N., Pears, M. A., Sharp, A. A., and Shields, M. J.: Megaloblastic erythropoiesis in acquired hemolytic anemia, Blood **17**:351, 1961.
376. Wilmers, M. J., and Russell, P. A.: Autoimmune haemolytic anaemia in infant treated by thymectomy, Lancet **2**:915, 1963.
377. Witebsky, E.: Ehrlich's side chain theory in the light of present immunology, Ann. N. Y. Acad. Sci. **59**:168, 1954.
378. Worlledge, S. M.: Annotation; autoantibody formation association with methyldopa (Aldomet) therapy, Brit. J. Haemat. **16**:5, 1969.
379. Worlledge, S. M., Carstairs, K. C., and Dacie, J. V.: Auto-immune haemolytic anaemia associated with a-methyldopa therapy, Lancet **2**:135, 1966.
380. Worlledge, S. M., and Rousso, C.: Studies in the serology of paroxysmal cold hemoglobinuria (P.C.H.) with special reference to its relationship with the P blood group system, Vox Sang. **10**:293, 1965.
381. Wyandt, H., Bancroft, P. M., and Winship, T. O.: Elliptic erythrocytes in man, Arch. Intern. Med. **68**:1043, 1941.
382. Young, L. E.: Hereditary spherocytosis, Amer. J. Med. **18**:486, 1955.
383. Young, L. E.: Hemolytic disorders; some highlights of twenty years of progress, Ann. Intern. Med. **49**:1073, 1958.
384. Young, L. E., Izzo, M. J., Altman, K. I., and Swisher, S. N.: Studies on spontaneous in vitro autohemolysis in hemolytic disorders, Blood **11**:977, 1956.
385. Young, L. E., Izzo, M. J., and Platzer, R. F.: Hereditary spherocytosis; clinical, hematologic and genetic features in 28 cases, with particular reference to the osmotic and mechanical fragility of incubated erythrocytes, Blood **6**:1073, 1951.
386. Young, L. E., Miller, G., and Swisher, S. N.: Treatment of hemolytic disorders, J. Chron. Dis. **6**:307, 1957.
387. Young, L. E., Platzer, R. F., Evin, D. M., and Izzo, M. J.: Hereditary spherocytosis; observations on the role of the spleen, Blood **6**:1099, 1951.
387a. Zail, S. S., and Joubert, S. M.: Starch gel electrophoresis of erythrocyte membranes in

hereditary spherocytosis, Brit. J. Haemat. **14:** 57, 1968.
388. Zalusky, R.: Drug-associated hemolytic anemia, Bull. N. Y. Acad. Med. **46:**427, 1970.
389. Zarkowsky, H. S., Oski, F. A., Sha'afi, R., Shohet, S. B., and Nathan, D. G.: Congenital hemolytic anemia with high sodium, low potassium red cells. I. Studies of membrane permeability, New Eng. J. Med. **278:** 573, 1968.
390. Zetterstrom, R., and Strindberg, B.: Sporadic congenital spherocytosis associated with congenital hypoplastic thrombocytopenia and malformations, Acta Paediat. **47:**14, 1958.
391. Zinkham, W. H., and Childs, B.: Effect of vitamin K and naphthalene metabolites on glutathione metabolism of erythrocytes from normal newborns and patients with naphthalene hemolytic anemia, Amer. J. Dis. Child. **94:**420, 1957.
392. Zinkham, W. H., and Childs, B.: A defect of glutathione metabolism in erythrocytes from patients with a naphthalene-induced hemolytic anemia, Pediatrics **22:**461, 1958.
393. Zinkham, W. H., and Diamond, L. K.: In vitro erythrophagocytosis in acquired hemolytic anemia, Blood **7:**592, 1952.
394. Zinkham, W. H., and Lenhard, R. E., Jr.: Metabolic abnormalities of erythrocytes from patients with congenital nonspherocytic hemolytic anemia, J. Pediat. **55:**319, 1959.
395. Zipursky, A.: Metabolic abnormalities of erythrocytes in hemolytic anemias, Ped. Clin. N. Amer. **9:**559, 1962.
396. Zuelzer, W. W., Mastrangelo, R., Stolberg, C. S., Paulik, M. D., Page, R. H., and Thompson, R. I.: Autoimmune hemolytic anemia; natural history and viral-immunologic interactions in childhood, Amer. J. Med. **49:**80, 1970.
397. Zuelzer, W. W., Stolberg, C. S., Page, R. H., Teruga, J., and Brough, A. J.: Etiology and pathogenesis of acquired hemolytic anemia, Transfusion **6:**438, 1966.

# 16 THE HEREDITARY HEMOGLOBINOPATHIES

The far-reaching observations of Pauling and associates,[370] which demonstrated that the sickling phenomenon was dependent upon an abnormal hemoglobin, stimulated an intense interest in human hemoglobin in normal and disease states. Rapidly accumulating information resulted in the identification of a large number of abnormal hemoglobins and showed that they were genetically controlled. This added information documented the concept that the clinical and pathologic features of many of the hereditary hemolytic disorders are basically conditioned by chemical and physical changes in the hemoglobin.[90,244,542,556]

The hemoglobinopathies comprise genetically determined disorders in which synthesis of normal adult hemoglobin is partially or completely suppressed causing the normal hemoglobin to be replaced by a hemoglobin variant including the fetal variety. Thalassemia is conveniently grouped with the hemoglobinopathies because of the large amounts of fetal hemoglobin replacing the normal adult type in patients with severe disease and the combination of fetal hemoglobin with other well-defined abnormal hemoglobins. No abnormal hemoglobin, however, has been described in patients with thalassemia.

The description of specific hereditary hemoglobinopathies necessitates a preliminary consideration of methods by which the abnormal hemoglobins are identified and an analysis of their genetic transmission.

For the laboratory evaluation of the hereditary hemoglobinopathies the following procedures are useful.
1. Smear for morphology; complete blood count, including reticulocytes
2. Sickle cell preparation
3. Tests for fetal hemoglobin
   a. Alkali denaturation
   b. Acid elution method of demonstrating fetal hemoglobin and distribution in red blood cells
4. Heat stability test for unstable hemoglobins
5. Incubation with brilliant cresyl blue for inclusion bodies in HbH disease
6. Heinz body preparation
7. Evidence of hemolysis
8. Osmotic fragility in hypotonic sodium chloride solution
9. Glutathione level—may be decreased in unstable hemoglobinopathies
10. Methemoglobin level; congenital methemoglobinemias due to enzyme deficiencies or HbM
11. Hemoglobin electrophoresis, $HbA_2$, HbF
12. Spectroscopy
13. Hybridization and recombination studies
14. Fingerprinting

Only those procedures will be discussed which are commonly employed in clinical laboratories.

**Methods for determining the hemoglobin types.** Differences between the hemoglobin of the human fetus and that of the adult have been known since 1886, when Korber[285] demonstrated that fetal hemoglobin was more resistant to denaturation by alkaline solutions than was the adult type. Two simple procedures have served to identify the fetal and other types of hemoglobins. Fetal hemoglobin is determined by the method of alkali denaturation, and the abnormal hemoglobins have been separated by the technique of electrophoresis.

*Alkali denaturation method for fetal hemoglobin (hemoglobin F).* The fetal hemoglobin content is determined by the "one point" denaturation technique described by Singer and co-workers.[458] With this technique, an approximate 10% hemoglobin solution is denatured for exactly 1 minute by N/12 NaOH, the reaction being halted and the denatured hemoglobin precipitated by the addition of 50%

saturated ammonium sulfate reagent. The hemoglobin concentration in the filtrate (undenatured) is determined photoelectrically, and the percentage of undenatured or alkali-resistant hemoglobin (fetal hemoglobin) is calculated.

Brinkman, Jonxis, and Huisman, using another alkali denaturation technique[84,266] in which readings are obtained from a curve constructed from sequential readings over a period of 12 minutes, show a variance with the 1-minute denaturation method of Singer and co-workers.[458] The former showed that, at high percentages of fetal hemoglobin, the results obtained with the 1-minute method are about 10% too low. This is attributed to the fact that incompletely denatured hemoglobin is removed by precipitation and filtration. At concentrations below 10% of fetal hemoglobin, this method is less accurate and more difficult to interpret. A combined alkaline denaturation and spectrographic method has also been described suitable for the range of 1 to 10% fetal hemoglobin and indicates its presence at the "trace level" (0.4 to 1%).[87]

To detect slight elevations of fetal hemoglobin as found in individuals heterozygous for beta-thalassemia, a modification of the technique of Singer and colleagues has been devised by Betke, Marti, and Schlicht[50] which is useful in the routine clinical laboratory. This method gives normal values for alkali-resistant hemoglobin in the 0.5 to 1% range but values in excess of 1.5% are clearly elevated.

*Acid elution method of demonstrating fetal hemoglobin in red blood cells.* Using a microspectrophotometric method, it was shown that hemoglobins A and F may be present in the same red cell and are apparently derived from hemoglobins synthesized in the same erythroblast.[322] The acid elution method demonstrating their simultaneous presence has been described previously (Chapters 1 and 3). The method is based on the lower solubility of alkali-resistant or fetal hemoglobin in an acid environment (citric-phosphate buffer). With this procedure hemoglobin F remains in the erythrocytes, whereas hemoglobins A, S, and C are eluted. Red cells that have lost their hemoglobin appear as pale-staining ghost forms, whereas those that contain fetal hemoglobin are largely intact and take the eosin stain.[278,279] The acid elution method tends to give higher fetal hemoglobin readings than assay by alkali denaturation. This procedure has also made it possible to identify small numbers of fetal erythrocytes found in the maternal circulation of many pregnant women. The details of the method and its modification have appeared in many papers.[97,170,279]

*Electrophoresis.* The migration of charged particles in an electrolyte solution which takes place when an electric current is passed through the solution is termed electrophoresis. In this process particles bearing positive charges migrate to the cathode while negatively charged particles move to the anode. This principle has provided a means by which plasma proteins and hemoglobin solutions exposed to an electric field under selected conditions are separated in accordance with their isoelectric points and the individual mobilities of each constituent. The speed and direction of forward migration depend upon the type of solution used to conduct the electric current, its pH, the ionic strength, and the strength of the electric current. A single amino acid substitution that alters the charge in any chain is usually sufficient to modify electrophoretic behavior of the whole molecule.

The moving boundary method of Tiselius, previously employed extensively, has been simplified with the use of paper electrophoresis. With the latter, a strip of filter paper properly prepared permits the differentiation of serum proteins and of hemoglobins according to their different velocities. In contrast to the use of acid pH (cacodylate buffer of pH 6.5) for the method of moving boundary electrophoresis, the filter paper method of zone electrophoresis employs an alkaline buffer of pH 8.6 in which negatively charged protein particles move toward the positive electrode (the anode). With the contemporary interest in the relationship of abnormal hemoglobins to the hereditary hemolytic anemias, paper electrophoresis has provided a readily accessible tool in the identification of the hemoglobins. This method incorporates certain basic features, which can be briefly outlined.

PAPER METHOD. In the paper method of electrophoresis the strip of paper is maintained in the horizontal position or is raised in the middle by suspension on one or more supporting rods. In either case, the paper is saturated with buffer solution, with the ends dipping into containers of the same solution. In the horizontal type of paper electrophoresis a length of filter paper wet with buffer solution rests on a plate of glass or plastic material with projecting points for support, with the overlapping

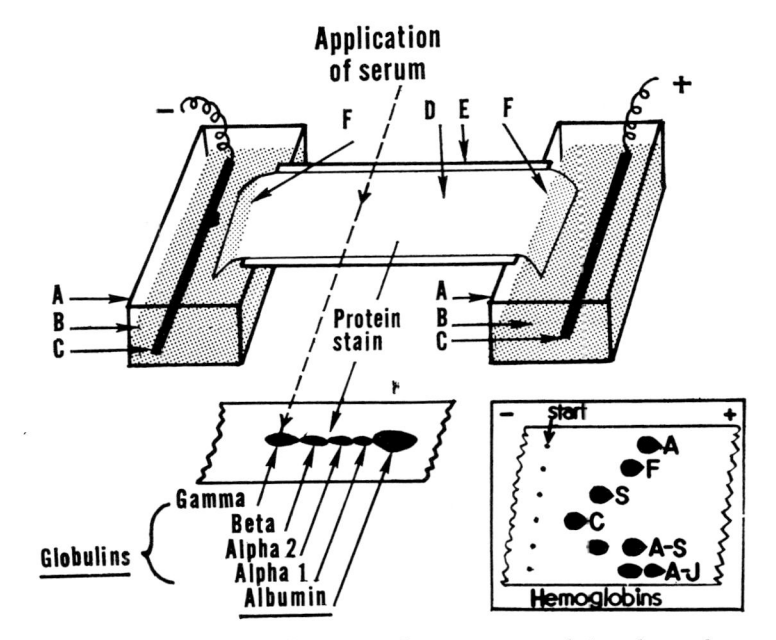

Fig. 32. Diagrammatic illustration of a type of apparatus used for electrophoresis and the results of electrophoretic separation of serum as revealed by protein stain. A, Glass or plastic buffer reservoirs. B, Buffer. C, Electrodes, connected to source of direct electrical current. D, Anticonvectant material, such as filter paper and cellulose acetate. E, Nonconducting support, such as glass or plastic. F, Ends of anticonvectant material (or wicks) in contact with buffer. Evaporation of buffer from the anticonvectant material during electrophoresis is prevented by covering the material with glass or plastic or by enclosing the entire assembly in a vapor-tight compartment. In the right lower corner is an insert of an electrophoretic pattern obtained with the same type of apparatus. Hemoglobin J, while uncommon, is included as an example of a fast hemoglobin. Hemoglobin is prepared for electrophoresis by washing and hemolyzing erythrocytes, after which insoluble materials are removed, leaving the hemoglobin in solution. Erythrophoresis is carried out by using the hemoglobin solution in the same manner as that for the analysis of serum. (From Tuttle, A. H.: Newer techniques in the investigation of blood disorders, Ped. Clin. N. Amer. 9:529, 1962.)

ends of the paper dipping vertically into troughs filled with the same solution. In adjacent compartments at each end are placed the respective electrodes. Before the solution is covered, minute quantities of the red cell hemolysate to be tested (prepared from the hemolysis of red cells in distilled water) are applied to the filter paper close to the cathodal end. In a solution of veronal buffer (pH 8.6, ionic strength of approximately 0.06, and a specified voltage and current flow) the various hemoglobins migrate toward the anode according to their individual mobilities. After an initial period of 2 to 3 hours the hemoglobins have separated sufficiently to be recognized, the length of the complete run (usually 4 to 6 hours) depending upon the particular requirements of the laboratory. At the end of the separation the strips are removed and dried, and amounts of each hemoglobin may be roughly estimated or accurately measured. Electrophoresis depends mainly on the charge carried by the protein molecule at the pH of the buffer and, to a much lesser extent, on the supporting and suspending media. (See Fig. 32.)

With the introduction of zone electrophoresis, in which various anticonvectant buffered bridging media are employed to connect wells of solution in which electrodes are immersed, the procedure has attained wide application to clinical problems. Although many anticonvectant bridging materials have been employed for investigative purposes, those of most general use in clinical laboratories include filter paper strips soaked in buffer, cellulose acetate, a synthetic polymer-polyacrylamide gel, agar gel, starch gel, and blocks of starch granules. Filter paper strips are readily available without tedious preparative techniques. Separate proteins can be stained and the strips can be retained as permanent records. A relative quantitation of separated stained proteins can be determined by photoelectric scanning. However, separation is not as definitive as with other techniques. Methods of elution are unsatisfactory and the strips will accommodate only small quantities, so that other methods are frequently necessary for analytical studies and quantitation. Agar gel is especially useful for identification of minor components of separate proteins by precipitation with specific antibodies (immunoelectrophoresis). The best resolution is obtained with starch gels, especially when the vertical method is employed. Starch gel is especially useful in identification of minor components of a mixture.[511] However, elution techniques satisfactory for clinical use are not available.

The starch gel electrophoretic technique of Smithies[485] is a sensitive and widely used method for resolving the complements of complex protein mixtures and is especially useful in the analysis of serum (i.e., haptoglobins) proteins. A modification of Smithies' technique has been devised for the analysis of serum, hemoglobin, and protein extracts.[319]

Starch block electrophoresis will accommodate larger quantities of a substance to be separated and can be cut into segments, from which elution is easily accomplished. It is of special value in harvesting of purified fractions for further studies and for quantitation. This technique and that of cellulose acetate, mentioned previously, are particularly useful in the measurement of hemoglobin $A_2$ which is so important in the diagnosis of thalassemia minor. The advantage of the latter technique is the more rapid separation of the bands. Both methods, however, are useful for routine hemoglobin electrophoresis.

**Designation of hemoglobin types.** Previously recommended nomenclature designated the capital letter A for normal adult hemoglobin, F for fetal hemoglobin, S for sickle cell hemoglobin, and consecutive letters of the alphabet for abnormal types in order of their identification. Currently, newly identified hemoglobin variants are named after the city or other geographic region in which they are discovered.

Case reports have established the importance of types C, D, and E, which occur in association with well-defined hematologic entities. The racial incidence of hemoglobins is exemplified by the predominance of the abnormal hemoglobins S, C, and D in Negroes and E in natives of Thailand.

The characterization of the various types of normal hemoglobin and their components are described in Chapter 4. The differences between these hemoglobins reside in the globin structure rather than in the heme. The various hemoglobins are differentiated by their mobilities on electrophoresis, by chromatographic and chemical determinations, and, in the case of fetal hemoglobin, by alkali denaturation and acid elution.

**Structure of the hemoglobin molecule: polypeptide content of globin.** In summarizing the normal hemoglobins the globin of the normal adult hemoglobin molecule (hemoglobin A) is made up of a pair of alpha peptide chains (alpha chains) linked with a pair of beta polypeptide chains (beta chains). The molecule of normal fetal hemoglobin (HbF), however, consists of a pair of alpha chains linked with another type of polypeptide chain—a pair of gamma chains.[399] The molecule of hemoglobin $A_2$ (Hb$A_2$) contains two alpha chains identical with those of HbA, but in a combination with a pair of polypeptide delta chains (Fig. 33).

The hemoglobins characteristic of two of the hemoglobinopathies are tetramers of a single polypeptide: hemoglobin H consists of four beta chains and Bart's hemoglobin of four gamma chains.

The abnormal hemoglobins are regarded as products of mutant genes at the alpha and beta loci. From genetic evidence, the production of four types of chains—alpha, beta, gamma, and delta—are under the control of sets of allelic genes at separate loci. Alpha, beta, gamma, and delta chains are chemically different. The synthesis of each type of chain is probably governed by a different set of genes so that one gene controls one polypeptide chain. Regulation of rates of synthesis may involve a genetic transition such as the changeover from hemoglobin F to hemoglobin A or, more precisely, from gamma to beta chains occurring late in fetal life and continuing in infancy.

Using Greek letters to designate the poly-

$$\text{Hb A} = 2 \text{ alpha, } 2 \text{ beta} = \alpha_2^A \, \beta_2^A$$

$$\text{Hb F} = 2 \text{ alpha, } 2 \text{ gamma} = \alpha_2^A \, \gamma_2^F$$

$$\text{Hb A}_2 = 2 \text{ alpha, } 2 \text{ delta} = \alpha_2^A \, \delta_2^{A2}$$

Fig. 33. Polypeptide chains of hemoglobin.

peptide chain and the superscript to denote the type of hemoglobin, normal hemoglobin and its two minor components may be designated as follows (Gerald and Ingram[182]):

HbA —alpha$_2^A$ beta$_2^A$
HbA$_2$—alpha$_2^A$ delta$_2^{A2}$
HbF —alpha$_2^A$ gamma$_2^F$

Thus, HbS (sickle cell hemoglobin) is designated as alpha$_2^A$ beta$_2^S$ since the affected polypeptide occurs in the beta chains. Bart's hemoglobin is written Hb Bart's—gamma$_4^F$, and HbH—beta$_4^A$.

A few abnormal hemoglobins such as hemoglobin I and hemoglobin Hopkins-2 have abnormal alpha chains, while the beta chains are structurally unaltered. These hemoglobins may, therefore, be designated HbI—alpha$_2^I$ beta$_2^A$; Hopkins-2—alpha$_2^{Ho2}$ beta$_2^A$.[240] A complete list of common and uncommon alpha and beta chain substitutions in the hemoglobin molecule are listed in Tables 21 to 23.

By dissociation and recombination by exposure of hemoglobin to media of low pH, it has been possible to demonstrate which polypeptide chains carry the abnormality in the test hemoglobin.[204] It has been possible by this method to demonstrate or confirm that the abnormalities of hemoglobin S, C, and G are on the beta chain and the abnormalities of hemoglobin I and Ho2 (Hopkins-2) are on the alpha chain.

It has been reported by Ingram[241] that more mutations are to be found in the beta peptide chain than in the alpha chain. The hemoglobins that are found with high frequency are all in the beta chain—hemoglobins S, C, E, and D$_{Punjab}$. The difficulties that would be encountered if the alpha chain were frequently involved are obvious, since the beta peptide chain contributes only to the formation of the adult hemoglobin, whereas the alpha chain is a component of adult and fetal hemoglobin and of hemoglobin A$_2$.[241]

In Chapter 1 the parallels between hemoglobin and protein synthesis are described according to the concepts of Jacob and Monod.[248] The structural genes are responsible for the molecular organization of protein and these are controlled by the operator and regulator genes. The operator gene reacts to a repressor substance which is produced by the regulator gene. The repressors can either be inactivated or activated. An example of this control is the switching off of HbF synthesis during the first year of life and its replacement by HbA synthesis.

While the genetic information is stored in nuclear DNA, the polypeptide chains (in this instance, the globin chains of hemoglobin) are manufactured in the cytoplasm. Protein is synthesized in the ribosomes which receive the information stored in nuclear DNA and conveyed through messenger RNA. Amino acids are activated to fit into position in the polypeptide chains and are conveyed to the ribosome by transfer RNA.[298]

*Electrophoretic mobility of the individual hemoglobins.* According to the specific conditions prescribed for paper electrophoresis of the common hemoglobin types, hemoglobins H and I move farthest toward the anode and C is the slowest, remaining near the starting point. Intermediate between A and C, in descending order of slower mobility, are the hemoglobins F, G, S, D, and E. Type F is imperfectly separated from type A unless F appears in great excess. Hemoglobins S and D have identical mobilities. In its homozygous form type G migrates at a single focus between types S and F and is differentiated from the latter by its lack of resistance to alkali denaturation.[431] The mobilities of types H and I, appearing closest to the anodal end of the filter paper, are greater than type A. Hemoglobin J[508] possesses an electrophoretic mobility between hemoglobins I and A. Electrophoretically HbA$_2$ runs identically with HbE but it can be separated by measuring the quantity. HbA$_2$ is usually not present in blood exceeding 5% of the total pigment. In HbE, the quantity of HbE present is nearly always far more than 20%. HbC is the slowest moving of all the hemoglobins. On electrophoresis HbC runs very near HbE or HbA$_2$ but can easily be separated by chromatography.[482]

The relative mobility rates are represented schematically in Fig. 34 and are shown electrophoretically in Fig. 35.

In the electrophoretic determination of serum proteins, separation also depends on the mobility of proteins in an electrical field. Here charged particles migrate in an electrolyte solution, with the rate of migration depending on their different surface charges and pH values above and below their isoelectric points. With application of the current, migration of the protein components proceeds as follows: albumin particles, which are smaller and more highly charged, migrate most rapidly followed by various globulins. In order of their decreasing mobility they are albumin, alpha and alpha-2 globulins, beta globulins, fibrinogen, and finally gamma globulin. (See Fig. 32.)

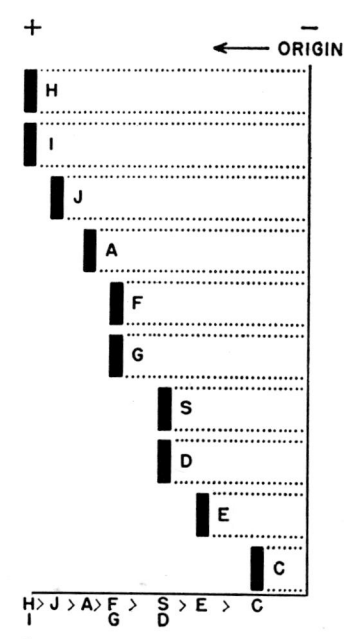

Fig. 34. Schematic representation of relative mobility of individual hemoglobin at pH 8.6. (From Smith, C. H.: The abnormal hemoglobins: clinical and hematologic aspects, J. Pediat. **50**:91, 1957.)

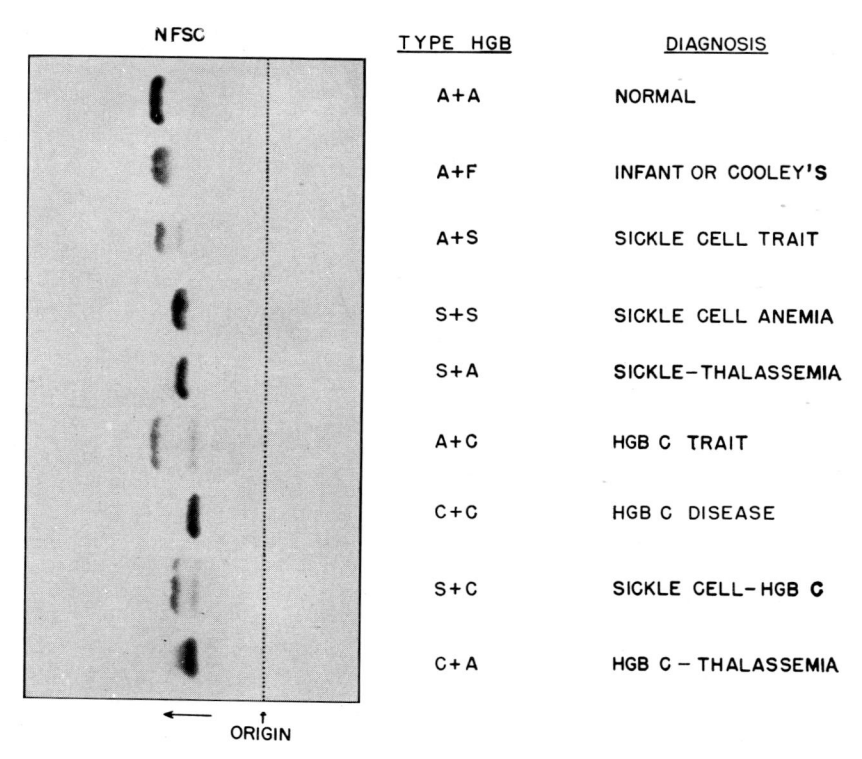

| TYPE HGB | DIAGNOSIS |
|---|---|
| A+A | NORMAL |
| A+F | INFANT OR COOLEY'S |
| A+S | SICKLE CELL TRAIT |
| S+S | SICKLE CELL ANEMIA |
| S+A | SICKLE-THALASSEMIA |
| A+C | HGB C TRAIT |
| C+C | HGB C DISEASE |
| S+C | SICKLE CELL-HGB C |
| C+A | HGB C - THALASSEMIA |

Fig. 35. Electrophoretic patterns of the common hereditary hemoglobinopathies. (From Smith, C. H.: The abnormal hemoglobins: clinical and hematologic aspects, J. Pediat. **50**:91, 1957.)

*Fetal hemoglobin.* Important biochemical differences exist between adult hemoglobin and the form elaborated by the human fetus during prenatal life. Although the heme component of the two hemoglobin molecules is similar, the structure and properties of globin and, possibly, of the heme-globin linkages are different. The property by which fetal hemoglobin is best known and most readily identified is its increased resistance to denaturation by alkaline solutions.

Fetal hemoglobin, which comprises 44 to 89% of the hemoglobin in the newborn infant,[428] decreases rapidly during the first year of life and is rarely demonstrable after the age of 30 months.[89] Following this period and in the child and adult, 2% represents the upper limit of normal. In certain of the chronic hereditary hemolytic disorders, fetal hemoglobin reappears in substantial amounts. Large quantities of fetal hemoglobin are synthesized in patients with sickle cell anemia (5 to 15%), severe Cooley's anemia (to a lesser extent), spherocytic anemia (usually less than 10%),[458] and aplastic anemia.[445] The highest concentrations of alkali-resistant hemoglobin are found in patients with severe Cooley's anemia in whom it may represent almost the entire hemoglobin content (12 to 100%). The reason for these excessive amounts of embryonic hemoglobin is unknown and cannot be correlated with the severity of the disease. Since multiple transfusions tend to depress hemoglobin production, true estimates of its concentration can be made only during treatment-free intervals or prior to the initiation of blood transfusions.[475]

Some of the acquired pathologic states which have been associated with increased levels of fetal hemoglobin include: megaloblastic anemia, congenital hypoplastic anemia, leukemia (acute and chronic myelogenous leukemia, erythroleukemia, acute lymphoblastic leukemia), sideroblastic anemia, metastatic carcinoma involving the bone marrow, and paroxysmal nocturnal hemoglobinuria.[359] Increased levels have also been found in pregnancy. In pernicious anemia, the level of HbF falls slowly to normal values with remission of the disease. Normal values are present in patients with iron-deficiency anemia and acquired hemolytic anemia.[458]

The presence of high concentrations of fetal hemoglobin in early infancy apparently suppresses formation of sickle hemoglobin[524] and hemoglobin C.[504] Sickling gradually increases after birth to reach maximal levels at 4 months of age.[526] The replacement of fetal cells which are incapable of being sickled by red cells formed during the early months of life which are capable of being sickled is more closely correlated with the drop of fetal hemoglobin than with the absolute percentage of hemoglobin S.[450] This state of high-level fetal hemoglobin and minimal sickle cell formation may serve as a protection against the probable dire effects of intracapillary sickling in utero where low oxygen tension prevails.

The explanation for the large quantities of fetal hemoglobin synthesized in these conditions may be due to mutant genes which block beta chain production and reactivate gamma chain production.[500]

*Hereditary persistence of fetal hemoglobin (the high fetal gene).* Fetal hemoglobin may be elevated in healthy adults to the extent of 6 to 33%. This anomaly, which occurs in families of African extraction, represents a persistence of fetal hemoglobin into adult life, perhaps as a partial failure of forming adult hemoglobin.[249] The high fetal hemoglobin component may occur in combination with hemoglobin A, S, or C and is allelic with genes for these hemoglobins. The F gene (high fetal), in combination with S or C hemoglobin, suppresses hemoglobin A formation completely. The F gene is either allelic with or closely linked to the locus for the S and C genes and for beta thalassemia[537] at a locus at which the structure of the beta chain of globin is determined.

In combination with hemoglobin A no hematologic abnormalities are present. The F (high fetal) gene is found unassociated with the usual findings in the thalassemia trait. When this abnormality occurs in persons who are heterozygous for hemoglobin S, there is also frequently little or no anemia. Exceptionally, a few patients with this combination (F-S) have had clinical manifestations characterizing the sickle cell disorder such as mild anemia, aseptic necrosis of the femoral head, and joint pains.[214] In a single case of interaction of the genes for hemoglobin C and high fetal gene, severe anemia resulted.[325]

Persons heterozygous for the fetal anomaly and for hemoglobin S have approximately 70% hemoglobin S and 30% hemoglobin F in their

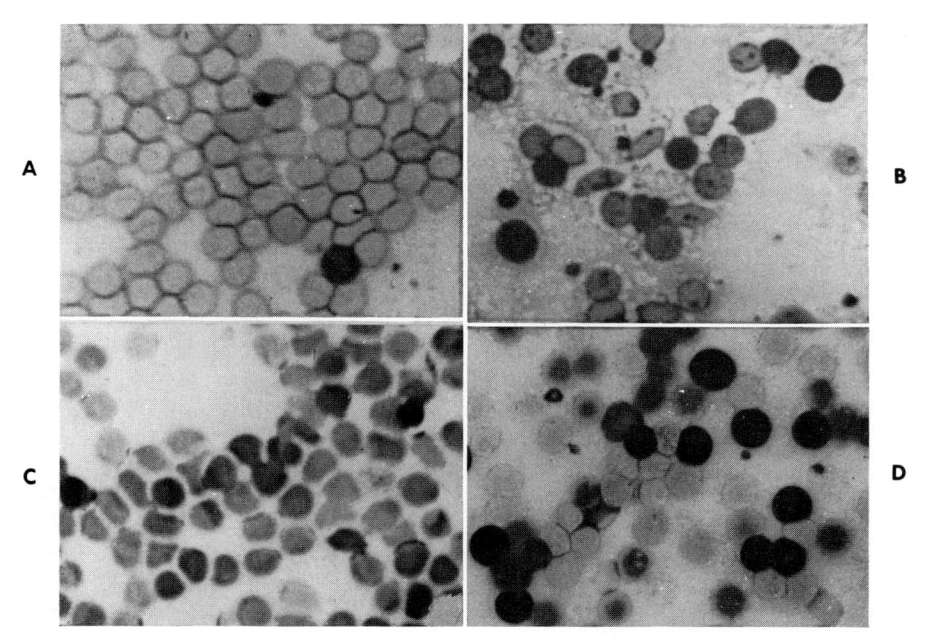

Fig. 36. Blood smear for fetal hemoglobin. **A,** Normal adult. **B,** Sickle cell anemia (S-S). **C,** Persistent F gene carrier. **D,** Mixture of cells of case presented in **C,** of cord blood, and of a normal adult. These smears obtained after acid elution demonstrate only occasional dark-stained cells containing fetal hemoglobin; the remainder are clear ghosts in **A,** containing adult hemoglobin. The heterogeneous distribution of fetal hemoglobin in homozygous sickle cell anemia in **B** is contrasted with its more or less uniform distribution of every cell in the high fetal gene type in **C.** (From Mitchener, J. W., Thompson, R. B., and Huisman, T. H. J.: Foetal haemoglobin synthesis in some haemoglobinopathies, Lancet 1:1169, 1961.)

red cell hemolysates, yet no evidence of a hemolytic disorder is present. In contrast, patients with homozygous sickle cell disease may have severe anemia at times when their red cell hemolysates contain these same proportions of hemoglobins S and F. This is explained by the fact that, in sickle cell anemia (S-S), hemoglobin F is heterogeneously distributed. In the combination of sickle hemoglobin with high fetal gene (S-F), there is a uniform distribution of hemoglobin F among the red cells. This uniform distribution of hemoglobin F among the red cells of the S-F heterozygotes, with high concentrations of fetal hemoglobin in each red cell, apparently prevents sickling of any of the cells at physiologic oxygen tensions so that the cells have a normal life-span. In homozygous sickle cell disease fetal hemoglobin is heterogeneously distributed so that many cells contain insufficient hemoglobin F to protect them from sickling in vivo. The cells containing the lowest concentrations of fetal hemoglobin are thus rapidly destroyed.[61,101] (See Fig. 36.)

The uniform distribution of fetal hemoglobin of the high fetal gene type present in substantial amounts in every cell, in contrast to the heterogeneously distributed fetal hemoglobin in homozygous sickle cell anemia, may be demonstrated by the acid elution method.[335]

Only one patient, apparently homozygous for the persistent fetal hemoglobin anomaly, has been discovered.[101] At 33 months there was no anemia, and no splenic enlargement, but marked abnormalities of the erythrocytes were present. The alkali-resistant fraction ranged between 87 and 92%.

Hereditary persistence of fetal hemoglobin has been reported in six Greek families.[164] In the Greek A-F heterozygotes the levels of HbF were below 20%, whereas in the Negro population reported by Conley and co-workers[101] the range was 17.3 to 33%, with a mean of 25.95%. The anemia is more severe, fetal hemoglobin is lower, and A$_2$ hemoglobin is higher in the Greek group of double heterozygotes for persistent HbF and beta thalassemia (thal-F heterozygote) than in the Negro group.

Chemical analysis of fetal hemoglobin from newborn infants has shown a heterogeneity in the gamma chains of this protein. At least two electrophoretically and chromatographically preparable fetal hemoglobin components have been observed. At a minimum these differ in the exchange of glycine and alanine in position 136 of the gamma chain and have been considered indicative of the presence of more than two such genetic loci. Fetal hemoglobin from thirty-two heterozygotes for the hereditary persistance of fetal hemoglobin demonstrated a marked heterogeneity at the molecular level despite a relatively uniform classic picture that is basically asymptomatic. It was concluded that this heterogeneity can be considered as additional evidence that multiple structural genes control the production of the gamma chain.

*Primitive hemoglobin (P).* Fetal hemoglobin is to be differentiated from the primitive type (P) that is found in early fetal life.[10] This hemoglobin, with an electrophoretic mobility on filter paper slower than those of the adult and fetal hemoglobins, prevails during the first half of embryonic life and is later replaced by fetal hemoglobin. The primitive hemoglobin is associated with severe hypoproteinemia and agammaglobulinemia, but its biologic significance awaits further study.[199] The presence of a special form of fetal hemoglobin in young human embryos is by no means settled. In another study, for instance, no embryonic human hemoglobin was found antedating hemoglobin F in the way hemoglobin F precedes hemoglobin A.[324] On the other hand, Huehns and co-workers[228] were able to detect two new fractions in the blood of human fetuses with a crown-rump length of less than 8.5 cm. Jonxis[264] suggested that the embryonic hemoglobins described earlier may correspond to one of those observed by Huehns.

*Cord blood hemoglobinopathies.* Bart's hemoglobin[3] is a protein made up of four gamma chains[235] appearing in infancy and is attributed to an interference with the alpha chain production on a genetic basis. As described by Minnich and associates,[332] this fast-moving hemoglobin has a slightly slower mobility than does HbJ on starch and paper electrophoresis at pH 8.6.

In a series of 449 Negro babies studied by Minnich and associates,[332] the cord blood of thirty-two newborn infants had Bart's hemoglobin (7.1%), forty-seven had HbS (10.5%), nine had HbC (2%), and two had HbD (0.4%). Of ninety cord bloods on Caucasian babies, one had 3.1% Bart's hemoglobin but no other abnormal hemoglobins. The amounts of hemoglobin Bart's are usually small, being 10% of total hemoglobin or less. This hemoglobin component decreases and often disappears by the time the infant is 3 months old. Hemoglobin Bart's rarely appears in older children or in adults.[296]

Hemoglobin Bart's was found in 4% of cord bloods of Chinese newborn infants and in 10% of those of Nigerian newborn infants.[139] In another series eleven Negro infants were shown to have high levels of hemoglobin Bart's in the neonatal period,[529] with none detectable after the age of 6 months. Some of the blood smears showed numerous target cells, microcytosis, and hypochromia, while other smears were normal.

Eng and associates[139] described a stillborn infant with hydrops with marked erythroblastosis in the circulating blood and organs and no evidence of immunization. The hemoglobin was largely Bart's, with a small amount of hemoglobin H. The fetus' condition could be interpreted as an example of homozygous alpha thalassemia. Both parents had the findings of heterozygous alpha thalassemia. Eng[139] described five additional cases of severe hydrops and erythroblastosis of the peripheral blood without immunization in association with a large amount of Hb Bart's. These cases were all of Chinese origin. The eight parents showed a microcytic blood picture, low A$_2$, and fetal hemoglobin. These patients with hydrops could fit into the category of homozygous alpha chain thalassemia. In all five cases the red cell showed sickling when left on a slide under a cover slip, despite the fact that no HbS was present. It is of interest that HbH, which contains four beta chains and no alpha chains, is found not infrequently in alpha chain thalassemia.

Another case of hydrops fetalis which probably resulted from homozygous alphathalassemia has been described.[378] This case was histologically indistinguishable from erythroblastosis fetalis, but no evidence of isoimmunization was present. Both parents had hypochromic microcytosis with normal HbA₂ levels, findings compatible with heterozygous alpha thalassemia.

Hemoglobin Alexandra moves on paper electrophoresis at alkaline pH more slowly than S and faster than HbE. This hemoglobin occurs in cord blood of newborn infants, decreasing steadily in concentration during the first few months and paralleling the rate of disappearance of hemoglobin F. No abnormal hemoglobin was found in either parent of an infant with Hb Alexandra.[163]

*Hereditary aspects.* One of the first steps in the diagnosis and appraisal of the degree of involvement in a patient with suspected hereditary hemoglobinopathy is the search for specific hemoglobins in the affected person and in other members of the family.

The principles relating to the familial distribution of the genes for the normal and abnormal hemoglobins conform to the basic principles of heredity. In the somatic cells of the body the genes are paired, one member of each pair being derived from one parent. The members of a pair of genes are termed alleles and occupy similar positions or loci on a pair of homologous chromosomes. The homozygous person receives an identical gene for the particular hemoglobin from both parents, whereas the heterozygous person receives different, contrasting, or alternate members of genes or alleles. In the homozygous state both genes of the pair are either normal or abnormal, and in the heterozygous individual one of the genes is normal and the other abnormal. In the case of abnormal hemoglobins the double heterozygous state is one in which the genes determining the two hemoglobins differ from each other. In exceptional cases of thalassemia–sickle cell disease and of hemoglobin C–thalassemia, patterns of genetic transmission other than multiple alleles are to be considered. These rare instances involve such chromosomal relationships as linkage in which genes are located in two different chromosomes, permitting independent transmission.

Comprehensive family pedigrees will frequently elucidate not only the hematologic picture of the patient but also that of other closely related persons who are asymptomatic or who have suffered from a mild but unexplained anemia. Numerous family studies have demonstrated that, with the exception of fetal hemoglobin, the genes responsible for the abnormal hemoglobins are alleles of those for normal hemoglobin.

The gene for any one of the abnormal hemoglobins may thus replace one or both genes for normal hemoglobin. When only one normal gene is replaced, the person is regarded as a carrier possessing a heterozygous hemoglobin trait. Homozygous or pure hemoglobin disease results when both genes for hemoglobin A are replaced by those of the same abnormal hemoglobin. With few exceptions, family studies have demonstrated that hemoglobins S, C, D, and E represent alleles of normal hemoglobin A.

*Relation of genetic composition to clinical-hematologic variations.* Expressivity of a gene refers to the variability of its expression in different persons and explains certain of the quantitative aspects observed in the inheritance of the abnormal hemoglobins. It has been postulated that the amount of a particular hemoglobin in a blood sample is influenced by interaction with the gene controlling another type of hemoglobin and with which it is combined. Thus, in a combination of Cooley's anemia and sickle cell disease the gene for Cooley's anemia permits the appearance of amounts of sickle cell hemoglobin as high as 80% in the offspring, despite the presence in the parent of less than 50% of this component. This augmenting influence, which is also seen in the interaction of the gene for Cooley's anemia with the genes for hemoglobin C or E, will be elaborated upon later.

The intensity of each syndrome varies from the asymptomatic or mild case, in which a single abnormal hemoglobin is present in the heterozygous state in combination with one of the two allelic genes for normal hemoglobin, to the severe case, in which two identical abnormal hemoglobins appear in the homozygous state (Table 20).

Intermediate grades of hemolytic disease are associated with the presence of two different abnormal hemoglobins—the mixed or double heterozygous state. Their simultaneous presence results in a hemolytic anemia of variable intensity together with moderate splenomegaly and peripheral blood changes characteristic of both diseases. Although a single dose of a gene for abnormal hemoglobin produces the trait or mild disease and a double dose the severe disease, the degree of clinical and hematologic changes cannot be exactly correlated

Table 20. Common abnormal hemoglobin syndromes

| Type | Diagnostic features of blood smear | Percent abnormal hemoglobin | Types of hemoglobin present |
|---|---|---|---|
| Sickle cell trait | Normocytic and normochromic red blood cells | 24 to 45% HbS | S—A |
| Sickle cell anemia (homozygous) | Normochromic or slightly hypochromic red blood cells; anisocytosis; poikilocytosis; polychromasia; target cells; sickle cells; occasional normoblasts | 80 to 100% HbS | S—S |
| Sickle cell–thalassemia disease | Large thin macrocytic cells; marked anisocytosis; basophilic stippling; nucleated red blood cells; moderate number of target cells; occasional sickled cells | 67 to 82% HbS | S—F—A |
| Homozygous hemoglobin C disease | Slightly microcytic or normocytic, normochromic red blood cells; large number of target cells | 100% HbC | C—C |
| Hemoglobin C trait | Normocytic, normochromic red blood cells; target cells may be absent or increased | 28 to 44% HbC | A—C |
| Sickle cell–hemoglobin C disease | Normochromic, slightly microcytic red blood cells; minimal anisocytosis and poikilocytosis, numerous target cells | HbS and HbC, each about 40 to 60% | S—C—F |
| Thalassemia–hemoglobin C disease | Microcytic, minimally hypochromic red blood cells; marked anisocytosis and poikilocytosis with oval cells, basophilic stippling, microspherocytes; target cells increased greatly | 29 to 93% HbC (usually 70 to 90%) | C—A |
| Thalassemia minor (trait) (heterozygous) | Hypochromic and microcytic red cells predominate, poikilocytosis, oval and cigarette-shaped forms, basophilic stippling; characteristic hypochromic macrocytes interspersed; usually increased levels of hemoglobin $A_2$ | None | A, $A_2$, and F rarely elevated |
| Thalassemia major (homozygous) | Hypochromic microcytes, scattered hypochromic macrocytes, large thin leaflike red cells (leptocytes), often wrinkled, target, oval, and cigarette-like forms, polychromasia, basophilic strippling, moderate target cells | 40 to 100% HbF | F—A |

with one particular mixture of abnormal hemoglobins. Thus, Cooley's anemia and sickle cell anemia, in both of which the homozygous state is represented, are more severe clinically and hematologically than either homogyzous hemoglobin C or E disease.

Prior to the discovery of abnormal hemoglobins it had been established that the gene responsible for Cooley's anemia or thalassemia occurs once in the heterozygous or mild disease and twice in the homozygous or severe disease. A similar pattern of inheritance was postulated for sickle cell disease[361]—i.e., that the gene responsible for sickling is present in the heterozygous sickle cell anemia. Exceptions to this genetic pattern—i.e., the failure to find similar recognizable blood changes in each parent of an affected child with either Cooley's anemia or sickle cell anemia—can now be explained by the presence of another unrelated abnormal hemoglobin in the dissimilar parent.

*Target cells.* Target cells are particularly prominent in the blood smear of patients with abnormal hemoglobins and often provide a clue to diagnosis. In the Negro patient this distinctive feature is particularly suggestive of the presence of abnormal hemoglobins.

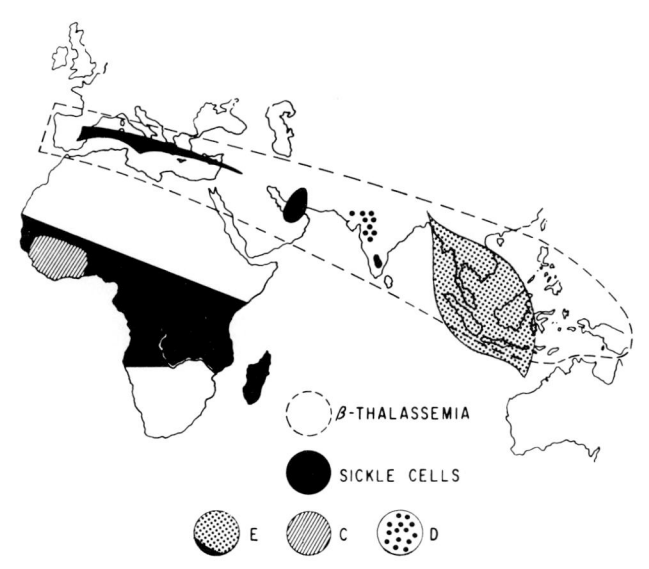

Fig. 37. World distribution of major hemoglobin abnormalities. (From Lehmann, H., Huntsman, R. G., and Ager, J. A. M.: The hemoglobinopathies and thalassemia. In Stanbury, J. B., Wyngaarden, J. B., and Fredrickson, D. S., editors: The metabolic basis of inherited disease, ed. 2, New York, 1966, McGraw-Hill Book Co. Copyright 1966 by McGraw-Hill Book Co. Used by permission of McGraw-Hill Book Co.)

Present in patients with both mild and severe Mediterranean anemia (usually up to 10%), target cells are further increased in patients with sickle cell anemia and appear in even larger numbers in persons with the genes for both Cooley's anemia and sickle cell anemia (microdrepanocytic or thalassemia–sickle cell disease) than in the person with only one of these genes for abnormal hemoglobin. In persons with sickle cell–hemoglobin C disease they are present to the extent of 40 to 90% of all red cells. It has been suggested that large numbers of target cells in the blood smear indicate the presence of hemoglobin C. Target cells are also increased in patients with hemoglobin E disease, perhaps less than in those with hemoglobin C disease. Few or none of these cells are noted in reported cases of sickle cell–hemoglobin D disease[498] or of hemoglobins G, H, I, and J.

**Syndromes associated with the abnormal hemoglobins.** Investigation of the physiochemical properties of the hemoglobin molecule has been particularly revealing in explaining the variability in the clinical, hematologic, and genetic aspects of sickle cell disease and Cooley's anemia. These studies have demonstrated that each of these diseases exist not only as the classic homozygous forms with well-known manifestations but also as variants. The latter, although less severe, nevertheless simulate sickle cell disease and Cooley's anemia clinically and hematologically. The differences can now be explained on the basis of the simultaneous presence of another hemoglobin. Thus the majority of abnormal syndromes to be described are initially diagnosed as either thalassemia or sickle cell disease.

The multiplicity of combinations of the abnormal hemoglobins in the heterozygous, double heterozygous, and homozygous states precludes a discussion confined exclusively to a single abnormal hemoglobin so that overlapping comments are inevitable.

**Geographic distribution of the abnormal hemoglobins.** The geographic distribution of the abnormal hemoglobins shows them to be associated with certain parts of the world and in certain races[294] (Fig. 37). Sporadic reports beyond these areas are not uncommon. HbS is found particularly in Africa in the West as well as the East, and in some distinct populations of the Near East and India. HbC is localized in West Africa (none seen in East Africa), HbD in India, and HbE among the peoples of southeast Asia, principally Thais,

Burmese, and Cambodians. HbH has been found more frequently among Chinese than any other group, although there are scattered reports of this abnormal hemoglobin among Greeks, Italians, Malayans, and other races. As the abnormal hemoglobins are characters that play an active part in natural selection, it has to be assumed that their incidence will rise or fall according to whether they are of selective value under definite environmental stresses.[294] No abnormal hemoglobin has as yet been isolated which is peculiar to the thalassemia patient. Thalassemia affects many of the peoples of the eastern hemisphere and has a widespread geographic distribution (Fig. 37). The specific areas and affected populations will be discussed in the section dealing with this disease.

*Factors involving alteration of oxygen affinity (heme-heme interaction, Bohr effect, and 2,3-diphosphoglycerate).* Before reviewing the various hemoglobinopathies, several factors involved in oxygen transport require definition, including heme-heme interaction, the Bohr effect, and the role of 2,3-diphosphoglycerate in its relation to the affinity of hemoglobin for oxygen.

In heme-heme interaction one heme communicates its state to another, eventually to the four heme groups of the hemoglobin molecule. In this process the oxygenation and deoxygenation of one heme facilitates the oxygenation and deoxygenation of the second, and so on until all four heme groups are oxygenated or deoxygenated. It would appear that, as each heme group accepts oxygen, it becomes progressively easier for the next heme group to take up oxygen.

Another factor visualized in oxygen dissociation curves is the Bohr effect, which implies the reciprocal binding of oxygen and hydrogen ions by deoxyhemoglobin and an increase in oxygen affinity with increasing pH. Thus acidosis decreases and alkalosis increases the affinity of hemoglobin for oxygen. An increase in temperature also decreases the affinity of hemoglobin for oxygen.

A recent rediscovery is the function of a substance within red cells that is involved in oxygen release to the tissues. This new information concerns an organic phosphate, 2,3-diphosphoglycerate (2,3-DPG), which is found in large amounts in red cells.[41,42,330] Primarily 2,3-DPG and secondarily ATP influence the release of oxygen to the tissues. Many studies have now demonstrated that oxygen dissociation from hemoglobin is facilitated by increased intraerythrocytic 2,3-DPG and ATP concentrations as a result of their preferential binding to deoxyhemoglobin; 2,3-DPG binds to the $\beta$ chain of deoxygenated hemoglobin and in so doing shifts the oxygen dissociation curve to the right, thus allowing more oxygen to be released for a given oxygen partial pressure.

Many clinical conditions can now be explained by the action of 2,3-DPG. Among these is the observation that a difference exists in the oxygen affinities of fetal and maternal blood (see Chapter 1). It has now been established that, although the concentration of 2,3-DPG in the two types of blood is not significantly different, the affinity of this phosphate for fetal deoxyhemoglobin is less than for the maternal pigment.[513] As a result, there is a lower oxygen affinity of the mother's blood as compared with that of the fetus, a difference which provides for the facilitated transport of oxygen from mother to fetus.

Blood stored for more than several days under conventional blood bank conditions demonstrates a significant increase in its oxygen affinity.[515] This phenomenon can now be explained by the fact that the increase in oxygen affinity can be traced to a fall in the red cell concentration of 2,3-DPG. However, when blood poor in 2,3-DPG is transfused into healthy recipients, a prompt increase in the level of 2,3-DPG occurs. Since the complete restoration to normal levels of 2,3-DPG may require 6 to 10 days, the high affinity for oxygen during this period may impair tissue oxygenation.[367] The level of red cell 2,3-DPG can be partially restored to normal by incubating the blood with inosine prior to transfusion.[5]

## SICKLE CELL DISEASE

*Sickle cell disease* is a comprehensive term used to include all those hereditary disorders whose clinical, hematologic, and pathologic features are related to the presence of sickle hemoglobin (hemoglobin S) in the red cells. Sickle cell disease is found primarily in Negroes. Relatively few cases have been reported in members of the white race. The majority of these cases occurred in persons of Italian, Greek, and Sicilian origin, suggesting an admixture of Negro blood with members of the Mediterranean races.[159]

The sickle cell trait is present in those persons who are heterozygous for the sickling character and represents the combination of the sickle cell gene and the gene for normal hemoglobin. In persons with sickle cell anemia the gene for sickling is present in the homozygous state and results from the inheritance of sickling genes from both parents. The presence of a gene for another abnormal type of hemoglobin or the gene for thalassemia should be suspected in a child with sickle cell anemia when the blood of only one of the parents shows the sickle trait.

*Sickling phenomenon.* The sickling abnormality is attributed to a mutant gene which is responsible for the synthesis of a type of hemoglobin different from normal hemoglobin. The red cells that sickle are biconcave disks indistinguishable from the normal erythrocytes containing no sickle hemoglobin. Although it had been shown previously[198] that the basic abnormality of the sickle red cell resided in the hemoglobin, Pauling and associates[370] demonstrated that the electrophoretic mobility of sickle cell hemoglobin differed from normal hemoglobin. They also pointed out that these differences were based upon the number and kind of ionizable groups located in the globin fraction of hemoglobin rather than in the heme and that this molecular abnormality was responsible for the varied phenomena characterizing sickle cell anemia.

Hemoglobins are also identified by examining the digested fragments of the hemoglobin molecules on a chromatogram. Of the 287 amino acids forming the polypeptide chain of a half-molecule of hemoglobin, a significant difference is observed in sickle and other hemoglobins as compared with normal hemoglobin. Ingram[238] found that normal and sickle hemoglobin differ in one portion of their polypeptide chains. In each "sickle peptide" having nine amino acids, valine replaces the normally occurring glutamic acid. This is presumably sufficient to alter the charge distribution on the surface of the molecule toward one favoring easy crystallization. Using the same method of trypsin and chymotrypsin digestin followed by "fingerprinting" of the peptide mixture, Ingram[239] also noted that the same glutamic acid of normal hemoglobin is replaced by the amino acid lysine in hemoglobin C disease. These findings with respect to both sickle cell hemoglobin and hemoglobin C reinforce the genetic evidence that these two mutations occur in similar places on the gene since they affect the same amino acid.[239] According to this concept, an altered gene is responsible for a corresponding alteration in the amino acid sequence of the protein with which it is identified.

A simple, rapid, and accurate test for hemoglobin S has been described,[21] demonstrating its specificity and selectivity.* This turbidimetric test is based upon the differential solubility of reduced hemoglobin S in certain hyperosmolar, inorganic buffers at a nearly neutral pH. Under these conditions hemoglobin S is insoluble, whereas hemoglobins $A_1$, $A_2$, $F_1$, C, and D are soluble. An opaque solution after mixing the blood specimen with the reagent was recorded as positive and a clear solution as negative. The method was found to be accurate using either venous anticoagulated blood or blood from a finger prick. Clear-cut results can be obtained in less than 3 minutes.

Fingerprinting consists of several steps. In the first step purified hemoglobin is split with the enzyme trypsin. Trypsin attacks only those peptide bonds to which arginine or lysine contributes the carbonyl group. This tryptic digestion fractures the polypeptide chains of protein into small peptide subunits. The second step is the separation of these peptides by high-voltage paper electrophoresis, and in the last step there is further separation by solvent chromatography. The resulting pattern of the separated peptides as it appears on the paper is referred to as a "fingerprint" of the protein. When the positions of the peptides from hemoglobin A (normal adult hemoglobin) were compared with those from hemoglobin S (sickle cell), it was found that, with one exception, all were identical. The latter, arbitrarily designated peptide 4, was isolated and found to contain eight amino acids; seven were identical in both hemoglobins A and S, but one, the sixth in the chain, was a glutamic acid residue in hemoglobin A, whereas it was valine in hemoglobin S. This amino acid substitution results in a more positively charged molecule which is reflected in electrophoretic mobility.

*Hybridization.* Human hemoglobin, which is composed of four polypeptide chains, can be dissociated into small subunits if it is made either acid (pH below 5) or alkaline (pH of 11 to

---

*Sickledex, Ortho Diagnostics, Rariton, N. J.

11.6).[245,520] These subunits consist of two polypeptide chains, either two alpha chains or two beta chains. When the pH is subsequently returned to neutrality the subunits recombine to form the normal molecule of four polypeptide chains (two alpha and two beta). Similarly, "hybrid" molecules can be found to determine whether an abnormality of the hemoglobin molecule resides in the alpha or beta chain. For example, when mixtures of HbA and HbS are exposed to dissociation of the globin chains and recombined by changing the pH, the subunits combine in random fashion. Some of the normal alpha chains will continue with normal beta subunits to form HbA and some of the normal alpha subunits will combine with the abnormal beta subunits to form HbS.[245,298,520] The properties of the "hybrid" HbS can then be identified by their electrophoretic mobility and behavior in chromatography. This technique has been employed to determine whether an unknown hemoglobin variant has an abnormal alpha or an abnormal beta chain.[298]

The intrinsic features of the sickling mechanism become apparent when hemoglobin is reduced, following exposure to low oxygen tensions or pH. The simplest method by which deoxygenation is accomplished is by placing a drop of blood under a sealed cover slip and observing the progressive increase in the number of sickle cells. Sickle hemoglobin is much less soluble than normal hemoglobin and even less so in the reduced state. Exposure to an environment of reduced oxygen tension causes sickle hemoglobin to become more viscous. This transformation is accompanied by intracellular crystallization[382] and tactoid formation.[202]

Concentrated stroma-free hemolysates prepared from the blood of patients with sickle cell anemia are extremely viscous when sickle hemoglobin is present in reduced states.[202] Increases in viscosity of the whole blood accompany the multiplication of sickled forms and contribute to slowing of the blood flow. The tactoid form represents an altered and orderly alignment of the abnormal hemoglobin molecules in the anoxic state producing the sickle and crescent forms.[202] The sickled erythrocyte has been described as a hemoglobin tactoid distorted by retained stroma.[203] Crystallization accounts for the high concentration of hemoglobin in sickle cells, attaining a mean corpuscular hemoglobin concentration of 50 to 60% in the crystals as compared with values of approximately 34% in the normal cell.[202]

The amount of gelling of reduced hemoglobin S involved in tactoid formation is influenced by the companion pigment particles which interact with it. Reduced hemoglobin must be sufficiently concentrated (above 10%) for gelling and tactoid formation to occur.[202] Actually, it has been shown that a minimum of 7% intraerythrocytic concentration of hemoglobin S pigment is needed to elicit the sickling phenomenon.[459] With lesser amounts the carrier may show a negative sickling test, but sickle hemoglobin may be demonstrable by electrophoresis. The presence of hemoglobin A in the heterozygous person with the sickle cell trait decreases the amount of hemoglobin S required for gel formation, and type C reduces this further. Sickling, therefore, depends not only upon the presence of hemoglobin S but also upon interaction with other hemoglobins. Type F hemoglobin, present in the homozygous patient with sickle cell anemia, exerts no significant influence on the gelling phenomenon.[462]

The sickling of the erythrocytes in patients with homozygous sickle cell anemia (S-S) and other forms of sickle cell disease (thalassemia–sickle cell and sickle cell–hemoglobin C disease) is rapid and assumes chiefly a filamentous form. In persons with the sickle cell trait, a holly leaf rather than the filamentous form predominates. The spicules of the holly leaf form represent the points of the tactoids.[381]

The sickle distortion is reversible so that the filamentous sickle cell which develops in an environment of lowered oxygen reverts to the normal discoid form when normal oxygen tension is restored. Oxygenation causes the crystallized hemoglobin S to go into solution again. Two types of sickle cells have been described: those reverting to the previously normal shape on exposure to oxygen and a smaller number which remain irreversible.[448] Sickle cells appearing on the blood smears of patients with sickle cell anemia are of the irreversible variety. The blood smear of persons with the sickle trait is devoid of sickle cells.

The substitution of a valine for a glutamic acid residue in position 6 of the beta chains of hemoglobin is the sole known abnormality in sickle cell anemia. All clinical manifestations of sickle cell disease are presumably attributable to the alteration in molecular structure and, consequently, to intravascular sickling of erythrocytes.[81] Hemoglobin S appears to be harmless and to function as satisfactorily as normal hemoglobin, except under conditions in which sickling formation occurs. When intravascular sickling is prevented, persons with 70% hemoglobin S in their red cell hemolysates display no evidence of anemia or disease and the life-span of their erythrocytes is normal.[101] On the other hand, even A-S erythrocytes sickle and are rapidly sequestered from the circulation of hypoxic individuals.

The clinical severity of various sickle hemoglobinopathies is directly related to the rate of increase of viscosity of blood during deoxygenation.[81] The principal determinants of the rate are the concentration of hemoglobin S in the red cell and the degree of interaction between hemoglobins when more than one major type was present. The viscosity of deoxygenated blood is directly related to the proportion of sickled red cells, the filamentous forms being associated with a greater viscosity than holly leaf forms.[81] The protective action of fetal hemoglobin in preventing destruction of the sickle cell has already been mentioned. It will be seen that sickle cells containing the lowest concentrations of fetal hemoglobin are rapidly destroyed, whereas those with high concentrations tend to persist in circulation.[192,507]

It is of interest that sickling may be demonstrated with the red cells of hemoglobin I,[15] Hb-Bart's,[139] HbC$_{Georgetown}$,[384] and HbC$_{Harlem}$[56] in the absence of HbS. It has been postulated that sickling in these cases does not result from attraction between complementary sites on adjacent hemoglobin molecules to form relatively insoluble long-chain polymers as with HbS, but perhaps from direct action on the stroma.

**Pathogenesis.** The varied manifestations of sickle cell anemia result from the insolubility of reduced sickle hemoglobin and the formation of sickle cells, which follows exposure to lowered oxygen tensions existing in the tissues. Although persons with the sickle cell trait heretofore had been regarded as uniformly asymptomatic, it is now known that occasionally they, too, are susceptible to the same difficulties as the homozygous patient in situations in which there is reduced oxygen tension such as occur in airplane flights.[303]

The entanglement and enmeshing of rigid and inflexible sickle cells with one another increases the internal friction of the suspension, resulting in an increased viscosity of the whole blood.[205] The sickling and increased blood viscosity combine to produce capillary stasis, the formation of masses and plugs of impacted red cells, thrombi, hemorrhage, vascular occlusion, infarction, and ischemic necrosis. Infection presumably increases plasma viscosity and results in an extreme degree of erythrostasis.

The formation of sickle cells increases vulnerability to mechanical fragility, especially as the hemoglobin is deoxygenated.[205] The shortened life-span of the cells during movement in the circulation and passage through organs results in hemolytic anemia. Selective sequestration and stagnation of sickle cells in the spleen[535] of the patient with sickle cell anemia probably results in their local destruction and for those cells that escape, increased intravascular hemolysis. The cells from patients with sickle cell trait and those from the patient with sickle cell anemia differ with regard to increased mechanical fragility. Mechanical fragility of the sickle cells of the patient with the trait begins to be affected at a level of deoxygenation at which the cells of the patient with the anemia already show a maximal increase. In general the in vitro behavior of sickle hemoglobin and sickle cells at reduced oxygen tensions are correlated with the severity of the clinical and hematologic features.[192]

Murayama[348] identified the presence of tubular rods of HbS in preparations of sickle cell hemolysates. From this observation he theorized that crumpling of sickle cells is caused by aggregation of HbS molecules into microtubules. The crumpling of disk-shaped erythrocytes into bizarre forms is considered the basic pathologic feature of sickle cell anemia. White[543] later found that glutaraldehyde promotes the sickling phenomenon, that the dense rods similar to those found in hemolysates do occur in the cytoplasm of sickled erythrocytes, and that the parallel orientation of the rods appears instrumental in crumpling erythrocytes containing HbS. Glutaraldehyde not only preserves the fine structure of sickle cells, but also appears to be an effective agent for promoting the sickling phenomenon. Sickled cells were filled with filaments and rods. The severity of erythrocyte distortion was closely related to the amount of HbS converted to the rod form and the extent of parallel association of the rods. Conversion of the entire mass of erythrocyte cytoplasm into a monotonous pattern of parallel rods is considered the end of the sickling process. The response of sickle cells to incubation with glutaraldehyde is grossly identical to the alterations which occur when susceptible erythrocytes are treated with sodium bisulfite or reduced oxygen tension. Only reticulocytes characterized by the presence of polyribosomes in their cytoplasm appeared to be spared from the sickling phenomenon.

Others[495] have shown that the sickling phenomenon is due to the intracellular formation of long slender crystals of reduced sickle hemoglobin. The rapid growth of these crystals causing tenting of the cell membrane may be responsible for the bizarre distortion of the erythrocytes.

The Murayama test is described as a specific tests for S hemoglobin.[355] The test depends on a feature of molecular structure: hydrophobic bonds formed between interacting tetramers by the number 6 valine, which is substituted for glutamic acid near the N-terminal end of each beta S globin chain. Basically, the red cells are thoroughly washed in physiological saline and a hemolysate is subsequently formed by adding water. The concentrated hemolysate is deoxygenated by exposing the surface to a flow of $CO_2$. Gel formation takes place at 37° C. and becomes liquid at 0° C. Only S hemoglobin or HbC$_{Harlem}$, a structural variant, gives a positive Murayama test. HbC$_{Georgetown}$, a non-S sickling hemoglobin, gels at 37° C. and remains gelled at 0° C. HbA and other nonsickling hemoglobins will not gel (sickle) at either 37° or 0° C. It has been suggested that the test should not be attempted when S hemoglobin is less than 15% of the concentrated hemolysate.

### Sickle cell trait

*Incidence and geographic distribution.* The sickle cell trait, representing the heterozygous state (hemoglobins A and S), occurs in approximately 7 to 9% of American Negroes.[350] A small number, about one in forty of those with sickling, show sickle cell anemia. The highest frequency of the trait has been reported from East Africa, where it varies from 30 to 45% in some Bantu tribes. The peak of the incidence falls somewhat toward the west coast of Africa, averaging 20 to 25% on the coast.[133] The high incidence of the sickle cell trait in several of the aborigine tribes of southern India has suggested that the sickle cell trait may have been carried from this area to Africa.[297]

In Ghana the commonest abnormal hemoglobin was hemoglobin S (19% of Southern Ghanians and 7% of Northern Ghanians); hemoglobin C had the highest world-wide frequency (20 to 21%).[284] In West Africa as a whole, the incidence of sickle cell trait has been stated as 20 to 30%. The commonest adult manifestations of sickle cell disease in West Africans are joint, muscular, and skeletal pains. Jaundice, severe anemia, and hepatosplenomegaly are often seen. Most young adult patients with HbSS "lose" their spleen because of siderofibrosis. Some have gross hepatosplenomegaly with spleens reaching the pelvis. Currently HbSS women live beyond the age of 25 years.

In the United States 1 in 12 of the total Negro population carries the sickle cell trait and the chance that both parents will carry the trait is about 1 in 144. Thus only about 0.7% of Negro families risk having children with the homozygous form of sickle cell anemia.

*Clinical and laboratory features.* The trait can be demonstrated in vitro by the ability of the erythrocytes to sickle when oxygen tension is lowered. This is accomplished by a variety of techniques, such as sealing a drop of fresh blood under a cover slip with petrolatum or, more rapidly, by mixing the blood with a reducing agent such as 2% sodium bisulfite. Sickling is slower in patients with the trait, and the red cells assume a holly leaf appearance rather than the typical elongated, pointed, and filamentous form observed in patients with sickle cell anemia. The amount of sickle cell hemoglobin in the blood of persons with the trait, as determined by electrophoresis, varies from 24 to 45% of the total hemoglobin.[536] The remainder is adult hemoglobin. HbF is not found in the trait after infancy. Target cells are present in small numbers, but the red cells in stained blood smears are predominantly normal. The red cells of healthy persons with the trait have a normal life-span.[74,461]

Persons with the trait are not anemic, show no physical abnormalities, and are usually asymptomatic. Splenic infarction resulting from vascular occlusion by sickled cells has been reported in patients with the sickle trait at moderate or high altitudes during flight.[102,103,127,339] Under severe conditions of deoxygenation, sickling crises also occur after a badly administered anesthetic and severe pneumonia. Incapability of concentrating urine normally,[275] gross hematuria,[80] acute pyelonephritis, priapism,[154] and retinal hemorrhage[213] have also been described occasionally in patients with the trait.

Not only are air travel and anaesthesia[283] probably dangerous to patients with sickle cell trait, but there may be particular hazards upon vigorous participation in athletic contest at higher altitudes. Jones and his associates[202] reported four sudden deaths in a group of 4,000 black military recruits undergoing vigorous physical training at an altitude of 4,060 feet. All were apparently healthy, had no family history of anemia, and originated from low-altitude areas. After varying types of exercise there was a loss of consciousness, shortness of breath, fainting, and, in one patient, no pulse or spontaneous respirations. Most occurred on the first day of training. The pathological features satisfied the criteria for sickle crises. In most of the cases classic microscopic findings of distended vessels packed with sickle cells and pooling of blood around splenic follicles were seen. It is likely that hypoxemia, acidosis, and excess lactate were present. Other factors that may lead to occlusive sickling crises were dehydration, high viscosity, and hypercoagulability. These authors[262] explain that in these cases the concomitant occurrence of hypoxia, acidosis, and accumulation of endogenous reducing agents was caused by the moderate-to-severe exercise after recent arrival at a relatively high altitude, thus precipitating sickling crises and sudden death.

There is probably no undue hazard to the recipient of small amounts of blood of sickle cell trait donors stored in the usual fashion.[274] One infant died, however, with massive intravascular sickling after an exchange transfusion with sickle cell trait blood.[518]

Because of these potential hazards, it would seem wise to identify individuals with the sickle cell trait before they are exposed to conditions in which an apparently benign condition is converted to one of a serious nature.[329]

In one study,[52] 1,000 Negro military recruits were screened with the new rapid differential solubility test for sickle cell hemoglobin (described on p. 366). A total of 75 had positive screening tests; 73 had sickle cell trait, 1 had sickle cell–hemoglobin C disease, and 1 had sickle–thalassemia disease. In this series the incidence of 7.5% of Hb-AS compares closely with the 7.2 to 9.4% in other series. There was no morbidity relative to their abnormal hemoglobin during their basic training, although these recruits were subjected to the same stress and environment as those associated with sudden death of the previously described cases.[262] It is possible that the four subjects previously reported had HbS levels above the maximum of 38% in the current series.

**Sickling and malaria.** Since the observations by Beet[40] that the sickle cell trait might protect the bearer from the effects of malaria, many studies have been carried out to test this hypothesis. According to this concept, the survival of persons with heterozygous sickle cell disease could offset the loss of persons with homozygous disease through malaria caused by *Plasmodium falciparum,* but not other malarial parasites, and thus maintain the high rates of sickling in malarious areas. Apparently, sickle hemoglobin is unsuitable for growth of *Plasmodium falciparum.* The malarial parasite has many of the enzyme systems that exist in the red blood cell and depends on some of the enzymes and metabolites of the red cell for its normal metabolism.[341] Thus, the loss of the sickle cell gene by early death of patients with homozygous sickle cell anemia is counterbalanced by the resistance of persons with the sickle cell trait to become infected with malaria. This concept of a selective or reproductive advantage for the person with heterozygous sickle cell disease over the normal person (balanced polymorphism) has also been extended to thalassemia, since many of the patients with this disease come from districts severely affected by malaria.[9]

More extended experience, however, based upon surveys in areas in which malaria and sickle cell disease prevail, including direct inoculation of *Plasmodium falciparum* into persons with and without sickle cells, has given conflicting evidence as to this protective relationship.[305] There is greater unanimity with respect to children—i.e., those who are heterozygous for the sickling gene (hemoglobin A-S) have a greater chance of surviving to reproductive age than do normal children when both are exposed to malarial infection.[393]

Although this subject is still controversial, it appears that possession of the sickle trait affords some degree of protection against infection with *Plasmodium falciparum.* The infection is of shorter duration and the parasite count is lower than in persons who do not possess the sickle cell trait.[134] Hence, those who are heterozygous for the sickle cell gene appear to have a selective advantage in regions in which malaria is common.

Luzzatto and co-workers[314] have shown that blood samples from children with the sickle cell trait (A-S heterozygotes) having acute malaria (*Plasmodium falciparum*), when incubated in vitro under anaerobic conditions, sickled in a linear function of time. The rate of sickling of parasitized cells was found to be two to eight times greater than that of nonparasitized cells within the same blood sample, indicating that parasitization of an A-S erythrocyte by *P. falciparum* substantially increases its probability to sickle. They suggested that once sickled, parasitized cells will be removed more effectively from the circulation by phagocytosis. This is probably the main mechanism whereby A-S heterozygotes are at a selective advantage against malaria.

### Sickle cell (drepanocytic) anemia

Sickle cell anemia is a hereditary form of hemolytic disease occurring almost exclusively in Negroes and is due to the presence in the red cells of sickle hemoglobin, the gene for which is present in the homozygous state. Its incidence in American Negroes is 0.3 to 1.3%.[350] The disease is marked by anemia, by painful and febrile episodes, occasionally by aplastic crises, and by a variety of manifestations due to distortion of the red cells. The clinical syndrome was first described by Herrick in 1910[215] in a Negro from the West Indies with chronic anemia in whose blood smear elongated and sickled cells were present. The bulk of hemoglobin (60 to 98% and in some series 80 to 100%) is of the S variety, with the remainder consisting of fetal (F) hemoglobin (usually 2 to 24%). Normal (A) hemoglobin is absent unless the patient has had a transfusion recently.

*Pathology.* The basic changes in the tissues and organs are due mainly to a combination of capillary stasis, obstruction by elongated and pointed sickle cells, thrombosis of small vessels, increased destruction of red cells, and hemosiderosis. Peripheral vascular spasm as a contributory factor in producing ischemic necrosis has been proposed.[276] The dilatation that follows allows these blood vessels to become engorged and packed with sickle cells. The bone marrow is hyperplastic from excessive erythrogenesis and blood stasis.[124] Of the nucleated cells in the marrow normoblasts predominate, but more primitive forms of the red cell series are also present. Only occasionally are sickled, nucleated erythrocytes observed.[124] Leukocytosis is marked and megakaryocytes are increased. Hyperplasia of the bone marrow is especially marked in children and accounts for the osteoporosis and subsequent expansion of the medullary spaces observed in the roentgenogram. Fat embolism secondary to necrosis of the bone marrow has been described.[521] Infarction of bone, followed by embolization of bone marrow and fat to various organs, is observed in patients with sickle cell–hemoglobin C disease as well as in those with sickle cell anemia.[447] Focal infarction of the marrow contributes to the bone pain of a crisis.[84] Aseptic necrosis of the femoral head has been related to thrombosis of blood vessels supplying the affected area.[77,503]

Hemosiderosis from increased hemolysis of the patient's cells and occasionally from transfusions is especially pronounced in the liver, bone marrow, lymph nodes, spleen, and kidney.

The spleen undergoes a series of changes progressing from congestive enlargement to fibrotic atrophy.[122] In younger people the spleen is slightly or moderately enlarged. The splenic pulp is a deep red color due to intense congestion and engorgement with sickle cells; the sinuses are compressed and infarcts are common. Thickening of the capsule and fibrous tissue organization subsequently follows in areas of organizing hemorrhage. The siderofibrotic lesions in persons with sickle cell anemia resemble the siderotic nodules or Gandy-Gamna bodies of the spleen which occur in persons with spherocytic anemia and portal hypertension.[120]

Of 115 patients with sickle cell anemia 1 to 36 years of age, twenty-one or 18% had splenomegaly. Two-thirds of those with enlarged spleen were in the first decade of life, although only one-third of the entire series was in that age group. In contrast to the increase of splenomegaly in patients of 10 years and under, only eight of seventy-eight patients over the age of 10 had splenomegaly, an incidence of 10%. In six children under 10 years of age splenomegaly was transient. In this group, the spleen edge became nonpalpable in a period of 6 months to 5½ years after it was felt.[528]

In the final stages of the disease the spleen is a shriveled and scarred mass, embedded in adhesions reflecting the replacement of the pulp by fibrous tissue. Atrophy from this sequence occasionally results in extremely small spleens (autosplenectomy). The size of the spleen, therefore, decreases as its vascularity diminishes, as the hemorrhages and infarcts become organized, and as fibrous tissue replaces the residual pulp.

The earliest lesion described in the evolution of splenic pathology is congestion of the reticular spaces with sickled erythrocytes and dilatation of the capillaries in the malpighian corpuscles.[120] Perivascular hemorrhages around the terminal arterioles became organized, producing thickening of the vessel walls and compromising the lumen. Infarcts are common and are surrounded by congestive pulp. Organization of infarcted areas by fibrous tissue results and the spleen undergoes progressive destruction and shrinkage resulting in a small wrinkled mass of fibrous tissue.

The peripheral blood smear in patients with splenomegaly contains low levels of irreversibly sickled cells. These cells are probably formed by prolonged anoxia or cycles of anoxia. The spleen with its sluggish circulation and low oxygen tension is well suited to production of irreversibly sickled cells. The low levels of irreversibly sickled cells in peripheral blood of patients with splenomegaly suggests that these cells formed in the spleen do not usually enter the general circulation. The spleen acts as a filter, removing these cells from the circulation. It has been postulated that the lower irreversibly sickled cells can be attributed to higher HbF levels in patients with splenomegaly.[441] Splenomegaly persists longer in patients with high levels of HbF; this is compatible with the theory that sickled cells are responsible for splenic infarction. A plausible hypothesis is that high levels of HbF determine low levels of irreversibly sickled cells, allowing persistence of splenomegaly. When hypersplenism occurs in children the decision is whether to perform splenectomy or await spontaneous atrophy. In such cases a low level of HbF suggests that spontaneous atrophy is likely to occur, whereas a high level of HbF suggests that splenectomy is indicated because splenic enlargement is likely to persist. Serjeant,[441] therefore, suggests that low levels of irreversibly sickled cells occur in patients with sickle cell anemia and splenomegaly. The HbF load appears to influence both the level of irreversibly sickled cells and persistence of splenomegaly. He suggests that low levels of the cells allow splenomegaly to persist and hence are the cause and not primarily the result of persistent splenomegaly.

Pearson and colleagues[379] described a state of "functional asplenia" in young children with sickle cell anemia. This term was used to indicate markedly impaired splenic reticuloendothelial function and was demonstrated by an isotopic scanning technique. They observed that the enlarged spleens of many young children with sickle cell anemia were incapable of clearing particles of about 1 $\mu$ in diameter from the blood. There were at least two indications that the physically enlarged spleens of infants and young children might be inactive.

This was based on the fact that in these children a syndrome of fulminant pneumococcal sepsis and meningitis was observed[414] similar to that seen in the postsplenectomy period.[470] Secondly, they noted Howell-Jolly bodies in capillary blood smears from such children. Such red cell inclusions are usually removed by the "pitting" function of the normal spleen. Their presence suggests a hematologic absence of the spleen. No splenic uptake of a specific colloid was noted in eleven of twelve children with sickle cell anemia, although many had enlarged spleens. Controls including children with sickle cell trait and HbS-C and HbS-thalassemia regularly demonstrated splenic uptake. Functional asplenia in children with sickle cell anemia is therefore defined as impaired splenic reticuloendothelial function despite clinical enlargement of the organ. The mechanism of functional asplenia has been ascribed to an abnormality of the splenic circulation—that is, the high viscosity of sinusoidal blood containing large numbers of sickled red cells could produce relative obstruction of flow. Another is reticuloendothelial blockade caused by saturation of phagocytic cells by particulate material.

In a further clarification of the concept of functional asplenia, Pearson and associates[373] noted that three children given infusions of fresh plasma showed no restoration of function. They concluded that functional aplenia probably is not a consequence of a contracted plasma volume or deficient opsonins or other humoral factors. Splenic function was restored, however, when transfusions of normal red cells were given. The best explanation was that the high viscosity of sickle cell blood causes a diversion of splenic blood flow through intrasplenic shunts, thus bypassing the phagocytic reticuloendothelial elements of the organ. When sickled cells are replaced by normal red cells through transfusion, splenic circulation and function are temporarily restored.

The liver is often markedly altered both in structure and in function. The liver is found enlarged and occasionally tender in many children with sickle cell anemia. Liver dysfunction and necrosis are brought about by severe impairment of hepatic flow due to the combined effects of anemia and capillary obstruction by masses of sickle cells and Kupffer cells distended with phagocytosed red cells. Focal necrosis, loss of liver cells, scarring, and cirrhosis (postnecrotic type)[487] characterize liver involvement.[190] Cholelithiasis due to increased destruction of red cells is not infrequently observed in patients with sickle cell anemia.[533] The incidence has been estimated to be from 6 to 37%.[32] The wide variations in incidence reflect the inclusion of patients under 10 years of age, in whom cholelithiasis is rare.[533] There is a relatively high frequency of gallstones in the form of bilirubin or pigment stones in patients with sickle cell disease. Some 30% of the patients with this disease have gallstones.[32] The diagnosis of cholelithiasis rests primarily on roentgenographic study. The radiopacity of calcium bilirubinate stones associated with hemolysis is proportionate to their calcium content and is unpredictable. It has been estimated that from 30 to 50% of patients with cholelithiasis, regardless of initial symptoms, will require gallbladder surgery within 20 years of the diagnosis.[32] Some patients with sickle cell anemia have been described with features indicative of the development of viral hepatitis.[33] Differentiation will require sequential liver function tests and a liver biopsy. Cirrhosis is frequently present in adults with sickle cell anemia.

The relatively high proportion of indirect-reacting bilirubin and absence of bile from the urine in most cases suggests that the jaundice, in the main, is attributable to increased red cell destruction.[190] In one case of a 33-year-old patient, however, the serum bilirubin was 112 mg. per 100 ml., of which 60 mg. was direct-reacting. The liver was large and of rubbery consistency, the gallbladder and bile ducts were normal, and no stones were found. The sinusoids were greatly engorged by red cells, many of which were sickled. Most of the red cells were found within enormously enlarged Kupffer cells. Hepatic dysfunction, unrelated to the severity of the anemia, is a common finding even in the younger and relatively asymptomatic cases.[221] In another young adult a similar elevation of bilirubin, especially of the direct-reacting type, occurred.[281] It was assumed that cholestatic jaundice resulted from increased bilirubin formation, decreased hepatic excretion due to dysfunction of the bile secretory apparatus, and possibly decreased urinary excretion of the bile pigment. Hepatic dysfunction is due to intravascular sickling with plugging and disruption of vascular integrity.

Severe liver disease has been reported in five patients 12 to 23 years of age whose direct bilirubin ranged from 20 to 50 mg./100 ml.[368] Progressive jaundice, marked elevation of alkaline phosphatase, and a leukemoid reaction were some of the features. The basis was vascular occlusion within the liver, ischemic parenchymal degeneration, fibrosis, and atrophy.

The kidney lesions in patients with severe sickle cell anemia are marked by congestion of glomerular capillaries and of tubular arterioles with sickle cells and by hemosiderosis and scarring. Hematuria is ascribed to congestion of small vessels, thrombosis, stasis, and infarction necrosis.[122] This complication may occur in homozygous sickle cell anemia, sickle cell trait, and sickle cell variant hemoglobinopathies.[437] Hematuria usually occurs in young adults. The sites of bleeding are evenly divided between the two sides.[8] Pain described as a dull ache in the flank, cramplike abdominal pain, and renal colic have been associated with gross hematuria.[394] Conservative measures such as bed rest and blood transfusions are uniformly recommended.

The kidney abnormalities have been summarized as follows[501]: histologic changes in the renal parenchyma characterized by initial glomerular engorgement and enlargement, which eventually give way to ischemia, fibrosis, and glomerular obliteration as well as to progressive development of edema, telangiectasis, fibrosis, scarring, and obliteration of the tubular elements in the medullary pyramids,[47] and, not infrequently, areas of focal pyelonephritis. Functional derangements include an inability to produce a concentrated urine during water deprivation and development of supernormal glomerular filtration rates. This probably represents a homeostatic compensatory effort (increased cardiac output) triggered by the anemia and aimed in part at bringing the effective erythrocyte flow through the renal parenchyma and other major organs to a normal level.[501] Enlargement and increased vascularity of the juxtamedullary glomeruli in older children may provide an anatomic basis for previously unexplained increased filtration rate.[47]

Excretory urography in eighteen children with sickle cell anemia revealed a high incidence of renal enlargement and collecting system deformity. With one exception none of the patients had histories of genitourinary symptoms or signs. Major kidney damage in sickle cell states is the result of intravascular sickling in the renal medulla.[386] VanEps and associates,[516] in microradioangiographic studies, found gross lesions of the vessels of the renal medulla with almost complete absence of vasa recta in sickle cell anemia and loss of normal bundle architecture in sickle cell trait and sickle cell–hemoglobin C disease. These findings suggested that the basic lesion in sickle cell nephropathy is obliteration of vasa recta leading to the observed abnormalities in concentrating function since these result from an intrinsic part of the countercurrent multiplication system of the long loops of Henle.

The nephrotic syndrome occurs not infrequently in children with sickle cell anemia.[29] Such children are almost totally resistant to therapy with the adrenal corticosteroids.[29] The pathogenesis of chronic renal insufficiency and the nephrotic syndromes in those patients is unknown.

Other mechanisms have been proposed for the renal defect in sickle cell anemia—i.e., the inability to elaborate a urine of appropriate hypertonicity.[304] Some of these include interference with the normal countercurrent mechanism, reduced permeability of the distal tubule, increased osmotic diuresis, decreased solute concentration within the medulla, and prolonged arterial oxygen desaturation. Infarction of the medulla (demonstrated on roentgenogram)[206] is still not regarded as sufficient explanation for the concentrating defect.

Enuresis is frequent in patients with sickle cell disease and is probably related to the events associated with hyposthenuria.[488] Excretion of excessive quantities of urine of low specific gravity by patients with sickle cell disease is well documented. From an early age, usually beginning at 4 to 5 years, many children with sickle cell anemia, sickle cell trait, or sickle cell abnormality in combination with other abnormal hemoglobins are unable to concentrate urine. In these patients early lesions of tubular scarring may explain the defects in renal concentrating ability. These children with sickle cell anemia drink large quantities of fluid, have serum of low osmolality, and void large quantities of urine.[422] In patients with sickle cell anemia, and to a lesser extent in those with sickle cell trait, the increased obligatory water loss is most likely the predominant factor responsible for enuresis and for nocturia. Efforts should be made to control the problem of enuresis by directing it to one of simple nocturia.[363]

Changes in the central nervous system are primarily intravascular, mainly due to thrombosis of small vessels in the meninges and cerebral cortex, resulting in hemorrhagic, degenerative, and atrophic changes.[232] These lesions, however, often fail to reveal thromboses. The striking findings are infarcts in the white matter and perivascular hemorrhages. The infarctions and small hemorrhages are apparently responsible for the varied neurologic findings.[20] Obliterative endarteritis of the cerebral vessels may also contribute to the causation of symptoms.[63]

Chronic leg ulcers occur in adolescents and adults, frequently in the lower third of the leg on the inner side just above the ankle.[316] They are usually punched out in appearance, single or multiple, and unilateral or bilateral. The histologic picture is that of chronic granulomatous ulcer.[94] There is no evidence that ulceration originates from thromboses due to the blocking of capillaries by sickled erythrocytes.[109] On the other hand, chronic leg ulcers have been attributed to the low temperatures in the superficial venous blood of the lower leg. In combination with sickling excessively high viscosity is produced, contributing to the severity of the thrombotic processes resulting in chronic leg ulcers.[418]

*Clinical features.* Sickle cell anemia is usually recognized during the preschool period. In half of the patients symptoms are present by 2 years of age,[525] although clinical manifestations are rare in the first 6 months of life. In a few recorded cases the disease has been diagnosed between 1 and 3 months of age.[146] In one series[438] the average age at onset of symptoms necessitating hospitalization ranged from 3 months to 15 years.

As already pointed out, excessive blood destruction and the pathologic tendency toward intravascular sickling, stasis, and thrombosis in various organ and tissue sites are responsible for the multiplicity of symptoms and the confusion with the other clinical syndromes. In children the most frequent complaints are joint, back, and abdominal pain, vomiting, fever, frequent upper respiratory infections, fatigability, and anorexia. Other less commonly encountered symptoms are headache, meningismus, dyspnea, weakness, epistaxis (without purpura), convulsions, lethargy, and listlessness. Episodes of acute abdominal pain may be severe, accompanied by fever, muscle spasm, nausea, vomiting, and leukocytosis.[316] These abdominal crises may have a fatal outcome and have been attributed to shock from massive sequestration of sickled red cells, plasma loss, and circulatory failure.[505]

The increased amounts of fetal hemoglobin in homozygous sickle cell disease apparently protect the erythrocytes from sickling, thereby reducing secondary clinical manifestations.[247] Regardless of the reason for the increase in fetal hemoglobin, its

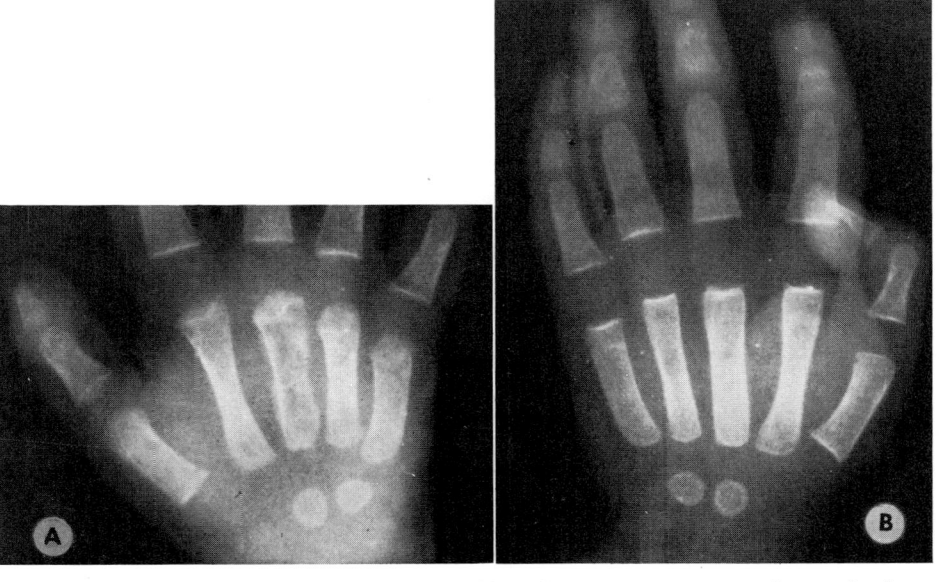

Fig. 38. Hand-foot syndrome in infants with sickle cell anemia. **A,** Note evidence of subperiosteal bone formation and areas of rarefaction in the body of the third metacarpal. **B,** Note complete regression after 1 month; these lesions are transitory.

occurrence in association with sickle cell disease appears to have an ameliorating effect on the clinical manifestations.

Central nervous system manifestations may be the initial complaints or may occur later in the disease. They may be erroneously diagnosed as meningitis, poliomyelitis, subdural hematoma, neoplasm, subarachnoid hemorrhage, and lead encephalitis. The lesions are multiple and their location is variable. The onset of symptoms is often sudden, with convulsions, meningeal signs, headache, aphasia, paralysis, urinary incontinence, and coma.[20] Pain in the extremities may be muscular or be based upon bone and joint involvement and often simulates osteomyelitis. Arthralgia may be severe. Inflamed and swollen joints occur but are infrequent. Localized swellings, presumably due to erythrostasis with sickle cells, develop over bony structures such as the jaw and long bones. Exacerbations of these complaints occur periodically and are often related to upper respiratory infections. In infants usually under 2 years of age dactylitis with marked pain and swelling of the hands and feet are occasionally observed (hand-foot syndrome, Fig. 38). Bony abnormalities are due to marrow hyperplasia, infarction, and osteomyelitis.[68] The hand-foot syndrome is caused by infarction of the short tubular bones of the hands and feet. The bony changes are due to absorption of the infarcted areas, resulting in radiolucent zones. Hyperemia surrounding the affected areas stimulates subperiosteal new bone formation. In 1,200 cases of sickle cell anemia in African infants in the Congo, 80% had the hand-foot syndrome.[289] This compares with an incidence of twenty cases in a series of 173 patients with the homozygous (S-S) disease and twenty cases of S-C disease in patients under 12 years of age in the United States.[527]

An infant with the typical roentgenographic and clinical features of the hand-foot syndrome has been reported who did not have sickle cell disease but a rare type of osteomyelitis due to group A beta-hemolytic streptococci.[200]

It has been stated that swelling of the hands and feet in a Negro infant in whom there is no readily apparent cause for the swelling warrants a suspicion of sickle cell anemia.[337] Abnormal roentgenologic findings do not appear for the first week or 10 days, are confined largely to the metacarpals and metatarsals, and extend infrequently to the phalanges. Abnormalities consist of blurring of the margins and a variable degree of rarefaction within the medullary cavities. Spontaneous regression occurs without residual signs.[246,510]

In sixty-four children under 1 year of age with sickle cell anemia, hepatomegaly, splenomegaly, and abdominal distention were the most common physical findings.[387] Jaundice, pallor, and dactylitis were each observed in 30% of the cases. Concurrent infection was common. Ten of the sixty-four patients, or 16%, died within the first year. The painful swollen hands and feet found in twenty-three patients were not always associated with radiographic evidence of dactylitis. Frank hemolytic or hyperhemolytic crises were a major finding.

A child 1½ years old with homozygous sickle cell anemia developed pneumococcal sepsis and meningitis. The fingers and toes became cyanotic 1 day after admission. The fingers then became gangrenous and several of the terminal phalanges sloughed off. X-ray examination of the hands and feet 4 weeks after the onset showed the typical findings of the hand-foot syndrome, involving all bones of the hands and feet. The course of the symmetrical gangrene could not be established, although infection, sickling, increased blood viscosity, vascular spasm, and cryoglobulinemia[87] may have been factors. Except for the skeletal defects the child recovered completely. Some of the clinical features resembled purpura fulminans. (See Chapter 27.)

Physical findings vary considerably and include marked pallor of the mucous membranes, greenish yellow discoloration of the scleras, lymphadenopathy, cardiac enlargement, and splenomegaly. Liver enlargement may be slight to moderate. The spleen, often slightly to markedly enlarged in children, atrophies with advancing age due to infarction and fibrosis. The incidence of splenomegaly has been found to be 33% in the first decade of life and 10% thereafter.[528] Although splenomegaly is not uncommon in patients with sickle cell anemia, it appears to be much more frequent in those with sickle cell–hemoglobin C disease and sickle cell–thalassemia disease. An enlarged spleen is often associated with shortened survival of transfused normal cells.[307] Less common are ascites, joint swelling, osteomyelitis, gallstones, and hemiplegia in patients with severe nervous system involvement. The veins of the retina may be dilated and tortuous; the arteries show this feature to a lesser extent.[201,308] Retinal hemorrhage has been observed.[213] Patients with hemoglobin S-S, S-C, or S-D disease, or S-thalassemia may show a dark red, comma-shaped, or corkscrew-shaped vascular fragment, found mainly in that part of the lower bulbar conjunctiva covered by the lid.[99] The vessel fragment is isolated from the rest of the conjunctival circulation. The lesion may represent sludged blood flow, with aneurysmal bulging of the vessel wall. Enlargement of the heart and the occurrence of apical systolic murmurs are indicative of hypertrophy and dilatation in response to prolonged anemia and anoxia.[280] Pericarditis is also noted. Episodes of bronchopneumonia occur commonly and are attributable both to infection and to pulmonary infarction. Cor pulmonale in older patients may be the consequence of multiple recurrent infarctions.[338]

In a survey of 305 patients with sickle cell anemia, hemoglobin S-C, and hemoglobin S-thalassemia, Robinson and Watson[414] noted that, in 87% of patients with proved bacterial meningitis and sickle cell anemia, the pneumococcus was the responsible organism. Of 252 patients with sickle cell anemia, fifteen had bacterial meningitis due to the pneumococcus organism. The majority of children were under 3 years of age. The authors suggested that the marked engorgement of the spleen and reticuloendothelial system by sickle erythrocytes and hemosiderin may produce blockade that results in a decreased phagocytic ability of the spleen.

Kabins and Lerner[269] reported four children with sickle cell hemoglobinopathies in whom fulminant pneumococcal infection occurred resembling that reported in splenectomized children, namely, that the illness proved fatal within a few hours of onset. They claimed that the rate of pneumococcal meningitis in children with hemoglobin SS disease was twenty times greater than in children without hemoglobinopathies. Two of the children had evidence suggestive of intravascular coagulation. The authors advised that children especially under the age of 6 years with a sickle cell hemoglobinopathy and an acute febrile illness should receive penicillin. They recommended further that at the first sign of change in sensorium, drop in blood pressure, or appearance of petechiae, the administration of oxygen, sodium bicarbonate, and probably heparin should begin.

Winkelstein and Drachman[546] studied the opsonizing activity for the pneumococcus with a phagocytic test using normal peripheral leukocytes incubated in normal serum and in serum from patients with sickle cell disease. Heat-labile serum opsonizing activity for the pneumococcus was markedly deficient in serum from the patients with a mean phagocytosis of 6.5%, whereas control children with AA$_2$ hemoglobin showed a mean value of 35.1%. It would seem that the same serum factor necessary for the phagocytosis of pneumococci was deficient in the serum of patients for sickle cell disease. Winkelstein and Drachman postulated that early in the infection a few pneumococci from the respiratory tract enter the circulation. Little or no antibody or opsonin is present in the serum. As a result, the spleen becomes the primary site of clearance for pneumococci from the circulation. Owing to the blockade due to plugging, thrombosis and infarction in the spleen, as well as lack of opsonin, ingestion by macrophages of the reticuloendothelial system is inefficient or ineffective. In the absence of adequate clearance, pneumococci lodge in other tissues and multiply. The lack of serum opsonin prevents adequate phagocytosis and killing when polymorphonuclear leukocytes migrate into the infected tissues.

The inability to concentrate urine normally is a feature of sickle cell anemia, and, to a lesser extent, the sickle cell trait.[156,275,288,554] In patients with sickle cell anemia the concentration defect is corrected by transfusion of normal red cells which is known to suppress intravascular sickling.[79,128,275] Hyposthenuria, however, can be reversed by red cell transfusion in young children but not in the older patients.[275] Children with sickle cell anemia are predisposed to *Salmonella* osteomyelitis.[224,231] The peculiar susceptibility to *Salmonella* osteitis of persons with sickle cell anemia has been attributed to diminished resistance of the gastrointestinal tract to invasion by pathogens.[211] Aseptic necrosis of the capital epiphysis of the femur and, less commonly, of the humerus occurs especially in older children and adults with homozygous sickle cell disease,[77,503] sickle cell–hemoglobin C disease, and sickle cell–thalassemia. The osseous lesions probably result from thromboses of the blood vessels supplying the affected areas, presumably due to the sickling phenomenon. Involvement of the femoral neck and head produces the clinical and pathologic picture of classic Legg-Perthes disease. Abnormal electroencephalograms are frequently observed in patients with sickle cell anemia and probably reflect blocking of the blood supply to various parts of the brain with varying damage to nerve cells.[223] It appears that sickle cell anemia in itself does not affect intellectual or psychologic functioning.[95] In contrast to its frequent presence in adults, chronic leg ulceration is rare in children.

The typical linear habitus with narrow hips and shoulders, decreased stature, increased upper dorsal kyphosis and lumbar lordosis, increased anteroposterior diameter of the chest, and hypogonadism are common in the adult patient. Many of these changes are also present in children, although to a lesser extent, unless the disease is severe in early life. Children often have a barrel-shaped chest, an enlarged and protruding abdomen, and thin extremities.[547]

There is a high degree of growth failure in boys and girls, delay in estrogen stimulation, delayed appearance of secondary sexual characteristics, and delay in the onset of menarche. Fertility is decreased and the incidence of abortion and premature delivery is increased.[257]

The increased susceptibility of patients with sickle cell anemia to serious infections with *Salmonella* has been difficult to explain. A group of patients with sickle cell anemia were immunized with *Salmonella* vaccines and their agglutinin titers studied.[411] The incidence and titers of preimmunization agglutinins to a large number of *Salmonella* antigens showed no significant differences between sickle cell anemia patients and controls. Patients immunized with various *Salmonella* vaccines also showed quantitatively and qualitatively normal responses of their immunoglobulins. Since the immune response was not found to be deficient, the increased incidence of severe *Salmonella* infections in these patients depends on other factors such as impaired phagocytosis and bone infarction associated with this disease. On the other hand, in the case of infection with *Plasmodium falciparum* malaria, the altered solubility of reduced hemoglobin S with consequent in vivo sickling probably interferes directly with the parasite's multiplication.

**Skeletal changes.** The skeletal abnormalities as revealed by roentgenographic examination are similar to those seen in patients with severe Cooley's anemia but are less marked and less common.[337] They are based upon marrow overgrowth resulting in osteoporosis, widening of the medullary spaces, and thinning of the cortices. These alterations are observed in the skull, vertebrae, long bones, hands, and feet. The skull changes consist of widening of the diploic spaces, external displacement of the outer table, and a hair-on-end appearance produced by the radial arrangement of the bony trabeculae so common in patients with Cooley's anemia. Skeletal changes are more frequent in adolescents and adults with sickle cell anemia than in children. In adult life the hematopoietic tissue is replaced by connective and osteoid tissue. New bone formation on the inner aspect of the cortex accounts for the thickening of the cortex and narrowing of the medullary cavity.[71] Osteoporosis, destruction, and collapse of the weakened vertebral bodies, especially in the lower thoracic and lumbar regions, cause compression deformities in both children and adults.[212]

**Blood.** The anemia is chronic, normochromic, and normocytic (derived from indices of hemoglobin, hematocrit, and red cell count), with signs of increased regenerative activity of the bone marrow. The blood smear shows round and oval cells, anisocytosis, poikilocytosis, polychromatophilia, microcytes, macrocytes, and a few spherocytes. Hypochromia is uncommon. Hyperchromia and polychromatophilia are less common. Macrocytosis appears when the anemia is severe. Sickled cells vary in number (0.5 to 25%) and are often surprisingly few in patients with severe disease. One of the standard deoxygenation techniques shows sickling to be complete and rapid in all red cells in patients with sickle cell anemia in contrast with slow development in the red cells of those with the sickle cell trait. Sickle cells (drepanocytes) are crescent or holly leaf shaped in appearance in persons with the sickle cell variants, but in those with the homozygous disease they are characteristically elongated, filamentous, pointed at each end, curved in the middle, and contain a full complement of hemoglobin. Target cells are increased in number. Nucleated red cells, chiefly normoblasts, vary from a few to many, especially in patients with pronounced anemia, and occur in the presence of pneumonia or other severe infections. Osmotic fragility is decreased, mechanical fragility increased,[205] and red cells have a shortened survival time.[74,461] (See Figs. 39 and 40.)

Hemolysis in sickle cell anemia is caused by an intracorpuscular defect. Contributing to hemolysis is the presence of varying numbers of irreversibly sickled cells. These are sickled cells that after exposure to oxygen remain in the sickled form and have lost the ability to return to normal.[443] The net synthesis of HbF is least in erythroid cells destined to become irreversibly sickled. Irreversibly deformed erythrocytes suffer preferential destruction.[48]

Bilirubin ranges from 1 to 3 mg. per 100 ml., with the major portion of the indirect type. The number of reticulocytes is increased, ranging from 5 to 25%. Excessive reticulocytosis indicates a superimposed acute infectious process or an immune hemolytic anemia. In one 18-month-old infant with a herpetic lesion, an added acquired hemolytic anemia was evidenced by a hemoglobin level of 4.6 gm. per 100 ml., reticulocytes of 78%, and a transient positive Coombs test.[509]

Patients with sickle cell anemia maintain a relatively stable hemoglobin concentration, with equilibrium between blood destruction and production established between 6 and 9 gm. per 100 ml. without transfusions. This stability is explained by the increased effective erythropoiesis in patients with this disease despite increased rates of destruction. By contrast in patients with thalassemia major there is less blood destruction but also less effective production—hence, the need for multiple transfusions.[148] The red cells range between 2 and 3.5 million per cubic millimeter. With an infection or aplastic crisis the hemoglobin may drop below 5 gm. per 100 ml. and the red blood count below 2 million per cubic millimeter.

The leukocytes range between 10,000 and 20,000 per cubic millimeter. A count of 30,000 or more occurs in patients with complications such as pneumonia and is associated with a marked shift to the left of polymorphonuclear neutrophils and the appearance of myelocytes. The platelet count is normal or slightly elevated. The sedimentation rate[67] is usually slow even in the presence of marked anemia because of the abnormal shape of the sickle cells and poor rouleaux formation. Coagulation studies reveal a correlation between advancing age and decreased liver function.[219] Maximal differences exist in Stuart factor (factor X), PTC (factor IX), fibrinogen, and moderate defects in prothrombin and factor VII. During crises there is increased fibrinolytic activity, a lytic factor that may be advantageous to the patient in a thrombotic crisis.

**Crises.** The symptomatic or clinical aspects

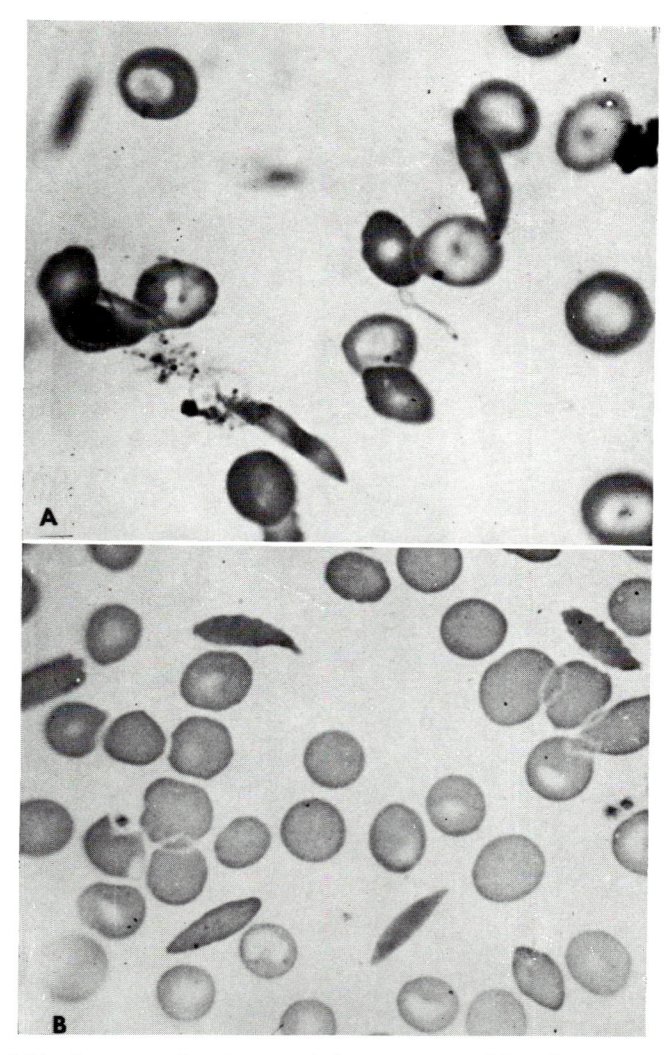

Fig. 39. Stained blood smears of patients with homozygous sickle cell anemia. Note elongated and narrow sickle cells with pointed ends. The nonsickled red cells vary in size and are round or oval. (**A** courtesy Dr. Ralph L. Engle, Jr., New York, N. Y.; **B** courtesy Dr. Ralph L. Engle, Jr., New York, N. Y., and Dr. David Lawrenz, Lakeville, Conn.)

of the crises in patients with sickle cell anemia are differentiated from the aplastic and hemolytic crises.

*Symptomatic or clinical crises.* With rare exceptions, a crisis is characterized by fever and severe pain in the joints, back, and extremities, usually without exacerbation of the anemia. At times these episodes are accompanied by a slight rise in hemoglobin concentration. The number of reticulocytes, serum bilirubin concentration, and excretion of urobilinogen in the urine and stool are not increased. This is the common type of crisis in patients with sickle cell anemia and is designated as the clinical and symptomatic type.[121] Plasma factors, more precisely some cryoprecipitable gamma globulin in the presence of cold agglutinins, can play a part in producing the painful osteoarthritic crisis of sickle cell disease. Cryoglobulinemia may seem to promote thromboses.[87] There is suggestive evidence that this type of crisis in childhood is

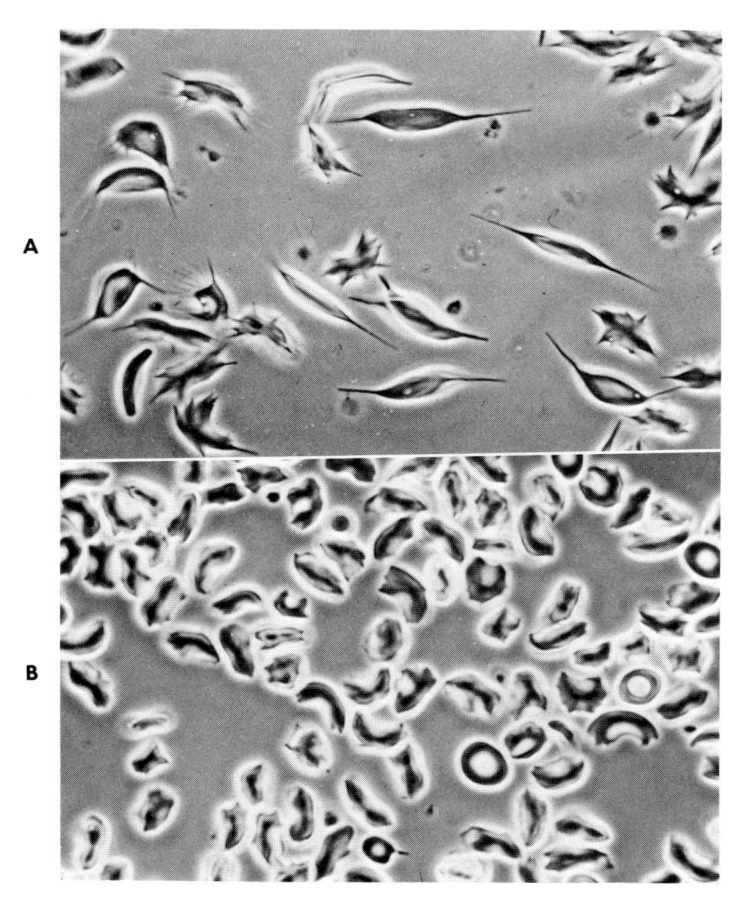

**Fig. 40.** Phase contrast microscopy of sickle cells in homozygous S-S disease, **A**, and heterozygous S-A trait, **B**. (Courtesy Dr. Julius Rutzky, Pontiac, Mich.)

associated with a sharp shrinkage of the plasma volume so that the peripheral hemoglobin concentration may actually be elevated. Furthermore, the anemic patient with this disease has a blood volume characteristically far in excess of the normal in periods of freedom from disability.[148,468] As would be expected in restoring expanded plasma levels during treatment with whole blood, plasma, or dextran, the hemoglobin level may actually drop. Sudden death occurring in infants and children during a severe crisis in sickle cell anemia has been reported.[254] The most striking necropsy finding in these patients was congestion of the internal organs with sickled erythrocytes.

*Aplastic and hemolytic crises.* The existence of a hemolytic crisis accompanied by a sudden destruction of blood and hyperfunctioning bone marrow in patients with sickle cell anemia has been challenged.[121] Others, however, have described authenticated cases of hemolytic and hyperhemolytic crises with pain, fever, increased rate of red cell destruction, anemia, normoblastemia, reticulocytosis, and a hyperplastic bone marrow.[434] The aplastic or aregenerative crisis, on the other hand, is well documented. It is characterized by a rapidly developing anemia due to the cessation of red cell production and the continued destruction of sickle cells in the circulation. However, hemolytic crises in patients with sickle cell anemia have occasionally been described in conjunction with an associated infection, such as pneumonia or septicemia, and are accompanied by severe pain in the back, abdomen, and extremities. A significant drop in red cells and hemoglobin and an increase in both the indirect serum bilirubin and reticulocyte count accompany these symptoms.[159]

Smits and her associates[486] have observed eight patients with sickle cell anemia who experienced a hemolytic crisis in each instance associated with reticulocytosis. Seven of these patients were found to be red cell glucose-6-phosphate dehydrogenase deficient. In each instance infection and/or a drug known to induce hemolysis in association with the enzyme defect alone could be implicated as the precipitating factor in the hemolytic episode. G-6-PD deficiency should therefore be considered as one of the etiologic factors in the hemolytic crises of sickle cell anemia.

Patients with sickle disease in painful crises usually have metabolic acidosis as manifested by significant reduction in plasma bicarbonate, $pCO_2$, and pH of venous blood. Following recovery from the crisis, there is a return to normal acid-base balance. For a given individual, there is an increase in the percentage of sickled cells at the time of pain, with fever and a decrease in sickled cells when the pain subsides.[30]

*Megaloblastic anemia.* Nutritional megaloblastic anemia has been reported in patients with sickle cell anemia and sickle cell–hemoglobin C disease, as in patients with other congenital hemolytic syndromes.[263] It has been attributed to an excessive need for folic acid, vitamin $B_{12}$, or both during periods of active growth and in the presence of pronounced erythropoiesis. A reversal to normoblastic erythropoiesis follows specific therapy. Transient episodes of megaloblastosis of the bone marrow occurred in a patient with sickle cell anemia complicated by an extracorpuscular hemolytic state.[364] In this patient a relative deficiency of hematopoietic factors could have resulted from the severe hemolytic process.

In another patient, a young adult, in whom a megaloblastic bone marrow developed, tissue stores of folic acid became so depleted that the daily oral administration of 1,000 μg of this vitamin was required until the bone marrow became normoblastic and serum folate reverted to normal.[309]

A 16-year-old Negro boy with sickle cell anemia experienced three episodes of folic acid deficiency accompanied by a megaloblastic bone marrow. Oral administration of a minimum of 500 μg of folic acid daily resulted in a satisfactory reticulocyte response and changed the bone marrow from megaloblastic to normoblastic.[11]

*Hypoplastic crisis.* Charney and Miller[88] pointed out that in sickle cell disease, in which the mean red cell life-span has been estimated to range from 6 to 21½ days, an aplastic episode can result in a precipitous fall in hemoglobin to as low as one-half the steady state level over a 2- to 7-day period. In their series, hyperhemolytic crises occurred with a hematocrit of 19% and reticulocyte counts of 13 to 38%. In nine cases the aplastic episodes were reticulocytopenic. Reticulocytopenia was self-limited and recovery was heralded by the appearance of large numbers of normoblasts in the peripheral blood. Since antecedent or current infection was not established in all cases, the authors postulate folic acid deficiency as a causative factor. Megaloblastic changes are known to occur in the bone marrow during red cell arrest in chronic hemolytic anemia.

With few exceptions,[383] the administration of folic acid usually does not result in any significant changes in peripheral blood values in sickle cell anemia. Since ascorbic acid is required for conversion of folic to folinic acid, its deficiency may conceivably lead to a reticulocytopenic episode in sickle cell anemia. At the present time the exact role of folic acid and ascorbic acid deficiency in the aplastic crises has still to be defined.

*Splenic-sequestration crisis.* In an occasional child with sickle cell anemia, usually in the first 3 years of life, a crisis is occasionally associated with sudden severe anemia and massive enlargement of the spleen. Transfusions result in remarkable shrinkage of the spleen. Since the resulting hemoglobin level is higher than could be accounted for by the amount of blood administered, the splenomegaly is interpreted as due to "pooling" of blood. The return of the sequestered or trapped blood following transfusions is accompanied by reduction in size of the spleen. If these episodes recur, splenectomy has been found effective in their prevention. Bleeding into the spleen has also been associated with thrombocytopenia in the young child with sickle cell anemia.[197]

The rapid loss of erythrocytes, splenomegaly, and shock can also occur during the late stages of pregnancy or in the early postpartum period in sickle cell–C disease, sickle-thalassemia, and homozygous sickle cell disease.[209,210] The loss of circulating erythrocytes is presumably the result of stagnation in various organs, particularly the spleen. Increased hemolysis occurs in areas of stasis.

*Diagnosis.* The demonstration of the sickling phenomenon in vitro prevents mistakes in diagnosis. The basic pathologic process accounts for diverse symptom complexes which simulate rheumatic fever, osteomyelitis, poliomyelitis, encephalitis,[476] and other neurologic disorders, and appendicitis and other acute surgical emergencies.

Although sickle cell anemia mimics rheumatic fever, especially when associated with joint pains, fever, and leukocytosis, the coexistence of the two diseases is rare,[385] but it has been reported on occasion.[514] Episodes in which the patient appears critically ill with abdominal pain, nausea, and vomiting may be severe and recurrent and extremely difficult to differentiate from a surgical condition requiring a laparotomy. The utmost conservatism must be exercised in management when it is established that the patient has sickle cell anemia. It is entirely possible, however, for the patient to suffer from the same surgical emergencies as persons without sickle cells. The combination of severe bone pain and fever requires differentiation from osteomyelitis. Except for the infrequent complications of *Salmonella* osteomyelitis and aseptic necrosis of the femoral and humeral capital epiphyses, osseous involvement requiring treatment is uncommon.

*Treatment.* Since there is no specific therapy, symptomatic and supportive measures are mainly relied upon.[292] The treatment of the patient with the painful or clinical crisis in whom anemia is not a major factor demands the most serious consideration. Bed rest, aspirin, codeine, or other analgesic and sedative drugs usually suffice to control symptoms in the average case. Use of oral hydration, intravenous infusions of glucose, or dilute electrolyte solutions increases blood volume and expedites mobilization of stagnant or trapped sickle cells.[433] Antibiotics are prescribed if infection is present. Hemodilution tends to overcome the shrinkage of plasma volume with which the crisis is associated and to restore it to precritical levels. The excessive plasma volume noted in patients who are not in crisis observed in a small number of cases[148,468] emphasizes the need for fluids. Plasma, dextran, and other plasma expanders[159,255] are useful in achieving this aim.

In contrast to patients with severe Cooley's anemia whose blood levels decline progressively unless supported by transfusions are patients with uncomplicated sickle cell anemia whose hemoglobin levels tend to stabilize between 6 and 9 gm. per 100 ml. without transfusions. Transfusions of packed cells are given for correction of severe anemia accompanying infection, for aplastic crisis, and for relief of extreme pain when other measures fail. Transfusions raise hemoglobin levels, increase the oxygen carrying capacity of blood, and reduce the number and concentration of sickle cells both by dilution and by the depressing action of blood supplements on hematopoiesis.[79,128,292,475]

The benefit of transfusions has been attributed to the effect of the transfused cells in reducing blood viscosity. Prophylactic "partial exchange transfusion" has been recommended[12] at 6- to 8-week intervals so as to maintain 15 to 40% circulating normal cells. This procedure was effective in five patients subject to recurrent crises, with resulting partial or moderate improvement. The treatment consisted of phlebotomy followed by a small transfusion.[12]

Limited exchange transfusion has also been given to patients for treatment of symptomatic crisis of sickle cell anemia.[65] Buffy coat-free, packed erythrocytes were used in therapy. Red cells were infused before and after a phlebotomy on successive days. This treatment ameliorates fever and bone pain, interrupts the cycle of hypoxia, vaso-occlusion, and organ injury by diluting autologous circulating erythrocytes containing sickle hemoglobin with those holding HbA; and raises the oxygen-carrying capacity of the blood with only a minor increase in blood volume.

Oxygen therapy is useful in combating severe anoxemia, especially in patients with congestive heart failure, but should only be employed for short periods of time. Continuous treatment with oxygen depresses bone marrow and aggravates the anemia.[396] Hyperbaric oxygenation decreases the percentage of circulating sickle cells, which remains low for prolonged periods after the patient is removed from the chamber.[290] There does not appear to be any striking remission of the sickle cell crisis and there was no tendency toward improved renal concentrating ability. Further observations are required to determine whether this is useful therapy in sickle cell anemia. A variety of agents, each designed to relieve the painful crisis through individual mechanisms, have been employed. These include Priscoline,[476] ACTH and cortisone,[436] intravenously administered sodium carbonate,[191] acetazolamide (Diamox),[208] phenothiazines,[377] and therapeutic defibrination with Arvin.[185] In one study[430] a trial of the rapid infusion of sodium bicarbonate gave no relief to the painful sickle cell crises. Painful swelling of the hands and feet has been satisfactorily treated in some clinics by steroids (methyl prednisolone) given in a dosage of 2 to 4 mg. repeated at intervals of 4 to 6 hours during a 24-hour period.[434] None of these agents has withstood the critical test of controlled clinical trials and thus their efficacy has never been established.[373a]

Long-term oral anticoagulant therapy to prevent painful crises by decreasing fibrin formation has resulted in a slight decrease in crises.[421] The mild improvement, however, was outweighed by an increase in the number of bleeding episodes. More extended trial is required with each of these methods of treatment before a definite opinion can be given as to their merit.

Cobaltous chloride may produce initial satisfactory hematopoietic responses, but these responses are not sustained. The serious disadvantage of the use of cobaltous chloride, in addition to such side effects as anorexia, nausea, and vomiting, is the depression of thyroid function.[195]

A treatment of priapism that has been suggested consists of aspiration of the corpora cavernosa in addition to intramuscular injections of diethylstilbestrol.[154]

Splenectomy in the treatment of patients with sickle cell anemia has had its advocates,[135,222,452] but it does not occupy the therapeutic position that it does in patients with hereditary spherocytosis and, to a lesser extent, Cooley's anemia. In one series of patients (Dickstein and Koop, quoted by Margolies[316]) with marked to moderate enlargement of the spleen, no major crises followed removal of the spleen. Since an enlarged spleen constitutes the main site of sickling, sequestration, and destruction of the sickled cells,[528] benefits from splenectomy should be substantial. Furthermore, removal of a large spleen increases the average erythrocyte survival time of the patient's red cells by one-third (a half-life of 3.1 days of $^{51}Cr$ presplenectomy as compared with a half-life of 11.4 days postsplenectomy).[490] Nevertheless, because of the natural tendency for the spleen to shrink in size and to atrophy, its removal is not advocated as a routine measure. Such removal should be reserved for the occasional patient who has a very large spleen and who requires excessive transfusions. In such patients normal red cells are presumably destroyed by the development of an extracorpuscular hemolytic defect.[307]

There is no contraindication to tonsillectomy when attacks of acute tonsillitis are frequent and associated with respiratory infections and a crisis. Preoperative transfusions and other safeguards are necessary.[159] The patient with sickle cell trait who is to have a tonsillectomy or other operative procedures should have a transfusion at least 1 week prior to remain well oxygenated. With the homozygous disease, transfusion at least 1 week prior to operation is advisable so that anoxia is prevented and old sickle cells in the circulation can be destroyed and their new formation suppressed.

*Urea therapy.* Recent uncontrolled studies[352a] have suggested that intravenous urea in invert sugar is effective in the treatment of acute vaso-occlusive crises in sickle cell disease. The proposed mechanism of action of urea was thought to be through the disruption of hydrophobic intermolecular bonds and the prevention of polymerization and aggregation of HbS. Oral urea[351a] has been used in a prophylactic program, but carefully controlled well-documented clinical trials will be required before the potential usefulness of this agent can be critically evaluated.

Since the maximum concentration of urea achieved in treated patients is approximately 30 to 50 mM., and since urea is rapidly cleared by the body, Cerami and Manning[78a] have presented an alternative explanation for the reported salutory effect of urea—that cyanate, in equilibrium with urea, is the active agent. They described an irreversible specific carbamylation reaction in which cyanate reacted with the alpha-amino group of the $NH_2$-terminl valine of HbS and inhibited sickling in vitro. Gillette, Manning, and Cerami[185a] have shown that the autologous survival of sickle cells treated in vitro with 50 mM. cyanate is prolonged toward the normal range. Since cyanate reacts with other proteins, de Furia and co-workers[115b] investigated the in vitro effect of cyanate on erythrocyte metabolism and function and found that glycolysis, ATP and 2,3-DPG stability, autohemolysis, and osmotic fragility were not affected and that potassium loss in carbamylated sickle cells was decreased. However, oxygen affinity of carbamylated cells was increased but 2,3-DPG reactivity, Bohr effect, and the buffering capacity of the blood were unaffected. Cyanate and similar compounds may have a potential clinical use in treating and preventing the anemia and painful crises of sickle cell disease.

*Prognosis.* The prognosis is very unfavorable, with a fatal outcome in many patients in childhood or early adult life. Death results from overwhelming infection, congestive cardiac failure, cerebral vascular accidents, and abdominal crises.[505] With the use of antibiotics, chemotherapy, transfusions, and oxygen in selected patients, life expectancy can be prolonged. Although it has been found that few survive the fourth decade,[85] increasing numbers of older persons will probably be encountered in North America in the future and a similar tendency in Africa as environmental conditions improve.[2,502] The outlook for the patient with the variants of sickle cell disease is more favorable than for the patient with homozygous sickle cell anemia.[111]

A study in Jamaica of sixty patients with sickle cell anemia over the age of 30 years showed that most of them were in full-time employment.[442] Twenty-one of the patients ranged in age from 40 to 60 years. Pains in the bones or joints, leg ulceration, and jaundice were the most frequent types of presentation, but only two patients had a hemoglobin considerably below 6 gm. per 100 ml. Most of the patients were well developed and of average height and, though the development of secondary sexual characteristics was delayed, there was an average of 2.6 pregnancies per patient. In almost all the patients the frequency and severity of painful crises had diminished with age. The liver edge was palpable in forty patients, and six (10%) had easily palpable spleens. In Jamaica, where the frequency of the HbS gene is about 11%, it can be calculated that approximately 0.32% of all children will have the disease.

## THALASSEMIA (COOLEY'S ANEMIA, MEDITERRANEAN ANEMIA, ERYTHROBLASTIC ANEMIA, HEREDITARY LEPTOCYTOSIS)

Thalassemia is a hereditary hemolytic disorder occurring predominantly in persons of Mediterranean origin and is characterized by abnormalities of red cell structure and hemoglobin synthesis resulting from a defect in erythropoiesis. The disorder ranges in severity from the asymptomatic trait to the severe form requiring frequent blood transfusions. In its severe form thalassemia combines the features of a refractory anemia with typical roentgenographic, clinical, and hematologic features.

Thalassemia includes a heterogeneous group of inherited syndromes that are characterized by a deficiency in the synthesis of normal adult hemoglobin. It has been estimated that there are approximately two million people in Italy alone who carry at least one thalassemia gene.[241]

Thalassemia major is the homozygous condition, and thalassemia minor represents the corresponding heterozygous state. A wide spectrum of hematologic phenotypes has been observed in both forms of the disease. Each is produced by mutations of a thalassemia-like nature and affect the alpha and beta chains contained in the globin of adult hemoglobin, leading to the broad designations of alpha and beta thalassemias. It is postulated that a thalassemia-like mutation is produced when one of the genes responsible for hemoglobin synthesis is rendered relatively or absolutely inactive.

Recently published volumes on the problems of Cooley's anemia[107,169] and the thalassemia syndromes[530] contain comprehensive discussions of the manifold facets of this disease.

Necheles and his associates[360] offer the following classification of the thalassemias, acknowledging that they consist not only of the commonly known beta thalassemia or Cooley's anemia but also of a number of closely related variants. These variants, currently defined as a group of syndromes, are characterized by a genetically determined diminished synthesis of one or another of the polypeptide chains constituting normal hemoglobin.

    I. Alpha thalassemia
        A. Silent H gene
        B. Alpha-thalassemia gene

    1. Severe
    2. Mild
  II. Beta-thalassemia
    A. Classic high $A_2$ variety
      1. Severe
      2. Mild
    B. High F variant (delta-beta-thalassemia)
    C. High F–high $A_2$ variant
  III. Delta-thalassemia
  IV. Thalassemia-like syndromes
    A. Hereditary persistence of fetal hemoglobin
    B. Lepore-like hemoglobin

*History.* In 1925 and in 1927 Cooley and associates[104,105] drew attention to an anemia that had heretofore been regarded as belonging to the heterogeneous group of von Jaksch's anemia but which possessed such well-defined features as to constitute a definite clinical entity. Outstanding features were its anemia, icterus, familial aspects, characteristic facies, skeletal changes, splenomegaly, and the appearance of large numbers of circulating normoblasts in the peripheral blood. Because of the latter aspect, the disease was initially termed erythroblastic anemia. From studies of the families of patients with the severe disease, it soon became apparent that the siblings and the parents all possessed the features of the disease in mild form.

The history of van Jaksch's anemia and "anemia pseudoleucaemica" has been recently reviewed by Lehndorff.[301] In 1889 and 1890 von Jaksch described a severe anemia associated with enlargement of spleen, liver, and lymph nodes, a marked leukocytosis with a scattering of myelocytes, and other early forms. It eventually became apparent that this syndrome was descriptive of varied blood responses to rickets, congenital syphilis, iron-deficiency anemia, infection, and acute leukemia. Von Jaksch's anemia has now lost its identity as a specific disease.

*Nomenclature.* The designation of thalassemia for Mediterranean or Cooley's anemia has shown increasing usage with the recognition of the abnormal hemoglobins. Soon after the original description by Cooley and Lee[104] of the group of patients whose condition ("erythroblastic anemia") was characterized by anemia, icterus, splenomegaly, erythroblastosis, and bone changes, Whipple and Bradford[540] proposed the term "thalassemia." This designation was derived from the Greek "thalass" for "the sea," which to a Greek meant the Mediterranean. Although there may be some reservations with regard to its derivation,[114] it lends itself to the terminology indicating combination with various abnormal hemoglobins and to qualification as to the degree of severity. Since to Thomas Cooley goes the credit for discovery of this disease, the severe form which he first described may also be distinguished as Mediterranean (Cooley's) anemia.

*Race and incidence.* The majority of patients have a Mediterranean ancestry, most commonly Italian, Syrian, and Greek. In Italy the highest prevalence is in the lower Po valley in northeastern Italy around Ferrara[51] and in southern Italy. The Italian islands of Sicily and Sardinia, the island of Corsica, and the islands of Cyprus and Crete have large concentrations of affected persons, probably due to inbreeding.[72] The disease has been reported in a variety of non-Mediterranean races with wide geographic distribution. It has been found among the Chinese (spreading from Canton and Hong Kong) and other Orientals, Asiatic Indians, Egyptians, Britains,[39,73] Germans, Bukharan and Kurdistan Jews,[323,389] Negroes,[23] and Mexicans, to mention only a few.[453] In some areas of Thailand[333] the incidence is high and represents one of the most common forms of hemolytic anemia. Its spread from areas adjoining the Mediterranean Sea by Greek traders in commerce, colonizations, and explorations may account for the present-day frequency with which this disease is found in southern Asia.[72] It would seem that mass migrations carried the genetic defect eastward to China from a single focus in the northern Mediterranean.[92] There is still the possibility, however, that spontaneous mutations arising in a number of areas account for the widespread nature of the thalassemia gene. If the frequency with which the mild type of Cooley's anemia is encountered in New York City is an indication of its extent among persons of Mediterranean origin in other parts of the United States, this condition is extremely prevalent. In New York City persons with the mild or severe disease are already separated by several generations from those originally born in southern Italy and Greece. Neel and Valentine,[362] on the basis of known incidence of the severe form, computed the mild form as occurring in approximately 4% of

**Figs. 41 and 42.** Schematic representation of genetic transmission in Cooley's anemia. "Th" is a gene for thalassemia (Cooley's anemia, Mediterranean anemia); "th" is the contrasting normal allele. The designation of "Th-th" is the heterozygote, a simplification of current terminology for the trait or mild form of the disease. "Th-Th" is the homozygote (severe disease, Mediterranean anemia), and "th-th" is the normal individual.

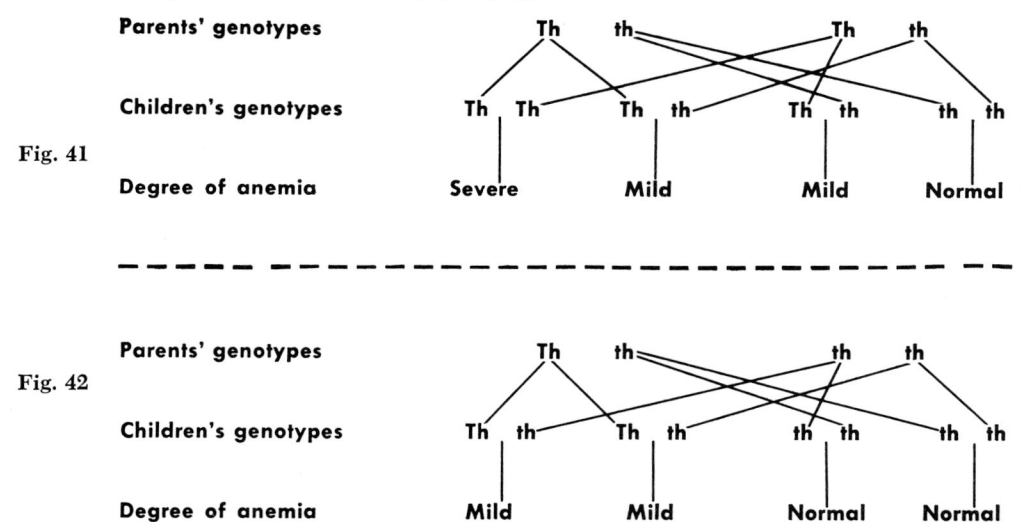

**Fig. 41.** Inheritance of the severe type of beta-thalassemia when both parents are heterozygous. (From Smith, C. H.: The abnormal hemoglobins: clinical and hematologic aspects, J. Pediat. **50:**91, 1957.)

**Fig. 42.** Inheritance of the mild type of beta-thalassemia when one parent is heterozygous and the other normal. (From Smith. C. H.: The abnormal hemoglobins: clinical and hematologic aspects, J. Pediat. **50:**91, 1957.)

adult Italians in the city of Rochester, N. Y. The bulk of Italians immigrated to the United States from the southern part of their country in the later half of the nineteenth century and the beginning of the twentieth.[171] It is in the offspring of this group in New York City that the largest number of cases of Cooley's anemia occur.

According to Lehmann and associates,[300] thalassemia is most commonly found in Asia and should no longer be regarded as having originated in the Mediterranean region. Cases observed in Turks, Persians, and Kurdistan Jews and even those in India might be related to cases among Mediterranean populations, but this explanation fails to account for thalassemia in Thailand. The Chinese cases originate from the area around Canton and Hong Kong, and numerous observations have been made in Indonesia, the Philippines, and New Guinea.

Since the Second World War 158,000 Greeks and 300,000 Italians have migrated to Australia (Australian Immigration, 1966) from regions in which the frequency of thalassemia minor ranges from 2 to 20%.[115] A reasonable estimate of the frequency for thalassemia minor in Greek and Italian migrants is about 4 to 5%, and calculations give 1 in 1,500 as the frequency of thalassemia major among the offspring of Greek × Greek or Italian × Italian marriages so that of the 14,000 such children born in Australia in 1964 there would be nine cases. If all migrants married Australians no cases would be produced.

*Genetic transmission.* The person with the trait or mild disease who functions as a carrier is heterozygous for a gene which when homozygous produces the severe disease. The gene for thalassemia has a varying expressivity for the grade of anemia, and sometimes it is difficult to separate the moderate from the severe type, hematologically (Figs. 41 and 42). The presence of the trait in only one parent of a child with the severe disease should prompt a search for the sickle cell trait, hemoglobin C disease, or hemoglobin E disease in the other parent and for the combined disease with the different hemoglobins in the patient.

The same selective advantage that the sickling trait possesses with respect to suboptimal growth of malarial parasites in red blood cells has been suggested for thalassemia.[341] The geographic distribution and severe loss of thalassemia genes suggest the possibility of a selective advantage of the trait to malaria. Data collected in Sardinia suggest very strongly that thalassemia heterozygotes are indeed protected against malaria.[341]

*Effect of the gene for thalassemia upon other hemoglobins.* The gene for thalassemia either interferes with the normal suppression of fetal hemoglobin or the latter is formed in place of the more difficult synthesis of the adult type of pigment. The presence of excessive amounts of hemoglobin S, C, and E in combination with thalassemia may reflect a compensatory replacement of normal hemoglobin, the synthesis of which is retarded by the gene for thalassemia. As has been already postulated, these increased concentrations may also reflect the potentiating effect of the gene for thalassemia on the formation of abnormal hemoglobin. Exception to this principle has been found in connection with a thalassemia gene associated with a low $A_2$ hemoglobin percentage which fails to interact with the genes for hemoglobin S, C, and E. This contrasts with the more common interacting thalassemia gene, which is responsible for an elevated $A_2$ component.[98]

*Clinical types.* The disease presents a wide and continuous spectrum of severity designated at each extreme as thalassemia major for the severe type and thalassemia minor for the mild type. In the affected person these correspond to the homozygous and heterozygous states, respectively. In both the major and minor types there are also varying grades of severity. Thus, thalassemia minor embraces forms which are asymptomatic without anemia (termed the trait or thalassemia minima) and the minor type per se which is usually associated with mild to moderate anemia. Patients with thalassemia minor or minima, being heterozygotes, remain true to type and never develop the severe disease. Italian writers refer to Rietti-Greppi-Micheli disease as a heterozygous type much less severe than thalassemia major and described by them as hemolytic icterus with increased red cell osmotic resistance to fragility.[349]

*Thalassemia intermedia.* The homozygous disease, in which each parent is heterozygous for thalassemia, falls into two classifications on the basis of grade of severity—the intermediate (moderate) type, in which the patients function effectively without transfusions, and the severe type, in which the patients require multiple blood supplements to maintain hemoglobin levels compatible with normal activity. In contrast to the severely affected patients, those in the intermediate group (5 to 10%) are able to maintain concentrations of hemoglobin ranging from 7 to 10 gm. per 100 ml. without treatment. In a group of thirteen such patients ranging in age from 11 months to 50 years, fetal hemoglobin percentages ranged from 15 to 85%.[143] Values for serum iron were normal or increased. Latent iron-binding capacities were markedly diminished or absent. The spleen in these cases was enlarged, ranging from 4 cm. below the costal margin to the level of the iliac crest. The distinction from the severe homozygous form was that the hemoglobin values (7 to 10 gm. per 100 ml.) were maintained in the absence of routine supportive transfusion therapy. In the intermediate group the disorder becomes clinically manifest later in childhood as compared with the severe homozygous disease in which transfusions are required during the first year of life. Necheles and colleagues[359] postulated that patients with thalassemia intermedia have less depression of beta-chain synthesis. It is in this group that a high incidence of extramedullary hematopoietic masses occur[144] (see p. 396). With advancing age cardiac failure also becomes manifest.[355] The patient reported initially at 19 years of age[465] now 49 years of age is under continuous care for recurrent cardiac failure. In another patient 41 years of age,[27] in addition to cardiac failure and diabetes mellitus associated with iron overload, there was evidence of hypopituitarism, porphyrinuria, and dipyrroles. The latter was interpreted as being due to a severe degree of ineffective erythropoiesis. On the other hand, patients with the intermediate type are observed in whom the disease is quiescent for many years until, quite suddenly, transfusions are required. This occurs following infections or exposure to noxious agents or for no apparent reason. From this point on, the need for transfusions may become so urgent that splenectomy is necessary.

The concept of thalassemia intermedia has been broadened to apply to a clinical designation for hematologic disease of varying grades of severity between thalassemia major and minor.[376] From such a standpoint, thalassemia intermedia is genetically heterogeneous. Cases have been placed in this category that result from the interaction of thalassemia with a variety of abnormal hemoglobin genes[499] and with variants such as the Lepore hemoglobin.[374] Although we have chosen to limit the intermediate form of thalassemia to homozygous patients requiring minimal treatment, cases presumably heterozygous have been described with severe anemia requiring transfusions.[376] This occurred in two adult Negro brothers with moderate hepatosplenomegaly who showed striking differences in $A_2$ and fetal hemoglobin levels. To explain the occurrence of severe thalassemia in heterozygous individuals, it has been suggested that non-genetic factors, such as environment, might modify biochemical expression of the genes governing thalassemia.[100] Extreme caution and close hematologic scrutiny of the parents of such pedigrees are essential before the intermediate form of thalassemia can be ascribed to a heterozygous individual.

The gross facial disfigurement of patients with thalassemia intermedia will yield to operative correction. The premaxilla can be contoured, sectioned, and reduced with apparent safety to the maxillary segment. Bleeding is no great problem. Correction of facial asymmetry and malocclusion by surgery has been successful.[268]

In the patient discussed by Nathan and Gibson[355] with thalassemia intermedia, the uric acid rose to 17 mg. per 100 ml. with pain in the hip attributed to gout. Another patient thought to have septic arthritis proved to have episodes of gout due to hyperuricemia with thalassemia. The hyperuricemia in these cases was attributed to ineffective erythropoiesis in the bone marrow and throughout the reticuloendothelial system. One of the effects of the high cellular turnover associated with massive cell destruction is hyperuricemia with gout, a complication also observed in other myeloproliferative disorders including polycythemia vera and leukemia. In the first case mentioned, a large intrathoracic mass 12 cm. in diameter had risen from the sixth rib. This mass was formed from a herniation or extrusion of the marrow tissue through a defect in the cortex of the rib. It remained in continuity with the medullary cavity and the capsule was formed from the periosteum. Histologic examination showed marked hypercellularity of the marrow mainly secondary to erythroid hyperplasia but with some increase in the myeloid precursors as well.

Occasionally one encounters cases of thalassemia intermedia in which one parent demonstrates the hematological criteria of the heterozygous form of thalassemia and in which the other parent appears normal. When the normal parent reveals no other form of hemoglobinopathy, it is still possible that the beta chain can be deficient. Such a mild beta-thalassemia gene was described by Schwartz.[429] He reported a family of Albanian descent in which the father of two children with a mild form of thalassemia intermedia had normal red cell morphology and normal level of hemoglobins $A_2$ and F, whereas the mother had elevated hemoglobin $A_2$. The children had hemoglobin F levels of less than 12%, unusual for thalassemia major in which levels of up to 100% are occasionally found. Blood samples were incubated with L-leucine-$^{14}$C to determine production of alpha and beta chains in reticulocytes. The decrease in beta-chain synthesis in the two siblings was less than that usually observed in thalassemia major. In the father and four of his relatives was found a degree of impairment of beta-chain production characteristic of heterozygous beta-thalassemia, despite the lack of the usual criteria of this disorder (decreaesd osmotic fragility in hypotonic saline, hypochromic macrocytes, microcytes, poikilocytosis, red cell stippling, and elevated $HbA_2$). In this family the interaction of this "silent" form of beta-thalassemia in the father and high hemoglobin $A_2$ in the mother resulted in thalassemia major of reduced severity in two of their children.

*Fetal hemoglobin in patients with thalassemia.* In patients with the severe disease, an extraordinary percentage of the circulating hemoglobin is of the alkali-resistant or fetal type, with values ranging from 40 to 100%.[310, 400, 553] In parents and asymptomatic siblings with the trait of the disease, fetal hemoglobin lies within the normal range (less than 2%).

It has been postulated that the common form of thalassemia in which fetal hemoglobin is produced in excess (beta-thalassemia) results from a mutation in which the production of beta-polypeptide chains required for adult hemoglobin synthesis is sharply curtailed.

With the decreased beta chain production there is a compensatory increase in the delta chain ($HbA_2$) and gamma chain (HbF) production.

Except for the marked elevation of fetal hemoglobin, no specific abnormal hemoglobin has been described in patients with this disease. No relationship has been demonstrated between the amount of fetal hemoglobin in an individual patient and the severity of the disease. It has been suggested that the increase in fetal hemoglobin stems from interference by the gene for thalassemia with the synthesis of adult hemoglobin so that reversion to fetal hemoglobin formation results. In several infants 1 and 2 months of age in whom clinical and hematologic features were already indicative of thalassemia major, fetal hemoglobin exceeded the elevated levels normally found at this age.[146] These observations indicate that the high level of fetal hemoglobin synthesis is a continuous process from fetal to adult life and that interference with the formation of normal adult hemoglobin is a permanent feature of the severe disease.

In a family with two siblings with Cooley's anemia, the cord blood of a subsequent newborn was examined.[270] Red cell morphology was normal for the newborn period. Fetal hemoglobin was 90%. At 2 months the hemoglobin was 8.4 gm./100 ml., with 90% fetal hemoglobin. At 3 months the fetal hemoglobin was 50% and hypochromic microcytes were present. The rate of beta chain synthesis was low at birth and did not rise at age 3 months. In contrast the rate of beta chain synthesis in normal infants was considerably higher at birth and rapidly increased during the first month of life. These results indicate that, in the infant who develops beta-thalassemia, low beta chain production can be detected on the first day of life.

With electrophoresis, fetal hemoglobin, when present in substantial amounts, can be demonstrated as a slower component than normal hemoglobin and almost continuous with it.

Leucine is present in all the peptide chains of hemoglobin A and F, whereas isoleucine is present in hemoglobin F but not in hemoglobin A. Marks and Burka[318] found that isoleucine is incorporated by polyribosomes of cells of thalassemic and nonthalassemic subjects in comparable amounts. (Polyribosomes are ribosomes with sedimentation coefficients greater than 100 S). However, polyribosomes in cells from thalassemic patients have significantly lower capacity to incorporate leucine than polyribosomes from nonthalassemic cells. In thalassemia, the defect in protein synthesis involves, therefore, a selective impairment of forming hemoglogin A. More precisely, the primary defect in subjects with thalassemia major consists of a decreased capacity to synthesize beta chains. The alpha chains formed in excess and not needed are rapidly destroyed. The demonstration that the synthesis of hemoglobin F proceeds at a similar rate in cells from thalassemic and nonthalassemic subjects may indicate that the decrease in beta-chain synthesis (which occurs in thalassemia) is not responsible for an increase in gamma-chain formation. A possible explanation is the persistence in thalassemia of early precursor erythroid cells which retain the capacity for gamma-chain synthesis beyond the stage at which fetal hemoglobin is normally made. If, in addition to the altered maturation, there is a defect in beta-chain synthesis, as in the thalassemia syndromes, a greater increase in the proportion of hemoglobin F results.[318]

Further evidence has been provided, showing that a defect in beta-chain synthesis exists in thalassemia. After incubation of reticulocytes with radioactive amino acid, the specific activity of the beta chain of globin from the blood of patients with thalassemia was consistently lower than that of the alpha chain.[216] The alpha chain consistently incorporated more carbon-14 per amino acid residue than the beta chain. In subjects without this disorder, the specific activity of the beta chain was always equal to or higher than that of the alpha chain.

In the heterozygous form of the persistent fetal gene and thalassemia (thal-F), the alkali-resistant hemoglobin may rise to over 65%. In this case fetal hemoglobin is quite uniformly distributed among the red cells.[101] In homozygous thalassemia with the same percentage of fetal hemoglobin the distribution of the pigment is strikingly heterogeneous in the red cells. In the former (high fetal gene) there is little evidence of anemia; in the latter it is very severe. The mild hemolytic disorder in the thal-F heterozygotes is presumably attributable to the thalassemia components since the homozygote for hereditary persistence of fetal hemoglobin displays no evidence of increased blood destruction.

**Pathogenesis.** Defective synthesis of normal hemoglobin with an increased percentage of fetal hemoglobin, impaired fabrication of circulating erythrocytes,[497] and increased hemolysis of the defective cells have been implicated in the causation of the disease. As presently conceived, thalassemia includes a group of inherited syndromes that are characterized by a deficiency in the synthesis of structurally normal hemoglobin A. In these syndromes, the common phenotypic expression is a hypochromic, microcytic anemia of varying severity.[371] It has been demonstrated in patients with severe Cooley's anemia that the problem of establishing equilibrium compatible with normal activity is greatly exaggerated by the inability of erythropoiesis to compensate for the accelerated rate of red cell destruction, and this inadequacy is greater than that in patients with other hemolytic anemias.[149] This accounts for the greater need for transfusion in patients with thalassemia than in those with sickle cell anemia in whom production is more effective. There is evidence that heme synthesis may be impaired by a relatively slow rate of protoporphyrin synthesis and by a partial block in the combination of protoporphyrin and iron.[26,194]

Hypochromia and microcytosis, despite abundance of iron stores, have suggested to many observers a block in the synthesis of hemoglobin as a major factor in the pathogenesis of this disease. The views commonly held are, however, that the mechanism of this disorder consists of a primary defect in the rate of synthesis of the globins rather than in heme synthesis. It has been originally suggested that the thalassemia genes cause inefficient production of polypeptide chains, possibly due to abnormal amino acid composition.[243] However, analysis of the amino acid content of individual tryptic peptides of the polypeptide chains in thalassemia has revealed no structural abnormalities. It is now thought, therefore, that the defect in the thalassemia syndromes appears to reside in the quantity of hemoglobin synthesis and is not associated with a qualitatively abnormal product.[178] Interference at the level of the genetic regulatory system results in structurally normal hemoglobin A being made at a reduced rate.

The thalassemias demonstrate differences in synthesis of four polypeptide chains—the alpha, beta, gamma, and delta chains. Each chain is chemically different and governed by a different set of structural genes. Thalassemia represents a mutation that results in subnormal production of hemoglobin $A_1$ and, more specifically, a severe block in the synthesis of the beta-polypeptide chains (beta thalassemia). This leads to a diminished concentration of hemoglobin $A_1$ and allows for the compensatory or relative increases of hemoglobin F (alpha$_2$ gamma$_2$) and $A_2$ (alpha$_2$ delta$_2$), neither containing beta chains.

As a result of abnormalities of hemoglobin synthesis, large quantities of hemoglobin are produced in a hyperplastic marrow, but the red cells undergo premature destruction in the marrow (ineffective erythropoiesis).

With the oral administration of radioactive glycine, it has been shown that the incorporation of glycine into the hemoglobin of patients with thalassemia major may be delayed and decreased, whereas labeling of stercobilin is accelerated and increased. This has been interpreted to mean that delivery of the erythrocytes to the peripheral blood is ineffective and that stercobilin formation increases as a result of abortive heme synthesis.[194] The defect in heme synthesis explains in part the hypochromia in the presence of an abundance of iron. It has also been shown that immature erythrocytes in thalassemia do not form heme from glycine as well as cells from other hemolytic anemias. The lesion is probably located in the conversion of glycine to delta-aminolevulinic acid.[153]

The delta-aminolevulinic acid dehydrase and heme synthetase activity in bone marrow aspirates was greatly reduced in thalassemia major as compared with the levels found in patients with pernicious anemia, iron deficiency anemia, and autoimmune hemolytic anemia.[494] These findings also suggest that a defect in heme synthesis exists in thalassemia. The only basic phenotypic expression of the thalassemia gene, however, is the reduction of globin synthesis and all other alterations are secondary to it. It is a reasonable hypothesis that a failure in globin synthesis could lead to an excess of heme which by a negative "feedback" mechanism results in a decrease in the activity of specific enzymes taking part in heme formation.[318]

The difficulty in the patient with homozygous thalassemia is that he is unable to maintain an adequate supply of functional erythrocytes despite an intense stimulation of erythropoiesis which results in marked bone marrow hyperplasia.[354] The red blood cells that are formed have an abnormally short life-span which is, in part, a consequence of their rapid destruction in the spleen. The anemia results, therefore, from excessive production of abnormal erythyrocytes. The turnover of hemoglobin precursors is markedly elevated so that their effective utilization is low—hence, a state of ineffective erythropoiesis.

One of the explanations given for thalassemia[242] is the presence of defective alpha and beta chain messenger RNA molecules that block a sufficient number of ribosomes so as to decrease the hemoglobin synthesis. Microcytic cells that are formed are later destroyed, resulting in a severe hemolytic anemia, which in turn touches off the maturation of red cells still conditioned to produce fetal hemoglobin. Ineffective hemoglobin synthesis in this disease leads to the piling up of heme within the red cells. This in turn by a feedback mechanism leads to the accumulation of breakdown products of heme including large quantities of iron.

In erythroid cells of patients with beta-thalassemia major,[317] the rate of synthesis of beta chains is on the average only one-fifth the rate of synthesis of the alpha chains. In subjects with beta-thalassemia minor, a lesser depression in beta-chain synthesis has been observed.[317] Bank and associates[22] proposed as the pathogenesis of beta-thalassemia "a basic genetic defect due to a series of unknown mutations which leads to the production of either decreased or defective mRNA for beta chains. This in turn leads to an absolute decrease in beta-chain production that is proportioned for the gene dose." Alpha chains are present in relative excess and those not utilized in HbA and HbF synthesis are unstable and may precipitate in the cells containing them. The excessive alpha chains become part of the inclusion bodies, resulting in preferential destruction of these red cells and are responsible for the hemolytic manifestations of beta-thalassemia. In contrast to beta-chain synthesis, gamma-chain synthesis relative to that of alpha-chain synthesis rises with thalassemic erythroid maturation. This most likely results from the preferential survival of those cells producing the most gamma chains.[62] There is also evidence in the studies of Fuhr and co-workers[173] that a defect exists at the level of the ribosome–messenger RNA complex. This defect involves an accumulation of ribosomal subunits and the presence of an inhibitor of protein synthesis.

Nathan[354a] has recently reviewed a number of studies utilizing cell-free systems in which globin chain synthesis was quantified. Defects in ribosome function, initiation factors, or supernatant factors were not detected. In similar investigations Nienhuis and Anderson[362a] and Benz and Forget[43a] have shown that the messenger RNA derived from beta-thalassemic reticulocytes, as compared to that derived from sickle cell reticulocytes, produced much less beta chain than alpha chain. These studies indicate that the quality or quantity of messenger RNA in patients with beta-thalassemia is diminished. Yet to be determined is whether or not defective beta chain synthesis in beta-thalassemia is due to the production of unstable beta messenger RNA which fails to interact with polyribosomes or to decreased production of a normal messenger. Schwartz[429a] has shown that the beta/alpha synthetic ratio in the marrow of heterozygotes for beta-thalassemia is approximately 1.0, a normal value, and that the ratio decreases to 0.5 in the peripheral blood reticulocytes, lending further support to the contention that messenger RNA is unstable.

*Pathology.* The anatomic changes in thalassemia reflect the abnormalities that characterize the disease—i.e., increased destruction of structurally defective red cells, increased regeneration with erythropoietic hyperplasia of the bone marrow, extramedullary hematopoiesis, deposition of excessive iron in tissues resulting from hemolysis of transfused red cells and the patient's own red cells, and the long-term effect of chronic hypoxia.

The skeletal structures contain abundant brown-red and chocolate-colored marrow; the bony trabeculae are thinned and often the site of new bone formation. The spleen is firm, hard, and greatly enlarged. The pulp is abundant; cellular and fibrotic tissue is increased. Extensive hematopoiesis is noted, chiefly of the red cell series and, to a lesser extent, of other myeloid elements. The follicles are atrophied.[35] Whipple and Bradford[539] first described the presence of large, pale mononuclear cells having a frothy or granular appearance and a small vesicular nucleus in the spleen and bone marrow of Cooley's anemia. These they termed foam cells. Later, it was shown that the foamy appearance is due to the accumulation of an acidic mucopolysaccharide of the chondroitin sulfuric acid type in the cytoplasm of the histiocytic cell giving an intense red coloration with the periodic acid–Schiff reaction.[440] A possible source of the mucopolysaccharide is from the destruction of the abnormal erythroid cells, late erythroblasts, and normoblasts.

In a young adult 24 years of age Gandy-Gamna bodies were observed in the portal spaces of the liver and lymph nodes. These bodies appeared as structures resembling iron-calcium deposits. Siderofibrotic lesions of this type are also found in sickle cell anemia.

In some patients visceral siderosis and fibrosis of the liver and pancreas are especially marked. The liver parenchyma is divided by broad irregular bands of fibrous tissue into nodules of varying sizes. Extreme hemosiderosis is diffuse throughout the liver so that iron pigment often fills the cytoplasm of the cells. Hepatic cells regenerate and show much less pigmentation. In the pancreas extensive and diffuse interlobular and intralobular fibrosis is frequently observed, with a similar division of the parenchyma into nodules. The anatomic changes in the liver and pancreas are frequently identical with those characterizing idiopathic hemochromatosis.[136] Lymph nodes show pigmentation and are also the site of increased erythropoiesis.

Hemosiderin deposits are especially marked in the liver, spleen, and pancreas and are also found in the thyroid, parathyroid, and adrenal glands, distal convoluted tubules of the kidneys, bronchial glands, gonads, lymph nodes, lungs, and myocardium.[540] The heart is dilated and hypertrophied, showing dense hemosiderotic staining of the myocardium, interstitial fibrosis, and hypertrophy of the myocardial fibers.

In a study of the marrow of patients with thalassemia minor, Block[54] found a slight and probably significant increase in erythroblasts which, with the moderate increase in intramedullary hemolysis, indicates that the rate of effective red cell production was slightly decreased. In thalassemia intermedia he found that the number of erythroblasts in the marrow was grossly increased. Here 90 to 100% of the marrow in two cases consisted of hematopoietic tissue, most of which was erythroblastic. This was accompanied by an even greater increase in intramedullary hemolysis, suggesting that the rate of effective erythropoiesis is about half of the normal.

**Clinical features.** The clinical features of thalassemia major and thalassemia minor are discussed separately.

*Thalassemia major.* Thalassemia major begins insidiously in infancy and is sufficiently developed in most patients to be recognized clinically in the latter half of the first year of life. Pallor, diarrhea, fever, poor feeding, and an enlarged spleen in children of Mediterranean origin lead to suspicions of the diagnosis. The severely anemic patient presents a pathognomonic facial appearance, including prominent frontal and parietal bosses, enlargement of the head, prominent malar eminences, depression of the bridge of the nose, puffy eyelids, a mongoloid slant of the eyes, often with an epicanthal fold, enlargement of the superior maxilla exposing the upper teeth, a muddy yellow complexion and icteric tint to the conjunctivae. Other characteristic features are small stature and hypogonadism. Hypertrophy of the upper maxilla may lead to eventual marked malocclusion, especially involving the frontal central incisors.[72] (See Figs. 43 and 44). Many of these patients have frequent epistaxis, some severe and prolonged enough to require packing by an otolaryngologist to control the bleeding or a transfusion to replace the acute blood loss.

Lymphadenopathy is occasionally noted. The abdomen protrudes when splenomegaly becomes prominent, especially in the younger child. Splenomegaly is progressive, and abdominal enlargement becomes disabling. Initially the liver is enlarged to a lesser degree but becomes markedly enlarged, especially after splenectomy. Chronic leg ulcers are rare occurrences.[106,155,369] Gallstones are uncommon under 10 years of age,[473] but as with other hemolytic anemias are likely to develop as patients grow older.[117] Nosebleeds are frequent. Pathologic fracture of the femur is an infrequent complication and is due to cortical atrophy. Pressure atrophy of the cortical and spongiosa develops, due to overgrowth and expansion of the hyperplastic marrow. With prolonged and intensive transfusion therapy the clinical evidence of hemosiderosis is superimposed on the manifestations of chronic anemia. The patient with Cooley's anemia who has had frequent transfusions shows a deep brown pigmentation and darkening of the skin due to increased amounts of melanin in the epidermis and hemosiderin in the dermis.[302] The skin gives a tanned, bronzed coloration with fine, dark, stippled-like freckles.

Cardiac dilation and enlargement and hemic murmurs are common. Asymptomatic cardiac enlargement begins in late childhood and slowly increases. Pericarditis of the acute, benign, nonspecific type has been described in patients with severe Cooley's anemia, especially those who have had splenectomy.[321,470,493] In all of these patients the pericarditis was self-limited and ended in complete recovery. The basis for this peculiar susceptibility is unknown. Children with Cooley's anemia whose hemoglobin levels are markedly lowered undergo prolonged effort with surprisingly little disability. Headache, precordial and bone pain, listlessness, and anorexia appear when the hemoglobin levels drop below 7 gm. per 100 ml. and are relieved by transfusions. Enlargement of the kidneys attributed to tubular dilation has been found in a large number of patients with thalassemia major.[196]

THE HEREDITARY HEMOGLOBINOPATHIES 393

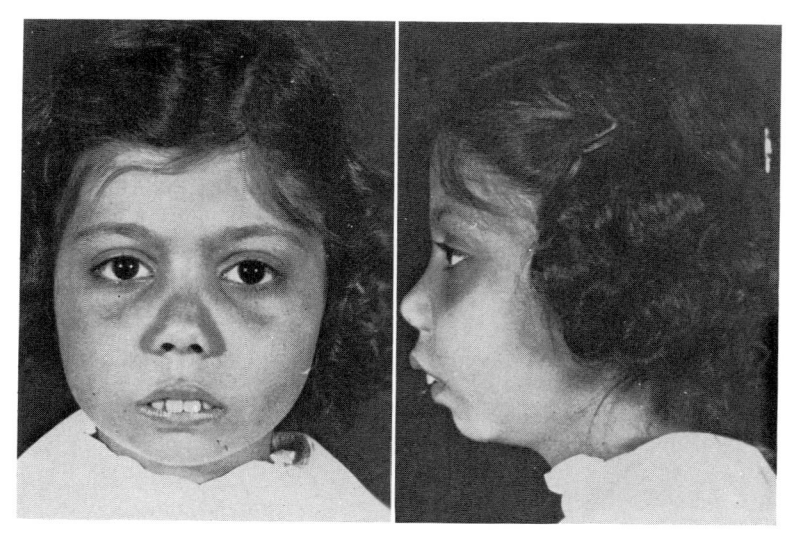

Fig. 43. Characteristic facies in severe Cooley's anemia (thalassemia major). Note prominent malar eminences, depression of the bridge of the nose, slight oblique appearance of eyes, and enlargement of superior maxilla with protrusion of lip upward exposing upper teeth.

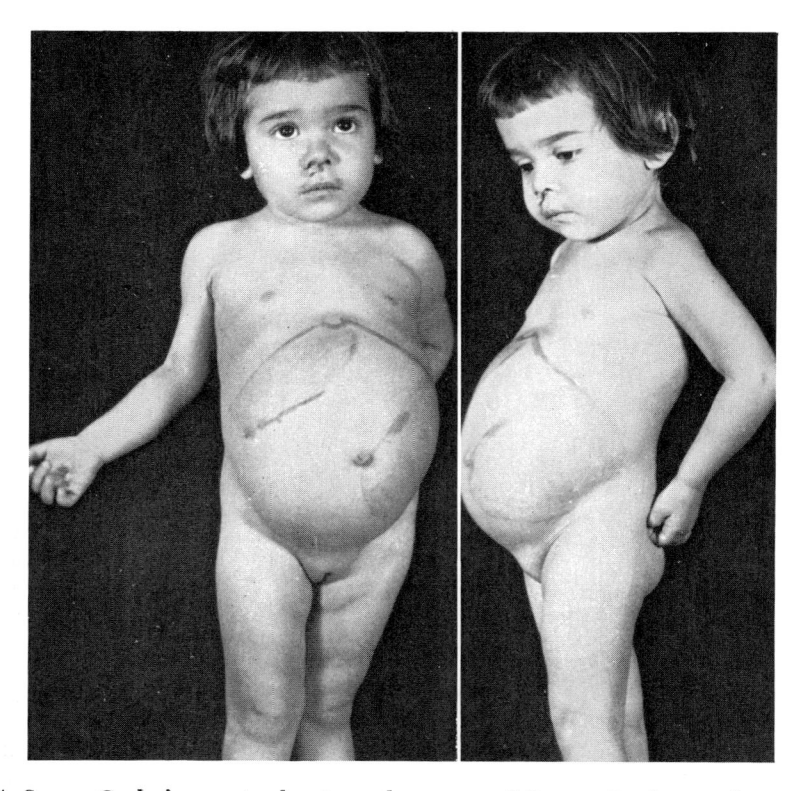

Fig. 44. Severe Cooley's anemia showing enlargement of liver and spleen and protrusion of abdomen. Facies is similar to that of patient shown in Fig. 43.

*Thalassemia minor.* The patient with the trait is asymptomatic and the disease goes unnoticed, usually being detected in the course of a family survey when a sibling is suspected of having the severe disease. Persons with the trait or mild type do not show the cardiac murmur, enlargement of the heart, or bone and joint pain of the severe type. Patients with mild or moderate anemia are often treated for iron-deficiency anemia until the lack of response to therapy prompts a blood examination and the true diagnosis is disclosed. Those with the mild disease show no facial abnormalities and minimal skeletal changes. In persons with the moderate or mild disease the spleen may be enlarged slightly or not at all.

**Growth and maturation.** In patients with thalassemia minor, growth is normal. In some patients growth and maturation of the skeleton are retarded, and Caffey[72] regards patients with Cooley's anemia as the best examples of skeletal dwarfism and infantilism caused by chronic anemia. Children with the severe disease grow normally until about the age of 8 to 10 years, at which time their growth rate undergoes marked retardation so that they attain a very short final height. Secondary sexual characteristics develop later than in the normal population. Normal menses are rare and cease several months to several years after the onset.

In the majority of severely affected male patients bone age is normal early and is delayed after 6 or 7 years of age.[143] Maturation of bone eventually occurs, if survival is sufficiently prolonged. As for height age after being normal or close to normal in the early years, height becomes retarded in the preadolescent and adolescent, rarely reaching a median normal height age prior to death. From limited observations, male intermediate patients are not retarded through adolescence and finally reach a normal height. Among female patients linear height tends to fall below normal in both severe and intermediate patients in the preadolescent and adolescent periods. Both groups are capable, however, of attaining low normal final statures. Bone age is retarded in both and is grossly in proportion to height age. Final bone maturation may be attained by both female groups.

Pituitary failure is not uncommon in hemochromatosis.[496] Four of fifteen adult patients investigated had severe pituitary deficiency by both clinical and laboratory criteria and five had evidence of a partial defect, with failure of at least one trophic hormone. The pituitary failure appears to be due to iron deposition in the anterior pituitary and is not related to the severity of liver disease or to the degree of abnormality of either iron or estrogen metabolism. Nine of the fifteen patients had diabetes mellitus and required insulin. In a recent report[27] a man with thalassemia intermedia and iron overload was described who presented with hypogonadism. Complete investigation showed him to have hypopituitarism. Comparable problems relating to pituitary dysfunction and iron overload in thalassemia major and intermedia in relation to growth and sexual function are under current investigation.

The status of sexual maturity was studied in our clinic of children with thalassemia major. Of twelve girls ranging in age between 13 and 26½ years, three were sexually mature. This was judged by the following criteria: the presence or absence of menses, breast tissue development, the presence or absence of pubic and/or axillary hair. Two others previously had had menses, which have ceased. One girl has had irregular menses but outwardly appeared physically immature. Six girls never had menses. There appeared to be no apparent correlation of sexual maturity with age of most of the recipients of transfusions, transfusion regimen, or medications received. All were transfused before 3 years of age. Nine males, their ages ranging between 14 and 25 years, were included in this survey. Sexual maturation was determined by the following criteria: presence of pubic, axillary, or facial hair, size of the penis, rugation, darkening and enlargement of the scrotum, deepening of the voice, and presence of acne. Of the nine males, four were considered sexually mature, fulfilling these criteria, and four had no physical evidence of beginning maturational changes. One male (aged 26 years) who had been maintained on oral testosterone daily for the past year showed evidence of only scanty pubic hair. As with the girls, there appeared no correlation of sexual maturity with the age of onset of transfusions or transfusion regimen.

**Skeletal changes.** The skeletal changes as revealed by roentgenographic examination in persons with Cooley's anemia reflect the overactivity and overgrowth of the bone marrow.[72] (Fig. 45). Extreme marrow hyperplasia results in osteoporosis, widening of the medullary spaces, thinning of the cortex, trabecular atrophy, coarse reticulation with regeneration of new bone which is a later development in the disease, and thickening of the skull. The frontal bone is the site of early and marked thickening. Overgrowth of the marrow in the para-

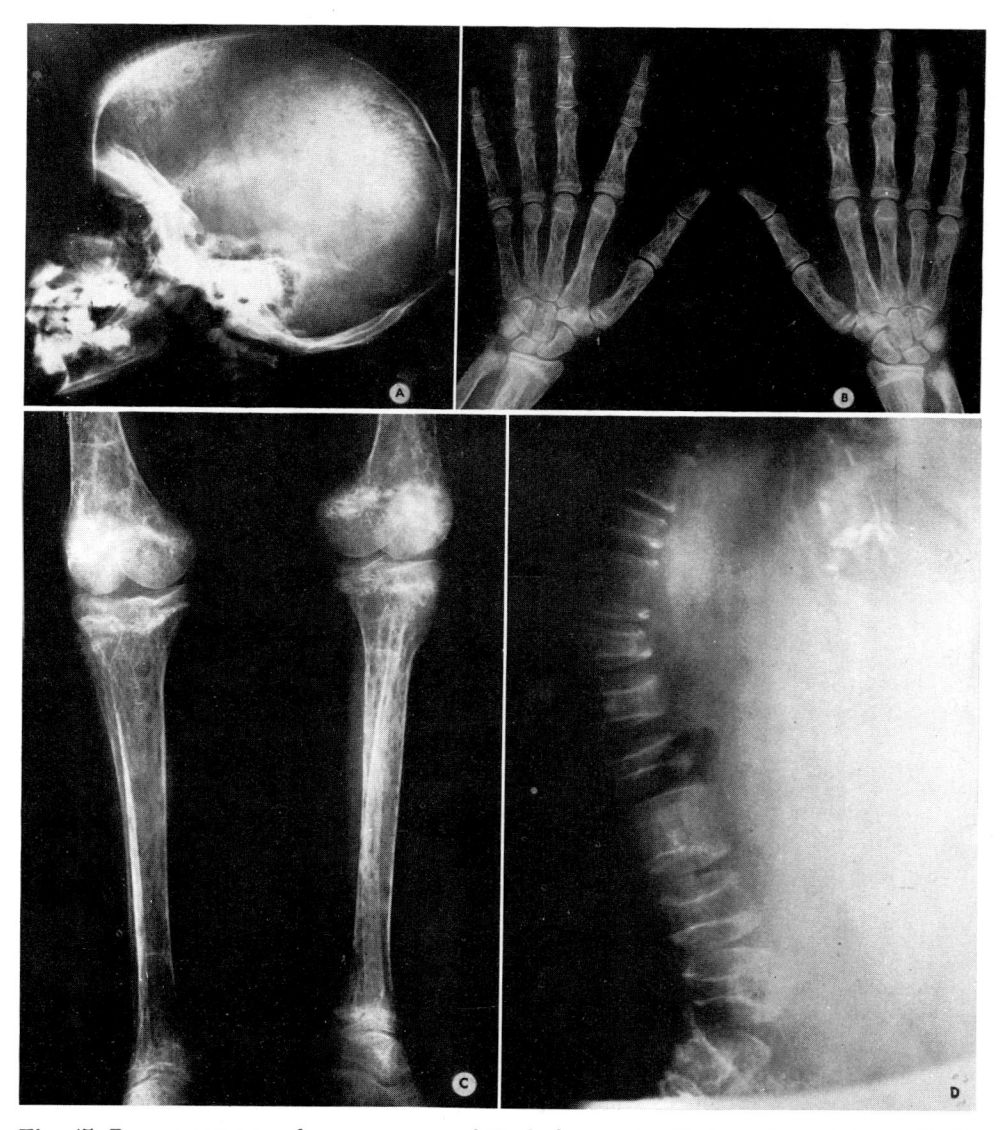

Fig. 45. Roentgenograms of a severe case of Cooley's anemia (thalassemia major). A, Skull, showing enlarged diploic space which is fairly granular, mottled, or striated; note "hair-on-end" appearance. Marked rarefaction of hands and wrists, B, and of lower extremities, C. D, Note compression of vertebral bodies.

nasal sinuses and mastoids interferes with their pneumatization and occasionally completely suppresses it.[72] Lateral views of the skull show an enlarged diploic space which is finely granular, mottled, or striated. Appearing between the tables and the skull, the perpendicular striations which seem to extend beyond the outer atrophied table give the appearance of "hair standing on end." The earliest skeletal changes are observed in the small bones, particularly in the metacarpals and metatarsals, revealing osteoporosis and expansion of the medullary cavities, producing a rectangular rather than a normal concave appearance. Cortical thinning may be so extreme as to result in pathologic fractures. Premature fusion of the epiphyses in the long bones of the extremities is a relatively common finding in patients with homozygous thalassemia who are more than 10 years of age. The anomaly was encountered

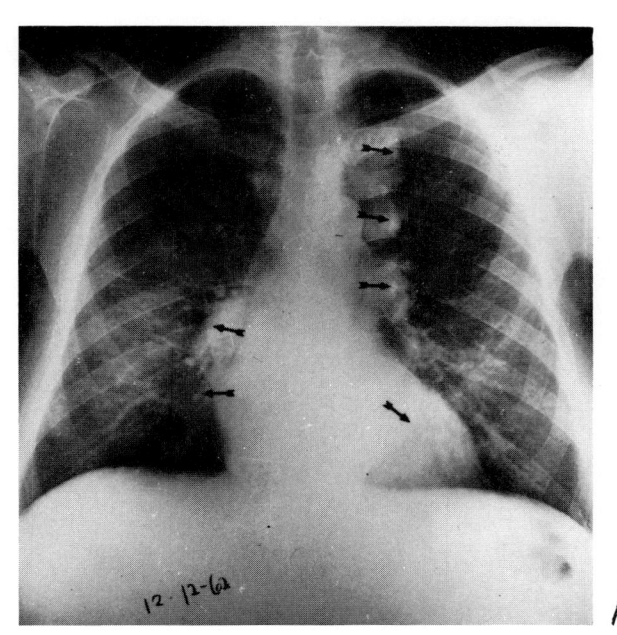

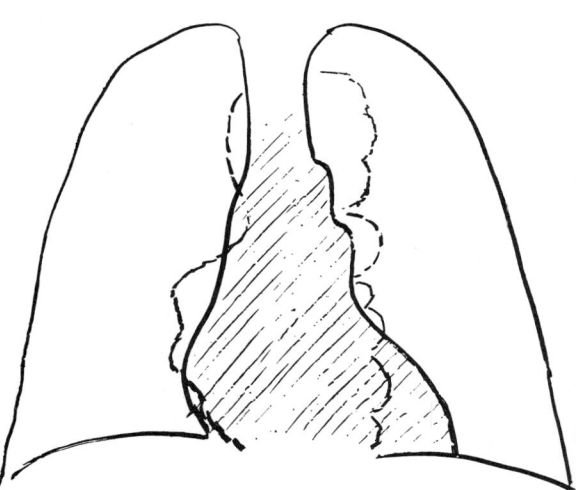

**Fig. 46.** Heterotopic bone marrow in thalassemia major (chest x-ray film and schematic drawing). Intrathoracic masses of bone marrow occupy paravertebral spaces. The masses lie lateral to the vertebral bodies and project through the intercostal spaces. These masses consist of compensatory extramedullary hematopoietic tissue. Patient, now 49 years of age, was originally reported at 19 years of age.[466] Course has been an intermediate type of thalassemia, requiring splenectomy as an adult. Few transfusions have ever been required, since hemoglobin level is usually mantained at 8 to 9 gm. per 100 ml.

in eleven of seventy-nine cases surveyed, with an incidence of 23% in patients older than 10 years. The sites of predilection were the proximal end of one or both humeri and the distal end of one or both femurs.[110]

The character and degree of the bone changes are modified significantly with age. In older children the bone lesions regress in the more distal portions of the skeleton (hands, arms, and legs), whereas with advancing age red marrow is replaced normally with fatty marrow. The characteristic changes described in the hands and other peripheral areas are thus diminished and may disappear at puberty.[70] On the contrary, in the skull, spine, and pelvis, which are sites of active and persistent red marrow formation, the roentgenographic changes become more conspicuous.[70,72] Compression of the vertebrae, quite common in patients with sickle cell anemia, is rare in those with Cooley's anemia. Severe reticulation and rarefaction of the vertebral bodies are not uncommon. Localized tumors of red marrow in the generally hyperplastic marrow have been described. Costal osteomas giving the appearance of large bony masses in the thorax without external signs of tumor have been described.[72,113] In one of the patients, the mass proved to be a large shell of bone containing red marrow and blood.[72] (See Fig. 46.) In the patient with the trait or mild form of the disease, skeletal changes are absent.

A variety of bony masses have been described in patients with the intermediate form of thalassemia.[144] These masses often lie lateral to the vertebral bodies occupying the entire thoracic paravertebral space. In a 63-year-old adult with the same form of thalassemia, a tumor mass of hematopoietic tissue was resected from the posterior mediastinum which extended from the level of the sixth to the eleventh rib.[282] In another patient 53 years of age[446] round paraspinal masses were present in the superior and inferior mediastinum. Paravertebral masses were also noted in two adults with thalassemia intermedia presumably on a heterozygous basis.[376] These multiple intrathoracic posterior mediastinal masses represent extramedullary he-

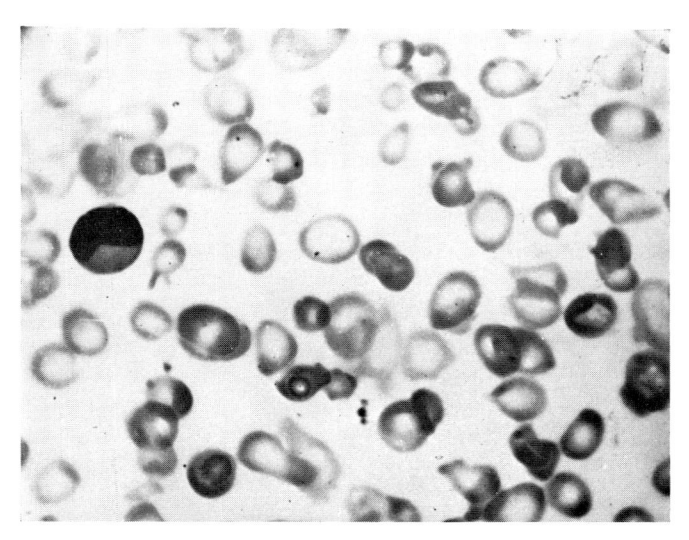

Fig. 47. Photomicrograph of blood smear of patient with severe Cooley's anemia (thalassemia major), pre-splenectomy. Note microcytes, hypochromic macrocytes, anisocytosis, and poikilocytosis. Many of the red cells appear fragmented.

matopoiesis in individuals with chronic hemolytic anemia whose blood levels, although decreased, are maintained at a steady state without the need for transfusion. These paravertebral masses are not confined to thalassemia but have also been described in hereditary spherocytosis.

It is generally believed that the bone lesions in thalassemia are caused principally by hyperplasia of the marrow, the overactive marrow widening the medullary space and the increased medullary pressure causing osteoporosis. Recent studies, however, suggest that the osteoporotic lesions in thalassemia are probably not actively related to hyperplasia of the bone marrow but probably the result of faulty metabolism which affects ossification.[96] Hyperprolinemia and hyperprolinuria are found in thalassemic children.[506] Hydroxyproline constitutes approximately 14% of the amino acid residual of collagens, and 95% of collagen is found in bones. It is as yet not clear whether hyperprolinemia and hyperprolinuria found in children are related to the osteoporosis present in these patients.

*Blood picture.* The blood picture in patients with thalassemia major and in those with thalassemia minor provides important clues to the diagnosis of these diseases.

*Thalassemia major.* The anemia is pronounced and of a hypochromic, microcytic type similar to that seen in patients with severe iron deficiency. The hemoglobin ranges between 5 and 9 gm. per 100 ml. and the red cell count between 2.5 and 3.5 million per cubic millimeter. These values are obtained soon after diagnosis before any transfusions have been given and, in those patients under treatment, after a prolonged interval following transfusion so there is no admixture with donor blood. In patients with the intermediate homozygous type the hemoglobin stabilizes between 7 and 10 gm. per 100 ml. without the need for transfusions. The reduction in hemoglobin level and hematocrit is proportionally greater than the reduction in the number of red cells, as occurs in patients with iron deficiency. The erythrocytes show polychromatophilia, marked hypochromia, anisocytosis, and poikilocytosis and are often fragmented. (See Fig. 47.)

Although microcytes predominate, the most important cells for diagnostic purposes are the large pale erythrocytes interspersed among them which contain irregularly distributed clumps of hemoglobin, with the intervening areas apparently possessing staining defects. These cells are extremely thin and leaflike, and in wet preparations their edges fold over and the several layers thus formed possess a remarkable transparency. In the stained smear the combination of scattered hemoglobin and the thinness of the cells result in bizarre and wrinkled shapes. (See Fig. 48.) The abnormal thinness of the red cells in this disease has led to its designation as hereditary leptocytosis.

A nonspecific macrocytic cell commonly

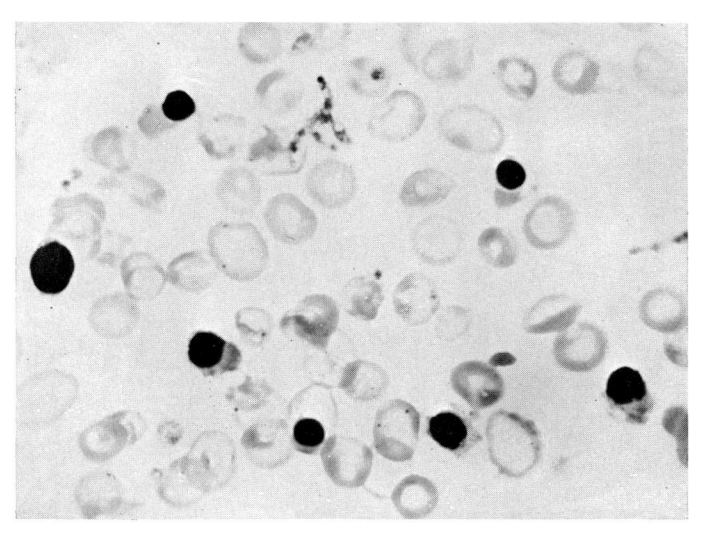

Fig. 48. Blood smear of patient with severe Cooley's anemia, post-splenectomy. Note excessive size and abnormal thinness of red cells, marked hypochromia, and large number of normoblasts.

Table 21. Polypeptide structure of normal hemoglobins and the more common hemoglobin A variants and their amino acid defects

| Hemoglobins | Abnormal polypeptide chain | Schematic representation | | Amino acid defect and localization | Designation indicating substituted amino acid | |
|---|---|---|---|---|---|---|
| Normal | | | | | | |
| A | — | Alpha$_2^A$ | Beta$_2^A$ | None | | |
| A$_2$ | — | Alpha$_2^A$ | Delta$_2^{A_2}$ | None | | |
| F | — | Alpha$_2^A$ | Gamma$_2^F$ | None | | |
| Abnormal | | | | | | |
| C | Beta | Alpha$_2^A$ | Beta$_2^C$ | Lysine replaces glutamic acid in residue 6 | Alpha$_2^A$ | Beta$_2^{6\ lys}$ |
| E | Beta | Alpha$_2^A$ | Beta$_2^E$ | Lysine replaces glutamic acid in residue 26 | Alpha$_2^A$ | Beta$_2^{26\ lys}$ |
| G$_{San\ José}$ | Beta | Alpha$_2^A$ | Beta$_2^G$ | Glycine replaces glutamic acid in residue 7 | Alpha$_2^A$ | Beta$_2^{7\ gly}$ |
| H | — | Beta$_4^A$ | | Polypeptide chain is normal but hemoglobin composed of four identical polypeptide chains | | |
| Bart's | — | Gamma$_4^F$ | | | | |
| I | Alpha | Alpha$_2^I$ | Beta$_2^A$ | Aspartic acid replaces lysine in residue 16 | Alpha$_2^{16\ asp}$ | Beta$_2^A$ |
| S | Beta | Alpha$_2^A$ | Beta$_2^S$ | Valine replaces glutamic acid in residue 6 | Alpha$_2^A$ | Beta$_2^{6\ val}$ |
| Lepore | Delta | Alpha$_2^A$ | Delta$_2^{Lepore}$ | | | |

Table 22. Less common hemoglobinopathies and abnormal polypeptide chain

| Hemoglobin | Schematic representation | |
|---|---|---|
| *Abnormal beta chain* | | |
| D beta | Alpha$_2^A$ | Beta$_2^D$ |
| D gamma; D Punjab | Alpha$_2^A$ | Beta$_2^D$ |
| G Galveston | Alpha$_2^A$ | Beta$_2^{G\ Galveston}$ |
| J | Alpha$_2^A$ | Beta$_2^J$ |
| N | Alpha$_2^A$ | Beta$_2^N$ |
| O | Alpha$_2^A$ | Beta$_2^O$ |
| P | Alpha$_2^A$ | Beta$_2^P$ |
| *Abnormal alpha chain* | | |
| D$_\alpha$ St. Louis | Alpha$_2^{D\ St.\ Louis}$ | Beta$_2^A$ |
| K | Alpha$_2^K$ | Beta$_2^A$ |
| Q | Alpha$_2^Q$ | Beta$_2^A$ |
| Hopkins No. 2 | Alpha$_2^{Ho2}$ | Beta$_2^A$ |
| Norfolk | Alpha$_2^{Norfolk}$ | Beta$_2^A$ |

found both in patients with the severe form and in those with mild forms of thalassemia is the target cell. This erythrocyte has been so named[31] because of its deeply stained center and periphery which are arranged in concentric light and dark zones. Another macrocyte is a round or sometimes oval cell with a narrow rim of hemoglobin of varying thickness with a large zone of central achromia in which only a faintly stained island of hemoglobin is occasionally noted.

Nucleated red cells are almost invariably found and constitute one of the most characteristic findings of the disease. The size and maturity of these cells vary, but most often they are typical normoblasts and mature micronormoblasts with pyknotic nuclei. Normoblasts vary from a few to large numbers, sometimes equaling or exceeding the leukocytes numerically. Erythroblastosis is extremely marked after splenectomy and constitutes a distinctive postoperative feature.

Red cells containing Howell-Jolly bodies are infrequently observed in patients with an intact spleen. Polychromasia and basophilic stippling are present but are less marked in patients with the severe type than in those with the mild type of Cooley's anemia because of the lack of hemoglobin. Reticulocytes are increased and range from 2 to 8%.[466] Moderate leukocytosis is present, with white cell counts ranging from 15,000 to 30,000 per cubic millimeter, but the upper level may be exceeded.

Granulocytes predominate and myelocytes are common. The platelet count is generally normal. Moderate leukopenia and, to a lesser extent, thrombocytopenia are occasionally observed and attributed to hypersplenism[328] or suppression by multiple transfusions. The bone marrow in severe cases shows primitive erythroid cells and a predominance of basophilic normoblasts, microblasts, and pronormoblasts.

The percentage of hemoglobin A$_2$ is very variable in thalassemia major and an elevated level is by no means always found.[530] In several reports a low or normal HbA$_2$ level has been noted in association with high HbA$_2$ levels in both parents. It has been pointed out, however, that the amount of HbA$_2$ when related to that of HbA is increased in cases of thalassemia major with high levels of HbF. Thus an individual with a high HbF shows a reduced HbA and a disproportionately higher HbA$_2$.

Large, usually single, inclusions having the staining properties of Heinz bodies have been described in the red cells in thalassemia major.[161,162,312] Their frequency is greatest in the normoblasts, either circulating ones or those found in the bone marrow and decreasing sharply in the more mature cells. These inclusions supposedly represent precipitated hemoglobin, very likely uncombined alpha chains. These chains represent aggregates of the excess of alpha chains of the hemoglobin molecule which have remained uncombined due to deficiency in the beta chains and have not been taken up by gamma or delta chains. Splenectomy facili-

**Table 23.** List of known hemoglobin substitutions and deletions*

| α-Chain variants ||| β-Chain variants |||
|---|---|---|---|---|---|
| Residue no. | Amino-acid substitution | Name | Residue no. | Amino-acid substitution | Name |
| 5 | Ala→Asp | J Toronto | 2 | His→Tyr | Tokuchi |
| 12 | Ala→Asp | J Paris | 6 | Glu→Val | S |
| 15 | Gly→Asp | J Oxford | 6 | Glu→Lys | C |
| 16 | Lys→Glu | I | 6 or 7 | Glu→deleted | Leiden |
| 22 | Gly→Asp | J Medellin | 7 | Glu→Gly | San José |
| 23 | Glu→Gln | Memphis | 7 | Glu→Lys | Siriraj |
| 23 | Glu→Val | G Audhali | 9 | Ser→Cys | Porto Alegre |
| 23 | Glu→Lys | Chad | 14 | Leu→Arg | Sogn |
| 30 | Glu→Gln | G Chinese | 16 | Gly→Asp | J Baltimore |
| 43 | Phe→Val | Torino | 16 | Gly→Arg | D Bushman |
| 47 | Asp→Gly | L Ferrara | 22 | Glu→Ala | G Coushatta |
| 47 | Asp→His | Hasharon | 22 | Glu→Lys | E Saskatoon |
| 50 | His→Asp | J Sardegna | 23 | Val→deleted | M Freiburg |
| 51 | Gly→Arg | Russ | 25 | Gly→Arg | G Taiwan Ami |
| 54 | Gln→Arg | Shimonoseki | 26 | Glu→Lys | E |
| 54 | Gly→Glu | Mexico | 28 | Leu→Pro | Genova |
| 57 | Gly→Asp | Norfolk | 30 | Arg→Ser | Tacoma |
| 58 | His→Tyr | M Boston | 35 | Tyr→Phe | Philly |
| 68 | Asn→Lys | G Philadelphia | 42 | Phe→Ser | Hammersmith |
| 68 | Asn→Asp | Ube II | 43 | Glu→Ala | G Galveston |
| 78 | Asn→Lys | Stanleyville II | 46 | Gly→Glu | K Ibadan |
| 80 | Leu→Arg | Ann Arbor | 47 | Asp→Asn | G Copenhagen |
| 84 | Ser→Arg | Etobicoke | 56 | Gly→Asp | J Bangkok |
| 85 | Asp→Asn | G Norfolk | 58 | Pro→Arg | Dhofar |
| 87 | His→Tyr | M Iwate | 61 | Lys→Glu | N Seattle |
| 90 | Lys→Asn | Broussais | 61 | Lys→Asn | Hikari |
| 92 | Arg→Gln | J Cape Town | 63 | His→Tyr | M Saskatoon |
| 92 | Arg→Leu | Chesapeake | 63 | His→Arg | Zürich |
| 102 | Ser→Arg | Manitoba | 67 | Val→Glu | M Milwaukee |
| 112 | His→Gln | Dakar | 67 | Val→Ala | Sydney |
| 114 | Pro→Arg | Chiapas | 69 | Gly→Asp | J Cambridge |
| 115 | Ala→Asp | J Tongariki | 73 | Asp→Asn | Korle Bu |
| 116 | Glu→Lys | O Indonesia | 6 | Glu→Val ⎫ | C Harlem |
| 136 | Leu→Pro | Bibba | 73 | Asp→Asn ⎭ | |
| 141 | Arg→Pro | Singapore | 76 | Ala→Glu | Seattle |
| 141 | Arg split off on hemolysis in plasma | Koellicker | 77 | His→Asp | J Iran |
| | | | 79 | Asp→Asn | G Accra |
| | | | 87 | Thr→Lys | D Ibadan |
| | | | 88 | Leu→Pro | Santa Ana |
| | | | 90 | Glu→Lys | Agenogi |
| | | | 91 | Leu→Pro | Sabine |
| | | | 92 | His→Tyr | M Hyde Park |
| | | | 94 | Asp→Asn | Oak Ridge |
| | | | 95 | Lys→Glu | N |
| | | | 91-95 or 92-96 or 93-97 | [Leu, His, Cys, Asp, Lys] deleted | Gun Hill |

*From Lehmann, H., and Carrell, R. W.: Variation in the structure of human haemoglobin, with particular reference to the unstable haemoglobins, Brit. Med. Bull. **25**:14. 1969.

Table 23. List of known hemoglobin substitutions and deletions—cont'd

| α-Chain variants ||| β-Chain variants |||
|---|---|---|---|---|---|
| Residue no. | Amino-acid substitution | Name | Residue no. | Amino-acid substitution | Name |
| | | | 98 | Val→Met | Köln |
| | | | 99 | Asp→His | Yakima |
| | | | 99 | Asp→Asn | Kempsey |
| | | | 102 | Asn→Thr | Kansas |
| | | | 113 | Val→Glu | New York |
| | | | 120 | Lys→Glu | Hijiyama |
| | | | 121 | Glu→Lys | O Arab |
| | | | 121 | Glu→Gln | D Punjab |
| | | | 126 | Val→Glu | Hofu |
| | | | 130 | Tyr→Asp | Wien |
| | | | 132 | Lys→Gln | K Woolwich |
| | | | 136 | Gly→Asp | Hope |
| | | | 143 | His→Asp | Hiroshima |
| | | | 145 | Tyr→His | Rainier |

| γ-Chain variants ||| δ-Chain variants |||
|---|---|---|---|---|---|
| Residue no. | Amino-acid substitution | Name | Residue no. | Amino-acid substitution | Name |
| 5 | Glu→Lys | F Texas I | 2 | His→Arg | $A_2$ Sphakia |
| 6 | Glu→Lys | F Texas II | 12 | Asn→Lys | $A_2$ N.Y.U. |
| 12 | Thr→Lys | F Alexandra | 16 | Gly→Arg | $A_2$ (or $B_2$) |
| 121 | Glu→Lys | F Hull | 22 | Ala→Glu | $A_2$ Flatbush |
| | | | 136 | Gly→Asp | $A_2$ Babinga |

tated their detection because of the increased number of nucleated red cells in the blood and the removal of the inclusions or cells containing them.

The inclusion bodies in thalassemia are observed predominantly in reticulocytes and younger cells. Nathan and Gunn[356] suggested that the precipitation of excess alpha chains predisposes beta thalassemic red cells to premature removal from the circulation. Precipitated alpha chains presumably give rise to Heinz bodies which may be removed by the pitting function of the spleen. Many small fragmented and distorted red cells in nonsplenectomized thalassemia major blood may arise from fragmentation of intracellular precipitates secondary to splenic passage.[464] Nathan and Gunn[356] have also pointed out that the increased membrane cation permeability of the thalassemic cell may hasten ultimate hemolysis of the remaining portion of the red cells by predisposing them to colloid osmotic lysis. In essence, the imbalance in globin synthesis (alpha chains produced in excess and beta chains suppressed) represents an important pathophysiological consequence of the precipitation of uncombined alpha polypeptide chains.[357,406]

The largest number of alpha chains detectable by electrophoresis have been observed in samples from splenectomized homozygous beta thalassemias.[162]

Aplastic crises have been described comparable to those in patients with spherocytic anemia and other hemolytic anemias resulting in erythroid marrow hypoplasia and reticulocytopenia.[253] These episodes of hypoplasia of erythrocyte precursors may occur both in patients with the severe or major forms of thalassemia major and with the intermediate forms the disease. Since intermediate patients do not receive regular transfusions, they may demonstrate sudden, serious increases in anemia when hypoplasia occurs. An intermediate patient who at other times maintains a hemoglobin concentration of 8 gm. per 100 ml. without transfusions, may suffer a drop in hemoglobin to 3 gm. per 100 ml. following mild upper respiratory infection.

A folic acid deficiency may occur without the appearance of megaloblasts. In this case the hematologic and clinical response to large doses of folic acid may be accompanied by painful erythropoietic crises caused by an acute increase in erythroid cell division with an attendant painful expansion in the intramedullary erythroid mass.[253] Folic acid deficiency with and without the megaloblastic changes in the bone marrow and with the presence of formiminoglutamicaciduria following histidine loading have also been reported.[313,351,413] The extent to which anemia is altered by folic acid administration will be described in the section on treatment.

Clearance studies in thalassemia major show depleted folate stores irrespective of age group.[517] Plasma levels of folate following oral folate administration are lower than in normal controls. The values in the age group over 12 years are significantly lower than in the younger group, suggesting that hemochromatosis occurring with increasing age impairs folate absorption.

Contrary to the normal decrease in antigen "i" from birth and a reciprocal increase in "I" in the adult, in thalassemia major, antigen "i" is constantly increased regardless of age.[184] This finding is attributed to the intense proliferative activity of the erythroid marrow and is not correlated with the large amount of fetal hemoglobin in this disease.

The osmotic fragility is strikingly abnormal. The red cells are markedly resistant to hemolysis in hypotonic sodium chloride solution so that in some instances they are not entirely hemolyzed even in distilled water. The thinness of the red cells renders them capable of absorbing more water than normal before disruption. The serum bilirubin is usually slightly elevated, ranging from 1.5 to 3 mg. per 100 ml. When the upper limit is exceeded, hepatitis, cholelithiasis, or a hemolytic crisis should be considered. The serum iron is increased and the iron-binding protein is fully saturated.[149,469]

The frequent occurrence of epistaxis in patients with thalassemia major often prompts a study of the coagulation mechanism. Coagulation data show similar findings to those found in patients with liver disease of any etiology—i.e., lowered PTC (factor IX), PTA (factor XI), factors V and VIII, and prothrombin.[217,220] The one abnormality that appears to exist in the greatest number of patients is the decrease of PTA (factor XI). Patients who often had the greatest difficulty with epistaxis had no significant coagulation defects. Mild impairment of the coagulation mechanism appeared between 7 and 10 years of age. In only the rare patient are the coagulation abnormalities of sufficient degree to warrant consideration of fresh frozen plasma or specific concentrate therapy prior to surgery. A general correlation exists between the coagulation status and the other parameters for measuring hepatic function, both deteriorating in older patients.

*Thalassemia minor.* The essential features consist of hypochromic microcytes and macrocytes, basophilic stippling, oval and target cells, and, less frequently, polycythemia[465-467] with or without slight anemia. Osmotic fragility is greatly decreased, even in the absence of anemia. Included in the diagnosis of thalassemia minor is the elevation of the slow minor component of hemoglobin $A_2$. As will be noted in a later section of this chapter, in these patients the $A_2$ fraction using starch block electrophoresis exceeds 3%. Fetal hemoglobin levels are usually normal. In the occasional case in which the $A_2$ fraction is normal or below 3% the fetal hemoglobin percentage is often elevated.[550,557] This combination (low $A_2$ and elevated fetal hemoglobin percentage) is not confined to Negroes, but has been observed in Italians as well.[101] In a rare case both the $A_2$ and fetal hemoglobin percentages are elevated.[375] $HbA_2$ may be reduced in the patient with thalassemia minor suffering from iron deficiency.[522]

Out of this complexity, two genetic subtypes of thalassemia need to be emphasized. These have been designated as $A_2$-thalassemia and F-thalassemia by Fessas.[160] In the heterozygotes of the former type there is an elevation of hemoglobin $A_2$ with normal or only slightly elevated values of fetal hemoglobin. In F-thalassemia trait hemoglobin $A_2$ is normal in amount and the fetal hemoglobin is elevated. The latter is to be distinguished from the heterozygotes with hereditary persistence of fetal hemoglobin (high-F syndrome). In one series[175] the F-thalassemia heterozygotes showed 8 to 36% fetal hemoglobin. The presence of microcytosis and morphologically abnormal red cells and a heterogenous distribution of fetal hemoglobin among the red cells characterizes the F-thalassemia heterozygote. In hereditary persistence of fetal hemoglobin trait, fetal hemoglobin ranges from 12 to 38% and is homogeneously distributed in red cells of normal morphology.

The congenital malformations associated with the $D_1$-trisomy syndrome provide a clue to the linkage of foci for $A_2$ hemoglobin, carbonic anhydrase,

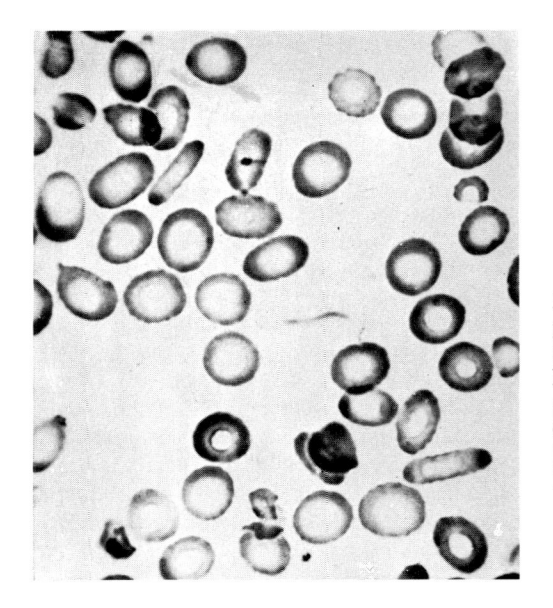

Fig. 49. Photomicrograph from blood smear of patient with the mild type of Cooley's anemia (thalassemia minor). Note anisocytosis, poikilocytosis, hypochromic macrocytes, microcytes, and oval, elongated, and rodlike cells. (×900.) (From Smith, C. H.: Detection of mild types of Mediterranean [Cooley's] anemia, Amer. J. Dis. Child. 75:505, 1948.)

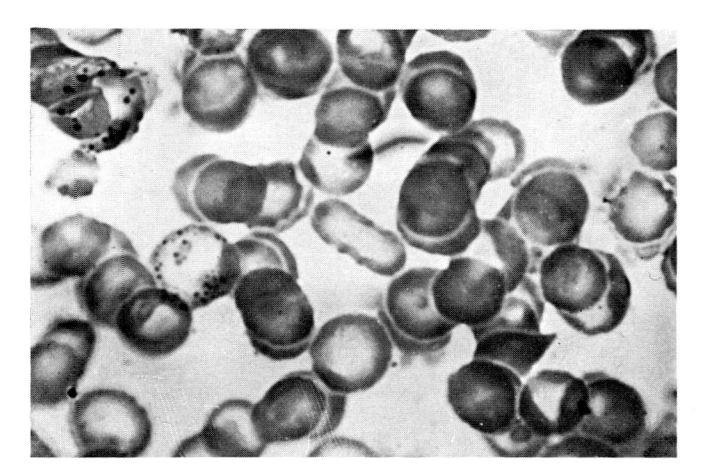

Fig. 50. Photomicrograph from patient with mild type of Cooley's anemia. Smear slightly overstained to demonstrate stippling. (×900.)

and fetal hemoglobin. In this syndrome an abnormally high fetal hemoglobin in the neonatal period is associated with a decreased $HbA_2$ concentration, an absence of carbonic anhydrase, and abnormalities in the polymorphonuclear leukocytes. These findings suggest the genetic linkage of the structural genes for carbonic anhydrase and the delta chain of $HbA_2$.[183]

The occurrence of morphologic changes of the red cells, far in excess of anemia, constitutes a fundamental principle in the detection of thalassemia minor. The hemoglobin level in patients with thalassemia minor is above 9 gm. per 100 ml. Since the mean corpuscular volume (MCV) of red cells represents the ratio between the volume of packed cells and the erythrocyte count, the smaller calculated value results from the increased numbers of red cells per cubic millimeter in relation to the normal or slightly lowered volume of packed red cells. Hypochromic and microcytic red cells predominate, simulating the blood smear of patients with iron-deficiency anemia. Varying degrees of poikilocytosis and anisocytosis are seen, but the distinguishing feature is the interspersal of hypochromic macrocytes, giving the smear a macrocytic appearance in many cases. Target cells appear in fewer than half of the patients; oval cells and cylindrical or cigarette-shaped forms are common. For unexplained reasons patients with the trait or mild anemia frequently show slight eosinophilia. (See Figs. 49 and 50.)

Excessive numbers of erythrocytes with punctate basophilia are sometimes sufficiently pronounced to suggest lead poisoning. Occasionally, they are equally common in the sibling and one of the parents. Elevated red cell counts exceeding 6 million per cubic millimeter are occasionally noted in children, but are most common in adults and are regarded as a compensatory physiologic response. Normoblasts and myelocytes are not present; reticulocytes seldom exceed 5%. We have seen several children with thalassemia minor whose hemoglobin during childhood ranged between 9 and 10 gm. per 100 ml. and showed a spontaneous rise to 12 and 13 gm. during adolescence. Occasionally, this change was accompanied by an elevated red blood cell count. The blood smear, however, still demonstrated the typical morphologic features of thalassemia. These changes are explained on the basis of the marked elevations of hemoglobin and red cells, at times of a polycythemic level, which occasionally appear in the normal adolescent.

Erythropoietic hyperplasia of the bone marrow is less marked than in patients with thalassemia major. Bone marrow rarefaction of varying degree is noted in the skull, lumbar spine, ribs, and bones of the elbow in persons carrying the thalassemia trait and may be attributed essentially to normoblastic hyperplasia in the bone marrow.[444,465] The skull has been found to be affected more often than other bones studied. Lateral skull films show a slightly enlarged diploic space which appears fairly granular or mottled[466] or a patchy hairbrush appearance[444] and not of the extensive nature found in the advanced forms of thalassemia. Polychromatic and pyknotic normoblasts are common.[14] The serum iron and latent iron-binding capacity are normal. Fetal hemoglobin levels are usually normal.

Beta thalassemia minor, the heterozygous state, is characterized by hypochromia, hypochromic macrocytes and microcytes, and an elevated percentage of hemoglobin $A_2$. There is a relative deficiency of beta chain production in this condition, though not as marked as that seen in the homozygous state. Total hemoglobin in this type of heterozygous beta thalassemia is usually normal or slightly increased. Other types of heterozygous thalassemia have been observed: those with elevated $HbA_2$ and normal red cell morphology, those with high levels of HbF as well as $HbA_2$, and the "silent" carrier of beta thalassemia in which red cell morphology and hemoglobins $A_2$ and F are normal despite a decrease in beta-chain synthesis (Schwartz).[429]

*Hemosiderosis and hemochromatosis.* Any disorder that depends upon transfusions as the mainstay of treatment is subject to increased iron deposition. In common with other refractory and chronic hemolytic anemias, iron stores accumulate from both the degradation of hemoglobin (250 mg. in each 500 ml. of blood) and increased iron absorption from the diet by the gastrointestinal tract. Another significant source is from the accelerated destruction of the patient's own defective red cells. In patients with severe Cooley's anemia widespread visceral hemosiderosis and fibrosis frequently coexist, although there is no uniformity about the progression from the former to the latter.[136] It has been suggested that the development of true hepatic cirrhosis and fibrosis of the pancreas which characterizes hemochromatosis depends upon the intervention of accessory factors such as combined hypoxia in addition to large iron deposits.[226] Both conditions prevail in patients with severe Cooley's anemia—hence, the concern about the development of hemochromatosis. With the advancing age of the child and progressive iron deposition, patients will occasionally manifest diabetes and other clinical and pathologic features identical with those of endogenous hemochromatosis. One of the serious complications of Cooley's anemia is irreversible heart failure. While myocardial siderosis may play an etiologic role, this association is by no means clear. In a study of iron deposition in acquired iron-storage disease such as thalassemia[424] no correlation was noted between the amount of iron histochemically demonstrated in the myocardium and conduction system or the amount of quantitatively analyzed myocardial iron and the presence of antemortem arrhythmias and conduction disturbances. In all hearts scarring was essentially moderate to heavy in the sinoatrial node and myocardium, but less marked in the atrioventricular node and bundle of His. The degree of scarring in each structure did not parallel the density of iron deposits found there. It was concluded that factors other than the presence of iron alone are responsible for the cardiac arrhythmias and conduction defects associated with iron-storage disease. On the other hand, in another patient with thalassemia major[27] histologic examination of the myocardium showed heavy iron deposition in the muscle fibers and it was "hard to believe that the deposits did not contribute to the intractable terminal myocardial failure."

In cases of thalassemia major with long survival following multiple transfusions, cirrhosis of the liver develops late.[548] The large amounts of intracellular iron in the liver are attributed primarily to persistently high intestinal absorption. The basis of iron absorption is the persistence in thalassemia major of a hyperactive but ineffective erythropoiesis which is a potent factor controlling iron absortion.[58,497] The additive factor of marked anemia is significantly involved since the amount of iron absorbed can be reduced by transfusion which concomitantly suppresses hematopoiesis.[152] Others[25] have found in homozygous thalassemia a wide variation (5 to 65%) in the absorption of iron when given as hemoglobin iron. The patient with heterozygous thalassemia, they found, absorbed as much iron as adult controls when iron is given as hemoglobin or ferrous sulfate.

The marked right ventricular hypertrophy in transfusion hemochromatosis may be due to a combination of siderotic myocardial degeneration and iron in alveolar septa, interfering with gaseous exchange and anemia.[548]

The development of precipitating antibodies against serum protein isoantigens in transfused thalassemia patients is a relatively common phenomenon, but it is not rare in other patients receiving multiple transfusions.[55] The frequency of precipitin formation to lipid-containing serum protein, on the other hand, appears to be higher in transfused patients with thalassemia than in other transfused patients. There is no apparent correlation between formation of antibodies to lipoproteins and to white blood cells, red blood cells, and platelets. Transfused thalassemic patients have also been shown to have agglutinating antibodies against the Gm groupings of gamma globulin.[7]

The association of hepatic cirrhosis with iron accumulation occurring in classic hemochromatosis and in thalassemia with multiple transfusions and long survival are uniformly impossible of reproduction experimentally by administering iron by oral or parenteral route.

There is clear evidence that excessive absorption from the intestine may continue irrespective of the body store of iron if the marrow is active, but this does not occur if the marrow is hypocellular.[152] It has been claimed that iron absorbed from the intestine is potentially fibrogenic, whereas that originating from repeated transfusions is initially located in the reticuloendothelial system and in this site appears to exert little, if any, toxic effects.[75] Redistribution into parenchymal cells may occur, but is a slow process and is usually apparent only in those patients who have received many transfusions over a relatively long period. Toxic factors, malnutrition, and anemia may be factors in the development of the pathologic changes of hemochromatosis.[57]

In thalassemia electron microscopy shows an increase of hemosiderin and dispersed ferritin molecules and the presence of crystalline ferritin in the liver, spleen, and bone marrow. Quite frequently one sees ferritin and iron micelles in the mitochondria.[49]

Idiopathic hemochromatosis of nonthalassemic origin has been described in a 13-year-old boy. Excessive iron storage was also found in three younger siblings. Also present in the patient were atrophic genitalia, hepatosplenomegaly, and congestive heart failure. Marked improvement followed removal of excess iron by phlebotomy and a chelating agent.[380]

*Red cell survival.* The red cells of the patient with the severe disease transfused into a normal recipient show a half-life of about 25 days as compared with the mean half-life of about 62 days attained with normal erythrocytes.[271] The shortened survival is also noted by the injection of the patient's own red cells labeled with $^{51}$Cr into his own circulation. By this method about 20% of the red cells have a life-span of only several days and the remainder of about 30 days.[19] The survival time of erythrocytes from patients with the trait transfused into normal recipients falls within the normal range.[271] On the other hand, in another study in which $^{51}$Cr and $^{59}$Fe were employed,[375] a shortened half-life in six of nine adults with thalassemia minor (mean half-life of 22 days as compared with normal range of 25 to 35 days) was among the findings. In addition, hyperplasia of the marrow, increased plasma iron turnover, and poor iron utilization were also noted. "Ineffective erythropoiesis"[497] appears, therefore, to play a role in the pathogenesis of the anemia of the heterozygous as well as the homozygous patient with thalassemia. This is further confirmed by a case report of chronic jaundice in a patient of nine years with thalassemia minor.[415]

Ineffective erythropoiesis with increased hemolysis, primarily in the marrow, resulted in chronic hyperbilirubinemia (3.1 to 6 mg. per 100 ml. total serum bilirubin). Ineffective erythropoiesis which characterizes thalassemia major implies the production of red cells so defective as to be destroyed within the bone marrow and thus never reach the extramedullary circulation. Destruction of immature erythrocytes laden with aggregates of alpha chains may be destroyed by marrow macrophages, and some after sequestration by the peripheral reticuloendothelial system upon release from the marrow. Also a fraction of defective hemoglobin may be expelled from otherwise intact red cells (erythrocyte pitting) as the red cell rids itself of unneeded cellular components such as nucleus, mitochondria, and ribosomes.[406]

The difficulties of classification within the group of thalassemia minor are illustrated in two adults with thalassemia minor, both with elevated $HbA_2$, in whom a fully saturated plasma-iron binding capacity and slightly enlarged spleen and liver coexisted with hemosiderin deposition in the liver parenchyma.[59] In one subject the anemia was attributed to impaired erythropoiesis, while in the other there was a shortening of the red cell life-span.

The use of $^{51}Cr$ in determining the longevity of red cells is not impaired by the fact that accelerated rates of $^{51}Cr$ elution takes place from hemoglobin solutions containing excessive amounts of fetal hemoglobin such as occur in cord blood and in the blood of patients with severe Cooley's anemia. This does not take place, however, from *intact red cells* containing large amounts of fetal hemoglobin.[150]

To what extent the neutral mucopolysaccharide found in red cells[14] of patients with severe Cooley's anemia contributes to their shortened life-span is unknown.

A study of three adult thalassemia patients given labeled glycine revealed that the turnover rate of hemoglobin F is slower than that of hemoglobin A in thalassemia.[174] The difference is achieved through the longer survival in the circulation of those red cells containing relatively greater amounts of fetal hemoglobin. The persistence of fetal hemoglobin in thalassemia may, therefore, occur for other reasons than as a compensatory phenomenon. It may be the result of natural selection operating on two populations of red cells, the F-rich cells achieving a position of advantage over the A-rich cells through their better survival.[174]

In thalassemia trait $^{51}Cr$ survival of red cells was normal. In subjects with G-6-PD deficiency the red cell life-span is in the order of 100 days.[46] This slight reduction is fully compensated by a corresponding increase in red cell production. A parallel might be drawn with normal red cell survival in sickle-cell trait and a reduced red cell survival in the homozygous sickle patient.

*Diagnosis.* Thalassemia major possesses so many distinctive features that the diagnosis is rarely overlooked. The association of the characteristic facies, skeletal changes, massive splenomegaly, severe anemia, markedly hypochromic and distorted red cells, stunted growth, and, usually, Mediterranean parentage separates this disease from other hemolytic anemias. Osmotic fragility is decreased, and sickling and spherocytosis are absent. The diagnosis is confirmed by examination of the blood of the patient's parents which shows decreased osmotic fragility, basophilic stippling, hypochromic microcytes and macrocytes, oval cells, and elevated $HbA_2$. The child who shows only moderate anemia with many of the clinical features of the severe disease often represents a combination of both sickle cell disease and thalassemia. The marked normoblastemia noted in the blood of patients with severe Cooley's anemia has led to confusion with di Guglielmo's disease, a rare entity in childhood. The occurrence of this erythroid proliferative disorder in a child with thalassemia has been described.[365] Clinical jaundice is uncommon in thalassemia minor and has been attributed to hemolysis of erythroid cells in the bone marrow.[415]

Thalassemia minor resembles iron deficiency so closely that the two are usually indistinguishable. The blood smears are identical and show large numbers of hypochromic microcytes, moderate stippling, and oval and target forms. The diagnosis is made by elimination since there are no pathognomonic features as are observed in patients with thalassemia major. Frequently, a diagnosis of thalassemia minor is suggested when a patient believed to have iron-deficiency anemia has not responded to iron therapy. The discovery in at least one parent of a blood picture similar to that of the patient, an abnormal percentage of $A_2$ hemoglobin, and a normal serum iron content

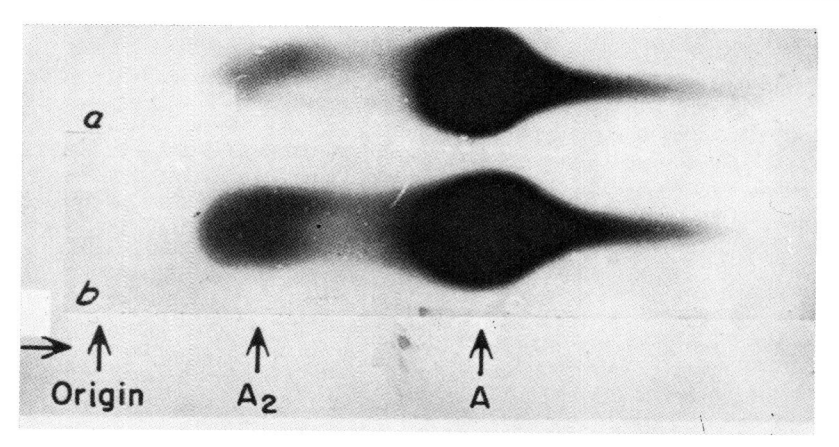

Fig. 51. Starch block electrophoresis of a normal hemolysate, a, and hemolysate with an increased amount of $A_2$ hemoglobin from a patient with known thalassemia minor, b.[218]

as contrasted with a low serum iron content in patients with iron-deficiency anemia establish the diagnosis of thalassemia minor. In the adult patient, thalassemia minor may co-exist with pernicious anemia[108] or megaloblastic states.[188]

In infants with thalassemia major, target cells and hypochromia are noted at birth. At the age of 2 or 3 months, normoblasts appear in the peripheral blood. The rate of fall of HbF concentration is much slower than in normal infants.[146] The increased uptake of $^{59}Fe$ is a specific character of the homozygous thalassemic reticulocytes and is present in the first weeks of life.[425]

Iron deficiency is common in females with beta thalassemia minor[54] and is best diagnosed by the lack of iron in the marrow. Recognition of the iron deficiency is important because it inhibits the elevation of $A_2$ hemoglobin necessary for diagnosis and because patients improve with iron therapy.[54]

*Starch block electrophoresis of hemoglobin in the diagnosis of the thalassemia trait.* When hemoglobin analyses are performed by paper electrophoresis at a pH of 8.6, two subtypes of normal hemoglobin are found. In addition to the main component, $A_1$, slow and fast components appear which are designated as $A_2$ and $A_3$, respectively. By the Tiselius moving boundary method performed at pH of 6.5, $A_2$, in contrast to its reaction during paper electrophoresis, migrates faster than $A_1$.[460]

An alternate method in which a starch block prepared from potato starch powder is substituted and hemolysates prepared in an identical manner as in the paper method are used provides electrophoretic patterns of diagnostic value in patients with thalassemia.[179,287,460]

The starch block suspended in an arbitrarily set volume of barbital buffer at a pH of 8.6 (ionic strength, 0.05) is covered with Parafilm and transferred to a cold room where electrophoresis is carried out at 4° C. at a specified voltage and current flow. Three major hemoglobin fractions can be readily observed—$A_3$, $A_1$, and $A_2$—in order of their speed of migration toward the anode. The $A_2$ component resembles hemoglobin E in electrophoretic mobility. The percentage of each component of A is obtained by elution from the respective areas of the block and determined spectrophotometrically. $A_2$ is found in a concentration of approximately 1 to 3% in the blood of normal persons. Levels in excess of 3.1% have been shown to have diagnostic value for the thalassemia trait.[267,374] (See Fig. 51.)

Another method in common use for separation and quantification of abnormal hemoglobins including estimation of $HbA_2$ is the cellulose acetate membrane technique. These methods have supplanted a paper method for measuring $HbA_2$.[218]

$HbA_2$ is practically absent at birth and does not reach adult levels until the age of 6 months.[332]

Rieder and Weatherall[403] summarized the reported variations of hemoglobin $A_2$. Elevated levels of hemoglobin $A_2$ are found not only in many individuals with thalassemia minor, but also in some patients with pernicious anemia in relapse and in some persons heterozygous for hemoglobin Zürich. Reduced levels are encountered in the newborn child, in some patients with anemia due to iron deficiency, and in persons with hereditary persistence of fetal hemoglobin. In the course of their studies they found that in the reticulocyte, hemoglobin $A_2$ synthesis is retarded before that of hemoglobin A.

A variant of hemoglobin $A_2$, called hemoglobin $B_2$, which is linked genetically to the beta-chain locus, has been described.[78] This is designated as alpha$_2{}^A$ delta$_2{}^B$. It is a minor, slow-moving fraction and related to $A_2$. In $B_2$ carriers the amount of $A_2$ is decreased to one-half its normal value, i.e., from 2.5 to 1.2%, while $B_2$ is present in the same low amount.[78] The sum of the two minor, slow-moving fractions adds up to normal values of $A_2$. It is of interest that when $B_2$ is present in a thalassemia heterozygous carrier, the values of both fractions are doubled and their sum is the high level of $A_2$, approximately 5%, typical of the thalassemia trait.[78,233] The hemoglobin fraction $B_2$ is allelic to $A_2$. $B_2$ is present in about 2% of the Negro population of the state of Georgia. In fourteen members of twenty-six cases of a family from Surinam, a double heterozygosity (for thalassemia and for the abnormal, minor component HbB$_2$) was demonstrated.[233] Inheritance indicated two different alleles (HbB$_2$ and beta thalassemia), each being present in an opposite member. An abnormal minor hemoglobin has been discovered in four heterozygous members of a Negro family.[293] This hemoglobin seems to be a variant from another delta-chain abnormality (HbA$_2{}^1$ or HbB$_2$) which migrates to the cathode on electrophoresis at pH 8.1. It is probably identical with hemoglobin-Flatbush as observed on starch gel electrophoresis at alkaline pH.[392]

$A_2$ is increased in patients with thalassemia minor, with a range of 2 to 9% and a mean of 5.11 ± 1.36, which exceeds the mean value in patients with thalassemia major and other miscellaneous diseases.[286] The elevation of the $A_2$ component serves, therefore, to distinguish patients with thalassemia minor from normal persons. Maximal values have occasionally been found in patients with intermediate forms of thalassemia and rarely in those with the severe disease. It should be emphasized that although the majority of patients with thalassemia minor showed elevated $A_2$ concentrations, a small percentage possess a normal concentration of this component. In this connection it has been pointed out[98] that the thalassemia gene that is not associated with an elevated $A_2$ fraction may also be responsible for the failure to interact with the gene for sickling, hemoglobin C, and hemoglobin E.

Two types of thalassemia based on phenomena of "interaction" and "noninteraction" fall into focus. These have been alluded to previously in discussing the effect of the gene for thalassemia upon other hemoglobins. In some families (noninteracting group) with a mixed heterozygosity for thalassemia and hemoglobins S and C, for instance, the abnormal hemoglobin (S or C) will account for approximately 40 to 50% of the total and hemoglobin A continues to be produced. In other families (interacting group) the abnormal hemoglobin amounts to 70 to 80% of the total, the remaining hemoglobin is fetal in type, and no hemoglobin A is produced. In the interacting families the amount of hemoglobin $A_2$ is abnormally elevated and fetal hemoglobin is normal. In noninteracting thalassemias hemoglobin $A_2$ is not elevated and very little fetal hemoglobin is found.

The thalassemia types have been classified further into beta thalassemia, in which beta-chain production is in short supply and alpha chains are unaffected. Beta thalassemia interacts with hemoglobins S, C, and E; hemoglobins F and $A_2$ are elevated since alpha-chain production is unimpaired. In alpha thalassemia, in which alpha-chain production is impaired, hemoglobin $A_2$ is not elevated, interaction with hemoglobins S, C, and E is nonexistent, but interaction does take place with abnormal alpha-chain hemoglobin (HbI and HbHpk[11]). In alpha thalassemia, Hb Bart's is often found at birth. Alpha thalassemia is commonly found in families of hemoglobin H disease and is particularly persistent in southeastern Asiatics and in the Negro.

*Course and prognosis.* Patients with thalassemia minor live normally regardless of the mild anemia. The outlook for patients with thalassemia major is poor, but the course is not a uniform one and depends upon the grade of severity of the disease encountered in the individual patient. As has been stated previously, thalassemia major falls into two classifications: the severe type, in which the patients require transfusions to maintain hemoglobin levels commensurate with normal activity, and a less severe one, the so-called intermediate type, in which patients function effectively without transfusions, maintaining hemoglobin levels of approximately 7 to 9 gm. per 100 ml. This separation can usually be made clinically, but transitional cases occur in which hemoglobin concentrations of patients requiring frequent transfusions subsequently stabilize at adequate levels without further treatment. On the other hand, patients with intermediate disease are observed who require no transfusions until there is exposure to infection or other noxious agents and more frequently for no apparent reason. From this point on, transfusions may be required so frequently that splenectomy is considered necessary.

Multiple transfusions at carefully spaced intervals, splenectomy in selected patients, and the liberal use of antibiotics permit a better prognosis for longevity in patients with thalassemia major than had heretofore been considered. The effect of these combined measures on ultimate longevity still has to be determined, especially in patients with the intermediate type of disease. In either classification, it is rare for severely affected patients to survive beyond the third decade. Among the patients with thalassemia major in our series, the oldest survivor is 28. In the group of patients with the intermediate type of disease there are five ranging in age from 30 to 51 years. One of these, now 49 years of age, originally reported when he was an adolescent,[465] has five children. This patient's spleen was removed at 31 years of age because of the sudden development of a hemolytic component after a burn, necessitating periodic transfusions. Until the recent onset of complications thought to be secondary to iron overload, the hemoglobin concentration had been stabilized at 9 to 10 gm. per 100 ml. without transfusions, although the blood smear still shows marked normoblastemia and other typical red cell changes characteristic of severe Cooley's anemia.

The frequently made statement that thalassemia major is almost always fatal before puberty no longer holds within the accepted definition of this term. It is difficult, however, to designate the precise period of puberty in these patients, since the development of sexual maturity is greatly retarded. In thalassemia intermedia the linear growth is normal. Bone and clinical evidences of maturation are occasionally slightly delayed. In thalassemia major, growth in early childhood is normal. In adolescence, physical, roentgenographic, and clinical evidences of adrenarche are usually absent. In three of thirteen female patients menses ceased in two after 4 years. Only one of eighteen males with thalassemia major had evidence of adrenal or gonadal maturation.[147]

Whereas infection was responsible for the death of many children with severe Cooley's anemia in the years before antibiotics were available, victims now succumb to heart failure. Although long-term transfusions prolong the lives of these patients, they are nevertheless responsible in large part for increased tissue iron. That excessive absorption of iron is also important as a cause of hemosiderosis is emphasized in those patients with thalassemia who have received minimal transfusions and eventually succumbed to heart disease.[136] In large part, cardiac complications are related to the heavy deposition of iron in the myocardium and are comparable in this respect to a similar incidence in idiopathic hemochromatosis.[166] Once heart failure sets in, it is irreversible, and the median duration of life from the onset of symptoms is approximately 1 year. The initial sign of a threatening cardiac nature in the asymptomatic patient is prolonged auricular-ventricular conduction (P-R interval) and the appearance of atrial premature contractions. With manifest heart failure, more serious atrial, as well as ventricular, arythmias recurred.

Acute benign nonspecific pericarditis has been described in thalassemia, especially among patients who have been splenectomized.[470] In all patients the pericarditis was self-limited and ended in complete recovery. The basis for this peculiar susceptibility is unknown.

Cardiac involvement and acquired hemochromatosis were observed in forty-one patients, thirty-nine with thalassemia major and two with aregenerative anemia.[142] Nineteen of the forty-one patients had pericarditis, twenty-six had congestive cardiac failure, and ten patients suffered from both. In late childhood, asymptomatic but progressive cardiac enlargement and electrocardiographic abnormalities appeared. The cardiac complications occurred in this setting, usually in the second decade. The average age at onset of pericarditis, 11 years, was a little earlier than that for heart failure, 16 years. On postmortem examination widespread iron deposition and fibrosis in the tissue characteristic of hemochromatosis were observed. These changes were especially marked in the liver, pancreas, gonads, thyroid, pituitary, and adrenal tissues. The kidneys, mucosa of the gastrointestinal tract, lymph nodes, and spleen were similarly affected. The heart showed widespread infiltration, destruction, and fibrosis of the myocardium.

***Treatment.*** There is no specific treatment for patients with severe Cooley's anemia. Iron, copper, liver, extracts from the spleen, pancreas, and adrenal gland and other endocrine products, steroids, large dosages of vitamin B components, plasma and cell extracts, and x-ray therapy have all been used without effect. Since only questionable improvement has been reported with cobalt,[45] it is not employed in routine treatment. Cooley's anemia represents a hypochromic microcytic anemia in which iron therapy is without value, as would be expected from the abundant iron stores already present.

***Transfusions.*** Transfusions are mainly relied upon as treatment for patients with thalassemia, and when they are excessive splenectomy is necessary. Hemoglobin and red blood cell levels in children with severe Cooley's anemia continue to decline progressively so that supportive transfusions are required to keep the patients asymptomatic under the stress of normal activity. Usually, this necessitates the administration of blood at 2- to 3-week intervals to maintain minimal levels. Transfusions, however, required to support adequate hemoglobin levels carry the inherent drawback of increased iron deposition from degraded hemoglobin. The hemoglobin level at which transfusions are indicated cannot be arbitrarily fixed but varies with the associated signs and symptoms in the individual patient. As a guide to management, patients with severe Cooley's anemia do not require transfusions until hemoglobin levels drop between 6.5 and 7.5 gm. per 100 ml., at which point clinical symptoms frequently set in.

In our experience, maintaining hemoglobin levels below 6 gm. per 100 ml. is potentially hazardous from the standpoint of developing heart failure. In patients with established cardiac difficulties the hemoglobin level should be maintained above 9 or 10 gm. per 100 ml. to prevent hypoxia. In addition to transfusion hemosiderosis, another deterrent to excessive blood administration is the possibility that multiple transfusions may depress endogenous hemoglobin synthesis and red cell function.[475]

At present, among those attending our transfusion clinics are eleven patients followed from early infancy who are now 18½ to 28 years of age. They receive one to two units of packed cells (usually frozen) every 2 weeks to maintain hemoglobin levels of 8.5 gm. per 100 ml. These patients attend college or are profitably employed in some phase of industry.

Under current trial is an investigation of the long-term clinical effects of maintaining hemoglobin levels above the usual 7.5 to 8 gm. per 100 ml. range in the severely affected child. It has been claimed that the increased hemoglobin concentrations will permit the patient to grow taller, show less hepatosplenomegaly, eliminate fractures, and, most important, lessen cardiac enlargement.[552] Still to be determined is whether the transient alleviation of chronic hypoxia by increased amounts of blood will retard the development of hemochromatosis and relieve cardiac musculature of the catastrophic effects of excessive iron deposition.

In a number of studies divergent opinions are expressed as to the value of a high-level transfusion program. Johnston and colleagues[258] found that growth retardation was evident only after the fourth year of life and that it was unrelated to pretransfusion hemoglobin levels. Brook and associates[66] observed that high-level transfusions depress prepubertal growth velocity, that they serve no advantages, and that they may be deleterious. They considered that, as far as growth is concerned, transfusions should be given in order to maintain well-being, and hemoglobin should be maintained at not less than 6.6 gm./100 ml. Beard and co-workers,[36] on the other hand, found striking clinical improvement with regression of abnormal cardiac symptoms and signs in patients in whom a hemoglobin level of over 10 gm./100 ml. had been maintained. Chelating agents were used to minimize iron loading. They concluded that the rationale for long-term intensive transfusion therapy is based on the assumption that it is the degree of anemia rather than the degree of iron loading which results in eventual heart failure and death. Kattamis and associates[273] concurred in these findings—namely, that the growth of thalassemic children during the first decade largely depends on maintaining fairly high hemoglobin levels. It is during this period that hypoxia is the main factor retarding growth and such a state is prevented by elevated levels of hemoglobin. In older children iron overload may be responsible for the delayed growth spurt. Growth retardation may be hormonal in view of the massive hemosiderosis of the pituitary, adrenal, thyroid, and gonads at necropsy.[168]

In another study,[259] the effect upon bone growth was measured when the hemoglobin level was maintained at 9 gm./100 ml., as compared with 7 gm. by varying the frequency of transfusions.

The midshaft of the second metacarpal bone as well as the cortical layer were measured by radiogram. Increased cortical bone breadth and periosteal deposition occurred with the higher hemoglobin level and apparently resulted from the decrease in excessive hematopoiesis produced by more frequent transfusion.

Until specific treatment becomes available, the most serious problem encountered in the patient with severe Cooley's anemia is the prevention and control of congestive heart failure. Treatment consists of the usual means of combating heart failure and appropriate therapy for arrhythmias—i.e., digitalization, diuretics, low salt diet, etc. In addition, small transfusions of packed red cells are given. At present there is no effective measure to rid the heart of excessive iron. Mobilization of iron stores achieved by repeated phlebotomies in patients with idiopathic hemochromatosis is precluded in patients with Cooley's anemia because of the constant need for maintaining adequate hemoglobin levels.

In addition to the previously described cardiac, hepatic, orthopedic, and growth abnormalities in thalassemia major, other metabolic and endocrine dysfunctions have been recently recognized in the later stages of the disease with progressive hemachromatosis. These include hyperuricemia resulting in gouty arthritis[368a] and renal stones, hypoparathyroidism,[173a] hypothyroidism, hyponatremic alkalosis, and diabetes mellitus with all of its consequences. Awareness of these complications and appropriate replacement therapy may contribute to prolonging patients' survival.

Chelating agents that increase urinary excretion of iron are important in the treatment of patients with conditions such as severe Cooley's anemia in whom massive iron loads exist.[166] Several effective chelating agents have been investigated. Fahey and associates[157] reported an appreciable urinary excretion of iron in patients with primary and secondary hemochromatosis (including thalassemia major) following intravenous or intramuscular administration of trisodium calcium diethylenetriaminepentaacetate (DTPA). Muller-Eberhard and co-workers[346] have confirmed the efficacy of this agent in thalassemia major with secondary hemochromatosis. As much as a sixteen-fold increase in excretion of iron (up to 40 mg. per 24 hours) and a three and one-half-fold increase in excretion of copper were achieved (with a dosage of 20 to 25 mg. per kilogram by intramuscular injection). This agent was effective in removal of iron, particularly in the older patients with secondary hemochromatosis. A possible hazard was the concomitant increased urinary excretion of magnesium, resulting in reduced plasma magnesium.

Deferoxamine (previously designated as desferrioxamine B), another chelating agent, is employed in the form of methane sulfonate under the name of Desferal. It interacts with trivalent iron to form ferrioxamine B. During this reaction the iron ion becomes enveloped in the deferoxamine. The resultant complex is soluble in water and passes readily through the kidney.

Deferoxamine belongs to the sideramines and is obtained from the actinomycetes. It has a strong affinity for trivalent iron and is thus able to take up iron from hemoglobin or from the more important iron-containing enzymes. The long chain of deferoxamine coils itself aronnd the iron atom so that the latter is thoroughly embedded. This agent has a selective action for iron and does not exert any untoward effects on serum electrolytes and other heavy metal ions, particularly the trace elements. Deferoxamine is prepared for intramuscular injection by dissolving 500 mg. of crystals in 1 ml. of sterile water and is given intramuscularly.

Deferoxamine, because of its marked specificity for iron, promises to be the most useful chelating agent yet available. Repeated intramuscular injections have been well tolerated and are not painful. This compound has been effectively used in hemochromatosis, thalassemia, liver cirrhosis, aregenerative anemia, and pulmonary hemosiderosis.[24,237,326,549]

In thalassemia major it is usually the older patient who demonstrates the most satisfactory excretion of iron. The dosage in one series[145] was 12 to 13 mg. per kilogram, given intramuscularly and rounded off to the nearest 500 mg. In the older child the dosage ranges from 500 to 1,000 mg. daily. The daily urinary excretion cannot be predicted with accuracy, but in a series of eight patients from 5 to 17 years of age it ranged from approximately 3 to 23 mg. per 24 hours. Others[237] have found in patients with iron overload that the urinary excretion varied from 2.5 to 24.1 mg. per gram of deferoxamine per 24 hours, with a maximum iron excretion of 53 mg. per 24 hours.

The effectiveness of deferoxamine in increasing iron output in thalassemia major has been confirmed in more recent studies. In some instances it was observed to cause a reticulocytosis. Even with a dosage of 1,000 mg. daily in two

12-hour 500 mg. doses, resulting in an excretion of 4.52 mg./day (amounting to 135 mg./month), the iron output lags behind iron intake. Most children receive at least 500 ml. blood monthly with an average iron content of 250 mg. This reflects the futility of trying to remove significant amounts of iron from patients who require repeated transfusions. Intravenous infusion of deferoxamine at the time of each blood transfusion has been suggested but the slight risk of development of cataract following prolonged therapy with deferoxamine necessitates periodic ophthalmic screening. Skin pigmentation was often decreased and subjective feelings of improvement have been reported.

Another effective method of mobilizing and removing excess iron in heavily iron-laden thalassemic children is to use large doses of DTPA between transfusions with daily injections of deferoxamine.[483,484]

It remains to be demonstrated whether either of these drugs or their combination will result in a reversal of tissue damage, particularly when cardiac musculature is affected. It is doubtful whether the patient with thalassemia major who is dependent on multiple transfusions can be adequately depleted of iron stores. For the patient with the intermediate form of the disease who only periodically requires transfusions, prolonged chelation may be more promising, but further trial is necessary. Although reports of this chelating agent have demonstrated minimal evidence of toxicity,[237] its use must still remain on an experimental basis. It is also possible that animal experimentation and prolonged trial in patients with hemochromatosis when long-term administration is necessary may disclose secondary deleterious tissue changes.

The use of deferoxamine in the therapy of acute iron poisoning was discussed in Chapter 12.

Folic acid deficiency which occurs in many patients with thalassemia major is not necessarily associated with a megaloblastic marrow. Treatment with oral folic acid in adequate dosage, regardless of the state of erythroid maturation, leads to a normal blood folic acid level and decreased excretion of formiminoglutamic acid, an early increase in nucleated red cells and reticulocytes, but not to a rise in hemoglobin concentration.[351] Only rarely does folic acid cause a significant decrease in transfusion requirements. In our own experience transfusion needs were reduced in two patients with thalassemia of the intermediate type who had briefly experienced a hypersplenic episode during which transfusions were required.

The precise dosage of folic acid has varied with the age of the patient and the severity of the anemia. It has been prescribed in a dosage of 0.5 mg. to 10 mg. daily, given orally.

*Splenectomy.* In the severely affected person the need for splenectomy is clearly indicated when transfusion requirements are progressively increased and when the spleen becomes massive and burdensome, causing discomfort and symptoms due to pressure. Although efforts are made in the immediate presplenectomy period to vary the number and size of transfusions so as to defer splenectomy, the blood requirements nevertheless become so extreme that decision for the operation is usually forced.[472]

At this time there will usually be abundant evidence that a hemolytic factor has developed which shortens the life of normal transfused cells. When there is doubt, labeling donor cells with radioactive chromium will establish the rate at which transfused blood is being destroyed. Although the increasing need for transfusions before splenectomy and the sharp reduction afterward confirms the elevation of an extracorpuscular hemolytic component, it does not appear to alter the basic disease significantly.[474] Retardation of growth and the incidence of congestive heart failure are not altered by removal of the spleen. From available data splenectomy appears more effective in the older child, but this may reflect a genetically milder disease permitting postponement until puberty. Another explanation is that slowing of growth and diminished metabolic needs in adolescence permit the establishment of erythropoietic equilibrium at levels compatible with well-being without supplementation by transfusions. Despite the preference to delay splenectomy until adolescence, it is frequently necessary to remove the spleen of the younger patient because of excessive transfusion needs.

Recent experience has demonstrated a potential hazard of severe and overwhelming infection following splenectomy in patients with Cooley's anemia and other dyscrasias in childhood.* While the pneumococcus appears to be the predominant organism in the collected experience of various reports, *Escherichia coli* is a frequent offender in Cooley's anemia. In

---

*See references 187, 236, 277, 471, and 472.

comparison with the numbers of splenectomies, the incidence is avowedly small. Nevertheless, close supervision for several years postoperatively is essential so that appropriate treatment may be instituted immediately in the event of an infection. Broad-spectrum antibiotics have been prescribed as a continuous prophylactic measure during the first 2 years after splenectomy, when infections are most common. With the known limitations of providing a totally effective drug, penicillin, 200,000 units given daily by mouth, is in use in many clinics.[471]

There is no contraindication to tonsillectomy in patients with Cooley's anemia. Irradiation is effective in treatment of lymphatic hyperplasia of the nasopharynx.[315] Minor coagulation defects may coexist with structural and functional abnormalities of the liver.

Under investigation in treatment of thalassemia is a trial of allogeneic marrow transplants.[420] While no definitive results have been obtained, there is fragmentary evidence that bone marrow may become adaptable in time.

A more rational form of therapy has been postulated.[356] Extracts containing normal messenger RNA might eventually be "manipulated in such manner as to replace the alleged defective messenger which occludes the polyribosomes of the thalassemic cell," and also the development of "efforts to reduce the production of alpha chain units in Cooley's anemia and of beta chains in HbH disease."

*Alpha-thalassemia*

Another less common type of thalassemia, is alpha-thalassemia, in which the production of alpha chains is almost completely suppressed. Since both HbF and $HbA_2$, in common with HbA, contain alpha chains, no compensating or relative increase of HbF and $HbA_2$ is possible.[174] Inherited deficiencies in the production of alpha chains in the alpha-thalassemia result in an excess of the complementary chains —beta, gamma, and delta. Bart's hemoglobin, which contains four gamma chains, and H hemoglobin, containing four beta chains, each devoid of alpha chains, may be found in pedigrees of alpha-thalassemia.

*Alpha-thalassemia major.* In this form both alpha chain genes are affected and neither is able to produce an adequate quantity of alpha chains. The homozygous state is incompatible with fetal survival. Infants with almost 100% Hb Bart's are stillborn at 34 to 36 weeks of gestation and have generalized hydrops, ascites, and hepatic enlargement. Where some alpha chains are formed, a small portion of HbF and lesser amounts of HbA are synthesized.[298] Some traces of HbH ($\beta_4$) are always present because beta chain production has already commenced. The peripheral blood of alpha-thalassemia major reveals severe erythroblastosis, reticulocytosis, and many target cells. The reported cases of alpha-thalassemia major originate from the Far East.[530] It is of interest that HbH ($\beta_4$) and Hb Bart's ($\delta_4$) are associated with the clinical findings of thalassemia despite their remarkably increased oxygen affinity.[391]

The level of Hb Bart's in the neonatal period serves as a useful guide to the degree of alpha chain deficiency so that several types of alpha-thalassemia have been defined.[531] Whereas infants with almost 100% Hb Bart's do not survive, infants with 20 to 30% Hb Bart's at birth do survive and develop moderately severe thalassemia associated with similar quantities of HbH as they grow older. The reason that HbH ($\beta_4$) may be found without Hb Bart's ($\delta_4$) in the milder case is that gamma chain production may have almost terminated when the patient was investigated for hemoglobin abnormalities. In the absence of gamma chain production no Hb Bart's will be formed.

The patients with homozygous alpha-thalassemia reported from Thailand died either in utero or soon after birth.[523] Placentas are larger than normal and friable. Hepatomegaly is much more pronounced than splenomegaly, in contrast to the reverse findings in hydrops fetalis due to hemolytic disease in the newborn.

The parents of these severely affected infants show minimal hematological changes and are assumed to be alpha-thalassemia carriers, but are clinically indistinguishable from normal.[298]

*Alpha-thalassemia minor.* The heterozygous state for alpha-thalassemia is very difficult to detect in adult life. It is not certain that the alpha-thalassemia in which Hb Bart's is found in the 5 to 15% range is the same entity as that in Southeast Asia and Africa.[531] The hydrops picture is not seen in Negroes, although 1 to 2% of American Negroes carry this amount of Hb Bart's in the neonatal period.[531] Hb Bart's

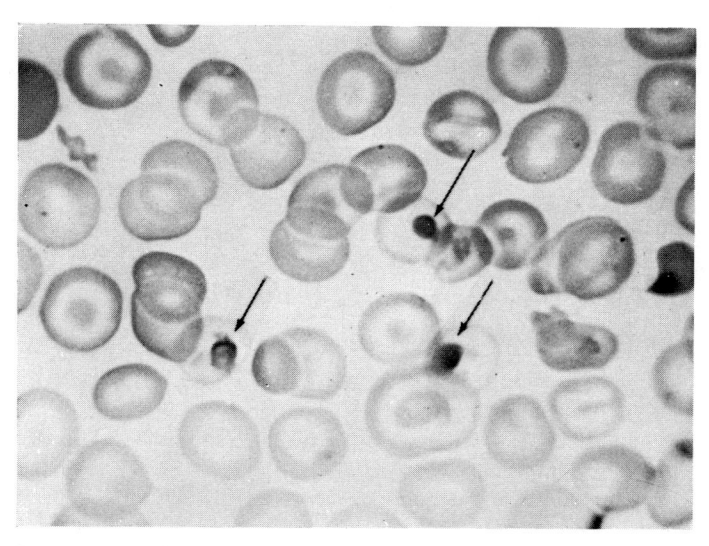

Fig. 52. Blood smear from a patient with hemoglobin H disease (post-splenectomy). Note inclusion bodies in three erythrocytes. (Courtesy Dr. Ralph L. Engle, Jr., New York, N. Y.)

usually disappears by the age of 6 months, although a trace may be found beyond the first year. It is usually associated with aniso- and poikilocytosis, mild hypochromia, and target cells. These are probably heterozygotes for alpha thalassemia. The presence of Bart's hemoglobin in the neonate is probably indicative of the heterozygous state of alpha thalassemia. Macrocytosis of red cells and evidences of increased resistance to hypotonic sodium chloride solution are also present. Eventually Hb Bart's and HbH disappear from the blood.

It has been pointed out that infants born with Hb Bart's of 5 to 15% or 1 to 2% represent two classes of carrier of alpha-thalassemia genes. The neonate in the former group shows red cell stigmata of thalassemia; the latter, with a smaller percentage of Hb Bart's, shows no red cell changes.[523] In either case the parents show minimal or none of the blood features of the alpha-thalassemia trait and may be indistinguishable from normal.[298] It may be said that the heterozygous alpha thalassemia is the least severe of all the thalassemias.[295]

### Hemoglobin H

Three members of a Chinese family were found to have a hypochromic microcytic anemia with blood smears resembling thalassemia. The electrophoretic pattern revealed an abnormal hemoglobin migrating more rapidly than normal hemoglobin (A). Other features included refractoriness to iron therapy, reticulocytosis, poikilocytosis, intraerythrocytic inclusion bodies, decreased osmotic fragility, a shortened red cell survival, and splenomegaly.[265,409] Marked anisocytosis, target cells, polychromatophilia, basophilic stippling, bilirubinemia, and the rapid development of intraerythrocytic inclusion bodies upon incubation, especially if exposed to supravital dyes such as brilliant cresyl blues, are additional characteristics. (See Fig. 52.) Hemoglobin H in reported cases varied from 2.5 to 40% of the total,[408] fetal hemoglobin was slightly increased, and the remainder was normal hemoglobin. It is of interest that this fast-moving hemoglobin did not appear in either parent and that the father and daughter of one of the affected patients showed red cell changes consistent with thalassemia minor.[409] In all subsequent reports the same failure to find hemoglobin H in either parent was observed.

A similar blood picture interpreted as hemoglobin H–thalassemia disease has been described in two unrelated middle-aged Filipino men. Hemoglobin analysis in these cases also revealed a major component of normal hemoglobin and a minor component of hemoglobin H. Fetal hemoglobin was normal.[340]

Increasing numbers of patients with hemoglobin H in combination with thalassemia minor (hemoglobin H–thalassemia) have been observed.[189,334,342,551] Cases of hemoglobin H

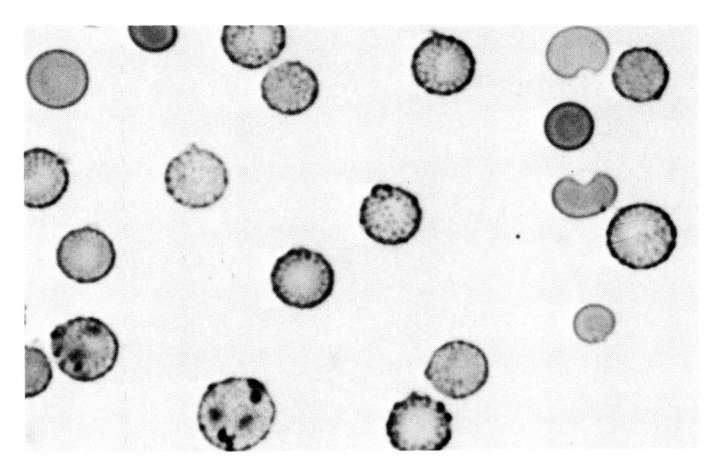

Fig. 53. Blood smear from patient with hemoglobin H disease. Finely stippled and larger dense inclusion bodies are identified after incubation with 1% brilliant cresyl blue. (Courtesy Dr. Denis R. Miller, New York, N. Y.)

have been found not only in Chinese and Filipinos, but also in Thai, Greek, Italian, and Swedish patients. Although devoid of hemoglobin H, parents and siblings in these reports present evidence of the thalassemia trait as well as of intraerythrocytic inclusion bodies resembling Heinz bodies. Further testing for increases of $A_2$ hemoglobin is necessary to confirm the diagnosis of thalassemia minor in these patients.[207] In a Sardinian patient with HbH the $A_2$ hemoglobin component was decreased.[125] Relatives were found to exhibit the hematologic features of the thalassemia trait, but the $A_2$ value was not increased. In addition to HbH the thalassemia trait was probably also present, and the low $A_2$ in the patient and family characterizes alpha-thalassemia.

Chronic hypochromic microcytic anemia associated with the presence of intraerythrocytic crystals and hemoglobin H has been described. The parents did not show the abnormal hemoglobin H in their blood. The family was partly of Chinese and partly of Indonesian origin.[140]

Hemoglobin H has a unique chemical composition for it contains no alpha-polypeptide chains, only beta chains. It is a tetramer of beta chains analogous to Hb Bart's, which is a tetramer of gamma chains. HbH is therefore designated as $\beta_4{}^A$.

Splenectomy may be of benefit in improving exercise tolerance, elevation of hemoglobin level, and erythrocyte mean life-span. However, hemolytic crises may still occur. Erythrocyte survival indicates a life-span of 40 to 45 days ($^{51}Cr$ method) before splenectomy, which increases to normal following this procedure. Splenectomy aids in the survival of erythrocytes with inclusions, but the contained HbA presumably retains its function in oxygen transport.[408]

Hemoglobin H with red cell inclusion bodies was noted in an adult with chronic myeloid leukemia.[38] The explanation offered for the presence of HbH was that a leukemic state sometimes led to an imbalance of hemoglobin chain synthesis, resulting in an excess of beta chains, which combine to form HbH as in the case of alpha-thalassemia.

HbH disease can be diagnosed in the laboratory by the following criteria: a blood film appearance suggestive of thalassemia, decreased osmotic fragility of the red cells, the finding of inclusions typical of HbH in the majority of red cells after incubation with brilliant cresyl blue at 37° C., and the presence of a fast-moving hemoglobin (10 to 30% of the total) on zone electrophoresis at pH 7.7[545] (Figs. 52 and 53).

Evidence has been presented indicating that at a red cell age of 40 to 45 days HbH denatures and precipitates, forming intraerythrocytic inclusions. These cells are rapidly removed by the spleen. HbH has a lower solubility in the deoxygenated state and precipitates reversibly, regardless of cell age. In the capillary bed random erythrocyte destruction takes place.[408]

The oxygen affinity of HbH is approximately ten times that of hemoglobin A.[43] Hemoglobin H shows no Bohr effect. (The ability of $CO_2$ to shift the slope of oxyhemoglobin dissociation curve to the right is known as the Bohr effect.) It is, therefore, concluded that the alpha-beta chain interactions rather than direct interactions between the hemes are essential for the normal oxygen affinity of hemoglobin A.

Ingram and Stretton[243] have given several explanations for the polymerization of beta chains. The somewhat abnormal beta chains of HbH with an unusual tendency to polymerize are formed in excess of alpha chains, which are being produced at either a normal or reduced rate due to the effect of an alpha-thalassemia gene. Another explanation is that normal beta chains are being produced in excess of alpha chains, which in turn are being produced at a markedly reduced rate because of the effect of two alpha-thalassemia genes. It is of interest that trace amounts of Hb Bart's have been demonstrated in adult cases of HbH.[229] If the formation of HbH and Hb Bart's is due to diminished alpha-chain production, it would be expected that Hb Bart's carriers at birth would develop HbH after cessation of HbF production. In the families of patients with Hb Bart's and HbH, interaction with the gene for alpha-thalassemia seems to be in evidence.

There is an approximately twofold greater $^{51}Cr$ specific activity of tagged HbH than HbA.[372] This is due to the presence in HbH of the four beta chains in comparison with the two beta chains in HbA. It is presumed that $^{51}Cr$ is tagged primarily to beta chains. Fetal hemoglobin, which has no beta chains, binds $^{51}Cr$ weakly and is rapidly eluted.

## High hemoglobin F-thalassemia

HbF-thalassemia is the most commonly observed variant of delta-beta thalassemias. Diagnosis of this trait is made by observing the hematological abnormalities of the thalassemia trait, normal or low levels of $HbA_2$, increased levels of fetal hemoglobin, and heterogenous distribution of HbF in the red cells. The HbF thalassemic gene causes a relatively mild disease. In most patients there is a late onset of the clinical manifestations, normal or almost normal growth, only minor bone and facial deformities, and moderate splenomegaly.[491] Transfusions are rarely required. HbF-thalassemia is usually explained as a mutation resulting in a complete deficiency of $\beta$ and $\alpha$ chains, together with continuation of $\gamma$ chain synthesis. According to another concept, the origin of the high F variant known as delta-beta thalassemia has its basis in the proximity of the delta and beta chain loci to each other on the same chromosome.[298] In this case a secondary beta thalassemia may interfere with the activity of the delta chain resulting in a beta thalassemia blood picture with a depressed $HbA_2$.

F-thalassemia has been observed in the heterozygous state, in combination with other hemoglobin abnormalities, with $\beta$ thalassemia, and in the homozygous form. In these cases (delta-beta thalassemia) HbF is elevated in the range of about 10 to 20% and is distributed unevenly over the red cell population.[317] In those heterozygous for hereditary persistence of HbF, levels of fetal hemoglobin may range up to 30% and HbF in this condition is distributed uniformly over the red cell population.

## Homozygous hemoglobin C disease

Homozygous hemoglobin C disease is a rare condition occurring principally in Negroes and occasionally in Caucasians.

***Essential features.*** Anemia is absent or mildly hemolytic, the reticulocyte count is normal or slightly increased, and bilirubin may be slightly elevated—features indicative of a compensated hemolytic process. The red cells are normocytic or slightly microcytic and normochromic, normoblasts appear occasionally, and tetragonal crystals of hemoglobin have been observed in 2% of the erythrocytes in one patient.[123] Red cells show a decreased osmotic fragility. Moderate erythrocytic hyperplasia is present in the bone marrow. The striking feature of the blood film is the large number of target cells estimated at 40 to 90% of all erythrocytes. Paper electrophoresis reveals 100% hemoglobin C, which has the slowest mobility rate of all hemoglobins tested by this technique. With rare exceptions fetal hemoglobin is not elevated above normal levels. As in patients with other hereditary hemolytic syndromes, the red cells of patients with homozygous hemoglobin C disease injected into a normal recipient show a shortened survival. The exponential type of survival time curve indicates the random destruction of red cells regardless of their age.[504] Splenomegaly is either moderate or very marked. Abdominal pain, arthralgia, jaundice, and cholelithiasis are uncommon. The prognosis is good and transfusions are rarely necessary. Splenectomy is occasionally carried out for relief of symptoms relating to pain over the splenic area.[123]

Hemoglobin C is less soluble than HbA in red cells, in hemolysates, and in dilute phosphate buffer. Red cells from patients with homozygous HbC (CC) disease exhibit aberrant physical properties which suggest that the cells are more rigid than normal erythrocytes.[32] These small dense cells are exceptionally rigid and probably are even more susceptible to fragmentation and sequestration. Increased rigidity of CC cells, by acceleration of their fragmentation, may be responsible for formation of microspherocytes. Microspherocytes are destroyed as they attempt to traverse the microcirculation, either by fragmentation or phagocytosis, or as a result of increased susceptibility to osmotic lysis.

*Hemoglobin C trait*

The combination of hemoglobins A and C is found in the asymptomatic carrier who is identified by the reaction of his blood to electrophoresis and the presence of numerous target cells in the blood smear. In the person with the trait the C pigment varies from 28 to 44%, sickling is absent, fetal hemoglobin is normal, and a mild hypochromia may be present. Recent studies[388] have shown that red cell survival was mildly shortened in patients with hemoglobin C trait, in contrast with earlier studies of a normal survival time.[534] While the presence of large numbers of target cells is regarded as the only hematologic abnormality, a moderately severe microcytic, normochromic anemia has been reported in patients with hemoglobin C trait.[480] Although the heterozygous individual is usually without symptoms, unilateral, renal hematuria and spotty areas of bone infarction in the dental roentgenograms have occasionally been noted.[480] The hemoglobin C trait is detected in about 2% of the American Negro population.[480]

*Hereditary elliptocytosis and hemoglobin C trait.* Two children in a Negro family were found to have both elliptocytosis and hemoglobin C. Each of these factors was traced to the respective parents. In one child some of the target cells associated with the hemoglobin C trait were elliptical, indicating the combined genetic effects in the same cells. Anemia in one child was corrected by iron, and the red cell survival was normal. The combination of elliptocytosis and hemoglobin C trait does not show a summation effect.[16]

*Hemoglobin C variant with sickling properties.* In four members of a Negro family spanning three generations an abnormal hemoglobin showing two distinct bands, type A and what appeared to be type C hemoglobins, was demonstrated.[384] This type of HbC produces sickling yet contains no sickle hemoglobin. It is designated as HbC$_{Georgetown}$ to designate its geographic origin. There was no anemia attributable to the presence of this hemoglobin trait. The red cells were found to sickle consistently with 2% sodium metabisulfite and in sealed coverslip preparations with reduced oxygen tension. Sickling has been reported in the absence of sickle hemoglobin in HbC$_{Harlem}$,[56] in the presence of a large amount of hemoglobin Bart's,[137,138] and in a case of thalassemia-hemoglobin I disease.[15] By fingerprinting it was determined that in this type of HbC an amino acid substitution of lysine for glutamic acid was found to occur at the seventh residue of the beta-polypeptide chain instead of the sixth position as in HbC.

*Hereditary persistence of fetal hemoglobin and hemoglobin C (C-F heterozygotes).* In this combination the spleen may be palpable and the blood may show numerous target cells, some resembling spherocytes. The incidence of the high fetal gene in the Memphis Negro is slightly less than 0.2%.[325] The alkali resistant hemoglobin was found in one series to range from approximately 28 to 30% and hemoglobin concentrations, 11.7 to 15 gm. per 100 ml.[101] Red cell survival was shortened. As in all combinations with persistent fetal hemoglobin the latter is fairly uniformly distributed among red cells.[449] Hemoglobin A was not detected in the hemolysates. The mild hemolytic disorder was attributable to the high concentration of HbC in the erythrocytes, but the mechanism by which this abnormal hemoglobin shortens the life-span of red cells is unknown.

*Hemoglobin D*

Hemoglobin D is a rare hemoglobin which possesses an electrophoretic mobility identical with sickle hemoglobin. It is distinguished by its much higher solubility in reduced form than the latter in a comparable physical state. In contrast to homozygous hemoglobin S disease, gelling, tactoid formation, and sickling are absent. Homozygous hemoglobin D disease has rarely been reported.[53,91] The anemia is slight, target cells are numerous, osmotic resistance to hypotonic saline solution is increased, and the erythrocyte life-span is shortened.

The person with the trait (hemoglobins A and D) is asymptomatic and reveals no quantitative blood changes and no sickling. He can only be identified by the presence of hemoglobin D. Hemoglobin D is not uncommon among American Negroes, with a reported incidence of 0.4%.[91] Occasional cases have been found among American Indians.[186] Foci of hemoglobin D prevalence have been described in Algerian Moslems and Indians of north central India.[91]

Three samples of hemoglobin D have been examined, coming, respectively, from a Turkish Cypriot ($D_{alpha}$), from Gujerati ($D_{beta}$), and the third from a Punjab ($D_{gamma}$ now called $D_{Punjab}$).[44] Each variety carries a chemical charge in a different part of the hemoglobin molecule. In all three varieties no sickling of the red cells was seen with the usual test, thus showing that no sickle hemoglobin was present. By trypsin digestion and "fingerprinting," these three varieties may be separated.[44] There is evidence that what was designated as hemoglobin $D_{St.\ Louis}$ is probably identical with hemoglobin $G_{Philadelphia}$.[241] The occurrence of the same type hemoglobin D in widely separated geographic localities (i.e., in Punjab, North Carolina, Chicago, Portugal, and Cyprus) has aroused great interest among those interested in deducing the origins and movements of populations that carry this abnormality.

## Hemoglobin E disease

Hemoglobin E disease was discovered during an investigation of a group of severely anemic patients from Thailand whose clinical and hematologic characteristics closely resembled those of patients with severe thalassemia. In some of these patients a mild course and survival into adult life suggested deviation from the uniformly severe case of thalassemia. A significant feature was the presence of the trait of thalassemia in only one parent instead of in both, which was to be expected in the usual case of the severe disease in a child. Investigation revealed that these patients possessed an additional hemoglobin designated as compound E which was also present in the second parent. With paper electrophoresis it was possible to demonstrate that hemoglobin E had a mobility intermediate between hemoglobin C and hemoglobin S. Further studies[93,353] revealed the several categories of pure or homozygous hemoglobin E disease, hemoglobin E trait (hemoglobin A plus hemoglobin E), and thalassemia–hemoglobin E disease. A survey in connection with these studies revealed that hemoglobin E was found in 13% of persons of Thai extraction, but was not detected in any of the racially unmixed Chinese in that area.

**Homozygous hemoglobin E disease.** The clinical features include easy fatigability, mild arthralgia, and occasionally icterus. In the small group of cases in this category, the spleen was slightly enlarged in only one patient and the liver in another. The hemoglobin level is moderately lowered, the erythrocyte levels are normal, reticulocytes are not increased, and target cells are numerous (25 to 60%). Red cell constants indicate a microcytic hypochromic anemia. The red cells show an increased resistance to hemolysis in hypotonic saline solutions. The bone marrow shows a mild erythrocytic hyperplasia. Paper electrophoresis reveals 94 to 98% hemoglobin E and up to 6% fetal hemoglobin.[93]

**Hemoglobin E trait.** Persons with the trait are asymptomatic. Blood values are normal and target cells are not observed. Paper electrophoresis reveals two components: normal hemoglobin A and hemoglobin E. Normal amounts of fetal hemoglobin are demonstrated by alkali denaturation.

## Hemoglobin G

Hemoglobin G pigment moves more slowly than hemoglobin A and faster than hemoglobin S, corresponding electrophoretically to the area in which fetal hemoglobin is found.[131,132] Its mobility coincides with fetal hemoglobin or migrates somewhat more slowly. Hemoglobin G is not alkali resistant and can be differentiated from fetal hemoglobin in this manner.[431]

A variety of hemoglobin G specimens have been identified from different parts of the world. In accordance with standard nomenclature the following HbG varieties can be listed: $G_{San\ Jose}$, with beta-peptide chain abnormality, and $G_{Philadelphia}$, $G_{Honolulu}$, $G_{Bristol}$, with alpha-chain abnormalities. Three abnormal hemoglobins identified as HbG by their electrophoretic mobility and performance in resin chromatography have been discovered in three healthy unrelated Negroes in Texas.[60] The three G hemoglobins have a substitution in the forty-third residue of the beta chain, glutamic acid being replaced by alanine. They are designated as HbG$_{Galveston}$, HbG$_{Port\ Arthur}$, and HbG$_{Texas}$. An alpha chain mutant G$_{Baltimore}$ has been described.[402] On paper electrophoresis at pH 8.6 this component showed a mobility similar to that of HbS and HbG$_{Philadelphia}$. Mutation involved a substitution of histidine for aspartic acid in the tryptic peptide IX of the alpha-polypeptide chain.

*Hemoglobin G trait.* In a family from the African Gold Coast in which the parents were homozygous for hemoglobins A and G, respectively, nine siblings were heterozygous (A-G), as expected.[131,132] These persons with the trait presented no clinical or hematologic abnormalities.

*Homozygous hemoglobin G disease.* The father of the aforementioned family (GG) was asymptomatic and did not have anemia (hemoglobin, 13.9 gm. per 100 ml.), and the blood smear was free of abnormalities. Fetal hemoglobin was not present, reticulocytes were 2%, and the serum bilirubin level was normal.[131,132]

*Hemoglobin G–sickle cell disease.* With heterozygous hemoglobin G–sickle cell disease, a moderately severe hemolytic anemia occurs with splenomegaly, sickling, increased osmotic resistance to hypotonic sodium chloride solution, and a blood picture resembling sickle cell–thalassemia disease.[431]

*Hemoglobin G–thalassemia.* An Italian patient with hemoglobin G–thalassemia possessed a blood picture and clinical findings somewhat more severe than those of patients with thalassemia minor. The hemoglobin was 10 gm. per 100 ml. and the smear revealed hypochromic red cells, target cells, and basophilic stippling. Other features included no elevation in fetal hemoglobin, slight reticulocytosis, a palpable spleen, and moderately hyperplastic bone marrow. The red cell survival was about two-thirds of the normal.[489] In an American family of Italian origin, hemoglobin G, hemoglobin S, and thalassemia occurred together.[432] Hemoglobin G did not appear clinically important taken alone or in combination with hemoglobin S or thalassemia.

## Hemoglobin I

A hemoglobin with a mobility more rapid than normal hemoglobin A was detected in several members of a Negro family. The affected persons were asymptomatic and showed no hematologic abnormalities.[419] This hemoglobin was present in equal amounts with hemoglobin A. Differences in mobility between hemoglobin H and hemoglobin I were not apparent at a pH of 8.6 but were clearly distinguishable at a pH of 6.5.

Hemoglobin I was also found in six members of another Negro family. The amount of hemoglobin I in the affected members ranged from 15 to 35%.[506] The amino acid substitution was shown to occur in the sixteenth residue of the alpha chain, lysine being substituted by aspartic acid.[347]

In a Negro woman in whom 70% concentration of HbI was demonstrated together with HbA with no sickle hemoglobin, sickling was produced when the blood was mixed with 2 to 4% sodium metabisulfite and, more consistently, with the more concentrated solution. The changes were not completely reversible nor could sickling be observed with simple deoxygenation as in a coverglass preparation. The sickling in this case was not due to the formation of tactoids or to gelation of abnormal hemoglobin, but to a direct chemical action on red cell stroma modified in some manner by the presence of HbI in excessive concentration.[15]

The high percentage of the abnormal hemoglobin (70% HbI) suggests that this patient had more than a simple hemoglobin trait. In a trait the normal adult hemoglobin should be present in more than 50% of the total hemoglobin. Excessive amounts of HbI in this case suggested the simultaneous presence of an interacting thalassemia gene. A complete family study could not be carried out. Three children showed moderate to severe hypochromic anemia, with one child reacting to iron therapy. Consequently a double heterozygous condition for HbI and for thalassemia was suspected.

## Hemoglobin J

Hemoglobin J, observed in a Negro family, was shown to have a more rapid electrophoretic mobility at a pH of 8.6 than normal adult hemoglobin but a slower mobility than the next component I. It was found in combination with normal hemoglobin. Sickling was absent, and no hematologic or physical abnormalities were found.[256,508]

Two hemoglobin types have been observed in Liberian natives—one with a mobility corresponding to hemoglobin J and the other between hemoglobin J and A. No cytologic abnormalities were found in either patient.

## Hemoglobin M

Methemoglobin is formed when hemoglobin, in its deoxygenated state, is oxidized to the ferric form. Methemoglobin is unable to serve as a respiratory pigment because in its ferric state iron cannot combine with oxygen. There are several categories of different etiology producing methemoglobinemia and cyanosis: the abnormal endogenous formation of oxidizing substances, a hereditary defect in the enzyme system normally responsible for maintaining hemoglobin in the reduced state, and the dominant transmission of an abnormality in hemoglobin itself—the hemoglobin M group of pigments.

Methemoglobinemia may, therefore, be caused in several ways. The common form due to the excessive formation of methemoglobin is caused by drugs and chemicals (see Chapter 17). More uncommon is the diminished reconversion of methemoglobin to hemoglobin due to a deficiency in the methemoglobin reductase enzyme system. The great majority of instances of methemoglobinemia resulting from an inherited enzyme deficiency are caused by a malfunction of NADH-dependent methemoglobin reductase or diaphorase.[298] These two types deal with normal globin. On the other hand, an abnormality of the globin part of the hemoglobin molecule permits the heme groups to exist only in the ferric state and are known collectively as the hemoglobins M. These hemoglobins result when the heme group, which is normally protected from external aqueous environment by being inserted into a well-protected pocket lined by hydrophobic chains from the neighboring amino acid residues, loses some of the protection.

The designation of hemoglobin M was proposed[456] for a spectroscopically abnormal methemoglobin first described by Hörlein and Weber[225] in a family with hereditary methemoglobinemia. They showed that the cyanosis was due to the presence of methemoglobin with an unusual spectral characteristic which was attributable to abnormality of the globin. Subsequently, Gerald[176] found that the hemoglobin from a patient with hemoglobin M disease could be resolved into two components identified electrophoretically and spectroscopically—one as hemoglobin A and the other as hemoglobin M.

In this disease two of the iron atoms of some of the hemoglobin molecules are in the oxidized (methemoglobin) state instead of being in the usual reduced state. This methemoglobin derivative of hemoglobin is incapable of combining with molecular oxygen, thus leading to clinical symptoms of cyanosis.[241]

Several hemoglobin M types have been described in which new amino acids replace the normal amino acids of polypeptide chains.[177] To explain an anomaly of the spectroscopic behavior of methemoglobin involving the globin segment of hemoglobin, it was postulated that the replaced amino acids occurred structurally in the proximity of the heme group. The new amino acid being near the heme group could then react with it, affecting its spectroscopic behavior. The hemoglobin M varieties with amino acid differences are $HbM_{Boston}$, $HbM_{Saskatoon}$, and $HbM_{Milwaukee}$. The first involves an abnormality of the alpha chain, the other two of the beta chain. In $HbM_{Boston}$ tyrosine replaces histidine in position 58, in $HbM_{Saskatoon}$ tyrosine replaces histidine in position 63, and in $HbM_{Milwaukee}$ glutamic acid replaces valine in position 67.[177] Two unrelated patients with hemoglobin M disease have also been reported.[158]

The cyanosis is, therefore, due to hemoglobin with a defective globin component.[158] It has been pointed out that when the defect is in the hemoglobin alpha chain, the fetal hemoglobin is also abnormal and the patient is cyanotic from birth. When the defect is in the beta chain, the patient is protected for the first few months.

In contrast to the therapeutic effect of methylene blue and ascorbic acid in patients with the established forms of congenital and of drug-induced types of methemoglobinemia in converting the pigment back to normal hemoglobin, methemoglobinemia due to hemoglobin M is unaffected by this therapy. Patients with the abnormal hemoglobin M have approximately 15 to 20% of the total pigment in the form of methemoglobin and are seemingly unaffected by its presence.[227]

## Miscellaneous abnormal hemoglobins

Several additional hemoglobinopathies reported from isolated areas thus far have only local significance. They are characterized by the following mobilities on the basis of paper electrophoresis at pH 8.6. Hemoglobin K moves faster than hemoglobin A and is so closely attached to the latter that it appears as its prolongation.[3,69] The abnormal component moves slower than hemoglobin J. Hemoglobin L[2] migrates between hemoglobin S and hemoglobin G. Hemoglobin N[3] moves faster than hemoglobin J but more slowly than hemoglobin H. Hemoglobin O[141] migrates between hemoglobin S and hemoglobin E. Hemoglobin Q[129,519] migrates in largest part between hemoglobin A and hemoglobin S, the remainder consisting of hemoglobin H. In contrast to patients with other hemoglobins listed in the miscellaneous category, the patient with hemoglobin Q disease suffered with a hypochromic anemia refractory to treatment.

Stanleyville I and II refer to two abnormal pigments found in the Belgian Congo that resemble HbD.[119] No sickling is noted. While on paper electrophoresis they behave like HbS or HbD, differences are found on chromatography at pH 6.

In addition to the "fast" hemoglobins (I, J, K, and N) others have been described. At pH 8.6 two abnormal hemoglobins found in Negroes have a mobility equal to HbI, Hopkins-1, and a second, Hopkins-2, comparable with HbJ.[481] Hopkins-2 has a locus on a different chromosome than that of A, S, and C, and may not be allelomorphic with these hemoglobins. Both Hopkins-1 and Hopkins-2, are mutational alterations in the alpha chain. Another fast hemoglobin, Norfolk, discovered in a purely English family, is similar but not identical with HbJ.[4] In Hb$_{Norfolk}$, glycine in position 57 in the alpha-peptide chain is replaced by aspartic acid.[13] This hemoglobin, a rare mutant, shows no physiologic abnormality. In contrast to HbM$_{Milwaukee}$, in which the new carboxyl side chain near the iron atom forms a strong, abnormal ferric complex, the carboxyl side chain of the new aspartic acid residue in hemoglobin Norfolk is apparently not in the right position to form such a complex.[241] A new minor component called hemoglobin Norfolk$_2$ has also been described.[241] Another fast moving hemoglobin in the general position of HbI on paper electrophoresis at pH 8.6, and more definitely established in starch gel electrophoresis as migrating slightly slower than Hb Bart's, has been designated as Hb$_{Mexico}$.[311] It is probably an alpha-chain variant.

HbP was first reported from Galveston, Texas, in the blood of a Negro woman,[426] and later from the Belgian Congo.[118] Its mobility lies between that of HbG and HbS on paper electrophoresis at pH 8.6.[118]

### SICKLE CELL VARIANTS
*Sickle cell–thalassemia disease (microdrepanocytic anemia)*

Sickle cell–thalassemia disease (microdrepanocytic anemia) accounts for most of the cases of sickle cell disease in white persons (usually of Greek or Italian origin), although it has been reported in American Negroes.[451] Such a patient usually inherits the gene for thalassemia from one parent and the gene for sickle cell hemoglobin from the other. Rare exceptions[454] include instances in which one parent with sickle cell–thalassemia disease (the other parent being normal) transmits both of the abnormal factors to the offspring. In another instance a normal offspring resulted from one parent with the combined disease and the other normal. Electrophoretic studies reveal the presence of sickle, normal, and occasionally fetal hemoglobin. The percentage of sickle hemoglobin ranges from 65 to 80% (in one patient 90%), which is less than the 75 to more than the 85% present in homozygous sickle cell anemia.[343] Hemoglobin analyses by electrophoresis and alkali denaturation have demonstrated that sickle cell–thalassemia disease consists of hemoglobins S, A, and F or hemoglobins S and A. Homozygous sickle cell anemia, on the other hand, consists exclusively of sickle and fetal hemoglobins, the latter in amounts of 2 to 24%.[463] The higher percentage of sickle hemoglobin in the offspring than in the parent with the trait (25 to 45% hemoglobin S) reflects the potentiating effect of the associated thalassemia gene. The disproportionate amount of hemoglobin S, despite its presence in only one parent, may also stem from the depression of normal hemoglobin synthesis by the thalassemia gene with corresponding increase of the abnormal hemoglobin. The clinical manifestations of the combined disease represent predominantly a sickle type of hemolytic anemia although of lesser severity than the homozygous sickle cell disease.

*Essential features.* The blood smear shows thin hypochromic macrocytes, poikilocytosis, marked anisocytosis, oval cells, basophilic stippling, and less frequently, normoblasts (Fig. 54). The increase in target cells exceeds that

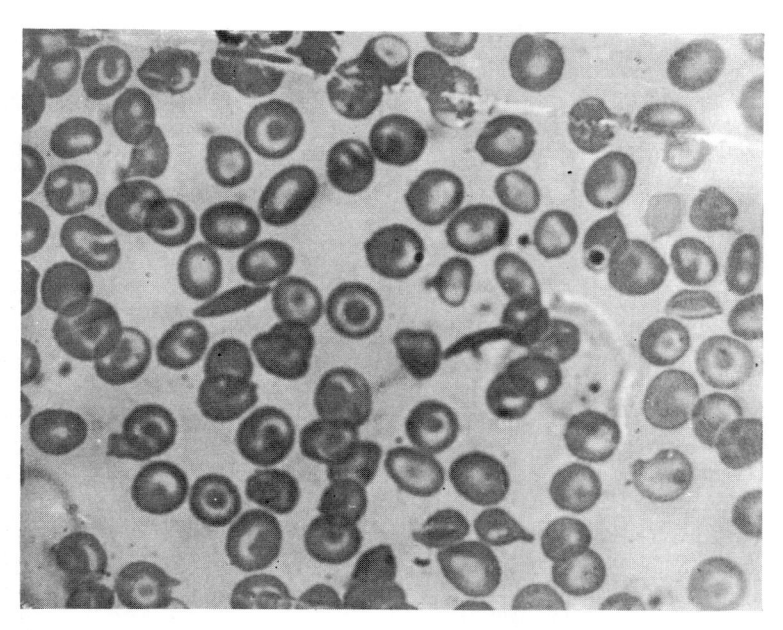

Fig. 54. Blood smear from a patient with sickle cell–thalassemia disease. Note hypochromic red cells and target and sickle cells. (×1020.)

in patients with sickle cell anemia. Sickle cells are few in number in the fixed smear but are increased at times to 100% in sickle cell preparations. Osmotic fragility is decreased. Clinically and hematologically, the disease presents itself as a moderate form of Cooley's anemia, rarely of sickle cell anemia. Anemia is moderate, with hemoglobin levels of 6 to 9 gm. per 100 ml., usually about 8 gm. per 100 ml., and red cells number approximately 3 million per cubic millimeter. Red cell constants indicate a microcytic hypochromic anemia as occurs in patients with thalassemia. The other sickle cell variants show normochromic, normocytic red cell constants as in homozygous (S-S) sickle cell anemia.

Although pulmonary dysfunction may be a factor in some patients with S-S and S-C disease, the unsaturation of arterial blood has been explained by assuming that the abnormal hemoglobins have a reduced affinity for oxygen in vivo.[416] This defect manifests itself as a displacement of the in vivo oxyhemoglobin dissociation curve to the right in patients whose red blood cells contain no hemoglobin A. Recent studies show that increased levels of intracellular 2,3-DPG are responsible for the decreased oxygen affinity.[83]

*Clinical findings.* The clinical manifestations are less severe than in patients with either sickle cell anemia or thalassemia major. Crises are rare, but abdominal, bone, and joint pain and, at times, unexplained fever occur. Severe cases are occasionally observed, as in patients with sickle cell anemia. Jaundice is mild and splenomegaly is mild to moderate. Aseptic necrosis of the head of the femur has also been reported.[395] Splenomegaly is much more common than in patients with sickle cell anemia, but not so marked as in those with thalassemia major. Hepatomegaly may be of significant degree. Patients with this disease are recognized because of anemia and, later in childhood, splenomegaly, unlike those with thalassemia major in whom these features are already advanced in the first year of life. Treatment depends upon severity. In severe cases multiple transfusions are needed and splenectomy rarely if blood requirements are high. Patients with mild cases require no treatment. Prognosis is better than in patients with homozygous sickle cell anemia.

Among American Negroes, the disease has an incidence of 0.5 to 2%.

### Sickle cell–hemoglobin C disease

The simultaneous presence of the sickle cell gene and the gene for hemoglobin C results in a type of sickle cell disease second in frequency only to classic sickle cell anemia among American Negroes.[439] The evidence derived from genetic studies strongly points to the association of these genes as alleles or close linkage upon the same chromosomes.[390]

The clinical manifestations are usually of lesser severity than those in patients with homozygous sickle cell anemia but are extremely variable, ranging from an asymptomatic state to severe disability. Some of those patients heretofore regarded as having milder cases of sickle cell anemia probably belong in the category of hemoglobin S-C disease. Crises are of lesser severity and are infrequent, hepatomegaly is usually present, and splenomegaly is moderate or marked. Fatigue, dyspnea, jaundice, migratory arthralgia, and recurrent abdominal pain may be present. Pregnancy seems to aggravate the clinical and hematologic signs and carries a greater risk than classic sickle cell (S-S) anemia. Hematuria, aseptic necrosis of the head of the femur, and splenic infarction during aerial flights have been described in hemoglobin S-C disease.[477] The course varies markedly in different patients and in individual patients.[512] Hematuria and vitreous hemorrhages occur more frequently in S-C disease than in homozygous sickle cell disease since they are complications at an age not attained by most patients with sickle cell anemia.[410] The primary pathologic changes are, however, referable to the presence of S hemoglobin.

In a group of 117 Nigerian patients with HbS-C disease a number of bizarre clinical features were based on changes consequent to marrow hyperplasia, bone infarction, and bone infections: flattening of the vertebral bodies, avascular hip changes with coxa vara, focal areas of hip disintegration, *Salmonella* arthritis, and, in children under 10 years, dactylitis.[34] Bone infarction in S-C disease resulting from vascular stasis, local anoxia, and thrombosis has been held responsible for painful symptoms of this disease. Pulmonary infarction is often heralded by bone pain. The latter, which may precede pulmonary symptoms, denotes infarction within the marrow. Small particles of necrotic marrow having gained access to a vein have been described in pulmonary vessels at autopsy.[398]

The anemia is usually of a mild, normochromic type, and the red cells vary slightly in size, being either normal or decreased in volume. The hemoglobin level rarely falls below 8 gm. per 100 ml., usually ranging from 9 to 10 gm. per 100 ml., and red cells range between 3.5 and 4.5 million per cubic millimeter. Anisocytosis and poikilocytosis are occasionally noted in patients with severe disease. Crises are associated with normoblastosis, reticulocytosis, and increased numbers of white cells in the peripheral blood. The reticulocyte count generally is normal or slightly elevated, serum bilirubin is normal, and osmotic fragility is decreased. Erythroid hyperplasia which characterizes the bone marrow is not so marked as in the bone marrow of patients with homozygous sickle cell anemia.[272] The absence of anemia in many children reflects compensatory hyperactivity of the bone marrow and is indicated by an increased reticulocyte level. Ferrokinetic measurements demonstrate a hemolytic process.[344] Sickle cells are few or absent in the blood smear, but rapid and complete sickling occurs in sealed fresh preparations. Target cells are numerous, averaging 60% (40 to 85%). This feature is of some significance since excessive numbers of target cells in the blood smear of a patient with a mild form of sickle cell anemia should arouse suspicion of the coexistence of hemoglobin C.

In this disorder in which the patient is heterozygous for both abnormal hemoglobins, each of the components may be regarded as equally divided,[423] although hemoglobin C may range from 37 to 67%. Fetal hemoglobin has been found in amounts up to 7%. Transfusions may be required in episodes of severe hemolytic anemia, and splenectomy has been employed in some of the patients in whom splenic infarction developed during flight.[478]

HbO$^{Arab}$ (alpha$_2$, beta$_2$ $^{121\ Glu\ \to\ Lys}$) was found in 25 members of four apparently unrelated Negro families in the West Indian island of Jamaica.[331] In each family the propositus had HbS-O disease. Two cases had been mistakenly diagnosed as HbS-C disease. Two persons heterozygous for both HbC and HbO$^{Arab}$ were found in these families and HbO$^{Arab}$ beta thalassemia in another relative. Oxygen dissociation studies on red cells containing HbS-O showed a lowered oxygen affinity comparable to that found in homozygous sickle cell anemia and outside the range for subjects with HbS-C disease. The clinical course and symptomatology of HbS-O disease are more severe than those of HbS-C disease. In the laboratory HbS-O disease may be mistaken for HbS-C disease in areas where HbS-C disease is expected to occur. Techniques other than filter paper electrophoresis, such as starch-gel electrophoresis, may be required to identify HbO$^{Arab}$.

### Sickle cell–hereditary spherocytosis

Sicklemia in combination with congenital spherocytosis has been observed with improvement of the anemia following splenectomy.[116] Sickling remained unaffected with a residual blood pattern showing the sickle cell trait (hemoglobin A-S). Each of the constitutional red cell defects (spherocytes and sickling) could be traced to individual patients.[260,320,477] Although the genes for sickling and spherocytosis are nonallelic, in one of our patients both defects were inherited from the same parent.

Hereditary spherocytosis should be considered in Negro patients with sickle cell trait when hemolytic anemia of any degree is demonstrated. The occurrence of cholelithiasis, splenomegaly, and moderate anemia with sickle cell trait led to the diagnosis of associated hereditary spherocytosis.[541] Symptoms were relieved following splenectomy and cholecystostomy.

### Hereditary spherocytosis, sickling, and thalassemia

An American Negro family has been described[98] in whom was found the genes responsible for three inherited abnormalities of the erythrocytes: spherocytosis, a thalassemia-like trait, and the sickling phenomenon. One patient was the possessor of the three abnormal genes. Two (spherocytosis and sickling) were observed in examining the blood, whereas the presence of the third (thalassemia) was inferred from its occurrence in two of the patient's children. The $A_2$ hemoglobin in this family was not increased. Analysis of the family pedigree suggests an independent and nonallelic segregation of the genes for each condition. Four cases of hereditary spherocytosis associated with sickle cell trait in a Negro family have been reported.[417] Splenectomy was performed in three of the subjects with alleviation of the anemia. This study suggested that the genes for spherocytosis and sickling are nonallelic and are not closely linked.

### Sickle cell–hemoglobin D disease

The patients with sickle cell–hemoglobin D disease are white persons in whom the coexistence of hemoglobins S and D results in a moderately severe hemolytic process similar to that observed in patients with sickle cell anemia.[13,479] However, one patient reveals the sickle cell trait and the other the trait of hemoglobin D. The blood count reveals a moderate anemia, with a hemoglobin level of about 8 to 9 gm. per 100 ml. of blood, and a red cell count of approximately 2.5 million per cubic millimeter. The peripheral blood may show poikilocytosis, anisocytosis, polychromasia, and occasionally nucleated red cells. In two reported patients[498] the red cells were increased in size. A few partially sickled cells are found in the fixed smear. With sickling tests the holly leaf or slow variety of sickling occurs rather than the filamentous or rapid variety found in patients with classic sickle cell anemia. Target cells are infrequent. Up to 12% fetal hemoglobin has been found. The liver and spleen may not be palpable or both organs may be greatly enlarged. Sickle cell–hemoglobin D disease has been reported in an 18-year-old Negro male.[326]

The mobility of hemoglobins S and D on starch gel electrophoresis at pH 8.6 is similar. Differentiation is possible on agar gel electrophoresis at pH 6.0. Furthermore, hemoglobin D is more soluble than hemoglobin S in a hypertonic saline solution.

## THALASSEMIA VARIANTS
### Thalassemia–hemoglobin C disease

Thalassemia–hemoglobin C disease usually occurs in Negroes and exceptionally in white persons. The anemia varies in intensity; it may be mild, rarely severe—in which case a hemoglobin level of 7 to 9.5 gm. per 100 ml. is observed. In the latter instance it runs the course of a severe chronic hypochromic microcytic anemia, although milder than that in patients with the homozygous thalassemia disease. Usually, however, there is no anemia and reticulocyte count is not elevated. Osmotic fragility may be normal, but in a few cases increased resistance to hypotonic saline solution has been noted. The blood smear shows many target cells (20 to 60%), anisocytosis and poikilocytosis, and an appreciable number of microspherocytes (Fig. 55).[151,555] Since the percentage of target cells in patients with severe Cooley's anemia is usually less than 10%, the finding of an unusually large percentage of these cells should lead one to suspect a hemoglobin variant of this disease. Reticulocytes number 2 to 5%. Fetal hemoglobin is not elevated. Hepatosplenomegaly is either absent or moderate. The disease results from the interac-

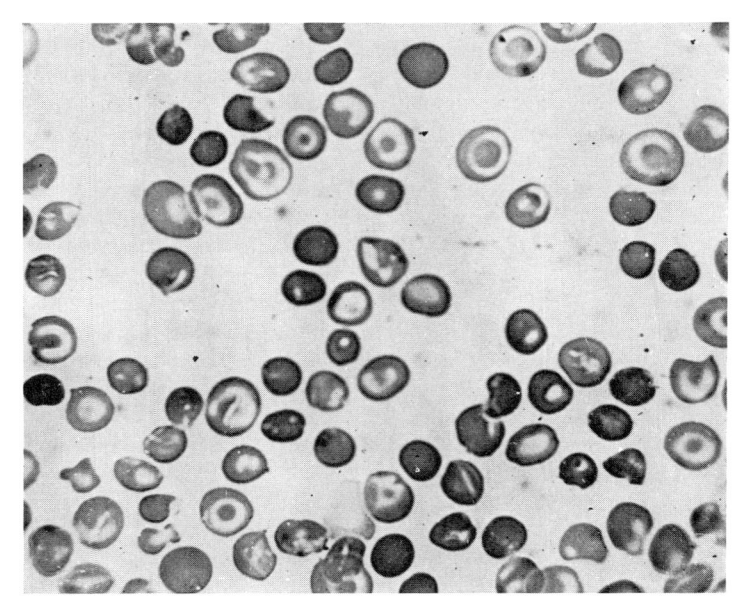

Fig. 55. Blood smear from patient with thalassemia–hemoglobin C disease. Note large number of target cells and microspherocytes. (From Erlandson, M., Smith, C. H., and Schulman, I.: Thalassemia–hemoglobin C disease in white siblings, Pediatrics 17:740, 1956.)

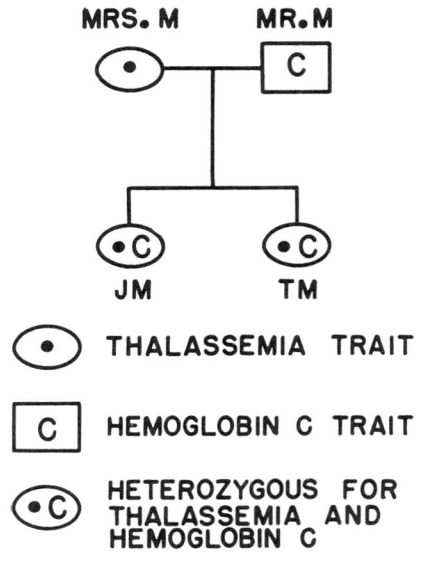

Fig. 56. Example of a family pedigree showing genetic transmission of double heterozygosity for two different sets of genes—thalassemia and hemoglobin C. (From Smith, C. H.: The abnormal hemoglobins: clinical and hematologic aspects, J. Pediat. 50:91, 1957; based on data from Erlandson, M., Smith, C. H., and Schulman, I.: Thalassemia–hemoglobin C disease in white siblings, Pediatrics 17:740, 1956.)

tion of the genes for sickling and thalassemia inherited from respective parents bearing the trait (Fig. 56). In this combination, also, hemoglobin C usually is present in an amount greatly in excess of that found in the parent and reflects the effect of coexistence with the thalassemia gene.[151,457] In the reported patients[151,457,555] hemoglobin C ranged from 29 to 93%.

*Thalassemia—hemoglobin E disease*

Thalassemia–hemoglobin E disease[93,499] represents a severe hemolytic syndrome simulating thalassemia major so closely as to be indistinguishable from it except that the course may be somewhat milder. Most cases of the combined disease have their onset in infancy, although medical attention may not be sought until adolescence. Fatigue, dyspnea on effort, joint pains, pallor, and jaundice occur frequently. The abdomen is markedly protuberant, the extremities are wasted, and jaundice varies in severity. Splenomegaly may be massive, and hepatomegaly is less marked. The patients are of small stature and present a facial appearance with mongoloid features similar to those of patients with classic Cooley's anemia.

Hematologic examination reveals a microcytic, hypochromic, hemolytic anemia, with markedly lowered hemoglobin and red cell values. The reticulocyte count is elevated. The blood smear coincides with that of the patients with the correspondingly severe Cooley's anemia. In some patients the stained blood smear reveals target cells numbering 5 to 20% of the red cells and a small number of spherocytes. Although osmotic fragility starts in more concentrated solutions of sodium chloride than is normal, fragility is not complete until the lowest dilutions are reached. Nucleated red cells are prominent in the blood smear. The bone marrow, like that in patients with thalassemia major, shows marked erythrocytic hyperplasia. Hemoglobin analysis shows a mixture of hemoglobins E and F, with the former comprising 60 to 80% of the total and fetal hemoglobin the remainder. When complete studies have been available, one parent possessed hemoglobin E, and the other showed hematologic evidences of the thalassemia trait.

Three patients in two Turkish families showed HbE to range from 83 to 87.5%, HbF from 6.5 to 10%, the remainder consisting of HbA.[6] Thalassemia–hemoglobin E disease is considered characteristic of peoples in southeastern Asia. Only sporadic cases are found outside this region. It is believed that the Turks emigrated for several centuries from central Asia to Asia Minor and intermarriage with the people of India and the Far East occurred during this period. Hemoglobin E trait was probably transmitted to the Greek population by admixture with the Turks during the period of the Ottoman Empire.

Transfusions are necessary in many of the younger children, but for the entire group they are not so urgent as in patients with thalassemia major. Splenectomy in many of these patients has been of benefit in promoting growth and better general health.

*Thalassemia and persistent fetal hemoglobin (thal-F heterozygotes)*

In a family in which persistent fetal hemoglobin and beta-chain thalassemia coexisted, four individuals inherited both abnormalities (thal-F heterozygotes) and demonstrated 67 to 70% fetal hemoglobin and 30 to 33% HbA.[538] The blood smears showed microcytosis, poikilocytosis, anisocytosis, and target cells, but revealed no significant anemia. Fetal hemoglobin was quite uniformly distributed among the red cells in the thal-F cases. Homozygous thalassemia with the same quantitative proportions of fetal and adult hemoglobin would show profound anemia and irregular distribution of fetal hemoglobin among the red cells.[101] The mild hemolytic disorder in the thal-F heterozygotes is presumably due to thalassemia, since the homozygote for hereditary persistence of fetal hemoglobin gives no evidence of increased blood destruction.[538]

Variants of thalassemia with hemoglobins G and H are described elsewhere in this book.

*Thalassemia–Lepore hemoglobin*

In the patient with the Lepore trait, the blood picture resembles that of the patient with the trait of thalassemia (slight hypochromia, microcytosis, and leptocytosis) except for a low content of $A_2$ hemoglobin. The abnormal (Lepore) hemoglobin is detected by starch electrophoresis and not by paper electrophoresis. At a pH of 8.6 it migrates in the region of sickle hemoglobin. It represents 10 to 12% of the total pigment. In the cases reported,[180] patients inherited the Lepore and the thalassemia traits from the respective parents. The Lepore trait-thalassemia trait interaction results in a moderately severe hemolytic anemia with marrow hypertrophy, secondary bone changes, and moderate splenomegaly, often not so extreme as in patients with thalassemia major. The hemoglobin level ranges between 6 and 10 gm. per 100 ml., and the erythrocyte morphology resembles that of thalassemia, consisting of marked microcytosis, hypochromia, and many target cells.[374] Frequently the combination of Hb Lepore with beta thalassemia results in severe disability which clinically and on routine hematologic examination closely resembles beta thalassemia major. The hemolysates, however, will show Hb Lepore 5 to 10%, with 70 to 95% HbF; $HbA_2$ is usually reduced.[299]

Barkhan and associates[28] noted in a case of the Lepore trait that on starch block electrophoresis the extra hemoglobin migrated a shade faster than HbS but behind HbF. The major component was HbA. In their case, the abnormal component constituted 9%, $HbA_2$ was low (1.7% of the total hemoglobin), and no fetal hemoglobin was found. This hemoglobin pattern, negative sickling test, and a thalassemia-like blood picture are characteristic of the Lepore trait. The Lepore heterozygotes are clinically well. The homozygous form of hemoglobin Lepore is associated with a severe hemolytic state with large amounts of HbF and the absence of HbA and $HbA_2$.[17,165] In the homozygote state reported by Duma and associates,[130] Hb Lepore was found in the quantity of 8.6%, the rest of the hemoglobin being HbF with a small quantity of HbA. No $HbA_2$ was present. The combination of sickle cell hemoglobin and hemoglobin Lepore was observed in two members of an Italian family. In the same family in a 6-year-old child hemoglobin Lepore was combined with the thalassemia trait. This child, who was initially diagnosed as thalassemia major and later splenectomized, revealed a small amount of hemoglobin Lepore and 17% of fetal hemoglobin.[455]

Chemical studies of the hemoglobin Lepore initially indicated that it resembled the hemoglobin $A_2$ molecule (alpha$_2$ delta$_2$).[181] Recent studies have clarified the structure and genetics of the hemoglobin Lepore. It must be remembered that the synthesis of the four polypeptide chains (alpha, beta, gamma, and delta) entering into the structure of the three normal human hemoglobins (adult, fetal, and $A_2$) is controlled by four separate structural loci, two of which (the beta and delta loci) are closely linked. Baglioni[17] showed that the N-terminal section of the nonalpha chain of hemoglobin Lepore corresponds to the N-terminal of the delta chain, while the C-terminal part corresponds to the C-terminal of the beta chain. The Lepore trait may be regarded as an abnormality in the "structural gene" in which there is coexistence in a single person of beta thalassemia and of an abnormal hemoglobin (hemoglobin Lepore), the latter containing a chain made up of both the delta and beta chains. Hemoglobin Lepore therefore contains, besides two alpha chains, two polypeptide chains containing sections of both the delta and beta chains. These findings have been confirmed in another study.[28] Baglioni[17] suggested that the composite peptide chain arises as a result of a nonhomologous crossing over between the beta and delta genes.

In the large series of Hb Lepore carriers (56 of 115 members of nine families investigated), only a small number of them originate from the focus where there is a high frequency of thalassemias, whereas the larger number are from the central and western part of Macedonia.[130]

*Thalassemia trait with simultaneous inheritance of one $A_2$-thalassemia gene and one F-thalassemia gene*

Two thalassemia heterozygotes have been described, one of which is designated as $A_2$-thalassemia (hemoglobin $A_2$ is elevated with normal or only slightly elevated values of fetal hemoglobin) and the other F-thalassemia trait (hemoglobin $A_2$ is normal in amount and fetal hemoglobin elevated). The latter may show the excessive amounts of fetal hemoglobin approximating those found in hereditary persistence of fetal hemoglobin (high-F syndrome). The genetic combination of F-thalassemia trait and $A_2$-thalassemia has been reported in a Greek family. In this family fifteen out of twenty-nine direct descendants were found to have thalassemia trait in association with large quantities of fetal hemoglobin (8 to 36%).[175] All showed minimal alterations of red cell morphology.

In two brothers these two types of thalassemia trait combined to produce a syndrome of minimal anemia with little or no hemoglobin A in the peripheral blood (fetal hemoglobin 94 to 98.8% and $A_2$ 1.1 to 1.2%, respectively). A significant feature of the combination of $A_2$-thalassemia and F-thalassemia is the extraordinary concentration of hemoglobin F present. With minimal anemia it parallels in the amount of fetal hemoglobin the severe anemia of homozygous thalassemia.

The high fetal hemoglobin in this family could be differentiated from the hereditary persistence of fetal hemoglobin in which microcytosis and significant aberrations in morphology are absent. Furthermore, the distribution of fetal hemoglobin among the red cells in the individuals with the combined $A_2$-thalassemia gene and F-thalassemia was characteristically heterogeneous as compared with the uniform distribution of increased amounts of fetal hemoglobin among the red cells in hereditary persistence of fetal hemoglobin.

## HEREDITARY HEINZ BODY ANEMIAS—UNSTABLE HEMOGLOBIN HEMOLYTIC ANEMIAS

Hereditary Heinz body anemia is a mild chronic hemolytic anemia, usually diagnosed by the presence of large inclusions in the red cells resembling Heinz bodies following splenectomy.[112,193] The salient features are a hemolytic anemia presenting from infancy in the heterozygote, and the presence of red cell inclusion bodies (Heinz bodies) from shortly after birth not necessarily associated with drug administration. For this reason the diseases in this group are often described as hereditary or congenital Heinz body anemias. They are inherited in a mendelian pattern with presentation in the heterozygote. There is no record of the homozygote with this condition.[251] The clinical effects of the abnormal gene may be mild to severe.

The congenital Heinz body hemolytic anemias have been summarized by Jacob[251] as consisting of the following features: "a chronic hemolytic anemia, the presence of circulating red cells with inclusion (Heinz) bodies, more obvious after splenectomy and frequently the excretion of urine darkened by accumulation of pyrrolic pigments termed dipyrolles." Regardless of their instability in vivo, the unstable hemoglobins are all precipitated by incubation at 50° C. for brief periods, and in doing so a mass of typical coccoid Heinz bodies results. Heme loss occurs concomitantly with the instability of hemoglobin. The disease is most often transmitted as an autosomal dominant trait. Actual heme depletion has been demonstrated in many of these hemoglobins during their precipitation into Heinz bodies. During the early phases of denaturation of hemoglobin by phenylhydrazine, Heinz bodies are generated in the interior of red cells. The electron microscope study of Rifkind and Danon[407] demonstrated that Heinz bodies later coalesce, migrate, and finally attach themselves to the red cell membrane. It was also shown that Heinz body–containing red cells become trapped in the spleen while passing through the small apertures in basement membrane separating the cords from sinusoids.[407]

It has only recently been realized that from the heterogeneous group of the hereditary Heinz body anemias one disorder could be identified possessing definitive characteristics which was designated as the unstable hemoglobin hemolytic anemias. A dark and sometimes mahogany-brown to even black urine is due to abnormal dipyrrolmethene pigments, probably derived from degraded hemoglobin, and liberated into the bloodstream as a result of intravascular hemolysis. A mild, chronic, hemolytic anemia often dates back to childhood. Jaundice may be continuous and anemia may be slight or marked. Prior to splenectomy a large number of red cells show punctate basophilia. In nonsplenectomized cases small Heinz bodies develop in blood incubated for 24 to 48 hours under sterile conditions. Splenectomy provides no clear clinical benefit, but does seem to improve the red cell life-span and in some cases results in a decreased transfusion requirement. After splenectomy, marked anisocytosis, contracted and crenated red cells, and Heinz bodies make their appearance. Such mutant unstable hemoglobins can also be recognized by their tendency to flocculate when hemolysates are heated to 50° C. for brief periods.[76] The globin of the unstable hemoglobins precipitates because it is no longer stabilized by firm heme-globin bonding.[76] The instability of the hemoglobin molecule leads to an accumulation of methemoglobin[76] even when a normal metabolic mechanism for its reduction is present. The clinical effects of the abnormal gene may be mild to severe. The disease is hereditary and based on a dominant gene of varying penetrance.

Jacob and Winterhalter[250] found that mutant, unstable hemoglobins precipitate as Heinz bodies in circulating red blood cells, resulting in their premature hemolysis. Heme-containing alpha chains accumulate in solution during Heinz body formation, but heme loss occurs predominantly from mutant beta chains which then precipitate.[250] This mechanism of Heinz body formation applies to most but not all unstable hemoglobins. The heme-depleted polypeptide chains in this disease are partially uncoiled and form the bulk of

Heinz body precipitates. Presumably the resulting excessively freed hemes are excreted as the dark urinary "dipyrrolic" pigments characteristic of congenital Heinz body hemolytic anemia.[250,252] The striking feature is the presence of inclusion bodies in 60 to 80% of the red cells of patients[76] following splenectomy. The presence of an enlarged spleen may give rise to secondary thrombocytopenia.[76] Certain amino acid substitutions occurring in the globin polypeptide chains in the vicinity of the heme pocket diminish the avidity of globin for its hemes.[358] This feature is illustrated in the following unstable hemoglobins.[250]

Köln—$\beta^{98}$ valine ⟶ methionine
Zürich—$\beta^{63}$ histidine ⟶ arginine
Hammersmith—$\beta^{42}$ phenylalanine ⟶ serine
Genoa—$\beta^{28}$ leucine ⟶ proline
Sydney—$\beta^{67}$ valine ⟶ alanine
Santa Ana—$\beta^{88}$ leucine ⟶ proline
Seattle—$\beta^{76}$ alanine ⟶ glutamic acid

In the light of recent studies of the enzymopathies involving the hexose monophosphate shunt and the unstable hemoglobins, both of which are characterized by Heinz body inclusions in erythrocytes, the number of cases of idiopathic Heinz body anemia have markedly decreased. There are, however, hereditary Heinz body anemias which refer to a condition that cannot be included in either of these categories and that belong to one of the as yet undifferentiated anemias which can best be characterized as idiopathic Heinz body anemia.[252]

Heinz bodies were produced experimentally in the red cells of rats fed diets containing phenacetin and acetic-4-chloranilide, the contaminant found in phenacetin.[427] These erythrocytes containing Heinz bodies were removed from the circulation predominantly by the spleen, and in splenectomized rats the Kupffer cells were the major sites of red cell sequestration. It was suggested that the sequence of red cell destruction seems to be that after the red cell containing the Heinz body is engaged in the Kupffer cells, it is hemolyzed within single membrane-bound structures (lysosomes, phagocytic vacuoles). The only indication that phagocytosis and destruction of red cells have occurred is the presence of single membrane-bound structures containing hemosiderin, at times associated with myelin figures.

In another study the fate of Heinz body-containing red blood cells in the spleen was studied with an electron microscope.[291] Marked distribution of red blood cells occurred within the cords of Billroth and the sinusoids, as the erythrocytes passed among relatively fixed structures of the red pulp and the sinusoidal basement membrane. Splenic macrophages were capable of "pitting" Heinz bodies from erythrocytes. "Pitting" was accomplished by red pulp macrophages engulfing the Heinz body regions of red blood cells. Within phagocytic cells conversion of ingested red blood cells to hemosiderin occurred within lysosomes.

From the list of approximately twenty presently identified unstable hemoglobins,[76] several of the well documented will be reviewed. As was stated, many of the variants (unstable hemoglobins) have amino acid substitutions in the region of the heme pocket. Such substitutions weaken the heme-globin linkage, since heme provides stability to the globin moiety of the molecule. The globin denatures only if the heme is allowed to escape.[76] The abnormal hemoglobin is put under further stress in some cases when methemoglobin-forming drugs are given. The unstable hemoglobin is identified in the laboratory when the hemolysate is heated to 50° C. for brief periods and flocculation occurs. Unstable hemoglobin usually amounts to only 10 to 30% of the total hemoglobin in the circulating red cells in affected heterozygous subjects.[544] Hemoglobin Hammersmith differs in being present in large amounts (35 to 40%) of the hemoglobin as determined by heat instability. The large number of Heinz bodies following splenectomy can be explained by the function of the spleen in removing inclusions from red cells without necessarily destroying the blood cell harboring these bodies.[107]

### Hemoglobin Zürich

Hemoglobin Zürich represents an inherited anomaly of hemoglobin in which hemolytic episodes follow the ingestion of sulfonamide. Severe hemolytic anemia may be accompanied by the development of erythrocytic inclusion bodies. The abnormality in Hb Zürich has been identified as a substitution of arginine for histidine in position 63 of the beta chain.[345] There appears to be no evidence of any complex formation of the arginine side chain with the iron atom of the heme group. Hb Zürich is therefore not to be considered as being harmful in the same sense as a hemoglobin of the M type abnormality.[241]

In Hb Zürich 25% of the hemoglobin is unstable but of a relatively less marked variety.

In this disorder the hemolysis is milder, probably due to the position and size of the amino acid substitution and its interaction with the amount of unstable hemoglobin synthesized.[544]

This hemoglobin moves more slowly than HbA, its electrophoretic mobility being intermediate between HbA and HbS.[172] The abnormal hemoglobin was observed in fifteen members over four generations of a large Swiss family. An abnormality in the beta chain tends to shorten the red cell survival in the heterozygote. No homozygotes are known. This anomaly was discovered during the search for an intrinsic red cell defect that could account for a severe hemolytic anemia after sulfanilamide therapy. The anomaly is harmless, unless the red cells are challenged by sulfonamide drugs or related compounds. The severe hemolytic episodes are characterized by the appearance of unusually large inclusion bodies, visible with both supravital and Giemsa stains. The mechanism of action is unknown. There are no defects in the erythrocyte enzymes, although they resemble the hemolytic changes produced by glucose-6-phosphate dehydrogenase deficiency. The drugs affecting hemoglobin Zürich–containing erythrocytes induce the formation of Heinz bodies and consequent hemolysis of the cells of all ages, including reticulocytes.

A second family with Hb Zürich was discovered in Maryland and was revealed by hemolytic crises when sulfonamides were administered.[404] It was determined that a crises was not due to mediation of erythrocyte glucose-6-phosphate dehydrogenase deficiency or to HbH disease. In this family six members from three generations were found to be heterozygous for Hb Zürich. In vivo and in vitro studies showed that Hb Zürich is synthesized at a rate almost equal to that of HbA, although its concentration in blood is less than half that of HbA, suggesting preferential loss or destruction of Hb Zürich. Precipitates of hemoglobin appeared in red cell hemolysates exposed to brilliant cresyl blue and other redox dyes. Although the same changes occurred with HbA, the rate of precipitation was much less.

*Hemoglobin Köln disease*

Hb Köln is perhaps the most thoroughly investigated of the unstable hemoglobins and probably the most common of this group of diseases.[261] The abnormal fraction of the hemolysate (about 20%) shows the presence of the substitution of a valine residue by methionine in position 98 of the beta chain. The small amount of hemoglobin Köln synthesized has been found to be due to a deficiency in the synthesis of $\beta$ Köln-chains.[544] In the majority of cases the disease presents as a mild hemolytic anemia which is well compensated. Fatigue, jaundice, and the occasional passage of dark urine commonly occur. Attacks of deep jaundice might be accompanied by fever and anemia. Splenomegaly may account for a secondary thrombocytopenia. The great majority of the red cells are normal in appearance with some hypochromia, a few irregularly contracted cells, and macrospherocytes. On starch gel electrophoresis a smeared band appears behind HbA. On in vitro incubation there is increased hemolysis which is reduced upon the addition of glucose.[76] There is a slight reduction in the osmotic fragility of the red cells. Five members of a family have been reported[261] who had a hemolytic anemia attributable to Hb Köln. It became apparent that they were a branch of a larger family with the same disorder. Splenectomy[544] provides clinical improvement in some cases. Although the results are often disappointing it finds a definite place in the therapy of hereditary anemia with unstable hemoglobins, including Hb Köln disease.[544]

Although most cases of Hb Köln disease have demonstrated an autosomal dominant mode of inheritance, the occurrence of the disorder as a spontaneous mutation has been reported.[330a] The increased oxygen affinity (low p50 $O_2$) of Hb Köln[115a] contributes to the well-compensated hemolytic state observed in patients in whom decreased oxygen delivery to the tissues results in increased erythropoietin production, enhanced erythropoiesis, and often normal or near-normal values of red cell mass.

*Hemoglobin Seattle*

Mild to moderate chronic hemolytic anemia in a mother and her two sons was found to be associated with the presence of about 40% abnormal hemoglobin of rapid electrophoretic mobility diagnosed as Hb Seattle.[230] Hb Seattle was found to be unstable in vitro, due to a replacement of alanine by glutamic acid at position 76 of the beta chain. The hemolytic anemia is likely caused by the presence of this unstable hemoglobin. Studies on the oxygen equilibrium and erythropoietic responses in patients with Hb Seattle indicate that a greater proportion of oxygen per red cell is released to the tissues and accordingly a lessened erythropoietic response would be expected.[492] The anemia in patients with Hb Seattle is mainly caused by the lessened secretion of erythropoietin due to the increased release of oxygen by the abnormal pigment. It is of interest that the mother was not jaundiced, did not pass red or brown urine, and had impalpable liver and spleen.

*Other unstable hemoglobins*

The hemolytic anemia is mild in Hb Sydney disease, severe in Hb Hammersmith disease, and moderate in Hb Santa Ana disease.[366] Another unstable hemoglobin, Gun Hill,[401] has been reported in two members of a Caucasian family who were heterozygous for the abnormal hemoglobin. Evidence of mild chronic hemolysis was found in both individuals. There is a deletion of five amino acids in the beta chains of Hb Gun Hill. This results in impaired heme binding and the abnormal molecule lacks half the expected number of heme groups.

## HEMOGLOBIN VARIANTS ASSOCIATED WITH ALTERED OXYGEN AFFINITY

A number of hemoglobin variants have been reported exhibiting increased oxygen affinity. They release a smaller proportion of oxygen per red cell to the tissues when compared with the normal. These hemoglobins are Hb Chesapeake, Capetown, Yakima, Kempsey, Hiroshima, and Rainier and have all been associated with polycythemia. Leukocytosis, thrombocytosis, and splenomegaly have been absent.[532] The erythrocytosis is benign since the clinical syndrome has been found in well subjects who were beyond middle age.[391] The first of these was reported by Charache and associates,[86] who noted the association of erythrocytosis with hemoglobin Chesapeake, an alpha-chain variant which was found to have increased oxygen affinity. Hb Capetown is also an alpha-chain variant; the remainder—Yakima, Kempsey, Hiroshima, and Rainier—are beta-chain variants. These individuals release less oxygen to the tissues at normal hemoglobin levels. The resulting hypoxia stimulates erythropoietin production and resulting polycythemia. The "shift to the left" of the oxygen dissociation curve is similar to the curve obtained from newborn infants.[532] There are moderate increases of hematocrit ranging from 45 to 55%, with a proportionate rise in the red cell count and hemoglobin levels. The similarity in the blood picture by these different hemoglobin variants depends on the position of their particular amino acid substitutions.[532]

In contrast, studies on oxygen equilibrium in patients with Hb Seattle indicate decreased oxygen affinity, and a greater proportion of oxygen per red cell is released to the tissues.[230] Measured erythropoietin levels in patients with Hb Seattle were minimal for the levels of their hematocrit. It appears that the increased availability of oxygen in these patients permits normal tissue oxygenation at a hemoglobin level that is lower than normal.

Hemoglobin Kansas is a beta-chain variant in which cyanosis is caused by the markedly increased dissociation of oxygen from hemoglobin with a resulting increased concentration of deoxyhemoglobin.[391,397] This form of cyanosis does not result in tissue hypoxia and is of cosmetic importance only.

## REFERENCES

1. Aach, R., and Kissane, J.: A patient with sickle cell anemia surviving forty-eight years, Amer. J. Med. 48:226, 1970.
2. Ager, J. A. M., and Lehmann, H.: Haemoglobin L, a new haemoglobin found in a Punjabi Hindu, Brit. Med. J. 2:142, 1957.
3. Ager, J. A. M., and Lehmann, H.: Observations on some "fast" haemoglobins: K, J, N, and "Barts," Brit. Med. J. 1:929, 1958.
4. Ager, J. A. M., and Lehmann, H.: Haemoglobin "Norfolk," Brit. Med. J. 2:539, 1958.
5. Åkerblom, O., deVerdier, C. H., Garby, L., and Högman, C.: Restoration of defective oxygen-transport function of stored red blood cells by addition of inosine, Scand. J. Clin. Lab. Invest. 21:245, 1968.
6. Aksoy, M., Cetingil, A. I., Kocabalkan, N., Sestakof, D., Aladag, T., Secer, F., and Bostanci, N.: Thalassemia-hemoglobin E disease in Turkey, with hypersplenism in one case, Amer. J. Med. 34:851, 1963.
7. Allen, J. C., and Kunkel, H. G.: Antibodies to genetic types of gamma globulin after multiple transfusions, Science 139:418, 1963.
8. Allen, T. D.: Sickle cell disease and hematuria; a report of 20 cases, J. Urol. 91:177, 1964.
9. Allison, A. C.: Protection afforded by sickle-cell trait against subtertian malarial infection, Brit. Med. J. 1:290, 1954.

10. Allison, A. C.: Notation for hemoglobin types and genes controlling their synthesis, Science **122**:640, 1955.
11. Alperin, J. B.: Folic acid deficiency complicating sickle cell anemia; a study on the response to titrated doses of folic acid, Arch. Intern. Med. **120**:298, 1967.
12. Anderson, R., Cassell, M., Mullinax, G. L., and Chaplin, H., Jr.: Effect of normal cells on viscosity of sickle-cell blood, in vitro studies and report of six years' experience with a prophylactic porgram of "partial exchange transfusions," Arch. Intern. Med. **111**:286, 1963.
13. Arends, T., Layrisse, M., and Rincon, A. R.: Sickle cell—haemoglobin D disease in a Portuguese child, Acta Haemat. **22**:118, 1959.
14. Astaldi, G., Ronanelli, E. G., Bernardelli, E., and Strosselli, E.: An abnormal substance present in the erythroblasts of thalassemia major; cytochemical investigations, Acta Haemat. **12**:145, 1954.
15. Atwater, J., Schwartz, I. R., Erslev, A. J., Montgomery, T. L., and Tocantins, L. M.: Sickling of erythrocytes in patient with thalassemia-hemoglobin-I-disease, New Eng. J. Med. **263**:1215, 1960.
16. Avery, M. E.: Hereditary elliptocytosis and hemoglobin C trait; a report of two cases, Bull. Johns Hopkins Hosp. **98**:184, 1956.
17. Baglioni, C.: The fusion of two peptide chains in hemoglobin Lepore and its interpretation as a genetic deletion, Proc. Nat. Acad. Sci. **48**:1880, 1962.
18. Baglioni, C.: A chemical study of hemoglobin Norfolk, J. Biol. Chem. **237**:69, 1962.
19. Bailey, I. S., and Prankerd, T. A. J.: Studies in thalassemia, Brit. J. Haemat. **4**:150, 1958.
20. Baird, R. L., Weiss, D., Ferguson, A., French, J., and Scott, R.: Studies in sickle cell anemia. XXI. Clinico-pathological aspects of neurological manifestations, Pediatrics **34**:92, 1964.
21. Ballard, M. S., Radel, E., Sakhadeo, S., and Schorr, J. B.: A new diagnostic test for hemoglobin S, J. Pediat. **76**:117, 1970.
22. Bank, A., Braverman, A. J., and Marks, P. A.: Globin chain-synthesis in thalassemia, Ann. N. Y. Acad. Sci. **165**:231, 1969.
23. Banks, L. O., and Scott, R. B.: Thalassemia in Negroes; report of a case of Cooley's anemia in a Negro child, Pediatrics **11**:622, 1953.
24. Bannerman, R. M., Callender, S. T., Hardisty, R. M., and Smith, R. S.: Iron absorption in thalassemia, Brit. J. Haemat. **10**:490, 1964.
25. Bannerman, R. M., Callender, S. T., and Williams, D. L.: Effect of desferrioxamine and DTPA in iron overload, Brit. Med. J. **2**:1573, 1962.
26. Bannerman, R. M., Grinstein, M., and Moore, C. V.: Haemoglobin synthesis in thalassemia; in vitro studies, Brit. J. Haemat. **5**:102, 1959.
27. Bannerman, R. M., Keusch, G., Kreimer-Birnbaum, M., Vance, V. K., and Vaughan, S.: Thalassemia intermedia, with iron overload, cardiac failure, diabetes mellitus, hypopituitarism and prophyrinuria, Amer. J. Med. **42**:476, 1967.
28. Barkhan, P., Stevenson, M. E., and Pinker, G.: Haemoglobin Lepore trait; an analysis of the abnormal haemoglobin, Brit. J. Haemat. **10**:437, 1964.
29. Barnett, H. L., and Bernstein, J.: Clinical pathological conference, J. Pediat. **73**:936, 1968.
30. Barreras, L., and Diggs, L. W.: Bicarbonates, pH and percentage of sickled cells in venous blood of patients with sickle cell crisis, Amer. J. Med. Sci. **247**:710, 1964.
31. Barrett, A. M.: Special form of erythrocyte possessing increased resistance to hypotonic saline, J. Path. Bact. **46**:603, 1938.
32. Barrett-Connor, E.: Cholelithiasis in sickle anemia, Amer. J. Med. **45**:889, 1968.
33. Barrett-Connor, E.: Sickle cell disease and viral hepatitis, Ann. Intern. Med. **69**:517, 1968.
34. Barton, C. J., and Cockshott, W. P.: Bone changes in hemoglobin SC disease, Amer. J. Roentgen. **88**:523, 1962.
35. Baty, J. M., Blackfan, K. D., and Diamond, L. K.: Blood studies in infants and in children; erythroblastic anemia, Amer. J. Dis. Child. **43**:667, 1932.
36. Beard, M. E. J., Necheles, T. F., and Allen, D. M.: Intensive transfusion therapy in thalassemia major, Pediatrics **40**:912, 1967.
37. Beaven, G. H., Ellis, M. J., and White, J. C.: Studies on human foetal haemoglobin. I. Detection and estimation, Brit. J. Haemat. **6**:1, 1960.
38. Beaven, G. H., Stevens, B. L., Drance, N., and White, J. C.: Occurrence of haemoglobin H in leukaemia, Nature **199**:1297, 1963.
39. Beaven, G. H., Stevens, B. L., Ellis, M. J., White, J. C., Bernstock, L., Masters, P., and Stapleton, T.: Studies in foetal haemoglobin. IV. Thalassemia-like conditions in British families, Brit. J. Haemat. **10**:1, 1964.
40. Beet, E. A.: Sickle-cell disease in the balovale district of Northern Rhodesia, E. African M. J. **23**:75, 1946.
41. Benesch, R.: How do small molecules do great things? New Eng. J. Med. **280**:1179, 1969.
42. Benesch, R., Benesch, R. E., and Yu, C. D.: Reciprocal binding of oxygen and diphosphoglycerate by human hemoglobin, Proc. Nat. Acad. Sci. **59**:526, 1968.

43. Benesch, R. E., Ranney, H. M., Benesch, R., and Smith, G. M.: Chemistry of the Bohr effect. II. Some properties of hemoglobin H, J. Biol. Chem. 236:2926, 1961.
43a. Benz, E. J., Jr., and Forget, B. G.: Defect in messenger RNA for human hemoglobin synthesis in beta thalassemia, J. Clin. Invest. 50:2755, 1971.
44. Benzer, S., Ingram, V. M., and Lehmann, H.: Three varieties of human haemoglobin D, Nature 182:852, 1958.
45. Berk, L., Burchenal, J. H., and Castle, W. B.: Erythropoietic effect of cobalt in patients with and without anemia, New Eng. J. Med. 240:754, 1949.
46. Bernini, L., Latte, B., Siniscalco, M., Piomelli, S., Spada, U., Adinolfi, M., and Mollison, P. L.: Survival of [51]Cr-labelled red cells in subjects with thalassemia trait or G-6-PD deficiency or both abnormalities, Brit. J. Haemat. 10:171, 1964.
47. Bernstein, J., and Whitten, C. F.: A histologic appraisal of the kidney in sickle cell anemia, Arch. Path. 70:407, 1960.
48. Bertles, J. F., and Milner, P. F. A.: Irreversibly sickled erythrocytes; a consequence of the heterogeneous distribution of hemoglobin types in sickle-cell anemia, J. Clin. Invest. 47:1731, 1968.
49. Bessis, M. C., and Breton-Gorius, J.: Iron metabolism in the bone marrow as seen by electron microscopy; a critical review, Blood 19:635, 1962.
50. Betke, K., Marti, H. R., and Schlicht, I.: Estimation of small percentages of foetal haemoglobin, Nature 184:1877, 1959.
51. Bianco, I., Moutalenti, G., Silvestroni, E., and Siniscalco, M.: Further data on genetics of microcythaemia or thalassemia minor and Cooley's disease or thalassemia major, Ann. Eugenics 16:299, 1952.
52. Binder, R. A., and Jones, S. R.: Prevalence and awareness of sickle cell hemoglobin in a military population; determination of a rapid screening method, J.A.M.A. 214:909, 1970.
53. Bird, G. W. G., and Lehmann, H.: Haemoglobin D in India, Brit. Med. J. 1:4, 1956.
54. Block, M.: Histopathologic studies in beta thalassemia minor and intermedia, Ann. N. Y. Acad. Sci. 165:126, 1969.
55. Blumberg, B. S., Alter, H. J., Riddell, N. M., and Erlandson, M. E.: Multiple antigenic specificities of serum lipoproteins detected with sera of transfused patients, Vox Sang. 9:128, 1964.
56. Bookchin, R. M., Nagel, R. L., and Ranney, H. M.: Structure and properties of hemoglobin $C_{Harlem}$, a human hemoglobin variant with amino acid substitutions in 2 residues of the beta-polypeptide chain, J. Biol. Chem. 242:248, 1967.
57. Bothwell, T. H., and Finch, C. A.: Iron metabolism, Boston, 1962, Little, Brown & Co.
58. Bothwell, T. H., Pirezio-Birdi, G., and Finch, C. A.: Iron absorption; factors influencing absorption, J. Lab. Clin. Med. 51:24, 1958.
59. Bowdler, A. J., and Huehns, E. R.: Thalassemia minor complicated by excessive iron storage, Brit. J. Haemat. 9:13, 1963.
60. Bowman, B. H., Oliver, C. P., Barnett, D. R., Cunningham, J. E., and Schneider, R. G.: Chemical characterization of three hemoglobins G, Blood 23:193, 1964.
61. Bradley, T. B., Jr., Brawner, J. N., III, and Conley, C. L.: Further observations on an inherited anomaly characterized by persistence of fetal hemoglobin, Bull. Johns Hopkins Hosp. 108:242, 1961.
62. Braverman, A. J., and Bank, A.: Changing rates of globin chain synthesis during erythroid cell maturation in thalassemia, J. Molec. Biol. 42:57, 1969.
63. Bridgers, W. H.: Cerebral vascular disease accompanying sickle cell anemia, Amer. J. Path. 15:353, 1939.
64. Brinkman, R., and Jonxis, J. H. P.: The occurrence of several kinds of haemoglobin in human blood, J. Physiol. 85:117, 1935.
65. Brody, J. I., Goldsmith, M. H., Park, S. K., and Soltys, H. D.: Symptomatic crises of sickle cell anemia treated by limited exchange transfusion, Ann. Intern. Med. 72:327, 1970.
66. Brook, C. G. D., Thompson, E. N., Marshall, W. C., and Whitehouse, R. H.: Growth in children with thalassaemia major and effect of two different transfusion regimens, Arch. Dis. Child. 44:612, 1969.
67. Bunting, H.: Sedimentation rates of sickled and non-sickled cells from patients with sickle cell anemia, Amer. J. Med. Sci. 198:191, 1939.
68. Burko, H., Watson, J., and Robinson, M.: Unusual bone changes in sickle-cell disease in childhood, Radiology 80:957, 1963.
69. Cabannes, R., and Buhr, J. L.: L'hémoglobine K.; identification, incidences biologiques et pathologiques, Sang 29:201, 1958.
70. Caffey, J.: Cooley's erythroblastic anemia; some skeletal findings in adolescents and young adults, Amer. J. Roentgen. 65:547, 1951.
71. Caffey, J.: Pediatric x-ray diagnosis, Chicago, 1956, Year Book Medical Publishers, Inc.
72. Caffey, J.: Cooley's anemia; a review of the roentgenographic findings in the skeleton, Amer. J. Roentgen. 78:381, 1957.
73. Callender, S. T., Mallett, B. J., and Lehmann, H.: Thalassemia in Britain, Brit. J. Haemat. 7:1, 1961.
74. Callender, S. T. E., Nickle, J. F., Moore, C.

V., and Powell, E. O.: Sickle-cell disease; studied by measuring the survival of transfused red blood cells, J. Lab. Clin. Med. 34:90, 1949.
75. Cappell, D. F., Hutchinson, H. E., and Jowett, M.: Tranfusional siderosis; the effects of excessive iron deposits on the tissue, J. Path. Bact. 74:245, 1957.
76. Carrell, R. W., and Lehmann, H.: The unstable haemoglobin haemolytic anaemias, Seminars Hemat. 6:116, 1969.
77. Carrington, H. T., Ferguson, A. D., and Scott, R. B.: Studies in sickle-cell anemia. XI. Bone involvement simulating aseptic necrosis, Amer. J. Dis. Child. 95:157, 1958.
78. Ceppellini, R.: Physiological genetics of human blood factors. In Wolstenholme, G. E. W., and O'Connor, C. M., editors: Ciba Foundation Symposium on biochemistry of human genetics, Boston, 1959, Little, Brown & Co.
78a. Cerami, A., and Manning, J. M.: Potassium cyanate as an inhibitor of the sickling of red blood cells *in vitro*, Proc. Nat. Acad. Sci. 68:1180, 1971.
79. Chaplin, H., Jr., Keitel, H. G., and Peterson, R. E.: Hematologic observations on patients with sickle cell anemia sustained at normal hemoglobin levels by multiple transfusions, Blood 11:834, 1956.
80. Chapman, A. Z., Reeder, P. S., Friedman, I. A., and Baker, L. A.: Gross hematuria in sickle cell trait and sickle cell hemoglobin C disease, Amer. J. Med. 19:773, 1955.
81. Charache, S., and Conley, C. L.: Rate of sickling of red cells during deoxygenation of blood from persons with various sickling disorders, Blood 24:25, 1964.
82. Charache, S., Conley, C. L., Waugh, D. F., Ugoretz, R. J., Spurrell, J. R., and Gayle, E.: Pathogenesis of hemolytic anemia in homozygous hemoglobin C disease, J. Clin. Invest. 46:1795, 1967.
83. Charache, S., Grisolia, S., Fiedler, A. J., and Hellegers, A. E.: Effect of 2,3-diphosphoglycerate on oxygen affinity of blood in sickle cell anemia, J. Clin. Invest. 49:806, 1970.
84. Charache, S., and Page, D. L.: Infarction of bone marrow in the sickle cell disorders, Ann. Intern. Med. 67:1195, 1967.
85. Charache, S., and Richardson, S. N.: Prolonged survival of a patient with sickle cell anemia, Arch. Intern. Med. 113:844, 1964.
86. Charache, S., Weatherall, D. J., and Clegg, J. B.: Polycythemia associated with a hemoglobinopathy, J. Clin. Invest. 45:813, 1966.
87. Charmot, G., Reynaud, R., and Bergot, J.: Cryoglobulinaemia and cold agglutinins in painful crisis of sickle cell anaemia, Lancet 2:540, 1963.

88. Charney, E., and Miller, G.: Reticulocytopenia in sickle cell disease, Amer. J. Dis. Child. 107:450, 1964.
89. Chernoff, A. I.: Studies on abnormal hemoglobins; persistence of fetal hemoglobin in the erythrocytes of normal children, Pediatrics 9:469, 1952.
90. Chernoff, A. I.: The human hemoglobins in health and disease, New Eng. J. Med. 253:322, 365, 415, 1955.
91. Chernoff, A. I.: The hemoglobin D syndromes, Blood 13:116, 1958.
92. Chernoff, A. I.: The distribution of the thalassemia gene; a historical review, Blood 14:899, 1959.
93. Chernoff, A. I., Minnich, V., Na-Nakorn, S., Tuchinda, S., Kashemsant, C., and Chernoff, R. R.: Studies on hemoglobin E; the clinical and genetic characteristics of the hemoglobin E syndromes, J. Lab. Clin. Med. 47:455, 1956.
94. Chernoff, A. I., Shapleigh, J. B., and Moore, C. V.: Therapy of chronic ulceration of the legs associated with sickle cell anemia, J.A.M.A. 155:1487, 1954.
95. Chodorkoff, J., and Whitten, C. F.: Intellectual status of children with sickle cell anemia, J. Pediat. 63:29, 1963.
96. Choremis, C., Liakakos, D., Tseghi, C., and Moschovakis, C.: Pathogenesis of osseous lesions in thalassemia, J. Pediat. 66:962, 1965.
97. Clayton, E. M., Feldhaus, W. D., and Phythyon, J. M.: The demonstration of fetal erythrocytes in the presence of adult red blood cells, Amer. J. Clin. Path. 40:487, 1963.
98. Cohen, F., Zuelzer, W. W., Neel, J. V., and Robinson, A. R.: Multiple inherited erythrocyte abnormalities in an American Negro family; hereditary spherocytosis sickling and thalassemia, Blood 14:816, 1959.
99. Comer, P. B., and Fred, H. L.: Diagnosis of sickle-cell disease by ophthalmoscopic inspection of the conjunctiva, New Eng. J. Med. 271:544, 1964.
100. Conley, C. L.: Letter to the editor, Blood 22:235, 1963.
101. Conley, C. L., Weatherall, D. J., Richardson, S. N., Shepard, M. K., and Charache, S.: Hereditary persistence of fetal hemoglobin; a study of 79 affected persons in 15 Negro families in Baltimore, Blood 21:261, 1963.
102. Conn, H. O.: Sickle-cell trait and splenic infarction associated with high altitude flying, New Eng. J. Med. 251:417, 1954.
103. Cooley, J. C., Peterson, W. L., Engle, C. E., and Jernigan, J. P.: Clinical triad of massive splenic infarction, sicklemia trait, and high altitude flying, J.A.M.A. 154:111, 1954.
104. Cooley, T. B., and Lee, P.: A series of cases

104. of splenomegaly in children with anemia and peculiar bone changes, Trans. Amer. Pediat. Soc. 37:29, 1925.
105. Cooley, T. B., Witwer, E. R., and Lee, P.: Anemia in children with splenomegaly and peculiar changes in the bones; report of cases, Amer. J. Dis. Child. 34:347, 1927.
106. Cooper, C. D., and Wacker, W. E. C.: The successful therapy with streptokinase-streptodornase of ankle ulcers associated with Mediterranean anemia, Blood 9:241, 1954.
107. Crosby, W. H.: Normal functions of the spleen relative to red blood cells; a review, Blood 14:399, 1959.
108. Crosby, W. H., and Sacks, H. J.: The coincidence of Mediterranean anemia and pernicious anemia in a young Sicilian, Blood 4:1267, 1949.
109. Cummer, C. L., and La Rocco, C. G.: Ulcers of the legs in sickle cell anemia, Arch. Dermat. 42:1015, 1940.
110. Currarino, G., and Erlandson, M. E.: Premature fusion of epiphyses in Cooley's anemia, Radiology 83:656, 1964.
111. Dacie, J. V.: The haemolytic anaemias, congenital and acquired, New York, 1954, Grune & Stratton, Inc.
112. Dacie, J. V., Grimes, A. J., Meisler, A., Steingold, L., Hemsted, E. H., Beavan, G. H., and White, J. C.: Hereditary Heinz-body anaemia; a report of studies on five patients with mild anaemia, Brit. J. Haemat. 10:388, 1964.
113. Dameshek, W.: "Target cell" anemia; an erythroblastic type of Cooley's erythroblastic anemia, Amer. J. Med. Sci. 200:445, 1940.
114. Dameshek, W.: "Thalassemia" or what's in a name, Blood 10:293, 1955.
115. Danks, D.: Thalassemia; immigration and eugenics, Australian Ped. J. 4:156, 1968.
115a. de Furia, F. G., and Miller, D. R.: Oxygen affinity in hemoglobin Köln disease, Blood 39:398, 1972.
115b. de Furia, F. G., Miller, D. R., Cerami, A., and Manning, J. M.: The effects of cyanate in vitro on red blood cell metabolism and function in sickle cell anemia, J. Clin. Invest. 51:566, 1972.
116. De Torregrosa, M. V., Ortiz, A., and Vargas, D.: Sickle cell-spherocytosis associated with hemolytic anemia, Blood 11:260, 1956.
117. Dewey, K. W., Grossman, H., and Canale, V. C.: Cholelithiasis in thalassemia major, Radiology 96:385, 1970.
118. Dherte, P., Lehmann, H., and Vandepitte, J.: Hemoglobin P in a family in the Belgian Congo, Nature 184:1133, 1959.
119. Dherte, P., Vandepitte, J., Agar, J. A. M., and Lehmann, H.: Stanleyville I and II, Brit. Med. J. 2:282, 1959.

120. Diggs, L. W.: Siderofibrosis of the spleen in sickle cell anemia, J.A.M.A. 104:538, 1935.
121. Diggs, L. W.: The crisis in sickle cell anemia; hematologic studies, Amer. J. Clin. Path. 26:1109, 1956.
122. Diggs, L. W., and Ching, R. E.: Pathology of sickle cell anemia, South. M. J. 27:839, 1934.
123. Diggs, L. W., Krauss, A. P., Morrison, D. B., and Rudnicki, R. P. T.: Intraethryrocytic crystals in a white patient with hemoglobin C in an absence of other types of hemoglobin, Blood 9:1172, 1954.
124. Diggs, L. W., Pulliam, H. N., and King, J. C.: The bone changes in sickle cell anemia, South. M. J. 30:249, 1937.
125. Dittman, W. A., Haut, A., Wintrobe, M. M., and Cartwright, G. E.: Hemoglobin H associated with an uncommon variant of thalassemia trait, Blood 16:975, 1960.
126. Diwany, M., Gabr, M., El Hefni, A., and Mokhtar, N.: Desferrioxamine in thalassaemia, Arch. Dis. Child. 43:340, 1968.
127. Doenges, J. P., Smith, E. W., Wise, S. P., and Breitenbucher, R. P.: Splenic infarction following air travel and associated with the sickling phenomenon, J.A.M.A. 156:955, 1954.
128. Donegan, C. C., Jr., MacIlwaine, W. A., and Leavell, B. S.: Hematologic studies on patients with sickle cell anemia following multiple transfusions, Amer. J. Med. 17:29, 1954.
129. Dormandy, K. M., Lock, S. P., and Lehmann, H.: Haemoglobin Q-alpha-thalassemia, Brit. Med. J. 1:1582, 1961.
130. Duma, H., Efremov, G., Sadikario, A., Teodosijev, D., Mladenovski, B., Vlaski, R., and Andreeva, M.: Study of nine families with haemoglobin-Lepore, Brit. J. Haemat. 15:161, 1968.
131. Edington, G. M., and Lehmann, A.: Haemoglobin G.; a new haemoglobin found in a West African, Lancet 2:173, 1954.
132. Edington, G. M., Lehmann, H., and Schneider, R. G.: Characterization and genetics of haemoglobin G, Nature 175:850, 1955.
133. Editorial: Sickle-cell anemia in Africa, Brit. Med. J. 2:433, 1952.
134. Editorial: Sickling and malaria, Brit. Med. J. 2:310, 1955.
135. Egdahl, R. H., Martin, W. W., and Hilkovitz, G.: Splenectomy for hypersplenism in sickle cell anemia, J.A.M.A. 186:745, 1963.
136. Ellis, J. T., Schulman, I., and Smith, C. H.: Generalized siderosis with fibrosis of liver and pancreas in Cooley's (Mediterranean) anemia, Amer. J. Path. 30:287, 1954.
137. Eng, L-I. L.: Haemoglobin "Bart's" and the

sickling phenomenon, Nature **191**:1314, 1961.
138. Eng, L-I. L.: Alpha-chain thalassemia and hydrops fetalis in Malaya; report of five cases, Blood **20**:581, 1962.
139. Eng, L-I. L., Gie, L. H., Ager, J. A. M., and Lehmann, H.: α-thalassemia as a cause of hydrops foetalis, Brit. J. Haemat. **8**:1, 1962.
140. Eng, L-I. L., Hin, P. S., Kong, K. L., and Endenburg, P. M.: Chronic hypochromic microcytic anaemia associated with haemoglobin H, Acta Haemat. **18**:156, 1957.
141. Eng, L-I. L., and Sadono: Haemoglobin O (Buginese X) in Sulawesi, Brit. Med. J. **1**:1461, 1958.
142. Engle, M. A., Erlandson, M. E., and Smith, C. H.: Late cardiac complications of chronic, severe refractory anemia with hemochromatosis, Circulation **30**:698, 1964.
143. Erlandson, M. E., Brilliant, R., and Smith, C. H.: Comparison of sixty-six patients with thalassemia major and thirteen patients with thalassemia intermedia; including evaluations of growth, development, maturation and progress, Ann. N. Y. Acad. Sci. **119**:727, 1964.
144. Erlandson, M. E., Currarino, G., and Smith, C. H.: Thalassemia intermedia; a phenotypic variant of homozygous thalassemia with prolonged survival and development of intrathoracic masses, American Pediatric Society, 74th annual meeting. Seattle, Wash., June 16-18, 1964.
145. Erlandson, M. E., Golubow, J., Wehman, J., and Smith, C. H.: Removal of iron from patients with secondary hemochromatosis, Blood **22**:815, 1963.
146. Erlandson, M. E., and Hilgartner, M.: Hemolytic disease in the neonatal period and early infancy, J. Pediat. **54**:566, 1959.
147. Erlandson, M. E., New, M., Brilliant, R., and Smith, C. H.: Maturation in chronic anemias, The Society for Pediatric Research Program and Abstracts, 35th annual meeting, May 4-6, 1965, Philadelphia, Pa.
148. Erlandson, M. E., Schulman, I., and Smith, C. H.: Studies on congenital hemolytic syndromes; rates of destruction and production of erythrocytes in sickle cell anemia, Pediatrics **25**:629, 1960.
149. Erlandson, M. E., Schulman, I., Stern, G., and Smith, C. H.: Studies of congenital hemolytic syndromes; rates of destruction and production of erythrocytes in thalassemia, Pediatrics **22**:910, 1958.
150. Erlandson, M. E., Schulman, I., Walden, B., and Smith C. H.: Chromium[51] elution from hemoglobin and intact erythrocytes of adults, infants and patients with Cooley's anemia, Proc. Soc. Exp. Biol. Med. **99**:173, 1958.

151. Erlandson, M., Smith, C. H., and Schulman, I.: Thalassemia-hemoglobin C disease in white siblings, Pediatrics **17**:740, 1956.
152. Erlandson, M. E., Walden, B., Stern, G., Hilgartner, M. W., Wehman, J., and Smith, C. H.: Studies in congenital hemolytic syndromes. IV. Gastrointestinal absorption of iron, Blood **19**:359, 1962.
153. Erlandson, M. E., Wehman, J., Stern, G., Hilgartner, M., and Smith, C. H.: Heme synthesis in thalassemia; defect in conversion of glycine to delta-aminolevulinic acid, Amer. J. Dis. Child. **102**:590, 1961.
154. Erman, S., and Bloomberg, H. H.: Priapism in sickle cell anemia treatment by estrogenic hormone, J. Urol. **84**:345, 1960.
155. Estes, J. E., Farber, E. M., and Stickney, J. M.: Ulcers of the leg in Mediterranean disease, Blood **3**:302, 1948.
156. Etteldorf, J. N., Smith, J. D., Tuttle, A. H., and Diggs, L. W.: Renal hemodynamic studies in adults with sickle cell anemia, Amer. J. Med. **18**:243, 1955.
157. Fahey, J., Rath, C. E., Princiotto, I., Brick, I. B., and Rubin, M.: Evaluation of trisodium calcium diethylenetriaminopenta-acetate in iron storage disease, J. Lab. Clin. Med. **57**:436, 1961.
158. Farmer, M. B., Lehmann, H., and Raine, D. N.: Two unrelated patients with congenital cyanosis due to haemoglobinopathy M, Lancet **2**:786, 1964.
159. Ferguson, A. D., Carrington, H. T., and Scott, R. B.: Studies in sickle cell anemia; a clinical review, M. Ann. D. C. **24**:517, 1955.
160. Fessas, P.: Haemoglobin C in a Greek family. In Beta-chain thalassemia. In Lehmann, H., and Betke, K., editors: Haemoglobin-colloquium, Stuttgart, 1962, Georg Thieme Verlag, p. 60.
161. Fessas, P.: Inclusion of hemoglobin in erythroblasts and erythrocytes of thalassemia, Blood **21**:21, 1963.
162. Fessas, P., and Loukopoulos, D.: Alpha-chain of human hemoglobin; occurrence in vivo, Science **143**:590, 1964.
163. Fessas, P., Mastrokalos, N., Fostripoulos, G., Vella, F., Ager, J. A. M., and Lehmann, H.: New variant of human foetal haemoglobin, Nature **183**:30, 1959.
164. Fessas, P., and Stamatoyannopoulos, G.: Hereditary persistence of fetal hemoglobin in Greece; a study and a comparison, Blood **24**:223, 1964.
165. Fessas, P., Stamatoyannopoulos, G., and Karaklis, A.: Hemoglobin "pylos"; study of a hemoglobinopathy resembling thalassemia in the heterozygous, homozygous and double heterozygous state, Blood **19**:1, 1962.
166. Finch, S. C., and Finch, C. A.: Idiopathic hemochromatosis, an iron storage disease;

iron metabolism in hemochromatosis, Medicine 34:381, 1955.
167. Fink, H.: Problems in Cooley's anemia, Ann. N. Y. Acad. Sci. 119:369, 1964.
168. Fink, H.: Transfusion hemachromatosis in Cooley's anemia, Ann. N. Y. Acad. Sci. 119: 680, 1964.
169. Fink, H.: Second conference on the problems of Cooley's anemia, Ann. N. Y. Acad. Sci. 165:5, 1969.
170. Finn, R., Harper, D. T., Sallings, S. A., and Krivans, J. R.: Transplacental transfusion, Transfusion 3:114, 1963.
171. Foerster, R. F.: The Italian emigration of our times, Cambridge, Mass., 1919, Harvard University Press, chap. 17.
172. Frick, P. G., Hitzig, W. H., and Betke, K.: Hemoglobin Zurich. I. A new hemoglobin anomaly associated with inclusion bodies after sulfonamide therapy, Blood 20:261, 1962.
173. Fuhr, J., Natta, C., Marks, P. A., and Bank, A.: Protein synthesis in cell-free systems from reticulocytes of thalassemic patients, Nature 224:1305, 1969.
173a. Gabriele, O. F.: Hypoparathyroidism associated with thalassemia, South. Med. J. 64: 115, 1971.
174. Gabuzda, T. G., Nathan, D. G., and Gardner, F. H.: The turnover of hemoglobins A, F and $A_2$ in the peripheral blood of three patients with thalassemia, J. Clin. Invest. 42: 1678, 1963.
175. Gabuzda, T. G., Nathan, D. G., and Gardner, F. H.: Thalassemia trait: Genetic combinations of increased fetal and $A_2$ hemoglobins, New Eng. J. Med. 270:1212, 1964.
176. Gerald, P. S.: The electrophoretic and spectroscopic characterization of Hgb M, Blood 13:936, 1958.
177. Gerald, P. S.: The clinical implication of hemoglobin structure, Pediatrics 31:780, 1963.
178. Gerald, P. S.: The thalassemia syndromes, biochemical, genetic and clinical considerations, combined Staff Clinic Conference, Amer. J. Med. 36:919, 1964.
179. Gerald, P. S., and Diamond, L. K.: The diagnosis of thalassemia trait by starch block electrophoresis of the hemoglobin, Blood 13: 61, 1958.
180. Gerald, P. S., and Diamond, L. K.: A new hereditary hemoglobinopathy (Lepore trait) and its interaction with thalassemia trait, Blood 13:835, 1958.
181. Gerald, P. S., Efron, M. L., and Diamond, L. K.: A human mutation (the Lepore hemoglobinopathy) possibly involving two "cistrons," Amer. J. Dis. Child. 102:514, 1961.
182. Gerald, P. S., and Ingram, V. M.: Recommendations for the nomenclature of hemoglobins, Blood 19:124, 1962.

183. Gerald, P. S., Walzer, S., and Diamond, L. K.: Location of the genetic elements controlling the hematologic changes in the $D_1$ trisomy, Blood 24:836, 1964.
184. Giblett, E. R., and Crookston, M. C.: Agglutinability of red cells by anti-i in patients with thalassemia major and other hematological disorders, Nature 201:1138, 1964.
185. Gilles, H. M., Reid, H. A., Odultoa, A., Ransome-Kuti, O., Lesi, F., and Ransome-Kuti, S.: Arvin treatment for sickle cell crisis, Lancet 2:542, 1968.
185a. Gillette, P., Manning, J. M., and Cerami, A.: Increased survival of sickle cell erythrocytes after treatment in vitro with sodium cyanate, Proc. Nat. Acad. Sci. 68:271, 1971.
186. Githens, J. H., Knock, H. K., and Hathaway, W. E.: Prevalence of abnormal hemoglobins in American Indian children, J. Lab. Clin. Med. 57:755, 1961.
187. Gofstein, R., and Gellis, S. S.: Splenectomy in infancy and childhood, Amer. J. Dis. Child. 91:566, 1956.
188. Goldberg, M. A., and Schwartz, S. O.: Mediterranean anemia in a Negro complicated by pernicious anemia of pregnancy, Blood 9: 648, 1954.
189. Gouttas, A., Fessas, P. H., Tsevrenis, H., and Xefteri, E.: Description d'une nouvelle variété, d'anémie hémolytique congénitale, Sang 26:911, 1955.
190. Green, T. W., Conley, C. L., and Berthong, W.: The liver in sickle cell anemia, Bull. Johns Hopkins Hosp. 92:99, 1953.
191. Greenberg, M. S., and Kass, E. H.: Studies on the destruction of red blood cells; observations on the role of pH in the pathogenesis and treatment of painful crisis in sickle-cell disease, Arch. Intern. Med. 101:355, 1958.
192. Griggs, R. C., and Harris, J. W.: The biophysics of the variants of sickle-cell disease, Arch. Intern. Med. 97:315, 1956.
193. Grimes, A. J., Meisler, A., and Dacie, J. V.: Congenital Heinz body anaemia; further evidence on the cause of Heinz-body production in red cells, Brit. J. Haemat. 10:281, 1964.
194. Grinstein, M., Bannerman, R. M., Vavra, J. D., and Moore, C. V.: Hemoglobin metabolism in thalassemia; in vivo studies, Amer. J. Med. 29:18, 1960.
195. Gross, R. T., Kriss, J. P., and Spaet, T. H.: The hematopoietic goitrogenic effects of cobaltous chloride in patients with sickle cell anemia, Pediatrics 15:284, 1955.
196. Grossman, H., Dische, M. R., Winchester, P. H., and Canale, V.: Renal enlargement in thalassemia major, Radiology 100:645, 1971.
197. Haggard, M. E., and Schneider, R. G.:

Sickle cell anemia in the first 2 years of life, J. Pediat. **58**:785, 1961.
198. Hahn, E. V., and Gillespie, E. B.: Sickle cell anemia; report of a case greatly improved by splenectomy, Arch. Intern. Med. **39**:233, 1927.
199. Halbrecht, I.: Studies on the different types of hemoglobin in the blood of the newborn and fetus, with special reference to the new embryonic (primitive) hemoglobin; Sixth International Congress of the International Society of Hematology, Boston, 1956, p. 433.
200. Haltalin, K. C., and Nelson, J. D.: Hand-foot syndrome due to streptococcal infection, Amer. J. Dis. Child. **109**:156, 1965.
201. Harden, A. S.: Sickle cell anemia, changes in the vessels and in the bones, Amer. J. Dis. Child. **54**:1045, 1937.
202. Harris, J. W.: Studies on the destruction of red blood cells; molecular orientation in sickle cell hemoglobin solutions, Proc. Soc. Exp. Biol Med. **75**:197, 1950.
203. Harris, J. W.: The role of physical and chemical factors in the sickling phenomenon. In Tocantins, L. M., editor: Progress in hematology, vol. 2, New York, 1959, Grune & Stratton, Inc., p. 47.
204. Harris, J. W.: The red cell production, metabolism destruction; normal and abnormal, Commonwealth Fund, Cambridge, Mass., 1963, Harvard University Press.
205. Harris, J. W., Brewster, H. H., Ham, T. H., and Castle, W. B.: Studies on the destruction of red blood cells; the biophysics and biology of sickle-cell disease, Arch. Intern. Med. **97**:145, 1956.
206. Harrow, B. R., Sloane, J. A., and Liebman, N. C.: Roentgenologic demonstrations of renal papillary necrosis in sickle-cell trait, New Eng. J. Med. **268**:969, 1963.
207. Hedenberg, F., Muller-Eberhard, U., Sjolin, S., and Wranne, L.: Haemoglobin H and inclusion-body anaemia in a Swedish family, Acta Pediat. **47**:652, 1958.
208. Henderson, A. B., Crockett, E. J., and Wright, C. H.: Effect of carbonic anhydrase inhibitors on course of sickle cell disease, Arch. Intern. Med. **104**:68, 1959.
209. Henderson, A. B., Potts, E. B., Burgess, D., and White, F.: Sickle-cell thalassemia disease and pregnancy; a case study, Amer. J. Med. Sci. **244**:605, 1962.
210. Henderson, A. B., Prince, A. E., and Greene, J. B.: Sickle-cell disease variants and pregnancy; pathophysiologic report, New Eng. J. Med. **264**:1276, 1961.
211. Hendrickse, R. G., and Collard, P.: Salmonella osteitis in Nigerian children, Lancet **1**:80, 1960.
212. Henkin, W. A.: Collapse of the vertebral bodies in sickle cell anemia, Amer. J. Roentgen. **62**:395, 1949.
213. Henry, M. D., and Chapman, A. Z.: Vitreous hemorrhage and retinopathy associated with sickle-cell disease, Amer. J. Ophthal. **38**:204, 1954.
214. Herman, E. C., and Conley, C. L.: Hereditary persistence of fetal hemoglobin, Amer. J. Med. Sci. **241**:215, 1961.
215. Herrick, J. B.: Peculiar elongated and sickle-shaped red blood corpuscles in a case of severe anemia, Arch. Intern. Med. **6**:517, 1910.
216. Heywood, J. D., Karon, M., and Weissman, S.: Amino acids; incorporation into alpha and beta chains of hemoglobin by normal and thalassemic reticulocytes, Science **146**:530, 1963.
217. Hilgartner, M. W., Erlandson, M. E., and Smith, C. H.: The coagulation mechanism in patients with thalassemia major, J. Pediat. **63**:36, 1963.
218. Hilgartner, M. W., Erlandson, M. E., Walden, B. S., and Smith, C. H.: A comparison of the paper and starch-block electrophoretic methods for determination of $A_2$ hemoglobin, Amer. J. Clin. Path. **35**:26, 1961.
219. Hilgartner, M. W., Horowitz, H., Ferguson, A., and Smith, C. H.: Studies of the coagulation mechanism in patients with sickle-cell anemia, Amer. J. Dis. Child. **102**:591, 1961.
220. Hilgartner, M. W., and Smith, C. H.: Coagulation studies as a measure of liver function in Cooley's anemia, Ann. N. Y. Acad. Sci. **119**:631, 1964.
221. Hilkovitz, G., and Jacobson, A.: Hepatic dysfunction and abnormalities of the serum proteins and serum enzymes in sickle-cell anemia, J. Lab. Clin. Med. **57**:856, 1961.
222. Hilkovitz, G., and Martin, W. W., Jr.: Sickle-cell anemia; comment on diagnosis and a report on splenectomy in two sisters, Arch. Intern Med. **108**:109, 1961.
223. Hill, F. S., Hughes, J. G., and Davis, B. C.: Electro-encephalographic findings in sickle cell anemia, Pediatrics **6**:277, 1950.
224. Hook, E. W., Campbell, C. G., Weens, H. S., and Cooper, G. R.: Salmonella osteomyelitis in patients with sickle cell anemia, New Eng. J. Med. **257**:403, 1957.
225. Hörlein, H., and Weber, G.: Über chronische familiäre Methämoglobinämie und eine neue Modifikation des Methämoglobins, Deutsche med. Wchnschr. **73**:476, 1948.
226. Howell, J., and Wyatt, J. P.: Development of pigmentary cirrhosis in Cooley's anemia, Arch. Path. **55**:423, 1953.
227. Hsia, D. Y-Y.: Inborn errors of metabolism, Chicago, 1959, Year Book Medical Publishers, Inc.
228. Huehns, E. R., Dance, N., Beaven, G. H.,

Keil, J. V., Hecht, F., and Motulsky, A. G.: Human embryonic haemoglobins, Nature 201:1095, 1964.
229. Huehns, E. R., Flynn, F. V., and Butler, E. A.: The occurrence of haemoglobin 'Bart's' in conjunction with haemoglobin H, Brit. J. Haemat. 6:388, 1960.
230. Huehns, E. R., Hecht, F., Yoshida, A., Stamatoyannopoulos, G., Hartman, J., and Motulsky, A. G.: Hemoglobin-Seattle ($A^2\beta_2^{76gluc}$); an unstable hemoglobin causing chronic hemolytic anemia, Blood 36:209, 1970.
231. Hughes, J. G., and Carroll, D. S.: Salmonella osteomyelitis complicating sickle cell disease, Pediatrics 19:184, 1957.
232. Hughes, J. G., Diggs, L. W., and Gillespie, C. E.: The involvement of the nervous system in sickle cell anemia, J. Pediat. 17:166, 1940.
233. Huisman, T. H., Punt, K., and Schaad, J. D. G.: Thalassemia minor associated with hemoglobin-$B_2$ heterozygosity; a family report, Blood 17:747, 1961.
234. Huisman, T. H. J., Schroeder, W. A., Dozy, A. M., Shelton, J. R., Shelton, J. B., Boyd, E. M., and Apell, G.: Evidence for mutiple structural genes for the gamma-chain of human fetal hemoglobin in hereditary persistence of fetal hemoglobin, Ann. N. Y. Acad. Sci. 165:320, 1969.
235. Hunt, J. A., and Lehmann, H.: Haemoglobin "Bart's"; a foetal haemoglobin without alpha chains, Nature 184:872, 1959.
236. Huntley, C. C.: Infection following splenectomy in infants and children, Amer. J. Dis. Child. 95:477, 1958.
237. Hwang, Y. F., and Brown, E. B.: Evaluation of deferoxamine in iron overload, Arch. Intern Med. 114:741, 1964.
238. Ingram, V. M.: Gene mutations in human haemoglobin; the chemical difference between normal and sickle-cell haemoglobin, Nature 180:326, 1957.
239. Ingram, V. M.: Chemistry of the abnormal human haemoglobins, Brit. M. Bull. 15:27, 1959.
240. Ingram, V. M.: Gene evolution and the haemoglobins, Nature 189:704, 1961.
241. Ingram, V. M.: The hemoglobins in genetics and evolution, New York, 1963, Columbia University Press.
242. Ingram, V. M.: A molecular model for thalassemia, Ann. N. Y. Acad. Sci. 119:485, 1964.
243. Ingram, V. M., and Stretton, A. O. W.: The genetic basis of the thalassemia disease, Nature 184:1903, 1959.
244. Itano, H. A., Bergren, W. R., and Sturgeon, P.: The abnormal human hemoglobins, Medicine 35:121, 1956.
245. Itano, H. A., and Robinson, E.: Properties and inheritance of hemoglobin by assymetric recombination, Nature 184:1468, 1959.
246. Ivy, R. E., and Howard, F. H.: Sickle-cell anemia with unusual bone changes, J. Pediat. 43:312, 1953.
247. Jackson, J. F., Odom, J. L., and Bell, W. N.: Amelioration of sickle cell disease by persistent fetal hemoglobin, J.A.M.A. 177:867, 1961.
248. Jacob, F., and Monod, J.: Genetic regulatory mechanisms in synthesis of proteins, J. Molec. Biol. 3:318, 1961.
249. Jacob, G. F., and Raper, A. B.: Hereditary persistence of foetal haemoglobin production and its interaction with sickle-cell trait, Brit. J. Haemat. 4:138, 1958.
250. Jacob, H. S., and Winterhalter, K.: Unstable hemoglobins; the role of heme loss in Heinz body function, Proc. Nat. Acad. Sci. 65:697, 1970.
251. Jacob, H. S.: Mechanisms of Heinz body formation and attachment to red cell membrane, Seminars Hemat. 7:341, 1970.
252. Jacob, H. S., Brain, M. C., Dacie, J. V., Carrell, R. W., and Lehmann, H.: Abnormal haem binding and globin SH group blockade in unstable haemoglobins, Nature 218:1214, 1968.
253. Jandl, J. H., and Greenberg, M. S.: Bone-marrow failure due to relative nutritional deficiency in Cooley's hemolytic anemia; painful "erythropoietic crises" in response to folic acid, New Eng. J. Med. 260:461, 1959.
254. Jenkins, M. E., Scott, R. B., and Baird, R. L.: Studies in sickle cell anemia. XVI. Sudden death during sickle cell anemia crises in young children, J. Pediat. 56:30, 1960.
255. Jenkins, M. E., Scott, R. B., and Ferguson, A. D.: Studies in sickle cell anemia; blood volume relationships and the use of a plasma extender in sickle cell disease in childhood; a preliminary report, Pediatrics 18:239, 1956.
256. Jim, R. T. S., and Yarbro, M. T.: Hemoglobin J in a healthy Hawaiian-Chinese-Caucasian male, Blood 15:285, 1960.
257. Jimenez, C. T., Scott, R. B., Henry, W. L., Sampson, C. C., and Ferguson, A. D.: Studies in sickle cell anemia. XXVI. The effects of homozygous sickle cell disease on the onset of menarche, pregnancy, fertility, pubescent changes and body growth in Negro subjects, Amer. J. Dis. Child. 111:497, 1966.
258. Johnston, F. E., Hertzog, K. P., and Malina, R. M.: Longitudinal growth in thalassemia major, Amer. J. Dis. Child. 112:396, 1966.
259. Johnston, F. E., and Roseman, J. M.: The effects of frequent transfusions upon bone loss in thalassemia major, Ped. Res. 1:479, 1967.
260. Jones, B., and Klingberg, W. G.: Hemoglo-

bin S-hereditary spherocytosis, J. Pediat. **54:** 375, 1959.
261. Jones, R. V., Grimes, A. J., Carrell, R. W., and Lehmann, H.: Köln haemoglobinopathy; further data and a comparison with other hereditary Heinz body anaemias, Brit. J. Haemat. **13:**394, 1967.
262. Jones, S. R., Bender, R. A., and Donowho, E. M., Jr.: Sudden death in sickle cell trait, New Eng. J. Med. **282:**323, 1970.
263. Jonsson, U., Roath, O. S., and Kirkpatrick, C. I. F.: Nutritional megaloblastic anemia associated with sickle cell states, Blood **14:** 535, 1959.
264. Jonxis, J. H. P.: The development of hemoglobin, Ped. Clin. N. Amer. **12:**535, 1965.
265. Jonxis, J. H. P., and Delafresnaye, J. F., editors: Abnormal haemoglobins, Springfield, Ill., 1959, Charles C Thomas, Publisher.
266. Jonxis, J. H. P., and Huisman, T. H. J.: The detection and estimation of fetal hemoglobin by means of the alkali denaturation test, Blood **11:**1009, 1956.
267. Josephson, A. M., Masri, M. S., Singer, L., Dworkin, D., and Singer, K.: Starch block electrophoretic studies of human hemoglobin solutions; results in cord blood, thalassemia and other hemolytic disorders; comparison with Tiselius electrophoresis, Blood **13:**543, 1958.
268. Jurkiewicz, M. J., Pearson, H. A., and Furlow, L. T., Jr.: Reconstruction of the maxilla in thalassemia, Ann. N. Y. Acad. Sci. **165:** 437, 1969.
269. Kabins, S. A., and Lerner, C.: Fulminant pneumococcosuria and sickle cell anemia, J.A.M.A. **211:**467, 1970.
270. Kan, Y. W., and Nathan, D. G.: The diagnosis of beta thalassemia on the first day of life, Abstracts 38th Annual Meeting Soc. Ped. Research Program, May 3-4, 1968, p. 122.
271. Kaplan, E., and Zuelzer, W. W.: Erythrocyte survival studies in childhood; studies in Mediterranean anemia, J. Lab. Clin. Med. **36:**517, 1950.
272. Kaplan, E., Zuelzer, W. W., and Neel, J. V.: Further studies on hemoglobin C; the hematologic effects of hemoglobin C alone and in combination with sickle cell hemoglobin, Blood **8:**735, 1953.
273. Kattamis, C., Touliatos, N., Haidas, S., and Matsaniotis, N.: Growth of children with thalassaemia; effect of different transfusion regimens, Arch. Dis. Child. **45:**502, 1970.
274. Kaufman, M., Steier, W., Applewhaite, F., Ruggiero, S., and Ginsberg, U.: Sickle-cell trait in blood donors, Amer. J. Med. Sci. **249:**56, 1965.
275. Keitel, H. G., Thompson, D., and Itano, H. A.: Hyposthenuria in sickle cell anemia; a reversible renal defect, J. Clin. Invest. **35:** 998, 1956.
276. Kimmelstiel, P.: Vascular occlusion and ischemic infarction in sickle cell disease, Amer. J. Med. Sci. **216:**11, 1948.
277. King, H., and Shumacker, H. B., Jr.: Splenic studies; susceptibility to infection after splenectomy performed in infancy, Amer. J. Surg. **136:**239, 1952.
278. Kiossoglov, K. A., Wolman, I. J., and Garrison, M., Jr.: Fetal hemoglobin containing erythrocytes. I. Counts of cell stained by the acid elution method compared with alkali denaturation measurements, Blood **21:**553, 1963.
279. Kleihauer, E., Braun, H., and Betke, K.: Demonstration von fetalem Hämoglobin in den Erythrocytin eines Blutausstrichs, Klin. Wchnschr. **35:**637, 1957.
280. Klinefelter, H. F.: The heart in sickle cell anemia, Amer. J. Med. Sci. **203:**34, 1942.
281. Klion, F. M., Weiner, M. J., and Schaffner, F.: Cholestasis in sickle cell anemia, Amer. J. Med. **37:**829, 1964.
282. Knoblich, R.: Extramedullary hematopoiesis presenting as intrathoracic tumors; report of a case in a patient with thalassemia minor, Cancer **13:**462, 1960.
283. Konotey-Ahulu, F. I. D.: Anaesthetic deaths and the sickle cell trait, Lancet **1:**267, 1969.
284. Konotey-Ahulu, F. I. D.: Patterns of clinical haemoglobinopathy, E. African Med. J. **46:** 149, 1969.
285. Korber, E.: Cited by Bischoff, H. Z.: Resistance of human hemoglobin with especial regard to infants, Ztschr. ges. exper. Med. **48:** 472, 1926.
286. Kunkel, H. G., Ceppelini, R., Muller-Eberhard, U., and Wolf, J.: Observations on the minor basic hemoglobin component in the blood of normal individuals and patients with thalassemia, J. Clin. Invest. **36:**1615, 1957.
287. Kunkel, H. G., and Wallenius, G.: New hemoglobin in normal adult blood, Science **122:**288, 1955.
288. Kunz, H. W., Pratt, E. I., Mellin, G. W., and Cheung, M. W.: Impairment of urinary concentration in sickle cell anemia, Pediatrics **13:**352, 1954.
289. Lambotte, C.: Hand-foot syndrome in sickle-cell disease, Letters to the editor, Amer. J. Dis. Child. **104:**200, 1962.
290. Laszlo, J., Obenour, W., Jr., and Saltzman, H. A.: Effects of hyperbaric oxygenation on sickle syndrome, South. Med. J. **62:**453, 1969.
291. Lawson, N. S., Schnitzer, B., and Smith, E. B.: Splenic ultrastructure in drug-induced

Heinz body hemolysis, Arch. Path. **87**:491, 1969.
292. Leavell, B. S.: Treatment of sickle cell anemia, Arch. Intern. Med. **94**:801, 1954.
293. Lee, R. C., and Huisman, T. H. J.: A variant of hemoglobin A$_2$ found in a Negro family, Blood **24**:495, 1964.
294. Lehmann, H.: Distribution of thalassemia and abnormal hemoglobin, Proc. Sixth International Congress Tropical Medicine and Malaria **6**:378, 1959.
295. Lehmann, H.: Thalassemia, Acta Haemat. **36**:256, 1966.
296. Lehmann, H., and Ager, J. A. M.: The hemoglobinopathies and thalassemia. In Stanbury, J. B., Wyngaarden, J. B., and Fredrickson, D. S., editors: The metabolic basis of inherited disease, Student Edition, New York, 1960, McGraw-Hill Book Co.
297. Lehmann, H., and Cutbush, M.: Sickle cell trait in southern India, Brit. M. J. **1**:404, 1952.
298. Lehmann, H., and Huntsman, R. G.: Man's haemoglobins, Philadelphia, 1966, J. B. Lippincott Co.
299. Lehmann, H., and Huntsman, R. G.: The haemoglobinopathies. In Woodruff, A. W., editor: Alimentary and haematological aspects of tropical disease, London, 1970, Edward Arnold (Publishers) Ltd.
300. Lehmann, H., Huntsman, R. G., and Ager, J. A. M.: The hemoglobinopathies and thalassemia. In Stanbury, J. B., Wyngaarden, J. B., and Fredrickson, D. S., editors: The metabolic basis of inherited disease, ed. 2, New York, 1966, McGraw-Hill Book Co.
301. Lehndorff, von H.: Anaemia Pseudoleucaemia Infantum "Jaksch-Hayem," Helvet. Pediat. Acta **18**:1, 1963.
302. Lerner, A. B.: Melanin pigmentation, Amer. J. Med. **19**:902, 1955.
303. Levin, W. C.: "Asymptomatic" sickle cell trait (editorial), Blood **13**:904, 1958.
304. Levitt, M. F., Hauser, A. D., Levy, M. S., and Polimeros, D.: The renal concentrating defect in sickle cell disease, Amer. J. Med. **29**:611, 1960.
305. Liachowitz, C., Elderkin, J., Guichirit, I., Brown, H. W., and Ranney, H. M.: Abnormal hemoglobins in the Negroes of Surinam, Amer. J. Med. **24**:19, 1958.
306. Liakakos, D., Karpouzas, J., and Agathopoulos, A.: Hyperprolinemia and hyperprolinuria in thalassemia, J. Pediat. **73**:419, 1968.
307. Lichtman, H. C., Shapiro, H., Ginsberg, V., and Watson, R. J.: Splenic hyperfunction in sickle cell anemia (abstr.), Amer. J. Med. **14**:516, 1953.
308. Lieb, W. A., Geeraets, W. J., and Guerry, D., III: Sickle-cell retinopathy; ocular and systemic manifestations of sickle-cell disease, Acta Ophthal. Suppl. **58**:7, 1959.
309. Lindenbaum, J., and Klipstein, F. A.: Folic acid deficiency in sickle-cell anemia, New Eng. J. Med. **269**:875, 1963.
310. Liquori, A. M.: Presence of fetal hemoglobin in Cooley's anemia, Nature **167**:950, 1951.
311. Lisker, R., Ruiz-Reyer, G., and Loria, A.: studies on several genetic hematologic characteristics of the Mexican population. IV. The finding of a fast hemoglobin component (hemoglobin Mexico) in an Indian family, Blood **22**:342, 1963.
312. Loukopoulos, D., and Fessas, P.: The distribution of hemoglobin types in thalassemic erythrocytes, J. Clin. Invest. **44**:231, 1965.
313. Luhby, A. L., and Cooperman, J. M.: Folic-acid deficiency in thalassemia major, Lancet **2**:491, 1961.
314. Luzzatto, L., Nwachuko-Jarrett, E. S., and Reddy S.: Increased sickling of parasitised erythrocytes as mechanism of resistance against malaria in the sickle-cell trait, Lancet **1**:319, 1970.
315. Manning, M. D., and D'Angio, G. J.: Irradiation of the nasopharynx in children; a survey of patients 5-20 years after treatment for lymphatic hyperplasia, Clin. Radiol. **18**:173, 1967.
316. Margolies, M. P.: Sickle cell anemia; composite study and survey, Medicine **30**:357, 1951.
317. Marks, P. A.: Thalassemia syndrome; biochemical, genetic and clinical aspects, New Eng. J. Med. **275**:1363, 1966.
318. Marks, P. A., and Burka, E. R.: Hemoglobin A and F; formation in thalassemia and other hemolytic anemias, Science **144**:552, 1964.
319. Marsh, C. L., Joleff, C. R., and Payne, L. C.: A rapid micromethod for starch-gel electrophoresis, Amer. J. Clin. Path. **41**:217, 1964.
320. Martin, W. W., Jr., Kough, R. H., and Branche, G. C., Jr.: Hereditary spherocytosis—sicklemia in the Negro; case report and study of a Negro family having multiple instances of hereditary spherocytosis, Blood **14**:688, 1959.
321. Master, J., Engle, M. A., Stern, G., and Smith, C. H.: Cardiac complications of chronic, severe, refractory anemia with hemochromatosis. I. Acute pericarditis of unknown etiology, J. Pediat. **58**:455, 1961.
322. Matioli, G., and Thorell, B.: Kinetics of alkali denaturation of hemoglobin in a single erythrocyte, Blood **21**:1, 1963.
323. Matoth, Y., Shamir, Z., and Freundlich, E.: Thalassemia in Jews from Kurdistan, Blood **10**:176, 1955.

324. Matsuda, G., Schroeder, W. A., Jones, R. T., and Weliky, N.: Is there any "embryonic" or "primitive" human hemoglobin? Blood **16**: 984, 1960.
325. McCormick, W. F., and Humphreys, E. W.: High fetal-hemoglobin C disease; a new syndrome, Blood **16**:1736, 1960.
326. McCurdy, P. R.: Clinical and physiologic studies in a Negro with sickle-cell hemoglobin D disease, New Eng. J. Med. **262**:961, 1960.
327. McDonald, R.: Deferoxamine and D.T.P.A. in thalassemia, J. Pediat. **69**:563, 1966.
328. McElfresh, A. E., Sharpsteen, J. R., and Akabane, T.: Secondary hypersplenism occurring in a seven-month-old infant with thalassemia major, J. Pediat. **47**:347, 1955.
329. Mentzer, W. C., Lubin, B. H., and Nathan, D. G.: Screening for sickle-cell trait and G-6-PD deficiency, New Eng. J. Med. **282**: 1155, 1970.
330. Miller, D. R., and Lichtman, M. A.: Clinical implications of altered activity of hemoglobin for oxygen. In Weed, R. I., editor: Hematology for internists, Boston, 1971, Little, Brown and Co.
330a. Miller, D. R., Weed, R. I., Stamatoyannopolous, G., and Yoshida, A.: Hemoglobin Köln disease occurring as a fresh mutation; erythrocyte metabolism and survival, Blood **38**: 715, 1971.
331. Milner, P. F., Miller, C., Grey, R., Seakins, M., DeJong, W. W., and Went, L. N.: Hemoglobin O$^{Arab}$ in four Negro families and its interaction with hemoglobin S and hemoglobin C, New Eng. J. Med. **283**:1417, 1970.
332. Minnich, V., Cordonnier, J. K., Williams, W. J., and Moore C. V.: Alpha, beta and gamma hemoglobin polypeptide chains during the neonatal period with description of a fetal form of hemoglobin D$_a$-St. Louis, Blood **19**: 137, 1962.
333. Minnich, V., Na-Nakorn, S., Chongchareonsuk, S., and Kochaseni, S.: Mediterranean anemia; a study of thirty-two cases in Thailand, Blood **9**:1, 1954.
334. Minnich, V, Na-Nakorn, S., Tuchinda, S., Pravit, W., and Moore, C. V.: Inclusion body anemia in Thailand (hemoglobin H-thalsemia disease), Proceedings of Sixth Congress of International Society of Hematology, New York, 1958, Grune & Stratton, Inc., p. 743.
335. Mitchner, J. W., Thompson, R. B., and Huisman, T. H. J.: Foetal haemoglobin synthesis in some haemoglobinopathies, Lancet **1**: 1169, 1961.
336. Moeschlin, S., and Schnider, U.: Treatment of primary and secondary hemochromatosis and acute iron poisoning with a new, potent iron-eliminating agent (desferrioxamine-B), New Eng. J. Med. **269**:57, 1963.
337. Moseley, J. E.: Patterns of bone change in sickle cell states, J. Mount Sinai Hosp. **26**: 424, 1959.
338. Moser, K. M., and Shea, J. G.: The relationship between pulmonary infarction, cor pulmonale and the sickle states, Amer. J. Med. **22**:561, 1957.
339. Motulsky, A. G.: Sicklemia, J.A.M.A. **155**: 388, 1954.
340. Motulsky, A. G.: Genetic and haematological significance of haemoglobin H, Nature **178**: 1055, 1956.
341. Motulsky, A. G.: Metabolic polymorphisms and the role of infectious diseases in human evolution, Human Biol. **32**:38, 1960.
342. Motulsky, A. G., Hebenstreit, W., Lonn, L., Erikson, N., and Paeth, G. W.: Hemoglobin H-thalassemia disease and further studies on the interaction of thalassemia with Hb C and S, Proceedings of Sixth Congress of International Society of Hematology, New York, 1958, Grune & Stratton, Inc., p. 729.
343. Motulsky, A. G., Paul, M. H., and Durrum, E. L.: Paper electrophoresis of abnormal hemoglobins and its clinical applications, Blood **9**:897, 1954.
344. Movitt, E. R., Mangum, J. F., and Porter, W. R.: Sickle cell-hemoglobin C disease quantitative determination of iron kinetics and hemoglobin synthesis, Blood **21**:535, 1963.
345. Muller, C. J., and Kingma, S.: Haemoglobin Zürich: $\alpha_2^A \beta^{63Arg}$, Biochim. et Biophys. Acta **50**:595, 1961.
346. Muller-Eberhard, U., Erlandson, M. E., Ginn, H. E., and Smith, C. H.: Effect of trisodium calcium diethylenetriaminepentaacetate on bivalent cations in thalassemia major, Blood **22**:209, 1963.
347. Murayama, M.: Chemical difference between normal human haemoglobin and haemoglobin-I, Nature **196**:276, 1962.
348. Murayama, M.: Molecular mechanism of red cell "sickling," Science **153**:145, 1966.
349. Muro, P. D., and Leonardi, G.: Hemopathic Mediterranean syndrome, Acta Med. Scand. **138**:362, 1950.
350. Myerson, R. M., Harrison, E., and Lohmuller, H. W.: Incidence and significance of abnormal hemoglobins; report of a series of 1,000 hospitalized Negro veterans, Amer. J. Med. **26**:543, 1959.
351. Naiman, J. L., Oski, F. A., and Diamond, L. K.: Thalassemia, Amer. J. Dis. Child. **106**: 234, 1963.
351a. Nalbandian, R. M.: Molecular aspects of sickle cell hemoglobin, Springfield, Ill., 1971, Charles C Thomas, Publisher.

352. Nalbandian, R. M., Henry, R. L., Nichols, B. M., Camp, F. R., Jr., and Wolf, P. L.: Molecular basis for a simple, specific test for S hemoglobin; the Murayama test, Clin. Chem. 16:945, 1970.
352a. Nalbandian, R. M., Schultz, G., Lusher, J. M., Anderson, J. W., and Henry, R. L.: Sickle cell crisis terminated by intravenous urea in sugar solution; a preliminary report, Amer. J. Med. Sci. 261:309, 1971.
353. Na-Nakorn, S., Minnich, V., and Chernoff, A. I.: Studies on hemoglobin E; the incidence of hemoglobin E in Thailand, J. Lab. Clin. Med. 47:490, 1956.
354. Nance, W. E.: Genetic control of hemoglobin synthesis, Science 141:123, 1963.
354a. Nathan, D. G.: Thalassemia, New Eng. J. Med. 286:586, 1972.
355. Nathan, D. G., and Gibson, J. M.: Thalassemia in a 48-year-old man, New Eng. J. Med. 278:782, 1968.
356. Nathan, D. G., and Gunn, R.: Thalassemia; the consequences of unbalanced hemoglobin synthesis, Amer. J. Med. 41:815, 1966.
357. Nathan, D. G., Stossel, T. B., Gunn, R. B., Zarkowsky, H. S., and Laforet, M. T.: Influence of hemoglobin precipitation on hemoglobin metabolism in alpha and beta thalassemia, J. Clin. Invest. 48:33, 1969.
358. Necheles, T. F., and Allen, D. M., Heinzbody anemias, New Eng. J. Med. 280:203, 1969.
359. Necheles, T. F., Allen, D. M., and Finkel, H. E.: Clinical disorders of hemoglobin structure and synthesis, New York, 1969, Appleton-Century-Crofts.
360. Necheles, T. F., Allen, D. M., and Gerald, P. S.: The many forms of thalassemia; definition and classification of the thalassemia syndromes, Ann. N. Y. Acad. Sci. 165:5, 1969.
361. Neel, J. V.: The inheritance of sickle cell anemia, Science 110:64, 1949.
362. Neel, J. V., and Valentine, W. N.: The frequency of thalassemia, Amer. J. Med. Sci. 209:568, 1945.
362a. Nienhuis, A. W., and Anderson, W. F.: Isolation and translation of hemoglobin messenger RNA from thalassemia, sickle cell anemia, and normal human reticulocytes, J. Clin. Invest. 50:2458, 1971.
363. Noll, J. B., Newman, A. J., and Gross, S.: Enuresis and nocturia in sickle cell disease, J. Pediat. 70:965, 1967.
364. Oliner, H. L., and Heller, P.: Megaloblastic erythropoiesis and acquired hemolysis in sickle-cell anemia, New Eng. J. Med. 261:19, 1959.
365. Olshin, I., and Sawitsky, A.: Familial thalassemia and erythremic myelosis, Pediatrics 22:250, 1958.
366. Opfell, R. W., Lorkin, P. A., and Lehmann, H.: Hereditary non-spherocytic haemolytic anaemia with post-splenectomy inclusion bodies and pigmenturia caused by an unstable haemoglobin Santa Ana-$\beta^{88}$ ($F_4$) leucine →proline, J. Med. Genet. 5:292, 1968.
367. Oski, F. A., and Delivoria-Papadopoulos, M.: The red cell, 2,3-diphosphoglycerate, and tissue oxygen release, J. Pediat. 77:941, 1970.
368. Owen, D. M., Aldridge, J. E., and Thompson, R. B.: An unusual hepatic sequela of sickle cell anemia; a report of five cases, Amer. J. Med. Sci. 249:175, 1965.
368a. Paik, C. H., Alavi, I., Dunea, G., and Weiner, I.: Thalassemia and gouty arthritis, J.A.M.A. 213:296, 1970.
369. Pascher, F., and Keen, R.: Ulcers of the leg in Cooley's anemia, New Eng. J. Med. 256:1220, 1957.
370. Pauling, L., Itano, H. A., Singer, S. J., and Wells, J. C.: Sickle cell anemia, a molecular disease, Science 110:543, 1949.
371. Pearson, H. A.: Newer concepts in the genetics of the thalassemias, Ped. Clin. N. Amer. 9:635, 1962.
372. Pearson, H. A., Cone, T. E., Jr., and Vertries, K. M.: Site of binding of chromium[51] to adult and fetal hemoglobins, Amer. J. Dis. Child. 102:598, 1961.
373. Pearson, H. A., Cornelius, E. A., Schwartz, A. D., Zelson, J. H., Wolfson, S. L., and Spencer, R. P.: Transfusion-reversible functional asplenia in young children with sickle-cell anemia, New Eng. J. Med. 283:334, 1970.
373a. Pearson, H. A., and Diamond, L. K.: The critically ill child; sickle cell disease crises and their management, Pediatrics 48:629, 1971.
374. Pearson, H. A., Gerald, P. S., and Diamond, L. K.: Thalassemia intermedia due to interaction of Lepore trait with thalassemia trait; report of three cases, Amer. J. Dis. Child. 97:464, 1959.
375. Pearson, H. A., McFarland, W., and King, E. R.: Erythrokinetic studies in thalassemia trait, J. Lab. Clin. Med. 56:866, 1960.
376. Pearson, H. A., and Noyes, W. D.: Thalassemia intermedia; cases in Negro siblings with unusual differences in minor hemoglobin components, Blood 23:829, 1964.
377. Pearson, H. A., and Noyes, W. D.: Failure of phenothiazines in sickle cell anemia, J.A.M.A. 199:33, 1967.
378. Pearson, H. A., Shanklin, D. R., and Brodine, C. R.: Alpha-thalassemia as cause of nonimmunological hydrops, Amer. J. Dis. Child. 109:168, 1965.
379. Pearson, H. A., Spencer, R. P., and Cornelius, E. A.: Functional asplenia in sickle-cell

anemia, New Eng. J. Med. 281:923, 1969.
380. Perkins, K. W., McInnes, I. W. S., Blackburn, C. R. B., and Beal, R. W.: Idiopathic haemochromatosis in children; report of a family, Amer. J. Med. 39:118, 1965.
381. Perosa, L., Ramunni, M., Bini, L., and Manganelli, G.: The genesis of sickle cell morphology, Acta haemat. 18:255, 1957.
382. Perutz, M. F., and Mitchison, J. M.: State of haemoglobin in sickle-cell anaemia, Nature 166:677, 1950.
383. Pierce, L. E., and Rath, C. E.: Evidence for folic acid deficiency in the genesis of anemic sickle cell crisis, Blood 20:19, 1962.
384. Pierce, L. E., Rath, C. E., and McCoy, K.: A new hemoglobin variant with sickling properties, New Eng. J. Med. 268:862, 1963.
385. Plachta, A., and Spier, R. D.: The coexistence of rheumatic heart disease and sickle cell anemia; review of the literature and report of case, Amer. J. Clin. Path. 22:970, 1952.
386. Plunket, D. C., Leikin, S. L., and LoPresti, J. M.: Renal radiologic changes in sickle cell anemia, Pediatrics 35:955. 1965.
387. Porter, F. S., and Thurman, W. G.: Studies of sickle cell disease, diagnosis in infancy, Amer. J. Dis. Child. 106:35, 1963.
388. Prindle, K. H., and McCurdy, P. R.: Red cell life-span in hemoglobin C disorders (with special reference to hemoglobin C trait), Blood 36:14, 1970.
389. Ramot, B., Abrahamov, A., Frayer, Z., and Gafni, D.: The incidence and types of thalassemia-trait carriers in Israel, Brit. J. Haemat. 10:155, 1964.
390. Ranney, H. M.: Observations on the inheritance of sickle cell hemoglobin and hemoglobin C, J. Clin. Invest. 33:1634, 1954.
391. Ranney, H. M.: Clinically important variants of human hemoglobin, New Eng. J. Med. 282:144, 1970.
392. Ranney, H. M., Jacobs, A. S., Bradley, T. B., Jr., and Cordova, F. A.: A "new" variant of haemoglobin $A_2$ and its segregation in a family with Hb-S, Nature 197:164, 1963.
393. Raper, A. B.: Sickling in relation to morbidity from malaria and other diseases, Brit. Med. J. 1:965, 1956.
394. Redman, J. F., and Mobley, J. E.: Sickle cell disease; renal colic and microscopic hematuria, J. Urol. 100:594, 1968.
395. Reich, R. S., and Rosenberg, N. J.: Aseptic necrosis of bone in Caucasians with chronic hemolytic anemia due to combined sickling and thalassemia traits, J. Bone Joint Surg. 35-A:894, 1953.
396. Reinhard, E. H., Moore, C. V., Dubach, R., and Wade, L. J.: Depressant effects of high concentrations of inspired oxygen on erythrocytogenesis, J. Clin. Invest. 23:682, 1944.
397. Reissman, K. R., Ruth, W. E., and Nomura, T.: A human hemoglobin with lowered oxygen affinity and impaired heme-heme interactions, J. Clin. Invest. 40:1826, 1961.
398. Reynolds, J.: Roentgenographic and clinical appraisal of sickle cell-hemoglobin C disease, Amer. J. Roentgen. 88:512, 1963.
399. Rhinesmith, H. S., Schroeder, W. A., and Pauling, L.: A quantitative study of hydrolysis of human DNP-globin; the number and kind of polypeptide chains in hemoglobin A, J. Amer. Chem. Soc. 79:4682, 1957.
400. Rich, A.: Studies on the hemoglobin of Cooley's anemia and Cooley's trait, Proc. Nat. Acad. Sci. 38:187, 1952.
401. Rieder, R. F., and Bradley, T. B., Jr.: Hemoglobin Gun Hill; an unstable protein associated with chronic hemolysis, Blood 32:355, 1968.
402. Rieder, R. F., and Naughton, M. A.: Hemoglobin $G_{Baltimore}$: a new abnormal hemoglobin and an additional individual with four hemoglobins, Bull. Johns Hopkins Hosp. 116:17, 1965.
403. Rieder, R. F., and Weatherall, D. J.: Studies on hemoglobin biosynthesis; asynchronous synthesis of hemoglobin A and hemoglobin $A_2$ by erythrocyte precursors, J. Clin. Invest. 44:42, 1965.
404. Rieder, R. F., Zinkham, W. H., and Holtzman, N. A.: Hemoglobin Zürich, clinical, chemical and kinetic studies, Amer. J. Med. 39:4, 1965.
405. Rifkind, R. A.: Heinz body anemia; an ultrastructural study. II. Red cell sequestration and destruction, Blood 26:433, 1965.
406. Rifkind, R. A.: Destruction of injured red cells in vivo, Amer. J. Med. 41:711, 1966.
407. Rifkind, R. A., and Danon, D.: Heinz body anemia; an ultrastructural study. I. Heinz body formation, Blood 25:885, 1965.
408. Rigas, D. A., and Koler, R. D.: Decreased erythrocyte survival in hemoglobin H disease as a result of abnormal properties of hemoglobin H; the benefit of splenectomy, Blood 18:1, 1961.
409. Rigas, D. A., Koler, R. D., and Osgood, E. E.: Hemoglobin H; clinical, laboratory, and genetic studies of a family with a previously undescribed hemoglobin, J. Lab. Clin. Med. 47:51, 1956.
410. River, G. L., Robbins, A. B., and Schwartz, S. O.: S-C hemoglobin; a clinical study, Blood 18:385, 1961.

411. Robbins, J. B., and Pearson, H. A.: Normal response of sickle cell anemia patients to immunization with Salmonella vaccine, J. Pediat. 66:877, 1965.
412. Robinson, A. R., Zuelzer, W. W., Neel, J. V., Livingstone, F. B., and Miller, M. J.: Two "fast" hemoglobin components in Liberian blood samples, Blood 11:902, 1956.
413. Robinson, M. G., and Watson, R. J.: Megaloblastic anemia complicating thalassemia major, Amer. J. Dis. Child. 105:275, 1963.
414. Robinson, M. G., and Watson, R. J.: Pneumoccocal meningitis in sickle cell anemia, New Eng. J. Med. 274:1006, 1966.
415. Robinson, S., Vanier, T., Desforges, J. F., and Schmid, R.: Jaundice in thalassemia minor; a consequence of "ineffective erythropoiesis," New Eng. J. Med. 267:523, 1962.
416. Rodman, T., Close, H. P., Cathcart, R., and Purcell, M. K.: The oxyhemoglobin dissociation curve in the common hemaglobinopathies, Amer. J. Med. 27:558, 1959.
417. Rodriguez, S., Leikin, S., Bullock, W. H., and Booker, C.: Hereditary spherocytosis and sickle cell trait in the Negro, J. Pediat. 68:589, 1966.
418. Rubenstein, E.: Studies on the relationship of temperature in sickle cell anemia, Amer. J. Med. 30:95, 1961.
419. Rucknagel, D. L., Page, E. B., and Jensen, W. N.: Hemoglobin I; an inherited hemoglobin anomaly, Blood 10:999, 1955.
420. Russell, P. S., and Winn, H. J.: Transplantation, New Eng. J. Med. 282:896, 1970.
421. Salvaggio, J. E., Arnold, C. A., and Banov, C. H.: Long term anticoagulation in sickle cell disease; a clinical study, New Eng. J. Med. 269:182, 1963.
422. Saxena, V. H., Scott, R. B., and Ferguson, A. D.: Studies in sickle cell anemia. XXV. Observations on fluid intake and output, J. Pediat. 69:220, 1966.
423. Schell, N. B., and McGinley, J. M.: Sickle-cell hemoglobin C disease, Amer. J. Dis. Child. 91:38, 1956.
424. Schellhammer, P. F., Engle, M. A., and Hagstrom, J. W. C.: Histochemical studies of the myocardium and conduction system in acquired iron-storage disease, Circulation 25:631, 1967.
425. Schettini, F.: Diagnosis of thalassemia major in the first months of life, Ann. N. Y. Acad. Sci. 165:387, 1969.
426. Schneider, R. G., and Haggard, M. E.: Haemoglobin P (the 'Galveston' type), Nature 182:322, 1958.
427. Schnitzer, B., and Smith, E. B.: Observations of phagocytized red cells containing Heinz bodies, Arch. J. Clin. Path. 46:538, 1966.
428. Schulman, I., Smith, C. H., and Stern G. S.: Studies on the anemia of prematurity, Amer. J. Dis. Child. 88:567, 1954.
429. Schwartz, E.: The silent carrier of beta thalassemia, New Eng. J. Med. 281:1327, 1969.
429a. Schwartz, E.: Heterozygous beta thalassemia; balanced globin synthesis in bone marrow cells, Science 167:1513, 1970.
430. Schwartz, E., and McElfresh, A. E.: Treatment of painful crises of sickle cell disease; a double blind study, J. Pediat. 64:132, 1964.
431. Schwartz, H., and Spaet, T. H.: Hemoglobin G; a fifth abnormal hemoglobin, Clin. Res. Proc. 3:51, 1955.
432. Schwartz, H. C., Spaet, T. H., Zuelzer, W. W., Neel, J. V., Robinson, A. R., and Kaufman, S. F.: Combinations of hemoglobin G, hemoglobin S and thalassemia occurring in one family, Blood 12:238, 1957.
433. Scott, R. B.: In Gellis, S. S., editor: Year book of pediatrics, Series 1957-1958, Chicago, 1957, Year Book Medical Publishers, Inc., p. 294.
434. Scott, R. B.: Sickle cell anemia; pathogenesis and treatment, Ped. Clin. N. Amer. 9:649, 1962.
435. Scott, R. B.: Sickle cell anemia—high prevalence and low priority, New Eng. J. Med. 282:164, 1970.
436. Scott, R. B., Banks, L. O., Jenkins, M. E., and Crawford, R. P.: Studies in sickle-cell anemia; clinical manifestations of sickle-cell anemia in children, J. Pediat. 39:460, 1951.
437. Scott, R. B., and Ferguson, A. D.: Studies in sickle cell anemia. XXVII. Complications in infants and children in the United States, Clin. Pediat. 5:403, 1966.
438. Scott, R. B., Ferguson, A. D., Jenkins, M. E., and Clark, H. M.: Studies in sickle-cell anemia; further observations on the clinical manifestations of sickle-cell anemia in children, Amer. J. Dis. Child. 90:682, 1955.
439. Scott, R. B., and Jenkins, M. E.: Studies in sickle-cell anemia, sickle-cell hemoglobin C disease, Amer. J. Dis. Child. 90:35, 1955.
440. Sen Gupta, P. C., Chatterjea, J. B., Mukherjee, A. M., and Chatterji, A.: Observations on foam cells in thalassemia, Blood 16:1039, 1960.
441. Serjeant, G. R.: Irreversibly sickled cells and splenomegaly in sickle-cell anaemia, Brit. J. Haemat. 19:635, 1970.
442. Serjeant, G. R., Richards, R., Barbor, P. R. H., and Milner, P. F.: Relatively benign sickle-cell anaemia in 60 patients aged over 30 in the West Indies, Brit. Med. J. 3:86, 1968.
443. Serjeant, G. R., Serjeant, B. E., and Milner, P. F.: The irreversibly sickled cell; a deter-

minant of hemolysis in sickle cell anaemia, Brit. J. Haemat. **17**:527, 1969.
444. Sfikakis, P., and Stamatoyannopoulos, G.: Bone changes in thalassemia trait; an x-ray appraisal of 55 cases, Acta Haemat. **29**:193, 1963.
445. Shahidi, N. T., and Diamond, L. K.: Alkali-resistant hemoglobin in aplastic anemia of both acquired and congenital types, New Eng. J. Med. **266**:117, 1962.
446. Sheba, C., Goodman, R. M., and Shahin, N.: A Bucharan Jewish family with thalassemia re-evaluated after twenty years, Proc. Tel-Hashomer Hosp. **3**:98, 1964.
447. Shelley, W. M., and Curtis, E. M.: Bone marrow and fat embolism in sickle cell anemia and sickle cell-hemoglobin C disease, Bull. Johns Hopkins Hosp. **103**:8, 1958.
448. Shen, S. C., Fleming, E. M., and Castle, W. B.: Studies on the destruction of red blood cells; irreversibly sickled erythrocytes; their experimental production in vitro, Blood **4**:498, 1949.
449. Shepard, M. K., Weatherall, D. J., and Conley, C. L.: Semi-quantitative estimation of the distribution of fetal hemoglobin in red cell populations, Bull. Johns Hopkins Hosp. **110**:293, 1962.
450. Shields, G. S., Lichtman, H. C., Messite, J., and Watson, R. J.: Studies in sickle cell disease; quantitative aspects of sickling in the newborn period, Pediatrics **22**:309, 1958.
451. Shields, G. S., Wethers, D., Gavis, G., and Watson, R. J.: Hemoglobin-S-thalassemia disease, Amer. J. Dis. Child. **91**:485, 1956.
452. Shotton, D., Crockett, C. L., Jr., and Leavell, B. S.: Splenectomy in sickle cell anemia; report of a case and review of the literature, Blood **6**:365, 1951.
453. Silver, H. K.: Mediterranean anemia in children of non-mediterranean ancestry, Amer. J. Dis. Child. **80**:767, 1950.
454. Silvestroni, E., and Bianco, I.: Genetic aspects of sickle-cell anemia and microdrepanocytic disease, Blood **7**:429, 1952.
455. Silvestroni, E., Bianco, I., and Baglioni, C.: Interaction of hemoglobin Lepore with sickle cell trait and microcythemia (thalassemia) in a Southern Italian family, Blood **25**:457, 1965.
456. Singer, K.: Hereditary hemolytic disorders associated with alterations of the hemoglobin molecule, Amer. J. Med. **18**:633, 1955.
457. Singer, K., Chapman, A. Z., Goldberg, S. R., Rubenstein, H. M., and Rosenblum, S. A.: Studies on abnormal hemoglobins; a new syndrome, hemoglobin C-thalassemia disease, Blood **9**:1023, 1954.
458. Singer, K., Chernoff, A. I., and Singer, L.: Studies on abnormal hemoglobin, Blood **6**:413, 1951.
459. Singer, K., and Fisher, B.: Studies on abnormal hemoglobins; electrophoretic demonstration of type S (sickle cell) hemoglobin in erythrocytes incapable of showing the sickle cell phenomenon, Blood **8**:270, 1953.
460. Singer, K., Josephson, A. M., Singer, L., Heller, P., and Zimmerman, H. S.: Studies of abnormal hemoglobins; hemoglobin S-thalassemia disease and hemoglobin C-thalassemia disease in siblings, Blood **12**:593, 1957.
461. Singer, K., Robin, S., King, J. C., and Jefferson, R. N.: The life span of the sickle-cell and the pathogenesis of sickle-cell anemia, J. Lab. Clin. Med. **33**:975, 1948.
462. Singer, K., and Singer, L.: Studies on abnormal hemoglobins; the gelling phenomenon of sickle cell hemoglobin; its biologic and diagnostic significance, Blood **8**:1008, 1953.
463. Singer, K., Singer, L., and Goldberg, S. R.: Studies on abnormal hemoglobin; sickle cell-thalassemia disease in the Negro, the significance of S + A + F and S + A patterns obtained by hemoglobin analysis, Blood **10**:405, 1955.
464. Slater, L. M., Muir, W. A., and Weed, R. I.: Influence of splenectomy on insoluble hemoglobin inclusion bodies in beta thalassemic erythrocytes, Blood **31**:766, 1968.
465. Smith, C. H.: Mediterranean (Cooley's) anemia in a youth of nineteen years observed since early childhood, J. Pediat. **20**:370, 1942.
466. Smith, C. H.: Familial blood studies in cases of Mediterranean (Cooley's) anemia; diagnosis of the trait or mild form of the disease, Amer. J. Dis. Child. **65**:681, 1943.
467. Smith, C. H.: Detection of mild types of Mediterranean (Cooley's) anemia, Amer. J. Dis. Child. **75**:505, 1948.
468. Smith, C. H.: Transfusions in pediatric practice; indications and limitations, Pediatrics **17**:596, 1956.
469. Smith, C. H., Erlandson, M. E., Schulman, I., and Stern, G.: Serum iron and iron-binding capacity of the serum in children with severe Mediterranean (Cooley's) anemia, Pediatrics **5**:799, 1950.
470. Smith, C. H., Erlandson, M. E., Schulman, I., and Stern, G.: Hazard of severe infections in splenectomized infants and children, Amer. J. Med. **22**:390, 1957.
471. Smith, C. H., Erlandson, M. E., Stern, G., and Hilgartner, M. W.: Postsplenectomy infection in Cooley's anemia; an appraisal of the problem in this and other blood

disorders with consideration of prophylaxis, New Eng. J. Med. **266**:737, 1962.
472. Smith, C. H., Erlandson, M. E., Stern, G., and Schulman, I.: The role of splenectomy in the management of thalassemia, Blood **15**:197, 1960.
473. Smith, C. H., and Morgenthau, J. E.: Cholelithiasis in severe Mediterranean (Cooley's) anemia, Blood **6**:1147, 1951.
474. Smith, C. H., Schulman, I., Ando, R. E., and Stern, G.: Studies in Mediterranean (Cooley's) anemia; clinical and hematologic aspects of splenectomy, with special reference to fetal hemoglobin synthesis, Blood **10**:582, 1955.
475. Smith, C. H., Schulman, I., Ando, R. E., and Stern, G.: Studies in Mediterranean (Cooley's) anemia; the suppression of hematopoiesis by transfusion, Blood **10**:707, 1955.
476. Smith, E., Rosenblatt, P., and Bedo, A. V.: Sickle-cell anemia crisis; report on seven patients treated with Priscoline, J. Pediat. **43**:655, 1953.
477. Smith, E. W., and Conley, C. L.: Clinical features of the genetic variants of sickle-cell disease, Bull. Johns Hopkins Hosp. **94**:289, 1954.
478. Smith, E. W., and Conley, C. L.: Sicklemia and infarction of the spleen during aerial flight, Bull. Johns Hopkins Hosp. **96**:35, 1955.
479. Smith, E. W., and Conley, C. L.: Sickle cell-hemoglobin-D disease, Ann. Intern. Med. **50**:94, 1959.
480. Smith, E. W., and Krevans, J. R.: Clinical manifestations of hemoglobin C disorders, Bull. Johns Hopkins Hosp. **104**:17, 1959.
481. Smith, E. W., and Torbert, J. V.: Study of two abnormal hemoglobins with evidence of a new genetic locus for hemoglobin formation, Bull. Johns Hopkins Hosp. **101**:38, 1958.
482. Smith, I.: Chromatographic and electrophoretic techniques. Vol. 2, Zone electrophoresis, New York, 1960, Interscience Publishers, Inc.
483. Smith, R. S.: Iron excretion in thalassemia major after administration of chelating agents, Brit. Med. J. **2**:1577, 1962.
484. Smith, R. S.: Chelating agents in the diagnosis and treatment of iron overload in thalassemia, Ann. N. Y. Acad. Sci. **119**:776, 1964.
485. Smithies, O.: An improved procedure for starch-gel electrophoresis; further variation in the serum protein of normal individuals, Biochem. J. **71**:585, 1959.
486. Smits, H. L., Oski, F. A., and Brody, J. I.: The hemolytic crisis of sickle cell disease; the role of glucose-6-phosphate dehydrogenase deficiency, J. Pediat. **74**:544, 1969.
487. Song, Y. S.: Hepatic lesions in sickle cell anemia, Amer. J. Path. **33**:331, 1957.
488. Soster, G., and Oski, F. A.: Enuresis in sickle cell anemia, Amer. J. Dis. Child. **113**:311, 1967.
489. Spaet, T. H.: Personal communication, New York.
490. Sprague, C. C., and Paterson, J. C. S.: Role of the spleen and effect of splenectomy in sickle cell disease, Blood **13**:569, 1958.
491. Stamatoyannopoulos, G., Papayannopoulou, T., Fessas, P., and Motulsky, A. G.: The beta-delta thalassemias, Ann. N. Y. Acad. Sci. **165**:25, 1969.
492. Stamatoyannopoulos, G., Parer, J. T., and Finch, C. A.: Physiologic implications of a hemoglobin with decreased oxygen affinity (hemoglobin Seattle), New Eng. J. Med. **28**:915, 1969.
493. Stanfield, J. B.: Acute benign pericarditis in thalassemia major, Proc. Royal Soc. Med. **55**:236, 1962.
494. Steiner, M., Baldini, M., and Dameshek, W.: Enzymatic defects of heme-synthesis in thalassemia, Ann. N. Y. Acad. Sci. **119**:548, 1964.
495. Stetson, C. A., Jr.: The state of hemoglobin in sickled erythrocytes, J. Exp. Med. **123**:341, 1966.
496. Stocks, A. E., and Martin, F. I. R.: Pituitary function in haemochromatosis, Amer. J. Med. **45**:839, 1968.
497. Sturgeon, P., and Finch, C. A.: Erythrokinetics in Cooley's anemia, Blood **12**:64, 1957.
498. Sturgeon, P., Itano, H. A., and Bergren, W. R.: Clinical manifestations of inherited abnormal hemoglobins; the interactions of hemoglobin S with hemoglobin D, Blood **10**:389, 1955.
499. Sturgeon, P., Itano, H. A., and Bergren, W. R.: Clinical manifestations of inherited abnormal hemoglobins; interaction of hemoglobin E and thalassemia trait, Blood **10**:396, 1955.
500. Sturgeon, P., Schroeder, W. A., Jones, R. T., and Bergren, W. R.: The relation of alkali-resistant haemoglobin in thalassemia and abnormal haemoglobin syndromes to foetal haemoglobin, Brit. J. Haemat. **9**:438, 1963.
501. Sweeney, M. J., Dobbins, W. T., and Etteldorf, J. N.: Renal disease with elements of the nephrotic syndrome associated with sickle cell anemia, J. Pediat. **60**:42, 1962.
502. Sydenstricker, V. P., Kemp, J. A., and Metts, J. C.: Prolonged survival in sickle cell disease, Amer. Practitioner **13**:584, 1962.

503. Tanaka, K. R., Clifford, G. O., and Axelrod, A. R.: Sickle cell anemia (homozygous S) with aseptic necrosis of the femoral head, Blood 11:998, 1956.
504. Thomas, E. D., Motulsky, A. G., and Walters, D. H.: Homozygous hemoglobin C disease; report of a case with studies on the pathophysiology and neonatal formation of hemoglobin C, Amer. J. Med. 18:832, 1955.
505. Tomlinson, W. J.: Abdominal crisis in uncomplicated sickle cell anemia; a clinicopathologic study of 11 cases with a suggested explanation of their cause, Amer. J. Med. Sci. 209:722, 1945.
506. Thompson, O. L., Moreland, H. J., Smith, G. W., Bowman, B. H., Alexander, M. J., and Schneider, R. G.: A family with hemoglobin I, Blood 22:313, 1963.
507. Thompson, R. B., Mitchner, J. W., and Huisman, T. H. J.: Studies on the fetal hemoglobin in the persistent high Hb-F anomaly, Blood 18:267, 1961.
508. Thorup, O. A., Itano, H. A., Wheby, M., and Leavell, B. S.: Hemoglobin J, Science 123:889, 1956.
509. Todd, R. McC., and O'Donohue, N. V.: Acute acquired haemolytic anaemia associated with herpes simplex infection, Arch. Dis. Child. 33:524, 1958.
510. Trowell, H. C., Raper, A. B., and Welbourn, H. F.: The natural history of homozygous sickle-cell anaemia in Central Africa, Quart. J. Med. 26:401, 1957.
511. Tuttle, A. H.: Newer techniques in the investigation of blood disorders; electrophoresis and red cell labelling with radioisotopes, Ped. Clin. N. Amer. 9:527, 1962.
512. Tuttle, A. H., and Koch, B.: Clinical and hematological manifestations of hemoglobin CS disease in children, J. Pediat. 56:331, 1960.
513. Tyuma, I., and Shimizu, K.: Different responses to organic phosphates of human fetal and adult hemoglobin, Arch. Biochem. 129:404, 1969.
514. Uzsoy, N. K.: The coexistence of rheumatic heart disease and sickle cell anemia, Amer. J. Med. Sci. 246:462, 1963.
515. Valtis, D. J., and Kennedy, A. C.: Defective gas-transport function of stored red-blood cells, Lancet 1:119, 1954.
516. VanEps, L. W. S., Pinedo-Veels, C., Vries, G. H., and de Konig, J.: Nature of concentrating defect in sickle-cell nephropathy; microradioangiographic studies, Lancet 1:450, 1970.
517. Vats, T., Canale, V. C., and Lanzkowsky, P.: Folate metabolism in thalassemia major, Amer. Ped. Soc., 79th Annual Meeting, Program and Abstracts, p. 61, April 30-May 3, 1969.
518. Veiga, S., and Vaithianathan, T.: Massive intravascular sickling after exchange transfusion with sickle cell trait blood, Tranfusion 3:387, 1963.
519. Vella, F., Wells, R. H. C., Ager, J. A. M., and Lehmann, H.: A haemoglobinopathy involving haemoglobin H and a new (Q) haemoglobin, Brit. Med. J. 1:752, 1958.
520. Vinograd, J. R., Hutchinson, W. D., and Schroeder, W. A.: $C^{14}$-hybrids of human hemoglobins. II. The identification of the aberrant chain in human hemoglobin S, J. Amer. Chem. Soc. 81:3168, 1959.
521. Wade, L. J., and Stevenson, J. D.: Necrosis of the bone marrow with fat embolism in sickle cell anemia, Amer. J. Path. 17:47, 1941.
522. Wasi, P., Disthasongchan, P., and Na-Nakorn, S.: The effect of iron deficiency on the levels of hemoglobin A and E, J. Lab. Clin. Med. 71:85, 1968.
523. Wasi, P., Na-Nakorn, S., Pootrakol, S., Sookanek, M., Disthasongchan, P., Pornpatkul, M., and Panich, V.: Alpha- and beta-thalassemia in Thailand, Ann. N. Y. Acad. Sci. 165:60, 1969.
524. Watson, J., Stahman, A. W., and Bilello, F. P.: The significance of the paucity of sickle cells in newborn Negro infants, Amer. J. Med. Sci. 215:419, 1948.
525. Watson, R. J.: Hereditary anemias, Bull. N. Y. Acad. Med. 30:106, 1954.
526. Watson, R. J.: Hemoglobins and disease. In Snapper, I., and Dock, W., editors: Advances in internal medicine, vol. 8, Chicago, 1956, Year Book Medical Publishers, Inc., p. 305.
527. Watson, R. J., Burko, H., Megas, H., and Robinson, M.: The hand-foot syndrome in sickle-cell disease in young children, Pediatrics 31:975, 1963.
528. Watson, R. J., Lichtman, H. C., and Shapiro, H. D.: Splenomegaly in sickle cell anemia, Amer. J. Med. 20:196, 1956.
529. Weatherall, D. J.: Abnormal haemoglobins in the neonatal period and their relationship to thalassemia, Brit. J. Haemat. 9:265, 1963.
530. Weatherall, D. J.: The thalassaemia syndromes, Philadelphia, 1965, F. A. Davis Co.
531. Weatherall, D. J.: The genetics of the thalassemias, Brit. Med. Bull. 25:24, 1969.
532. Weatherall, D. J.: Polycythemia resulting from abnormal hemoglobins, New Eng. J. Med. 280:604, 1969.
533. Weens, H. S.: Cholelithiasis in sickle cell anemia, Ann. Intern. Med. 22:182, 1945.
534. Weinstein, I. M., Spurling, C. L., Klein,

H., and Necheles, T. F.: Radioactive sodium chromate for the study of survival of red cells. III. The abnormal hemoglobin syndromes, Blood 9:1155, 1954.
535. Weissman, R., Jr., Hurley, T. H., Harris, J. W., and Ham, T. H.: Studies on the function of spleen in the hemolysis of red cells in hereditary spherocytosis and sickle-cell disorders, J. Lab. Clin. Med. 42:965, 1954.
536. Wells, I. C., and Itano, H. A.: Ratio of sickle-cell anemia hemoglobin to normal hemoglobin in sicklemics, J. Biol. Chem. 188:65, 1951.
537. Went, L. N., and MacIver, J. E.: Thalassemia in the West Indies, Blood 17:166, 1961.
538. Wheeler, J. T., and Krevans, J. R.: The homozygous state of persistent fetal hemoglobin with thalassemia, Bull. Johns Hopkins Hosp. 109:217, 1961.
539. Whipple, G. H., and Bradford, W. L.: Racial or familial anemia of children associated with fundamental disturbances of the bone and pigment metabolism, Amer. J. Dis. Child. 44:336, 1932.
540. Whipple, G. H., and Bradford, W. L.: Mediterranean disease-thalassemia, J. Pediat. 9:279, 1936.
541. Whitaker, J. A., Windmiller, J., Vietti, T., and Sartain, P.: Hereditary spherocytosis associated with sickle trait and cholelithiasis, J. Pediat. 63:65, 1963.
542. White, J. C., and Beaven, G. H.: A review of the varieties of human haemoglobin in health and disease, J. Clin. Path. 7:175, 1954.
543. White, J. G.: The fine structure of sickled hemoglobin in situ, Blood 31:561, 1968.
544. White, J. M., and Brain, M. C.: Defective synthesis of an unstable haemoglobin; haemoglobin Köln ($\beta^{98}$ Val-Met), Brit. J. Haemat. 18:195, 1970.
545. White, J. M., and Jones, R. W.: Management of pregnancy in a women with HbH disease, Brit. Med. J. 4:473, 1969.
546. Winkelstein, J. A., and Drachman, R. H.: Deficiency of pneumococcal serum opsonizing activity in sickle-cell disease, New Eng. J. Med. 279:459, 1968.
547. Winsor, T., and Burch, G. E.: Habitus of patients with active sickle cell anemia of long duration, Arch. Intern. Med. 76:47, 1945.
548. Witzleben, C. L., and Wyatt, J. P.: The effect of long survival on the pathology of thalassemia major, J. Path. Bact. 82:1, 1961.
549. Wöhler, F.: The treatment of hemochromatosis with desferioxamine, Acta Haemat. 30:65, 1963.
550. Wolff, J. A., and Ignatov, V. G.: Heterogeneity of thalassemia major, Amer. J. Dis. Child. 105:234, 1963.
551. Wolff, J. A., Michaels, R. H., and Von Hofe, F. H.: Hemoglobin H-thalassemia disease, Blood 8:492, 1958.
552. Wolman, I. J.: Transfusion therapy in Cooley's anemia; growth and health as related to long-term hemoglobin levels; a progress report, Ann. N. Y. Acad. Sci. 119:736, 1964.
553. Zannos, L.: Studies on the resistance of haemoglobin to alkali, Acta paediat. 42:305, 1953.
554. Zarafonetis, C. J. D., McMaster, J. D., Molthan, L., and Steiger, W. A.: Apparent renal defect in sicklemic individuals, Amer. J. Med. Sci. 232:76, 1956.
555. Zuelzer, W. W., and Kaplan, E.: Thalassemia-hemoglobin C disease; a new syndrome presumably due to the combination of the genes for thalassemia and hemoglobin C, Blood 9:1047, 1954.
556. Zuelzer, W. W., Neel, J. V., and Robinson, A. R.: Abnormal hemoglobins. In Tocantins, L. M., editor: Progress in hematology, vol. 1, New York, 1956, Grune & Stratton, Inc., p. 91.
557. Zuelzer, W. W., Robinson, A. R., and Booker, C. R.: Reciprocal relationship of hemoglobin $A_2$ and F in beta chain thalassemia; a key to genetic control of hemoglobin F, Blood 17:393, 1961.

# 17 POLYCYTHEMIA, METHEMOGLOBINEMIA, SULFHEMOGLOBINEMIA, AND MISCELLANEOUS ANEMIAS

## POLYCYTHEMIA

Polycythemia refers to an increase in the number of red blood cells, in the hemoglobin level, and in the hematocrit per unit volume of blood which is substantially in excess of normal values. Several types of polycythemia may be differentiated: *true or absolute polycythemia,* in which the total number of red cells (red cell mass) in the circulating blood is increased, and *relative polycythemia,* resulting from shrinkage of the total plasma volume, in which the red cell volume remains normal.

True polycythemia may be further classified into *primary polycythemia,* polycythemia vera of unknown etiology, and *secondary polycythemia,* in which there is an increase in total volume of red cells in response to a recognizable cause. The latter includes conditions in which oxygen saturation of arterial blood is lowered, pathologic states involving the central nervous system, and abnormalities of the hemoglobin molecule associated with increased oxygen affinity or of pigment metabolism. Except in persons with polycythemia due to hemoconcentration, the blood volume is increased chiefly as a result of augmentation of circulating red cells.

The alkaline-phosphatase activity in the polymorphonuclear cell serves as a differential test between the two types of polycythemia. A strongly positive test is observed in persons with leukemoid reactions due to polycythemia vera, and a negative test signifies myelogenous leukemia. Secondary polycythemia unassociated with a leukemoid response falls within the range of normal.[45,89]

### Relative polycythemia

Relative polycythemia is observed in persons with conditions of hemoconcentration associated with marked loss of body fluids, as occurs in patients with diarrhea, vomiting, severe burns, profuse sweating, and dehydration from water deprivation. The "polycythemia of stress" occurring in anxiety states in adults is also due to reduced blood volume.[37,87] In patients with relative polycythemia, the white blood cells and platelets are normal.

### Primary polycythemia (polycythemia vera, erythremia, Vaquez-Osler disease)

Primary polycythemia is a specific disease of unknown etiology characterized by cerebral and cardiovascular symptoms, a peculiar reddish purple color of the skin, bloodshot eyes, visual disturbances, thrombosis and hemorrhage, and usually splenomegaly. This disease occurs in middle and old age and is extremely rare in childhood.[43,81] The bone marrow is hyperplastic; total blood cell formation is increased with a marked elevation of red cells, hemoglobin level, and hematocrit, as well as of leukocytes and platelets. Hemorrhagic and thromboembolic phenomena in this disease are attributed to hypervolemia, increased red cell mass with resultant sluggish blood flow, thrombocytosis, and ineffective clot formation.[2,137] Studies with $^{59}$Fe show increased hemoglobin formation within normal iron pathways.[4] The total blood volume is strikingly increased. Intravenously administered radioactive phosphorus is the treatment of choice. The disease is chronic, progressive, and ultimately fatal. The absence of splenomegaly and, particularly, normal white cell and platelet counts rule out polycythemia vera.

*Benign familial polycythemia.* Benign familial polycythemia is another type of primary polycythemia which occurs more frequently in children than does polycythemia vera. Recently, a number of abnormal hemoglobins associated with increased oxygen affinity and a leftward shift of the oxygen dissociation curve have been identified. These include Hb Chesapeake,[27] Hb Yakima,[102] Hb Rainier,[128] Hb Ypsilanti,[64,117] Hb Kempsey,[111] Hb Hiroshima,[69] and Hb J Capetown.[15] The altered oxygen affinity in these hemoglobinopathies stimulates increased erythropoietin secretion and increased erythropoiesis and results in polycythemia. The patient, one or more siblings, and in some cases a parent manifest an elevated hemoglobin level (up to 27 gm. per 100 ml.), red cell count (10 million per cubic millimeter), and hematocrit (82%) without evidence of underlying cardiopulmonary insufficiency. There is no splenomegaly or other physical sign except for a ruddy countenance and deeply injected conjunctivae. The red cell mass is increased, but the leukocyte and platelet counts are normal, thus differing from polycythemia vera.[9,99] Red cell survival may sometimes be prolonged to explain the polycythemia rather than increased red cell production.[82] The condition may be asymptomatic or it might be associated with minor manifestations of headache, lethargy, occasionally dizziness, and easy fatigability.[1] No treatment is needed; the prognosis is favorable.

## Secondary polycythemia (erythrocytosis, erythrocythemia, compensatory polycythemia)

The term secondary polycythemia signifies an increase in the total volume of red cells in response to a recognizable cause. Secondary polycythemia is most commonly found in infancy and childhood in patients with cyanotic congenital heart disease due to shunts from the pulmonary circuit. The mixture of unsaturated venous blood and arterial blood results in a lowered oxygen saturation. The hemoglobin ranges between 15 and 25 gm. per 100 ml., the red count between 5.5 and 9 million, and the hematocrit between 65 and 85%, paralleling the red cell counts.[3] The mean red cell volume is usually higher than in normal children of corresponding age and weight, ranging between 80 and 110$\mu^3$.[149] The polycythemia serves as an extremely effective compensatory mechanism until the hematocrit reaches levels of 80% or more. At this point the disadvantages of coexisting high blood viscosity outweigh the advantages of the increased available oxygen which polycythemia provides.[98,118] The response of the bone marrow to the persistent anoxic stimulus which accounts for the polycythemia is probably mediated by erythropoietin.[68] It is of interest that a hemoglobin concentration which is regarded as normal for the average child may represent a state of hypochromic anemia in the young patient with cyanotic heart disease and erythrocytosis. Iron therapy corrects the hypochromic anemia and is responsible for a further increase in the red cell count, hemoglobin level, and hematocrit. In the patient with polycythemia associated with cyanotic congenital heart disease, there is no persistence of fetal hemoglobin and, in contrast to polycythemia vera, the leukocyte and platelet counts are not increased. Following operative correction of tetralogy of Fallot, reticulocytes are diminished to a very low point, and urobilin excretion is greatly increased. Both mechanisms, a virtual cessation of blood formation and, to an even greater extent, blood destruction, contribute to a reduction of the preoperative polycythemia.[78]

Lowered arterial oxygen saturation also prevails in patients with chronic pulmonary disease because of imperfect oxygenation of the blood in the lungs with resulting polycythemia as in patients with emphysema and fibrosis. Compensatory polycythemia occurs in persons living in areas at high altitudes where the partial pressure of oxygen is reduced and in those with methemoglobinemia and sulfhemoglobinemia in whom the oxygen-carrying capacity of the red blood cells is compromised by the presence of these pigments. The clinical manifestations of chronic mountain sickness, which occurs in persons living at high altitudes, resemble those of polycythemia.[97] In rare cases those persons living for long periods at great elevations may develop all the hematologic and physical features of polycythemia vera. Not only is there erythroid but also marked megakaryocytic hyperplasia. The greatly increased number of platelets in such cases is a prominent feature of primary, rather than of secondary, polycythemia.[93] Other causes of secondary polycythemia include brain tumors such as cerebellar hemangioblastomas, Cushing's syndrome, kidney tumors (particularly hypernephroma[34]), hydronephrosis,[59] and often cobalt therapy.

Abnormally high erythrocyte values in the neonatal period in excess of normal for this period have been described in conjunction with anorexia and nervous system signs and symptoms.[150] Polycythemia also may occur as a complication of congenital adrenal hyperplasia[65] in the newborn infant in whom levels of hemoglobin and hematocrit may be so high as to require phlebotomies.

Boys and girls from 10 to 18 years of age often normally show maximal hemoglobin values of 16 to 18 gm. per 100 ml. and red cell counts of 5.5 to 6.5 million per cubic millimeter. These peak values simulating polycythemia recede in subsequent years. A form of benign polycythemia associated with hypertension but not with splenomegaly, leukocytosis, or thrombocytosis indicative of polycythemia vera has been described in white males of early middle age.[119] This syndrome, described originally by Gaisböck, may have its origin in those adolescents in whom, for some reason, the polycythemia does not normally recede.

The role of puberty in influencing the rate of hemoglobin production is manifested in the significant difference in hemoglobin concentrations between adults and children in various anemias. It has been our experience, for instance, that in thalassemia minor the hemoglobin rises to normal values and the red blood cell count to normal or polycythemic levels in the male adolescent. Despite improvement in blood values, the poikilocytosis and stippling characteristics of the younger patient persist. Shahidi and Clatanoff[121] in a long-term follow-up of two male siblings with hereditary nonspherocytic hemolytic anemia noted marked hematologic improvement in the older boy during puberty, whereas the younger brother, who was prepubescent, remained anemic. While the erythrocyte life-span was the same in both patients, the total nucleated erythron was greater in the older boy, namely, increased hemoglobin was synthesized. The significant differences in hemoglobin concentrations between adults and children was also documented in larger groups of those with hereditary nonspherocytic (associated with G-6-PD deficiency) and spherocytic hemolytic anemia. These observations suggested that puberty in males plays an important role in compensation of the hemolytic process possibly resulting from erythroid stimulation by androgens produced endogenously.

## METHEMOGLOBINEMIA

Iron normally exists in the ferrous state in the iron porphyrin complex of the heme portion of the hemoglobin molecule. Methemoglobin is formed when hemoglobin in its deoxygenated state is oxidized to the ferric form. In this state iron cannot combine with oxygen, and, when methemoglobin is produced in significant amounts it reduces the oxygen-combining capacity of the blood which is thus incapable of transporting oxygen. Methemoglobinemia is characterized by intense cyanosis due to the presence of methemoglobin in the circulating red blood cells in concentrations substantially above normal.

Primary, or congenital, and secondary, or drug-induced, methemoglobinemia are the two major types of this condition. In patients with a less common form of congenital methemoglobinemia the defect lies in the globin component and is therefore included in the discussion of abnormal hemoglobins (hemoglobins M) (Chapter 16). Primary, or congenital, methemoglobinemia can be further characterized on a hereditary basis as either recessive, due to an enzyme deficiency, or dominant, due to a hemoglobinopathy.

*Pathogenesis.* Methemoglobin is being formed continuously in the red cells and is simultaneously reduced to hemoglobin by one or more enzymes in the erythrocytes so that the content of methemoglobin within the red cells is less than 2% of the total hemoglobin.[13] The mean value for methemoglobin has been given as 2.2% in premature infants, between 1 and 1.5% in newborn infants and children in the first year of life, and below 1% thereafter.[84] The enzyme system responsible for normally reducing methemoglobin to hemoglobin is dependent upon the integrity of the erythrocyte and is associated with the glycolytic process.[13] The effects of the formation of methemoglobin are twofold. First, methemoglobin as such becomes unavailable for transport of oxygen. Second, the presence of methemoglobin renders the dissociation curve of the residual oxyhemoglobin less S shaped and more hyperbolic. Indeed, this change causes a shift of the dissociation curve of the residual oxyhemoglobin to the left. The total effect is a lowered capacity for unloading oxygen to the tissues and, hence, a tissue susceptibility to anoxia.[13,38]

Relatively small amounts of methemoglobin approximating 15% of the total hemoglobin are sufficient to produce cyanosis. The relative capacity of the pigments to produce cyanosis of comparable intensity has been given as 5 gm. of reduced hemoglobin per 100 ml. of blood, 1.5 gm. of methemoglobin per 100 ml. of blood, and less than 0.5% of sulfhemoglobin.[54]

Cardiovascular mechanisms for increasing the oxygen supply to the tissues are called into play when the concentration of methemoglobin exceeds 40% of the blood pigments. At levels exceeding 60%, ataxia, prostration, and unconsciousness occur. Failure of an oxygen supply necessary for sustaining life could be expected to result when the methemoglobin concentration reaches about 85%.[13]

Methemoglobinemia results clinically either from an inborn error of metabolism in which the intracellular enzymes normally reducing methemoglobin are deficient or from the effect of chemical or therapeutic agents which oxidize hemoglobin at a rate beyond the capacity for its reduction.

A variety of mechanisms are usually present that are capable of reducing methemoglobin as it is formed, mainly through the medium of methemoglobin reductases. Erythrocytes appear to contain two enzymatic systems that catalyze reduction of methemoglobin to hemoglobin—one utilizes DPNH (reduced diphosphopyridine nucleotide) and the other TPNH (reduced triphosphopyridine nucleotide). The former coenzyme results from anaerobic glycolysis and the latter from the pentose phosphate shunt or oxidative pathway.[143] The energy of the mature erythrocyte is derived primarily from anaerobic glycolysis and glucose oxidation via the oxidative pathway. Reduction of methemoglobin occurs only when glucose or lactate is present, and the rate of reduction in vitro is greater when methylene blue is added.

*Congenital (familial) methemoglobinemia*

Congenital (familial) methemoglobinemia is caused by a congenital absence of a reducing factor in the erythrocytes which is responsible for the reconversion of methemoglobin to hemoglobin in normal red cells. The defect is often familial,[18] transmitted as a recessive. Patients with this disease suffer from a deficiency of the flavoprotein, coenzyme factor 1 (diaphorase 1), which acts as a carrier in the conversion of methemoglobin to hemoglobin.[62] This enzyme deficiency results in an accumulation of methemoglobin in the red cells. The shift to the left of the oxygen dissociation curve is not always observed.[44] Without treatment the majority of these patients tend to reach equilibrium at about 40% methemoglobin in the blood.[54] Most patients show persistent diffuse cyanosis which is generalized but particularly marked in the fingers, toes, buccal mucous membranes, lips, nose, cheeks, and conjunctivae. Clubbing of the fingers does not occur. There is no anemia, but mild compensatory polycythemia may develop. Patients are usually asymptomatic except for occasional headaches and in older persons poor exercise tolerance may be noted. Usually, there is no physical disability even with strenuous exercise. Life expectancy is unaffected. Congenital methemoglobinemia may be confused initially with cyanotic congenital heart disease. The absence of signs of heart disease and spectroscopic examination of the blood reveal the diagnosis of methemoglobinemia.

A case of methemoglobinemia has been described that followed a dominant rather than the usual recessive inheritance. This variant was at first ascribed to an inability to utilize glucose for the reduction of methemoglobin.[129] The defect was later demonstrated, however, to be caused by the inadequate synthesis of glutathione.[130] The deficiency of this essential co-factor apparently results in an impairment of triosephosphate dehydrogenase activity. This in turn resulted in an insufficient reduction of DPN, which is an essential component of DPNH-dependent methemoglobin reductase. This variant of methemoglobinemia differs from the two groups of hereditary methemoglobinemia—the recessive type, which is based on enzyme deficiency, and methemoglobin M disease, which is due to an abnormal globin within the hemoglobin molecule.

*Congenital methemoglobinemia associated with hemoglobin M*

The defect in congenital methemoglobinemia associated with hemoglobin M lies in the globin component (Chapter 16). Methemoglobin constitutes 15 to 25% of the total hemoglobin in affected persons. They live normal lives and are undisturbed by cyanosis. Ascorbic acid and methylene blue exert no effect on the methemoglobin or cyanosis.

*Drug-induced methemoglobinemia*

Various compounds activate the oxidation of hemoglobin from the ferrous to the ferric state, forming methemoglobin. These direct oxidants include nitrites, chlorates, and quinones,[13] and prominent among these compounds are aniline and its derivatives sulfanilamides, acetanilid, phenacetin, bismuth subnitrate, and potassium chlorate. In infancy and childhood the offenders are marking ink, shoe dies, certain red wax crayons,[113] well water containing nitrates from the soil, meat containing a high nitrate content,[103] and furniture polish containing nitrobenzene.[92] Nitrate from contaminated water from shallow wells used in infant feeding mixtures is converted to nitrite in the bowel and, on absorption, causes methemoglobinemia.[35,50,52] The absorption of aniline dye from marking ink on diapers and other articles of infants' clothing has been responsible for outbreaks of methemoglobinemia in nurseries which frequently affect premature infants.[49,73,80,109] Similar poisoning from aniline dyes results from cutaneous absorption from freshly dyed shoes and blankets. Methemoglobinemia has also been produced in young infants by the application of ointments containing benzocaine.[148] Intracorpuscular methemoglobin and sulfhemoglobin have been noted in the course of hemolytic anemia caused by large doses of sulfonamides and toxic agents.[36] Heinz bodies and contracted red cells have been noted in the blood smears of affected patients.

### Features common to methemoglobinemia

*Diagnosis.* Methemoglobinemia is suspected when there is a definite history of ingestion of or exposure to a toxic substance when cyanosis exists in the absence of evidence of cardiac or respiratory dysfunction. The diagnosis is supported if a sample of venous blood retains the characteristic chocolate brown color after vigorous shaking with air for 15 minutes. Methemoglobin has a well-defined absorption band spectroscopically at 630 m$\mu$ which disappears on the addition of 5% solution of potassium cyanide. A striking feature is the intensive, peculiarly grayish cyanosis that develops within 1 to 2 hours after ingestion of the toxic substance. The discoloration progresses rapidly until the skin and mucous membranes become almost black in color.[92] In mild cases the child is fully conscious and in no distress. In severe cases the patient has considerable anoxemia and dyspnea and develops circulatory failure.

*Treatment.* Patients with mild cases of acquired methemoglobinemia recover spontaneously upon withdrawal of the toxic substance. In a patient with disease of any degree of severity treatment should be initiated immediately. Methylene blue acts as a specific antidote, converting methemoglobin to hemoglobin. The recommended dosage for infants is 2 mg. per kilogram of body weight; for older children, 1.5 mg. per kilogram; and for adults, 1 mg. per kilogram. It is readily available in ampules of 1% solution, the solution being given by slow intravenous injection. Treatment may be repeated if methemoglobinemia recurs. Ascorbic acid orally or parenterally also reduces methemoglobin, but the conversion takes place more slowly and therefore is not practical in urgent cases.

In patients with hereditary methemoglobinemia, orally administered methylene blue or ascorbic acid may be given over prolonged periods to combat cyanosis and particularly associated symptoms such as headache. Ascorbic acid in an oral dosage of 500 mg. given to a 12½-year-old boy caused a significant drop in methemoglobin concentration.[136] Intravenous methylene blue acts more promptly, but a gradual return to the original methemoglobinemia is inevitable when therapy is terminated.

Toxic effects have been observed when methylene blue is given in excessive dosage.[67] These consist of a generalized bluish gray skin discoloration which may persist for 3 to 4 days and of an acute hemolytic anemia which may become manifest about 1 week later. The anemia may be of sufficient severity to require transfusions.

### Methemoglobinemia in young infants

The susceptibility of young infants to the development of methemoglobinemia upon exposure to certain toxic agents has been shown to be due to a deficient reduction of methemoglobin in the red cells.[116] Well water containing a high percentage of nitrates causes methemoglobinemia in formula-fed infants even though their parents, drinking the same water, remain normal.[35,116]

The differences in the reactions of the infants and their parents are explained by observations that the erythrocytes of cord blood reduce significantly less methemoglobin than do those of adult controls in the presence of lactate, lactate and methylene blue, or glucose. The normal in vivo pathway for reduction of methemoglobin has been shown to be dependent upon the generation of reduced diphosphopyridine nucleotide (DPNH).[62] The red cells of the young infant have difficulty in reducing hemoglobin, presumably on the basis of a transient deficiency of either DPNH-dependent methemoglobin reductase or of one of the enzymes responsible for its generation.[115,116]

## SULFHEMOGLOBINEMIA

Sulfhemoglobin is a pigment not normally present in the body. It is inert as an oxygen carrier. The combination of inorganic sulfides with hemoglobin in vivo results in its formation.[54] Sulfhemoglobinemia often accompanies methemoglobinemia. Once sulfhemoglobin is formed, it is stable and irreversible, disappearing after 3 to 4 months when the affected red cells are destroyed. In contrast to methemoglobin, methylene blue and ascorbic acid are of no value in converting sulfhemoglobin to hemoglobin. The absorption band of sulfhemoglobin is at 618 m$\mu$ and is unaltered by the addition of potassium cyanide solution.

Enterogenous cyanosis, formerly of great interest, refers to an ill-defined clinical syndrome characterized by attacks of cyanosis, headache, abdominal pain, and bowel dysfunction (either diarrhea or constipation). Sulfhemoglobinemia is frequently present, often associated with methemoglobinemia. In constipated patients sulfhemoglobinemia is attributed to the absorption of an enterogenous oxidizing agent such as hydrogen sulfide.

Cyanosis due to sulfhemoglobinemia which was both congenital and familial has been described in a newborn infant.[96] In another case cyanosis due to sulfhemoglobinemia occurred in a 5-year-old child with nonspecific gastroenteritis to whom a triple sulfonilamide had been given in the course of prolonged administration of a sulfur tonic.[53]

## MISCELLANEOUS ANEMIAS
### Anemia of chronic renal insufficiency

Anemia is a well-known accompaniment of chronic renal failure, irrespective of the type of lesion causing it. It occurs in patients with primary diseases of the kidney, such as acute and chronic glomerulonephritis, chronic pyelonephritis, and congenital polycystic kidneys or in those with diseases possessing renal components such as lupus erythematosus. Within limits, the degree of anemia varies with the level of nitrogen retention.

*Pathogenesis.* The two main factors concerned with the pathogenesis of chronic renal failure are depression of erythropoiesis and increased red cell destruction. Inadequate marrow response is evident from the poor utilization of intravenous injections of radioactive iron.[41,55,79,91] The actual factor responsible for erythroid depression is still unknown, but a toxic retention product remains a possibility. Hydremia has also been considered to explain the anemia based on a normal red cell volume with increased plasma volume so that the anemia is more apparent than real.[133] This may be contributory but many patients with massive edema have little or no anemia. There are indications also that kidney disease interferes with erythropoiesis by retarding the elaboration or activation of an erythropoietic stimulating factor produced by the normal kidney.[68,75,105]

Utilizing a fluorescent antibody technique, sheep erythropoietin was localized in the capillary walls of the glomerular tufts, suggesting that erythropoietin is either produced or stored in these cells.[56] Many observations agree that erythropoietin is absent from the plasma of anemic uremic patients, suggesting that the anemia is chiefly due to this lack which is responsible for diminished blood production.[86,100] In contrast, erythrocytosis has been demonstrated in patients with renal tumors or other structural abnormalities of the kidney.[101] Caution has been expressed in interpreting the low plasma erythropoietin levels as the causative factor in uremia, emphasizing that further investigation is needed to determine if this is, indeed, the essential mechanism of producing erythroid failure. One has to determine whether the plasma erythropoietin levels are low in uremic patients because of the lack of functioning renal tissue, or because of the uremic state with its other metabolic abnormalities.[86]

Transfusion of the red cells of the patient or of a normal donor into the patient's circulation reveals a shortened life-span for both types of cells.[26,41,46,79,91] The most marked hemolysis as judged by shortened red cell survival occurs during the period of increasing uremia and azotemia. It is assumed that rapidly progressive anemia in the absence of detectable blood loss is caused by an extracorpuscular hemolytic factor.[91] In patients with stationary chronic renal failure normal donor cells show no shortened survival. Increased destruction of red cells in patients with chronic disease carries a poor prognosis.[79] Erythrocytes from patients with severe renal failure are normal as measured by their normal life-span when injected into healthy recipients,[91] indicating the absence of an intracorpuscular defect. It seems likely, therefore, that a combination of depressed erythropoiesis and increased cell destruction is manifest in some stage of chronic nephritis.

Blood loss from epistaxis and gastrointestinal bleeding may contribute to the anemia, since a hemorrhagic tendency is not uncommon in persons with chronic nephritis. Although changes in bleeding time and tourniquet test are found in patients with renal failure, the most consistent disturbances occur in relation to platelet numbers and their thromboplastic function, and the plasma factors of the blood.[88] Cheney and Bonnin[28] found that the occurrence of hemorrhagic signs in uremia is more closely related to reduced levels of platelet thromboplastic function (PTF) than to any other blood coagulation defect. There appeared to be a significant linear relation between platelet thromboplastic factor functions and blood urea nitrogen level. Defects were also found in stable factor (factor VII) and in capillary integrity. Thrombocytopenia is common in some series of cases[110] but not in others. From the standpoint of bleeding conditions associated with renal disease, a complete investigation of the coagulation status is required, with particular reference to platelet number and function.

In discussing the anemia of chronic renal disease, Erslev[47] states that the conditions which cause chronic renal disease may interfere with the normal production and survival of red blood cells in a number of ways. Defective iron reutilization results in a suboptimal rate of red blood cell production. Iron for hemoglobin synthesis may be in short supply because of defective iron reutilization or because of frequent blood loss from the gastrointestinal or gynecologic tracts. The concentration of most coagulation factors is not reduced in uremia and the platelet count is merely moderately reduced in about 20% of cases. In the majority of cases of uremia, the cause of the bleeding appears to be due to impaired platelet function. Platelet aggregating ability and platelet factor 3 release are depressed. Bleeding time is prolonged and platelet adhesion to glass beads or aggregation after exposure to adenosine diphosphate (ADP) is subnormal. The pathogenesis of the bleeding tendency is inadequately explained but it is improved by dialysis.

The combined effect of a shortening of red blood cell life-span, decreased iron utilization, decreased responsiveness to erythropoietin, and increased blood loss results in an increased demand for red blood cells. In chronic renal disease, the kidney fails to release an adequate amount of erythropoietin and the anemia remains uncorrected. In a few patients with the nephrotic syndrome, an excessive urinary loss of transferrin may lead to impaired delivery of iron to the bone marrow. In patients undergoing intensive dialysis therapy, there is a loss not only of blood and iron but of folic acid. Folic acid is dialyzed and easily lost in the dialysis fluid. Erslev[47] concludes that "the actual level of anemia experienced depends (1) on the demands for red blood cells caused by the effect of azotemia on red cell production and red cell survival; (2) on the residual capacity of the kidneys to produce erythropoietin; and possibly (3) on the effect of extrarenal erythropoietin."

*Laboratory findings.* The anemia is usually normochromic and normocytic; occasionally it is microcytic or macrocytic. Contracted and deformed erythrocytes assuming a triangular shape and fragmented and distorted cells described as poikilocytes, helmet or burr cells have also been observed.[36] Reticulocytes may be reduced in numbers[21] or slightly to moderately increased,[91] the levels probably depending upon the degree of associated hemolysis. Anemia occurs in practically all patients with any significant degree of azotemia.[21] Hemoglobin levels average 8 to 9 gm. per 100 ml. in patients with moderate azotemia[21] but drop to 4 and 5 gm. as nitrogen retention increases. The white blood cells may be normal in number or slightly increased. Erythrocyte glycolytic activity and the concentration of erythrocyte adenosine triphosphate and 2,3-DPG are increased. These abnormalities result from hyperphosphatemia.[90] The oxygen dissociation curve is shifted to the right.[140] Platelets are present in normal or decreased numbers.

*Bone marrow.* The bone marrow is normal or moderately hypercellular in the majority of patients but becomes mildly hyperplastic with excessive nitrogen retention.[21] In a series of thirty patients with uremia, Gasser[60] found no relation between the degree of azotemia and the percentage of erythroblasts in the marrow. Both hypoplasia and hyperplasia of erythroid elements coexisted with all grades of azotemia. In five children with renal disease in whom erythroid elements of the bone marrow numbered less than 1%, four showed congenital malformations of the kidney. The remaining patient suffered from the acute hemolytic-uremic syndrome,[61] consisting of sudden severe hemolytic anemia (hemoglobin, 2.6 gm. per 100 ml.), a positive Coombs test, renal failure (nonprotein nitrogen, 137 to 222 mg. per 100 ml.), thrombocytopenia, hemorrhage, and convulsions. Despite the clinical similarity to thrombotic thrombocytopenic purpura, there was no microscopic evidence of this disease. Bilateral renal cortical necrosis was found at postmortem examination.

***Diagnosis.*** Chronic renal failure is to be considered in any child with prolonged and undiagnosed normochromic and normocytic anemia, especially when there is no response to iron therapy. Earlier in the course of the disease the urinary abnormalities may be minimal and easily overlooked, and the blood pressure readings may be equivocal. In one such patient the sole anatomic defect was the presence of medullary cysts in otherwise normal-sized kidneys.[125] Other cases of congenital cysts of the renal medulla have been reported,[51] some designated as the medullary sponge kidney.[107] Anemia and a rise in nitrogenous products will also be found in patients with congestive heart failure and impaired renal function. Temporary depression of renal function, azotemia, and anemia also follow severe hemorrhage from the stomach and duodenum.[40]

Three sisters were reported who at 4, 7½, and 9 years of age, respectively, presented with anemia and were found to be uremic.[5] They progressed rapidly to death from renal failure. Autopsy on one of these children showed the typical pathological features of medullary cystic disease. The carrier state was represented in the mother by an inability to concentrate urine. A review of these cases has been reported by Giselson and colleagues[63] under the heading of renal medullary cystic disease or familial juvenile nephronophtisis. They reported on two siblings with this disorder—one who died at 17 years of age, and a brother in good physical condition at 15 years of age—and concluded that the first signs and symptoms are due to either proximal or distal tubular insufficiency. Tubular proteinuria and osteodystrophy or defective urine concentrating ability may be found in the first stages of the disease. The results of this family study are in accordance with the assumption that this disorder is inherited as an autosomal recessive trait.

***Treatment.*** Since the severity of the anemia depends upon the degree and duration of nitrogen retention, there can be no lasting improvement with any type of treatment unless renal function is improved. It does not respond to oral or parenteral iron, liver extract, folic acid, or vitamin $B_{12}$. Transfusion with packed cells remains the treatment of choice for symptomatic relief. Fresh blood is preferable because of a possible coexisting hemolytic element especially in the patient with advanced disease. Specific therapy for bleeding will depend upon the coagulation factor involved. Platelet-rich plasma or concentrates and judicious use of steroids may be helpful in platelet reduction or their defective function. Vitamin K and fresh or fresh frozen plasma may be necessary for the improvement of coagulation defects. The bone marrow may compensate to the point of stabilizing the hemoglobin so that transfusions are no longer necessary. Oral cobaltous chloride has been advocated in the treatment of anemia of chronic renal disease.[58] Although oral cobaltous chloride therapy temporarily increases erythropoiesis and hemoglobin synthesis, serious toxic complications have prevented its widespread clinical use.

### Anemia of infection

With the advent of antibiotics and other modern therapeutic measures, anemia due to infection has become relatively infrequent. Its incidence, though small, usually involves persons with chronic rather than acute infections. Severe anemias coexisting with infection are usually hemolytic in nature and have been observed in connection with sepsis due to streptococci, staphylococci, and pneumococci. Sepsis in the newborn period, for instance, may provoke an anemia with evidences of intense blood destruction. Acute hemolytic anemias occur also in patients with selected viral infections, such as virus pneumonia, infectious mononucleosis, influenza, and Coxsackie virus A infections.[36] In the large majority of patients, however, overt hemolysis rarely accompanies an acute infection and, when it does occur, suggests unusual susceptibility of the patient.[36] Slight degrees of increased blood destruction insufficient to give clinical manifestations are a more common occurrence. Aplastic anemia has also been known to occur in infants and children with severe infections.

Anemia due to chronic infections may be associated with a variety of disease conditions such as pneumonia, empyema, tuberculosis, bacterial meningitis and particularly Hemophilus influenza, rheumatic fever, osteomyelitis, pyelonephritis, wound infections, brucellosis, subacute bacterial endocarditis, and intestinal parasites. The anemia of rheumatic fever may be due to many factors: decreased erythropoiesis, shortened survival of red cells,[112] and, in the early phase, an increase in plasma volume with a transient decrease in hematocrit values due to dilution. Mild infections do not provoke anemia unless they are prolonged or recurrent. As a rule, infections of less than one month's duration manifest no significant anemia.[144] Once anemia develops it gradually increases in severity with the progression of infection but eventually stabilizes.

*Pathogenesis.* Although the mechanism of the anemia of infection has not been completely elucidated, there is convincing evidence that toxic depression of erythropoiesis and shortened survival of the red blood cells contribute to its pathogenesis.

It will be remembered that the heme portion of hemoglobin is a metal complex consisting of iron in the center of a porphyrin structure. The underlying porphyrin of the hemoglobin molecule is termed protoporphyrin.[144] Coproporphyrin, uroporphyrin, and protoporphyrin represent the most important naturally occurring porphyrins. Coproporphyrin is usually the predominant porphyrin in the urine and feces. Human erythrocytes contain free coproporphyrin as well as free protoporphyrin. In patients with the anemia of chronic infection an excess of free protoporphyrin and coproporphyrin in the red cells and increased urinary coproporphyrin may be interpreted as an inability to synthesize completely the heme portion of the hemoglobin molecule.

The decreased rate of the erythrocyte production is due to a quantitative defect in the conversion of protoporphyrin into hemoglobin. The increased amounts of free coproporphyrin and protoporphyrin in the red cells of patients with anemia of chronic infection are in agreement with this concept.[83] The anemia of infection has also been regarded as a disturbance of iron as well as of porphyrin metabolism. In patients with infectious states iron is absorbed normally and leaves the plasma rapidly. Iron administered intravenously also increases the serum iron transiently, being diverted to the tissues and thus rendered not readily available for hemoglobin formation.[42]

In addition to depression of erythropoiesis, a hemolytic factor has been demonstrated as shown by a shortened red cell life-span in patients with a variety of chronic infectious disorders.[20] A decreased red cell survival has been noted in children with acute rheumatic fever.[112] The fact that the bone marrow is unable to compensate for the moderate increase in the red cell destruction is further evidence that erythropoiesis is depressed.[20]

*Blood findings and other laboratory data.* The anemia due to chronic infection is rarely severe. The hemoglobin usually ranges between 8 and 11 gm. per 100 ml. with a corresponding reduction in the number of red cells. The anemia is usually of a normochromic, normocytic type, but when protracted it tends to become microcytic and hypochromic, in which case slight anisocytosis and poikilocytosis are also present. Reticulocyte counts are normal or reduced. The serum bilirubin is normal, and other evidences of blood destruction are lacking, despite the shortened life-span of the red cells. The bone marrow shows no hypoplasia; rather the cellularity is normal or increased. If the bone marrow is hyperplastic, there is an increase in the granulocytic elements and, at times, of less mature erythroid elements.[120] The excessive granulopoiesis of the marrow often is manifested in the younger patient by marked leukocytosis which may reach the intensity of a leukemoid reaction often out of proportion to the nature or degree of infection. Hypoferremia is present; the serum iron is markedly lowered, and the serum iron-binding capacity is moderately reduced.[24] The serum copper, the free erythrocyte protoporphyrin and coproporphyrin, and coproporphyrinuria are increased. The levels of haptoglobin, an acute phase reactant, may be elevated or normal, even in patients with concomitant hemolysis.

*Clinical features.* Pallor is indicative of the anemia, but the predominant symptoms and physical signs are those of the basic infection. Chronic anemia in children, especially when accompanied by an increased sedimentation rate, requires a search for an underlying infection. The course and prognosis are determined by the nature of the causative infectious process rather than of the anemia.

*Treatment.* The anemia is corrected with subsidence of the basic disease and the elimination of the focus of infection. Iron therapy is unnecessary, for this substance is abundantly available in the tissues. Liver extract, vitamin $B_{12}$, folic acid, and other antianemia agents are without value. Increased erythropoiesis and hemoglobin synthesis have been reported with the administration of cobaltous chloride,[11] but undesirable side effects such as nausea, vomiting, and goiter limit its usefulness. Blood transfusions are given for their supportive effects when the hemoglobin level drops below 8 gm. per 100 ml., especially in the event of debilitating signs and, also, when surgical intervention is contemplated.

### Anemia of acute hemorrhage

*Etiology.* Acute blood loss may be primarily external or internal into the tissues, organs, or body cavities. The severity of the anemia and symptomatology depend upon the amount and rate of blood loss. Anemia may result from trauma, hemophilia, thrombocytopenic purpura, sudden rupture of esophageal varices in portal hypertension, and gastrointestinal ulceration, in the course of leukemia, and in the newborn infant from premature placental separation, rupture of a placental blood vessel, incision or rupture of the placenta itself, and faulty tying or clamping of the umbilical cord.

*Blood picture.* Immediately following the hemorrhage, the blood volume is reduced, and until it is restored the levels of hemoglobin and red blood cells may be deceptively high because of vasoconstriction and stasis. During the next 1 to 3 days when the blood volume is restored by the entrance of tissue fluids into the circulation, blood values decrease and give a true indication of the extent of blood loss. On the first day there is a transient polymorphonuclear leukocytosis with a shift to the left of these cells, the appearance of myelocytes, and an increase in the number of platelets. The anemia is normochromic and normocytic.

The number of reticulocytes increase on the second to the third day, reaching maximal levels from the fifth to seventh day, and terminating by the tenth to the fourteenth days. The persistence of reticulocytosis is indicative of continued bleeding. Polychromatophilia and normoblasts appear with severe hemorrhage. During active regeneration there is a tendency toward macrocytosis. The increase in hemoglobin and red cells is often followed by a lag in hemoglobin synthesis due to a deficiency of building materials existing prior to the hemorrhagic episode. Blood production is proportional to the amount of iron available in the stores or after iron ingestion. The intensity of the stimulus is inversely proportional to the anemia, depending upon normal bone marrow capacity.[33] In the absence of adequate iron stores the anemia becomes hypochromic and microcytic. Under favorable conditions and depending upon the size of the blood loss, normal values are reached in 4 to 8 weeks. The bone marrow shows a normoblastic hyperplasia during the regenerative period. Alimentary azotemia occurs in patients with massive hemorrhage in the gastrointestinal tract, frequently from a bleeding peptic ulcer.[32] The elevation of blood urea nitrogen is due to the absorption of digested hemoglobin.

*Clinical features.* Unless blood loss is rapid and extensive, there are few symptoms. With significant hemorrhage clinical signs are related to the fall in blood pressure and blood volume. Pallor, faintness, cold, sweating, restlessness, tachycardia, rapid breathing, and shock are characteristic. In the newborn infant posthemorrhagic anemia with a rapid fall in hemoglobin, pallor, weakness, loss of muscle tone, and limpness are pronounced. Mild jaundice is noted when blood is sequestered in tissues and body cavities, as in the patient with a large cephalhematoma.

*Treatment.* The immediate steps in treatment are the control of hemorrhage and restoration of blood volume to offset the reduction in blood pressure. Transfusions, preferably of whole blood, are indicated to restore both blood volume and the deficit of hemoglobin and erythrocytes. Less blood than the calculated amount lost (Chapter 7) is given initially to avoid suddenly overtaxing the depleted cardiovascular system. Iron is prescribed for at least 2 months to secure optimal hemoglobin synthesis.

### Chronic hemorrhagic anemia

*Etiology.* Chronic hemorrhagic anemia is due to repeated overt hemorrhages or concealed small hemorrhages, frequently from the same sources responsible for a single massive hemorrhage previously described. The gastrointestinal tract is most commonly affected, with bleeding from ulcerations, gastritis induced by aspirin therapy, anomalies such as a Meckel's diverticulum, polyps, esophageal varices in portal hypertension at times associated with bleeding from hemorrhoidal vessels, bleeding into the lungs in idiopathic pulmonary hemosiderosis, coagulation disorders, severe epistaxis, idiopathic thrombocytopenic purpura, hookworm disease, and genitourinary bleeding.

*Clinical and laboratory features.* Pallor, irritability, and anorexia occur with markedly lowered hemoglobin and red cell levels. The anemia varies with the duration and intensity of bleeding. The blood picture is typically that of an iron-deficiency anemia. As iron stores are depleted a hypochromic microcytic anemia develops. Reticulocytes rarely exceed 5%. Bone marrow activity is slightly increased to the extent of a mild to moderate normoblastic hyperplasia. The white blood count is normal. In patients with persistent anemia, examination of the stools for occult blood is mandatory.

*Treatment.* The source of bleeding must be localized. Iron is prescribed as for patients with nutritional iron-deficiency anemia. Transfusions are given only exceptionally to patients in whom greatly lowered blood values have persisted over long periods and, preoperatively, to those being prepared for surgical eradication of a Meckel's diverticulum or other congenital anomalies.

## Vitamin deficiencies and anemia

Many of the vitamins, especially those of the B group, are concerned with some phase of erythropoiesis. Although this relationship can be demonstrated experimentally in animals, only deficiencies of vitamin $B_{12}$ and folic acid have been definitely found to provoke anemia in man.

*Vitamin A.* A severe anemia (hemoglobin, 6.7 gm. per 100 ml.; red cells, 2,710,000 per cubic millimeter) was noted in an allergic child whose diet contained no vitamin A supplement. The anemia and other symptoms of vitamin A deficiency promptly responded to large doses of vitamin A.[10]

*Riboflavin ($B_2$).* A mild anemia has been observed in swine[145] and dogs[127] with riboflavin-deficient diets. Riboflavin deficiency resulting from a riboflavin-deficient diet and a riboflavin antagonist, galactoflavin, produces a normochromic, normocytic anemia and reticulocytopenia.[85] The total leukocyte counts, platelet, and differential counts remain within normal limits. The bone marrow is characterized by a selective hypoplasia of the erythroid precursors. Pronormoblasts commonly show prominent vacuolization of both cytoplasm and nucleus. This blood picture confined to depletion of erythroid elements resembling the entity known as pure red cell anemia was restored to normal by riboflavin administration. The anemia of riboflavin deficiency is distinct from other anemias related to deficiencies of the other B vitamins. Deficiencies of vitamin $B_{12}$ and folic acid are associated with megaloblastic anemias; the pyridoxine-responsive anemia is hypochromic and microcytic. Administration of riboflavin is associated with a prompt decrease in the M:E ratio due to an increase principally in the number of late nucleated erythroid elements.[6]

*Nicotinic acid (niacin).* The relationship of nicotinic acid to anemia has not been established. Pellagra is associated with deficiency of nicotinic acid and other nutritional factors. Anemia is inconstantly associated with this disease. It can be microcytic, normocytic, or macrocytic[72] and probably results from multiple nutritional deficiencies rather than from nicotinic acid deficiency per se. It is of interest that a patient with hypochromic anemia in the tropics who was refractory to iron therapy responded to nicotinic acid.[57]

*Pyridoxine (vitamin $B_6$).* Nutritional microcytic anemia due to pyridoxine deficiency has been produced in a number of animals, notably in dogs, pigs,[23] and rats.[123] The anemia is characterized by irregular reticulocytosis, normoblastemia, polychromatophilia, bone marrow hyperplasia, elevated plasma iron levels, and hemosiderosis of the liver, spleen, and bone marrow. Although normoblastic marrow hyperplasia occurs most often, in a small number of cases the bone marrow is megaloblastic. The anemia fails to respond to iron or copper but is relieved by synthetic pyridoxine,[25,146] which also mobilizes the iron deposits from the tissues. With iron-enriched diets the absorption of iron is increased during pyridoxine deficiency, resulting in hemosiderosis of the liver and spleen and high serum iron values.[147] Pyridoxine deficiency rarely occurs in man. However, an infant with severe hypochromic, microcytic anemia induced by pyridoxine deprivation responded promptly to parenteral and oral administration of the vitamin.[126] Occasionally, anemias refractory to the common antianemia agents have responded to pyridoxine. In one adult, refractory hypochromic anemia and abnormalities in tryptophan metabolism were simultaneously corrected by the injection of pyridoxine.[71] In another patient with hypochromic anemia reported on from the tropics in whom there was no diarrhea or steatorrhea, a satisfactory response was obtained with pyridoxine.[57] A moderate recovery from anemia was observed in a patient with severe hypochromic anemia and hemochromatosis following the administration of pyridoxine.[134] The disturbance in pyridoxine metabolism was unassociated with any disturbance in tryptophan metabolism. Intermittent pyridoxine deficiency has also been described in man with recurrent episodes of severe red cell hypochromasia, microcytosis, and a high serum iron.[48] These abnormalities were corrected by the administration of pyridoxine. It is of interest that the hematologic picture in pyridoxine deficiency closely simulates Cooley's anemia.

Several patients have been described with microcytic, hypochromic anemia, hyperferremia, and hemosiderosis with complete or almost complete correction of all abnormalities after the administration of vitamin $B_6$, even in small doses.[12,77,108] The bone marrow shows no abnormality of megakaryocytes or leukocytes; hence, vitamin $B_6$ does not appear to be necessary for the development or maturation of granulocytes or thrombocytes. Interruption of pyridoxine therapy may result in reticulocytopenia, a reduction in the concentration of hemoglobin, and a decrease in free erythrocyte protoporphyrin. Reinstitution of pyridoxine therapy was followed by reticulocytosis. In other cases only a partial remission resulted. Cases of pyridoxine-responsive anemia have been reported in siblings.[95] Patients with sideroachrestic anemia may also respond partly or adequately to the administration of pyridoxine. In an adult,[114] prompt reticulocytosis followed the daily oral administration of 5 mg. of pyridoxine. Relapse in this patient occurred between 12 and 14 weeks after discontinuing the initial course of therapy. In most patients relapse occurs between 2 and 4 months after the drug is discontinued. The precise dosage of pyridoxine in this form of anemia has not been established, although the minimum has been estimated in adults to be between 1.5 and 2.5 mg. per day.

Pyridoxine-responsive anemia usually does not appear to result from a dietary deficiency of pyridoxine. The amount of pyridoxine necessary to produce a response is frequently greater than the ordinary dietary requirement. It is for this reason that the hematologic condition responding to pyridoxine is described as pyridoxine-responsive anemia. The pathogenesis seems to be due to a defect in hemoglobin synthesis involving a failure to form porphobilinogen and to utilize iron.

Bickers and associates[12] summarize the activity of vitamin $B_6$ and also provide an explanation for the marked hemoglobin deficiency seen in vitamin $B_6$-deficient animals and in human beings with pyridoxine-responsive anemia. Vitamin $B_6$ is composed of three compounds—pyridoxine, pyridoxal, and pyridoxamine—each of which may be metabolized to the active form, pyridoxal-5-phosphate. The latter compound serves as a coenzyme for a variety of reactions, involving decarboxylation and transamination, and is essential in heme formation, being a participant in the formation of delta-aminolevulinic acid from glycine and succinic acid. Biochemical evidence of vitamin $B_6$ deficiency is manifested by increased urinary excretion of xanthurenic acid, kynurenin, and kynurenic acid, as well as a failure to convert tryptophan to N-methylnicotinamide.

*Vitamin C and the anemia of scurvy.* In the scorbutic infant the anemia is hypochromic and microcytic; in the adult it is normocytic or slightly macrocytic. The bone marrow presents no constant picture in scurvy. The cellularity may be reduced, normal, or increased, the reaction being usually normoblastic. Although anemia is a common finding in patients with scurvy, it has not been exactly determined in what manner a lack of vitamin C (ascorbic acid) interferes with hematopoiesis. In Chapter 13 it is shown that vitamin C plays a part in folic acid metabolism and that its deficiency contributes to the etiology of the anemia. Accelerated blood destruction also has been noted in patients with scurvy.[135] Contributing to the anemia is the loss of blood from hemorrhages characteristic of the disease. Anemia develops in scurvy in spite of adequate supplies of iron, vitamin $B_{12}$, and folic acid.[19] The total white blood cell count, differential count, and platelet count are usually normal. Moderate leukopenia and thrombocytopenia may be present in patients with scurvy. Treatment with ascorbic acid corrects the anemia promptly, resulting in an elevated reticulocyte count in 4 to 6 days.

The results of ferrokinetic measurements, carried out in the adult Bantu with scurvy and in scorbutic guinea pigs indicate that there is no major impairment in iron transport when ascorbic acid deficiency is present.[16] Iron absorption is greater than normal in ascorbic acid deficiency, probably in response to an increased erythropoietic activity of between two and three times normal. The plasma iron is lower than normal in scorbutic subjects, with a prompt rise when ascorbic acid is given. Erythropoiesis is, therefore, effective in scurvy, which is reflected in the elevated reticulocyte count to the same degree as the plasma iron turnover. The anemia present in the scorbutic Bantu results from hemolysis and/or hemorrhage greater than the marrow's capacity to respond.[16]

**Vitamin E deficiency.** Anemia regularly develops in the rhesus monkey when it is deprived of vitamin E. The anemia is accompanied by granulocytosis, an increased concentration of bone marrow deoxyribonucleic acid, and a prompt reticulocytosis following vitamin E administration. The anemia seems to be due primarily to inadequate erythropoiesis. In addition, the bone marrow of the deficient monkey shows the presence of multinucleated erythroid percursors without megaloblastic changes.[106] Multinucleated erythroid cells are present in a variety of severe anemias in man, but are most commonly found in megaloblastic cases.

Low serum tocopherol levels and susceptibility to peroxide hemolysis have been shown to exist in premature infants for many months unless corrected by the administration of vitamin E.[104] With a 10-day course of tocopherol therapy the hemoglobin rose in a group of deficient premature infants from an average hemoglobin of 7.6 to 9.8 gm. per 100 ml., while the reticulocyte count decreased from 8.3 to 3.9%. In other studies no difference was found in hemoglobin levels in tocopherol deficient prematures and in those infants whose tocopherol levels had been repleted. A multiplicity of factors including vitamin E deficiency, increased content of polyunsaturated fatty acids in the diet and the red cell membrane, glutathione peroxidase deficiency, and iron therapy may be operative in the etiology of the anemia associated with prematurity. In a review of vitamin E, Silber and Goldstein[124] concluded that there is as yet no evidence to support a hematologic effect of vitamin E in adult man, and that to date no proof is available for any clinical benefit of tocopherol in vitamin E—deficient adults.

## Anemia of hypothyroidism

A mild normocytic or macrocytic, normochromic anemia usually accompanies untreated hypothyroidism. The hemoglobin ranges between 8 and 11 gm. per 100 ml., and the red cell count ranges between 3.5 and 4.5 million per cubic millimeter. The bone marrow is hypocellular.[149] Fatty bone marrow confined to the long bones has been described in persons with cretinism.[14] The yellow color of the skin in hypothyroidism is due to carotinemia—not to excessive bilirubin.[14] When uncomplicated, the anemia of hypothyroidism is undoubtedly due to lack of production. The anemia probably represents an adjustment to the decreased metabolic demands of the body.[70] In older persons, rarely in children, the anemia is macrocytic or hypochromic and microcytic, resulting from superimposed deficiency of $B_{12}$ or iron. The finding of a megaloblastic bone marrow indicates vitamin $B_{12}$ deficiency, in which case a hematopoietic response is expected with vitamin $B_{12}$ therapy.[131,132] With iron depletion for any reason the administration of iron is necessary. Without these complications, as is usually the case in hypothyroidism in childhood, the anemia is refractory but responds to thyroid. The response may be slow and consistent with readjustments to oxygen supply and demand. With iron depletion for any reason the anemia is hypochromic and microcytic and additional treatment with iron is necessary.

Spontaneous hypothyroidism is another condition in which both latent and overt pernicious anemia is not uncommon.[132] It is of interest that achlorhydria was present in 46% of a series of adult patients with this condition. To what extent achlorhydria is a factor in the causation of iron deficiency frequently accompanying cretinism in infancy is still to be determined.

Clinical and experimental evidence suggests that the thyroid has a definite influence in hematopoiesis.[89] Removal of the thyroid gland in rabbits results in a moderate and persistent anemia of the macrocytic type.[122] The anemia in persons with hypothyroidism may be regarded as an effect upon the bone marrow of the sluggish oxidation that occurs in all tissues.

## Blood changes in lead poisoning

Lead intoxication, except for industrial cases, is relatively common in infants and children, with its highest incidence between the ages of 12 and 36 months.[30] Children are more susceptible to lead intoxication than adults. It is acquired from a variety of sources, such as repeated ingestion of chips of peeling lead paint from walls, plaster, window sills, frames, repainted toys, furniture, and lead nipple shields and the inhalation of lead fumes from the burning of battery casings. The essential diagnostic features include dense bands at the ends of the long bones and metallic flecks in the large bowel observed on roentgenograms, increased content of lead in the urine (over 0.1 mg. per liter in 24 hours) and blood (0.06 mg. per 100 ml.),[31] bluish black and stippled "leadlines" on the gingival margins, increased excretion of coproporphyrin and delta-aminolevulinic acid in the urine, history of pica for paint and plaster, and definitive blood changes.

Among the important hematologic changes are basophilic stippling, moderate reticulocytosis, polychromatophilia, microcytic and hypochromic anemia, anisocytosis and poikilocytosis, and an increased number of target cells. The anemia is usually mild, but the hemoglobin level may range from 5 to 10 gm. per 100 ml.[31] Anemia is brought about by the toxic effect of the lead upon hematopoiesis in the marrow and by an increased hemolysis of circulating red blood cells. The phenomenon of stippling has been attributed to the primary effect of lead upon the red cell precursors of the bone marrow rather than upon the red cells in the peripheral blood.[94] As hemoglobinization of normoblasts becomes defective, the stippling increases. That stippled red cells are removed by the spleen is evident by their increase in the circulation after administering a lead salt to a splenectomized animal.[94]

The disturbance in hemoglobin synthesis stems from the effect of lead in preventing the incorporation of iron in the protoporphyrin nucleus of heme with resultant excretion of excessive coproporphyrin in the urine (essentially coproporphyrin III) and the accumulation of free protoporphyrin within the red cell.[138] This excess of free protoporphyrin in the erythrocytes accounts for their red fluorescence when thin wet-preparations of blood of patients with lead poisoning are examined under ultraviolet light.[141] Another and earlier explanation has been given for the accelerated destruction of red cells in the peripheral blood. In vitro studies have shown that lead injures the surface of the red cell, altering its cation flux and rendering the cell inelastic, brittle, and susceptible to fragmentation by mechanical trauma although red cell osmotic fragility is decreased.[8] The brittle cells are short-lived and readily destroyed in the circulation. Probably multiple factors enter into the pathogenesis of anemia and red cell stippling in lead poisoning.

Ferrokinetics are normal. The rate of removal of iron from plasma and the uptake of iron by the erythron are essentially unaffected in subjects with lead intoxication, in spite of a low hematocrit and bone marrow erythroid hyperplasia. The defect lies rather in the improper synthesis of porphobilinogen from delta-amino-levulinic acid and impaired production of heme from protoporphyrin and iron.[17] Red cell hypochromia, despite adequate iron stores, results from the depression of hemoglobin synthesis and is exaggerated by its lag behind red cell formation.[74] Other biochemical abnormalities useful in the diagnosis include increased content of erythrocyte delta-aminolevulinic acid and decreased delta-aminolevulinic acid dehydrogenase activity.[139]

Stippling occurs in patients with many kinds of anemias but may be sufficiently pronounced in those with the mild form of Cooley's anemia to simulate lead poisoning. The basophilic granules, however, are often larger and coarser in persons with lead poisoning than in those with other anemias. The stippled cell had been interpreted as a reticulocyte in which the basophilic material has been altered by lead.[142] Stippling has also been ascribed to the injurious effect of lead on the ribonucleic acid of the young erythrocyte and its precipitation by Wright's stain to give the characteristic punctate basophilic appearance.[138] Many stippled red cells give a positive iron reaction.[94] Chisolm[29] reviewed a number of studies which demonstrated the presence of mitochondria in basophilic stippled cells. Basophilic granulations in these cells are composed of aggregations of ribonucleic acid surrounding mitochondria. The presence of mitochondria gains significance because of the intracellular localization of various steps in heme synthesis. Mature mammalian erythrocytes that contain no mitochondria cannot synthesize the heme precursors. In lead poisoning, on the other hand, both the inhibition of essential enzymatic steps and the increased capacity to synthesize heme precursors are present because of the persistence of mitochondria in stippled cells. Stippling is composed either wholly or in part of ribonucleoproteins. According to Jensen and associates,[76] the ribosomes of cells from animals with lead intoxication have a greater propensity to form aggregates and therefore to result in stippling. They also observed that the association of nonheme iron with basophilic stippling is usually the consequence of the presence of two separate morphologic structures within the cell which may not be resolved or separated from each other in light or phase microscopy, but may be distinguished by the use of electron microscopy. The bone marrow shows erythroid hyperplasia and stippling of the red cell precursors. No constant changes have been observed in the total white blood cell count or platelet count.[22] Because iron deficiency may antedate or coexist with lead intoxication, iron therapy is required in addition to deleading measures.

The free passage of lead across the placenta has been demonstrated in many animal species.[7] Exposure to heavy concentrations of lead during pregnancy increased the rate of spontaneous abortions. Infants of a mother with lead poisoning may be undersized, show delayed growth and dentition, and have a high postnatal incidence of convulsions and nervous system disorders. The fetal risk is maximal in the first trimester. In one report[7] treatment of lead poisoning during the eighth month of pregnancy resulted in delivery of a normal infant 4 weeks after therapy was given to the mother.

## REFERENCES

1. Abildgaard, C. F., Cornet, J. A., and Schulman, I.: Primary erythrocytosis, J. Pediat. 63:1072, 1963.
2. Abraham, J. P., Ulutin, O. N., Johnson, S. A., and Caldwell, M. J.: A study of the defects in the blood coagulation mechanism in polycythemia vera, Amer. J. Clin. Path. 36:7, 1961.
3. Adams, F. H., and Cunningham, S. C.: Further studies on the blood of children with cyanotic heart disease with special reference to the hemoglobin, J. Pediat. 41:424, 1952.
4. Aggeler, P. M., Pollycove, A, Hoag, S., Donald, W. C., and Lawrence, J. H.: Polycythemia vera in childhood; studies of iron kinetics with $Fe^{59}$ and blood clotting factors, Blood 17:345, 1961.
5. Alexander, F., and Campbell, S.: Familial uremic medullary cystic disease, Pediatrics 45:1024, 1970.
6. Alfrey, C. P., and Lane, M.: The effect of riboflavin deficiency in erythropoiesis, Seminars Hemat. 7:49, 1970.
7. Angle, C. R., and McIntire, M. S.: Lead poisoning during pregnancy, Amer. J. Dis. Child. 108:436, 1964.
8. Aub, J. C., Fairhall, L. T., Minot, A. S., and Reznikoff, P.: Lead poisoning, Medicine 4:1, 1925.
9. Auerbach, M. L., Wolff, J. A., and Mettier, S. R.: Benign familial polycythemia in childhood; report of two cases, Pediatrics 21:54, 1958.
10. Bass, M. H., and Caplan, J.: Vitamin A deficiency in infancy, J. Pediat. 47:690, 1955.
11. Berk, L., Burchenal, J. H., and Castle, W. B.: Erythropoietic effect of cobalt in patients with and without anemia, New Eng. J. Med. 240:754, 1949.
12. Bickers, J. N., Brown, C. L., and Sprague, C. C.: Pyridoxine responsive anemia, Blood 19:304, 1962.
13. Bodansky, O.: Methemoglobinemia and methemoglobin producing compounds, Pharmacol. Rev. 3:144, 1951.
14. Bomford, R.: Anaemia in myxoedema, Quart. J. Med. 7:495, 1938.
15. Botha, M. C., Beale, D., Isacs, W. A., and Lehmann, H.: Haemoglobin J-Cape Town-$\alpha_2^{92\ Arg \rightarrow Gln}\beta_2$, Nature 212:792, 1966.
16. Bothwell, T. H., Bradlow, B. A., Jacobs, P., Keeley, K., Kramer, S., Seftel, H., and Zail, S.: Iron metabolism in scurvy with special reference to erythropoiesis, Brit. J. Haemat. 10:50, 1964.
17. Boyett, J. D., and Butterworth, C. E.: Lead poisoning and hemoglobin synthesis; report of a study of fifteen patients with chronic lead intoxication, Amer. J. Med. 32:884, 1962.
18. Breakey, V. K. St. G., Gibson, Q. H., and Harrison, D. C.: Familial idiopathic methaemoglobinaemia, Lancet 1:935, 1951.
19. Bronte-Stewart, B.: The anaemia of adult scurvy, Quart. J. Med. 22:309, 1953.
20. Bush, J. A., Ashenbrucker, H., Cartwright, G. E., and Wintrobe, M. M.: The anemia of infection; the kinetics of iron metabolism in the anemia associated with infection, J. Clin. Invest. 35:89, 1956.
21. Callen, I. R., and Limarzi, L. R.: Blood and bone marrow studies in renal disease, Amer. J. Clin. Path. 20:3, 1950.
22. Cantrow, A., and Trumper, M.: Lead poisoning, Baltimore, 1944, The Williams & Wilkins Co.
23. Cartwright, G. E.: Dietary factors concerned in erythropoiesis, Blood 2:111, 1947.
24. Cartwright, G. E., and Wintrobe, M. M.: The anemia of infection; a review. In Dock, W., and Snapper, I., editors: Advances of internal medicine, vol. 5, Chicago, 1952, Year Book Medical Publishers, Inc., p. 165.
25. Cartwright, G. E., Wintrobe, M. M., and Humphreys, S.: Studies on anemia in swine due to pyridoxine deficiency, together with data on phenylhydrazine anemia, J. Biol. Chem. 153:171, 1944.
26. Chaplin, H., and Mollison, P. L.: Red cell life span in nephritis and in hepatic cirrhosis, Clin. Sci. 12:351, 1953.
27. Charache, S., Weatherall, D., and Clegg, J.: Polycythemia associated with hemoglobinopathy, J. Clin. Invest. 45:813, 1966.
28. Cheney, K., and Bonnin, J. A.: Haemor-

rhage, platelet dysfunction and other coagulation defects in uraemia, Brit. J. Haemat. 8:215, 1962.
29. Chisolm, J. J., Jr.: Disturbances in the biosynthesis of heme in lead intoxication, J. Pediat. 64:174, 1964.
30. Chisolm, J. J. Jr., and Harrison, H. E.: The exposure of children to lead, Pediatrics 18:943, 1956.
31. Chisolm, J. J., Jr., and Harrison, H. E.: The treatment of acute lead encephalopathy in children, Pediatrics 19:2, 1957.
32. Chunn, C. F., and Harkins, H. N.: Alimentary azotemia, Amer. J. Med. Sci. 201:745, 1941.
33. Coleman, D. H., Stevens, A. R., Jr., Dodge, H. T., and Finch, C. A.: Rate of blood regeneration after blood loss, Arch. Intern. Med. 92:341, 1953.
34. Conley, C. L., Kowal, J., and D'Antonio, J.: Polycythemia associated with renal tumors, Bull. Johns Hopkins Hosp. 101:63, 1957.
35. Cornblath, M., and Hartmann, A. F.: Methemoglobinemia in young infants, J. Pediat. 33:421, 1948.
36. Dacie, J. V.: The haemolytic anaemias, congenital and acquired, New York, 1954, Grune & Stratton, Inc.
37. Dameshek, W.: Stress erythrocytes (editorial), Blood 8:282, 1953.
38. Darling, R. C., and Roughton, F. J. W.: The effect of methemoglobin on the equilibrium between oxygen and hemoglobin, Amer. J. Physiol. 137:56, 1942.
39. Daughaday, W. H., Williams, R. H., and Daland, G. A.: The effect of endocrinopathies on the blood, Blood 3:1342, 1948.
40. De Gruchy, G. C.: Clinical haematology in medical practice, Springfield, Ill., 1958, Charles C Thomas, Publisher.
41. Desforges, J. F., and Dawson, J. P.: The anemia of renal failure, Arch. Intern. Med. 101:326, 1958.
42. Dubach, R., Moore, C. V., and Minnich, V.: Studies in iron transportation and metabolism; utilization of intravenously injected radoactive iron for hemoglobin synthesis, and an evaluation of the radioactive iron method for studying iron absorption, J. Lab. Clin. Med. 31:1201, 1946.
43. Dystra, O. H., and Halbertsma, T.: Polycythemia vera in childhood; report of a case with changes in the skull, Amer. J. Dis. Child. 60:907, 1940.
44. Eder, H. A., Finch, C., and McKee, R. W.: Congenital methemoglobinemia; a clinical and biochemical study of a case, J. Clin. Invest. 28:265, 1949.
45. Editorial: Polycythemia, Lancet 1:189, 1959.
46. Emerson, C. P., and Burrows, B. A.: The mechanism of anemia and its influence on renal function in chronic uremia, J. Clin. Invest. 28:779, 1949.
47. Erslev, A. J.: Anemia of chronic renal disease, Arch. Intern. Med. 126:774, 1970.
48. Erslev, A. J., Lear, A. A., and Castle, W. B.: Pyridoxine-responsive anemia, New Eng. J. Med. 262:1209, 1960.
49. Etteldorf, J. N.: Methylene blue in the treatment of methemoglobinemia in premature infants caused by marking ink, J. Pediat. 38:24, 1951.
50. Ewing, M. C., and Mayon-White, R. M.: Cyanosis in infancy from nitrates in drinking water, Lancet 1:931, 1951.
51. Faigel, H. C.: Congenital cysts of the renal medulla, Amer. J. Dis. Child. 107:277, 1964.
52. Faucett, R. L., and Miller, H. C.: Methemoglobinemia occurring in infants fed milk diluted with well water of high nitrate content, J. Pediat. 29:593, 1946.
53. Fichter, E. G.: Sulfhemoglobinemia, Amer. J. Dis. Child. 88:749, 1954.
54. Finch, C. A.: Methemoglobinemia and sulhemoglobinemia, New Eng. J. Med. 239:470, 1948.
55. Finch, C. A., Gibson, J. G., II, Peacock, W. C., and Fluharty, R. G.: Iron metabolism, utilization of intravenous radioactive iron, Blood 4:905, 1949.
56. Fisher, J. W., Taylor, G., and Porteous, D. D.: Erythropoietin localization in the glomeruli of sheep kidney using a fluorescent antibody technique, Blood 24:846, 1964.
57. Foy, H., and Kondi, A.: Hypochromic anemias of the tropics associated with pyridoxine and nicotinic acid deficiency, Blood 13:1054, 1958.
58. Gardner, F. H.: The use of cobaltous chloride in the anemia associated with chronic renal disease, J. Lab. Clin. Med. 41:56, 1953.
59. Gardner, F. H., and Freymann, J. G.: Erythrocythemia (polycythemia) and hydronephrosis; report of a case with radio-iron studies, with recovery after nephrectomy, New Eng. J. Med. 259:323, 1958.
60. Gasser, C.: Aplasia of erythropoiesis, acute and chronic erythroblastopenias or pure (red cell) aplastic anaemias in childhood, Ped. Clin. N. Amer. 4:445, 1957.
61. Gasser, C., Gautier, E., Steck, A., Siebenmann, R. E., and Oechslin, R.: Hämolytischurämische Syndrome, bilaterale Nierenrindennekrosen bei akuten erworbenen hämolytischen Anämien, Schweiz. med. Wchnschr. 85:905, 1955.
62. Gibson, Q. H.: The reduction of methemoglobin in the red cells and studies on

the cause of idiopathic methemoglobinemia, Biochem. J. 42:13, 1948.
63. Giselson, N., Heinegard, D., Holmberg, L-G., Lindstedt, E., Lindstedt, G., and Scherstén, B.: Renal medullary cystic disease or familial juvenile nephrophthisis; a renal tubular disease, Amer. J. Med. 48:174, 1970.
64. Glynn, K. P., Penner, J. A., and Rucknagel, D. L.: Familial erythrocytosis; a description of three families, one with hemoglobin Ypsilanti, Ann. Intern. Med. 69:769, 1968.
65. Gold, A. P., and Michael, A. F., Jr.: Congenital adrenal hyperplasia associated with polycythemia, Pediatrics 23:727, 1959.
66. Goldberg, A. F.: Acid phosphatase activity in Auer bodies, Blood 24:305, 1964.
67. Goluboff, N., and Wheaton, R.: Methylene blue induced cyanosis and acute hemolytic anemia complicating the treatment of methemoglobinemia, J. Pediat. 58:86, 1961.
68. Gordon, A. S.: Hemopoietine, Physiol. Rev. 39:1, 1959.
69. Hamilton, H. B., Iuchi, I., Miyaji, T., and Shibata, S.: Haemoglobin Hiroshima ($\beta^{143}$ histidine—aspartic acid); a newly identified fast moving beta chain variant associated with increased oxygen affinity and compensatory erythemia, J. Clin. Invest. 48:525, 1969.
70. Harris, J. W.: The red cell; production, metabolism, destruction; normal and abnormal, Cambridge, Mass., 1963, Commonwealth Fund, Harvard University Press.
71. Harris, J. W., Price, J. M., Whittington, R. M., Weisman, R., Jr., Horrigan, D. L., and Cleveland, O.: Pyridoxine responsive anemia in the adult human, J. Clin. Invest. 35:709, 1956.
72. Harrison, T. R.: Principles of internal medicine, ed. 4, New York, 1962, McGraw-Hill Book Co., p. 542.
73. Howarth, B. E.: Epidemic of aniline methaemoglobinaemia in newborn babies, Lancet 1:934, 1951.
74. Hutchison, H. E., and Stark, J. M.: The anaemia of lead poisoning, J. Clin. Path. 14:548, 1961.
75. Jacobson, L. O., Goldwasser, E., Fried, W., Plzak, L.: Role of the kidney in erythropoiesis, Nature 179:633, 1957.
76. Jensen, W. N., Moreno, G. D., and Bessis, M. C.: An electron microscopic description of basophilic stippling in red cells, Blood 25:933, 1965.
77. Jones, N. F., and Hutt, M. S. R.: Observations on a case of pyridoxine-responsive anaemia, Lancet 1:1199, 1961.
78. Josephs, H. W.: The mechanism of the reduction of red cells and hemoglobin following operation for tetralogy of Fallot, Bull. Johns Hopkins Hosp. 86:1, 1950.
79. Joske, R. G., McAlister, J. M., and Prankerd, T. A. J.: Isotope investigations of red cell production and destruction in chronic renal disease, Clin. Sci. 15:511, 1956.
80. Kagan, B. M., Mirman, B., Calvin, J., and Lundeen, E.: Cyanosis in premature infants due to aniline dye intoxication, J. Pediat. 34:574, 1949.
81. Kellman, L.: Primary polycythemic manifestations, Amer. J. Dis. Child. 58:146, 1939.
82. Knock, H. L., and Githens, J. H.: Primary erythrocytosis of childhood, Amer. J. Dis. Child. 100:189, 1960.
83. Krammer, A., Cartwright, G. E., and Wintrobe, M. M.: The anemia of infection; studies on free erythrocyte coproporphyrin and protoporphyrin, Blood 9:183, 1954.
84. Kravitz, H., Elegant, L. D., Kaiser, E., and Kagan, B. M.: Methemoglobin values in premature and mature infants and children, Amer. J. Dis. Child. 91:1, 1956.
85. Lane, M., and Alfrey, C. P., Jr.: The anemia of human riboflavin deficiency, Blood 25:432, 1965.
86. Lange, R. D., and Gallagher, N. I.: The clinical and experimental observations on the relationship of the kidney to erythropoietin production. In Jacobson, L. O., and Doyle, M., editors: Erythropoiesis, New York, 1962, Grune & Stratton, Inc.
87. Lawrence, J. H., and Berlin, L. I.: Relative polycythemia—polycythemia of stress, Yale J. Biol. Med. 24:498, 1952.
88. Leikin, S. L.: Hematologic aspects of renal disease, Ped. Clin. N. Amer. 11:667, 1964.
89. Leonard, B. J., Israels, M. C. G., and Wilkinson, J. F.: Alkaline phosphatase in the white cells in leukaemia and leukemoid reactions, Lancet 1:289, 1958.
90. Lichtman, M. A. and Miller, D. R.: Erythrocyte glycolysis, 2, 3-diphosphoglycerate and adenosine triphosphate concentration in uremic subjects; relationship to extracellular phosphate concentration, J. Lab. Clin. Med. 76:267, 1970.
91. Loge, J. P., Lange, R. D., and Moore, C. V.: Characterization of the anemia associated with chronic renal insufficiency, Amer. J. Med. 24:4, 1958.
92. MacDonald, W. P.: Methaemoglobinaemia resulting from poisoning in children, M. J. Australia 1:145, 1951.
93. Marlow, A. A., and Fairbanks, V. F.: Polycythemia vera in an eleven-year-old girl, New Eng. J. Med. 263:950, 1960.
94. McFadzean, A. J. S., and Davis, L. J.: On the nature and significance of stippling in

lead poisoning, with reference to the effect of splenectomy, Quart. J. Med. 18:57, 1949.
95. Medal, L. S., Elizondo, J., Gallardo, J. T., and Gittler, C.: Pyridoxine-responsive anemia; report of 2 cases in brothers and a review of the literature, Blood 17:547, 1961.
96. Miller, A. A.: Congenital sulfhemoglobinemia, J. Pediat. 51:233, 1957.
97. Monge, C.: Chronic mountain sickness, Physiol. Rev. 23:166, 1953.
98. Nadas, A. S.: Pediatric cardiology, Philadelphia, 1957, W. B. Saunders Co.
99. Nadler, E. B., and Cohn, I.: Familial polycythemia, Amer. J. Med. Sci. 198:41, 1939.
100. Naets, J. P.: The role of the kidney in erythropoiesis, J. Clin. Invest. 39:102, 1960.
101. Nixon, R. K., O'Rourke, W., Rape, C. E., and Korst, D. R.: Nephrogenic polycythemia, Arch. Intern. Med. 106:797, 1960.
102. Novy, M. J., Edwards, M. J., and Metcalf, J.: Hemoglobin Yakima. II. High blood oxygen affinity associated with compensatory erythrocytosis and normal hemodynamics, J. Clin. Invest. 46:1848, 1967.
103. Orgeron, J. D., Martin, J. D., Caraway, C. T., Martine, R. M., and Hauser, G. H.: Methemoglobinemia from eating meat with high nitrite content, Pub. Health Rep. 72:189, 1957.
104. Oski, F. A., and Barness, L. A.: Vitamin E deficiency; previously unrecognized cause of hemolytic anemia in premature infants, J. Pediat. 70:211, 1967.
105. Penington, D. C.: The role of erythropoietic hormone in anaemia, Lancet 1:301, 1961.
106. Porter, F. S., Fitch, C. D., and Dinning, J. S.: Vitamin E deficiency in the monkey. IV. Further studies of the anemia with emphasis on bone marrow morphology, Blood 20:471, 1962.
107. Potter, E. L., and Osathanondh, V.: Medullary sponge kidney; two cases in young infants, J. Pediat. 62:901, 1963.
108. Raab, S. O., Haut, A., Cartwright, G. E., and Wintrobe, M. M.: Pyridoxine-responsive anemia, Blood 18:285, 1961.
109. Ramsay, D. H. E., and Harvey, C. C.: Marking-ink poisoning; an outbreak of methemoglobin cyanosis in newborn babies, Lancet 1:910, 1959.
110. Rath, C. E. Maillard, J. A., and Schreiner, G. E.: Bleeding tendency in uremia, New Eng. J. Med. 257:808, 1957.
111. Reed, C. S., Hampson, R., Gordon, S., Jones, R. T., Novy, M. J., Brimhall, B., Edwards, M. J., and Koler, R. D.: Erythrocytosis secondary to increased oxygen affinity of a mutant hemoglobin; hemoglobin Kempsey, Blood 31:623, 1968.

112. Reinhold, J.: The survival of transfused red cells in acute rheumatic fever with reference to a latent haemolytic mechanism, Arch. Dis. Child. 29:201, 1954.
113. Rieders, F., and Brieger, H.: Mechanism of poisoning from wax crayons, J.A.M.A. 151:1490, 1953.
114. Rosenberg, S. J., and Bennett, J. M.: Pyridoxine-responsive anemia, New York State J. Med. 69:1430, 1969.
115. Ross, J. D.: Deficient activity of DPNH-dependent methemoglobin diaphorase in cord blood erythrocytes, Blood 21:51, 1963.
116. Ross, J. D., and Desforges, J. F.: Reduction of methemoglobin by erythrocytes from cord blood; further evidence for deficient enzyme activity in the newborn period, Pediatrics 23:718, 1959.
117. Rucknagel, D. L., Glynn, K., and Smith, J.: Hemoglobin Ypsi, characterized by increased oxygen affinity, abnormal polymerization and erythremia, Clin. Res. 15:270, 1967.
118. Rudolph, A. M., Nadas, A. S., and Borges, W. H.: Hematologic adjustments to cyanotic congenital heart disease, Pediatrics 11:454, 1953.
119. Russell, R. P., and Conley, C. L.: Benign polycythemia; Gaisböck's syndrome, Arch. Intern. Med. 114:734, 1964.
120. Saifi, M. F., and Vaughan, J. M.: The anaemia associated with infection, Brit. Med. J. 1:35, 1948.
121. Shahidi, N. T., and Clatanoff, D. V.: The role of puberty in red-cell production in hereditary haemolytic anaemias, Brit. J. Haemat. 17:335, 1969.
122. Sharpe, J. C., and Bisgard, J. D.: The relation of the thyroid gland to hematopoiesis, J. Lab. Clin. Med. 21:347, 1936.
123. Shen, S. C., Wong, P. Y. C., and Oguro, M.: Experimental production of pyridoxine deficiency anemia in rats, Blood 23:679, 1964.
124. Silber, R., and Goldstein, B. D.: Vitamin E and the hematopoietic system, Seminars Hemat. 7:40, 1970.
125. Smith, C. H., and Graham, J. B.: Congenital medullary cysts of the kidneys with severe refractory anemia; report of a case, Amer. J. Dis. Child. 69:369, 1945.
126. Snyderman, S. E., Holt, L. E., Jr., Carretero, R., and Jacobs, K.: Pyridoxine deficiency in the human infant, Amer. J. Clin. Nutrition 5:200, 1953.
127. Spector, H., Maass, A. R., Michaud, L., Elvehjem, C. A., and Hart, E. B.: The role of riboflavin in blood regeneration, J. Biol. Chem. 150:75, 1943.
128. Stamatoyannopoulos, G., Yoshida, H., Adamson, J., and Heinenberg, S.: Hemoglobin

Rainier ($\beta^{145}$ tryosine-histidine); alkali resistant hemoglobin with increased oxygen affinity, Science **159**:741, 1968.
129. Townes, P. L., and Lovell, G. R.: Hereditary methemoglobinemia; a new variant exhibiting dominant inheritance of methemoglobin A, Blood **18**:18, 1961.
130. Townes, P. L., and Morrison, M.: Investigation of the defect of a variant of hereditary methemoglobinemia, Blood **19**:60, 1962.
131. Tudhope, G. R., and Wilson, G. M.: Anaemia in hypothroidism; incidence, pathogenesis and response to treatment, Quart. J. Med. **29**:513, 1960.
132. Tudhope, G. R., and Wilson, G. M.: Deficiency of vitamin $B_{12}$ in hypothyroidism, Lancet **1**:703, 1962.
133. Verel, D., Turnbull, A., Tudhope, G. R., and Ross, J. H.: Anaemia in Bright's disease, Quart. J. Med. **28**:491, 1959.
134. Verloop, M. C., and Rademaker, W.: Anaemia due to pyridoxine deficiency in man, Brit. J. Haemat. **6**:66, 1960.
135. Vilter, R. W., Woolford, R. M., and Spies, T. D.: Severe scurvy; a clinical and hematologic study, J. Lab. Clin. Med. **31**:609, 1946.
136. Waisman, H. A., Bain, J. A., Richmond, J. B., and Munsey, F. A.: Laboratory and clinical studies in congenital methemoglobinemia, Pediatrics **10**:293, 1952.
137. Wasserman, R. L., and Gilbert, H. S.: Surgery in polycythemia vera, New Eng. J. Med. **269**:1226, 1963.
138. Watson, R. J., Decker, E., and Lichtman, H. C.: Hematologic studies of children with lead poisoning, Pediatrics **21**:40, 1953.
139. Weissberg, J. B., Lipschutz, F., and Oski, F. A.: δ-aminolevulinic acid dehydrogenase activity in circulating blood cells, New Eng. J. Med. **284**:565, 1971.

140. Whaun, J. M., Delivoria-Papadopoulos, M., Henderson, L., Weissberg, J., and Oski, F. A.: Red cell phosphate and hemoglobin oxygen affinity in uremia, New Eng. J. Med. **281**:966, 1969.
141. Whitaker, J. A., and Vietti, T. J.: Fluorescence of the erythrocytes in lead poisoning in children; an aid to rapid diagnosis, Pediatrics **24**:734, 1959.
142. Whitby, L. E. H., and Britton, C. J. C.: Relation of stippled cell and polychromatic cell to reticulocyte, Lancet **1**:1173, 1933.
143. White, A., Handler, P., and Smith, E. L.: Principles of biochemistry, ed. 3, New York, 1964, McGraw-Hill Book Co.
144. Wintrobe, M. M.: Clinical hematology, ed. 5, Philadelphia, 1961, Lea & Febiger.
145. Wintrobe, M. M., Buschke, W., Follis, R. H., Jr., and Humphreys, S.: Riboflavin deficiency in swine, Bull. John Hopkins Hosp. **75**:102, 1944.
146. Wintrobe, M. M., Follis, R. H., Jr., Miller, M. H., Stein, H. J., Alcayaga, R., Humphreys, S., Suksta, A., and Cartwright, G. E.: Pyridoxine deficiency in swine, Bull. Johns Hopkins Hosp. **72**:1, 1943.
147. Wirtshafter, Z. T., and Walsh, J. R.: Pyridoxine deficiency versus undernutrition, Arch. Path. **77**:239, 1964.
148. Wolff, J. A.: Methemoglobinemia due to benzocaine, Pediatrics **20**:915, 1957.
149. Wolman, I. J.: Laboratory applications in clinical pediatrics, New York, 1957, McGraw-Hill Book Co.
150. Wood, J. L.: Plethora in the newborn infant associated with cyanosis and convulsions; a review of postnatal erythropoiesis, J. Pediat. **54**:143, 1959.

# 18 LEUKOCYTES—CELL TYPES

The origin of white blood cells has been described elsewhere in conjunction with blood formation in the embryo (Chapter 1). These cells differ from the erythrocytes in the absence of hemoglobin and in the possession of a nucleus. They are larger than erythrocytes, ranging from $8\mu$ for the small lymphocytes to $15\mu$ for the largest monocytes. These colorless corpuscles constitute the most important elements in the body's defenses against invading microorganisms.

The leukocytes possess an extensive enzymatic apparatus of which specific uses have not been entirely explored. They contain enzymes such as glucuronidase, acid and alkaline phosphatase, and esterase and biologically important substances of nonenzymatic nature such as glutathione, glucuronic acid, histamine, and glycogen.[137]

*Growth and multiplication.* As in the red blood cells, growth and multiplication of the leukocytes are closely identified with the nucleic acid components of the cytoplasm and nucleus. Deoxyribonucleic acid (DNA) is found in the chromatin of the cell nucleus and ribonucleic acid (RNA) in the cell cytoplasm and nucleolus. These two substances can be differentiated by the cytochemical Fuelgen test for deoxyribonucleic acid. Following mild hydrolysis with hydrochloric acid and treatment with reduced fuchsin, a red color is produced with the dye if deoxyribose is split off.[227]

Folic acid (pteroylglutamic acid—PGA) and folinic acid (citrovorum factor), its biologically more active form, are indispensable in the synthesis of deoxyribonucleic acid of the cell nucleus. In the treatment of patients with leukemia it will be seen that analogues of folic acid and of some of the nucleic acid components such as the purines act as antimetabolites. By gaining entrance into the cells, they block enzyme systems and interfere with their growth.

The functional demands of each of the white blood cells vary in relation to local tissue changes in health and disease. The white blood cells require a rich oxygen supply for growth and development, in contrast to anoxic conditions required for optimal erythropoiesis.[66] When white blood cells are rapidly destroyed as in patients with leukemia with excessively high white cell counts, large amounts of uric acid are liberated. In patients with acute leukemia being treated with steroids, for instance, serious disturbances of kidney function may result.

A, B, and $Rh_o(D)$ antigens have been demonstrated on human leukocytes, particularly the neutrophil. The antigens are not related to the secretor status of the leukocyte donor, nor are such antigens transferred to leukocytes by means of incubation with plasma of a strong secretor.[4]

*Chemotactic factors.* The functional demands for each type of the white blood cells vary with local tissue changes. The stimulus for each type of cell is largely chemotactic. The direction toward which a cell migrates is influenced by the presence of foreign particles, infecting organisms, or substances elaborated from the site of tissue injury. This property is manifested chiefly by granulocytes, monocytes, and eosinophils but not by lymphcytes. The rapid disintegration of cells requires a cycle of compensatory and regenerative mechanisms for their replacement. Under pathologic conditions such as pyogenic infections, the nucleic acid and other products of tissue destruction serve as a stimulus for proliferation. A leukocytosis-promoting factor which stimulates a discharge of granulocytes from the bone marrow has been isolated in inflammatory exudates. Other products produce leukopenia so that the leukocytic level observed at any one time depends upon the interaction of these opposing factors.[151]

The presence of another substance in normal plasma which expels granulocytic leukocytes from the bone marrow into the blood and to some of the organs has been described. This substance represents the expulsion factor which mediates the delivery of polymorphonuclear leukocytes to the circulation to replace those destroyed.[228]

Particularly in infants the bone marrow may produce sufficiently large numbers of myeloid cells to constitute a leukemoid blood picture in the course of a severe infection. In less severe infections in the younger patients, abnormal responses may also occur, producing a leukocytosis out of proportion to the stimulus.

The stimulus for production of a particular leukocyte varies with each type of cell and depends upon the nature of the chemical substances liberated from the affected tissues. Certain infections stimulate production of polymorphonuclear leukocytes, whereas others may depress them.

*Glucose-6-phosphate dehydrogenase in leukocytes.* Some interrelationship exists between the enzyme glucose-6-phosphate dehydrogenase (G6PD) in red cells and white blood cells and between the enzyme in white cells and hemolytic disease. Marked reduction in the mean level of G6PD activity of leukocytes has occasionally been noted in persons with the erythrocyte defect,[202] but this association is not constant.[145] Others have reported low normal values in white cells in Negro males and subnormal values in Caucasian males with the severe red cell defect.[144] The same inconsistency was found in two families of Greek and Spanish ancestry, suggesting some interrelationship between G6PD activity in red and white blood cells but not sufficiently marked to be a consistent manifestation of a single trait.[215]

Decreased activity of glycolytic enzymes in the leukocytes of patients with hereditary hemolytic anemias associated with deficiencies of erythrocyte enzymes have been reported in triose phosphate isomerase deficiency,[217] phosphoglucose isomerase deficiency,[187] and phosphoglycerate kinase deficiency.[242] Patients with triose phosphate isomerase deficiency appear to have an unusual susceptibility to infection, but impaired phagocytic activity or leukocyte function has yet to be demonstrated in the enzyme-deficient leukocytes.[243]

The reduced glutathione (GSH) content of normal leukocytes was found by one method ("alloxan 305" procedure) to be 5.2 mg. per $10^{10}$ white blood cells.[199] No differences from normal levels were found in patients susceptible to agranulocytosis.

*Functions—phagocytosis and antibody formation.* The polymorphonuclear leukocytes, monocytes, and other reticuloendothelial cells contribute to the body defenses by their motility and their capacity for ingesting and destroying invading bacteria and discharging granulocytes from the bone marrow.[151] Most of the white blood cells are capable of ameboid movement and obey chemotactic stimuli. They play a part in the defense of the body by phagocytic and immunologic means. The ingestion of a particle by living cells is termed phagocytosis. Ameboid mobility of the granulocytes and monocytes may be quantitatively evaluated and serves as an index of their viability.[136] Neonatal leukocytes obtained from cord blood have been found to have lower ameboid and phagocytic activities when compared to maternal leukocytes and those of other adults.[44,148,161] This inferiority would indicate an inherent functional difference corresponding to that found in other organs and systems. The relationship to immunity in the neonatal period has still to be determined.

Metchnikoff, in originally coining the name phagocyte (eating cell), pointed out that this cell was richly endowed with a variety of ferments, enabling it to perform the task of engulfing microorganisms and other cells and substances. Recent information has supplemented this concept by the discovery that in mammalian polymorphonuclear leukocytes there were digestive enzymes and some antibacterial substances which are sequestered within cytoplasmic granules or lysosomes.[112,251] The lysosome is a subcellular structure containing a large number of granules within a specialized membrane. There are over a dozen proteolytic and hydrolytic enzymes confined within the lysosomes, including ribonuclease, deoxyribonuclease, cathepsins, glycosidases, sulfatases, and phosphatases. These enzymes are discharged when needed, directly into or about the digestive vacuole surrounding engulfed material. The phagocytized material eventually undergoes dissolution. The discharge of lytic enzymes may interfere with metabolism of the host and cell death follows.[195]

Macrophages refer to the monocytic cells which ingest not only bacteria but also large particles such as red blood cells. Lymphocytes

Table 24. Serum immunoglobulin changes in disease*

|  | IgG (G) | IgA (A) | IgM (M) |
|---|---|---|---|
| Immunoglobulin disorders |  |  |  |
|    Lymphoid aplasia | – – – | – – – | – – – |
|    Agammaglobulinemia | – – – | – – – | – – – |
|    Selective IgG, IgA deficiency | – – – | – – – | N or + + |
|    Selective IgA, IgM deficiency | N | – – – | – – – |
|    An-IgA-globulinemia | N | – – – | N |
|    Ataxia telangiectasia | N | – – – | N |
| Multiple myeloma, macroglobulinemia |  |  |  |
|    G (IgG)-myeloma | + + + | – – | – – |
|    A (IgA)-myeloma | – – | + + + | – – |
|    M-macroglobulinemia (Waldenström) | – | – | + + + |
|    Bence-Jones proteinuria | – | – | – |
| Gastrointestinal protein loss | – – | – – | – – |
| Nephrotic syndrome | – – | – | N |
| Infection |  |  |  |
|    Pulmonary tuberculosis | + | N | N |
|    Trypanosomiasis | N(+) | N(+) | + + + |
| Lupus erythematosus | + + | + | + |
| Rheumatoid arthritis | + | + | + |
| Hepatic disease |  |  |  |
|    Laennec's cirrhosis | + + | + + + | N |
|    Biliary cirrhosis | N | N | + + |
|    Acute hepatitis | + | + | + |
|    Hepatoma | N | N | – |
| Leukemia, lymphoma, etc. |  |  |  |
|    Acute lymphoblastic leukemia | N | – | N |
|    Chronic lymphocytic leukemia | – | – – | – – – |
|    Acute myeloblastic leukemia | N | N | N |
|    Chronic myelocytic leukemia | N | – | N |
|    Hodgkin's disease | N | N | N |

*From Fahey, J. L.: Antibodies and immunoglobulins. II. Normal development and changes in disease, J.A.M.A. **194**:257, 1965.
Key: N signifies normal; –, – –, and – – – signify progressively more severe reduction below normal; +, + +, and + + + signify progressively greater increases above normal.

possess slight phagocytic powers but participate more actively in the elaboration of antibodies.[105] These immune substances are associated with the gamma globulin of blood plasma. In the course of their disintegration, cytoplasm which contains gamma globulin is released in the lymph and blood. The rate of lymphocytic dissolution has been attributed to hormonal control—more specifically through the medium of pituitary-adrenocortical secretions.[72,253]

Plasma cells, like lymphocytes to which they are related, are also associated with antibody formation. Evidences of this function are the increased numbers of plasma cells in persons with hyperglobulinemia, their deficiency in those with agammaglobulinemia, and the high concentration of ribonucleic acid in the cytoplasm. Severe impairment of immunologic response and decreased resistance to infection in agammaglobulinemia are associated with a sharp decrease of plasma cells (Table 24).[93]

*Chemotaxis and opsonins.* In the process of phagocytosis several precursors are called into operation.[73] Chemotaxis is involved in the initial events in the inflammatory response and includes a series of segmental steps in which phagocytic cells migrate into an area which contains the inflammatory stimulus. Humoral factors that play a part include local release of histamine, bradykinin, and other components of the plasminogen-kinin system which affect vascular dilation, concentration, margination, and emigration of leukocytes.[73]

Opsonization follows chemotaxis and precedes the engulfment of bacteria. Opsonins interact with particles and not the phagocyte. Opsonins include IgG and IgM antibodies and complement components. Engulfment during phagocytosis depends upon the recognition of either antibody alone (IgG) or antibody (IgM)-complement complexes ($C^{1,4,2,3}$). In contrast to the monocyte, the neutrophil requires both complement ($C^{1,4,2,3}$) and IgG for rosette formation and erythrophagocytosis.[119] These globulins coat the bacterial surfaces and render them more susceptible to phagocytosis. In the absence of opsonins, some phagocytosis may occur, but at a markedly diminished rate. Following appropriate opsonization, the sequence of events involves surface attachment, engulfment, and formation of a phagocytic vacuole, followed by degranulation (the lysis of leukocyte granules which release their contents into the phagocytic vacuole). The latter will be discussed in the section that follows on chronic granulomatous disease.

*Chronic granulomatous disease of childhood.* The disease now called chronic granulomatous disease of childhood was originally described by Berendes, Bridges, and Good[21] and by Landing and Shirkey[133] as a disease in which severe bacterial infections resulted ultimately in death despite the most vigorous antibiotic treatment. With few exceptions of its occurrence in girls, the condition is practically always confined to boys and is regarded as an X-linked hereditary disease.

In 1966, Holmes and colleagues[117] demonstrated for the first time that polymorphonuclear neutrophils from children with chronic granulomatous disease were unable to kill certain bacteria after ingestion. Characteristic of this disease is that the patient's granulocytes ingest staphylococci and certain gram-negative bacteria normally but do not kill them. All the factors in this phenomenon are still unknown but information about many features is now available.

Chronic granulomatous disease is usually clinically apparent before 2 years of age. The most constant features are recurrent and severe bacterial infections of the skin, lymph nodes, lungs, bones, and liver. Lymphadenopathy, hepatosplenomegaly, and chronic eczematoid dermatitis are common physical signs. Children all receive intensive antibiotic treatment for the recurrent severe infections until one eventually proves fatal, usually before the age of 10. Autopsy findings include multiple pulmonary and reticuloendothelial granulomatosis and histiocytic infiltration of lymph nodes, liver, spleen, and bone marrow.[143]

Phagocytosis of bacteria is associated with the rupture of the leukocyte granules during their degeneration when their contents are discharged into the phagocytic vacuole containing the ingested organisms.[45,50] Leukocyte granules contain a variety of antibacterial agents, among which are hydrolytic enzymes from lysosomes, cationic proteins, phagocytin, and myeloperoxidase. Klebanoff and White[130] found that the ability of leukocytes in chronic granulomatous disease to kill certain organisms depends on bacterial formation of the hydrogen peroxide required for an antimicrobial system in the leukocytes; this is mediated by myeloperoxidase in the presence of a halide. The leukocytes of children with chronic granulomatous disease can destroy organisms which generate hydrogen peroxide such as streptococci and pneumococci. Staphylococci, on the other hand, produce catalase, which destroys hydrogen peroxide and survives in leukocytes with the disease.[201] The defect in bacterial killing does not appear to indicate impaired phagocytosis, but following ingestion of the bacteria prolonged intracellular survival occurs. Impaired degranulation by the diseased leukocytes after phagocytosis was suggested at one time, but normal degranulation has now been demonstrated in typical cases of chronic granulomatous disease.[128]

The biochemical events associated with intracellular killing of ingested bacteria include increases in oxygen consumption, in hexose-monophosphate shunt activity, and in hydrogen peroxide production. Normal leukocytes in vitro reduce nitroblue tetrazolium (NBT) dye to purple formazan during phagocytosis of polystyrene particles.[14] Baehner and Karnofsky[13] found that the polymorphonuclear neutrophils from patients with chronic granulomatous disease of childhood are deficient in NADH oxidase and have diminished postphagocytic hydrogen peroxide production.[116] Hydrogen peroxide is probably essential for normal intracellular killing by polymorphonuclear neutrophils. The defect in hydrogen peroxide production may explain the abnormal bactericidal activity of polymorphonuclear neutrophils from patients with chronic granulomatous disease. The deficiency of leukocyte NADH oxidase, with resultant failure to kill ingested bacteria (i.e. staphylococci), is felt to be responsible for recurrent suppurative infections which occur in children with chronic granulomatous disease. Leukocytes fail to increase oxygen consumption with phagocytosis or to reduce nitroblue tetrazolium dye.

A simplified screening test has been described for the diagnosis of chronic granulomatous disease.[124] Normal phagocytes suspended in plasma when mixed with latex particles for ingestion and nitroblue tetrazolium dye will reduce the dye to a blue color. The reaction depends on the release of enzymes from the phagocytic lysosomal granules and the cell cytoplasm after phagocytosis. Since such release is deficient in patients with chronic granulomatous disease, no blue color develops in the tube. This test can be used to identify heterozygous carrier mothers of male offspring who showed the recessive sex-linked trait. The carrier mothers themselves are not usually susceptible to infection. Nitroblue tetrazolium (NBT) dye reduction by leukocytes of patients receiving prednisone was significantly reduced.[156] The exact mechanism of corticosteroid action remains unknown. Polymorphonuclear leukocytes (PMN) from patients with chronic granulomatous disease of childhood phagocytize *C. albicans* normally but are unable to kill the intracellular organisms.[175] Johnston and Janeway[125] differentiate between phagocytosis in which the body clears itself of bacterial infection and resistance to infection by fungi and viruses, which depends primarily on the integrity of the small lymphocyte. They emphasize that a normal child usually has an absolute neutrophil count of more than 1,200 to 1,500 cells per cu. mm. Values below these may be associated with furunculosis, cellulitis, and pneumonia. If a child has recurrent bacterial infection with an appropriate leukocytosis, then chronic granulomatous disease should be considered. An abnormality of delayed hypersensitivity may be determined by appropriate skin testing with *Monilia albicans* extract or other reagents such as PPD, streptokinase-streptodornase, or mumps antigens according to a definitive program. In addition, quantitative determinations of IgG, IgA, and IgM should be made. A summary of diagnostic considerations in a child with frequent infections is offered by the writers.

It has been pointed out that the NBT test cannot at present be used in neonates because of falsely positive reactions, and it is not reliable in patients with phagocytic defects.[188] Inasmuch as this test is concerned primarily with neutrophils, a severe neutropenia may also limit its usefulness. Another limitation of the test is the fact that it does not identify the causative organisms or the sites of infection.

A case of Job's syndrome—a variant of chronic granulomatous disease—was described in a 5-year-old girl, the red-haired, fair-skinned child of dark-skinned, dark-haired immigrants from Southern Italy. No underlying disease was discovered to account for her recurrent "cold" suppurative infections due to pyogenic staphylococci. The patient's polymorphonuclear neutrophils failed to reduce nitroblue tetrazolium dye. Streptococci could, however, be handled normally.[15]

***Rebuck skin-window; study of leukocytic functions in vivo.*** The method described by Rebuck[203] is used for evaluating the morphological events comprising the inflammatory cycle in man. In essence, this method consists of scrapping off the epidermis and applying an antigenic irritant as the inflammatory agent. The site usually chosen is either the volar surface of the forearm or the anterior surface of the thigh, although any other convenient region may be employed. The skin is shaved and cleaned with alcohol. With a sterile scalpel or razor blade the epithelium is scraped away from an area of 3 or 4 mm. in diameter. A small amount of bleeding is to be desired as evidence that the corium has actually been denuded. A solution or suspension of the desired nonlethal inflammatory agent is applied to the denuded corium; a drop of DPT, purified tuberculin protein, typhoid vaccine, or egg white may be applied as the antigenic irritant with a platinum loop. The lesion is then immediately covered with a sterile, chemically clean cover slip, which is in turn surmounted by a square of cardboard, cut slightly larger than the cover slip. The cardboard is covered by surgical adhesive tape, approximately 2 by 4 inches. The cells of the inflammatory exudate migrate to the undersurface of the cover slip, flattening themselves out as they do so. In 30 to 60 minutes the cover slip is removed and rapidly dried; at the same time, another sterile cover slip is placed over the same lesion, and the process is repeated as often as desired at timed intervals. In this way a series of permanent, fixed preparations of in vivo samplings of the cellular exudates is obtained. The cover slips exhibit a single layer of exudative cells on their undersurfaces. The cover slips having been rapidly dried, are stained with a standard May-Grünwald-Giemsa or Wright-Giemsa stain.

In the normal child the events of the inflammatory cycle induced either by simple mechanical or by antigenic stimulation are as follows.[186] There is an initial infiltration of histogenous mononuclear cells (histiocytes), beginning within 30 minutes; subsequent polymorphonuclear infiltration begins 30 minutes to 1 hour after irritation, and reaches a maximum during the next 3 to 4 hours. Beginning 4 to 6 hours after initiation of the inflammatory process, infiltration of small mononuclear cells indistinguishable from small, medium, and large circulating lymphocytes begins. During the subsequent 12 hours these cells undergo a dramatic cytomorphogenesis to become the hematogenous polyblasts and macrophages of the acute inflammatory process.

In neutropenic states, for example, no neutrophilic cells were present during the entire 48 hours in which the inflammatory process was studied. Lymphocytes and monocytes, although present in the blood, were deficient in the window.

In demonstrating the factors required for mononuclear chemotaxis, it is worthy of note that the prior appearance of neutrophilis is requisite for the accumulation of mononuclear cells in Rebuck windows in patients with cyclic neutropenia.[73]

*Autophagic vacuoles.* Human erythrocytes and circulating reticulocytes are the sites of membrane-enclosed bodies with the fine structural characteristics of cytolysosomes or autophagic vacuoles. These vacuoles correspond to the lysosomes of leukocytes and constitute an intracellular digestive system disposing of redundant cellular material (such as cytoplasmic organelles, iron particles, and segments of erythrocytic cytoplasm) of red cells.[129] Their lysosomal nature is substantiated by the demonstration of acid phosphatase activity. The autophagic vacuoles appear to be instrumental in the disposal of mitochondria, ribosomes, and other material present particularly in circulating reticulocytes.

The autophagic vacuoles are increased in normal individuals without spleens or in those with abnormalities of erythropoiesis. They were most abundant in splenectomized persons with associated hematologic disorders.[129]

*Muramidase (lysozyme).* Muramidase was originally named lysozyme by its discoverer, Alexander Fleming,[88] because of its remarkable capacity to lyse or dissolve cell walls of certain bacteria. It has a widespread distribution throughout the animal and bacterial worlds. Lysozyme presumably originates not only from granulocytes and monocytes in blood but also from tissue macrophages, and is released from these cells to appear in serum, nasal and lacrimal secretions, and various body fluids. Leukocyte muramidase is derived from the release of this enzyme from the white cells. The major portion of this enzyme in the serum is derived from the breakdown of senescent leukocytes. In infections, however, the concentrations of muramidase in sera are increased with increases in leukocyte muramidase, suggesting release from viable cells.

In the blood, muramidase is measurable in the serum, neutrophils, monocytes, and macrophages. Lymphocytes, basophils, eosinophils, erythrocytes, and platelets contain little or none. Serum muramidase may be considered a rough index of leukopoiesis both in the normal state and in proliferative diseases involving myeloid and monocytic cells. Increased values have been reported in infections, tuberculosis, and acute and chronic myelocytic and monocytic leukemia. The highest values are found in acute myelomonocytic leukemia and untreated megaloblastic anemia with neutropenia.

Lysozyme is excreted in large quantities in urine. The occasional increase in serum or urinary lysozyme concentrations occurs in some patients with multiple myelomas, sarcomatosis, Hodgkin's disease, and typhoid fever.

Osserman and Lawlor[181] reported that patients with monocytic and myelomonocytic leukemia excrete large quantities of lysozyme in the urine. Later it was shown that these patients also have hypokalemia.[171] Serial measurements of serum muramidase activity may be of value in determining the efficiency of antileukemic treatment in monocytic and myelocytic leukemia, with highest values in acute myelomonocytic leukemia. In leukemia, enzyme values appear to return to normal when complete remissions are attained, while increased serum activity persists with incomplete marrow remissions. It has been stated that the results of serial serum muramidase determinations in acute leukemia indicate that such assays may provide at least as much information as serial bone marrow examinations in acute lymphocytic, myelomonocytic, and monocytic leukemia, and appear of little value in acute myelocytic leukemia.[194,257] (This subject is discussed again in Chapter 22.)

*Erythrophagocytosis.* Phagocytosis also plays an important role in the removal of damaged or altered erythrocytes from the peripheral blood.

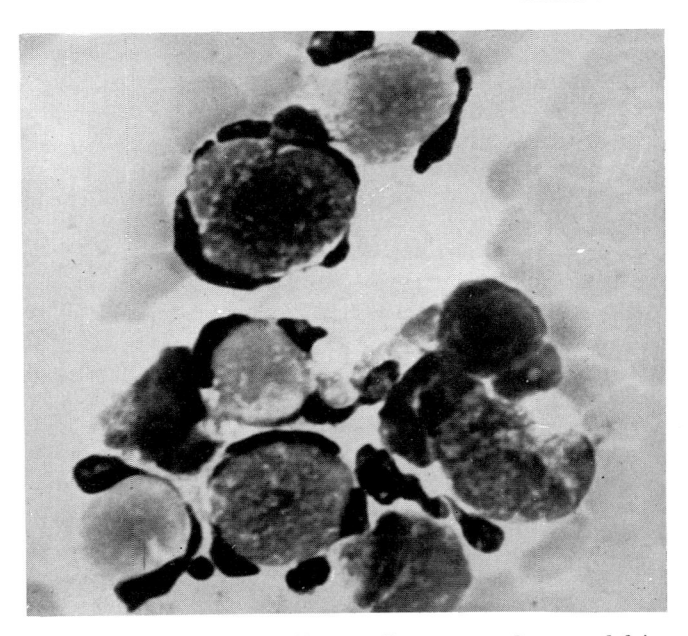

Fig. 57. L.E. cells. Polymorphonuclear cells (usually segmented neutrophils) containing homogeneous nuclear material with nucleus displaced to one side. (×1100.) (From Holman, H. R.: Systemic lupus erythematosus, J. Pediat. 56:109, 1960.)

Polymorphonuclear neutrophils and monocytes which have ingested intact red blood cells occasionally can be observed. They have been noted in patients with hemolytic disease of the newborn, idiopathic acquired hemolytic anemia, leukemia, chemical poisoning, paroxysmal cold hemoglobinuria, typhoid fever, and other infections. In the blood of a 2-year-old child with leukemia many promyelocytes showed erythrophagocytosis.[240] In children with acquired hemolytic anemia, marked erythrophagocytosis was observed when the buffy coat of the blood had been previously incubated at 37° C. for 1 hour.[265] Erythrophagocytosis noted in the peripheral blood and in the spleen of patients with hemolytic anemia has also been related to the opsonic activity of autoantibodies altering the surface of the red cells.[30]

*L.E. phenomenon.* Phagocytosis is also exemplified by the L.E. cell (Fig. 57), which constitutes an important diagnostic feature of disseminated lupus erythematosus, a febrile disease of unknown etiology characterized by malaise, fever, skin lesions, polyserositis, arthralgia, cardiac manifestations, and renal damage. A common feature is a biologically false-positive serologic reaction for syphilis.[160,167,168] A palpable spleen and enlargement of superficial lymph nodes have been observed in an appreciable number of patients but are inconstant features. Of aid in diagnosis is the demonstration of L.E. cells from preparations of the blood and bone marrow.

A normochromic, normocytic anemia with a hemolytic component is present in 3 to 5% of patients. Leukopenia and an increased number of nonsegmented neutrophils are seen in about one-third of the patients at initial examination and increase subsequently to about one-half at some time in the course of the disease.[152] Platelets may be reduced to the degree of simulating thrombocytopenic purpura. With present methods of treatment, including steroids, patients are kept free of symptoms for a considerable length of time. Progressive renal failure constitutes the major problem.

An important diagnostic test for disseminated lupus erythematosus is the demonstration of the L.E. cell described by Hargraves.[104] The L.E. phenomenon is an in vitro reaction which depends upon the presence of a nucleolytic factor and active phagocytic cells that are attracted to the lysed nuclear material which it later engulfs.

The L.E. cell is a segmented neutrophil (rarely a monocyte) which has phagocytized an amorphous mass derived most often from the nucleus of polymorphonuclear leukocytes or lymphocytes. Swelling and loss of structure of chromatin material results, with the lysed nuclear mass acting as a foreign body. This material is chemotactic and attracts phagocytic cells which engulf it. The cell, usually a neutrophil, contains this nuclear mass and because of its size pushes the nucleus of the phagocytizing cell to one side, thus only partially surrounding the inclusion body.

The ingested nuclear material varies in staining reaction from light pink to dark purple. It is stained by basic dyes and is Feulgen-positive, indicating its nuclear origin.

The L.E. rosette results from the attempt of a cluster of leukocytes to phagocytize simultaneously a single large mass of extracellular nuclear material. The presence of a plasma factor is indicated by the development of L.E. cells after incubating the plasma or serum of patients with systemic lupus erythematosus with the buffy layer from bone marrow or peripheral blood of normal persons.

The factor responsible for the L.E. phenomenon in patients with disseminated lupus erythematosus is associated with the gamma globulin fraction of the plasma. There are many explanations for the interaction between L.E. factors and the nucleus of cells. According to one theory, the L.E. plasma factor induces specific chemical changes in leukocytic nuclei (i.e., the depolymerization of deoxyribonucleic acid) so that these altered nuclei are later ingested by other leukocytes to form L.E. cells. An alternate theory explains nucleophagocytosis on the basis of antinuclear autoantibodies which correspond to the L.E. serum factor of the patient's plasma. There is evidence that the L.E. factor is a gamma globulin which acts as an antibody and combines directly with the cell nuclei and nuclear nucleoproteins.[114,115] It is now known that there are many antibodies found in this disease which are directed against a variety of cellular constituents. While both 7S and 19S antinuclear antibodies occur in systemic lupus erythematosus, the L.E. cell antibody has been shown to be a 7S antibody with specificity for nucleoprotein, requiring both DNA and histone.[170]

In one study antinuclear antibodies were found in 91.5% of serum samples from patients with systemic lupus erythematosus and in 25% of the patients with rheumatoid arthritis and other collagen diseases.[200] That both hereditary factors as well as environmental agents are involved in systemic lupus erythematosus is the finding of antinuclear antibodies in 58% (25 of 43 families) of the relatives of these patients. In another series[83] antinuclear antibodies were found in 42% (38 of 90) of relatives of patients with systemic lupus erythematosus and in 47% (18 of 38) of relatives of patients with rheumatoid arthritis.

That an immunologic mechanism may be responsible for the nucleophagocytosis of the L.E. phenomenon is suggested by the associated evidence of autoimmune hemolytic anemia, leukopenia, and thrombocytopenia in this disease and by the experimental production in vitro of L.E. cells.[154]

Placental transmission of the L.E. factor to the newborn infant has been reported. The L.E. test remains positive in the infant's blood until about 7 weeks of age and then becomes negative. It is not surprising that this factor, being a gamma globulin, can pass the placental barrier. In one case a newborn infant delivered of a mother with signs of subacute systemic lupus erythematosus developed a severe hemolytic anemia, leukopenia, and thrombocytopenia.[218] Complete restitution occurred at 3½ months of age, following treatment with blood transfusions and prednisone.

In other observations nucleophagocytosis produced experimentally by mixing antileukocytic serum with leukocytes from the same source resulted in structures resembling L.E. cells.[263] According to this hypothesis, the L.E. plasma factor constitutes an "autoimmune" substance which stimulates antileukocyte antibody. In the presence of the L.E. factor white cells are sensitized and phagocytized by other leukocytes,[86] and a high antibody serum would be responsible for both the ultimate development of L.E. cells and the formation of rosettes.[264]

Nucleolysis which is fundamental in the L.E. phenomenon must be distinguished from the nonspecific nucleophagocytosis. An example of the latter is the tart cell. This cell is occasionally found in normal bone marrow and in persons with pathologic conditions such as lymphoblastoma, multiple myeloma, pulmonary infection, and metastatic carcinoma.[106] The distinguishing feature between the L.E. cell and the tart cell is the difference in the morphologic appearance of the respective inclusion bodies. In the L.E. cell the inclusion body is amorphous and is characterized by the absence of visible chromatin material. In the tart cell the engulfed material can be readily identified as a cell nucleus resembling most often the nucleus of a lymphocyte. The L.E. cell must therefore be differentiated from other cells of nonspecific conditions in which an intact nucleus with a normal chromatin pattern is phagocytized. The significance of the tart cell is obscure. Hargraves,[104] who first described both the L.E. cell and the tart cell, emphasized the fact that the latter is usually a histiocyte whereas the former is almost always a neutrophilic polymorphonuclear leukocyte. Furthermore, he stated that the inclusion body of the L.E. cell is usually a homogeneous purple-staining mass with no visible chromatin pattern.

The engulfment of nuclei and nuclear fragments of other cells is commonly observed in specimens of heparinized bone marrow of normal persons and patients with conditions other than systemic lupus erythematosus.

Few positive results have been reported if these criteria are adhered to in patients with conditions other than systemic lupus erythematosus.[212] The L.E. cells, however, have been reported in patients with penicillin reactions, and the possibility of the association of this phenomenon with hypersensitivity has been suggested.[246] Positive L.E. tests have been reported infrequently in a variety of conditions such as leukemia, Hodgkin's disease, lymphosarcoma, and, with greater regularity, in rheumatoid arthritis and allergic reactions, particularly to drugs.[118]

L.E. cells should be sought for in patients with unexplained fever, leukopenia, thrombocytopenia, hemolytic anemia, arthritis, nephrotic syndrome, and uremia in which the etiology is obscure.[152] In children, protracted polyarthralgia, fever, and leukopenia should lead to suspicion of disseminated lupus erythematosus and a search for L.E. cells. The characteristic scaly eruption of erythematosus over the bridge of the nose and extending to the malar prominences in a butterfly fashion may not always be conspicuous. It may reappear on exposure to sunlight and with the cessation of steroids and corticotropin therapy. Occasionally, patients with autoimmune (acquired) hemolytic anemia and idiopathic thrombocytopenic purpura may develop overt manifestations of disseminated lupus erythematosus with positive L.E. tests following splenectomy.[57]

*Lupus erythematosus.* Tests for several simple methods of demonstrating L.E. cells and rosettes with and without the use of anticoagulants have been devised. In each of these the patient supplies all necessary elements for producing L.E. cells: the L.E. factor, nuclear material with which the L.E. factor can react, and the phagocytic cell. Thus, the use of white blood cells from blood or bone marrow of normal persons is eliminated. These tests are carried out with anticoagulants[147] or with the use of clotted blood.[210,236] With the latter, caution must be exercised in distinguishing tart cells (damaged nuclear material engulfed by phagocytic cells) from L.E. cells. Extracellular material may appear in L.E. preparations in the form of homogeneous round bodies known as hematoxylin bodies.[7] They are remnants of injured nuclei closely resembling the inclusions in L.E. cells. L.E. cells and hematoxylin bodies have been reported in naturally occurring skin lesions of systemic lupus erythematosus.[258]

*Life-span of leukocytes.* The life-span of the leukocytes has been divided into three phases: the hemopoietic phase, extending from the development of the primitive cell to its delivery into the circulation; the intravascular phase, the period within the circulation; and the extravascular phase, the period of time the leukocyte spends in the viscera and in the tissues. The segment within the circulation therefore must be viewed in relation to the larger extravascular areas. The lung, liver, spleen, gastrointestinal tract, striated muscle, and kidney have been implicated as leukocyte removal sites.[26] The pulmonary circulation, particularly, represents a sizeable reservoir of leukocytes and platelets that may be readily discharged into the circulation under proper stimulation. The lungs are optimally located to deliver large quantities of leukocytes and platelets into the circulation more rapidly than are the bone marrow, spleen, liver, or other hemopoietic sites.[27]

Various techniques have been used to estimate the life-span of the white blood cells, but they have not yielded consistent results. One of these methods[182] utilizes the incorporation of radioactive phosphorus into the deoxyribonucleic acid of the leukocytes. The majority of the labeled granulocytes enter the bloodstream from the bone marrow at an age of 6 days and survive in the circulation for about 9 days. By the same technique two groups of labeled lymphocytes were differentiated—one with a mean age of less than 10 days and the majority with a mean age of about 100 to 200 days. It has been shown that sufficient lymphocytes enter the bloodstream through the thoracic duct to replace those circulating in the peripheral blood several times.[196] When lymphocytes in dogs were labeled by means of [32]P, specific activity reached a peak on the fourth day. These findings were consistent with a short maturation time for the lymphocyte and a short intravascular time.[196]

The life-span of eosinophils and basophils is approximately 8 to 12 days.[178] The life-span of 3 days or less has been given for the granulocyte series in patients with granulocytic leukemia[179] and about 30 days for the lymphocytes in patients with chronic lymphocytic leukemia,[177] both obtained by radioactive phosphorus labeling of the white blood cells with subsequent DNA extraction. In persons recovering from acute toxic leukopenia, approximately 14 days may be required for maturation of primitive myeloblasts to the four- or five-lobed polymorphonuclear neutrophil.[65] The Pelger-Huët anomaly of the granulocytic leukocytes (poor segmentation and condensation of the nuclear chromatin, described later in this chapter) has been employed as a biologic tag to determine the survival time of the transfused neutrophils in the peripheral blood.[213] Most of the cells disappeared within 6 to 8 hours, and none were found after 49½ hours. These results are comparable to those in a series[150] in which 80 to 85% of the leukemic leukocytes tagged in vivo with a radioactive chromium were removed from the circulation within 24 hours. Some cells persisted for as long as 5 days.

*Leukoagglutinins.* In persons with leukopenic syndromes, substances acting upon leukocytes have been detected which are comparable to the antibodies present in the serum of patients with thrombocytopenia and acquired hemolytic anemias. In the serum from a patient with agranulocytic angina, Moeschlin and Wagner[165] demonstrated leukocyte-destroying factors which were active in vivo and in vitro. Drugs such as Pyramidon combine with a protein in the serum, forming an antigen which causes sensitization and antibody formation. The antibody becomes attached to the leukocytes which are agglutinated and destroyed when they come in contact with the antigen.[166] The serum of such a patient not only agglutinates normal human leukocytes in vitro but also produces a rapid fall of the white blood count when it is injected into a normal person. The destruction of agglutinated leukocytes occurs in vivo, probably in the lung capillaries.[3]

Agglutination and destruction of circulating leukocytes have a wide application. These processes have also been assumed to occur in persons with infection such as primary atypical pneumonia, cyclic agranulocytosis, and pancytopenic states and in newborn infants with transitory granulocytopenia.[138] In a family with multiple cases of neonatal neutropenia, one ending fatally, a potent leukoagglutinin was found in the maternal serum which agglutinated leukocytes obtained from the father and all three children, but failed to agglutinate the mother's own cells.[132] Two cases of neonatal leukopenia due to leukoagglutinins have been reported.[103] The isoimmunization in the mother had probably been due to previous pregnancies and blood transfusions. A similar family with three cases of neonatal neutropenia has also been reported.[33] During the mother's last pregnancy, leukocyte antibody titers were found to be rising. At delivery the titer was 1:512, when leukolysins and passive transfer of antibody to the fetus in the cord blood were also demonstrated. The original sensitization was attributed to prior transfusion with the husband's whole fresh blood. The difficulty of always correlating the presence of agglutinins with neutropenia is the observation by Payne and co-workers[191] that transplacental passage of leukocyte agglutinins from sensitized mothers to newborn infants did not induce significant leukopenia or neutropenia.[191] Bone marrow exhaustion follows peripheral depletion of injured or agglutinated granulocytes.

Leukocyte agglutinins may be detected by adding serum of an affected person to a suspension of leukocytes as completely free of red cells and platelets as possible.[62] The leukoagglutinin may manifest itself as an isoantibody, an autoantibody, or an allergic antibody in the patient with drug hypersensitivity. Since the serum substance destroys the patient's own leukocytes, an autoantibody analogous to the antibody against the red cells in patients with acquired hemolytic anemia appears to be involved. An electrophoretic method that correlates with the leukoagglutinin technique has been described for the detection of leukocyte antibody.[77] Fetal-maternal leukocyte incompatibility and the development of leukoagglutinins have been incriminated in infants with transfusion reactions and neonatal agranulocytosis. In one series 18% of the 406 gravid women developed leukoagglutinins during pregnancy.[189] With increasing parity, the proportion of women immunized did not differ significantly. The possibility that frequent transfusions of blood may lead to the development of leukocyte antibodies and their involvement in febrile transfusion reactions has been reported.[35,190]

A variety of methods is now available for the study of leukocyte and platelet antibodies.[239] They consist of macroscopic agglutination methods, a modified Coombs-type platelet antibody test, including the antiglobulin consumption test,[61] and quantitative micromethods, including the use of activated antigens.

Terasaki and associates[234] reported lymphocytotoxic antibodies in serum specimens from patients with systemic lupus erythematosus and rheumatoid arthritis. These cytotoxic antibodies characteristically reacted with a temperature optimum of 15° C. as was found earlier with serums from patients with infectious mononucleosis, rubella, and rubeola. The lymphotoxin found in systemic lupus was cytotoxic to autologous lymphocytes in twenty-four of thirty-two specimens tested. It is possible that viruses may cause alterations in the cell membrane causing lymphocytes to form antibodies against the slightly altered antigens. These antibodies may then cross-react with normal antigens present in the lymphocytes.

## TYPES OF WHITE CELLS

The leukocytes present in the normal blood comprise three main groups: the granulocytic or myeloid series, the lymphocytes, and the monocytes. The bone marrow and lymph nodes give rise to granulocytes and lymphocytes, respectively. Monocytes originate from a reticular cell of the reticuloendothelial tissues present principally in the lymph nodes and spleen and to some extent in the bone marrow and other organs. The individual types of white cells differ from one another in structure and function.

### Granulocytic or myeloid series

For practical purposes, development of leukocytes may be regarded as proceeding in definitive lines: the myeloblast gives rise to myelocytes and granulocytes, the lymphoblast to lymphocytes, and monoblasts to monocytes. It has already been pointed out that primitive cells of both red and white cell series possess similar structural and staining characteristics and, in their maturation, reveal many common features. The immature forms of all white cells (the myeloblast, lymphoblast, and monoblast) are not found in the peripheral blood of the normal person, but their differentiation assumes importance in persons with leukemia in whom they infiltrate both bone marrow and blood.

*Granulopoiesis—maturation compartments.* The concept of the total picture of granulopoiesis embraces a physiologic steady state, with cells originating primarily in the bone marrow and eventually entering the blood. It has been described[85] as comprising three phases: the first relates to the turnover of granulocytes in the blood; the second concerns the granulocytes delivered from the marrow reserve and maturation compartment; and the third phase concerns the cells originating in the proliferative compartment of the marrow. The blood granulocyte pool comprises two subunits: the circulating granulocyte pool and the marginal granulocyte pool. The marginal pool consists of cells adhering or marginated along the capillary and venous beds and approximates in numbers the freely circulating granulocytes. The marginated pool may also be sequestered in various organ capillaries. The circulating and marginal beds are in continuous interchange. From the circulation, the neutrophilic granulocytes reach the tissues, where their defensive function is performed. In the bone marrow granulopoiesis may be subdivided into four stages: the stem cell compartment in which myeloblasts are formed; the proliferating cell compartment where the myeloblasts, promyelocytes, and most of the myelocytes undergo mitosis; the maturation or differentiating compartment where myelocytes and metamyelocytes mature; and the reserve or storage compartment, containing a mass of mature granulocytes, which provides an available supply of cells for the peripheral blood when needed. This compartment is composed of fully segmented, mature neutrophilic leukocytes which usually account for approximately one-third of the granulocyte population.

To summarize, the renewal of granulocytes requires active proliferation within a stem cell pool, sequential movements from this pool into the proliferating pool, then the maturation pool, and, finally, movement into the peripheral blood.[47,49] Leukokinetics (dynamics of leukocyte production)[10] refers to movement of granulocytes from their mitotic or proliferative pool, and, in sequence, through the maturation, storage, marginal, and circulating granulocyte pools. Following administration of H³-thymidine to patients with a variety of hemopoietic conditions, the emergence and pattern of labeling of neutrophilic granulocytes may be studied in peripheral blood leukocytic concentrates. The emergence time of neutrophilic segmented granulocytes (time from H³-thymidine injection to the first appearance of labeled segmented forms in the peripheral blood) was found to vary in steady state equilibrium from 96 to 144 hours.[89]

Using appropriate label (diisopropylfluorophosphate, DF³²P) to tag granulocytes in vitro and return them to the donor, it is observed that one-half of the labeled cells are removed in 6.6 hours. The average time granulocytes spend in the circulation is 9 hours. The turnover rate in the various pools (mitotic, maturation, and storage) of the bone marrow ranges from 159 to 256 hours. The life-span of granulocytes up to their entrance into the tissues is estimated as 6½ to 11 days.[149]

The mean half-time disappearance of in vivo–labeled granulocytes from the circulation is 7.2 hours in contrast to the in vitro value of 6.7 hours.[41] The mean time required for myelocytes to divide, mature, and appear in the blood is 11.4 days. The mean generation time of the myelocytes is estimated to be not more than 2.9 days. It was demonstrated by in vivo studies that DF³²P-labeled cells move directly from the total blood granulocyte pool to inflammatory exudates, without dilution by unlabeled bone marrow or tissue granulocytes. There is as yet no experimental evidence to indicate that cells pass from the blood to the bone marrow or return from the tissues to the blood.

The granulocyte reserves of the bone marrow may be estimated by the intravenous administration of endotoxin[146,235] (purified lipopolysaccharide extract from *Salmonella abortus equi*). Endotoxin acts on hematopoietic tissues to stimulate an initial leukopenia followed by a leukocytosis. The ability of endotoxin to produce agranulocytosis involves the release of mature granulocytes, primarily from the marrow granulocyte reserves. Endotoxin affects the hematopoietic system by causing a shift of circulating granulocytes into the marginated pool and an influx of cells from the bone marrow into the blood.[198] A significant increase in circulating granulocytes was observed in all hematologically normal children. Poor to absent granulocytic responses were seen in children with aplastic anemia and acute leukemia.[235]

*Myeloblast—differentiation from lymphoblast.* In the patient with the common form of acute leukemia differentiation is usually directed toward distinguishing between the myeloblast and the lymphoblast. Morphologic characterization, however, frequently does not permit definite classification into either category. Myeloblasts refer to any cell of the granulocytic series having fine chromatin structure and no specific granules. Usually, nucleoli are visible. In patients with some forms of acute leukemia in whom sufficient numbers of promyelocytes justify the classification of the early forms of myeloblasts, smaller primitive cells are found which are designated as micromyeloblasts. The latter seldom contain nucleoli, but they can be distinguished from lymphocytes by their finely meshed chromatin. Red-staining, bar-shaped structures known as Auer bodies are found in the cytoplasm of monocytes, myelocytes, and myeloblasts but not in the cytoplasm of lymphoblasts. When the chromatin is more reticular and particularly when some folding of the nucleus is apparent, the cell is recognized as a myelomonoblast.[29]

Lymphoblasts may have a more sharply defined nuclear membrane, a coarser chromatin network, and a smaller number of nucleoli than myeloblasts have, but these features are not always detectable. The associated presence of substantial numbers of younger lymphocytes (prolymphocytes) and mature lymphocytes or promyelocytes and later myelocytes suggests a more definitive classification of the predominating immature cells as either lymphoblasts or myeloblasts. Both types of blast cells possess certain common fundamental diagnostic features. They are usually round, large (15 to 20$\mu$ in diameter), and uniform in size. The narrow zone of the cytoplasm is basophilic and frequently vacuolated, and the nuclear pattern is distinctive. Instead of masses of dense basichromatin, such as are found in the mature cells, the chromatin stains lightly and is finely granular and stippled or sievelike and shows the presence of nucleoli. In the absence of cytologic differences the primordial cell is usually classified as a stem cell.

The morphologic differences between the myeloblast and lymphoblast, when stained by Wright's method, are listed in Table 25.[84] In

Table 25. Morphologic differences between the myeloblast and lymphoblast

|  | Myeloblast | Lymphoblast |
|---|---|---|
| Cytoplasm | Abundant | Scanty |
| Nuclear membrane | Smooth and thin | Dense |
| Chromatin | Fine network; finely divided particles | Coarse and some aggregation |
| Nucleoli | 2 to 5 | 1 to 2 |
| Nucleolar membrane | Indefinite | Distinct |
| Mitochondria (supravital staining) | Fine; spherical; scattered diffusely in cytoplasm | Larger, oval, thicker than myeloblast; frequently clustered about nucleus or scattered through cytoplasm |

acute leukemia of childhood the predominate blast cells usually favor the designation of lymphoblasts. Monoblasts are difficult to distinguish from myeloblasts and their diagnosis depends upon the presence of the more mature monocytes resembling them in the abundant granular gray-blue cytoplasm and in the characteristic folded and indented nucleus.

In differentiating the myeloblast, promyelocyte, and metamyelocyte the degree of DNA synthesis may be determined by autoradiographic techniques utilizing tritiated thymidine to label DNA. Maximal DNA synthesis occurs in the myeloblasts, less in the promyelocytes, and least in the myelocytes. The metamyelocyte does not synthesize DNA, and mitoses are not seen. Hence, the metamyelocyte is a nondividing cell.[49]

**Promyelocytes (progranulocytes) and myelocytes.** Promyelocytes are the same size or larger than myeloblasts. A nomenclature committee sponsored by the American Society of Clinical Pathologists and the American Medical Association[87] recommended the term progranulocyte for cells of the granulocytic series which have a nuclear structure too coarse for that of a blast cell and which have not developed discernible specific granules. This terminology has not been followed in the present text because it is difficult to identify this cell, and because in the bulk of descriptions the cell more mature than the myeloblast is the promyelocyte which does contain granules. The cytoplasm is deeply basophilic and may be abundant or confined to a narrow margin around the nucleus. The nuclei are round, the chromatin is coarser, and the nucleoli are not so numerous or so sharply demarcated as those in the myeloblast. In contrast to the myeloblast, which is devoid of granules, promyelocytes and myelocytes are granular. In the promyelocyte the granules are relatively few (the earliest forms have no more than ten granules), stain deep red to dark blue, and increase in number as the cell matures. A few granules overlie the nucleus.

The shift from promyelocyte to myelocyte is a gradual one and often difficult to separate into sharply defined categories. According to Sabin's classification, promyelocytes contain ten granules in early stages and a moderate number in a later stage, but the maximal numbers are not present until the myelocyte stage is reached. Furthermore, the granules in the promyelocyte cannot be differentiated into neutrophils, eosinophils, or basophils. Starting with the promyelocyte and continuing to the most mature granulocytes, the granules are peroxidase-positive and serve as an important feature in differentiating the granulocyte from the myeloblast.

Myelocytes are about the same size or smaller than the promyelocyte. The nuclei, which stain reddish purple, are large, round, oval, flattened on one side, or somewhat kidney shaped and are eccentrically placed. Nucleoli are indistinct and less numerous than those in the more primitive cells. Within the reddish purple cytoplasm are numerous dark granules which are scattered throughout and also cover the nucleus. As the myelocytes mature, the granules assume a definitive neutrophilic, eosinophilic, and basophilic character. Each of these cells in turn becomes a progenitor of the respective fully mature granulocytes.

Myelocytes frequently appear in the circulating blood of infants and young children in response to severe infection and hemolytic anemias marked by leukocytosis. Because of the more active response of the bone marrow in younger persons, the presence of small numbers of late myelocytes usually does not have the same connotation that it has in older persons. Occasionally, however, the leukocytosis and outpouring of young cells in children in response to infections may be sufficiently extreme to constitute a leukemoid reaction.

***Metamyelocyte or juvenile form.*** Metamyelocytes are smaller than the myelocyte, and the nucleus is oval and horseshoe shaped in older forms. The chromatin strands are coarse but not so deeply stained as those in more mature cells. The nuclear membrane is sharply defined as is that in the polymorphonuclear cell, and nucleoli are not observed. The cytoplasm is less basophilic than that in the myelocyte, and an eosinophilic cast predominates. The granules are smaller, stain less deeply, and are clearly differentiated as neutophilic, eosinophilic, and basophilic. Ameboid motion initially observed in the late myelocytes is definitely established in the metamyelocyte and characterizes the more mature cells to follow. The cytoplasm and nucleus may not develop evenly so that precise classification as to late myelocyte and metamyelocyte is not always possible.

***Polymorphonuclear granulocytes.*** The mature granulocytes are described as polymorphonuclear cells because of the lobulation of the nucleus and are further classified as neutrophils, eosinophils, and basophils according to their reaction with the ordinary Romanowsky stains.

***Neutrophils.*** The polymorphonuclear neutrophil measures 9 to $12\mu$, with an average diameter of $10\mu$. The cytoplasm is faintly pink, and minute granules which fill the cell stain pink or violet. The nucleus consists of coarsely condensed chromatin strands which stain deep purple.

The nucleus is of two types—nonsegmented and segmented, according to the absence or presence of lobulation. Segmented neutrophils, which normally number 60 to 65% of the white blood cells, are mature cells in which the nucleus consists of two to five lobes connected by a thin strand of chromatin. The nonsegmented cells number 4 to 5% of the total number of white cells and are variously designated as staff or stab cells. They are slightly smaller than metamyelocytes, in which the nucleus fails to segment presumably due to toxic or other influences. Irregular condensation occurs in the nucleus of these cells, with a pyknotic area at each end. Constriction of the nucleus in the middle or in other areas leads to odd-shaped segmented forms. In the cells of persons with some infections the nucleus is short, narrow, bent on itself, and deeply stained. Granulation in these cells is usually neutrophilic but may be eosinophilic or basophilic.

An inherited anomaly of leukocytes characterized by isolated giant neutrophils with multilobed nuclei has been described.[63] Several members of this family possessed these cells, which measured $16.9\mu$, on the average, compared with the normal of $12.7\mu$. No impairment of health resulted from this anomaly.

A family has been reported in whom the neutrophilic nuclei showed constitutional hypersegmentation.[241] Of twenty-one subjects, thirteen displayed hypersegmentation. This type of hypersegmentation is inherited as a simple dominant and is permanent. It should be differentiated from the nuclear hypersegmentation pattern in pernicious anemia and folic acid deficiency in which there is normally no hereditary pattern.

"LEFT AND RIGHT SHIFTS" (ARNETH COUNT; COOKE AND SCHILLING COUNT). According to Arneth's theory, the nucleus of the polymorphonuclear cell becomes more segmented with age. The round or oval nucleus of the myelocyte becomes more indented as the cell matures, with increasing segmentation in progressively older cells. As modified by Cooke and Schilling and in accordance with present usage, "a shift to the left" implies the presence in the bloodstream of immature forms consisting of large numbers of band forms. This shift is noted in infections, toxic states, and hemorrhage, with the extent of the shift proportional to the extent of the disturbance. In patients with mongolism without infection there is a shift to the left in lobe count. In younger persons severe infections are often accompanied by the additional presence of myelocytes and metamyelocytes. The blood smear of patients with pernicious anemia, sprue, and megaloblastic anemia of infancy, on the other hand, demonstrate a shift to the right. In these conditions, many of the granulocytes may be abnormally large and show hypersegmentation of their nuclei. Here, too, the lobes may vary in size, and the chroma-

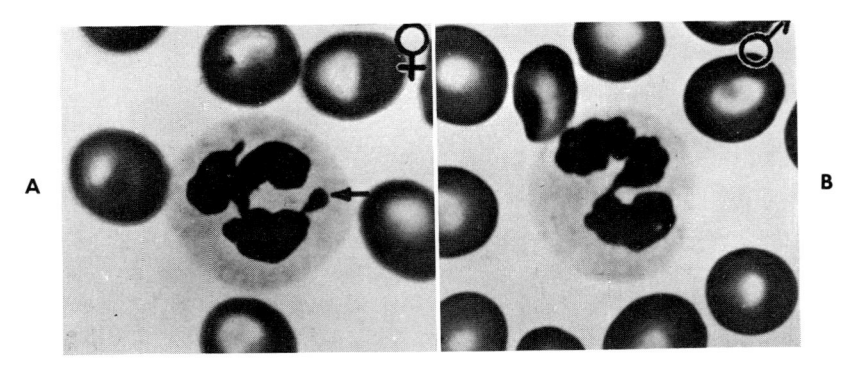

Fig. 58. A, Neutrophil in a blood film from a chromosomal female illustrating the accessory nuclear lobule that is present in an average of 2 to 3% of neutrophils in females. B, A similar accessory nuclear lobule does not occur in neutrophils of chromosomal males. (×1800.) (From Grumback, M. M., and Barr, M. L.: In Pincus, G., editor: Recent progress in hormone research, vol. 14, New York, 1958, Academic Press, Inc.)

tin is not so uniformally homogeneous as in normal cells.

In contrast to the concept of increased nuclear segmentation with age are the observations based on the emergence time and labeling of polymorphonuclear neutrophils following administration of ³H-thymidine.[89] Using this technique, the number of segments of neutrophilic granulocytes was found to be unrelated to cell age. However, band forms were found in the circulation about 24 hours earlier than segmented forms, suggesting that they are younger and perhaps that some are acceptable to the blood while others continue to mature to segmented forms. No distinct difference was found in the maturation and emergence time between the granulocytes with two or more segments.

SEX DIFFERENCE IN NEUTROPHILS. A sex difference in the nuclear structure of the human polymorphonuclear neutrophilic leukocyte has been described.[64] In the female a solitary "drumstick" with a well-defined solid round head, 1.5μ in diameter, is joined by a single fine chromatin strand to one of the main lobes of the nucleus (Fig. 58). These structures are rarely found in the unsegmented forms or precursors. This distinctive nuclear appendage which has been confined to the female has been found in persons of all ages and in blood specimens from the umbilical cord.[233] These appendages are not to be confused with sessile nodules and related structures which are attached to the nucleus of the polymorphonuclear cell in both the male and female.

A small mass, usually adjacent to the nuclear membrane, which stains deeply with hematoxylin, Feulgen reagent, and thionine, is known as the sex chromatin or Barr body.[8] It has been shown to be present in 80 to 90% of the somatic cells of the normal female.

*Eosinophils.* The eosinophil is a polymornuclear granulocyte the same size or a little larger than the neutrophil and possesses a bilobed or band-formed nucleus. The cytoplasmic granules are large, coarse, and spherical, have an affinity for the eosin stain, and take a bright reddish orange or deep red stain. The granules are scattered through the cytoplasm and superimposed on the nucleus. Eosinophils are less motile and more fragile than neutrophils. They represent 1 to 4% of the total number of leukocytes and possess a life-span of 6 days.[79]

Charcot-Leyden crystals are formed in conditions associated with marked eosinophilia. Ayres and Starkey[11] have shown that lowering of the surface tension is necessary for the formation of Charcot-Leyden crystals from eosinophils. They offer evidence that synthetic detergents of the anionic, cationic, and nonionic types result in the rapid and constant formation of Charcot-Leyden crystals from eosinophils. They postulate that Charcot-Leyden crystals are crystalline proteins derived only from the nucleus of the eosinophil. According to them Charcot-Leyden crystals are formed mainly in the sputum of asthmatics and in areas of allergic inflammation containing eosinophils as well as in other conditions in which eosinophils are prominent.

Despite a more potent oxidative response during phagocytosis, eosinophils ingest microorganisms less efficiently and kill bacteria less effectively than do polymorphonuclear leukocytes.[12]

EOSINOPHILIA. Eosinophilia occurs in patients with several well-defined groups of diseases in which there is an increase in eosinophils above 5% or 500 per cubic millimeter. Following is a list of conditions in which eosinophilia occurs.

  Allergic disorders
    Bronchial asthma
    Hay fever
    Urticaria
  Skin diseases
    Eczema
    Psoriasis
    Scabies
    Erythema neonatorum
  Parasitic infections
    Trichinosis
    Ascaris
    *Echinococcus* disease
    Visceral larva migrans
  Pulmonary eosinophilia
    Eosinophilic pneumonitis (Löffler's syndrome)
    Prolonged pulmonary eosinophilia
    Tropical eosinophilia
    Pulmonary eosinophilia with asthma
  Blood disorders
    Eosinophilic leukemia
    Hodgkin's disease
    Recovery phase of acute infectious lymphocytosis
    Postsplenectomy
    Eosinophilic leukemoid reaction
  Irradiation
  Familial eosinophilia
  Miscellaneous infections and disorders
    Scarlet fever
    Chorea
    Drugs and chemicals
    Benzol poisoning
    Camphor, phosphorus, etc.
    Periarteritis nodosa
    Metastatic neoplasms

From the time when it was first demonstrated that foreign materials such as parasitic extracts were chemotactic for eosinophils, the relationship of these cells to diseases of sensitization has been amply confirmed. The number and proportion of eosinophils are greatly increased in patients afflicted with various types of allergy, with parasitic infection, especially by nematodes, and following anaphylactic reactions. The eosinophil is the only cell that is known to respond specifically during states of hypersensitivity, becoming attached to shock tissues.[226] The cell, being phagocytic for foreign substances, is a part of the body defenses.

Intravenous inoculation of *Trichinella* larvae into rats is followed by eosinophilia, with a peak of 6 days. Reinjection of the parasites 20 days later results in an enhanced eosinophil response. Eosinophilia appears to share common features with recognized immune phenomena.[81] The earlier onset and augmented height of the eosinophil response to second larval challenge seems analogous to the increase in number of antibody-forming cells known to characterize the response to a subsequent administration of well-known antigens. This phenomenon may also indicate that the eosinophilia accompanying trichinosis may be an immune phenomenon.

A condition observed in pediatric practice which is associated with eosinophilia is visceral larva migrans. This entity refers to infection with dog and cat ascarids (*Toxocara canis* and *Toxocara catis*, respectively) and should be considered in the differential diagnosis of febrile illnesses associated with eosinophilia. A history of eating dirt or of exposure to dogs and cats in the home in patients with eosinophilia suggests visceral larva migrans associated with *Toxocara* infection. It represents an imperfect adaptation of the parasite to the host so that its life cycle in the latter is not completed. The eggs reach the soil through fecal contamination where within weeks they develop to infective-stage larvae. If ingested by a child, the larvae migrate through the intestinal wall via the vascular system and reach the liver, lungs, brain, eye, and other organs. Instead of completing the migration back to the intestine as in the normal dog or cat host, they either become encysted and are destroyed or continue to migrate through the tissues.[225]

Although liver biopsy may reveal characteristic larvae, the diagnosis should be considered in the absence of this examination in young exposed patients with persistent or marked eosinophilia, recurrent wheezing associated with pulmonary infiltration, hepatomegaly of undetermined nature, ocular disorders of obscure etiology, unexplained central nervous system disturbances, including convulsions, and hyperglobulinemia.[110] In a patient with a similar condition there was an additional finding of a marked and persistent elevation of the heterophil agglutinin titer with antibodies similar to those found in persons with serum sickness.[221] Cases previously described as allergic-hyperergic tissue responses resulting in disseminated visceral lesions[266] probably fit into this category as well.

Moderate eosinophilia with values of about 25% can persist with fluctuations for a period of years in children without any identifiable cause except allergic symptoms. A syndrome of extreme leukocytosis and eosinophilia (up to 84%) has been reported by Bass[17] in which children who were chronically affected had a favorable outcome. When a normal leukocyte count has been restored, a mild eosinophilia may persist. In the light of recent studies it is necessary to eliminate visceral larva migrans infection in patients with chronic eosinophilia.

Pulmonary involvement accompanied by eosinophilia occurs in a number of distinctive syndromes in which this combination exists. Löffler's syndrome, the best known of these, is a benign condition characterized by a patchy migratory infiltration which usually clears within a month. The accompanying eosinophilia reaches its peak in 3 to 4 days and usually disappears in 10 to 15 days. It is generally regarded as a response to an immune reaction taking place largely in the lungs. It has been suggested, however, that infiltrates in patients with Löffler's syndrome are due to the trapping of the eosinophils in the lung and not to an allergic pulmonary reaction.[78] It has been produced by infection with intestinal parasites, plant products, bacteria, and drugs.

Prolonged pulmonary eosinophilia, another syndrome described by Crofton and associates,[48] is to be considered when radiographic shadows and eosinophilia persist for prolonged periods and are more widespread than in patients with Löffler's syndrome. It lasts 2 to 6 months and longer before recovery sets in and is marked by extreme eosinophilia. In many of these patients there is a personal or family history suggestive of an allergic diathesis. Probable etiologic factors include hypersensitivity to drugs and bacterial and parasitic infection.

A young woman afflicted with recurrent respiratory distress, pulmonary infection, and pericarditis had a leukocytosis with an eosinophilia that at one time rose to 96%.[102] Her illness was characterized by cough, fever, sweats, malaise, and arthralgia in association with bilateral pulmonary infiltrations and the marked eosinophilia. Massive eosinophilic pericarditis occurred during the most severe episode. Bone marrow was hyperplastic with eosinophilia and megakaryocytosis. Selective periodic treatment with adrenocorticosteroids was extremely effective.

The term hereditary eosinophilia has been applied to a benign anomaly, probably due to a disordered regulation of eosinophil production.[173] Eosinophilia has been described in several generations of a family with its occurrence in well members. Hereditary eosinophilia is transmitted by an autosomal dominant mode of inheritance and is distinguished from cases of familial eosinophilia secondary to allergy or parasitic infections. The degree of eosinophilia varies among different families and among members of one family. Values of over 50% eosinophils have been noted in many of the families.

Tropical eosinophilia or "eosinophilic lung" occurs in the inhabitants of India and many tropical countries. In persons with this syndrome there is sometimes an initial stage of malaise, fever, coryza, and dry cough, the spleen may be palpable, and eosinophilia is marked. The roentgenogram shows a diffuse mottling throughout both lung fields, although sometimes the lesions are more localized. There may be an allergic background, but more recently it has been ascribed to a mite infection of the upper respiratory tract.

Patients with pulmonary eosinophilia with asthma include those in whom pulmonary infiltrations and eosinophilia are associated with symptoms incidental to chronic or recurrent bronchial asthma.

Patients with eosinophilic leukemia, in contrast to those with other forms of eosinophilia, show a marked relative and absolute increase in the circulating mature eosinophils which also infiltrate the tissues during the course of the disease. Patients with this type of leukemia respond for varying periods to ACTH and the steroid hormones.[69] They usually show no pulmonary changes of the magnitude described in patients with other conditions such as pulmonary eosinophilia, except when an associated pneumonia occurs. Evans and Nesbitt[80] reported on a patient who typifies others in whom the eosinophils showed a progressive immaturity as symptoms become more severe. Terminally, a large proportion of the cells were myeloblasts in both blood and bone marrow. During this period, however, in which the only abnormality is confined to excessive numbers of mature eosinophils, conditions other than leukemia are to be considered.

With the elimination of the major etiologic factors in causation, cases of chronic eosinophilia in which the blood response persists for many years before the blood count eventually returns to normal are still encountered in children with poorly defined allergies. This anomalous type of eosinophilia may occasionally herald serious organic disease.[111] A good prognosis is to be expected in patients with eosinophilia of undetermined origin if there is no associated anemia, leukocytosis, or marked elevation of the sedimentation rate. The cause, even in patients with marked leukocytosis and massive eosinophilia, may be benign.

Three adult patients (21 to 35 years of age) had white counts up to 81,000 per cu. mm., blood eosinophilia up to 98%, generalized cardiomegaly, intractable cardiac failure, renal dysfunction, and a short illness (11 to 26 months).[207] Necropsy showed in two of the patients severe mural endocardial fibrosis with superficial fibrin-platelet thrombi, myocardial scarring, vegetative valvular endocarditis, and eosinophilic hyperplasia of the bone marrow and spleen, without abnormal or leukemic myeloblasts. These features are similar to those documented in patients with Löffler's fibroplastic parietal endocarditis, and in "eosinophilic" leukemia without abnormal myelopoiesis. It was suggested that these two conditions are the same disease.

Magnesium deficiency in both intact and adrenalectomized rats is accompanied by an extremely high blood eosinophilia.[122] Massive infiltration of eosinophils into the lung and other organs has been observed.

EOSINOPENIA. Eosinopenia occurs following stress and has been related to the release of adrenocortical hormones. A prompt decrease occurs in circulating eosinophils in healthy persons following a single injection of adrenocorticotropic hormone. The eosinophilic response must be interpreted as a nonspecific stress reaction of the intact organism. Eosinopenia occurs after administration of ACTH, epinephrine, surgical operations, infections, cardiac failure, and any other conditions of stress.

The fall in the eosinophil count following injections of adrenocorticotropic hormone (ACTH) has become widely used as a test of adrenal function. In the Thorn test,[238] following the preinjection determination of the absolute eosinophil count, 25 mg. of ACTH is given intramuscularly to the child or adult, and the percentage decrease is measured in 4 hours. A reduction of 50% or more in the eosinophil count is presumptive evidence that the cortical tissue has the normal capacity to respond to stimulation. A significant fall in eosinophils, therefore, does not occur in patients with chronic adrenal insufficiency such as Addison's disease.

No such clear-cut results are obtained in the newborn infant. Apparently, dosages ranging from 5 to 10 mg. are necessary to provoke eosinopenic responses beyond the range of spontaneous changes.[260] Farquhar[81] found a normal response in the newborn infant with a decrement of 30% or greater when a 10 mg. dose was injected. On the basis of these observations the presence of physiologic transitory adrenal insufficiency in the newborn period depends upon the standardization of dosage. With adequate dosage, the response of the adrenal cortex is found to be normal in the majority of newborn and premature babies in the first days of life.[260]

*Basophils.* Basophils originate in the bone marrow and are regular constituents of the peripheral blood. The basophilic leukocytes contain two very significant compounds—heparin and histamine. These two agents are presumably released when the cell undergoes degranulation to participate in anaphylactic and lipemia-clearing reactions.[220] These cells are distinguished by the large, round, coarse, bluish black, and azurophilic granules which obscure the nucleus by their number. These granules are peroxidase negative and are situated above, below, and at each side of the relatively lightly staining nucleus. The nucleus is round, kidney shaped, and slightly lobulated. The cytoplasm stains faint pink to lilac. The basophil is motile and somewhat smaller than the mature neutrophil. The basophils number 0 to 0.5% in children and adults. All stages of leukocytic differentiation are demonstrable in bone marrow for basophilic white blood cells. They are increased in patients with chronic myeloid leukemia, polycythemia vera, chronic hemolytic anemia, Hodgkin's disease, smallpox, chickenpox, some cases of cirrhosis of the liver, after radiation, and following splenectomy. In patients with lobar pneumonia, acute rheumatic fever, or anaphylactoid purpura, the number of circulating basophils has been found to be low in the acute stage and high during recovery.[162]

*Tissue mast cells (tissue basophils).* The tissue mast cell is also a granular basophil which shows little motility as compared with the active basophils. The separation of the tissue mast cells from the circulating basophils has been a subject of controversy.[183,226] Both have in common metachromasia of the granules. The cytoplasm of the mast cells is filled with granules that stain well with methylene blue, Wright-Giemsa stain, or toluidine blue (1% toluidine blue in methyl alcohol). Mast cells are found in groups about blood vessels and in the connective tissue where they originate.

Tissue mast cells, however, can be differentiated from blood basophils and are not interchangeable with them. Tissue mast cells do not possess myeloid precursors as do basophilic leukocytes. Functionally, the two cells may have much in common in the production of several biologically active substances, especially in the associated content of heparin and histamine in their granules.[206] Serotonin (5-hydroxytryptamine) has also been isolated from the tissue mast cells. There is suggestive evidence that serotonin and histamine act in conjunction to cause capillary permeability, hyperemia, and edema which constitute the vascular response to acute inflammation.[214]

Morphologically, tissue mast cells can be differentiated from basophilic leukocytes. The former possesses a normal vesicular nucleus which is rarely indented, but the cytoplasmic contours vary widely, being round, irregularly oval, spindle, or star shaped. The bluish cytoplasm may be hidden because of the heavily packed granules. These do not overlie the nucleus as they do in the basophil. By contrast the blood basophils usually have a small cell body with a polymorphic or lobulated nucleus typical of leukocytes, and the granules tend to be irregularly distributed.[248] Accumulations of mast cells are observed in both the macular and papular type of urticaria pigmentosa, a dermatologic disorder occurring principally in childhood.

## *Lymphocytes*

Lymphocytes originate from lymphocytic tissue in many parts of the body, mainly from the lymph nodes, spleen, bone marrow, tonsils, thymus, Peyer's patches of the gastrointestinal tract, and liver. Considerable lymphocyte formation takes place in Peyer's patches. Lymphocytes enter the blood stream in two ways—indirectly through the thoracic duct, right lymph duct, or other lymphatic-venous communications, or directly through the walls of blood capillaries in lymphoid tissue. They are actively motile cells whose function in antibody formation has already been discussed. They are classified into large and small cell types, with the latter predominating. Large and intermediate forms of lymphocytes are assumed to be younger and less mature than small lymphocytes, but this premise is yet to be established.

Classically, lymphocytes have been defined as small round cells in the blood, lymph, lymphoid organs, and body fluids ranging in size from 5 to 17$\mu$. They represent a highly mobile population of cells widely distributed in the body which exhibit numerous functions vital to the mammalian organism. These small round cells may represent several lines of differentiation with highly different specialized functions.

Currently the body's immune system is conceived of as having two distinct cell populations arising from a common stem cell. One population is differentiated in the thymus and the other population is differentiated in a site not yet identified in man.[95,208] In the so-called thymus-dependent system, the stem cell comes under the influence of a microchemical environment in the thymus, inducing it to differentiate along a specific pathway—that of the small lymphocyte. The thymus-independent cells are responsible for the secretion of the immunoglobulins and the production of antibody. Clinically they defend the body against bacterial infection. The thymus-differentiated cells are responsible for delayed hypersensitivity, graft rejection, graft-versus-host reaction, and defense against viral and fungal infection. These cell-mediated immune responses are those reactions which may be transferred by lymphoid cells but not by serum.[100] Based on neonatal thymectomy experiments, the mediating cells are derived from a thymus-dependent population of lymphoid cells. Certain populations of lymphocytes represent a bulwark of defense against many infections.

The small mature lymphocytes found in the peripheral blood are of two types, though morphologically indistinguishable. A small population has a life-span of 3 to 4 days, while the larger proportion has a long life-span of 100 to 120 days.[159] There is evidence that many of the small lymphocytes which enter the blood from the thoracic duct have a long life-span. They are depleted by thymectomy and can be shown in labelling experiments to have been derived from the thymus. They are immunologically competent cells which can initiate immune reactions. According to Good,[96] the great majority of circulating lymphocytes and the bulk of the lymphocytes of the "recirculating readily mobilizable pool of lymphocytes do not appear to be involved in the synthesis of presently known immunoglobulins, but instead represent a pool of cells dependent upon the thymus for differentiation and development."

In the proposed classification of primary immunologic deficiencies, several syndromes that may be confused with each other are worthy of mention.[219]

1. Infantile sex-linked agammaglobulinemia (Bruton's disease)
2. Immune deficiency with thrombopenia and eczema (Wiskott-Aldrich syndrome)
3. Ataxia-telangiectasia
4. Autosomal recessive alymphocytic agammaglobulinemia (Swiss type agammaglobulinemia)
5. Thymic aplasia (DiGeorge's syndrome)

Recent investigations suggest that the thymus serves as the principal source of the small lymphocyte population of the blood, spleen, and lymph nodes.[6,38,141] According to this hypothesis, lymphoid elements of the thymus migrate early in life to seed other lymphopoietic organs. A second population of small lymphocytes may be unrelated in function to the thymus lymphocytes. According to a prevailing concept, the lymphocytes derived from the thymus form clones of immunologically competent cells—the so-called immunocytes.* The small lymphocyte is the most common lymphoid cell and can initiate an immunologic reaction, when given the appropriate stimulus. Alymphocytosis is based on a congenital atrophy or dysfunction of the thymus. In a case of alymphocytosis and agammaglobulinemia the thymus weighed less than 1 gram.[209]

*Small lymphocytes.* Small lymphocytes vary in size from 6 to 10μ in diameter, usually about the same size as red blood cells. They contain a well-defined, round, oval, or indented nucleus, with closely packed aggregates of chromatin which stains deep purple. The nucleus fills almost the entire cell with the periphery sharply defined and more heavily stained. The cells have a narrow rim of bluish cytoplasm which is often frayed and stains clear pale blue. Although the cytoplasm is usually devoid of granules in well-stained preparations, some of the cells contain a few distinct reddish purple or azurophilic granules of medium size. In thick smears the lymphocytes are spindle shaped with pointed projections of cytoplasm at opposite poles of the cell. This feature has no pathologic implications.

*Phytohemagglutinin.* Phytohemagglutinin (PHA), an extract of the red kidney bean, was originally employed for its erythrocyte-agglutinating ability in obtaining leukocytes from whole blood. Nowell[174] demonstrated that PHA initiates the transformation of lymphocytes from normal peripheral blood into large primitive basophilic "blast" cells capable of dividing. It has been postulated that this transformation may be the result of its action as an antigen, indicating the lymphocyte response to antibody production.[76] It is of interest that lymphocytes from chronic lymphatic leukemia give rise to few "blasts" when stimulated in tissue culture with PHA, whereas in acute leukemia the blast production is normal.[9] The transformation of lymphocytes into "blasts" was also depressed when blood was cultured from patients who had been irradiated.[155] There has been increasing evidence that the small lymphocytes under stimulation of phytohemagglutinins and other substances are able to proliferate and produce mitosis. Ribas-Mondo[205] has investigated the true sequence of DNA synthesis in the interphase nuclei of the proliferating lymphocytes. Utilizing phytohemagglutinin and autoradiographic techniques, he was able to demonstrate three patterns of DNA replication in the interphase nuclei of short term cultures.[205] Initially there was a light, homogeneous labelling in the whole nucleus and no labelling over the nucleolus. This phase was followed by heavy labelling equally distributed over the whole nucleus and nucleoli, and finally by labelling over the nucleoli and moderate labelling at the periphery of the nucleus. These three patterns of labelling appear consecutively during the process of DNA synthesis. Thus the nuclear and nucleolar associated chromatin replicates during the late stage of DNA synthesis. Recent studies suggest that the small lymphocyte cannot be considered as the final stage of maturation. Rather, it is regarded as a resting cell with the potential for undergoing enlargement,

---

*See references 23, 55, 56, 99, 158.

in which following appropriate stimulation both DNA replication and RNA synthesis occur. Cooper and Rubin[46] demonstrated that after exposure to phytohemagglutinin the earliest change in RNA lymphocyte metabolism was a decrease in total RNA. This was followed after 1 hour by a progressive increase in the rate of RNA synthesis, which continued for 24 hours. The early loss cannot be completely explained, but may be due to the primary effect of PHA treatment which results in the degradation of preexisting RNA.

Many studies have demonstrated the presence in the bone marrow of a pluripotent stem cell which is morphologically indistinguishable from the lymphocyte. With the possibility of the presence of lymphocytes which could have pluripotency in the marrow of patients with aplastic anemia, Humble[121] attempted a trial of PHA in humans with this disease. Initial reports showed a response in four patients in whom marrow hypoplasia was secondary to known causes. Later studies seem to indicate that patients with "idiopathic aplastic anemia" are less likely to respond to PHA therapy if at all. Hayes and Spurr[107] suggest that further studies are needed before definitive conclusions can be drawn as to the true value of this agent.

*Large lymphocytes.* Large lymphocytes vary from 10 to 15μ in size. The nucleus is larger than that in the small lymphocyte; it is round, slightly indented, and thickened at the margins, and the chromatin material is paler and not so markedly condensed as in the small lymphocyte. The cytoplasm is more abundant than in the small lymphocyte, frequently contains azurophilic granules, and the edges are frequently scalloped and stain clear light blue. A perinuclear clear zone is a differentiating feature.

*Young lymphocytes (prolymphocytes).* Prolymphocytes are occasionally found in normal blood and more frequently in the blood of children, especially those with chronic upper respiratory infections with associated tonsillar and cervical node enlargement. The cell is the same size as the large lymphocyte or is intermediate between the large cell and the small cell. The nucleus is less compact, with light spaces between the chromatin threads. The most important feature is the deep blue basophilic staining of the cytoplasm which is homogeneous and agranular.

During the first months of life small numbers of lymphocytes that resemble the abnormal cells found in patients with infectious mononucleosis are occasionally observed in the blood smears from normal infants. These cells, however, bear no relationship to this disease or to any other related condition. Scattered vacuoles may be found normally in the rim of deeply staining blue cytoplasm. These cells are to be differentiated from the heavily vacuolated cells, producing a foamy appearance characterizing the lymphocytes of infectious mononucleosis.

Atypical lymphocytes are not specifically diagnostic but occur in a wide variety of diseases, namely of suspected viral etiology, such as infectious mononucleosis, hepatitis, the posttransfusion syndrome, and drug sensitivities.[262]

**Lymphoblasts.** Lymphoblasts, from which the lymphocyte is derived, are characterized by a large round or oval nucleus, staining reddish purple with fine granular chromatin which is slightly coarser than that found in the nucleus of the myeloblast. One or two nucleoli are present in the lymphoblast, the nuclear membrane is well defined, and the cytoplasm is usually clear blue or deeply basophilic and nongranular.

### Monocytes

Monocytes, measuring from 13 to 20μ, are larger than most cells found in the peripheral blood. They represent 5 to 10% of the total circulating white blood cells. The monocyte is a motile cell with slow ameboid motion, in contrast to the more active neutrophil. The cytoplasm is abundant in relation to the nucleus and stains darker than the pink cytoplasm of neutrophils. The pseudopods are blunt. The cytoplasm is a dull gray, muddy blue color and is filled with large numbers of evenly spread fine, lilac or reddish blue granules, interspersed among which are a lesser number of unevenly distributed azurophilic granules and occasional vacuoles. The granules are peroxidase positive but in much lesser numbers and finer than those in the granulocytes. The gray-blue cytoplasm of the monocyte contrasts with the clear light blue of the lymphocyte.

The nucleus is somewhat eccentric and possesses a skeinlike or lacy structure which stains lighter than that of the lymphocyte or metamyelocyte. It has a loosely arranged chromatin with light spaces and grooves, in contrast to the clumped chromatin of the lymphocyte. The nucleus is indented, multilobulated, and convoluted and often presents a folded appearance. The nuclear folds with the heavier staining at their margins are characteristic of the monocyte. The monocyte phagocytoses red cells, cellular fragments, and the incompletely lysed nuclei of other cells as occurs in the formation of the tart cell.

The morphological events of vacuolization and degranulation appear to be similar for the polymorphonuclear and mononuclear phagocytes. The monocyte has the capacity for continued synthesis of new granules, the capacity to rid itself of bacterial products by exocytosis, and the ability to survive a phagocytic act, in contrast to the neutrophil, which usually dies.

The blood monocytes of mammals are phagocytic cells which are related to the phagocytic tissue macrophages of the reticuloendothelial system.[43] There is evidence that the mononuclear cells isolated from the peripheral blood or peritoneal cavity of mammals can differentiate into large cells resembling tissue macrophages. Mononuclear phagocytes take a variety of forms and physiologic properties such as sticking to glass, membrane ruffling, ingestion of fluid droplets (pinocytosis), or particles (phagocytosis) from the environment.[82] Several phases of these cells have been delineated in their life history: the immature forms arise from stem cells in the bone marrow; young adult forms (monocytes) then enter the blood and a short time later migrate into tissues; the tissue forms then undergo maturation to become macrophages.

In a schematic representation there are three compartments in which mononuclear phagocytes reside: in the bone marrow compartment, promonocytes proliferate and give rise to monocytes; in the peripheral blood compartment monocytes are transported from bone marrow to tissues; and in the tissue compartment mononuculear phagocytes become phagocytic macrophages.

Monocytes and fixed phagocytes of the reticuloendothelial system[222] play an important role in host susceptibility to and defense against viral pathogens. Macrophages remove antibody-neutralized virus from the circulation and degrade the antibody-virus complexes to low molecular weight metabolites. When viral replication in macrophages does occur, other mechanisms of host defense are summoned to combat the progress of the infection.

*Young monocyte (promonocyte).* Although the nucleus of the mature monocyte may be round, it is more likely to be so in the young monocyte. The cell is somewhat larger, and the cytoplasm is perhaps less granular and grayer than that in the older cell. The features are intermediate between those of the mature cell and the monoblasts.

*Monoblasts.* Monoblasts are difficult to differentiate from the corresponding myeloblasts and promyelocytes. The cells, possessing an irregular cell outline due to the presence of blunt pseudopodia, are nonmotile. The cytoplasm is deeply basophilic with a grayish blue cast, differing in this way from the blasts of other cell series. The cytoplasm contains dust-like reddish blue granules and vacuoles. The nucleus is large and round, often kidney shaped, horseshoe shaped, or convoluted like the mature cell. The chromatin is fine and lacy and stains lighter than that in the mature monocyte. Nucleoli may or may not be present. The peroxidase reaction is negative or poorly defined. The presence of monocytes and promonocytes in the same smear facilitates the diagnosis of the primitive monoblasts.

The Naegeli and Schilling types of acute monocytic leukemia[249] are described. In the Naegeli variety the myeloblast is regarded as the precursor of the monocyte, so that the leukemia is myelomonocytic. The peripheral blood shows a predominance of monocytes in various stages of maturity in association with myeloblasts and young myelocytes. Many of the monocytic precursors may be difficult to distinguish from myelocytes. In the Naegeli type the monocytic cell also has a markedly distorted nucleus with a polymorphous shape, the entire cell is extremely large, and the cytoplasm which is abundant is filled with fine purplish red granules smaller than the larger azure granules of the myelocytes. Scattered in the cytoplasm are small numbers of azure granules similar to those observed in the myelocyte.

The Schilling type is a true monocytic leukemia in which the reticuloendothelial cells have been transformed into monocytes. In this type the cells range from mature monocytes to monoblasts with only an occasional myelocyte. Many of the primordial cells are difficult to differentiate from lymphoblasts or myeloblasts, but the majority possess the characteristics of monoblasts. In some of these cells and particularly in the promonocytes, the nucleus is semitransparent, lacy, and folded on itself, and the deeper underlying folds are clearly visible. Promyelocytes and monocytes show a variable reaction with the peroxidase stain, some negative and others weakly positive. The Schilling type is often regarded as a variant of leukemic reticuloendotheliosis. It is the less common of the two types of monocytic leukemia.

*Monocytosis.* Monocytosis occurs in the recovery phase of acute infection, during the resolution process of pneumonia, in the acute phase of rheumatic fever, in active tuberculosis, in Boeck's sarcoidosis, in Hodgkin's disease, in protozoal infections such as malaria, in the recovery phase of agranulocytosis, and in disorders of lipid metabolism. A moderate increase in young monocytes may accompany the outpouring of the abnormal lymphocytes which characterize the blood picture in infectious mononucleosis. Increased numbers of monocytes often occur in children with mesenteric adenitis accompanying upper respiratory infections in contrast to the polymorphonuclear leukocytosis observed in those with appendicitis.

Cunningham and co-workers[52] demonstrated that the major effect of the tubercle bacillus was on the monocyte of the connective tissues and blood. The epithelioid cell of the tubercle has been proved to be an altered phase in the life cycle of the monocyte. According to this view, the lipoids of the tubercle bacillus are solely responsible for the monocyte-epithelioid proliferation and differentiation in patients with tuberculosis.[52,67] Whereas the tubercle bacillus grows and multiplies within the monocyte, lymphocytes are intimately connected with limiting the spread of the infection. In patients with tuberculosis the ratio of monocytes to lymphocytes in absolute numbers has been used to express the extent of invasion as compared to the degree of resistance. An increase in monocytes with an increase of the ratio of monocytes to lymphocytes indicates a serious prognostic sign; a lowering of the ratio with an increase in lymphocytes indicates a favorable sign.[223]

Others have observed that the changes in the monocyte-lymphocyte ratio are caused more often by a consistent decrease in lymphocytes during active disease and increase during healing than by the more irregular fluctuations of the monocytes. According to this view, a sounder interpretation of the clinical status of the tuberculosis process can be made by evaluating each cell type separately, especially the lymphocyte, than by calculating the monocyte-lymphocyte ratio.[157]

## Miscellaneous

*Histiocytes.* Histiocytes are occasionally seen in the peripheral blood and in the bone marrow. They are derivatives of the reticuloendothelial system and are also referred to as macrophages, clasmatocytes, and endothelial phagocytes. These cells are said to be related to monocytes, but this has not yet been established. They are larger than other cells of the peripheral blood. The nucleus is larger and lighter in color than that of either the monocyte or lymphocyte. The cell outline is irregular due to the pseudopodial formation of the cytoplasm. Many of the histiocytes are actively phagocytic; the cytoplasm is vacuolated and may contain intact red cells, remnants of other blood elements, and often peculiar reddish rodlike structures or granules. The granular form of histiocyte is also termed a Ferrata cell.

The histiocytes are increased in number in patients with chronic myelocytic leukemia, agranulocytosis, and virus disease, in the tissues of patients with Letterer-Siwe disease, and in patients exposed to radioactive materials and chemicals.

The group of interrelated conditions which include Letterer-Siwe disease (nonlipid histiocytosis), Hand-Schüller-Christian disease, and eosinophilic granuloma of bone has been regarded as variants of a single nonlipid disease[142] with differentiation on the basis of the age of the patient, the microscopic findings, and distribution of the lesions and more recently[140] as manifestations of a single infection of the reticuloendothelial system. The basic cellular components of the focal infiltration in this group are the histiocytes which are large mononuclear cells with abundant cytoplasm, often with evidence of marked phagocytic activity.

Letterer-Siwe disease occurs in infants as an acute, rapidly progressive malady in which there is widespread proliferation of the histiocytes throughout all of the reticuloendothelial system.[18] Distinctive cells have been identified in the bone marrow and in larger numbers in touch preparations of skin lesions,[169] thus serving as a readily available diagnostic aid. Occasionally, in patients with disease of long duration lipoid droplets are found in small amounts within the cytoplasm. In addition to the anemia, thrombopenia, and leukopenia found at some stage of the disease, hemohistiocytes may appear in the peripheral blood corresponding to the proliferating histiocyte of the tissues.[176]

In patients with Hand-Schüller-Christian disease (triad of diabetes insipidus, exophthalmos,

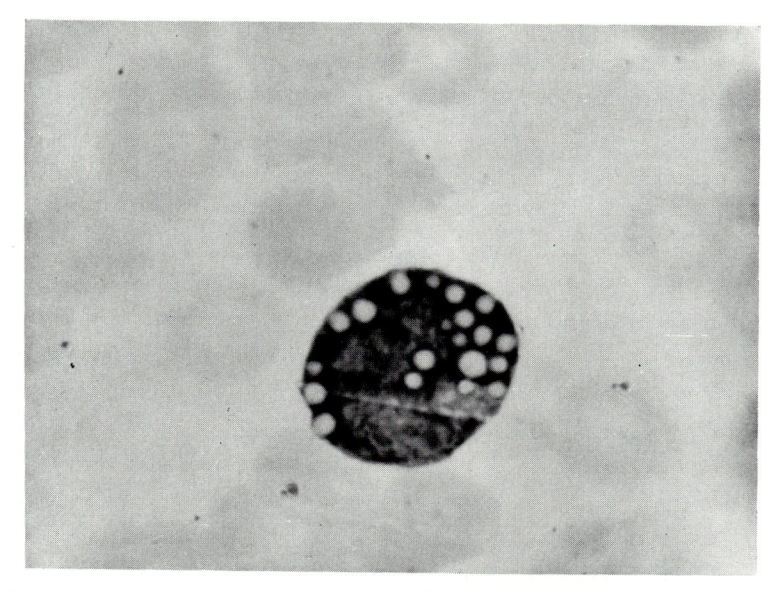

Fig. 59. Bone marrow from a 3-year-old child with multiple congenital anomalies and iron-deficiency anemia. Note cluster of globules in the cytoplasm of the plasma cell, the so-called Russell bodies. (×2400.)

and defects in the membranous bones), there is a tendency for the histiocytes to undergo lipidization, with the accumulation of cholesterol esters within them producing foam cells. Widespread skeletal involvement is common.

Eosinophilic granuloma, the mildest form of the group, occurs as a local lesion in bone and is characterized by sheetlike collections of histiocytes interspersed with a great many eosinophilic cells and an occasional foam cell (Chapter 25).

*Plasma cell (plasmacyte).* The plasma cell is larger than the lymphocyte and has a round, oval, or elongated shape with abundant intensely basophilic cytoplasm. Blue staining is deeper than that of the lymphocyte or any blast form. The nucleus is small and eccentrically placed with chromatin arranged in coarse clumped masses with a cartwheel distribution. A well-defined clear zone is present in the cytoplasm adjacent to the nucleus. The cytoplasm may contain sparse azure granules, but more important are the multiple tiny vacuoles giving the cell a foamy or spongy appearance. Occasionally, larger acidophilic globules occur singly or in groups. These cytoplasmic inclusions are known as Russell bodies and consist of mucoprotein. There is also abundant evidence that Russell bodies contain gamma globulin.[92] These structures can be found in the bone marrow of patients with plasmacytosis due to any cause and are often noted to be numerous within areas of chronic inflammation (Fig. 59). They are not the product of a degenerative process.[252]

Plasma cells are regarded by some as an independent series and by others as a form of lymphocyte.[153] In either case the mature cells are derived from plasmablasts with intermediate forms constituting young plasma cells. Plasma cells rarely appear normally in the peripheral blood but are present in the bone marrow, lymph nodes, spleen, and other areas. They are found in greatly increased numbers in the peripheral blood in patients with multiple myeloma, plasma cell leukemia, and, to a lesser extent, in measles, rubella, chickenpox, serum reactions, and skin disorders. The so-called myeloma cell is a derivative of the early plasma cell and shows the main features of the plasmablasts. During the first months of life the infant forms no plasma cells.[34] 19S globulins formed in the newborn baby are probably synthesized in a transitional cell, which is a precursor of mature plasma cells.[51]

It seems well established that plasma cells are primarily responsible for the synthesis of the antibody components of gamma globulin, perhaps to a greater extent than the lymphoid elements. In patients with agammaglobulinemia there is a failure of plasma cell proliferation. In biopsy specimens of lymph nodes in these patients no plasma cells or secondary follicle formation appears in response to injections of a bacterial vaccine, and no antibody is formed.[123] Good[94] failed to find plasma cells in the bone marrow of patients with agammaglobulinemia after infection and after the antigenic stimulation as occurs in normal children.

On the other hand, hypergammaglobulinemia is most often associated with an increase of plasma cells in the lymph nodes, spleen, and bone marrow. The concept that antibody and gamma globulin are produced by plasmacytes is given further support by the close correlation observed between the plasmacytic development in the bone marrow and increased gamma globulin production in patients suffering from acute rheumatic fever and in patients convalescent from streptococcal pharyngitis.[97] Abnormal protein formation and marked hyperglobulinemia occur in patients with plasmacytic malignancies such as multiple myeloma and plasma cell leukemia.

The plasmatic theory of the synthesis of antibodies is supported by the occurrence of plasma cell hyperplasia during immunization, discovery of antibodies in plasma cells through fluorescent microscopy or radioautography, marked globulinemia in plasmacytomas, and lack of plasma cells in cases of agammaglobulinemia.[237] Plasma cells are found in increased numbers of tissue lesions, bone marrow, lymph nodes, and peripheral blood in various hypersensitive states. In a mild case of serum sickness following an injection of equine tetanus antitoxin, plasmacytosis occurred, amounting to 30% of the white cells in the peripheral blood.[16] In four of eight other cases of serum sickness 1 to 3% of the white cells were plasma cells. All patients had 7S antibody, whereas 19S antibody was found in only two.

Plasma cell hepatitis[20] is a clinical syndrome observed predominantly in young females in which biopsy specimens of liver reveal microscopic evidence of postnecrotic cirrhosis and large numbers of plasma cells in the inflammatory infiltrate. Associated features are marked hyperglobulinemia and arthritis. This condition has been reported in a 12½-year-old girl with moderate hepatosplenomegaly and a weakly positive L.E. cell phenomena. A good clinical response to steroids was observed.[37] 6-Mercaptopurine has also been found effective in reducing the inflammatory response in this condition.[185]

*Türk's cell (Türk irritation cell).* Türk cells are the same size as plasma cells and are closely related to them. They may be identical with the plasma cell, an intermediate cell, or represent an atypical lymphocyte. The cytoplasm is nongranular and stains deeper blue than the plasma cell, and the nucleus is eccentric, but the chromatin is not cartwheel shaped. These cells are increased in number in the peripheral blood of patients with severe anemias, measles, rubella, agranulocytosis, and chronic infections, especially when associated with a marked leukocytosis.

*Rieder cells.* Rieder cells are lymphoblasts or myeloblasts in which the nucleus is deeply indented resembling lobulation. This conformation has been ascribed to the more rapid maturation of the nucleus than the cytoplasm.

*Auer bodies.* Auer bodies or rods are small or elongated slender rods that stain red, purple, or azurophilic with Wright's stain and are peroxidase positive. They are sometimes found singly or in larger numbers in the cytoplasm of myeloblasts, myelocytes, monoblasts, monocytes, and granular histiocytes (Ferrata cells) but not in the cytoplasm of lymphocytes or lymphoblasts. Most commonly, cells that contain Auer bodies are undifferentiated without granules in the cytoplasm, and their presence in such cells is suggestive of leukemia. (See Fig. 60.)

The peripheral leukocytes of three patients with acute myelogenous leukemia have been studied by combined electron microscopy and ultrastructural cytochemistry. Auer bodies present in immature granulocytes were found to contain specific evidence of acid phosphatase activity, indicating that Auer rods are lysosomes.[90,255] A number of observations were made which support the origin of Auer rods from azurophilic granules, which are known to be lysosomes.

## DEGENERATIVE AND TOXIC CYTOPLASMIC CHANGES

*Amato bodies.* Amato bodies are irregular pale blue-staining cytoplasmic clumps up to $2\mu$ in size. They occur in polymorphonuclear neutrophils in patients with various infections such as diphtheria, scarlet fever, pneumonia,

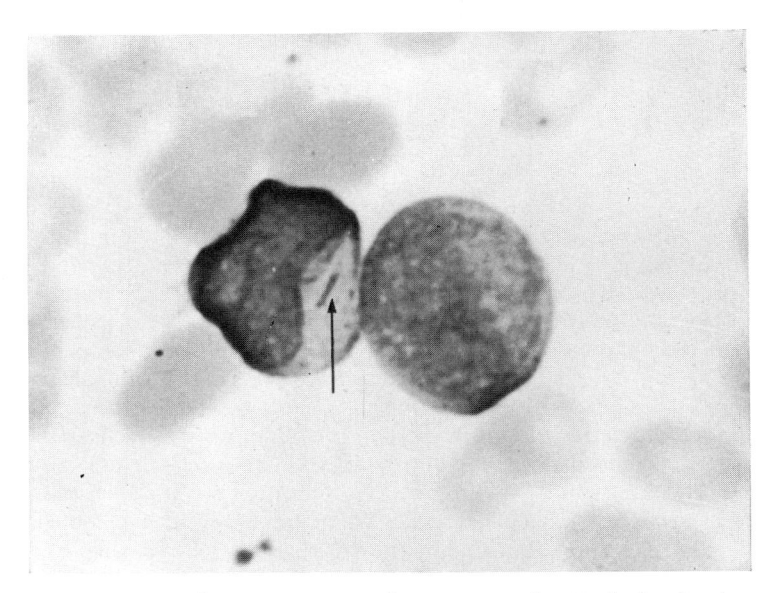

Fig. 60. Bone marrow smear from a patient with acute granulocytic leukemia. Arrow points to an Auer body in one of the promyelocytes. (×3600.) (Courtesy Dr. Richard T. Silver, New York, N.Y.)

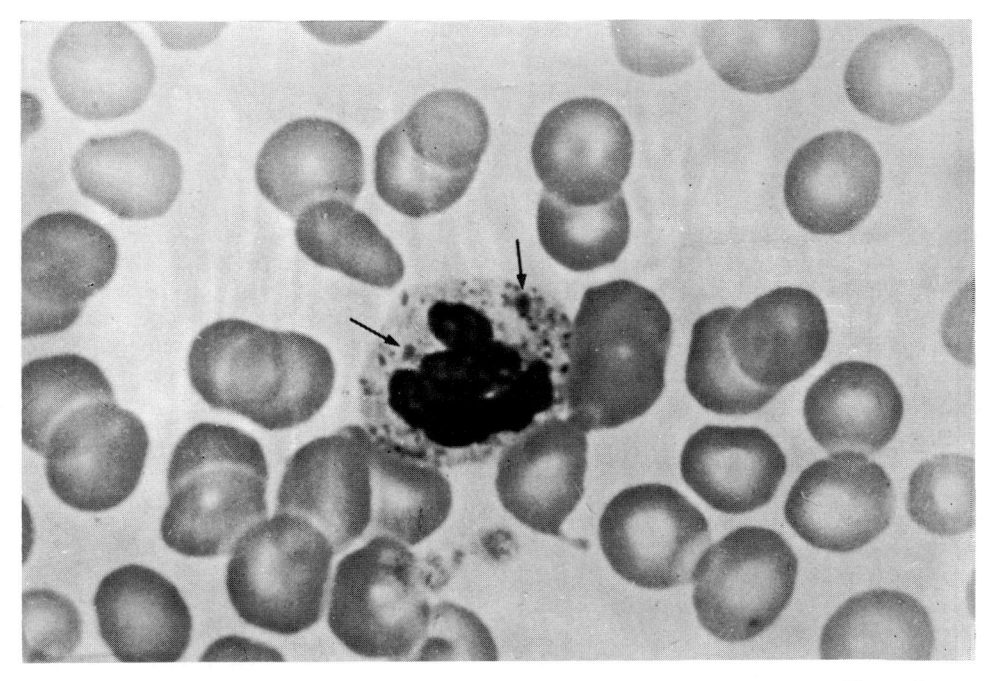

Fig. 61. Blood smear from an infant with meningitis. Arrows point to two Döhle inclusion bodies in neutrophil. These are small localized areas of bluish cytoplasm and probably represent defective maturation. (×2000.) (Courtesy Dr. Julius Rutzky, Pontiac, Mich.)

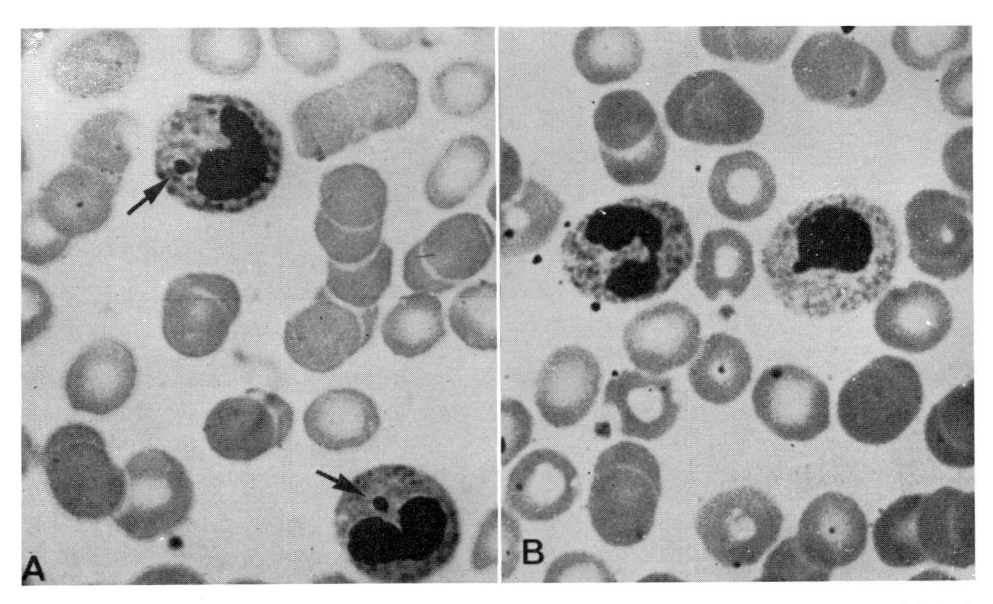

Fig. 62. Pelger-Huët anomaly in blood smear of 5-year-old girl. Note the characteristic bilobed nucleus of granulocytes in both illustrations. The nuclei have a rodlike, dumbbell, or "pince-nez" appearance and possess a coarse and lumpy chromatin structure. Arrows in **A** point to sex chromatin appendage, demonstrating its occurrence in this anomaly. (Courtesy Dr. Philip Lanzkowsky, New York, N.Y.)

and other coccal conditions and have been mistaken for inclusion bodies, possibly of etiologic significance. Amato bodies are probably the same as Döhle bodies. (See Fig. 61.)

*Toxic granules.* Toxic granules and vacuolization are also regarded as degenerative changes, occurring in the cytoplasm during acute infections. Excess vacuolization may be especially noticeable in patients with severe infections and in the blast cells of patients with leukemia. The toxic granules are deeply staining, irregularly distributed, coarse, basophilic granules that are peroxidase-negative and occur in segmented and nonsegmented polymorphonuclear neutrophils. They have been shown to be liquid droplets and not granules and represent a leukocyte that has undergone cloudy swelling.[98]

*Pelger-Huët phenomenon of granulocytes.* Pelger-Huët phenomenon of granulocytes is a hereditary anomaly characterized by partial or complete failure of segmentation of polymorphonuclear cells so that the number of nonsegmented cells is enormously increased. (See Fig. 62.) This benign anomaly may occur in heterozygous or homozygous form. The nucleus is usually broad and kidney shaped and sharply delimited, consisting of strands of intensely stained chromatin with the intervening spaces clear. The conglomerates are particularly prominent in the blunt end of the nucleus. Segmented cells with two and sometimes three lobes occur less frequently, but the clumping and condensation of chromatin are present in these cells as well. In the heterozygous form, the vast majority of the neutrophils have a nucleus with a rodlike, dumbbell, "pince-nez" appearance. These cells with bilobed nuclei and narrow bridge between the lobes account for 70% or more of the neutrophils.[135] Ten percent are nonsegmented. Almost all the neutrophils of the homozygote are of the bilobed form. The presence of the nonsegmented cells here does not represent a shift to the left as occurs in patients with infections and usually has no effect on health. This is a mature neutrophil and not equivalent to the myelocyte or metamyelocyte. The neutrophils, although morphologically abnormal, behave normally in all other respects.

In a patient with combined Pelger-Huët anomaly and addisonian pernicious anemia, an increase in nuclear segmentation occurred in response to megaloblastic erythropoiesis. With vitamin $B_{12}$ therapy the neutrophils once more assumed the characteristic bilobed form of the Pelger-Huët anomaly.[5] The sex chromatin appendage is often difficult to identify in the female with the anomaly. This anomaly is transmitted as a non–sex-linked mendelian dominant character.[213,244] The homozygous form may sometimes, not always, be lethal in man. An acquired form has been described in an adult with chronic myelogenous leukemia.[60] The Pelger-Huët anomaly has also been described as an acquired form in other myelopathies such as acute leukemia and myeloid metaplasia, especially following prolonged exposure to myelotoxic therapeutic agents.[71]

The Pelger-Huët anomaly was demonstrated in seven members of two generations of a Cape colored family in Africa. Two of the six female subjects in this series showed the presence of the sex chromatin appendage in normal numbers.[135]

*Nuclear projections.* An increased number of nuclear projections, distinct from Barr bodies, have been reported in infants with $D^1$ (13-15) trisomy syndrome[120] and in XO females with Turner's syndrome.[231]

*Russell bodies.* The cytoplasm of a plasma cell may contain prominent spherical hyaline bodies or globules which take an acidophilic stain (Fig. 59). These masses, termed Russell bodies, occur singly or in groups and are regarded as consisting of mucoprotein secreted by the parent cell. They appear in the plasma cell in myeloma and in plasma cell leukemia.[192]

*Hematogones.* Lymphocyte-like cells termed hematogones, regarded as blood cell precursors, are occasionally encountered in the bone marrow, rarely in the peripheral blood. In contrast to the large erythrogones (hemocytoblast), these cells resemble small lymphocytes in size and morphology. They differ from the lymphocytes to the extent that they possess a denser, more homogeneous, slightly purplish, dull, matlike nucleus, either with a narrow rim of cytoplasm or entirely devoid of it. Occasionally, the nucleus is partially or completely traversed by a fine cleft. The hematogones often present the appearance of naked nuclei and also differ from the nucleus of the normoblasts in their lighter staining. These cells are found occasionally in the blood of young infants but more frequently in the bone marrow in patients with pure red cell (chronic aregenerative) anemia,[224] lymphocytic leukemia, and, more particularly, giant follicular lymphoblastoma in whom increased numbers have been observed in both the peripheral blood and bone marrow.[211] The hematogone may be the same cell included in the classification of micromyeloblasts, undifferentiated primordial cells, or hemocytoblasts.

*Miscellaneous inclusion bodies.* Atypical granules or inclusion bodies have been described in all types of white blood cells, especially in granulocytes.

*Alder's anomaly.* Coarse, dark, azurophilic granules in the cytoplasm of the white cells, especially the neutrophils, occur as a rare hereditary anomaly without pathologic significance.[126]

*Döhle bodies.* Round or oval-shaped bodies of bluish cytoplasm either just visible or ranging in diameter to approximately 1 to $2\mu$ have been described in the cytoplasm of the polymorphonuclear neutrophil cells in patients with scarlet fever and other specific infections. They appear during the first day or two after a burn and often disappear when the skin is nearly completely covered.[250] Döhle bodies (Fig. 61) appear sky blue with Wright's stain. They are amorphous in shape but tend to be circular or elliptical in outline. Döhle bodies do not stain with fat and glycogen stains but appear red after staining with methyl-green pyronine, suggesting that they have a large ribonucleic acid content.[180] Döhle bodies may be observed in the myelocytes, metamyelocytes, band forms, neutrophilic leukocytes, eosinophils, and basophils. An increased number have been reported in the granulocytes of untreated patients with cancer and a marked increase during therapy with cyclophosphamide.[113] Amato bodies are probably the same as Döhle bodies.

Döhle bodies have been described in the neutrophilic leukocytes of normal gravid women.[1] In 500 blood films screened from uncomplicated pregnancies, all but nine exhibited Döhle bodies. The appearance of the Döhle bodies in normal pregnant women is without explanation.

*Chediak-Higashi anomaly of leukocytes.* This metabolic abnormality of the circulating leukocytes was described by Chediak in Cuba and Higashi in Japan and has been encountered in North America (Fig. 63). The anomaly consists of Döhle-like azurophilic granules ranging in size from 2 to $5\mu$ in diameter in the cytoplasm in all types of leukocytes in con-

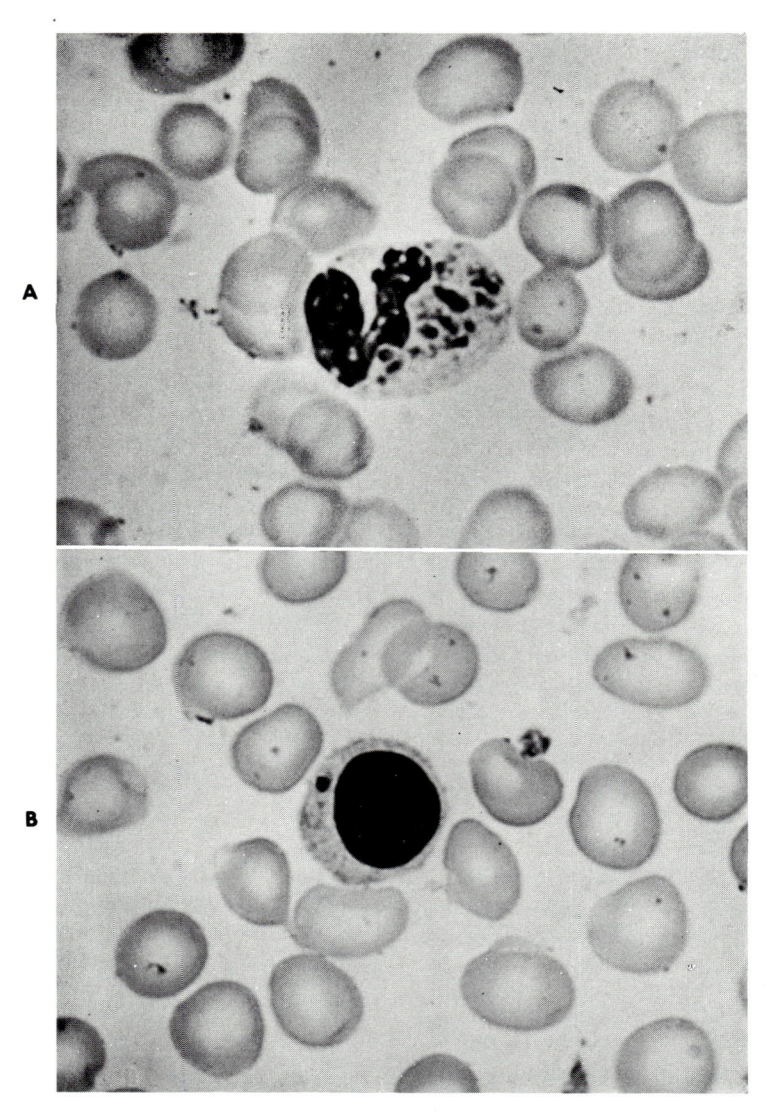

Fig. 63. Blood smear in Chediak-Higashi syndrome. **A,** Note pyknotic nucleus of polymorphonuclear leukocyte and abnormally large oval, fusiform, and irregularly shaped cytoplasmic granules. **B,** One such granule is also present in lymphocyte. (Courtesy Dr. Frederick H. von Hofe, East Orange, N.J.)

junction with abnormally formed or pyknotic nuclei. The inclusion bodies are usually larger and fewer in number than other types. In one report,[75] three to six large, irregular, slate-green masses were noted in the cytoplasm of the polynuclear neutrophils. In some cells they were smaller and more numerous. With electron microscopy and ultrastructure cytochemistry the massive leukocyte granules were shown to be giant lysosomes.[254] The hypopigmentation depends on the presence of giant melanosomes.[259] These inclusion bodies have also been described in patients with malignant lymphoma.[75] Massive leukocyte granules and inclusions have also been observed in erythrocytes.[74] This disorder may affect children of either sex and shows a recessive hereditary pattern,[216] fully manifest in homozygotes. The heterozygote carriers have been identified by abnormal granulations in the lympho-

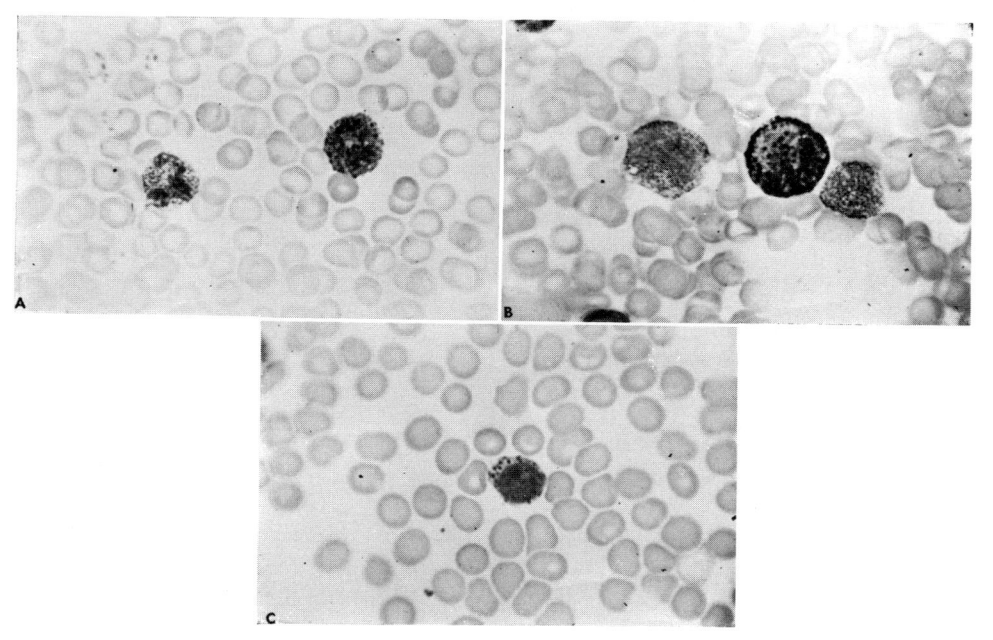

Fig. 64. Blood and bone marrow smears from a 3½-year-old boy with gargoylism (Hurler's syndrome). Heavy granulation (Reilly bodies) present in polymorphonuclear leukocytes of the peripheral blood, A, myelocytes of the bone marrow, B, and lymphocytes, C, are characteristic of this disease. These granules differ from toxic granulation and those found in the basophilic leukocytes. Although coarse granules are common, fine and medium granules may also be present. (Courtesy Dr. Ralph L. Engle, Jr., New York, N.Y.)

cyte. Chromosomal patterns are normal.[131] Consanguinity is common. The disease is characterized by semialbinism, photophobia, nystagmus, excessive sweating, pale optic fundi, hepatosplenomegaly, and generalized lymphadenopathy.[42,68] During the course of the disease, a progressive granulocytopenia ensues and patients suffer from recurrent infections, which ultimately result in death. Children usually die in early childhood but may survive until 5 to 10 years, then often die of a lymphoma-like disease. Patients rarely survive until early adult life, suffering only from neurological defects. Pathologically, histiocytes along with immature lymphoid cells infiltrate lymph nodes and spleen. In addition to the granulations the myeloid precursors in the bone marrow reveal extensive vacuolization and acidophilic inclusions.[28] A perivascular infiltrate of histiocytes has been noted in postmortem sections of brain.[184] Inclusions in histiocytes possess a lipid component.

The serum muramidase activities of four granulocytopenic patients with the Chediak-Higashi syndrome were strikingly elevated, indicating a markedly increased rate of granulocyte turnover.[28] Two of the patients, both with histologic and clinical evidence of the infiltrative phase of the syndrome, had intermittent hypersplenism represented by splenomegaly, thrombocytopenia, and hemolytic anemia with splenic sequestration. There was also indirect evidence consistent with intramedullary granulocyte destruction.

Hodgkin's disease developed in a girl 8 years, 9 months of age with the physical and hematologic stigmata of Chediak-Higashi syndrome.[230] A diagnosis of Hodgkin's disease was made following biopsy of a cervical lymph node. The peripheral blood smear showed numerous slate-gray cytoplasmic inclusions in about 50% of the polymorphonuclear leukocytes, which were peroxidase-positive.

*Reilly bodies and other inclusion bodies in gargoylism.* In patients with gargoylism (Hurler's syndrome, lipochondrodystrophy, Fig. 64), a rare disease of early childhood characterized by dull coarse cretinoid facies, dwarfism, skeletal deformities, clouding of the corneas, and mental retardation, fine and coarse blue-colored granules have been described by Reilly in some 60 to 90% of the granulocytes and their precursors in the bone marrow and occasionally in the lymphocytes and monocytes.[204,256] These granules are the same as those noted by Alder as a hereditary anomaly. Patients with gargoylism have been described in whom the abnormal inclusions were confined to the lymphocytes, the granulocytes being unaffected.[163]

In the lymphocytes of gargoylism the cytoplasmic inclusions also stain with May-Grunwald-Giemsa and metachromatically with toluidine blue.[164] These inclusions are described as distinct from those in polynuclear cells (Reilly bodies) and appear typically as deeply stained granules in the center of vacuoles, sharply defined against the surrounding cytoplasm. These staining reactions indicate that the inclusions consist of acid mucopolysaccharides and are correlated with the excessive excretion of this substance in the urine of many clinically diagnosed cases of gargoylism.[172]

In addition basophilic granules have also been described in the bone marrow, both extracellular and intracellular within large mononuclear cells, resembling histiocytes. In a few patients the granules are largely intracellular. However, in most cases they are dispersed throughout the particles of bone marrow, perhaps resulting from rupture of cells during preparation. The basophilic granules were described originally by Gasser[91] and more recently by Pearson and Lorincz[193] in the bone marrow of seventeen of eighteen patients with documented gargoylism (increased excretion of the acid mucopolysaccharides, chondroitin sulfuric acid B, and heparin monosulfuric acid). Thus, the coarse granulations once thought to be present solely in the circulating granulocytes of gargoylism have now also been found in lymphocytes as well as in bone marrow aspirates.

Mucopolysaccharides have now been identified by several investigators as chondroitin sulfuric acid B (dermatan sulfate) and in smaller amounts, heparitin sulfate (heparan sulfate). Of five patients with the Hurler syndrome,[22] three excreted increased amounts of both dermatan sulfate B and heparan sulfate and showed the advanced skeletal changes of the disease. The remaining two patients excreted heparan sulfate only and had small uncharacteristic bone changes.

The nature of the metabolic defect underlying the Hurler syndrome is unknown. Possibly it is due to an increased mucopolysaccharide production or a decreased breakdown or error in the synthesis of a mucopolysaccharide acceptor protein.[22]

Recent studies have demonstrated intracellular deposition of mucopolysaccharides in fibroblasts of patients with Hurler's and Hunter's disease[58] and have opened up possibilities for study of the metabolic defect[70] and the antenatal diagnosis of the disease.

*Cellular metachromasia.* Danes and Bearn[59] reported the presence of granules taking a metachromatic stain in the cytoplasm of fibroblasts cultured from the skin of patients with specific mucopolysaccharidosis. Skin fibroblasts available by biopsy are finely minced and established in culture and prepared by specified methods. Cellular metachromasia is evidenced by red cytoplasm after staining with toluidine blue O. Cells are scored as positive for metachromasia if there are pink or reddish-purple cytoplasmic granules or vacuoles.[232] Danes and Bearn suggested that the genetic defect that can be recognized in cell culture of skin fibroblasts from patients with Hurler and Hunter syndromes[58] might possibly be found in similar cultures from patients with other genetic mucopolysaccharidoses. Taysi and colleagues[232] found the test was positive for cystic fibrosis as well as in other conditions in cultures from pediatric patients unrelated to mucopolysaccharidoses. Although the specificity of metachromasia has been questioned as a means of identifying both heterozygous carriers and affected persons with mucopolysaccharidoses, it is important to emphasize the need for rigid attention to tissue culture techniques.[19] Further studies will determine the usefulness of metachromasia in diagnosis and genetic counseling.

In a comparison of the commonly used tests for the detection of Hurler's syndrome, the gross albumin turbidity test is the most reliable. (To 1.0 ml. urine add 2 drops of 5N HCL and 2.0 ml. of the acid-albumin reagent. The resulting turbidity is graded 0 to 4 after 10 minutes at room temperature.) The test was preferred to the toluidine spot test and carbazole test.[39]

*May-Hegglin anomaly.* The May-Hegglin anomaly is a rare condition characterized by platelet abnormalities in the peripheral blood and Döhle inclusion bodies in the granulocytes. The platelets are large and poorly granulated, although morphologically normal platelets may be present as well. Some platelets are cigar shaped and elliptic, although round forms predominate. More than one-third of the cases are thrombocytopenic.[180] The platelets measure up to 15µ in rare instances. The Döhle bodies, which are readily seen in the majority of neutrophil granulocytes, may be found in some of the eosinophils, basophils, and macrocytes and consist largely of ribonucleic acid. These bodies are fusiform or crescentic, with sharply defined borders situated most often near the periphery of the cell.

The anomaly is transmitted as a simple dominant.[247] While Amato and Döhle bodies have been regarded as identical, it is claimed that the cytoplasmic patches in the May-Hegglin anomaly are larger and more discrete and occur in a much larger percentage of cells. While the syndrome is usually symptomless, the anomaly has been found in association with severe and fatal purpura, presumably due to a maturation defect of megakaryocytes.[139] The May-Hegglin anomaly is often familial, with variable expressivity. A case has been reported in a 6-year-old girl, but the platelet count in the patient's mother and brother were normal.[180] In another case the anomaly appeared in thirteen subjects in three generations of one family.[247] In a mother and daughter with the May-Hegglin anomaly an identical chromosome abnormality was present, i.e., loss of most of the short arm of a chromosome.[36] However, the deletion was found in one member of the family without the May-Hegglin anomaly and was not found in an unrelated patient with the anomaly. These studies suggest that the chromosome abnormality is probably unrelated to the May-Hegglin anomaly.

*Tay-Sachs disease (infantile amaurotic familial idiocy).* Tay-Sachs disease is a hereditary disease of lipid storage in which the sphingolipid ganglioside accumulates in the cytoplasm of the neurones of the brain. Abnormal granules have been found in the leukocytes of several patients with this disease.[229] Course granules randomly scattered throughout the cytoplasm of leukocytes varying in number from a few to more than 100 have been noted. Their color ranges from light blue to dark purple and their size from a bare visibility to a diameter of $2\mu$, the average being about 0.5 mm. The granules appear similar to those of Alder's anomaly. More than 50% of the granulocytes and 5% of the mononuclear cells are affected.

*Other lipidoses and related diseases.* Vacuolated lymphocytes and monocytes have been observed in other sphingolipidoses, including Niemann-Pick disease, Gaucher's disease, and generalized gangliosidosis.[32] The polymorphonuclear leukocytes of patients with generalized gangliosidosis contain Reilly bodies.[134] In Wolman's disease,[261] associated with increased accumulation of cholesterol, vacuolated lymphocytes in the peripheral blood have been identified.

## CELL STAINS

*Romanowsky stains.* Romanowsky stains, of which Wright's stain is a modification, consist of a combination of methylene blue with eosin. Depending upon their acid and basic affinities, the red and blue structures of cells are identified in contrasting colors. The nuclei of white cells stain purplish blue, with clear separation of basichromatin and oxychromatin, neutrophil granules stain light pink or lavender, and the granules of eosinophils and basophils stain red and deeply azurophilic, respectively.

*Supravital staining.* Supravital staining[53] permits the examination of cytoplasmic structures of blood cells in the living motile state. In the combination employed, the mitochondria are stained by Janus green and the specific granules and vacuoles of the cytoplasm by neutral red dye. The nucleus and cytoplasm are left unstained, but the nuclear outlines are readily discerned. Mitochondria are most plentiful in the blast cells and decrease progressively as the cells mature, being reduced in the late myelocytes and frequently absent in the mature polymorphonuclear leukocyte, lymphocyte, and monocyte.

At times the blue-green stain may serve in differentiating the blast cells by the shape and size of the mitochondria and their location. In the myeloblast the mitochondria are numerous and extremely fine and are scattered diffusely or packed in a segment of the cytoplasm. In the lymphoblast they are short, thick, oval, or spherical and may be clustered around the nucleus or may be scattered diffusely. In the monoblast they exist as fine, slender rods scattered through the cell.

Motility is absent in the blast forms but is present in varying degrees of ameboid motion in the mature cells of the three series, most marked in the polymorphonuclear neutrophil. In the monocyte the supravital stain is particularly diagnostic since the neutral red bodies are characteristically clustered as a rosette in the indentation of the nucleus. Supravital staining does not replace fixed smear but serves as an adjunct in the differentiation of cells and as an aid in visualizing their physiologic activity.

*Peroxidase stain.* The presence of an oxidating ferment in the cytoplasm of myeloid cells provides an added means of differentiating these from other cells. In the commonly used techniques (such as the Goodpasture and the copper peroxidase method of Sato and Sekiya), this ferment causes the oxidation and precipitation of benzidine by hydrogen peroxide. Cells of the granulocytic series, including promyelocytes, give a strong peroxidase reaction as contrasted with lymphocytes, plasma cells, and red cells which are peroxidase negative. Monocytes show fewer and less well-defined peroxidase-positive granules than do granulocytes. The peroxidase reaction in myeloblasts may show faint localized positivity, occasionally accompanied by positively-staining Auer rods, but the reaction is less intense than in more mature myeloid cells. When used with the Sudan black B stain, in which myeloblasts stain positively, the peroxidase reaction is of diagnostic use in separating these cells from lymphoblasts.[108]*

*Miscellaneous stains.* Leukocyte alkaline phosphatase is an enzyme capable of hydrolyzing phosphorus from a wide variety of phosphomonoesters.[127] This enzyme is present in the cytoplasm of leukocytes of the granulocyte series and can be assayed chemically or roughly quantitatively by cytochemical staining. With histochemical methods the granules representing alkaline-phosphatase activity stain from a pale brown color to deep black. In blood from cases of infection, polycythemia vera, myelofibrosis, and leukemoid reactions, alkaline phosphatase staining is increased, whereas in acute and chronic myeloid leukemia and in paroxysmal nocturnal hemoglobinuria the reaction is decreased. The test is valuable, therefore, in distinguishing a nonleukemic myeloid (leukemoid) reaction from chronic myelocytic leukemia.

The presence of deoxyribonucleic acid can be demonstrated by a microchemical reaction known as Feulgen's nuclear reaction.[101] With Feulgen's stain leukocytes and nucleated red cells take up the stain according to the concentration of deoxyribonucleic acid in the nucleus. The clear definition of nucleoli (unstained spaces) is sometimes of help in differentiating lymphoblasts (1 to 2 nucleoli) from myeloblasts (2 to 4 nucleoli).

Methyl green–pyronine also stains, to some degree, the ribonucleic content of leukocytes.[197]

The periodic acid–Schiff reaction is widely used in hematology for demonstrating glycogen and related mucopolysaccharides.[109] Lymphocytes may stain positively with periodic acid-Schiff reagent.

*Phase contrast microscopy.* Phase contrast microscopy provides a useful technique by which the details of living cells can be examined. The papers by Ackerman and Bellios[2] and by Bessis,[24] among others, provide a background for this technique. Phase contrast intensifies relatively minute differences in optical density and permits the detection of intimate details of cells and cytoplasmic structures. It allows important structures of living cells to be examined—chromatin, mitochondria, the centrosome of the cell. Phase contrast allows the movements of the pseudopods of granulocytes to be examined in detail.[24] Granulocytes and monocytes are observed to spread on supporting surfaces and become objects which are easily identified. The centrosome, for instance, appears as a region more transparent than the surrounding cytoplasm and devoid of granules. In its neighborhood, however, the granules are arranged radially. Red cells examined with phase contrast microscopy reveal a scintillating effect, probably resulting from differences in thickness due to molecular movement. This scintillation disappears at the moment when the red cell of sickle cell anemia becomes rigid.[25] Phase contrast gives a very detailed image of the erythroblast. Platelets are seen so distinctly with this method that they can be counted directly on a special counting chamber.

## REFERENCES

1. Abernathy, M. R.: Döhle bodies associated with uncomplicated pregnancy, Blood 27: 380, 1966.
2. Ackerman, G. A., and Bellios, N. C.: A study of the morphology of living cells of blood and bone marrow in vital films with the

---

*For more extensive discussions and methods of peroxidase and related stains, see references 40, 54, and 109.

phase contrast microscope. I. Normal blood and bone marrow, Blood 10:3, 1955.
3. Ambrus, C. N., Ambrus, J. C., Johnson, G. C., Packman, E. W., Chernick, W. S., Back, N., and Harrisson, J. W. E.: Role of the lungs in regulation of the white blood cell level, Amer. J. Physiol. 178:33, 1954.
4. Anderson, R. E., and Walford, R. L.: Direct demonstration of A, B and Rh$_o$(D) blood group antigens on human leukocytes, Amer. J. Clin. Path. 40:239, 1963.
5. Ardeman, S., Chanarin, I., and Frankland, A. W.: The Pelger-Huët anomaly and megaloblastic anemia, Blood 22:472, 1963.
6. Arnason, B. G., Janković, B. D., and Waksman, B. H.: A survey of the thymus and its relation of lymphocytes and immune reactions, Blood 20:617, 1962.
7. Arterberry, J. D., Drexler, E., and Dubois, E. L.: Significance of hematoxylin bodies in lupus erythematosus cell preparations, J.A.M.A. 187:389, 1964.
8. Ashley, D. J. B.: The technic of nuclear sexing, Amer. J. Clin. Path. 31:230, 1959.
9. Astaldi, G., Massimo, L., Airo, R., and Mori, P. G.: Phytohaemagglutinin and lymphocytes from acute lymphoblastic leukaemia, Lancet 1:1265, 1966.
10. Athens, J., Haab, O. P., Raab, S. O., Mauer, A. M., Ashenbrucker, H., Cartwright, G. E., and Wintrobe, M. M.: Leukokinetic studies. IV. The total blood circulating and marginal granulocyte pools and granulocyte turnover rate in normal subjects, J. Clin. Invest. 40:989, 1961.
11. Ayres, W. W., and Starkey, N. M.: Studies on Charcot-Leyden crystals, Blood 5:254, 1950.
12. Baehner, R. L., and Johnston, R. B., Jr.: Metabolic and bacterial activity of human eosinophils, Brit. J. Haemat. 20:277, 1971.
13. Baehner, R. L., and Karnovsky, M. L.: Deficiency of reduced nicotinamide-adenine dinucleotide oxidase in chronic granulomatous disease, Science 162:1277, 1968.
14. Baehner, R. L., and Nathan, D. G.: Leukocyte oxidase; defective activity in chronic granulomatous disease, Science 155:835, 1967.
15. Bannatyne, R. M., Skowron, P. N., and Weber, J. L.: Job's syndrome; a variant of chronic granulomatous disease. Report of a case, J. Pediat. 75:236, 1969.
16. Barnett, E. V. Stone, G., Swisher, S. N., and Vaughan, J. H.: Serum sickness and plasmacytosis; a clinical, immunologic and hematologic analysis, Amer. J. Med. 35:113, 1963.
17. Bass, M. H.: Extreme eosinophilia and leukocytosis, Amer. J. Dis Child. 62:68, 1941.
18. Batson, R., Shapiro, J., Christie, A., and Riley, H. D., Jr.: Acute non-lipid disseminated reticuloendotheliosis, Amer. J. Dis. Child. 90:323, 1955.
19. Bearn, A. G., and Danes, B. S.: Metachromasia elaborated, New Eng. J. Med. 282:102, 1969.
20. Bearn, A. G., Kunkel, H. G., and Slater, R. J.: The problem of chronic liver disease in young women, Amer. J. Med. 21:3, 1956.
21. Berendes, H., Bridges, R. A., and Good, R. A:. Fatal granulomatosis of childhood; clinical study of a new syndrome, Minnesota Med. 40:309, 1957.
22. Berggord, I., and Bearn, A. G.: The Hurler syndrome; a biochemical and clinical study, Amer. J. Med. 39:221, 1965.
23. Berman, L.: The immunologically competent cell (immunocyte) system; an attempt at a delineation of the cellular relationships, Blood 21:246, 1963.
24. Bessis, M.: Phase contrast microscopy and electron microscopy applied to the blood cells, Blood 10:272, 1955.
25. Bessis, M., Bricka, M., Gorios-Breton, J., and Tabuis, J.: New observations on sickle cells with special reference to their agglutinability, Blood 9:39, 1954.
26. Bierman, H. R., Kelly, K. H., and Cordes, F. L.: The sequestration and visceral circulation of leukocytes in man, Ann. N. Y. Acad. Sci. 59:850, 1955.
27. Bierman, H. R., Kelly, K. H., Cordes, F. L., Byron, R. L., Jr., Polhemus, J. A., and Rappoport, S.: The release of leukocytes and platelets from the pulmonary circulation by epinephrine, Blood 7:683, 1952.
28. Blume, R. S., Bennett, J. M., Yankee, R. A., and Wolff, S. M.: Defective granulocyte regulation in the Chediak-Higashi syndrome, New Eng. J. Med. 279:1009, 1968.
29. Boggs, D. R., Wintrobe, M. M., and Cartwright, G. E.: The acute leukemias; analysis of 322 cases and review of the literature, Medicine 41:163, 1963.
30. Bonnin, J. A., and Schwartz, L.: The combined study of agglutination, hemolysis and erythrophagocytosis; with special reference to acquired hemolytic anemia, Blood 9:773, 1954.
31. Boyer, M. H., Basten, A., and Besson, P. B.: Mechanism of eosinophilia. III. Suppression of eosinophilia by agents known to modify immune responses, Blood 36:458, 1970.
32. Brady, R. O.: Genetics and the sphingolipidoses, Med. Clin. N. Amer. 53:827, 1969.
33. Braun, E. H., Buckwold, A. E., Emson, H. E., and Russell, A. V.: Familial neonatal neutropenia with maternal leukocyte antibodies, Blood 16:1745, 1960.

34. Bridges, R. A., Condie, R. N., Zak, S. J., and Good, R. A.: The morphologic basis of antibody formation development during the neonatal period, J. Lab. Clin. Med. 35:331, 1959.
35. Brittingham, T. E., and Chaplin, H., Jr.: Febrile transfusion reactions caused by sensitivity to donor leukocytes and platelets, J.A.M.A. 165:819, 1957.
36. Buchanan, J. G., Pearce, L., and Wetherley-Mein, G.: The May-Hegglin anomaly; a family report and chromosome study, Brit. J. Haemat. 10:508, 1964.
37. Bumbalo, T. S., Bellanti, J. A., and Terplan, K. L.: Plasma-cell hepatitis case; report with immunologic studies, Pediatrics 29:191, 1962.
38. Burnett, F. M.: The role of the thymus and related organs in immunity, Brit. J. Med. 2:807, 1962.
39. Carter, C. H., Wan, A. T., and Carpenter, D. G.: Commonly used tests in the detection of Hurler's syndrome, J. Pediat. 73:217, 1968.
40. Cartwright, G. E.: Diagnostic laboratory hematology, New York, 1968, Grune & Stratton, Inc.
41. Cartwright, G. E., Athens, J. W., and Wintrobe, M. M.: The kinetics of granulopoiesis in normal man, Blood 24:780, 1964.
42. Chediak, M. M.: Nouvelle anomalie leucocytaire de caractere constitutionnel et familial, Rev. Hèmat. 7:362, 1952.
43. Cline, M. J., and Lehrer, R. I.: Phagocytosis by human monocytes, Blood 32:423, 1968.
44. Coen, R., Grush, O., and Kauder, E.: Studies of bacterial activity and metabolism of the leukocyte in full-term neonates, J. Pediat. 75:400, 1969.
45. Cohn, Z. A., and Hirsch, J. G.: The isolation and properties of the specific cytoplasmic granules of rabbit polymorphonuclear leucocytes, J. Exp. Med. 112:983, 1960.
46. Cooper, H. L., and Rubin, A. D.: RNA metabolism in lymphocytes stimulated by phytohemagglutinin; initial response to phytohemagglutinin, Blood 25:1014, 1965.
47. Craddock, C. G.: The production, utilization and destruction of white blood cells. In Tocantins, L. M., editor: Progress in hematology, New York, 1962, Grune & Stratton, Inc.
48. Crofton, J. W., Livingstone, J. L., Oswald, N. C., and Roberts, A. T. M.: Pulmonary eosinophilia, Thorax 7:1, 1952.
49. Cronkite, E. P., and Fliedner, T. M.: Granulocytopoiesis, New Eng. J. Med. 270:1347, 1964.
50. Crowder, J. G., Martin, R. R., and White, A.: Release of histamine and lysosomal enzymes by human leucocytes during phagocytosis of staphylococci, J. Lab. Clin. Med. 74:436, 1969.
51. Cruchaud, A., Rosen, F. S., Craig, J. M., Janeway, C. A., and Gitlin, D.: The site of synthesis of the 19S gamma globulins in dysgammaglobulinemia, J. Exp. Med. 115:114, 1962.
52. Cunningham, R. S., Sabin, F. R., Sugiyama, S., and Kindwall, J. A.: Role of the monocyte in tuberculosis, Bull. Johns Hopkins Hosp. 37:231, 1925.
53. Cunningham, R. S., and Tompkins, E. H.: The supravital staining of normal human blood cells, Folia Haemat. 42:257, 1950.
54. Dacie, J. V., and Lewis, S. M.: Practical haematology, ed. 4, New York, 1968, Grune & Stratton, Inc.
55. Dameshek, W.: The thymus and lymphoid proliferation, Blood 20:629, 1962.
56. Dameshek, W.: "Immunoblasts" and "immunocytes"; an attempt at a functional nomenclature, Blood 21:243, 1963.
57. Dameshek, W., and Reeves, W. H.: Exacerbation of lupus erythematosus following splenectomy in "idiopathic" thrombocytopenic purpura and autoimmune hemolytic anemia, Amer. J. Med. 21:560, 1956.
58. Danes, B. S., and Bearn, A. G.: Hurler's syndrome; demonstration of an inherited disorder of connective tissues in cell culture, J. Exp. Med. 123:1, 1966.
59. Danes, B. S., and Bearn, A. G.: Cellular metachromasia; a genetic marker for studying the mucopolysaccharidosses, Lancet 1:241, 1967.
60. Darte, J. M., Dacie, J. V., and McSorley, J. G. A.: Pelger-like leucocytes in chronic myeloid leukemia, Acta Haemat. 12:117, 1954.
61. Dausset, J., Colombani, J., and Colombani, M.: Study of leukopenias and thrombocytopenias by the direct antiglobulin consumption test on leukocytes and/or platelets, Blood 18:672, 1961.
62. Dausset, J., Nenna, A., and Brecy, H.: Leukoagglutinins; leukoagglutinins in chronic idiopathic and symptomatic pancytopenia and in paroxysmal nocturnal hemoglobinuria, Blood 9:696, 1954.
63. Davidson, W. M., Milner, R. D. G., and Lawler, S. D.: Giant neutrophil leucocytes; an inherited anomaly, Brit. J. Haemat. 6:339, 1960.
64. Davidson, W. M., and Smith, D. R.: A morphological sex difference in the polymorphonuclear neutrophil leucocytes, Brit. M. J. 2:6, 1954.
65. Doan, C. A.: Neutropenic state; its significance and therapeutic rationale, J.A.M.A. 99:194, 1932.

66. Doan, C. A.: The white blood cells in health and disease, Bull. N. Y. Acad. Med. 30:415, 1954.
67. Doan, C. A., and Wiseman, B. K.: The monocyte, monocytosis and monocytic leukoses, Ann. Intern. Med. 8:383, 1934.
68. Donohue, W. L., and Bain, H. W.: Chediak-Higashi syndrome; a lethal familial disease with anomalous inclusions in the leukocytes and constitutional stigmata, Pediatrics 20:416, 1957.
69. Donohue, W. L., Snelling, C. E., Jackson, S. H., Keith, J. D., Chute, A. L., Laski, B., and Silverthorne, N.: Pituitary adrenocorticotropic hormone (ACTH) therapy in eosinophilic leukemia, J.A.M.A. 143:154, 1950.
70. Dorfman, A., and Matalon, R.: The Hurler and Hunter syndromes, Amer. J. Med. 47:691, 1969.
71. Dorr, A. D., and Moloney, W. C.: Acquired pseudo-Pelger anomaly of granulocytic leukocytes, New Eng. J. Med. 261:742, 1959.
72. Dougherty, T. F., and White, A.: Functional alterations in lymphoid tissue induced by adrenal cortical secretion, Amer. J. Anat. 77:81, 1945.
73. Douglas, S. D.: Analytic review; Disorders of phagocyte function, Blood 35:851, 1970.
74. Efrati, P., and Danon, D.: Electron-microscopical study of bone marrow cells in a case of Chediak-Higashi-Steinbrinck syndrome, Brit. J. Haemat. 15:173, 1968.
75. Efrati, P., and Jonas, W.: Chediak's anomaly of leukocytes in malignant lymphoma associated with leukemic manifestations; case report with necropsy, Blood 13:1063, 1958.
76. Elves, M. W., Roath, S., and Israels, M. C. G.: The response of lymphocytes to antigen challenge in vitro, Lancet 1:806, 1963.
77. Eng, G. D., and Leikin, S. L.: Electrophoretic studies of leukocyte antibodies. II. Study of clinical states, J. Lab. Clin. Med. 57:899, 1961.
78. Epstein, W. L., and Kligman, A. W.: Pathogenesis of eosinophilic pneumonitis (Löffler's syndrome), J.A.M.A. 162:95, 1956.
79. Essellier, A. F., Jeanneret, R. L., and Morandi, L.: The mechanism of glucocorticoid eosinopenia; contribution to the physiology of eosinophile granulocytes, Blood 9:531, 1954.
80. Evans, T. S., and Nesbit, R. R.: Eosinophilic leukemia; report of a case with autopsy confirmation; review of literature, Blood 4:603, 1949.
81. Farquhar, J. W.: The evaluation of the eosinopenic response to corticotrophin and cotisone in the newborn infant, Arch. Dis. Child. 30:133, 1955.
82. Fedorko, M. E., and Hirsch, J. G.: Structure of monocytes and macrophages, Seminars Hemat. 7:109, 1970.
83. Fennell, R. H., Jr., Maclachlan, M. J., and Rodnan, G. P.: The occurrence of antinuclear factors in the sera of relatives of patients with systemic rheumatic disease, Arthrit. Rheumat. 5:296, 1962.
84. Fessas, P., Wintrobe, M. M., Thompson, R. B., and Cartwright, G. E.: Treatment of leukemia with cortisone and corticotrophin, Arch. Intern. Med. 94:384, 1954.
85. Fieschi, A., and Sacchetti, C.: Clinical assessment of granulopoiesis, Acta Haemat. 31:150, 1964.
86. Finch, S. C., Ross J. F., and Ebaugh, F. G.: Immunologic mechanisms of leucocyte abnormalities, J. Lab. Clin. Med. 42:555, 1953.
87. First report of the Committee for Clarification of the Nomenclature of Cells and diseases of the Blood and Blood-forming Organs, Amer. J. Clin. Path. 18:443, 1948.
88. Fleming, A.: On a remarkable bacteriolytic element found in tissues and secretions, Proc. Roy. Soc. London. 93:3061, 1922.
89. Fliedner, T. M., Cronkite, E. P., Killman, S. A., and Bond, U. P.: Granulopoiesis. II. Emergence and pattern of labeling of neutrophilic granulocytes in humans, Blood 24:683, 1964.
90. Freeman, J. A.: Origin of Auer bodies, Blood 27:499, 1966.
91. Gasser, G.: In discussion of paper by Alder, A.: Konstitutionellbedingte Granulationsveränderungen der Leükocyten und Knochenveränderungen, Schweiz. med. Wchnschr. 80:1095, 1950.
92. Goldberg, A. F., and Deane, H. W.: A comparative study of some staining properties of crystals in a lympho-plasmocytoid cell and of amyloids; with special emphasis on their isoelectric points, Blood 16:1708, 1960.
93. Good, R. A.: Agammaglobulinemia, Bull. Univ. Minnesota Hosp. 26:1, 1954.
94. Good, R. A.: Studies on agammaglobulinemia; failure of plasma cell formation in the bone marrow and lymph nodes of patients with agammaglobulinemia, J. Lab. Clin. Med. 46:167, 1955.
95. Good, R. A.: Manipulating the "new immunology," J.A.M.A. 207:852, 1969.
96. Good, R. A.: The lymphocyte—an introduction, Seminars Hemat. 6:1, 1969.
97. Good, R. A., and Campbell, B.: Correlation of the plasmacytosis of the bone marrow with the modifications of the gamma globulin of the serum in rheumatic fever, Amer. J. Med. 9:330, 1950.
98. Gordin, R.: Toxic granulation in leukocytes; development and relation to cloudy swell-

ing, Acta Med. Scandinav. (supp. 270) 143: 1, 1952.
99. Gorman, J. G., and Chandler, J. G.: Is there an immunologically incompetent lymphocyte? Blood 23:117, 1964.
100. Gotoff, S. P.: Cell-mediated deficiency, J. Pediat. 78:379, 1971.
101. Greig, H. B. W.: A substitute for the Feulgen staining technique, J. Clin. Path. 12:93, 1959.
102. Hall, S. W., Kozak, M., and Spink, W. W.: Pulmonary infiltrates, pericarditis an eosinophilia; a unique case of pulmonary infiltration and eosinophilia syndrome, Amer. J. Med. 36:135, 1964.
103. Halvorsen, K.: Neonatal leucopenia due to fetomaternal leucocyte incompatibility, Acta Paedit. Scandinav. 54:86, 1965.
104. Hargraves, M. M., Richmond, H., and Morton R.: Presentation of two bone marrow elements; "tart" cell and "L.E." cell, Proc. Staff. Meet. Mayo Clin. 23:25, 1948.
105. Harris, S., and Harris, T. N.: Studies on the transfer of lymph node cells; effects of variation in the interval between the injection of antigen into the donor and collection of its lymph node cells, J. Exp. Med. 100:269, 1954.
106. Haserick, J. R., and Sundberg, R. D.: Bone marrow as diagnostic aid in acute disseminated lupus erythematosus; report on Hargraves' "L.E." cell, J. Invest. Dermat. 11:209, 1948.
107. Hayes, D. M., and Spurr, C. L.: Use of phytohemagglutinin to stimulate hematopoiesis in humans, Blood 27:78, 1966.
108. Hayhoe, F. G. J., Quaglino, D., and Doll, R.: The cytology and cytochemistry of acute leukaemias; a study of 140 cases, London, 1964, Her Majesty's Stationery Office.
109. Hayhoe, F. G. J., Quaglino, D., and Flemans, R. J.: Consecutive use of Romanowsky and periodic-acid-Schiff techniques in the study of blood and bone marrow cells, Brit. J. Haemat. 6:231, 1960.
110. Heiner, D. C., and Kevy, S. V.: Visceral larva migrans, New Eng. J. Med. 254:629, 1956.
111. Hildebrand, F. L., Christensen, N. A., and Hanlon, D. G.: Eosinophilia of unknown cause, Arch. Intern. Med. 113:129, 1964.
112. Hirsch, J. G.: Cinemicrophotographic observations on granule lysis in polymorphonuclear leukocytes during phagocytosis, J. Exp. Med. 116:827, 1962.
113. Hoga, T., and Laszlo, J.: Döhle bodies and other granulocytic alterations during chemotherapy with cyclophosphamide, Blood 20:668, 1962.
114. Holman, H.: Systemic lupus erythematosus; a review of certain recent developments in the study of this disease, J. Pediat. 56:109, 1960.
115. Holman, H. R., and Kunkel, H. G.: Affinity between the lupus erythematosus serum factor and cell nuclei and nucleoprotein, Science 126:162, 1957.
116. Holmes, B., Page, A. R., and Good, R. A.: Studies of the metabolic activity of leukocytes from patients with a genetic abnormality of phagocytic function, J. Clin. Invest. 46:1422, 1967.
117. Holmes, B., Quie, P. G., Windhorst, D. B., and Good, R. A.: Fatal granulomatous disease of childhood; an inborn abnormality of phagocytic function, Lancet 1:1225, 1966.
118. Howqua, J., and Mackay, I. R.: L. E. cells in lymphoma, Blood 22:191, 1963.
119. Huber, H., Douglas, S. D., and Fudenberg, H. H.: The IgG receptor; an immunological marker for the characterization of mononuclear cells, Immunology 17:7, 1969.
120. Huehns, E. R., Lutzner, M., and Hecht, F.: Nuclear abnormalities of the neutrophils in D (13-15) trisomy syndrome, Lancet 1:589, 1964.
121. Humble, J. G.: The treatment of aplastic anemia with phytohaemagglutinin, Lancet 1:1345, 1964.
122. Hungerford, G. F., and Karson, E. F.: The eosinophilia of magnesium deficiency, Blood 16:1642, 1962.
123. Janeway, C. A., and Gitlin, D.: The gamma globulins. In Levine, S. Z., editor: Advances in pediatrics, vol. 9, Chicago, 1957, Year Book Medical Publishers, Inc., p. 65.,
124. Johnston, R. B., Jr.: Screening test for the diagnosis of chronic granulomatous disease, Pediatrics 43:122, 1969.
125. Johnston, R. B., Jr., and Janeway, C. A.: The child with frequent infections; diagnostic considerations, Pediatrics 43:596, 1969.
126. Jordans, G. H. W.: Hereditary granulation anomaly of the leucocytes (Alder), Acta Med. Scandinav. 129:348, 1947.
127. Kaplow, L. S.: A histochemical procedure for localizing and evaluating leukocyte alkaline phosphatase activity in smears of blood and bone marrow, Blood 10:1023, 1955.
128. Kauder, E., Kahle, L. L., Moreno, H., and Partin, J. C.: Leukocyte degranulation and vacuole formation in patients with chronic granulomatous disease of childhood, J. Clin. Invest. 47:1753, 1968.
129. Kent, G., Minick, O. T., Voline, F. I., and Orfer, E.: Autophagic vacuoles in human red cells, Amer. J. Path. 48:831, 1966.
130. Klebanoff, S. J., and White, L. R.: Iodination defect in the leukocytes of a patient

with chronic granulomatous disease of childhood, New Eng. J. Med. 280:460, 1969.
131. Kritzler, R. A., Terner, J. Y., Lindenbaum, J., Magidson, J., Williams, R., Praisig, R., and Phillips, G. B.: Chediak-Higashi syndrome; cytologic and serum lipid observations in a case and family, Amer. J. Med. 36:583, 1964.
132. Lalezari, P., Nussbaum M., Gelman, S., and Spaet, T. H.: Neonatal neutropenia due to maternal isoimmunization, Blood 15:236, 1960.
133. Landing, B. H., and Shirkey, H. S.: Syndrome of recurrent infection and infiltration by viscera by pigmented lipid histiocytes, Pediatrics 20:431, 1957.
134. Landing, B. H., Silverman, F. N., Craig, J. M., Jacoby, M. D., Lahey, M. E., and Chadwick, D. L.: Familial neurovisceral lipidosis, Amer. J. Dis. Child. 108:503, 1964.
135. Lanzkowsky, P., Colussi, P., and McKenzie, D.: Pelger-Huët anomaly of the granulocytes in a Cape colored family, J. Pediat. 67:826, 1965.
136. Lapin, J., and Horonick, A.: Ameboid motility of human leukocytes, Blood 11:225, 1956.
137. Lawrence, J. S.: Physiology and functions of the white blood cells, J.A.M.A. 157:1212, 1955.
138. Lehndorff, H.: Transitorische Granulocytopenie beim Neugeborenen, Helvet. Paediat. Acta 6:173, 1951.
139. Leitner, S., Neumark, E., and Herres, P.: Panmyelopathy with Döhle bodies, thrombocytopenia and erythroblastosis (Hegglin's syndrome), Acta Haemat. (Basel) 11:321, 1954.
140. Lichtenstein, L.: Histiocytosis X; integration of eosinophilic granuloma of bone, "Letterer-Siwe disease," and "Schüller-Christian disease" as related manifestations of a single nosologic entity, Arch. Path. 56:84, 1953.
141. Maldonado, J. E., Bayrd, E. D., and Kiely, J. M.: The thymus gland and its relationship to the hematopoietic and immunologic systems; a review, Mayo Clinic Proc. 39:60, 1964.
142. Mallory, T. B.: Pathology; diseases of bone, New Eng. J. Med. 227:955, 1942.
143. Mandell, G. L., and Hook, E. W.: Leukocyte function in chronic granulomatous disease of childhood; studies on seventeen year old boy, Amer. J. Med. 47:473, 1969.
144. Marks, P. A., and Gross, R. T.: Erythrocyte glucose-6-phosphate dehydrogenase deficiency; evidence of differences between Negroes and Caucasians with respect to this genetically determined trait, J. Clin. Invest. 38:2253, 1959.
145. Marks, P. A., Gross, R. T., and Hurwitz, R. E.: Gene action in erythrocyte deficiency of glucose-6-phosphate dehydrogenase; tissue enzyme-levels, Nature 83:1266, 1959.
146. Marsh, J. A., and Perry S.: The granulocyte response to endotoxin in patients with hematologic disorders, Blood 23:581, 1964.
147. Mathis, H. B.: A simple office procedure for demonstrating lupus erythematosus cells in peripheral blood, Blood 6:470, 1951.
148. Matoth, Y.: Phagocytic and ameboid activities of the leukocytes in the newborn infant, Pediatrics 9:748, 1952.
149. Mauer, A. M., Athens, J. W., Ashenbrucker, H., Cartwright, G. E., and Wintrobe, M. M.: Leukokinetic studies. II. A method for labeling granulocytes in vitro with radioactive diisopropylfluorophosphate (DEP$^{32}$), J. Clin. Invest. 39:1481, 1960.
150. McCall, M. S., Sutherland, D. A., Eisentraut, A., and Lanz, H.: The tagging of leukemic leukocytes with radioactive chromium and measurement of the in vivo cell survival, J. Lab. Clin. Med. 45:717, 1955.
151. Menken, V.: The determination of the level of leukocytes in the blood stream with inflammation; a thermostable component concerned in the mechanism of leukocytosis, Blood 4:1323, 1949.
152. Michael, S. R., Vural, I. L., Bassen, F. A., and Schaefer, L.: Hematologic aspects of disseminated (systemic) lupus erythematosus, Blood 6:1059, 1951.
153. Michels, N. A.: The plasma cell, Arch. Path. 11:775, 1931.
154. Miescher, P.: Nucléophagocytose et phénomène L. E., Schwiez, med. Wchnschr. 83:1042, 1953.
155. Millard, R. E.: Effect of previous irradiation on the transformation of blood lymphocytes, J. Clin. Path. 18:783, 1965.
156. Miller, D. R., and Kaplan, H. G.: Decreased nitroblue tetrazolium dye reduction in the phagocytes of patients receiving prednisone, Pediatrics 45:861, 1970.
157. Miller, G. L.: Clinical significance of the blood in tuberculosis, New York, 1943, Commonwealth Fund.
158. Miller, J. F. A. P.: Immunological function of the thymus, Lancet 2:748, 1961.
159. Miller, J. F. A. P.: Annotation; the role of blood cells in immunity, Brit. J. Haemat. 16:331, 1969.
160. Miller, J. L., Brodey, M., and Hill, J. H.: Studies on significance of biologic false-positive reactions, J.A.M.A. 164:1461, 1957.
161. Miller, M. E.: Phagocytosis in the newborn infant; humoral and cellular factors, J. Pediat. 74:255, 1969.
162. Mitchell, B.: Basophilic leukocytes in chil-

dren in health and disease, Arch. Dis. Child. 33:193, 1958.
163. Mittwoch, U.: Abnormal lymphocytes in gargoylism, Brit. J. Haemat. 5:365, 1959.
164. Mittwoch, U.: Inclusions of mucopolysaccharides in the lymphocytes of patients with gargoylism, Nature 191:1315, 1961.
165. Moeschlin, S., and Wagner, K.: Agranulocytosis due to occurrence of leukocyteagglutinins (Pyramidon and cold agglutinins), Acta Haemat. 8:29, 1952.
166. Moeschlin, S., Meyer, H., Israels, L. B., and Tarr-Gloor, E.: Experimental agranulocytosis; its production through leukocyte agglutination by anti-leukocytic serum, Acta Haemat. 11:73, 1954.
167. Moore, J. E., and Lutz, W. B.: The natural history of systemic lupus erythematosus; an approach to its study through chronic biologic false positive reactors, J. Chron. Dis. 1:297, 1955.
168. Moore, J. E., Shulman, L. E., and Scott, J. T.: The natural history of systemic lupus erythematosus; an approach to its study through chronic biologic false positive reactors, J. Chron. Dis. 5:282, 1957.
169. Moore, T. D.: A simple technique for the diagnosis of nonlipid histiocytosis, Pediatrics 19:438, 1957.
170. Morse, J. H., Müller-Eberhard, H. J., and Kunkel, H. G.: Antinuclear factors and serum complement in systemic lupus erythematosus, Bull. N. Y. Acad. Med. (2nd ser.) 38:641, 1962.
171. Muggia, F. M., Heinemann, H. O., Farhangi, M., and Osserman, E. F.: Lysozymuria and renal tubular dysfunction in monocytic and myelomoncytic leukemia, Amer. J. Med. 47:351, 1969.
172. Muir, H., Mittwoch, U., and Bitter, T.: The diagnostic value of isolated urinary polysaccharides and the lymphocyte inclusions in gargoylism, Arch. Dis. Child. 38:358, 1963.
173. Naiman, J. L., Oski, F. A., Allen, F. H., Jr., and Diamond, L. K.: Hereditary eosinophilia; report of a family and review of the literature, Amer. J. Human Genet. 16:195, 1964.
174. Nowell, P. C.: Phytohemagglutinin; an initiator of mitosis in cultures of normal human leukocytes, Cancer Res. 20:462, 1966.
175. Oh, M-H. K., Rodey, G. E., Good, R. A., Chilgren, R. A., and Quie, P. G.: Defective condidacidal capacity of polymorphonuclear leukocytes in chronic granulomatous disease of childhood, J. Pediat. 75:300, 1969.
176. Orchard, N. P.: Letterer-Siwe's syndrome; report of a case with unusual peripheral blood changes, Arch. Dis. Child. 25:151, 1950.
177. Osgood, E. E., Li, J. G., Tivey, H., Duerst, M. L., and Seaman, A. J.: Growth of human leukemic leukocytes in vitro and in vivo as measured by uptake of $P^{32}$ in DNA, Science 114:95, 1951.
178. Osgood, E. E., Seaman, A. J., Tivey, H., and Regas, D. A.: Duration of life and of different stages of maturation of normal and leukemic leukocytes, Rev. Hèmat. 9:543, 1954.
179. Osgood, E. E., Tivey, H., Davison, K. B., Seaman, A. J., and Li, J. G.: Relative rates of formation of new leukocytes in patients with acute and chronic leukemias; measured by uptake of radioactive phosphorus in isolated desoxyribosenucleic acid, Cancer 5:331, 1952.
180. Oski, F. A., Naiman, L. R., Allen, D. M., and Diamond, L. K.: Leukocytic inclusions—Döhle bodies—associated with platelet abnormality (the May-Hegglin anomaly); report of a family and review of the literature, Blood 20:657, 1962.
181. Osserman, E. F., and Lawlor, D. P.: Serum and urinary lysozyme (muramidase) in monocytic and monomyelocytic leukemia, J. Exp. Med. 124:921, 1966.
182. Ottesen, J.: On the age of human white cells in peripheral blood, Acta Physiol. Scandinav. 32:75, 1954.
183. Padawer, J.: Studies on mammalian mast cells, Trans. N. Y. Acad. Sci. 19:690, 1957.
184. Page, A. R., Berendes, H., Warner, J., and Good, R. A.: The Chediak-Higashi syndrome, Blood 20:330, 1962.
185. Page, A. R., Condie, R. M., and Good, R. A.: Suppression of plasma cell hepatitis with 6-mercaptopurine, Amer. J. Med. 36:200, 1964.
186. Page, A. R., and Good, R. A.: Studies on cyclic neutropenia; a clinical and experimental investigation, Amer. J. Dis. Child. 94:623, 1957.
187. Paglia, D. E., Holland, P., Baughan, M. A., and Valentine, W. N.: Occurrence of defective hexosephosphate isomerization in human erythrocytes and leukocytes, New Eng. J. Med. 280:66 1971.
188. Park, B. H.: The use and limitations of the nitroblue tetrazolium test as a diagnostic aid, J. Pediat. 78:376, 1971.
189. Payne, R.: The development and persistence of leukoagglutinins in various women, Blood 19:411, 1962.
190. Payne, R., and Rolfs, M.: Further observations on leukoagglutinin transfusion reactions, Amer. J. Med. 29:449, 1960.
191. Payne, R., Rolfs, M. R., Tripp, M., and Weigle, J.: Neonatal neutropenia and leukoagglutinins, Pediatrics 33:194, 1964.
192. Pearse, A. G. E.: The nature of Russell bodies and Kurloff bodies, J. Clin. Path. 2:81, 1949.

193. Pearson, H. A., and Lorincz, A. E.: A characteristic bone marrow finding in the Hurler syndrome, Pediatrics 34:280, 1964.
194. Perillie, P. E., Kaplan, S. S., Lefkowitz, E., Rogoway, W., and Finch, S. C.: Studies of muramidase (lysozyme) in leukemia, J.A.M.A. 203:317, 1968.
195. Perry, S.: Biochemistry of the white blood cell, J.A.M.A. 190:918, 1964.
196. Perry, S., Craddock, C. G., Jr., Lutz, V., Crepaldi, G., and Lawrence, J. S.: Rate of production of $P^{32}$-labeled lymphocytes, Blood 14:50, 1959.
197. Perry, S., and Reynolds, J.: Methyl-green-pyronin as a differential nucleic acid stain for peripheral blood smears, Blood 11:1132, 1956.
198. Perry, S., Weinstein, I. M., Craddock, C. G., Jr., and Lawrence, J. S.: The combined use of typhoid vaccine and $P^{32}$ labeling to assess myelopoiesis, Blood 12:549, 1957.
199. Pisciotta, A. V., and Daly, M.: Studies on agranulocytosis. III. The reduced glutathione (GSH) content of leukocytes of normals and patients recovered from agranulocytosis, Blood 16:1572, 1960.
200. Pollak, V. E.: Antinuclear antibodies in families of patients with systemic lupus erythematosus, New Eng. J. Med. 271:165, 1964.
201. Quie, P. G.: Intracellular killing of bacteria, New Eng. J. Med. 280:502, 1969.
202. Ramot, B., Fisher, S., Szeinberg, A., Adam, A., Sheba, C., and Gafni, D.: A study of subjects with erythrocyte glucose-6-phosphate dehydrogenase deficiency. II. Investigation of leukocyte enzymes, J. Clin. Invest. 38:2234, 1959.
203. Rebuck, J. W., and Crowley, J. H.: A method of Rebuck; studying leukocytic functions in vivo, Ann. N. Y. Acad. Sci. 59:757, 1955.
204. Reilly, W. A.: The granules in the leukocytes in gargoylism, Amer. J. Dis. Child. 62:489, 1941.
205. Ribas-Mundo, M.: DNA replication patterns of normal human leukocyte cultures; time sequence of DNA synthesis in relation to the $H^3$-thymidine incorporation over the nucleolus, Blood 28:891, 1966.
206. Riley, J. F.: Heparin, histamine and mast cells, Blood 9:1123, 1954.
207. Roberts, W. C., Liegler, D. G., and Carbone, P. P.: Endomyocardial disease and eosinophilia; a clinical and pathologic spectrum, Amer. J. Med. 46:28, 1969.
208. Rosen, F. S.: The lymphocyte and the thymus gland; congenital and hereditary abnormalities, New Eng. J. Med. 279:643, 1968.
209. Rosen, F. S., Gitlin, D., and Janeway, C. A.: Alymphocytosis, agammaglobulinaemia, homografts and delayed hypersensitivity; study of a case, Lancet 2:380, 1962.
210. Rosenfeld, S., Swiller, A. I., and Morrison, M.: Simple method of demonstrating the L.E. cell by finger puncture, J.A.M.A. 155:568, 1954.
211. Rosenthal, K., Dreskin, O. H., Vural, I. L., and Zak, F. G.: The significance of hematogones in blood, bone marrow and lymph node aspiration in giant follicular lymphoblastoma, Acta Haemat. 8:368, 1952.
212. Ross, S. W., and Wells, B. B.: Systemic lupus erythematosus; a review of literature, Amer. J. Clin. Path. 23:139, 1953.
213. Rosse, W. F., and Gurney, C. W.: The Pelger-Huët anomaly in three families and its use in determining the disappearance of transfused neutrophils from the peripheral blood, Blood 14:170, 1959.
214. Rowley, D. A., and Benditt, E. P.: 5-hydroxytryptamine and histamine as mediators of the vascular injury produced by agents which damage mast cells in rats, J. Exp. Med. 103:399, 1956.
215. Sabine, J. C., Jung, E. D., Fish, M. B., Pestaner, L. C., and Rankin, R. E.: Observations on the inheritance of glucose-6-phosphate dehydrogenase deficiency in erythrocytes and in leucocytes, Brit. J. Haemat. 9:164, 1963.
216. Saraiva, L. G., Azevedo, M., Correa, J. M., Carvallo, G., and Prospero, J. D.: Anomalous panleukocytic granulation, Blood 14:1112, 1959.
217. Schneider, A. S., Valentine, W. N., Hattori, M., and Heins, H. L., Jr.: Hereditary hemolytic anemia with triosephosphate isomerase deficiency, New Eng. J. Med. 272:229, 1965.
218. Seip, M.: Systemic lupus erythematosus in pregnancy with haemolytic anaemia, leucopenia and thrombocytopenia, in the mother and her newborn infant, Arch. Dis. Child. 35:364, 1960.
219. Seligmann, M., Fudenberg, H. H., and Good, R. A.: Editorial. A proposed classification of primary immunologic deficiencies, Amer. J. Med. 45:817, 1968.
220. Shelley, W. B., and Juhlin, L.: Functional cytology of the human basophil in allergic and physiologic reactions; technic and atlas, Blood 19:208, 1962.
221. Silver, H. K., Henderson, P., and Contopoulos, A.: Extreme eosinophilia, increased blood heterophile-agglutination titer, and hyperglobulinemia, Amer. J. Dis. Child. 83:649, 1952.
222. Silverstein, S.: Macrophages and viral immunity, Seminars Hemat. 7:185, 1970.
223. Smith, C. H.: The leukocytic reaction in

224. tuberculosis of infancy and childhood, Amer. J. Med. Sci. **182**:221, 1931.
224. Smith, C. H.: The anemias of early infancy, J. Pediat. **16**:375, 1940.
225. Smith, H. D., and Beaver, P. C.: Visceral larva migrans due to infection with dog and cat ascarides, Ped. Clin. N. Amer. **2**:163, 1955.
226. Speirs, R. S.: Physiological approaches to an understanding of the function of eosinophils and basophils, Ann. N. Y. Acad. Sci. **59**:706, 1955.
227. Stedman, E., and Stedman, E.: The cytological interpretation of the Feulgen reaction, Biochem. J. **47**:508, 1950.
228. Steinberg, B., and Marten, R. A.: Plasma factor increasing circulatory leukocytes, Amer. J. Physiol. **161**:14, 1950.
229. Strouth, J. C., Zeman, W., and Merritt, A. D.: Leukocyte abnormalities in familiar amaurotic idiocy, New Eng. J. Med. **274**:36, 1966.
230. Tan, C., Etcubanas, E., Lieberman, P., Isenberg, H., King, O., and Murphy, M. L.: Chediak-Higashi syndrome in a child with Hodgkin's disease, Amer. J. Dis. Child. **121**:135, 1971.
231. Taylor, A. I.: 13-15 trisomy in arrhinencephaly, Lancet **1**:149, 1966.
232. Taysi, K., Kistenmacher, M. L., Punnett, H. H., and Mellman, W., Jr.: Limitations of metachromasia as a diagnostic aid in pediatrics, New Eng. J. Med. **281**:1108, 1969.
233. Tenczar, F. J., and Streitmatter, D. E.: Sex difference in neutrophils, Amer. J. Clin. Path. **26**:384, 1956.
234. Terasaki, P. I., Mottironi, V. D., and Barnett, E. V.: Cytotoxins in disease; autocytoxins in lupus, New Eng. J. Med. **283**:724, 1970.
235. Thatcher, L. G., and Smith, N. J.: Granulocyte responses of children to bacterial endotoxin, J. Pediat. **62**:484, 1963.
236. The lupus erythematosus test, queries and minor notes, J.A.M.A. **151**:1460, 1953.
237. Thiery, J. P.: Microcinematographic contributions to the study of plasma cells. In Wolstenholme, G. E. W., and O'Connor, C. M., editors: Cellular aspects of immunity, Boston, 1959, Little, Brown & Co.
238. Thorn, G. W., Forsham, P. H., Prunty, F. T. G. and Hills, A. G.: A test for adrenal cortical insufficiency; the response to pituitary adrenocorticotropic hormone, J.A.M.A. **137**:1005, 1948.
239. Tullis, J. R.: Leukocyte and thrombocyte antibodies; current concepts of their origin, identity and of significance, J.A.M.A. **180**:136, 1962.
240. Ullrich, O., and Wiedemann, H. R.: Promyelozyten-erythrophagie, Acta Haemat. **11**:134, 1954.
241. Underitz, E.: Eine neue Sippe mit Erblich-Konstitutioneller Hochsegmentierung der Neutrophilenkerne, Schweiz. Med. Wchnschr. **88**:1000, 1958.
242. Valentine, W. N., Hsieh, H-S., Paglia, D. E., Anderson, H. M., Baughan, M. A., Jaffe, E. R., and Garson, O. M.: Hereditary hemolytic anemia associated with phosphoglycerate kinase deficiency in erythrocytes and leukocytes, New Eng. J. Med. **280**:528, 1969.
243. Valentine, W. N., Schneider, A. S., Baughan, M. A., Paglia, D. E., and Heins, H. L., Jr.: Hereditary hemolytic anemia with triose phosphate isomerase deficiency; studies in kindreds with coexistent sickle cell trait and erythrocyte glucose-6-phosphate dehydrogenase deficiency, Amer. J. Med. **41**:27, 1966.
244. Van der Sar, A.: The Pelger-Huët familial nuclear anomaly of the leucocytes, Amer. J. Clin. Path. **14**:544, 1954.
245. van Furth, R.: Origin and kinetics of monocytes and macrophages, Seminars Hemat. **7**:125, 1970.
246. Walsh, J. R., and Zimmerman, H. J.: Demonstration of "L.E." phenomenon in patients with penicillin hypersensitivity, Blood **8**:651, 1953.
247. Wassmuth, D. R., Hamilton, H. E., and Sheets, R. F.: May-Hegglin anomaly; hereditary affection of granulocytes and platelets, J.A.M.A. **183**:737, 1963.
248. Waters, W. J., and Lacson, P. S.: Mast cell leukemia presenting as urticaria pigmentosa; report of a case, Pediatrics **19**:1033, 1957.
249. Watkins, C. H., and Hall, B. E.: Monocytic leukemia of the Naegele and Schilling types, Amer. J. Clin. Path. **10**:387, 1940.
250. Weiner, W., and Topley, E.: Döhle bodies in the leucocytes of patients with burns, J. Clin. Path. **8**:324, 1955.
251. Weissman, G.: Lysosomes, Blood **24**:594, 1964.
252. Welsh, R. A.: Electron microscopic localization of Russell bodies in human plasma cells, Blood **16**:1307, 1960.
253. White, A.: Influence of endocrine secretions on the structure and function of lymphoid tissue, Harvey Lect., p. 43, 1947-1948.
254. White, J. G.: The Chediak-Higashi syndrome; a possible lysosomal disease, Blood **28**:143, 1966.
255. White, J. G.: Fine structural demonstration of acid phosphatase activity in Auer bodies, Blood **29**:667, 1967.
256. Wiedemann, H. R.: Beiträge zur Pfaundler-Hurlerschen Krankheit, Ztschr. Kinderh. **70**:81, 1951.

257. Wiernick, P. H., and Serpick, A. A. Clinical significance of serum and urinary muramidase activity in leukemia and other hematologic malignancies, Amer. J. Med. 46:330, 1969.
258. Wilson, R. M., Abbott, R. R., and Miller, D. K.: The occurrence of L.E. cells and hematoxylin bodies in the naturally occurring cutaneous lesions of systemic lupus erythematosus, Amer. J. Med. Sci. 241:31, 1961.
259. Windhorst, D. B., Zelickson, A. S., and Good, R. A.: Chediak-Higashi syndrome; herereditary gigantism of cytoplasmic organelles, Science 151:81, 1966.
260. Wolman, B.: The function of the adrenal glands in the newborn, Arch. Dis. Child. 27:283, 1952.
261. Wolman, M. Sterk, V. V., Gath, S., and Frenkel, M.: Primary familial xanthomatosis with involvement and calcification of the adrenals, Pediatrics 28:742, 1961.
262. Woo, T. A., and Frenkel, E. P.: The atypical lymphocyte, Amer. J. Med. 42:923, 1967.
263. Zimmerman, H. J., Walsh, J. R., and Heller, P.: Production of nucleophagocytosis by rabbit and antileukocytic serum, Blood 8:651, 1953.
264. Zinkham, W. H., and Conley, D. D.: Some factors influencing the formation of L.E. cells; a method of enhancing L.E. cell production, Bull. Johns Hopkins Hosp. 98:102, 1956.
265. Zinkham, W. H., and Diamond, L. K.: In vitro erythrophagocytosis in acquired hemolytic anemia, Blood 7:592, 1952.
266. Zuelzer, W. W., and Apt. L.: Disseminated visceral lesions associated with extreme eosinophilia, Amer. J. Dis. Child. 78:153, 1949.

# 19 LEUKOPENIA AND LEUKOPENIC SYNDROMES

Leukopenia denotes the condition in which the number of circulating white blood cells is below 4,000 per cubic millimeter, without reference to the type of leukocyte involved. Except when the leukocyte count is exceedingly low and all types of white blood cells are reduced, leukopenia is usually due to a reduction in the neutrophils. Infrequently, the lymphocytes are markedly reduced, resulting in alymphocytosis.[17] On the other hand, in some instances there may be neutropenia without leukopenia. This is seen occasionally in serial white blood counts of patients with many conditions of protracted leukopenia, although the granulocytes are consistently reduced. In such an event the bulk of cells are made up of lymphocytes, occasionally with monocytes.

*Pathogenesis.* Leukopenia is brought about by a variety of mechanisms.[43,48] These include diminished manufacture of white blood cells as a result of simple inhibition (e.g., overwhelming infection, septicemia),[6] maturation arrest (i.e., agranulocytosis), aplasia of the marrow (i.e., aplastic anemia), damage or destruction of leukocyte-forming tissue (such as that caused by chemical and physical agents), destruction or inhibitory effect of the spleen on granulocytes (i.e., splenic neutropenia), or direct action on the peripheral blood by leukocyte agglutinins. A redistribution of the white cells conceivably also may cause peripheral leukopenia by withdrawing granulocytes from vascular channels to localized areas of pus formation. Replacement of the bone marrow by leukemic or neoplastic cells or by cells of entities such as Gaucher's or Hodgkin's disease results in leukopenia in some phase of the respective diseases. The cause is unknown but has been attributed to crowding of myeloid tissue or a disturbance of local metabolism by the rapid multiplication of invading cells. In some cases the concept of hypersplenism is involved.

Leukocyte agglutinating factors responsible for the production of agranulocytosis and leukopenia have been demonstrated in the serum of patients. The formation of antibodies capable of agglutinating white blood cells in the bloodstream has led to the concept of immunogranulocytosis or immunoleukopenia. This phenomenon is comparable to autoimmune mechanisms involved in the production of certain types of idiopathic hemolytic anemia and thrombopenic purpura. Antileukocyte activity has been demonstrated in the sera from patients with a wide variety of hematologic diseases with leukopenia, especially in those with a hyperplastic marrow.[76] The majority of these agglutinins are blood group specific, and a small percentage are nonspecific (globulins).[53] This agglutinating mechanism has been applied to the leukopenic effect of drugs and chemicals,[54] to idiopathic immunoneutropenia,[47] and to the development of the L.E. phenomenon in disseminated lupus erythematosus.[20] Transitory granulocytopenia of the newborn infant (neonatal agranulocytosis) has also been explained on the basis of immunoleukopenia.[45,55] Leukoagglutinins occur more frequently among persons who have had transfusions, especially repeated transfusions—hence the possibility that they represent antibodies to antigens of leukocytes.[60]

*Bone marrow.* Although the bone marrow reflects the state of granulopoiesis, the bone marrow findings cannot always be correlated with those in the peripheral blood. The combined examination is necessary, however, for interpretation and management of a leukopenic condition.

The bone marrow ranges from the normal to a maturation arrest at the promyelocytic level. The variability depends upon the stage, duration, and severity of the disease when the bone marrow is examined. Thus the peripheral leukopenia of severe infection may be unassociated with alteration of the bone marrow, and the reason for the leukopenia is unexplained. On the other hand, in patients with chronic neutropenia the bone marrow may reveal few myelocytes, promyelocytes, and infrequent myeloblasts with an increase in reticular cells, lymphoid cells, and plasma cells. In other cases a true maturation arrest occurs with striking hyperplasia of early myelocytes with a conspicuous absence of mature granulocytes.

*Tests for bone marrow function.* The injection of epinephrine is said to induce a redistribution of granulocytes in the blood by causing a shift from the "marginal" to the "circulating" pool. The following tests with pyrogens and etiocholanolone, on the other hand, measure the marrow granulocyte reserve and in leukopenia especially provide important information of the bone marrow components. In chronic benign granulocytopenia, for instance, the knowledge of existing reserves in the marrow of immature granulocytes contributes to a favorable prognosis.

The dose of Lipexal (Pyrexal, the purified extract from *Salmonella abortus equi*) is 0.8 to 5.0 mg./kg. given intravenously. The total granulocyte increment with this method is 2,800 to 8,500 cells per cu. mm.[38]

Another method for demonstrating bone marrow granulocyte reserves is by the use of etiocholanolone.[24] This substance is a naturally occurring steroid metabolite which has been shown to cause leukocytosis consisting of polymorphonuclear neutrophils after its intramuscular administration. The granulocytes mobilized in response to etiocholanolone come from the bone marrow reserve. The minimum time required for a myelocyte to mature to a polymorphonuclear neutrophil is 72 hours. Once the neutrophil stage is reached, cells usually remain in the bone marrow pool for 24 hours or more before release into the peripheral blood. These cells constitute the marrow granulocyte reserve and are available for mobilization to the functional pool. Etiocholanolone induces peripheral blood granulocytosis by stimulating the release of mature cells from the bone marrow granulocyte reserve.

An intramuscular dose of 0.2 mg. per kg. results in a mean maximum granulocyte increase of 9,100 cells per cu. mm. with a minimum increment of 2,600 cells per cu. mm.[78] Granulocytes reach a maximum approximately 12 hours after injection and then remain relatively constant for a subsequent 7 to 8 hours.

Bone marrow response to local stimuli can also be studied by the Rebuck skin-window (see Chapter 18). A modified method has been described.[83] On abrasions made in the forearm a drop of typhoid vaccine or purified tuberculin protein is placed, and the denuded areas are covered with Wright's stain and examined for cellular composition of the exudate. Normal controls show an exudate rich in polymorphonuclear leukocytes during the early hours of the test, followed by a predominately monocytic exudate. In two cases of chronic benign granulocytopenia the exudate was virtually acellular during the first few hours. Later, moderate numbers of monocytes appeared. In one, no granulocytes were seen at any time; in another, an occasional band form was noted.

The serum unsaturated $B_{12}$-binding capacity has also been demonstrated to serve as a simple index of the total blood granulocyte pool.[12]

*Causes.* These may be summarized as follows:

1. Infections
   a. Bacterial
   b. Viral
   c. Miscellaneous
      (1) Protozoal
      (2) Rickettsial
   d. Overwhelming
2. Chemicals, drugs, and physical agents
   a. Irradiation
   b. Therapeutic agents in systemic and blood diseases
3. Miscellaneous
   a. With blood disorders
      (1) Agranulocytosis
      (2) Aplastic anemia and leukemia
      (3) Hypoplastic anemia and leukopenia
      (4) Periodic (cyclic) neutropenia
      (5) Chronic hyoplastic neutropenia
      (6) Chronic benign granulocytopenia in childhood
      (7) Infantile genetic agranulocytosis
      (8) Neonatal agranulocytosis
   b. Involving the spleen
      (1) Primary and secondary splenic neutropenia
   c. Nutritional deficiencies
   d. Immunoneutropenia

*Infections.* A persistent leukopenia may indicate a serious prognosis in the presence of certain infections in which leukocytosis ordinarily is expected.[75] Its presence is, therefore, of diagnostic value in patients with bacterial infections such as typhoid, paratyphoid, and undulant fever, with certain virus diseases such as influenza, measles, rubella, and primary atypical pneumonia, with protozoal infections such as malaria, and with the early stage of rickettsialpox.

Review of a large series of cases of brucellosis reveals that anemia is not only uncommon but when present is usually mild.[68] In contrast, leukopenia is more frequent and occurs in 10 to 25% of patients. The leukopenia results from decreased numbers of granulocytes. Relative lymphocytosis and often an absolute increase in lymphocytes are found. Thrombocytopenia is rare.

Leukopenia is noted in about one-third of patients with disseminated lupus erythematosus on initial examination and develops subsequently in about one-half, sometimes in the course of the disease.[51] A moderate increase in nonsegmented neutrophils is seen in most patients.

*Chemicals, drugs, and irradiation.* Chemicals and drugs such as anticonvulsants, antimicrobial agents (i.e., chloramphenicol), antithyroid drugs (i.e., thiouracil and its derivatives), tranquilizers,[81] antihistimines (i.e., Pyribenzamine), and sulfonamides are occasionally associated with leukopenia and neutropenia. Exposure to physical agents such as irradiation and to chemicals such as antimetabolites, nitrogen mustards, Myleran, and 6-mercaptopurine, which are employed in the therapy of leukemia and neoplastic disease, can be expected to produce leukopenia and a hypoplastic bone marrow when given in sufficient dosage and over a variable length of time. Depending upon individual susceptibility and duration of exposure, benzol results in leukopenia, agranulocytosis, and a complete picture of aplastic anemia. In hypersensitive persons aminopyrine and related antipyrine may cause serious and even fatal leukopenia and agranulocytosis.

Attention has been focused on an increasing number of reports of agranulocytosis associated with the use of dipyrone. When the causal relationship between aminopyrine (Pyramidon) and agranulocytosis was established in 1935,[37] the use of this drug virtually stopped. Since this drug fell into disrepute certain of its derivatives, notably dipyrone which is the sodium sulfonate derivative of aminopyrine, came into use for its analgesic and antipyretic effects. However, seven deaths, three of them in children, have been attributed to its use.[30]

Not only do these chemicals exert a destructive effect upon myelopoietic cells in the bone marrow, but also, as stated previously with regard to drug-sensitive persons, agglutinins can account for peripheral destruction of leukocytes. According to this concept, bone marrow depletion and exhaustion result secondarily from the accelerated destruction of granulocytes in the peripheral blood.

The lymphocyte is the most radiosensitive of all white blood cells, and the most important change in the white blood cell picture after exposure to radiation is a reduction in the total number of these cells. This is principally due to a decrease in the number of granulocytes which numerically represent the majority of blood cells in the average human being.[44]

*Immunoneutropenia.* Within recent years there has been increasing evidence that cases of granulocytopenia due to a variety of causes may be associated with the formation of leukocyte antibodies. A large amount of literature and numerous methods demonstrating the presence of these antibodies have accumulated.[16,34,79]

Leukocyte agglutinins may be defined as serum factors which, under specified conditions, have the ability to agglutinate leukocytes in vitro. Leukocytes can be used from the individual whose serum is being examined for leukocyte agglutinins (autoagglutinins) or those from another person (isoagglutinins). Leukocyte agglutinins tend to occur with varying frequency after blood transfusions, pregnancy, injections of heterologous serum, in the serum of patients suffering from blood diseases or from splenomegalies, including infectious mononucleosis, leukemia, Hodgkin's disease, paroxysmal nocturnal hemoglobinuria, aplastic anemia, pernicious anemia, collagen diseases such as lupus erythematosus and rheumatoid arthritis, cirrhosis of the liver, chronic idiopathic neutropenia,[11] drug-induced neutropenia with aminopyrine,[54] and after viral infections such as virus pneumonia, hepatitis, and rubella.

The autoleukocyte and isoleukocyte antibodies act as agglutinins and lysins occurring in complete or incomplete forms, and may be complement fixing. A number of techniques have been developed for their demonstration. For technical simplicity the leukocyte agglutination test will prove to be most useful. Another relatively simple method is the antiglobulin consumption test in which leukocytes are exposed to antiglobulin serum and testing for diminution in titer of the antiglobulin serum. Other methods[14] are based on the consumption of complement, fluorescent antiglobulin technique, demonstration of lysis, and precipitation or opsonic activity.

*Miscellaneous.* The miscellaneous causes of leukopenia include a wide variety of conditions.

AGRANULOCYTOSIS. The incidence of fatal agranulocytosis is greater in adults than in children. Secondary neutropenia may occur following the administration of drugs or following infections which damage the bone marrow. Although the disease occurs primarily in adults, greater heed should be given this condition in childhood because of the increasing use of drugs and antimicrobial and antibiotic agents.

Agranulocytosis is an acute febrile disease with a high mortality rate characterized by leukopenia, pronounced reduction in neutrophils, and slight, if any, changes in the red blood cells or platelets. An important clinical feature is the necrotic lesions in the throat and elsewhere. Most cases of agranulocytosis are attributed to the effect of one of a number of drugs in a susceptible person.

The bone marrow usually shows a reduction in the total count of nucleated cells and a depression of the myeloid elements, leaving the red cell precursors and megakaryocytes relatively undisturbed. The pathologic changes in the bone marrow are extremely variable and depend upon the stage of the disease when bone marrow is aspirated. Following injury there is a gradual disappearance of the myeloblasts, promyelocytes, myelocytes, and metamyelocytes and, eventually, of the more mature neutrophilic cells. These elements are replaced in the bone marrow by plasma cells, reticuloendothelial elements, and lymphocytes. Occasionally, in this phase a proliferation of myeloblasts occurs. During recovery and in the patient with the mild form that has not progressed, the less mature myeloid forms reappear and are followed by the segmented neutrophilic cells.

Repeated bone marrow studies are required, however, to guard against a sudden shift to an immature level. In patients with mild injury both promyelocytes and myelocytes are present, and a marked reduction in the more mature elements and an increase in stem cells and lymphocytes require immediate withdrawal of the offending drug. The prognosis, therefore, is favorable if normal numbers of granulocytes are observed in the marrow and is unsatisfactory if only lymphocytes and plasma cells are present.

Since the bone marrow returns to normal before mature granulocytes are liberated in the peripheral blood, prognosis depends upon the cellular composition of the marrow. Except for antimicrobial agents and antibiotics, the effectiveness of the drugs usually prescribed for treatment of agranulocytosis must be correlated with the myelopoietic content of the marrow.

When penicillin or other antibiotics administered to combat infection are found to cause agranulocytosis, recovery from the agranulocytosis following their withdrawal probably is spontaneous and basically depends upon the ability of intrinsic factors supplied by the patient to stimulate granulopoiesis. Severe neutropenia, with a marked increase in the concentration of serum iron, has been reported in an infant receiving 1 gm. of methicillin (in the form of Staphcillin) daily.[49] These changes were reversed when the drug was discontinued.

LEUKOPENIA IN APLASTIC ANEMIA AND LEUKEMIA. In children a persistent neutropenic leukopenia with or without purpura frequently signifies the presence of aplastic anemia or leukemia. One of the most common features of childhood leukemia is the occurrence of leukopenia, with predominance of lymphocytes and a moderate anemia during the course of an unexplained low-grade fever associated with bouts of markedly elevated temperatures. Examination of the peripheral blood normally reveals a sparsity of platelets and occasionally immature white blood cells, whereas bone marrow examination usually demonstrates heavy infiltration with leukemic cells.

PANCREATIC INSUFFICIENCY AND BONE MARROW DYSFUNCTION. Bone marrow hypoplasia with anemia, neutropenia, and marked thrombocytopenia have been reported with pancreatic insufficiency.[71] Pulmonary involvement is absent and the sweat test is normal. The pancreatic insufficiency is unrelated to cystic fibrosis and the neutropenia is associated with bone marrow hypoplasia. Diarrhea and failure to thrive in infancy, elevation in fetal hemoglobin, inconstant galactosuria, and growth retardation are prominent features. Three patients were observed in one family. The neutrophils show a maturation arrest, as evidenced by increased numbers of band forms and polymorphonuclear leukocytes with minimal evidence of segmentation. The disease appears to have a much better prognosis than cystic fibrosis. Hematologic abnormalities did not respond to steroids and vitamin therapy.

In another small series, the patients exhibited an association of exocrine pancreatic insufficiency with variable neutropenia,[70] severe metaphyseal dysostosis, mainly of the hips, and dwarfism. The syndrome appears to be the most common form of exocrine pancreatic insufficiency in infants and children other than cystic fibrosis. Hematologists working in pediatric centers are now aware of this syndrome and are recognizing patients who are initially found to have neutropenia and/or anemia and occasionally thrombocytopenia. None of thirty-six patients whose cases have been reported died in infancy or childhood.

In a child 10 years of age with chronic granulocytopenia, the white count dropped to 850 cells per cubic millimeter on one occasion. The bone marrow, however, revealed scattered blast cells which did not appear in the peripheral blood for many months. During the entire period of early granulocytopenia, the hemoglobin and platelet levels were completely normal. It was not until months later that the full-blown picture of leukemia appeared in the peripheral blood and bone marrow.

HYPOPLASTIC ANEMIA AND LEUKOPENIA. Leukopenia may occur in patients with mild hypoplastic anemia. In one instance fatal idiopathic aplastic anemia occurred in first cousins, and a mild anemia and protracted leukopenia that extended from childhood into adult life was observed in a sister of one of them. In addition to oral ulceration, susceptibility to furunculosis and skin infiltration is common, with intervals of good health between episodes despite the persistent leukopenia. The bone marrow in these patients shows a greater proportion of myeloid cells of all grades of maturity. A similar bone marrow picture was observed in a child with persistent leukopenia and neutropenia in whom febrile episodes occurred when the leukopenia was most marked.

PERIODIC (CYCLIC) NEUTROPENIA. Periodic neutropenia is a rare condition characterized by extreme leukopenia due to the disappearance of neutrophilic granulocytes from the circulating blood at approximately 3-week intervals and occurring at any age period but frequently beginning in infancy and childhood. The agranulocytic periods last 10 days and are associated with the appearance of ulcers in the oral mucous membranes, fever, skin infections, and sore throat. Splenomegaly, adenopathy, arthralgia, abdominal pain, ischiorectal infections, lymphadenitis, and conjunctivitis have also been reported.[59,63] As in patients with other kinds of leukopenia, when the white count is lowest, mouth ulcerations, gingivitis, and often attacks of furunculosis are prone to appear.

In general, the fluctuations of the circulating neutrophils are a reflection of the cyclic changes in the bone marrow. The granulocytes and their precursors may disappear from the bone marrow before the onset of neutropenia and reappear just prior to the return of neutrophils in the peripheral blood.[59] Often, the bone marrow is depleted of mature forms, during the agranulocytic stage, but an abundance of early granulocytic forms constituting a "maturation arrest" is found.

Recurrent neutropenia has been described[56] in a patient with onset of disease in infancy marked by furunculosis, aphthous stomatitis, and fever, who was followed until death as a young adult. The 3-week cycle of neutropenia persisted, with the leukocytes during these episodes numbering 2,000 to 4,000 per cubic millimeter and the granulocytes 6 to 10%.

The pathogenesis of these syndromes, the reason for their periodicity, and the tendency for ulceration of the buccal mucosa have not been explained. No definite relationship to hormonal imbalance or the menstrual cycle has been established. It is not yet clear whether antileukocytic antibodies play a role in causation.[73]

Cyclic or periodic neutropenia is characterized by years of episodes of neutropenia or agranulocytosis, monocytosis, mucosal ulcer, malaise, and fever recurrent every 21 days and lasting 4 to 7 days, alternating with periods of health. These are sometimes grouped as the periodic diseases.[63]

The clinical manifestations nearly always appear before the age of 10 years and tend to recur regularly thereafter. The disease usually runs a benign course, although death due to infection may occur. Splenectomy or administration of adrenal corticosteroids produce slight improvement in some cases. More recently, clinical and hematological improvement followed therapy with testosterone.[9]

A monocytosis has been described in about half of the reported cases of cyclic neutropenia. Occasionally the monocytosis is so great that the total leukocyte count is maintained within normal limits. Morley and co-workers[57] reported twenty cases of cyclical neutropenia from five families. Anemia, eosinophilia, or thrombocytopenia occurred in several patients. The family studies suggest that the disease is transmitted as an autosomal dominant.

Although the disease is usually benign, it varies in severity and has even been fatal. Because of the upsets of hypogammaglobulinemia with cyclic neutropenia the levels of gamma globulin were estimated and found to be normal or increased. Eventually the cycles become less marked and the level at which the white blood cells stabilize may be very low or nearly normal.

CHRONIC HYPOPLASTIC NEUTROPENIA. In chronic hypoplastic neutropenia[73] the course is extremely chronic and marked by repeated infections involving the skin and oral cavity and frequently by symptom-free intervals. Splenomegaly of slight to moderate degree is present in all patients. The marked hypoplasia of granulocytic precursors of the bone marrow and the failure to respond to splenectomy differentiates this condition from primary splenic neutropenia in which granulocytic hyperplasia is present in the marrow and benefit is obtained by splenectomy.

In a case of leukopenia in a young adult, in vitro and in vivo tests indicated the presence of leukocyte agglutinins.[7] The bone marrow revealed normal cellularity and cytology of the elements, except for the fact that the white cell series showed no maturation beyond the stage of metamyelocytes. Splenectomy did not alter the leukopenic course of the blood counts. The leukopenia followed for 5 years has been that of a benign disease characterized only by repeated infections which have been easily controlled for the most part by antibiotics. The author points out that while the immunologic basis is not conclusively proved, there seems to be a parallel between this disease of white cells and idiopathic hemolytic anemia and thrombocytopenic purpura. In another young adult with a similar course, leukoagglutinins were not found.[10] Repeated bone marrow studies showed normal erythroid and megakaryocytic elements. During periods of agranulocytosis there were scattered myelocytes and promyelocytes but no cells maturing beyond this stage. For 1 month splenectomy produced reversion of the blood and bone marrow to normal but neutropenia soon returned.

CHRONIC BENIGN GRANULOCYTOPENIA IN CHILDHOOD. Chronic benign granulocytopenia with leukopenia has been reported frequently. The bone marrow in these patients is usually normal, but in some there is a disturbance in maturation of myelocytes to the segmented forms.[21]

In one small analyzed series[83] the striking feature of the bone marrow was the virtual absence of fully mature, segmented neutrophilic leukocytes which normally account for approximately one-third of the granulocytic population. By contrast the many mature cells, metamyelocytes and band forms, and, at times, earlier precursors were always plentiful. This led to the assumption that mature granulocytes are depleted by increased peripheral destruction, possibly enhanced by sequestration. Several of the patients showed transient leukocytosis associated with a left shift during natural febrile reactions following surgical trauma or acute infection. Between infections the children appeared healthy. The composition of the bone marrow in these cases could be interpreted as a chronic state of depletion of mature leukocytes with a compensatory increase in the marrow in the number of immature granulocytes of all classes. The increased rate of removal of leukocytes from the circulation was only moderate, but sufficient to produce neutropenia resulting in increased susceptibility to infection but not a total lack of resistance. On the other hand, in a 9-year-old girl with chronic granulocytopenia and recurrent infections, the granulocytopenia was attributed to an intrinsic intracellular defect probably on a congenital basis. In this case there was an active myelopoiesis, an accumulation of mature and perhaps hypermature neutrophilic granulocytes in the bone marrow, an impaired release of granulocytes to the blood, and a shortened blood granulocyte survival time.[39]

Spontaneous remissions with eventual recovery may occur in a period of months to years.[19,65,77] In some children there is a lowered resistance to infection, whereas in others neutropenia with leukopenia, which persists for years without causing ill health but with a transient rise of granulocytes with severe infection, is discovered as a chance finding. In one such child the granulocytes numbered below 10%, with white blood counts ranging from those observed in leukopenia to normal counts. This persisted from the ages of 2 to 7 years, with a complete and lasting remission following tonsillectomy. Rarely, chronic neutropenia occurs in several siblings of a family, ranging in severity from the mild to fatal case. Continuous treatment with antibiotics has been recommended as a means of rendering the child with chronic neutropenia free from infections.[50]

A form of this disease has been reported in adults whose course is marked by attacks of severe infection from relatively trivial causes. Cutaneous sepsis and inflammation of the gums, lips, mouth, and throat are common with free intervals of comparative good health.[2] The bone marrow varies from hypoplasia to hyperplasia.

A study of two brothers with chronic neutropenia, possibly caused by a deficiency in the plasma of a factor necessary for myelopoiesis, has been reported.[7] Transfusion of fresh plasma led to short-time normalization of myelopoiesis in one brother. The essential features, in addition to the neutropenia, were chronic gingivitis, delayed healing of cutaneous wounds, and recurring oral and pharyngeal infections.

"Myelokathexis" refers to a type of granulocytopenia in which there is an increased rate of intramedullary death and functional inferiority of mature granulocytes.[82] This phenomenon appeared to be responsible for the retention and accumulation of leukocytes within the bone marrow and a corresponding lack of cells in the circulating blood. In spite of a bone marrow showing abundant mature and hypersegmented polymorphonuclear leukocytes, their reduced viability and functional activity suggested that many of the granulocytes were undergoing death within the bone marrow and the remainder did not enter the peripheral blood as readily as in normal persons, because of reduced motility. Neither prednisone nor splenectomy had any effect on the blood picture. The persistent granulocytopenia was associated with a high degree of susceptibility to infections of the respiratory tract.

In a study of fifteen patients with severe absolute neutropenia of 1 to 19 years' duration, Kyle and Linman[40] found no bone marrow hypoplasia or splenomegaly to account for the neutropenia. The patients in this group showed no increase in frequency of infection. The neutropenia was chronic and did not respond to corticosteroids. This benign condition does not require therapy and should be recognized as such. Leukoagglutinins were found in only two patients. Rebuck skin-window showed a delayed, subnormal neutrophil level at 4 hours. In the differential diagnosis the following conditions were considered and eliminated: hypersplenism, cyclic neutropenia, chronic hypoplastic neutropenia, familial benign chronic neutropenia, and infantile genetic agranulocytosis. In their series, Kyle and Linman encountered no infections; this neutropenia may possibly belong in the group of immunoneutropenias.

Cutting and Lang[13] described a syndrome characterized by consistent neutropenia associated with normal to decreased leukocyte counts, with relative lymphocytosis, monocytosis, and variable eosinophilia. This syndrome occurs as a familial, benign chronic neutropenia and is inherited as a non-sex-linked dominant. The symptoms are mild. Therapeutic measures such as splenectomy and corticosteroids appear to be unnecessary once the diagnosis has been established. The bone marrow shows a normal cellularity. Granulopoiesis is well represented to the myelocyte stages, with a marked reduction in the more mature forms.

INFANTILE GENETIC AGRANULOCYTOSIS. A variant of chronic benign granulocytopenia in childhood is infantile genetic agranulocytosis in which a severe depletion of granulocytes, frequently with leukopenia, is transmitted on the basis of simple recessive inheritance.[36]

In this category are five cases of severe neutropenia of probable congenital origin described by MacGillivray and co-workers.[46] Severe skin sepsis was a prominent clinical feature. The peripheral blood often showed a monocytosis, eosinophilia, and sometimes a raised platelet count. The bone marrow revealed depression of neutrophil granulopoiesis and prominence of eosinophils. All patients had a raised serum gamma globulin. Three died in early infancy; two were alive in early adolescence, but were still neutropenic. The clinical and hematologic features were similar to "infantile genetic agranulocytosis" as described by Kostmann.[36] The condition varies in severity, and apparently patients given suitable antibiotic therapy may survive into adolescence. The cases in this group differ from other cases in their chronicity, high mortality, and the marrow appearance of depression of granulopoiesis.

A 4½-year-old white boy whose illness was classified as infantile genetic agranulocytosis revealed a hypercellular bone marrow affecting the white cell series only.[42] Granulopoiesis was markedly reduced and was represented by myelocytes and earlier forms. There was a complete absence of mature neutrophils and band forms. The blood film showed a neutropenia, lymphocytosis, and monocytosis with vacuolization of the monocytes and toxic granulation. Clinically the patient showed extreme susceptibility to infection.

A case resembling this syndrome, but without evidence of a genetic background,[1] was that of a 2-month-old girl who suffered from infection, starting soon after birth, and revealed an almost complete absence of neutrophilic myeloid elements in the peripheral blood and bone marrow. Death occurred at 5 months due to an overwhelming pulmonary infection. Monocytosis in this and other similar cases, sometimes as high as 50% of cells, has been considered a compensatory mechanism for the depleted phagocytic function. Hypergammaglobulinemia and bone marrow plasmacytosis have also been reported. In this group of cases the agranulocytosis may be associated with varying total numbers of white cells, ranging from leukopenia to moderate and marked leukocytosis.

NEONATAL AGRANULOCYTOSIS. Lubhy and Slobody[45] observed transient agranulocytosis in successive siblings in the neonatal period. Such a circumstance was explained by transplacental isoimmunization of the mother to a leukocyte factor of her infant in a manner analogous to Rh isoimmunization causing hemolytic disease of the newborn infant.[61] In these patients agranulocytosis persisted for 3 to 4 weeks, and in one of the infants it was accompanied by pulmonary infection. The predominance of neutrophilic myelocytes in the bone marrow may represent either a maturation arrest or a depletion of mature cells because of their increased agglutination and destruction in the peripheral blood.

Infants born to mothers with chronic neutropenia have revealed a transitory neutropenia which presumably was caused by the transplacental passage of a neutropenic factor.[74] In one case the mother's serum contained a demonstrable leukoagglutinin which could be transferred by a transfusion of plasma to a normal donor with a resulting severe neutropenia. The neonatal neutropenia persisted for 3 weeks. Hyperplasia of the granulocytic series with a maturation arrest at the myelocytic stage was present in the bone marrow of the affected infants.

In a newborn infant the association of neutropenia and sepsis caused by *Shigella alkalescens* prompted a consideration of the role of infection in the causation of the blood response.[64] Rossi and Brandt[64] pointed out the need for differentiating the causes of neutropenia in the newborn period. To be considered are sepsis of the newborn infant, transient granulocytopenia of the newborn infant, chronic benign neutropenia of infancy and childhood, infantile genetic agranulocytosis, isolated chronic neutropenia, splenic neutropenia, chronic idiopathic immunoneutropenia, and recurrent, cyclic, or periodic neutropenia. The additional role of transplacental acquired maternal leukoagglutinins in the neutropenia was postulated in this case when 8 months postpartum the mother's serum was found to contain agglutinins against the neutrophils of both the baby and the father. Smith and associates[72] suggested that neutropenia of infection may be due to the effect of endotoxin released as the gram-negative bacteria disintegrated.

Multiple cases of neonatal neutropenia occurring in one family were traced to a potent leukoagglutinin found in the maternal serum which agglutinated the leukocytes obtained from the father and three available children.[8,41] On the other hand, leukocyte agglutinins were absent in a patient with severe granulocytopenia associated with infection from 1 week of age which terminated fatally at 13½ months of age.[28] The serum electrophoretic pattern was normal. The bone marrow revealed an arrest at the myelocytic stage.

Female infants with congenital agranulocytosis have been reported.[38,51a] Eosinophilia and monocytosis were found in the blood and bone marrow. The bone marrows were devoid of neutrophilic myelocytes, metamyelocytes, and polymorphonuclear cells. The patients died from sepsis at the age of 7 weeks and 3 months, respectively. At autopsy neutrophils were not evident in any of the tissues examined.

Two white siblings of opposite sex have been reported,[3] both of whom died of congenital neutropenia. The authors suggested the designation of "lethal congenital neutropenia with eosinophilia." There was no plasma cell infiltration of bone marrow and other tissues.

SPLENIC NEUTROPENIA. Primary splenic neutropenia[80] is characterized by profound leukopenia and neutropenia, fever, ulcerations of the mucous membranes, susceptibility to infection, splenomegaly, and myeloid hyperplasia of the bone marrow in which there may be an associated depression of the red cells and platelets. This has been regarded as a form of hypersplenism in which the leukocytes are involved in splenic hyperactivity. Relief of all symptoms results from splenectomy. In patients with secondary splenic neutropenia, leukopenia occurs with disorders involving the spleen such as Banti's disease (portal hypertension), Gaucher's disease, lymphosarcoma, and Hodgkin's disease. It is not yet certain whether the leukopenia in the primary or secondary syndromes results from hypersequestration and hyperdestruction of granulocytes by and within the spleen or from inhibition by the spleen through a hormonal effect or by both mechanisms.

ALYMPHOCYTOSIS. Alymphocytosis is a rare fatal disease occurring in infants and young children[17] which is characterized by fever, hepatosplenomegaly, and leukopenia with an absolute reduction of all types of leukocytes, especially the lymphocytes. Pancytopenia occurs terminally. Postmortem examination reveals a widespread and generalized atrophy and necrosis of lymphoid tissue. Infection with *Candida albicans* (moniliasis) was a common factor in patients reported on.

The suspected presence of agammaglobulinemia in these cases based on pathologic findings[31] has been confirmed by later studies. It is now possible to separate patients with agammaglobulinemia into two groups. One group manifests a persistent lymphopenia and is characterized by the features outlined above for alymphocytosis—i.e., an unremitting course marked by pneumonia, moniliasis, and other infections usually beginning during the first 3 months of life and terminating fatally during the patient's infancy. These patients may demonstrate thymic alymphoplasia and lymphocytic hypoplasia of their tissues; the thymus is rudimentary and other lymphoid structures contain only sparse populations of small lymphocytes.* A child has been described with thymic alymphoplasia, congenital agammaglobulinemia, and congenital alymphocytosis in whom there was a decreased capacity to develop hypersensitivity (such as to *Candida albicans*) and a decreased capacity to reject homografts as has been shown for rats or mice thymectomized at birth.[23]

It is of interest that in major respects patients in this group correspond to the responses of the experimental animal. Thymectomy of the newborn rat[5] or mouse[52] results in severe lymphopenia, generalized deficiency of the small lymphocytes in all the lymphoid tissues and an increased susceptibility to infection, a remarkable tolerance to homografts, and a decreased capacity to develop delayed hypersensitivity.

To summarize, the first group of agammaglobulinemia includes the entity of thymic alymphoplasia.[22] This is a congenital anomaly manifested by a rudimentary thymus, the primitive structure being composed primarily of reticular cells or large thymocytes. It is totally lacking in Hassall's corpuscles, and is entirely devoid of lymphocytes or small thymocytes. This condition normally is accompanied by severe lymphopenia, a generalized marked paucity of lymphocytes in the tissues or lymphocytic hypoplasia, and an increased susceptibility to infection.

In the second group of patients of congenital agammaglobulinemia, symptoms often have a later onset, a more intermittent course of bacterial infections, and a variable leukocyte response marked only occasionally by transitory lymphopenia. Their lymphoid organs, including the thymus, contain more nearly normal numbers of lymphocytes.[23]

NUTRITIONAL DEFICIENCIES. In experimental animals nutritional deficiencies induce leukopenia and granulocytopenia. Leukopenia, granulocytopenia, and occasionally anemia develop in rats fed a purified diet deficient in riboflavin.[18] Folic acid corrects leukopenia, and granulocytopenia can be corrected by the administration of protein.[35] In patients in whom white blood cell regeneration was promoted

---

*See references 15, 22, 29, 52, and 69.

by dietary protein, granulocytes were found to react to a greater degree than lymphocytes and monocytes.[26]

In a study of the neutropenias in childhood, Kauder and Mauer[33] regarded their causation as due to decreased production, increased destruction, or a combination of these defects. Disorders of increased destruction could be separated into intracellular and extracellular mechanisms. Ineffective myelopoiesis was compared to the analagous process in abnormal erythropoiesis. They pointed out that after entering the blood from the bone marrow the neutrophil does not always stay in the circulation but may transiently marginate along vessel walls. These two components of the blood neutrophil population, the circulating and marginating, are about equal in size and are in constant equilibrium.[4]

Some assessment of neutrophil production can be obtained by study of the bone marrow. Relative decreases in marrow myeloid precursors are to be expected in conditions associated with decreased production and compensatory hyperplasia in those diseases characterized by increased cell destruction.

Pseudoneutropenia[33] results from instances where the marginating cells contribute a disproportionate percentage of the total blood granulocyte pool. The true situation could be suspected by demonstrating the mobilization of marginating neutrophils after injection of epinephrin. A more precise demonstration of this sequestration would result from measurement of these compartments with $DF^{32}P$-labeled neutrophils ($^{32}P$-tagged diisopropylfluorophosphate).

*Treatment.* In deciding on treatment, it must be remembered that many diseases such as leukemia, aplastic anemia, disseminated lupus erythematosus, and lymphosarcoma may be preceded by a period of prolonged and undiagnosed leukopenia. One child with neutropenia and repeated respiratory infections who was followed from 3 to 6 years of age eventually succumbed with a pathologic diagnosis of lymphosarcoma. In this patient splenectomy was unsuccessful in altering the blood picture.

The first steps in the treatment of neutropenia should aim toward the elimination of suspected drugs or chemicals and removal of the patient to an environment free from possible exposure to offending agents. In the event of recurrent infections, antibiotics should be prescribed to offset the effect of granulocytopenia, with the hope that myeloid tissue will regenerate spontaneously. Mouth ulcerations require urgent local treatment.

Etiologic agents are usually difficult to ascertain, and the problem of therapy is one of stimulating granulocytic proliferation. Unfortunately, such specific agents are not yet available, and treatment, on the whole, is unsatisfactory. Definitive treatment consists of prophylactic and therapeutic administration of antibiotics and the adrenocortical hormones and splenectomy. None of these measures significantly alters the blood picture of patients with the cyclic or other neutropenias, although ACTH, the steroid hormones, and splenectomy produce some degree of symptomatic relief, especially with respect to fever and oral ulcers. Pentnucleotide, liver extract, vitamins, and bone marrow extracts and leukocytic products have been ineffective in reversing leukopenia and granulocytopenia.[59]

Permanent and spontaneous remissions have been observed after prolonged periods of leukopenia, especially when recurrent infections have been mild. No clear-cut distinction can always be made between clinical syndromes that have in common leukopenia and granulocytopenia. Attempts are usually made to explain the leukopenia on the basis of splenic hyperactivity. Only in patients with primary splenic neutropenia, when all criteria are fulfilled, does removal of the spleen lead to complete recovery.[80] In other patients in whom the bone marrow shows a myelocytic hyperplasia without splenic enlargement, removal of the spleen only rarely results in improvement without altering the basic condition.[66]

## REFERENCES

1. Aarskog, D.: Infantile congenital aneutrocytosis, Arch. Dis. Child. **36**:511, 1961.
2. Adams, E. B., and Witts, L. J.: Chronic agranulocytosis, Quart. J. Med. **18**:173, 1949.
3. Andrews, J. R., McClellan, J. T., and Scott, C. H.: Lethal congenital neutropenia with eosinophilia occurring in two siblings, Amer. J. Med. **29**:358, 1960.
4. Athens, J. W., Raab, S. O., Haab, O. B., Mauer, A. M., Ashenbrucker, H., Cartwright, G. E., and Wintrobe, M.: Leukokinetic studies. III. The distribution of granulocytes in the blood of normal subjects, J. Clin. Invest. **40**:159, 1961.
5. Arnason, G., Janković, B. D., Waksman, B. H., and Wennersten, C.: Role of the thymus in immune reactions in rats. II. Suppressive effect of thymectomy at birth on reactions of

delayed (cellular) hypersensitivity and the circulating small lymphocyte, J. Exp. Med. 116:177, 1962.
6. Bigler, J. A., and Brennenmann, J.: Sepsis with leukopenia (agranulocytosis) in children; report of ten cases, Amer. J. Dis. Child. 40:515, 1939.
7. Bjore, J., Nelson, L. R., and Plum, C. M.: Familial neutropenia possibly caused by deficiency of a plasma factor, Acta Paediat. 51:497, 1962.
8. Braun, E. H., Buckwold, A. E., Emson, H. E., and Russell, A. V.: Familial neonatal neutropenia with maternal leukocyte antibodies, Blood 16:1745, 1960.
9. Brodsky, I., Reimann, H. A., and Dennis, L. H.: Treatment of cyclic neutropenia with testosterone, Amer. J. Med. 38:802, 1965.
10. Browne, E. A., and Marcus, A. J.: Chronic idiopathic neutropenia, New Eng. J. Med. 262:795, 1960.
11. Butler, J. J.: Chronic idiopathic immunoneutropenia, Amer. J. Med. 24:145, 1958.
12. Chikkappa, G., Corcino, J., Greenberg, M. L., and Herbert, V.: Correlation between various blood white cell pools and the serum $B_{12}$-binding capacities, Blood 37:142, 1971.
13. Cutting, H. O., and Lang, J. E.: Familial benign chronic neutropenia, Ann. Intern. Med. 61:876, 1964.
14. Dacie, J. V., and Lewis, S. M.: Practical haematology, ed. 3, New York, 1963, Grune & Stratton, Inc.
15. Dameshek, W.: The thymus and lymphoid proliferation (editorial), Blood 20:629, 1962.
16. Dausset, J., Colombani, J., and Colombani, M.: Study of leukopenias and thrombocytopenias by the direct antiglobulin consumption test on leukocytes and/or platelets, Blood 18:672, 1961.
17. Donohue, W. L.: Alymphocytosis, Pediatrics 11:129, 1953.
18. Endicott, K. M., Kornberg, A., and Ott, M.: Hemopoiesis in riboflavin deficient rats, Blood 2:164, 1947.
19. Fanconi, G.: Klinische demonstrationen, Ann. Paediat. 157:308, 1941.
20. Finch, S. S., Ross, J. F., and Ebaugh, F. G.: Immunologic mechanisms of leukocyte abnormalities, J. Lab. Clin. Med. 42:555, 1953.
21. Gasser, C.: Die Pathogenese der essentiellen chronischen Granulocytopenie im Kindesalter auf Grund der Knochenmarksbefunde, Helvet. paediat. acta 7:426, 1952.
22. Gitlin, D., and Craig, J. M.: The thymus and other lymphoid tissues in congenital agammaglobulinemia. I. Thymic alymphoplasia and lymphocytic hypoplasia and their relation to infections, Pediatrics 32:517, 1963.
23. Gitlin, D., Rosen, F. S., and Janeway, C. A.: The thymus and other lymphoid tissues in congenital agammaglobulinemia. II. Delayed hypersensitivity and homograft survival in a child with thymic alymphoplasia, Pediatrics 33:711, 1964.
24. Godwin, H. A., Zimmerman, T. S., Kimball, H. R., Wolff, S. M., and Perry, S.: The effect of etiocholanolone on the entry of granulocytes into the peripheral blood, Blood 31:461, 1968.
25. Greig, H. B. W.: A substitute for the Feulgen staining technique, J. Clin. Path. 12:93, 1959.
26. Guggenheim, K., and Buechler, S.: The effect of quantitative and qualitative protein deficiency on blood regeneration; white blood cells, Blood 4:958, 1954.
27. Hayhoe, F. G. J., Quaglino, D., and Fleman, S. R. J.: Consecutive use of Romanowsky and periodic-acid-Schiff techniques in the study of blood and bone-marrow cells, Brit. J. Haemat. 6:23, 1960.
28. Hedenberg, F.: Infantile agranulocytosis of probable congenital origin, Acta Paediat. 48:77, 1959.
29. Hitzig, W. H., and Willi, H.: Hereditäre lympho-plasmocytäre Dysgenesie "Alymphocytose mit Agammaglobulinämie," Schweiz. med. Wchnschr. 91:1625, 1961.
30. Huguley, C. M., Jr.: Agranulocytosis induced by dipyrone; a hazardous antipyretic and analgesic, J.A.M.A. 189:938, 1964.
31. Janeway, C. A., and Gitlin, D.: The gamma globulins. In Levine, S. Z., editor: Advances in pediatrics, vol. 9, Chicago, 1957, Year Book Medical Publishers, Inc., p. 65.
32. Kaplow, L. S.: A histochemical method for localizing and evaluating leukocyte alkaline phosphatase activity in smears of blood and marrow, Blood 10:1023, 1955.
33. Kauder, E., and Mauer, A. M.: Neutropenias of childhood, J. Pediat. 69:147, 1966.
34. Killmann, S. A.: Leukocyte agglutinins; properties, occurrence and significance, Springfield, Ill., 1960, Charles C Thomas, Publisher.
35. Kornberg, A. J., Daft, F. S., and Sebrell, W. H.: Granulocytopenia and anemia in rats fed diets of low casein content, Science 103:646, 1946.
36. Kostmann, R.: Infantile genetic agranulocytosis; a new recessive lethal disease in man, Acta Paediat. (supp. 105) 45:1, 1956.
37. Kracke, R. R., and Parker, F. P.: Relationship of drug therapy to agranulocytosis, J.A.M.A. 105:960, 1935.
38. Krill, C. E., and Mauer, A. M.: Congenital agranulocytosis, J. Pediat. 68:361, 1966.
39. Krill, C. E., Jr., Smith, H. D., and Mauer, A. M.: Chronic idiopathic granulocytopenia, New Eng. J. Med. 270:973, 1964.
40. Kyle, R. A., and Linman, J. W.: Chronic

idiopathic neutropenia; a newly recognized entity? New Eng. J. Med. 279:1015, 1968.
41. Lalezari, P., Nussbaum, M., Gelman, S., and Spaet, T. H.: Neonatal neutropenia due to maternal isoimmunization, Blood 15:236, 1960.
42. Lang, J. E., and Cutting, H. O.: Infantile genetic agranulocytosis, Pediatrics 35:596, 1965.
43. Lawrence, J. S.: Leukopenia; a discussion of its various modes of production, J.A.M.A. 116:478, 1941.
44. Lawrence, J. S., Adams, W. S., and Valentine, W. N.: White blood cell changes in clinical disorders, J.A.M.A. 150:454, 1952.
45. Lubhy, A. L., and Slobody, L. B.: Transient neonatal agranulocytosis in two siblings; transplacental isoimmunization to a leukocyte factor? Amer. J. Dis. Child. 92:496, 1956.
46. MacGillivray, J. B., Dacie, J. V., Henry, J. R. K., Sacker, L. S., and Tizard, J. P. M.: Congenital neutropenia; a report of five cases, Acta Paediat. 53:188, 1964.
47. Martensson, J., and Vikbladh, I.: Idiopathic immunoneutropenia; report of a case with leukocyte agglutinating factor in the serum, Blood 9:632, 1954.
48. Mauer, A. M.: White blood cell disorders, Ped. Clin. N. Amer. 9:739, 1962.
49. McElfresh, A. E., and Huang, N. N.: Bone-marrow depression resulting from the administration of methicillin; with a comment on the value of serum iron determination, New Eng. J. Med. 266:246, 1962.
50. McLean, M. M.: Chronic neutropenia, Arch. Dis. Child. 32:431, 1957.
51. Michael, S. R., Lutfi Vural, I., Bassen, F. A., and Schafer, L.: The hematologic aspects of disseminated (systemic) lupus erythematosus, Blood 6:1059, 1951.
51a. Miller, D. R., Freed, B. A., and Lapey, J. D.: Congenital neutropenia. Report of a fatal case in a Negro infant with leukocyte function studies, Amer. J. Dis. Child. 115:337, 1968.
52. Miller, J. F. A. P.: Role of the thymus in immunity, Brit. M. J. 2:459, 1963.
53. Moeschlin, S., and Schmid, E.: Investigation of leukocyte agglutination in serum of compatible and incompatible blood groups, Acta Haemat. 11:241, 1954.
54. Moeschlin, S., and Wagner, K.: Agranulocytosis due to the occurrence of leukocyte-agglutinins, Acta Haemat. 8:29, 1952.
55. Moeschlin, S., Meyer, H., Israels, L. G., and Tarr-Gloor, E.: Experimental agranulocytosis; its production through leukocyte agglutination by antileukocytic serum, Acta Haemat. 11:73, 1954.
56. Moncrieff, A.: Recurrent neutropenia, Arch. Dis. Child. 26:438, 1951.

57. Morley, A. A., Carew, J. P., and Baikie, A. G.: Familial cyclical neutropenia, Brit. J. Haemat. 13:719, 1967.
58. Page, A. R., Berendes, H., Warner, J., and Good, R. A.: The Chediak-Higashi syndrome, Blood 20:330, 1962.
59. Page, A. R., and Good, R. A.: Studies on cyclic neutropenia; a clinical and experimental investigation, J. Dis. Child. 94:623, 1957.
60. Payne, R.: Leukocyte agglutinins in human sera; correlation between blood transfusions and their development, Arch. Intern. Med. 99:587, 1957.
61. Payne, R., and Rolfs, M. R.: Fetomaternal leukocyte incompatibility, J. Clin. Invest. 37:1756, 1958.
62. Perry, S., and Reynolds, J.: Methyl-green-pyronin as a differential nucleic acid stain for peripheral blood smears, Blood 11:1132, 1956.
63. Reimann, H. A., and de Bernardinis, C. T.: Periodic (cyclic) neutropenia, an entity; a collection of sixteen cases, Blood 4:1109, 1949.
64. Rossi, J. P., and Brandt, I. K.: Transient granulocytopenia of the newborn associated with sepsis due to Shigella alkalescens and maternal leukocyte agglutinins, J. Pediat. 56:639, 1960.
65. Salmonsen, L.: Granulocytopenia in children, Acta paediat. 35:189, 1948.
66. Sandella, J. F.: Cyclic acute agranulocytosis; report of a case with improvement after splenectomy, Ann. Intern. Med. 35:1365, 1951.
67. Saraiva, L. G., Azevedo, M., Correa, J. M., Carvalho, G., and Prospero, J. D.: Anomalous panleukocytic granulation, Blood 14:1112, 1959.
68. Schirger, O., Nichols, D. R., Martin, W. J., Wellman, W. E., and Weech, L. A.: Brucellosis; experience with 224 patients, Ann. Intern. Med. 52:827, 1960.
69. Sherman, J. D., Adner, M. M., and Dameshek, W.: Effect of thymectomy on the golden hamster (Mesocricetus auratus). I. Wasting disease, Blood 22:252, 1963.
70. Shmerling, D. H., Prader, A., Hitzig, W. H., Giedion, A., Hadorn, B., and Kuhns, M.: Syndrome of exocrine pancreatic insufficiency, neutropenia, metaphyseal dysostosis and dwarfism, Helvet. Paediat. Acta 24:547, 1969.
71. Shwachman, H., Diamond, L. K., Oski, F. A., and Khaw, K. T.: The syndrome of pancreatic insufficiency and bone-marrow dysfunction, J. Pediat. 65:645, 1964.
72. Smith, R. T., Platou, E. S., and Good, R. A.: Septicemia of the newborn; current status of the problem, Pediatrics 17:549, 1956.
73. Spaet, T. H., and Dameshek, W.: Chronic

hypoplastic neutropenia, Amer. J. Med. 13:35, 1952.
74. Stefanini, M., Mele, R. H., and Skinner, D.: Transitory congenital neutropenia; a new syndrome, Amer. J. Med. 25:749, 1958.
75. Sturgis, C. C.: Syndromes associated with leukopenia; a general review of the subject (Trimble lecture), Clinics 1:492, 1942.
76. Tullis, J. L.: Prevalence, nature and identification of leukocyte antibodies, New Eng. J. Med. 258:569, 1958.
77. Vahlquist, B. C., and Anjou, H.: Granulocytopenia, chronic benign, Acta Haemat. 8:149, 1952.
78. Vogel, J. M., Yankee, R. A., Kimball, H. R., Wolff, S. M., and Perry, S.: The effect of etiocholanolone in granulocyte kinetics, Blood 30:474, 1967.
79. Walford, R. L.: Leukocyte antigens and antibodies, New York, 1960, Grune & Stratton, Inc.
80. Wiseman, B. K., and Doan, C. A.: Primary splenic neutropenia, Ann. Intern. Med. 16:1097, 1942.
81. Woodward, D. J., and Solomon, J. D.: Fatal agranulocytosis occurring during promazine (Sparine) therapy, J.A.M.A. 162:1308, 1956.
82. Zuelzer, W. W.: "Myelokathexis"—a new form of chronic granulocytopenia; report of a case, New Eng. J. Med. 270:699, 1964.
83. Zuelzer, W. W., and Bajoghli, M.: Chronic granulocytopenia in childhood, Blood 23:359, 1964.

# 20 LEUKOCYTOSIS, LEUKEMOID REACTIONS, AND LYMPHOCYTOSIS

## LEUKOCYTOSIS

Leukocytosis is the term used to designate an increase in the total number of white blood cells. Although such increase may be due to a preponderance of any one of the cellular elements, most often the term leukocytosis is used simply to imply an increase due to neutrophils. Neutrophilia is the preferable term and differentiates this form of leukocytosis from lymphocytosis, monocytosis, and eosinophilia.

### *Physiologic leukocytosis*

Leukocytosis is physiologic when it occurs without associated infection or other demonstrable pathologic lesions. The high leukocyte count of the newborn infant, with maximal values of 38,000 per cubic millimeter on the first day of life, is well known. The great majority of babies at this time have an average of 10,000 to 25,000 leukocytes per cubic millimeter, although much lower counts have been noted. The leukocytosis is initially due to a preponderance of polymorphonuclear neutrophils, mainly with a single-lobed or double-lobed nucleus. Trilobed forms appear about the ninth day to the second week.[13] Wide variations are found both between different infants and between different counts in the same baby. A pronounced drop at the end of the third or fourth day, with white blood cells averaging 12,000 per cubic millimeter, is maintained until the end of the first year. After the end of the second week lymphocytes predominate for the remainder of infancy.

Strenuous exercise, convulsive seizures, emotional disorders, fear and agitation, and pregnancy and labor have been associated with elevated leukocyte counts. Whether or not leukocytosis is attributable to digestion has not been demonstrated conclusively.[46]

### *Pathologic leukocytosis*

The extent of leukocytosis or leukopenia in patients with infection has been related to specific factors present in inflammatory exudates.[29] According to this concept, the leukocyte level in the bloodstream of patients with inflammatory conditions is the resultant of leukocytosis-promoting and leukopenic factors, respectively.

Usually, a neutrophilic leukocytosis with a shift to the left of the polymorphonuclear cells, eosinopenia, and lymphopenia point to infection. The reappearance of eosinophils and segmented neutrophilic leukocytes and the appearance of monocytosis indicate the recovery phase of an illness.[26]

Acute infections caused by cocci (staphylococci, streptococci, pneumococci, etc.) are the most common causes of a neutrophilic increase. Because of the tendency of the leukocytes to form pus, especially in localized areas, examination of the white blood cell count of patients with inflammatory conditions serves as a valuable clinical and diagnostic procedure.

Neutrophilic leukocytosis occurs in patients with pneumonia, scarlet fever, rheumatic fever, diphtheria, diabetic coma, azotemia, poisoning by chemicals and drugs such as lead, mercury, and camphor, acute hemorrhage, malignant neoplasms with metastases to the bone marrow, marked tissue destruction such as burns, and sudden hemolysis of red cells. In patients with dehydration the extent of leukocytosis is gauged by comparison with elevation of the hemoglobin level and red cell count.

Because of the great lability of the hematopoietic system in early life, the white blood cell response in younger patients may be disproportionate to the intensity of stimulation. Marked leukocytosis and an outpouring of immature cells into the peripheral blood may result from a moderate infection. In general, excessively high white blood cell counts or leukopenia associated with a shift to the left of the polymorphonuclear cells and toxic granulation indicates a serious outlook, especially if accompanied by excessive numbers of immature white cells and an absence of eosinophils.

## LEUKEMOID REACTIONS

Leukocytosis refers to white blood cell counts above the normal high of 11,000 per cubic millimeter, and leukopenia refers to counts under 4,000 per cubic millimeter. Leukemoid reactions are unusual blood responses[23] associated with exaggerated leukocytic reactions (approximately 50,000 per cubic millimeter and above) or the presence of immature white cells suggesting leukemia regardless of the leukocyte level,[7] without postmortem evidence of leukemia. Depending upon the cell type involved, leukemoid reactions may be classified as granulocytic (myeloid), lymphocytic, and monocytic. Most commonly, especially in younger patients, a leukemoid condition implies a hyperleukocytosis with a marked shift to immature neutrophilic granulocytes, myelocytes, metamyelocytes, occasional promyelocytes, and rarely myeloblasts. This response in infants is frequently associated with normoblasts in the peripheral blood. It is differentiated from leukemia by the absence of anemia, thrombocytopenia, hemorrhagic phenomena, splenomegaly, and lymphadenopathy and by the infrequent appearance of blasts.[17] Exceptionally, many of these features may be present in leukemoid reactions.[18] The clinical course, the transient period of the reaction without recurrence, bone marrow aspiration, and the absence of tissue infiltration usually rule out leukemia. The leukemoid process also lacks the characteristic gap or hiatus leukemicus between the blast forms and polymorphonuclear neutrophils with few or no transition forms such as myelocytes.

Another method of differentiation is by the measurement of alkaline phosphatase activity by histochemical and biochemical methods. A high cellular activity of this enzyme is found in the neutrophilic granulocytes of normal persons and of those with leukemoid reactions due to pyogenic infection, and negligible amounts are found in the leukocytes of those with chronic myelogenous leukemia.[22,53]

Alkaline phosphatase is confined to the neutrophil and its presence is believed to indicate maturity of the cell.[49] In the more fully differentiated members of the myeloid series, concentration of this enzyme may, therefore, be a biochemical expression of maturity. Although its precise function within the cell has not yet been clarified, leukocyte alkaline phosphatase apparently bears no relationship to serum alkaline phosphatase. Normally, the enzyme first appears in the myelocyte and increases in concentration as the cell matures.[37] In chronic granulocytic leukemia low values of alkaline phosphatase activity in the leukocytes are observed at the onset of illness, but the enzyme may appear in greater concentration with infection and remissions due to treatment.[28] Abnormally high values are found in Hodgkin's disease, infections, and leukemias other than chronic granulocytic leukemia. Acid phosphatase activity is present in Auer bodies, while alkaline phosphatase is absent.[15] This enzymatic activity is also found to be consistently very low in paroxysmal nocturnal hemoglobinuria. Low values are also found in patients with a variety of hematologic and nonhematologic diseases such as idiopathic thrombocytopenic purpura, myeloid metaplasia, infectious mononucleosis, pernicious anemia in relapse, collagen diseases, and refractory or aplastic anemia.[47]

It has been postulated that leukocyte alkaline phosphatase is controlled by a gene on chromosome 21.[1,50] This assumption was based on the high activity of this enzyme in children with mongolism (Down's syndrome), a condition characterized by trisomy for chromosome 21. This information together with the low alkaline phosphatase activity in chronic myelogenous (granulocytic) leukemia, in which there is a deletion of chromosomal material from one of the pair of No. 21 chromosomes, leads to the premise that one of the genetic loci for enzymes regulating leukocyte alkaline phosphatase activity may be present on the No. 21 chromosome in the human karyotype.[21,35]

It is of interest that lactic dehydrogenase is another enzyme showing changes in leukemia. It is consistently elevated in both untreated acute leukemia and chronic granulocytic leukemia, reverting to normal levels during remission.[52] Serum glutamic-oxalacetic transaminase levels are occasionally elevated in leukemia, especially in terminal phases.[52]

Hyperleukocytosis of the myeloid type occurs following pyogenic infection, metastatic carcinoma of bone, ulcerative colitis, severe hemorrhage, primary tuberculous infection in childhood, and acute tuberculosis at any age period (usually of the myeloid type),[51] in episodes of acute hemolysis in the course of an established chronic hemolytic anemia, or following infection or drug therapy.[19] Congenital leukemia may be difficult to differentiate from the leukemoid reaction occurring with sepsis in the newborn infant. A positive diagnosis of leukemia often cannot be made from the blood and bone marrow findings alone, and evidence of organ infiltration with white cell precursors is necessary. A leukemoid reaction with increased numbers of myelocytes, metamyelocytes, and nucleated red cells may appear during the early treatment phase of iron-deficiency anemia before hemoglobin concentrations are elevated.

A leukemoid reaction with a predominance of lymphocytes occurs in patients with whooping cough, chickenpox, and acute infectious lymphocytosis. In all of the patients with these conditions the majority of lymphocytes are normal, with small numbers of younger forms with deep blue cytoplasm. In patients with infectious mononucleosis the increase in total leukocytes is seldom more than 20,000 per cubic millimeter. Elevations above this number are exceptional, but the presence of diagnostic atypical lymphocytes readily separates this disease from leukemia.

Blood pictures similar to those of patients with myelocytic and lymphocytic leukemia[12] have been reported in patients with miliary tuberculosis. A leukemoid reaction with monocytosis may occur in patients with tuberculosis in childhood with a hematogenous spread. A count of 82,000 white blood cells per cubic millimeter with 44% monocytes has been reported in a 16-year-old boy with generalized tuberculous adenitis.[14]

In a group of 364 tuberculous patients who were previously untreated, anemia was present in 17%, leukocytosis (leukocyte count of more than 14,000 per cubic millimeter) in 3%, and leukopenia (leukocyte count of less than 3,500) in 1%. In twenty-four patients who had differential counts done, lymphocytosis was present in 3.8%, monocytosis in 35%, neutrophilia in 32%, and eosinophilia in 14%.[5]

## LYMPHOCYTOSIS

There are few conditions in which a significant increase in lymphocytes occurs so that they are responsible for a moderate or marked leukocytosis. An absolute lymphocytosis is found in patients with acute and chronic (nonspecific) infectious lymphocytosis, infectious mononucleosis, and pertussis and, to a lesser extent, in those with syphilis, tuberculosis, and hyperthyroidism. A relative increase in lymphocytes is common in patients with conditions with a decreased number of granulocytes. A relative lymphocytosis is associated with the leukopenia of measles, German measles, exanthema subitum, and brucellosis. It will be recalled that following the first week of life lymphocytes normally predominate until the fourth or fifth year of life, and a lymphocytosis occurring in this period must be evaluated from this standpoint. Occasionally, in infancy a marked lymphocytosis transiently accompanies an infectious or postinfectious state which cannot be assigned to a specific cause.

It has been pointed out that because of the normally higher leukocyte count below 6 months of age, different numerical criteria are necessary for the evaluation of blood counts in pertussis.[24] In a series of 180 hospital patients the number of leukocytes and of lymphocytes were said to be increased and suggestive of pertussis during the first half-year of life only when they exceeded 20,000 and 15,000 per cubic millimeter, respectively. For children over 6 months of age the upper limits of leukocytes and lymphocytes were 15,000 and 11,000 per cubic millimeter, respectively. Marked leukocytosis (more than 50,000 per cubic millimeter) was noted in only eight cases. In uncomplicated pertussis the erythrocyte sedimentation rate is usually normal or subnormal and does not seem to vary with the patient's age or the stage of the disease.

The relative number of each type of leukocyte is calculated from the leukocyte count and the percentage found in the peripheral smear. When for some reason the polymorphonuclear leukocyte percentage is decreased, the numbers of lymphocytes appear elevated. A relative lymphocytosis is thus associated with a neutropenia and should be differentiated from an absolute increase. Leukocytosis with a marked predominance of lymphocytes (an absolute increase) is characteristic of pertussis, infectious lymphocytosis, infectious mononucleosis, and lymphocytic leukemia. With viral infections, on the other hand, the increase in lymphocytes is only moderate and is usually based on a decrease in the percentage of polymorphonuclear leukocytes.

*Causes of lymphocytosis*
1. Infections
    a. Marked lymphocytosis (absolute)— acute infectious lymphocytosis, infectious mononucleosis, pertussis

b. Moderate lymphocytosis (relative)—measles, rubella, varicella, mumps, roseola infantum, brucellosis, and typhoid and paratyphoid fever
2. Chronic infections—tuberculosis, syphilis
3. Convalescence—especially after viral disease
4. Neoplasm—lymphoblastic leukemia
5. Physiologic—in infants a predominance of lymphocytes is normally present from fourth month to fourth year

In the pediatric age group an appraisal of lymphocytosis depends on the normal fluctuations within each group. Lymphocytes average 30% at birth, rise to 60% by the fourth to the sixth month, and remain at this level until the fourth year, when they drop to 50%. They decrease to 40% at the end of the sixth year, and then to 30% by the eighth year, which is also the adult value. Lymphocytosis has been designated[31] as an increase in the number of lymphocytes above 9,000 per cubic millimeter in infants and young children, 7,200 per cubic millimeter in older children, and 4,000 per cubic millimeter in adults.

In virus disorders not only may lymphocytes appear excessive, but atypical lymphocytes termed virocytes may appear in the peripheral blood. These are large cells of lymphocytic origin whose cytoplasm is moderately to deeply basophilic. They occasionally possess a few small vacuoles and the nucleus has a loose chromatin pattern. These cells should be differentiated from those of infectious mononucleosis whose cells also stain deeper blue with Wright's stain but whose cytoplasm is heavily vacuolated, giving it a distinctive foamy appearance. Virocytes appear in varying numbers in the blood of children with upper respiratory infections and in viral hepatitis, roseola infantum, and other virus diseases.

Recent investigations have shown that the small lymphocytes are a very heterogenous collection of cells of different origin and function.[32] Some are the immunologically competent, antigen-sensitive cells and are associated with the development of delayed hypersensitivity. On the basis of the incorporation of $^{32}P$ into the DNA of lymphocytes, Ottensen[36] found two populations of lymphocytes: about 20% had a mean age of 2 to 3 days, and 80% a mean age of 100 to 200 days. Gowans[16] found that there is a continuous circulation of lymphocytes between lymph channels and blood. Normal lymphocytes enter the blood through the thoracic duct or other lymphatic ducts and circulate for a relatively brief time, leave the vascular system again, and reenter by way of the lymph node structure. These may constitute the cuff of small lymphocytes which can be observed surrounding germinal centers in lymph nodes. The process of recirculation is in sharp contrast to the neutrophilic system, in which once the cells have left the blood they do not return. The fate of the larger and medium lymphocytes is not known, but they may have a life history quite distinct from the small lymphocyte.

It is thought[33] that stem cells from bone marrow migrate to the thymus and differentiate to thymus lymphocytes, from whence they may emigrate as immunologically competent cells. Alternately the thymus could produce a humoral substance capable of inducing competence in primitive stem cells (immunocompetent cell—antigen-sensitive cell—a cell which can be stimulated by antigen to either form antibodies or give rise to cells which produce antibodies). The lymphocytes in the recirculating pool are characterized by a long life-span. The majority of lymphocytes in the blood, entering from the thoracic duct and in the "cuff" of lymphocytes surrounding general arteries, appear to be the long-lived variety of lymphocytes.

*Acute infectious lymphocytosis*

**Definition.** Acute infectious lymphocytosis* is a specific entity of unknown etiology which is both infectious and contagious. It may occur sporadically or in epidemic form. The incubation period has been estimated to be between 12 and 21 days. It is characterized by hyperleukocytosis due to an increase in small mature lymphocytes in which the elevated blood levels persist for approximately 2 to 7 weeks. It is a benign infection, distinct from infectious mononucleosis, acute lymphoblastic and chronic lymphocytic leukemia, and miscellaneous infections associated with a lymphocytosis. The clinical signs and symptoms may be so mild as to escape attention, or the onset may be marked by varying degrees of constitutional reaction. A noteworthy feature is the absence of lymphadenopathy and enlargement of the spleen.

---

*See references 6, 8, 34, 42, 44, and 45.

*Age.* The highest incidence is in children from 1 to 14 years of age, with most of the recorded cases occurring during the first 10 years of life. Several cases have been reported in young adults.[10] In general, the height of the leukocyte count tends to vary inversely with the age of the patient.

*Etiology.* Attempts to identify a causative agent have thus far met with inconclusive results. Organisms obtained from routine nasopharyngeal cultures probably represent normal inhabitants or secondary invaders. They do not differ from the flora of patients exhibiting the usual hematologic response with similar respiratory infections. A bacterial or viral etiology has been postulated.[25] An adenovirus type 12 has been isolated from the upper respiratory tract of four children with a pertussis-like lymphocytosis.[34] In one of the patients the white cell count rose to 168,000 per cubic millimeter with a predominance of small mature lymphocytes. The additional finding of eosinophilia implicated acute infectious lymphocytosis rather than pertussis. The studies in this small series suggested that this agent is responsible for a pertussis-like illness with hematologic findings indistinguishable from, and diagnostic of, acute infectious lymphocytosis. This finding awaits confirmation in other cases.

In a recent epidemic[20] in a state school for retarded children in whom the white blood count ranged between 26,000 to 93,000 per cubic millimeter, the search for an etiology included a study of infectious and noninfectious agents. An enterovirus, presently untyped but resembling the Coxsackie A subgroup in physical, chemical, and host specificity, was isolated in 21% of the patients' stool specimens. Fourfold rises in neutralizing antibody against this enterovirus occurred in the sera of a significantly greater proportion of patients than in patient contacts. Since the disease often terminates with eosinophilia, stools were examined for intestinal parasites as an etiologic factor. *Giardia lamblia* was not an uncommon finding, but since it is a parasite which is ubiquitous in institutional children its relation to lymphocytosis remains in doubt.

*Epidemiology.* The disease occurs sporadically as multiple cases in families and in institutional epidemics.* It is therefore contagious but of a low degree of infectivity. It has been reported in North, Central, and South America, Europe, and Africa. In the epidemic reports the majority of patients were devoid of positive physical findings. According to some reports, the patients presented themselves with signs of respiratory infection or gastrointestinal distress, principally diarrhea.[38] In the epidemics the peak white blood cell counts in the individual patients ranged from 15,100 to 147,000 per cubic millimeter and the lymphocytes ranged from 63 to 97%. In a recent[20] epidemic, 4 months after investigation of the first case, hyperleukocytosis with lymphocytosis had developed in twenty-seven children.

*Pathology.* Microscopic examination of lymph nodes in the few patients studied[45] revealed the striking proliferation of the lining reticuloendothelium with almost complete blockage of the sinuses by masses of these cells and degeneration of the lymph follicles. In a 14-year-old boy complaining of recurring abdominal pain, surgical exploration revealed a normal appendix. One of a group of shotty nodes in the ileocecal mesentery revealed hyperplasia of the follicles, some of which showed hyalinization and prominence of the cells lining the sinuses.[42]

*Clinical features.* The condition at times may be so mild as to escape attention, or the onset may be marked in individual patients by varying degrees of constitutional reaction. Fever, upper respiratory infections, skin rashes, abdominal complaints, and meningoencephalitic manifestations may be present. Accidental discovery as the result of routine blood examinations is not uncommon, particularly in institutional epidemics. No consistent correlation is evident between the degree of leukocytosis and the severity of symptoms.

*Nasopharynx.* A feature common to most of the patients in whom any manifestations were present is mild infection of the upper respiratory tract. The throat may be deeply injected at the time of the initial examination, and a history of recent infection of the upper respiratory tract frequently is elicited.

*Nervous system.* Increasing experience has shown that acute infectious lymphocytosis should be considered in the diagnosis of an acute febrile illness in which there are symptoms suggestive of central nervous system involvement. Headache, irritability, vertigo, and

---
*See references 2, 11, 27, 38, 40, and 43.

pain and slight stiffness of the back of the neck may occur without other signs of meningitis. The spinal fluid may show a slight pleocytosis with variations in the type of predominating cell,[48] although a slight increase in lymphocytes has been reported when the spinal fluid count was positive. This disease may simulate poliomyelitis[3] and meningoencephalitis[6] since headache, stiffness of the neck, restlessness, fever, malaise, vomiting, sore throat, and identical spinal fluid changes may occur at the onset of both conditions. The blood counts readily separate both diseases. Differentiation between these conditions assumes particular importance when the symptoms occur during the summer and early fall.

*Skin.* A generalized morbilliform eruption and, less commonly, a herpetic eruption have been observed in patients during the first week of the disease.

*Abdomen.* Signs may be sufficiently pronounced to suggest an acute surgical condition with an elevated temperature, vomiting, and severe abdominal pain.[9,42] Diarrhea was the most prominent symptom in sixteen of twenty-eight patients in one epidemic.[38]

*Spleen and lymph nodes.* An important diagnostic criterion of infectious lymphocytosis is absence of significant enlargement of the spleen and lymph nodes. Preexisting cervical nodes, especially of the posterior chain, are usually sequelae of previous attacks of nasopharyngitis and are not directly related to the development of acute infectious lymphocytosis. Lymphadenopathy and enlargement of the spleen are absent, unless they existed prior to the onset of the disease.

**Incubation period.** Because the abnormal white cell counts are unexpectedly encountered in the course of routine blood examinations, the exact onset and duration of the leukocytic changes are unknown. It is therefore difficult to designate a precise incubation period. From the available cases thus far reported, it has been possible to fix the approximate length of the incubation period between 12 and 21 days.

**Laboratory findings.** Highly significant features of diagnostic import are observed among the laboratory findings.

*Blood.* The red cells, hemoglobin content, platelets, and sedimentation rate are normal if the disease is uncomplicated. When the constitutional reaction is severe, the hemoglobin content and the red blood cell count may drop to the lower limit of normal. The absence of anemia is an important diagnostic feature in differentiating this ailment from acute lymphoblastic and chronic lymphatic leukemia and from the lymphocytosis occurring in prolonged postinfectious states. No deviations in bleeding or clotting time have been observed.

The outstanding feature in patients with acute infectious lymphocytosis is the hyperleukocytosis with the relative and absolute increase in normal small mature lymphocytes (Figs. 65 and 66). White blood cell counts at the height of the disease are usually over 40,000 to 50,000 per cubic millimeter, with a maximum recorded level over 100,000 per cubic millimeter. In the reported institutional epidemics the peak white blood cell counts in the individual patients ranged from 15,000 to 147,000 per cubic millimeter and lymphocytes from 60 to 97%.[43] The lymphocytes are mainly the small variety and are of uniform size and normal structure. Only occasionally are slightly larger or intermediate types encountered, but these are also mature cells. The nucleus in these cells is condensed and possesses the coarse chromatin masses of the normal mature lymphocytes. These lymphocytes have also been referred to as overripe and have been described as being smaller than normal with a dark purple chromatic material in the nucleus and with very little cytoplasm.[30]

The duration of the markedly abnormal leukocytic reaction is usually 3 to 5 weeks and occasionally 7 weeks. An elevation in the percentage of eosinophilic leukocytes occurs frequently during the course of the disease, usually at or following the peak of leukocytosis.

*Bone marrow.* The myeloid elements and nucleated red cells are normal in number. In many patients the bone marrow shows an increase in the total number of nucleated cells and in the percentage of small mature lymphocytes; otherwise it is not abnormal.

*Heterophil agglutination (Paul-Bunnell) test.* The heterophil agglutination test is uniformly negative.

**Differential diagnosis** (*Table 26*). Lymphocytic reactions in childhood are difficult to interpret because a predominance of lymphocytes and a greater lability of the blood-forming mechanism are common to this age period. In the differentiation of acute infectious lymphocytosis, these physiologic hematopoietic responses, as well as certain specific conditions

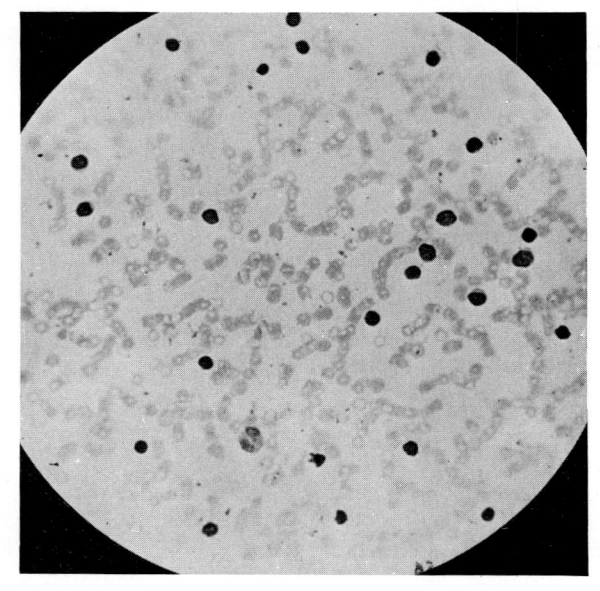

Fig. 65. Typical blood smear from a patient with acute infectious lymphocytosis. (×400.)

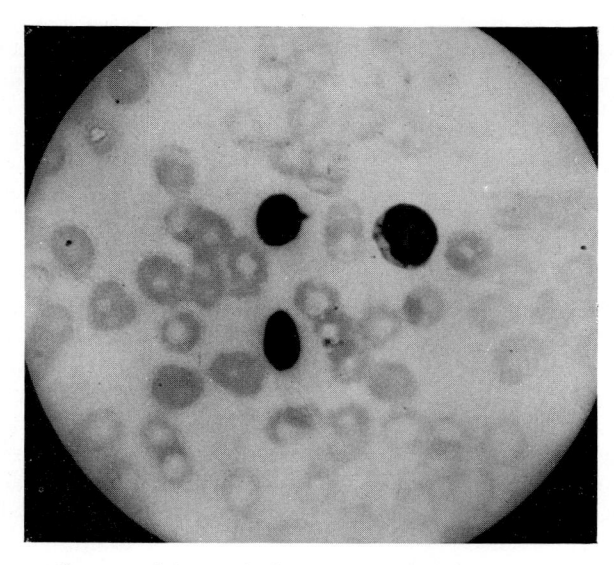

Fig. 66. Higher magnification of Fig. 65, showing that lymphocytes are mainly of the small variety and of uniform size and structure. Only occasionally are slightly larger or intermediate types encountered, but these are also mature. (×1000.) (From Smith, C. H.: Acute infectious lymphocytosis; a specific infection, J.A.M.A. 125:342, 1944.)

Table 26. Differential diagnosis of acute infectious lymphocytosis*

|  | Acute infectious lymphocytosis | Infectious mononucleosis | Acute lymphoblastic (stem cell) leukemia | Chronic lymphocytic leukemia |
|---|---|---|---|---|
| Age (usual incidence) | First decade | First 3 decades | First and second decades | After 45 yrs. |
| Fever and systemic symptoms | Occasionally present | Usually present | Variably present | Infrequent |
| Enlarged lymph nodes | Absent | Present | Present | Present |
| Splenomegaly | Absent | Present in 50% | Present | Present |
| Leukocytosis | Extreme | Moderate | Leukopenia to marked | Usually pronounced |
| Lymphocytosis | Present | Present | Present | Present |
| Types of lymphocytes, diagnostic cells | Normal, small | Atypical, abnormal | Lymphoblasts | Mature, small |
| Anemia | Absent | Rare | Present | Late in course |
| Thrombocytopenia | Absent | Rare | Present | Present |
| Bone marrow lymphocytes | Increased in number; normal, small | Occasionally atypical | Lymphoblasts predominate | Lymphocytes predominate |
| Heterophil agglutination | Negative | Positive | Negative | Negative |
| Prognosis | Uniformly favorable | Favorable with few exceptions | Uniformly fatal | Uniformly fatal |

*From Smith, C. H.: Advances in pediatrics, vol. 2, Chicago, 1947, Year Book Medical Publishers, Inc., p. 64.

in which the lymphocytes or their precursors are known to be increased, must be evaluated.

*Infectious mononucleosis.* Infectious mononucleosis is usually more severe and characterized by fever, sore throat, rash, rarely jaundice, enlargement and tenderness of the lymph nodes, and often splenomegaly. The febrile phase lasts for 1 to 3 weeks, but enlargement of the glands and spleen may persist. Acute infectious lymphocytosis, on the other hand, may run an asymptomatic course, or there may be transient sore throat, fever, and constitutional symptoms. Lymph nodes and spleen are not enlarged. The heterophil antibody reaction is usually positive in patients with infectious mononucleosis but is consistently negative in those with acute infectious lymphocytosis.

The blood picture constitutes the most important differential feature. In patients with infectious mononucleosis, the total white blood cell count usually does not exceed 20,000 per cubic millimeter, whereas acute infectious lymphocytosis is characterized by a hyperleukocytosis, with maximal levels frequently exceeding 50,000 cells per cubic millimeter. A more important feature of a hematologic differentiation rests in the morphologic appearance of the lymphocytes in the two conditions. In patients with acute infectious lymphocytosis the hyperleukocytosis is associated with a preponderance of small lymphocytes possessing a normal cytologic appearance. In those with infectious mononucleosis, however, the distinctive feature is the presence of characteristic atypical mononuclear cells. The variability of atypical lymphocytes and monocytes in persons with this disease contrasts sharply with the uniform size and normal structure of the cells in those with acute infectious lymphocytosis.

*Acute lymphoblastic (stem cell) leukemia.* The extreme leukocytosis and the predominance of lymphocytes in patients with acute infectious lymphocytosis have occasionally led to the erroneous diagnosis of acute lymphoblastic leukemia. Identification of the blast cell which is invariably found in a careful search of the blood smear of patients with leukemia is the distinguishing feature. The size of these cells varies from that of a small lymphocyte to twice that size. Lymphoblasts are usually round, large, and uniform in size, and the narrow zone of cytoplasm is basophilic and occasionally contains a few large vacuoles.

Even more distinctive is the nuclear pattern. In contrast with the masses of dense basichromatin found in the nucleus of the normal and large lymphocyte of the patient with acute infectious lymphocytosis, the nuclear chromatin of the lymphoblast stains lightly, is finely granular, stippled, or sievelike, and nucleoli are present. In patients with acute leukemia with a hyperleukocytosis of the magnitude found in those with acute infectious lymphocytosis, the blood exhibits not only large numbers of lymphoblasts but also a severe anemia and a decrease in platelets, and the spleen and lymph nodes are enlarged.

Examination of the bone marrow also serves to differentiate the two diseases. In acute lymphatic leukemia in children, bone marrow aspiration usually shows complete replacement of the bone marrow by blast or stem cells. In children with acute infectious lymphocytosis, on the other hand, the myeloid and erythroblastic elements are present in normal proportions, and the chief abnormality in many patients consists of an increased percentage of normal lymphocytes.

*Chronic lymphocytic leukemia.* The blood picture of patients with acute infectious lymphocytosis resembles that of those with chronic lymphocytic leukemia in respect to the white blood cells. In patients with either of these diseases there is a hyperleukocytosis with a preponderance of small mature lymphocytes and the bone marrow shows increased percentages of normal small lymphocytes and is cellular. The age incidence of the two diseases, however, is very different since chronic lymphocytic leukemia is a disease of older persons. In patients with chronic lymphocytic leukemia, the spleen and lymph nodes are enlarged, anemia and thrombocytopenia eventually develop, and the outcome is uniformly fatal, in contrast to the negative physical and hematologic findings and favorable prognosis in patients with acute infectious lymphocytosis.

*Leukemoid reactions.* The hyperleukocytosis of infectious lymphocytosis cannot be regarded as a leukemoid reaction of the lymphoid type. The absence of immature and atypical cells in the blood and bone marrow precludes this designation. Moreover, the leukemoid reaction resulting from infection is transitory; the lymphocytic response in patients with acute infectious lymphocytosis is protracted. Pertussis as a cause of the extreme leukocytosis and lymphocytosis can be excluded by the absence of cough and characteristic clinical manifestations.

*Miscellaneous infections.* A number of specific infections are associated with lymphocytosis. Typhoid fever, brucellosis, and tuberculosis should be excluded by appropriate tests.

*Pertussis.* During the latter part of the catarrhal period or early paroxysmal stage, the total leukocyte count rises to a level from 15,000 to 50,000 per cubic millimeter. Lymphocytes account for 70 to 90% of the total increase in the number of leukocytes. The leukocytosis and lymphocytosis exceed any other febrile illness except infectious lymphocytosis. In one series,[24] marked leukocytosis of more than 50,000 per cubic millimeter was found in only eight cases.

Available data render invalid the view that the lymphocytosis represents a peculiar individual response, the so-called constitutional lymphatic reaction. Patients with acute infectious lymphocytosis, afflicted with antecedent, concurrent, or subsequent illnesses such as acute otitis media or pneumonia, exhibit a neutrophilic response.

**Treatment and prognosis.** There is no specific therapy. Treatment is symptomatic and similar to that in patients with other acute infections of the upper respiratory tract. Because of the low infectivity of the condition, the large number of asymptomatic cases, and the brief span of constitutional reactions in the febrile cases, no isolation seems necessary. The prognosis in all cases has been uniformly excellent, and no sequelae have been observed.

It has been suggested that infectious lymphocytosis, which affects the hematopoietic system and in which the lymphatic system has at one time experienced such an extreme proliferative response, might be associated with long-term sequela such as leukemia. A follow-up 19 years after a thirty-one–case epidemic of infectious lymphocytosis in Wisconsin showed that, in the twenty-five persons located and examined, no significant after-effects could be associated with this illness.[4,39]

### Chronic nonspecific infectious lymphocytosis (low-grade fever syndrome)

*Clinical picture.* The symptom complex of chronic nonspecific infectious lymphocytosis is characterized by a persistent slight to moderate leukocytosis and a preponderance of lymphocytes. It is frequently encountered in pediatric practice[44] and is distinct from acute infectious lymphocytosis. Difficulties in diagnosis arise when an acute infection of the upper respiratory tract is followed for prolonged periods by a low-grade fever, with the temperature ranging from 99° F. up to and usually not exceeding 101° F. In addition to the protracted fever the symptom complex includes anorexia, pallor, irritability, fatigability, and abdominal pain localized to the region of the umbilicus. The fauces are injected, the tonsils, when present, are usually greatly hypertrophied, and postnasal discharge is frequent. At times, the superficial cervical lymph nodes are slightly enlarged. The heart and lungs are normal; there are no murmurs or other cardiac abnormalities. In infants and young children the spleen may be palpable, but this finding is inconstant, especially in older children. The age of incidence is usually from 6 months through 10 years, especially in the period from 3 to 6 years. Cases are less commonly observed between 3 and 6 months of age. In these infants moderate elevations of temperature (103° to 104° F.) frequently interrupt the usual course of low-grade fever (temperature up to 101° F.). Although these episodes are usually related to exacerbations of infection of the nasopharynx, other causes of lymphocytosis must be eliminated.

*Blood.* The accompanying slight to moderate leukocytosis and lymphocytosis usually persist for periods of months and sometimes a year or more. The total white blood cell counts usually range from 8,000 to 18,000, rarely reaching 20,000 per cubic millimeter, with 60 to 80% lymphocytes. White blood cell counts reaching 25,000 per cubic millimeter are frequently observed in infants under 6 months of age. The hemoglobin ranges between 10 and 11 gm. per 100 ml., and the platelets are normal in number. Lymphocytosis in this group of patients with chronic disease resembles that which occurs in postinfectious states in infants and children. Most of the lymphocytes are of the small mature type, structurally similar to those in patients with acute infectious lymphocytosis. Occasionally, cells of the larger variety are seen which are of normal shape and which possess a deeply basophilic cytoplasm and an eccentric nucleus which stains more intensely than that of the normal lymphocyte. The same depth of staining is observed in another type of lymphocyte which is about one and one-half times the size of a red cell and whose nucleus is round, oval, or slightly indented. In infants the zone of cellular cytoplasm is often wider and the basophilia deeper than in the corresponding cells of blood in older children. These larger cells are not specific, since they appear in increased numbers in the blood of young children during the active stage and convalescence of a large variety of infections and may occasionally be found in the blood of normal infants.

*Differential diagnosis.* Chronic nonspecific infectious lymphocytosis is not contagious and does not appear in epidemic form in contrast to acute infectious lymphocytosis. Moreover, the acute disease is usually asymptomatic, the blood reaction is comparatively short and well defined, hyperleukocytosis is marked, and the disease is not characterized at any age period by either lymphadenopathy or splenomegaly.

Chronic nonspecific infectious lymphocytosis is often confused with infectious mononucleosis, especially in young children, acute lymphoblastic leukemia, and acute rheumatic fever. Not only is the heterophil agglutinin test negative in the patient with chronic infectious lymphocytosis, but the lymphocytes lack the irregularity of shape and the abundant, frequently vacuolated, and foamy cytoplasm which are distinctive features of the cells of patients with infectious mononucleosis.

Acute lymphoblastic (stem cell) leukemia is differentiated by the presence of lymphoblasts, hyperleukocytosis, often leukopenia, anemia (hemoglobin below 10 gm. per 100 ml.), and thrombocytopenia. Marked lymphadenopathy and splenomegaly are additional confirmatory features but may be absent in the patient with early disease. Examination of the bone marrow serves to differentiate the two diseases unequivocally, although this procedure is rarely necessary.

Many of the patients are referred with a diagnosis of acute rheumatic fever because of a more or less continuous lowgrade fever, a failure to gain weight or loss of weight, fatigability, and abdominal pain. From the hematologic standpoint, acute rheumatic fever is usually associated with moderate leukocytosis with polymorphonuclear leukocytes as the predominant cell in contrast to chronic nonspecific infectious lymphocytosis in which lymphocytosis characterizes the blood smear. The sedimentation rate is markedly increased in patients with rheumatic fever and does not approach normal until some time after the fever and clinical signs have abated, whereas in those with chronic lymphocytosis the sedimentation rate is normal or only slightly increased for short intervals. Nosebleeds, the development of carditis, pains in the arms, legs, and joints, subcutaneous nodules, and erythematous rashes are other features present in patients with rheumatic fever and absent in those with lymphocytic diseases.

A disease identical with or similar to chronic infectious lymphocytosis has been reported as lymphocytic fever.[41] It occurs chiefly in children under 2 years of age with enlargement of the liver and spleen, slight lymphadenopathy, and a leukocytosis with a preponderance of small lymphocytes persisting for months and occasionally a year or more.

The lymphocytic blood picture in patients with chronic infectious lymphocytosis is a useful diagnostic aid in differentiating the abdominal pain, which may occur in both diseases, from surgical conditions and from nonspecific mesenteric lymphadenitis, which are associated with a neutrophilic response.

*Treatment and prognosis.* Chronic nonspecific infections lymphocytosis may be a source of anxiety to both parents and physician. It is, therefore, desirable to emphasize that the prognosis is entirely favorable, that treatment is symptomatic, and that subsidence of the disease depends upon relief of infection in the nasopharynx. Striking improvement often follows tonsillectomy, but tonsillectomy is not advocated as a routine measure.

Repeated temperature readings are unnecessary, and antibiotics are futile in altering the pattern of low-grade fever. Once the diagnosis is established, restriction of activities is unnecessary.

**REFERENCES**

1. Alter, A. A., Lee, S. L., Pourfar, M., and Dobkin, G.: Leukocyte alkaline phosphatase in mongolism, a possible chromosomal marker, Blood 22:165, 1963.
2. Barnes, G. R., Jr., Yannet, H., and Lieberman, R.: A clinical study of an institutional outbreak of infectious lymphocytosis, Amer. J. Med. Sci. 218:646, 1949.
3. Beloff, J. S., and Gang, K. M.: Acute poliomyelitis and acute infections lymphocytosis; their apparent simultaneous occurrence in summer camp, J. Pediat. 26:586, 1945.
4. Clement, D. H.: Reassurance regarding infectious lymphocytosis, Peditarics 41:597, 1968.
5. Corr, W. P., Jr., Kyle, R. A., and Bowie, E. J. W.: Hematologic changes in tuberculosis, Amer. J. Med. Sci. 248:709, 1964.
6. Crisalli, M., and Terragna, A.: La malattia di Smith (linfocitosi infettiva acuta), revisione della letteratura e presentazione di tre casi, Minerva Pediat. 10:849, 1958.
7. Custer, R. P.: An atlas of the blood and bone marrow, Philadelphia, 1949, W. B. Saunders Co.
8. Descovich, C., and Santarsierg, M.: La malattia di Smith (linfocitosi infettiva acuta), contributo clinico ed osservazioni su vertisette casi, Clinica Pediat. Bologne 45:233, 1963.
9. Duncan, P. A.: Acute infectious lymphocytosis, Amer. J. Dis. Child. 66:267, 1943.
10. Duncan, P. A.: Acute infectious lymphocytosis in young adults, New Eng. J. Med. 233:177, 1945.
11. Finucane, D. L., and Philips, R. S.: Infectious lymphocytosis, Amer. J. Dis. Child. 68:301, 1944.
12. Gardner, R. H., and Mettier, S.: Lymphocytic leukemoid reaction of the blood associated with miliary tuberculosis, Blood 4:767, 1949.
13. Garrey, W. E., and Bryan, W. R.: Variations in white blood cell counts, Physiol. Rev. 15:597, 1935.
14. Gibson, A.: Monocytic leukemoid reaction associated with tuberculosis and a mediastinal teratoma, J. Path. Bact. 58:469, 1946.
15. Goldberg, A. F.: Acid phosphatase activity in Auer bodies, Blood 24:305, 1964.
16. Gowans, J. L.: The life history of lymphocytes, Brit. M. Bull. 15:50, 1959.
17. Hill, J. M., and Duncan, C. N.: Leukemoid reactions, Amer. J. Med. Sci. 201:847, 1941.
18. Hilts, S. V., and Shaw, C. C.: Leukemoid blood reaction, New Eng. J. Med. 249:434, 1953.
19. Holland, P., and Mauer, A. M.: Myeloid leukemoid reactions in children, Amer. J. Dis. Child. 105:568, 1963.
20. Horowitz, M. S., and Moore, G. T.: Acute infectious lymphocytosis; an etiologic and epidemiologic study of an outbreak, New Eng. J. Med. 279:399, 1968.
21. King, M. J., Gillis, E. M., and Baikie, A. G.: The polymorph alkaline phosphatase in mongolism, Lancet 2:661, 1962.
22. Koler, R. D., Seaman, A. J., Osgood, E. E., and Vanbellinghen, P.: Myeloproliferative diseases; diagnostic value of the leukocyte alka-

line phosphatase test, Amer. J. Clin. Path. 30: 295, 1958.
23. Krumbhaar, E. B.: Leukemoid blood picture in various clinical conditions, Amer. J. Med. Sci. 172:519, 1926.
24. Lagergren, J.: The white blood cell count and the erythrocyte sedimentation rate in pertussis, Acta Paediat. 52:405, 1963.
25. Landolt, R. F.: Akute infektiöse Lymphocytosen in Kindesalter, Helvet, Paediat. Acta 2: 377, 1947.
26. Lawrence, J. S., Adams, W. S., and Valentine, W. N.: White blood changes in clinical disorders, J.A.M.A. 150:454, 1952.
27. Lemon, B. K., and Kaump, D. H.: Infectious lymphocytosis; report of epidemic in children, J. Pediat. 36:61, 1950.
28. Martinez-Maldonado, M., Menendez-Corrada, R., and Rivera de Sala, A.: Diagnostic value of alkaline phosphatase in leukocytes, Amer. J. Med. Sci. 248:175, 1964.
29. Menkin, V.: Leukocyte level in blood stream with inflammation, Blood 4:1323, 1949.
30. Meyer, L. M.: Acute infectious hymphocytosis, Amer. J. Clin. Path. 16:244, 1946.
31. Miale, J. B.: Laboratory medicine, hematology, ed. 3, St. Louis, 1967, The C. V. Mosby Co., p. 836.
32. Miller, J. F. A. P.: The role of blood cells in immunty, Brit. J. Haemat. 10:331, 1967.
33. Miller, J. F. A. P.: The thymus—yesterday, today and to-morrow, Lancet 2:1299, 1967.
34. Olson, L. C., Miller, G., and Hanshaw, J. B.: Acute infectious lymphocytosis presenting as a pertussis-like illness: its association with adenovirus type 12, Lancet 1:20, 1964.
35. O'Sullivan, M. A., and Pryles, C. V.: A comparison of leukocyte alkaline phosphatase determinations in 200 patients with mongolism and 200 "familial" controls, New Eng. J. Med. 268:1168, 1963.
36. Ottesen, J.: On the age of human white cells in the peripheral blood, Acta Physiol. Scand. 32:75, 1959.
37. Perry, S.: Biochemistry of the white blood cell, J.A.M.A. 190:918, 1964.
38. Peterman, M. G., Kaster, J. D., Gecht, E. A., and Lembert, G. L.: Epidemic of acute infectious lymphocytosis with diarrhea, Pediatrics 3:214, 1949.
39. Putnam, S. M., Moore, G. T., and Mitchell, D. W.: Infectious lymphocytosis; long-term follow-up of one epidemic, Pediatrics 41:588, 1968.
40. Reyersbach, G., and Lenert, T. F.: Infectious mononucleosis without clinical signs or symptoms, Amer. J. Dis. Child. 61:237, 1941.
41. Rosenbaum, S.: Febris lymphocytotica, Ann. Paediat. 152:117, 1938.
42. Ryder, R. J. W.: Acute infectious lymphocytosis, Amer. J. Dis. Child. 110:299, 1965.
43. Scalettar, H. E., Maisel, J. E., and Bramson, M.: Acute infectious lymphocytosis, Amer. J. Dis. Child. 88:15, 1954.
44. Smith, C. H.: Infectious lymphocytosis, Amer. J. Dis. Child. 62:231, 1941.
45. Smith, C. H.: Acute infectious lymphocytosis; specific infection; report of four cases showing its communicability, J.A.M.A. 125:342, 1944.
46. Sturgis, C. C., and Bethell, F. H.: Quantitative and qualitative variations in normal leukocytes, Physiol. Rev. 23:279, 1943.
47. Tanaka, K. R., Valentine, W. N., and Fredricks, R. E.: Disease or clinical conditions associated with low leukocyte alkaline phosphatase, New Eng. J. Med. 262:912, 1960.
48. Thelander, H. E., and Shaw, E. B.: Infectious mononucleosis, with specific reference to cerebral complications, Amer. J. Dis. Child. 61:1131, 1941.
49. Trubowitz, S., Feldman, D., Benante, C., and Hunt, V. M.: The alkaline phosphatase content of human leukocytes following marrow suppression by nitrogen mustard, J. Lab. Clin. Med. 22:259, 1958.
50. Trubowitz, S., Kirkman, D., and Mase, K. B.: The leukocyte alkaline phosphatase in mongolism, Lancet 2:486, 1962.
51. Twomey, J. J., and Leavell, B. S.: Leukemoid reactions to tuberculosis, Arch. Intern. Med. 116:21, 1965.
52. West, M., Heller, P., and Zimmerman, H. S.: Serum enzymes in disease. III. Lactic dehydrogenase and glutamic-oxaloacetic transaminase in patients with leukemia and lymphoma, Amer. J. Med. Sci. 235:689, 1958.
53. Wiltshaw, E., and Moloney, W. C.: Histochemical and biochemical studies in leukocyte alkaline phosphatase activity, Blood 10:1120, 1955.

# 21 INFECTIOUS MONONUCLEOSIS

***Definition.*** Infectious mononucleosis is an acute infectious disease of unknown etiology. It is usually benign, has a self-limited course, and is characterized by lymphocytosis with atypical lymphocytes in the peripheral blood, enlarged lymph nodes and spleen, and various other constitutional symptoms. In a large number of patients the serum reveals a high titer of agglutinins for sheep red cells.

***Historical.*** The earliest descriptions of the disease were by Filatov[29] in 1885 and by Pfeiffer[74] in 1889, who gave it the name glandular fever. The latter reported a symptoms complex in children marked by an acute onset and enlargement of the posterior cervical nodes, the liver, and spleen. Case reports of glandular fever appeared in the literature in increasing numbers, emphasizing the clinical aspects of the disease. In 1920 Sprunt and Evans[93] drew attention to its infective nature, described the changes in the peripheral blood characterized by an increase in mononuclear and other normal cells, and designated the disease as infectious mononucleosis. Soon afterward, Longcope[63] and Downey and McKinlay[21] provided an accurate morphologic description of the cells diagnostic of this disease. The three types of cells described by the latter are frequently referred to as Downey cells. Tidy and Daniel at this time[98] confirmed the significance of these cells and pointed out that glandular fever and infectious mononucleosis were identical conditions. From that time until the serologic studies were made, this disease received increasing recognition, and both the clinical features and blood picture became more sharply defined.

A basic contribution in the diagnosis of infectious mononucleosis was made in 1932 with the discovery by Paul and Bunnell[72] that the serum of patients with this disease agglutinated the washed erythrocytes of sheep in concentrations above a normal titer. These agglutinins are termed heterophil antibodies because the reaction is with antigens of a different species that has nothing to do with their development—in this case, sheep cells. The discovery stimulated renewed interest in this disease, particularly in its immunologic aspects, and provided a diagnostic criterion of great accuracy in a disease with such protean manifestations.

Interest in a possible viral etiology of infectious mononucleosis has recently been renewed by the reports[70] that a newly discovered member of the herpes virus group (called herpes-type virus [HTV] or Epstein-Barr virus [EBV]) first isolated in association with Burkitt's lymphoma in Africa[26] may be implicated. The Epstein-Barr (EB) virus which was originally seen in cell cultures derived from Burkitt's lymphoma has been implicated as the etiologic agent of infectious mononucleosis.[5] Many studies have demonstrated a rise in the EB virus antibody titer in patients with infectious mononucleosis. In spite of this association and even though a similar herpes-group virus has been found in cultures of peripheral leukocytes from patients with infectious mononucleosis, this virus is not yet established as the etiologic agent of either infectious mononucleosis or Burkitt's tumor.

Henle, Henle, and Diehl[42] demonstrated that patients with infectious mononucleosis acquired antibodies to the EB virus and implicated a herpes-like virus originally observed in continuous cell cultures derived from Burkitt's lymphomas by Epstein and associates.[27]

When EB virus was isolated from the serum of a laboratory technologist with infectious mononucleosis and from sera of a group of college students with the same disease and definite heterophil-antibody responses were investigated, antibodies to the EB virus were found which persisted during convalescence without loss of titer.

Certain epidemiologic features of infectious mononucleosis are indicated by the antibody patterns to the EB or herpes-like virus of Burkitt's lymphomas. The absence of antibody correlated well with susceptibility: of 268 entering college students whose sera lacked EB virus antibody, infectious mononucleosis developed in 15%; of 94 whose serum already contained antibody, none had clinical disease. EB virus antibody correlated well with heterophil antibody. It was present in the sera of all 135 patients who had heterophil antibody-positive infectious mononucleosis. It was felt by Evans and his associates[28,70] that EB virus is strongly implicated as a cause of infectious mononucleosis. On the other hand, viruses like the Epstein-Barr have also been found in cells cultured from lymphoid tissue of cancer patients and from the peripheral leukocytes of cases of myeloblastic and lymphoblastic leukemia, and have turned up in the sera of many perfectly healthy people. Clearly, infection with a virus like the EB organism is common and is sometimes associated with infectious mononucleosis. Whether this virus is an oncogenic agent or merely a latent "passenger" virus in tumors or whether it is activated by infectious mononucleosis remains to be determined. However, among the acute infections, EB antibodies appear to be specific for infectious mononucleosis.

In connection with EB virus antibodies in infectious mononucleosis is the observation that sera from patients with this disease may contain antinuclear antibodies, cold agglutinins with anti-i specificity, and cardiolipin-flocculating antibodies causing biological false positive tests for syphilis. Of twenty-one patients 13 to 34 years of age, antinuclear antibodies in low titer were found by immunofluorescence in fourteen.[53] The LE phenomenon, however, was never encountered in this group of patients.

*Pathology.* The focal cellular and perivascular infiltration with normal and abnormal lymphocytes in so many of the organs such as the liver, nervous system, kidneys, heart, and lungs accounts in large measure for the variety of clinical symptoms.

Atypical lymphocytes are not present in the bone marrow, although a shift to the left of polymorphonuclear neutrophils with increased numbers of myelocytes occasionally is observed. In the lymph nodes the nodal architecture is maintained, and marked proliferative activity of the pulp with packing by lymphocytes is present. Throughout the pulp, in the sinuses, and on the edges of the germinal centers, large numbers of the atypical mononuclear cells observed in patients with infectious mononucleosis have been described.[35]

Although infectious mononucleosis is a benign disease, many of its manifestations have been compared to those observed in malignant transformation of white cells. The atypical large lymphocytes of infectious mononucleosis have been shown to incorporate tritiated $^3$H-thymidine in vitro to a greater degree than do normal circulating leukocytes.[13,37] In one study in early infectious mononucleosis the mean percentage of labeled cells after 2 hours of incubation was more than thirty times the value for normal blood.[37] It increased to 10.5% after 4 hours. Normal values were reached when recovery was complete. Since thymidine is known to be a specific precursor of deoxyribonucleic acid, these findings indicate that the lymphocytes of infectious mononucleosis have a greater tendency to synthesize deoxyribonucleic acid than normal lymphocytes. This increase in thymidine labeling is shared by leukocytes from patients with acute and chronic granulocytic leukemia and the immature lymphocytes from certain patients with lymphoblastic leukemia. In other observations studying DNA (incubation with $^3$H-thymidine) and RNA ($^3$H-cytidine) synthesis in infectious mononucleosis, it was noted that active proliferation of atypical cells is restricted to an early period of the disease, whereas release of such atypical cells may continue for a considerable period.[25]

Increased levels of enzymes involved in folic acid metabolism and decreased glucose-6-phosphate dehydrogenase activity are found in leukocytes from patients with infectious mononucleosis when compared to leukocytes from normal subjects.[10] A high glycogen content is also found.[20]

*Clinical features.* The problem of diagnosis usually is resolved by combining the heterophil antibody test with the hematologic and clinical findings, especially since seronegative cases of this disease have occurred. In early stages of the disease the diagnosis is puzzling, since enlarged and tender lymph nodes, characteristic blood abnormalities, and a positive heterophil test often do not appear until the end of the first week or 10 days.

The involvement of the liver and, to a lesser extent, the peripheral and central nervous systems has been reported with sufficient frequency to serve as an accessory diagnostic feature. The causative agent has not yet been identified, although a virus etiology is suspected.[52] The disease appears in both epidemic and sporadic forms. It is infectious but manifests a low degree of contagiousness. It occurs at any age, most commonly in children and young adults and rarely in infants. The incubation period is given as 4 to 14 days.

The disease is marked by fever, sore throat, and epistaxis, frequently with acute tonsillitis, and often with generalized enlargement of the lymph nodes and spleen. The edge of the spleen is soft, and the organ is never greatly enlarged. The spleen is palpable in approximately 50% of patients. Other clinical features to attract attention include headache, vomiting, urticaria, rash, jaundice, periorbital edema, and pain referable to the external muscles of the eyes. Abdominal pain may be a predominant feature, and the signs and symptoms may simulate acute appendicitis. Appendectomies have been performed before the true nature of the condition was recognized.[96] Hematuria and rectal bleeding have been encountered[106] but are rare in children.

In a few instances an enanthem, consisting of pinhead-sized spots which darken in 3 to 4 days, appears on the palate. True petechiae numbering ten to several hundred clustered near the junction of soft and hard palate and more posteriorly close to the midline have also been described.[88] They appear 3 days to 10 weeks (usually between the fifth and seventeenth day of illness)[66] after the onset of symptoms and last 3 to 11 days. These have not been associated with a hemorrhagic diathesis. The petechial eruption is not specific for infectious mononucleosis but resembles the eruption in rubella, secondary syphilis, and meningococcemia.[66]

An exanthem occurs more frequently. The rash may be macular, maculopapular, purpuric, or morbilliform, resembling rubella. Rose spots simulating those found in patients with typhoid fever have also been observed. Urticaria as the only skin manifestation has been reported in several cases. Falsely positive serologic reactions for syphilis[80] have also been encountered occasionally in the first week of the disease but revert to negative between the third and tenth weeks. The incidence of a biologic false-positive serologic test for syphilis is extremely low (0.66% in one series).[45] In association with a rubelliform rash and lymphadenopathy, differentiation of syphilis from infectious mononucleosis may be difficult in the early weeks. In a series of 200 cases of infectious mononucleosis, five complications were observed: rupture of the spleen, facial nerve palsies, mild meningitis, salivary gland inflammation, and complete atrioventricular block.[44] Orchitis is another rare complication.[76,108]

In an 18-year-old girl the skin lesions were of a diffuse maculopapular eruption covering the entire body including the palms and soles. The rash later coalesced in scattered areas and on the face presented as a butterfly eruption. The white blood count rose to 21,900/cu. mm., of which 39% were cells typical of infectious mononucleosis. The heterophil titer rose to 1:440.

*Clinical types.* Although symptoms vary widely, they have been classified by some authors into several categories. The glandular or childhood type is marked by sore throat, fever, and generalized lymphadenopathy and frequently occurs in epidemics. In young adults the pharyngeal type is common and is marked by fatigue and sore throat, general malaise, low-grade fever, and slight to moderate enlargement of lymph nodes. In patients with the febrile type, the onset is sudden, often with prolonged typhoid-like fever, headaches, chills, and prostration, followed later by rash and lymph node and splenic enlargement. Less commonly, the onset is ushered in variously as an acute allergic reaction with angioneurotic edema, jaundice, the signs of meningoencephalitis, or a severe angina with a membrane on or near the tonsils that mimics diphtheria.

In some children the initial period of illness, extending for 5 to 7 days, may be marked by the temperature reaching levels of hyperpyrexia with no other abnormal physical signs than a slightly palpable spleen. There may be no complaints. Leukocytes range from 5,000 to 6,000 per cubic millimeter, with a predominance of polymorphonuclear neutrophils. After several days of fever a diffuse eruption resembling rubella may appear without the enlargement of the postauricular, postcervical, and occipital lymph nodes which marks this disease. At the end of a week, temperatures are lower, eruptions are fading, and a moderate leukocytosis with a predominance of lymphocytes and a substantial number of diagnostic cells of infectious mononucleosis is noted. Throughout the entire extent of the disease, symptoms and physical signs may be minimal.

In rare instances the early stages of infectious mononucleosis simulate leukemia both clinically and hematologically, and careful scrutiny of blood smears and heterophil antibody tests is needed to differentiate between the two conditions. Of the clinical features that have been enumerated, the presence of unexplained fever, posterior cervical adenopathy, pharyngitis, and a tonsillar exudate should prompt a careful examination of the blood smear for the atypical cells found in patients with infectious mononucleosis.

A child has been described with acute lymphoblastic leukemia who developed infectious mononucleosis during a remission maintained by 6-mercaptopurine.[57] Another case of infectious mononucleosis has been reported with the rare complication of a mass in the anterior mediastinum.[102] Spontaneous concurrent regression of both conditions occurred.

*Involvement of the nervous system.* The pathologic changes in patients with infectious mononucleosis are widespread and include changes in the central nervous system, in the liver, and, to a lesser extent, in the heart and spleen. Involvement of the nervous system has been increasingly recognized in children as well as in adults. It has been stated[54] that this disease should be considered in the differential diagnosis of encephalitis and meningitis, for which no specific cause has been found. The nervous system manifestations vary from intense headache, blurred vision, and stiffness of the neck to definite evidence of central nervous system involvement. Encephalitis, encephalomyelitis, serous meningitis, acute polyradiculoneuritis as observed in patients with the Guillain-Barré syndrome,[24] facial palsy, retrobulbar neuritis, and other signs of isolated or diffuse upper and lower motor neuron lesions have been described. Although the association of seizures with infectious mononucleosis is infrequent, this disease should be considered in the differential diagnosis of unexplained and ill-defined convulsive episodes.[59] Alterations in the spinal fluid may occur to the extent of a moderate pleocytosis, increased pressure, increase in mononuclear cells, and, less frequently, increased protein. Neurologic complications appear 2 to 4 weeks after the onset of infectious mononucleosis but may precede or occur concomitantly with it. Recovery from the neurologic complications is the rule, although permanent damage and even death from respiratory paralysis have been noted.[20] A fatal case in a 19-year-old male has been reported in which an infectious neuronitis involved almost all of the cranial and spinal nerve roots.[18]

*Involvement of the liver.* Increasing evidence supports the view that impaired liver function accompanies the majority of cases of this disease. Jaundice may occur as the initial symptom or later in the disease with enlargement of lymph nodes. More frequently, hepatitis in the absence of jaundice has been reported in many studies as revealed with the use of serial liver function tests. In an examination of sixty-two children with a presumptive diagnosis of infectious mononucleosis, Hsia and Gellis[51] have shown 84% to have abnormal liver function. It has been suggested, therefore, that tests for liver function such as enzyme studies, cephalin flocculation, thymol turbidity, and bromsulphalein retention be used to supplement other diagnostic tests for infectious mononucleosis. The serum alkaline phosphatase, SGOT, and SGPT may also be increased. Similarly, in patients suspected of having infectious hepatitis it may be advisable to test for heterophil antibodies. Patients, especially children, with infectious mononucleosis, however, recover quickly and completely, whereas the course of those with infectious hepatitis is more prolonged and complicated. The impaired liver function may also account for prolonged convalescence and for the easy exhaustion and weakness found especially in young adults, though less commonly in children. Pathologic examination of the liver reveals a varying picture—from a normal architecture to focal hepatitis with loss of liver cells, cellular infiltration by atypical mononuclear cells, dilatation and invasion of sinuses, areas of scattered focal necrosis, and enlarged portal lymph nodes. The usual course of hepatitis is 2 to 6 weeks, with a rapid return to normal.[69] In rare cases in young adults jaundice and death with hepatic coma and massive necrosis of the liver have been reported.[2] In one such patient whole lobules had degenerated; in other areas the more central hepatic cells showed the greater disintegration. In the portal tracts there were bands of abnormal mononuclear cells, lymphocytes, and a scattering of neutrophil polymorphonuclear leukocytes. The diffuse focal hepatitis varies in degree in different cases. Hepatic failure is an exceedingly rare cause of death in infectious mononucleosis.

*Involvement of the heart.* Cardiac complications occur infrequently, especially in childhood, and are detected by electrocardiographic and clinical examinations. These have been attributed to focal interstitial infiltrations of mononuclear cells and lymphocytes in the myocardium.[1] Fatal acute myocarditis with focal microscopic areas of necrosis and fragmentation of heart muscle fibers has been reported.[30] Although scattered necropsy reports have shown involvement of the myocardium, there is every evidence that valvular heart disease is a rare complication of infectious mononucleosis.[43] The changes observed on the electrocardiogram are transient and consist of lowering or inversion of the T waves in various leads and increased P-R interval. Since clinical examination infrequently reveals an affected heart, the correct interpretation of these electrocardiographic findings remains uncertain.[49] The first symptoms of infectious mononucleosis may be those of acute benign pericarditis.[36,91] Although patients with fatal nervous system involvement or splenic rupture are more likely to show definite myocarditis, chronic heart disease is not to be expected as a sequela in patients with infectious mononucleosis.

The rarity of cardiac complications in infectious mononucleosis was demonstrated in Hoagland's[46] series of 419 consecutive patients with this disease in whom no evidence of valvular or pericardial disease was observed. The only clinical manifestations of heart disease were the occasional palpitations and dyspnea with exertion. Electrocardiograms of 338 patients revealed abnormalities in only 6%. As a rule, tracings became normal within 4 weeks after onset of illness. Electrocardiography as a routine procedure was therefore not recommended. Only the rare patient with cardiac dysfunction was confined to bed.

*Rupture of the spleen.* Rupture of an enlarged spleen can occur spontaneously or as a result of trauma and has also been related to vigorous palpation of the abdomen. The liability to rupture is not encountered until the third week of illness and is due to the softness and friability of the spleen resulting from thinning of the capsule and dissolution of the trabeculae by lymphocytic infiltration.[14] Rupture of the spleen has, however, been reported as early as the fourth day after the onset of the disease[109] and may be accompanied by severe postoperative bleeding due to thrombocytopenia.[103]

*Laboratory findings.* Characteristic abnormalities are found in the peripheral blood and by serologic examination.

*Blood picture.* In the majority of patients the blood picture constitutes the most important diagnostic feature of infectious mononucleosis. The total white blood cell count usually ranges from 10,000 to 20,000 per cubic millimeter during the peak of the disease, in the second and third weeks, and exceeds the upper limit to 50,000 in rare cases. At such extreme levels it must be differentiated from acute infectious lymphocytosis. Leukocytosis usually accompanies fever and enlargement of the lymph nodes. The count, however, varies greatly, and leukopenia with white blood cell levels as low as 3,000 per cubic millimeter may mark the disease in its first week. Frequently, in young adults, the white blood cell count is normal, but clinical symptoms and the blood smear provide the clue to diagnosis.

The striking feature in the blood smear is the shift from an early normal or increased percentage of polymorphonuclear neutrophils to a predominance of the mononuclear elements to the extent of 50 to 90%. The term mononuclear cells was formerly applied to both monocytes and lymphocytes—hence the term infectious mononucleosis. The majority of abnormal cells are now known to be derivatives of the lymphocytic series and must be differentiated from the immature lymphocytes of leukemia. The atypical mononuclear cell in the blood of patients with infectious mononucleosis represents its distinctive feature. The identification of lymphocytes, however, has been verified by supravital staining (Fig. 67 and Plate 2). Monocytes may also be increased. The characteristic mononuclear cells, consisting mainly of lymphocytes, are larger than normal, their cellular edges are often ragged and irregular, and the cytoplasm is usually abundant, staining a darker blue with Wright's stain than do normal large lymphocytes. The cytoplasm contains fine or coarse azure granules, and one of the most striking features is the vacuolation. The vacuoles are of two types: they may be large and scattered in cells with abundant cytoplasm, or they may be smaller and more numerous. The combination of fine vacuolation and basophilia gives the cytoplasm a distinctive foamy appearance. (See Fig. 67.)

The nucleus of the cells in patients with infectious mononucleosis may be round, oval, or kidney shaped; occasionally, it is divided and often eccentrically placed. The Downey type I cell refers to the cells with dark blue

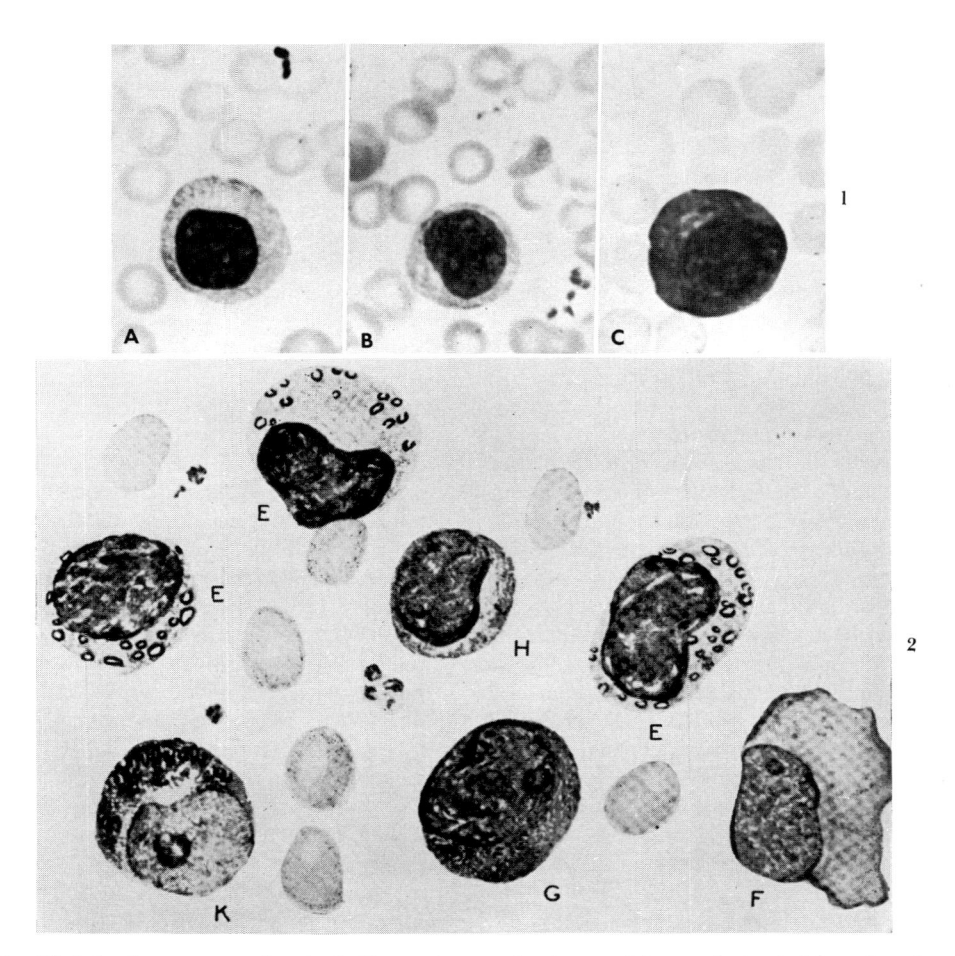

Fig. 67. Infectious mononucleosis, 1, Photomicrograph of several types of atypical lymphocytes found in the blood smear of patients with infectious mononucleosis. A and C possess a finely vacuolated cytoplasm giving a foamy appearance, exaggerated in C by the deep basophilia. The color of the cytoplasm with Wright's stain varies from a slate color to the deep blue of a plasma cell. The nuclear pattern in B is not so coarse as that in the other cells and is more immature, with finer strands of lighter staining chromatin. Several nucleoli are present. This cell resembles somewhat the lymphoblast and is often referred to as the Downey type III cell (see K in 2). (Courtesy Dr. Ralph L. Engle, Jr., New York, N. Y.)

2, Drawings of representative cells in the blood smear of patients with infectious mononucleosis. Although a number of different cell types usually appear in the blood smear at one time, especially at the height of the disease, all of these cells were not found together in any single case. F is a cell with irregular edges, eccentric nucleus, abundant cytoplasm, and concentration of basophilia in the periphery. A lightly staining perinuclear zone is observed in K. Deep basophilia of the cytoplasm is noticable in G, H, and K. Vacuolation of the cytoplasm is present in E and G. The finer vacuoles and deep basophilia in G give the cytoplasm a foamy appearance, an important diagnostic feature. Cells of type K occurred most infrequently. The nucleus of the K-type cell stains lightly and approaches in immaturity the nucleus of the lymphoblasts. (From Smith, C. H.: Infectious lymphocytosis, Amer. J. Dis. Child. 62:231, 1941.)

foamy cytoplasm and an irregular kidney-shaped nucleus. The Downey type II cell possesses larger amounts of light blue cytoplasm and an eccentrically placed nucleus of normal appearance. The diagnosis in the acute stages of infectious mononucleosis is made by the presence of one or another of the characteristic types of cells and by the assortment of unusual cells in the blood smear.

Occasionally, small numbers of large rounded cells with well-differentiated nuclei having a diffuse sievelike arrangement of chromatin and sometimes showing nucleoli and lightly basophilic cytoplasm, resembling reticuloendothelial cells, appear in the peripheral blood. The cells resemble lymphoblasts and are designated as Downey type III. They probably originate from areas of reticulum cell proliferation in affected lymph nodes.[22]

Schumacher and colleagues[84] studied the peripheral mononucleosis lymphocytes from eleven patients with infectious mononucleosis by electron microscopy. In comparison with normal lymphocytes, the mononucleosis lymphocyte showed significantly greater cell and cytoplasmic area, greater cell length, more nucleoli, polyribosomes, and compound vacuoles. Much evidence is available to show that the actual site of protein synthesis in the living cell is the polyribosome. The authors consider that infectious mononucleosis represents a disease which is characterized by a marked immunologic response to an antigenic stimulus. This stimulus may be the herpes-like virus and may be followed by a variable host response. A few cells in mononucleosis were seen that had features of both the lymphocyte and monocyte and were difficult to classify.

Just as agglutination may appear in higher titer in patients with diseases other than infectious mononucleosis, so have these atypical cells been noted in patients with a variety of conditions such as infectious hepatitis, virus pneumonia, German measles, measles, acute brucellosis, influenza, roseola infantum, and others.

Because of the increased incidence in so-called virus diseases, the atypical lymphocytes have been termed virocytes.[4,60,101] It is important to point out that the blood smears of young infants are particularly prone to show these cells in a number of nonspecific infections unrelated to infectious mononucleosis. In patients with conditions other than infectious mononucleosis, however, the abnormal mononuclear cells appear in much smaller numbers, rarely reaching 10%. At the height of the illness, the quantitative difference serves as a differential criterion. Eosinophilia has been observed during the acute stage of the disease, but is even more common during convalescence.

It has already been stated that the blood picture in the introductory stages may simulate leukemia. This confusion results from the occasional presence of immature cells resembling lymphoblasts (Downey type III cells), especially when they are observed in association with anemia, leukopenia, and thrombopenia. However, the eventual appearance of atypical lymphocytes in significant numbers provides an indication of the true nature of the process.

Stevens and associates[95] suggested that the intercurrent development of infectious mononucleosis is apt to be associated with transitory remission in the course of acute lymphocytic leukemia, indeed that this favorable effect may be more lasting in some cases with long survival. The development of infectious mononucleosis in the course of acute lymphocytic leukemia appears to have a favorable effect on the latter disease as determined from published cases. In addition, after convalescence these patients appear to have high titers to EB virus (EBV). When serial serum specimens were available, a secondary rise in antibody titer well after recovery from infectious mononucleosis was documented. This rise possibly is unique to the concurrence of these two diseases, since titers in patients without leukemia fall after recovery from infectious mononucleosis and remain relatively constant. Serum samples from patients with long survival after acute lymphocytic leukemia without a history of concurrent infectious mononucleosis were also assayed and found to have a geometric mean anti-EBV titer higher than various control groups. Further studies are required to evaluate this phenomenon.

The red blood cell count, hemoglobin concentration, platelet count, sedimentation rate, coagulation time, and bleeding time are usually normal. A mild anemia may attend convalescence. Exceptionally, thrombocytopenic purpura[3,62,71] and acute hemolytic anemia[40,97] have been reported during the course of infectious mononucleosis.

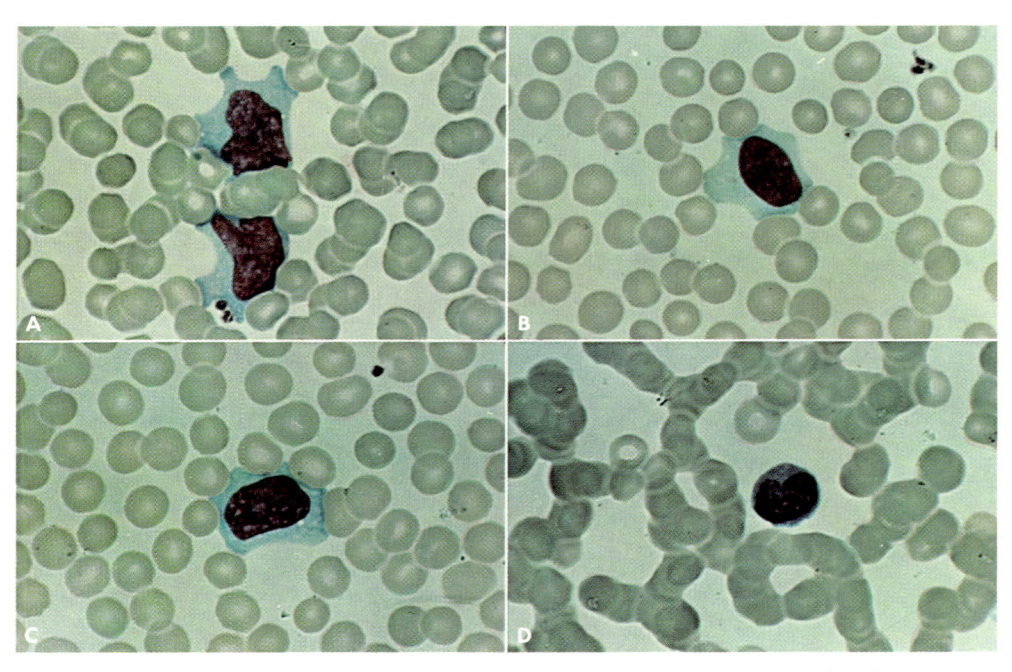

**Plate 2.** Atypical lymphocytes in infectious mononucleosis with characteristic abundant vacuolated cytoplasm, irregular cell margin, and pleomorphic nucleus containing nucleoli (**A**, **B**, and **C**). Other lymphocytes, **D**, are smaller, with clumped nuclear chromatin and intensely blue (see **K** in **2**). (Courtesy Dr. Ralph L. Engle, Jr., New York, N. Y.)

Acute hemolytic anemia occurring during the course of infectious mononucleosis is often associated with marked prostration, high fever, and deepening jaundice. The anemia may be of sufficient severity to necessitate splenectomy.[105] Uncommonly, a positive antiglobulin (Coombs) test,[40,50,81] cold agglutinins,[97] and autohemolysins indicative of an autoimmune mechanism have been present.

As with certain cases of idiopathic thrombocytopenia, the probable mechanism of thrombocytopenia in infectious mononucleosis and other viral infections is in part an immunologic one. Another explanation for the thrombocytopenia is alteration of the platelets by infection, rendering them autoantigenic or productive of a new antigen when combined with virus.[16,75] The duration of thrombocytopenia is from 4 to 22 days, with a return to a normal number of platelets within 2 months. Prednisone has been used effectively, as with other cases of thrombocytopenic purpura in childhood.[12]

It has been postulated that the etiologic factors, viral or bacterial, responsible for causing infectious mononucleosis may also injure the red cells or platelets directly or through antibody formation. Abnormal splenic function or hypersplenism may be involved similarly in causing a reduction in any of the formed elements of the blood in patients with infectious mononucleosis inasmuch as this disease is so often accompanied by splenomegaly.[3] Elevation of serum alkaline phosphatase is found especially in severe illness, but its causation is not clear. It cannot be attributed solely to obstructive interference with hepatic excretion of the enzyme.[7] A correlation is often observed between the occurrence of hyperglobulinemia, leukocytosis, and elevation of the serum alkaline phosphatase.

*Heterophil antibody (Paul-Bunnell) test.* There is no unanimity of opinion; however, a heterophil antibody titer of 1:112 is usually considered diagnostic although the critical level stated in various laboratories ranges from 1:56 to 1:1792. No correlation appears to exist between the heterophil antibody titer and the severity of the disease. The heterophil antibody test has been found positive in 60 to 90% of patients, and for that reason examination of the blood smear for atypical lymphocytes is still of paramount importance. The timing of tests is important, since the titer may be low in the first week and usually reaches a peak in the second and third weeks, in some instances, to extraordinary levels. An elevated titer may persist during convalescence, usually 2 to 5 months, sometimes 6 months and longer, after the symptoms subside. It may revert to normal, however, in 6 to 8 weeks. Repetition of tests, therefore, is important in doubtful cases, and increased positive reactions probably depend upon this factor. When venous blood is difficult to obtain, a fingertip microheterophil agglutinin technique has been described which compares favorably with the regular heterophil technique.[41]

According to Vahlquist and associates,[99] a positive Paul-Bunnell reaction is rare below 5 years of age, and this is explained by a defect in antibody formation during this period. Past this age, the reaction does not differ from adult cases with respect to intensity and duration of the serologic reaction.

Positive Paul-Bunnell reactions have been reported as early as the first year of life but only expectionally have such reactions been obtained on absorbed sera. Regarding reactions exceeding 1:20 or 1:32 after absorption as indicative of infectious mononucleosis Vahlquist and associates[99] did not find a single positive reaction below 5 years of age. Among patients 5 to 9 years of age, the reaction occurred in 8.8%, whereas among those 10 to 14 years old, it was positive in 26.4%. It is not known whether the reaction is rare in early years because of low incidence of infection or because of age-specific lack of ability to form heterophil antibodies. Conditions with a scattering of virocytes, such as those occurring in acute upper respiratory infection, chronic infectious lymphocytosis, and viral infections, are readily differentiated from infectious mononucleosis, which is characterized by an outpouring of large numbers of abnormal lymphocytes whether or not the Paul-Bunnell test is positive.

Recently vanFurth and co-workers[100] have shown that gamma globulins were synthesized by infectious mononucleosis cells in tissue culture.

MacKinney[65] has demonstrated that these cells produce heterophil antibodies. Tissue culture of peripheral blood leukocytes with $^{14}$C-leucine resulted in radioactive protein identified as immunoglobulin by immunoelectrophoresis, gel filtration, and immunoprecipitation. Radioactive heterophil antibody was detected by precipitin reaction with heterophil antigen. It was found in significant concentration in infectious mononucleosis cultures but not in normal controls.

*Differential agglutination tests.* Heterophil

**Table 27.** Scheme of differential agglutination

| Source of serum | Heterophil agglutinins after absorption by | |
|---|---|---|
| | guinea pig kidney | beef cells |
| Infectious mononucleosis | Present | Absent |
| Normal serum | Absent | Present |
| Serum sickness | Absent | Absent |

agglutinins against sheep cells are present in low titer in normal serum and after the injection of horse serum. These are the Forssman[31] type of antibodies which are distinct from those elaborated in patients with infectious mononucleosis. The fact that the Forssman[31] type of antibody combines actively with guinea pig kidney and does not react with beef red cells is employed in the diagnosis of infectious mononucleosis. The heterophil antibodies present in patients with serum sickness and in those with normal serum can be removed by absorption with guinea pig kidney, whereas antibodies in the serum of patients with infectious mononucleosis are not absorbed to the same extent. Although complete absorption with beef red cells is to be expected in patients with infectious mononucleosis, if at least one-fourth of the agglutinin titer remains after absorption with guinea pig kidney, the test is positive for infectious mononucleosis.[17] A titer of at least 1:30 following absorption is considered necessary for a diagnosis of infectious mononucleosis. In one series of 200 patients below 29 years of age, the characteristic heterophil antibody reactions were sheep cell agglutination of at least 1:56 in unabsorbed serum, a titer of at least 1:28 after absorption of serum with guinea pig kidney, and no agglutination after beef cell antigen absorption.[44]

Table 27 indicates the scheme of differential agglutination.

Absorption tests therefore add to the accuracy of the diagnosis, especially in patients with low titers. In clinical practice, however, these tests are frequently not undertaken when the blood smear and supportive clinical features confirm the diagnosis. In the presence of other unequivocal evidences of this disease, a negative serologic test does not rule out the diagnosis of infectious mononucleosis.

Forssman[31] discovered that the injection of emulsions of guinea pig organs into rabbits induced the formation of antibodies that would lyse sheep erythrocytes. The Forssman type antibodies react against an antigen widely spread in animal tissues—i.e., guinea pig, horse, dog, cat—and absent in tissues of man, ox, rat, etc. Guinea pig kidney is rich in the Forssman antigen, and beef red cells are deficient in this antigen. If sheep cell agglutinins are absorbed by a suspension of guinea pig tissue, then the antibodies are of the Forssman type. If the sheep cell agglutinins are not absorbed by guinea pig tissue but are removed by ox erythrocytes, then the antibodies are probably specific for the unknown agent, which causes infectious mononucleosis.

Absorption tests are especially pertinent in rare instances in which the Paul-Bunnell test has been found positive without the associated features of infectious mononucleosis. These include a variety of conditions in which an occasional patient may reveal a significant titer—e.g., infectious hepatitis, purpura, German measles, scarlet fever, sarcomas, upper respiratory infections, primary atypical pneumonia, monocytic and myelogenous leukemia, thrombocytopenic purpura,[94] and Hodgkin's disease.[82] In one series[92] elevated heterophil antibody titers (1:112 or more) were observed in 19% of patients with acute leukemia. This antibody was completely or almost completely absorbed by guinea pig kidney, demonstrating its relationship to the Forssman type in contrast to poor absorption in patients with infectious mononucleosis. No elevated heterophil antibodies were observed in this series in patients with chronic leukemia.

A sharp reduction in titer has been observed when enzyme (papain) treated sheep erythrocytes are mixed with the serum of patients with infectious mononucleosis.[68] In contrast, the serum of patients with an elevated heterophil antibody titer unrelated to infectious mononucleosis showed a conspicuous increase in reactivity with enzyme-treated sheep red cells as compared with their reactivity with untreated cells.

We have noted unabsorbed titers ranging

from 1:112 to 1:7168 in patients with thrombocytopenic purpura, severe Cooley's anemia, lymphoma, and cirrhosis of the liver and in children with regional ileitis.

Formalized horse red cells have been used as a rapid slide test for infectious mononucleosis.[47] It is claimed that the horse cell possesses a greater specificity for diagnosis than the presumptive heterophil test using sheep cells. An ox cell hemolysin test had also been employed as a check against the heterophil antibody test.[73]

Several studies have confirmed the reliability of the use of formalized horse red cells in the diagnosis of infectious mononucleosis. In one series the agglutination titer in the serum was higher with horse red cells than with sheep cells.[86] If absorptions with guinea pig, kidney, and ox red cells were done, the expected results were obtained: only the ox red cells removed the antibody against horse red cells from the serum of the patients suffering from infectious mononucleosis, while both absorbants removed the antibody from the serum of patients suffering with other diseases. In another study[6] comprising 372 patients with suspected infectious mononucleosis results showed the use of formalized horse red cells in the Monospot test (rapid slide test) to be simple and time-saving and of sufficient specificity for routine use in the general laboratory.

In one series[89] a microcapillary tube was substituted for the slide agglutination technique in screening tests on 296 individuals suspected of having infectious mononucleosis. The age range was from 3 months to 17 years. Here, too, the horse red cell agglutination reaction was found to be a reliable and simple screening test and produced only 0.6% false positives and 1.9% false negatives. It was emphasized that the horse cell agglutination reaction serves only as a screening test. Where other clinical findings are atypical or in disagreement with the test, then Davidsohn's differential test plus hematological evaluation should be performed for confirmation of the diagnosis. The study also confirmed previous observations that there were no positive sheep cell or horse cell agglutinations in patients under 1 year of age.

*Differential diagnosis.* The diverse clinical picture, the wide range of symptoms, and the pathologic lesions in patients with infectious mononucleosis may obscure the diagnosis and require a consideration of many diseases which it mimics. These include leukemia, acute infectious lymphocytosis, poliomyelitis, German measles, chronic upper respiratory infections, rheumatic fever, acute appendicitis, infectious hepatitis, pertussis, mumps, influenza, and lymphocytic choriomeningitis. About 7% of cases diagnosed as glandular fever, but giving a negative Paul-Bunnell reaction, are due to toxoplasmosis.[11] Usually, the enlargement of the lymph nodes and the spleen, sore throat, fever, numerous atypical lymphocytes in the blood smear, an increased titer of heterophil antibodies, and the absence of anemia, and of invasive blast cells in the marrow establish the proper diagnosis. Although infectious hepatitis and infectious mononucleosis resemble each other by liver function tests and in pathologic findings, infectious mononucleosis usually is associated with an increased heterophil antibody titer, and the number of patients with clinical jaundice is small.

It should also be pointed out that during the first months of life small numbers of lymphocytes occasionally are observed in the blood smears from normal infants which resemble the abnormal cells found in patients with infectious mononucleosis. These cells, however, bear no relationship to this disease or to any other related condition.

Infectious mononucleosis and acute lymphocytic leukemia can both present clinically with fever, leukocytosis, lymphadenopathy, splenomegaly, and morphologically abnormal lymphocytes in the peripheral blood. Although these conditions can easily be differentiated by bone marrow examination and their different clinical courses, both diseases may occur concurrently. In one group of four patients,[34] infectious mononucleosis preceded acute leukemia by 3 months in one case and occurred in three cases at various times during a hematologic remission. It appears probable that, as the course of acute lymphocytic leukemia becomes more prolonged by improved therapy, intercurrent illnesses such as infectious mononucleosis will be recognized with increasing frequency. Freedman and colleagues[34] also summarized the features of five previously documented cases involving the association of infectious mononucleosis and acute lymphocytic leukemia. In most cases the patient who had infectious mononucleosis had no evidence of leukemic activity.[57] The authors concluded that infectious mononucleosis is an intercurrent illness which is etiologically unrelated to acute leukemia.

**Prognosis.** In spite of the alarming nature of many of the symptoms, the prognosis is good except in rare patients with splenic rupture or superimposed infections. Fatal cases of infectious mononucleosis have occurred, however, without rupture of the spleen. They reveal a widespread involvement of lymphoid tissue and the presence of atypical mononuclear cells throughout a majority of the organs.[87]

In thirty autopsies of infectious mononucleosis at the Armed Forces Institute of Pathology, the three major causes of death were spontaneous rupture of the spleen (thirteen cases), Guillian-Barré syndrome (six cases), and hemorrhage from the nasopharynx or gastrointestinal tract (four cases). Secondary infection constituted the most common cause of death in the remaining seven patients.[64]

**Treatment.** The disease is self-limited, and no specific therapeutic measure has proved effective. Treatment is symptomatic, and reliance must be placed upon rest and supportive measures in view of involvement of various organs, especially the liver, nervous system, and heart.

In children complications are rare, although the overall incidence in all age groups has been approximated as 5%.[107] Antibiotics may be of value in patients with severe sore throat and in controlling secondary infections. Corticosteroids may be prescribed with caution in a number of complications in infectious mononucleosis. These include hemolytic anemia, thrombocytopenia, the severe anginose form of the disease, and severe nervous system complications. Cortisone and ACTH have been employed in diminishing the severity of the disease,[19] in respiratory distress,[77] in relieving allergic manifestations,[61] and in the treatment of meningoencephalitis.[33] It should be emphasized that the value of the steroid hormones in reducing constitutional symptoms must be balanced against the risk of disseminating a concomitant or occult bacterial infection.[8]

In a large number of cases severe pharyngeal inflammation and edema are prominent features of the disease, and in an exceptional case laryngeal stridor develops.[67] Although tracheotomy is rarely required, the degree of obstruction necessary to convert a markedly narrowed airway to an occluded one is slight.

For the patients with hemorrhagic manifestations due to thrombocytopenia, treatment with the adrenocortical steroids has been effective. Prednisone or prednisolone is given in comparable dosage to that of idiopathic thrombocytopenic purpura, i.e., 2 mg. per kilogram of body weight per day in divided dosage every 6 or 8 hours. It is rare that 60 mg. daily has to be exceeded. The use of corticosteroids in thrombocytopenia purpura secondary to infectious mononucleosis is definitely indicated, since the risk of intracranial hemorrhage is probably greater than any theoretical risk from treating a possible virus infection with steroids.[38] The basic disease, infectious mononucleosis, is not worsened by its use, although this observation does not serve as an indication for the routine use of corticosteroids in the absence of thrombocytopenia. Treatment for 5 to 7 days should effect an increase in platelets and the control of hemorrhage.[106] In very unusual cases splenectomy is necessary to control hemorrhage due to thrombocytopenia.[15] For patients with the rare complication of hemolytic anemia transfusions are given with or without the steroid hormones. In one patient in whom cortisone was ineffective, splenectomy was resorted to with a favorable response.[97]

A group of 100 patients was observed[83] and subjected to a variety of therapeutic programs, including chloroquine, prednisone, and antibiotics. From analysis of the fever, signs and symptoms, duration of illness, total hospital stay, and hospitalization after therapy, it was concluded that none of the drugs, with the possible exception of intravenous steroids, was beneficial in the treatment of the basic disease. For those patients with presumable secondary invaders in the tonsils and pharynx, appropriate antibiotics are of value, but only when the organism is determined by culture. Indiscriminate antibiotic treatment was to be avoided. Intravenous hydrocortisone appeared to be beneficial for only the severe anginose variety with airway obstruction. It was concluded from this study that the best treatment is symptomatic.

Bed rest in the acute febrile stages of the disease is considered important; usually this is a matter of 2 to 3 weeks. Activity is governed largely by the patient's fatigability. Persistently abnormal liver functions do not indicate that bed rest is required. In children and adolescents in the absence of fever, pharyngeal and tonsillar inflammation, or any complication, it is questionable whether drastic limitation of activities is ever required.

*Recurrences.* Although unquestionable recurrences have been reported, they are extremely rare[9,55] and frequently fail to demonstrate significant heterophil antibodies. However, a nonspecific rise in titer occurs some months after the initial attack, especially following an upper respiratory infection. Since atypical lymphocytes are known to persist for extended periods, recurrences may be erroneously diagnosed. More extensive experience is required with a combination of laboratory techniques, especially liver function tests, to rule out the influence of hepatitis as a causative factor in prolongation and chronicity of the disease or its recurrence.

*Febrile postcardiotomy syndrome with splenomegaly and atypical lymphocytes.* A clinical entity termed febrile postcardiotomy lymphocytic splenomegaly has been described in patients 3 to 7 weeks after open-heart surgery utilizing a pump oxygenator.[48,85,104] Fever has its onset 8 to 42 days after the operation, with splenomegaly somewhat later, and lymphocytes resembling those of infectious mononucleosis appear in the blood. In contrast to infectious mononucleosis, lymphoadenopathy is absent or minimal and pharyngitis is absent. A rise in heterophil agglutinin is rare. Hepatosplenomegaly and disturbed liver function are transient. The syndrome lasts about 1 month and subsides without specific therapy. The etiology is unknown, and recovery takes place in all cases.

World-wide reports have established posttransfusion mononucleosis as a frequent consequence of large-volume fresh blood transfusions.[90] Foster and Jack[32] reported that after open-heart surgery, posttransfusion mononucleosis developed in six patients who had cytomegalovirus complement-fixing antibody before operation. Three of them showed an appreciable antibody rise during the episode of mononucleosis, and cytomegalovirus was isolated from the leukocytes of another two. The cytomegalovirus in the blood of patients experiencing posttransfusion mononucleosis may be of endogenous as well as of exogenous derivation. Studies by Lang and his associates[58] also support an etiologic role for cytomegalovirus in the "postperfusion" or "postpump" syndrome. Virus was recovered from washed leukocytes or leukocyte-rich plasma. Cell-free plasma and erythrocytes did not yield virus.

A significant rise in the titer of complement-fixing antibodies to the cytomegalovirus strain "AD169" has been observed in patients with a mononucleosis-like disease without a positive heterophil agglutination test.[56] Leukocytosis, relative and absolute lymphocytosis, and the appearance of abundant atypical lymphocytes were features of the hematologic pattern.

This condition is to be differentiated from the postcardiotomy syndrome, which is an uncommon complication of heart surgery occurring after a latent period. It is identified by fever and pleuropericarditis,[23,78] elevated erythrocyte sedimentation rate, and spontaneous resolution. Arthralgia and tendency to relapse are less common features. Corticosteroid rapidly suppresses the disorder and, when used prophylactically, prevents its appearance. A hypersensitivity reaction in an immunologic sense, with positive tests for heart antibodies, has been demonstrated.[78]

Three instances of a syndrome resembling infectious mononucleosis were observed in young adults after splenectomy for idiopathic thrombocytopenic purpura.[79]

## REFERENCES

1. Allen, F. H., and Kellner, A.: Infectious mononucleosis; an autopsy report, Amer. J. Path. 23:463, 1947.
2. Allen, V. R., and Basa, B. H.: Fatal hepatic necrosis in glandular fever, J. Clin. Path. 16: 337, 1963.
3. Angle, R. M., and Alt, H. L.: Thrombocytopenic purpura complicating infectious mononucleosis; report of a case and serial platelet counts during the course of infectious mononucleosis, Blood 5:449, 1950.
4. Bakst, H., and Liebowitz, J.: Infectious mononucleosis; report of case with first appearance of significant numbers of heterophil antibodies and abnormal lymphocytes ("virocytes") in seventh week of illness, Amer. J. Med. 13:235, 1952.
5. Banatvala, J. E.: Infectious mononucleosis; recent developments, Brit. J. Haemat. 19: 129, 1970.
6. Basson, V., and Sharp, A. A.: Monospot; a differential slide test for infectious mononucleosis, J. Clin. Path. 22:324, 1969.
7. Barondess, J. A., and Erle, H.: Serum alkaline phosphatase activity in hepatitis of infectious mononucleosis, Amer. J. Med. 29: 43, 1960.

8. Beeson, P. B., Muschenheim, C., Castle, W. B., Harrison, T. R., Ingelfinger, F. J., and Bondy, P. K., editors: Year book of medicine, 1957-1958 series, Chicago, 1958, Year Book Medical Publishers, Inc.
9. Bender, C. E.: Recurrent mononucleosis, J.A.M.A. 182:156, 1962.
10. Bertino, J. R., Simmons, B. M., and Donohue, D. M.: Increased activity of some folic acid enzyme systems in infectious mononucleosis, Blood 19:587, 1962.
11. Beverley, J. K. A., and Beattie, C. P.: Glandular toxoplasmosis; a survey of 30 cases, Lancet 2:379, 1958.
12. Bloom, G. E., Canales, L., and Fairchild, J. P.: Thrombocytopenic purpura with infectious mononucleosis; two cases in children with review of the literature, Amer. J. Dis. Child. 106:415, 1963.
13. Bond, V. P., Fliedner, T. M., Cronkite, E. P., Rubini, J. R., Brecker, G., and Schore, P.: Proliferative potentials of bone marrow and blood cells studied by in vitro uptake of $H^3$-thymidine, Acta Haemat. 21:1, 1959.
14. Custer, R. P., and Smith, E. B.: The pathology of infectious mononucleosis, Blood 3:830, 1948.
15. Dameshek, W., and Grassi, M. A.: Infectious lymphadenosis and thrombocytopenic purpura; recovery after splenectomy, Blood 1:339, 1942.
16. Davidsohn, I., and Lee, C. L.: The laboratory in the diagnosis of infectious mononucleosis, Med. Clin. N. Amer. 46:225, 1962.
17. Davidsohn, I., Stern, K., and Kashiwagi, C.: The differential test for infectious mononucleosis, Amer. J. Clin. Path. 21:1101, 1951.
18. Davie, J., Clayton, C., and Little, S. C.: Infectious mononucleosis with fatal neuronitis, Arch. Neurol. 9:265, 1963.
19. Doan, J. K., and Weisberger, A. J.: Use of ACTH in infectious mononucleosis, Ann. Intern. Med. 38:1058, 1953.
20. Dolgopol, V. B., and Husson, G. S.: Infectious mononucleosis and neurological complications; report of a fatal case, Arch. Intern. Med. 83:179, 1949.
21. Downey, H., and McKinlay, C. A.: Acute lymphadenosis compared with acute lymphatic leukemia, Arch. Intern. Med. 32:82, 1923.
22. Downey, H., and Stasney, J.: The pathology of the lymph nodes in infectious mononucleosis, Folia Haemat. 54:417, 1936.
23. Dresdale, D. T., Ripstein, C. B., Guzman, S. V., and Greene, M. A.: Postcardiotomy syndrome in patients with rheumatic heart disease; cortisone as a prophylactic and therapeutic agent, Amer. J. Med. 21:57, 1956.
24. Eaton, O. M., Stevens, H., and Silver, H. M.: Respiratory failure in polyradiculoneuritis associated with infectious mononucleosis, J.A.M.A. 194:609, 1965.
25. Epstein, L. B., and Brecher, G.: DNA and RNA of circulating atypical lymphocytes in infectious mononucleosis, Blood 25:197, 1965.
26. Epstein, M. A., Achong, B. G., and Barr, Y. M.: Virus particles in cultured lymphoblasts from Burkitt's lymphoma, Lancet 1:702, 1964.
27. Epstein, M. A., Barr, Y. M., and Achong, B. G.: Studies with Burkitt's lymphoma, Wiestar Inst. Sympos. Monogr. 4:69, 1965.
28. Evans, A. S., Niederman, J. C., and McCollum, R. W.: Seroepidemiologic studies of infectious mononucleosis and EB virus, New Eng. J. Med. 279:1121, 1968.
29. Filatov, N. F.: Lectures on the acute infectious diseases of children, vol. 1, Moscow, 1885, A. Lang, p. 13.
30. Fish, M., and Barton, H. R.: Heart involvement in infectious mononucleosis, Arch. Intern Med. 101:636, 1958.
31. Forssman, J.: Die Herstellung hochwertiger spezifischer Schafhämolysine ohne Verwendung von Schafblut, Biochem. Ztschr. 37:78, 1911.
32. Foster, K. M., and Jack, I.: A prospective study of the role of cytomegalovirus in posttransfusion monoucleosis, New Eng. J. Med. 280:1311, 1969.
33. Frankel, E. P., Shiver, C. B., Jr., Berg, P., and Caris, T. N.: Meningoencephalitis in infectious mononucleosis; report of a case treated with cortisone, J.A.M.A. 162:885, 1956.
34. Freedman, M. H., Gilchrist, G. S., and Hammond, G. D.: Concurrent infectious mononucleosis and acute leukemia, J.A.M.A. 214:1677, 1970.
35. Gall, E. A., and Stout, H. A.: The histological lesion in lymph nodes in infectious mononucleosis, Amer. J. Path. 16:433, 1940.
36. Gardiner, C. C.: Acute pericarditis as the initial manifestation of infectious mononucleosis, Amer. J. Med. Sci. 237:352, 1959.
37. Gavosto, F., Pileri, A., and Marianni, G.: Incorporation of thymidine labelled with tritium by circulating cells of infectious mononucleosis, Nature 184:1691, 1959.
38. Gellis, S. S., editor: Year book of pediatrics, 1964-1965 series, Chicago, 1965, Year Book Medical Publishers, Inc.
39. Gilbraith, P., Mitus, W. J., Gollerkeri, M., and Dameshek, W.: The "infectious mononucleosis cell"; a cytochemical study, Blood 22:630, 1963.
40. Hall, B. D., and Archer, F. C.: Acute hemolytic anemia associated with infectious

mononucleosis, New Eng. J. Med. **249**:973, 1953.
41. Heemstra, J. G., and Stanage, W. F.: A fingertip, microheterophile agglutination technic, Pediatrics **23**:753, 1959.
42. Henle, G., Henle, W., and Diehl, V.: Relation of Burkitt's tumor-associated herpestype virus to infectious mononucleosis, Proc. Nat. Acad. Sci. **59**:94, 1968.
43. Hoagland, R. J.: Cardiac involvement in infectious mononucleosis, Amer. J. Med. Sci. **232**:252, 1956.
44. Hoagland, R. J.: The clinical manifestations of infectious mononucleosis; a report of 200 cases, Amer. J. Med. Sci. **240**:21, 1960.
45. Hoagland, R. J.: False-positive serology in mononucleosis, J.A.M.A. **185**:783, 1963.
46. Hoagland, R. J.: Mononucleosis and heart disease, Amer. J. Med. Sci. **248**:1, 1964.
47. Hoff, G., and Bauer, S.: A new rapid slide test for infectious mononucleosis, J.A.M.A. **194**:119, 1965.
48. Holswade, G. R., Engle, M. A., Redo, S. F., Goldsmith, E. I., and Barondess, J. A.: Development of viral diseases and a viral diseaselike syndrome after extracorporeal circulation, Circulation, **27**:812, 1963.
49. Houck, A. H.: Involvement of the heart in infectious mononucleosis (editorial), Amer. J. Med. **14**:261, 1953.
50. Houk, V. N., and McFarland, W.: Acute autoimmune hemolytic anemia complicating infectious mononucleosis, J.A.M.A. **177**:108, 1961.
51. Hsia, D. Y-Y., and Gellis, S. S.: Hepatic dysfunction in infections in children, Amer. J. Dis. Child. **84**:175, 1952.
52. Hunt, J. S.: The pathogenesis of infectious mononucleosis, Amer. J. Med. Sci. **228**:83, 1954.
53. Kaplan, M. E., and Tan, E. M.: Antinuclear antibodies in infectious mononucleosis, Lancet **1**:561, 1968.
54. Karpinski, F. E., Jr.: Neurologic manifestations of infectious mononucleosis in childhood, Pediatrics **10**:265, 1952.
55. Kaufman, R. E.: Recurrences in infectious mononucleosis, Amer. Pract. Digest Treat. **1**:673, 1950.
56. Klemola, E., and Kääriäinen, L.: Cytomegalovirus as a possible cause of a disease resembling infectious mononucleosis, Brit. Med. J. **2**:1099, 1965.
57. Lampkin, B. C., Canales, L., and Mauer, A. M.: Infectious mononucleosis with acute lymphoblastic leukemia, J. Pediat. **71**:876, 1967.
58. Lang, D. J., Sednick, E. M., and Willerson, J. T.: Association of cytomegalovirus infection with the post-perfusion syndrome, New Eng. J. Med. **278**:1147, 1968.
59. Lazar, H. P., Manfredi, R., and Hammond, J. H.: Seizures in infectious mononucleosis, Amer. J. Med. **21**:990, 1956.
60. Liebowitz, J.: Infectious mononucleosis, Modern Medical Monographs, vol. 5, New York, 1953, Grune & Stratton, Inc.
61. Liebowitz, S.: Infectious mononucleosis; report of a case presenting as acute anaphylactic shock treated with ACTH and cortisone, New York J. Med. **51**:2711, 1954.
62. Lloyd, P. C.: Acute thrombocytopenic purpura in infectious mononucleosis, Amer. J. Med. Sci. **207**:620, 1944.
63. Longcope, W. T.: Infectious mononucleosis (glandular fever) with a report of 10 cases, Amer. J. Med. Sci. **164**:781, 1922.
64. Lukes, R. J., and Cox, F. H.: Clinical and morphologic findings in 30 fatal cases of infectious mononucleosis, Amer. J. Path. **34**:586, 1958.
65. MacKinney, A. A.: Studies of plasma protein synthesis by peripheral cells from normal persons and patients with infectious mononucleosis, Blood **32**:217, 1968.
66. McCarthy, J. T., and Hoagland, R. J.: Cutaneous manifestations of infectious mononucleosis, J.A.M.A. **187**:153, 1964.
67. Meade, R. H., III: Laryngeal obstruction in children, Ped. Clin. N. Amer. **9**:233, 1962.
68. Muschel, L. H., and Piper, D. R.: Enzyme-treated red blood cells of sheep in the test for infectious mononucleosis, Amer. J. Clin. Path. **32**:240, 1959.
69. Nelson, R. S., and Darragh, J. H.: Infectious mononucleosis hepatitis; a clinicopathologic study, Amer. J. Med. **21**:26, 1956.
70. Niederman, J. C., McCollum, R. W., Henle, G., and Henle, W.: Infectious mononucleosis; clinical manifestations in relation to EB virus antibodies, J.A.M.A. **203**:205, 1968.
71. Pader, E., and Grossman, H.: Thrombocytopenic purpura in infectious mononucleosis, New York J. Med. **56**:1905, 1956.
72. Paul, J. R., and Bunnell, W. W.: The presence of heterophile antibodies in infectious mononucleosis, Amer. J. Med. Sci. **183**:90, 1932.
73. Peterson, E. T., Walford, R. L., Figueroa, W. G., and Dusholm, R.: Ox cell hemolysis in infectious mononucleosis and in other diseases, Amer. J. Med. **21**:193, 1956.
74. Pfeiffer, E.: Drusenfieber, Jahrb. Kinderh. **29**:257, 1889.
75. Radel, E. G., and Schorr, J. B.: Thrombocytopenic purpura with infectious mononucleosis, J. Pediat. **63**:46, 1963.
76. Ralston, L. S., Saiki, A. K., and Powers, W.

T.: Orchitis as complication of infectious mononucleosis, J.A.M.A. 173:1348, 1960.
77. Redmond, A. J.: Infectious mononucleosis treated with ACTH, New York J. Med. 54:3411, 1954.
78. Robinson, J., and Bridgen, W.: Immunological studies in the postcardiotomy syndrome, Brit. Med. J. 2:706, 1963.
79. Rosenberg, A., and Van Slyck, E. J.: A syndrome resembling infectious mononucleosis after splenectomy for idiopathic thrombocytopenic purpura, Ann. Intern. Med. 63:965, 1965.
80. Sadusk, J. F.: The skin eruption and false-positive Wassermann in infectious mononucleosis (glandular fever), Internat. Clin. 1:239, 1941.
81. Sawitsky, A., Papps, J. P., and Wiener, L. M.: The demostration of antibody in acute hemolytic anemia complicating infectious mononucleosis, Amer. J. Med. 8:260, 1950.
82. Schultz, L. E.: Heterophile antibody titer in diseases other than infectious mononucleosis, Arch. Intern. Med. 81:328, 1949.
83. Schumacher, H. R., Jacobson, W. A., and Bemiller, C. R.: Treatment of infectious mononucleosis, Ann. Intern. Med. 58:217, 1963.
84. Schumacher, H. R., McFeely, A. E., and Mangel, T. K.: The mononucleosis cell. III. Electron microscopy, Blood 33:833, 1969.
85. Seaman, A. J., and Starr, A.: Febrile postcardiotomy lymphocytic splenomegaly; a new entity, Ann. Surg. 156:956, 1962.
86. Seitanidis, B.: A comparison of the Monospot with the Paul-Bunnell test in infectious mononucleosis and other diseases, J. Clin. Path. 22:321, 1969.
87. Shinton, N. K., and Hawkins, C. F.: A fatal case of glandular fever, Lancet 2:708, 1956.
88. Shiver, C. B., Jr., and Frenkel, E. P.: Palatine petechiae, an early sign of infectious mononucleosis, J.A.M.A. 161:592, 1956.
89. Sigler, A. T.: Comparison of screening tests for infectious mononucleosis in children, Johns Hopkins Med. J. 126:312, 1970.
90. Smith, D. R.: Syndrome resembling infectious mononucleosis after open-heart surgery, Brit. Med. J. 1:945, 1964.
91. Soloff, L. A., and Zatuchni, J.: Infectious mononucleosis associated with symptoms of acute pericarditis, J.A.M.A. 152:1530, 1953.
92. Southam, C. M., Goldsmith, Y., and Burchenal, J. H.: Heterophile antibodies and antigens in neoplastic diseases, Cancer 4:1036, 1951.
93. Sprunt, T. P., and Evans, F. A.: Mononuclear leukocytosis in relation to acute infections ("infectious mononucleosis"), Bull. Johns Hopkins Hosp. 31:410, 1920.
94. Stefanini, M., and Adelson, E.: Studies on platelets; heterophile reaction due to Forssman antibody in patients with idiopathic and secondary thrombocytopenic purpura, Amer. J. Clin. Path. 22:1164, 1952.
95. Stevens, D. A., Levine, P. H., Lee, S. K., Sonley, M. J., and Waggoner, D. E.: Concurrent infectious mononucleosis and acute leukemia. Case reports. Review of the literature and serologic studies with the herpes-type (EB) virus, Amer. J. Med. 50:208, 1971.
96. Strauss, R.: Infectious mononucleosis simulating acute appendicitis with description of a specific lesion of the appendix, Amer. J. Clin. Path. 12:295, 1942.
97. Thurm, R. H., and Bassen, F.: Infectious mononucleosis and acute hemolytic anemia; report of two cases and review of the literature, Blood 10:841, 1955.
98. Tidy, H. L., and Daniel, E. C.: Glandular fever and infectious mononucleosis with an account of an epidemic, Lancet 2:9, 1923.
99. Vahlquist, B., Ekelund, H., and Tveteras, E.: Infectious mononucleosis and pseudomononucleosis in childhood, Acta Paediat. 47:120, 1958.
100. van Furth, R., Schuiti, H. R., and Higmans, W.: The formation of immunoglobulin by human tissues in vitro. IV. Circulating lymphocytes in normal and pathological conditions, Immunology 11:29, 1966.
101. Vaughan, J., and Greenberg, S. D.: The significance of atypical mononuclear leukocytes, J. Pediat. 60:177, 1962.
102. Waterhouse, B. E., and Lapidus, P. H.: Infectious mononucleosis associated with a mass in the anterior mediastinum, New Eng. J. Med. 277:1137, 1967.
103. Wetherall, J. H., and Oldfield, M. C.: Rupture of the spleen and thrombocytopenia in glandular fever, Lancet 1:636, 1963.
104. Wheeler, E. O., Turner, J. D., and Scannell, J. G.: Fever, splenomegaly and atypical lymphocytes; a syndrome observed after cardiac surgery utilizing pump oxygenator, New Eng. J. Med. 266:454, 1962.
105. Wilson, S. J., Ward, C. E., and Gray, L. W.: Infectious lymphadenosis (mononucleosis) and hemolytic anemia in a Negro, Blood 4:189, 1949.
106. Wintrobe, M. M.: Clinical hematology, ed. 4, Philadelphia, 1956, Lea & Febiger.
107. Wiseman, B. K.: The treatment of infectious mononucleosis, J. Chron. Dis. 6:347, 1957.
108. Wolnisty, C.: Orchitis as a complication of infectious mononucleosis, New Eng. J. Med. 266:88, 1962.
109. York, W. H.: Spontaneous rupture of the spleen; report of a case secondary to infectious mononucleosis, J.A.M.A. 179:178, 1962.

# 22 LEUKEMIA—GENERAL ASPECTS AND CLINICAL FEATURES

Leukemia is a disorder of the white blood cells of unknown etiology, usually with a fatal outcome. There are patients, however, who have had such prolonged remissions that their prognosis is undeterminable. It is generally considered to be a neoplastic change in the blood-forming tissues and is characterized by an uncontrolled and disorderly proliferation of leukocytes and their precursors with invasive tendencies. Although the white blood cells are usually present in excessive numbers in the circulating blood, they may be present in normal or reduced numbers. In either case immature or abnormal cells are present during a major part of the course of the disease.

It is of interest historically that, although cases of leukemia had been previously reported by others, credit for ascribing the altered state of the blood to an increase in the colorless cells rather than to pus and for naming the condition leukemia (white blood) goes to Virchow.[269]

Furth[98] has emphasized the essential identity between leukemia and neoplasms since in both conditions the immature cell has acquired an inability to respond to forces in the host normally regulating their maturation and proliferation. Many concepts, especially those relating to causation and treatment of leukemias in human beings, stem from animal experimentation, especially from experiments on leukemia in mice which is similar both pathologically and clinically to that in human beings.

No proof exists yet that leukemia in mice is identical with that in human beings, although similar effects result in increasing susceptibility following ionizing radiation and in the parallel therapeutic responses following administration of a variety of chemical agents. New mitotic poisons employed in the treatment of human patients have been obtained by screening in mice with experimentally produced leukemia.

*Classification of leukemia in childhood.* Leukemia is classified as acute or chronic and by the type of white blood cell predominating in the bone marrow and circulating blood. No rigid criteria can be applied for designating the exact duration of the disease. It is much more practical, especially since survival has been extended by chemotherapy, to employ the terms acute and chronic in relation to clinical severity and to qualify further as to the type of cell or cellular pattern predominating in the disease.

For the purposes of management, it is best to ascertain as closely as possible the type of leukemia involved. This will depend on smears taken from the peripheral blood and bone marrow and, where there is a problem in diagnosis, on bone marrow biopsy in addition to aspiration.

*Acute stem cell leukemia.* The predominant cell in the bone marrow and peripheral blood in the majority of patients with acute leukemia is usually primitive, and there is a virtual absence of cellular differentiation into myeloblastic or lymphoblastic types. The morphologic characteristics in these patients do not suggest any specific line of development. Although it is possible in rare cases to separate these immature cells, the term stem cell leukemia overcomes the difficulties of differentiation. The majority of these cells are often classified as lymphoblasts because of their resemblance to lymphocytes in their proximity (Figs. 68 and 69). It is for this reason that acute lymphoblastic leukemia frequently has been regarded as the most common form of leukemia in childhood. (For differentiation of cell types occurring in leukemia, see Chapter 18.) In the more recent reports, the terms granulocytic and lymphocytic are used for the leukemias instead of myelogenous and lymphatic leukemias.

*Granulocytic types.* Granulocytic types of leukemia encountered in children are of three types: acute myeloblastic or promyelocytic,

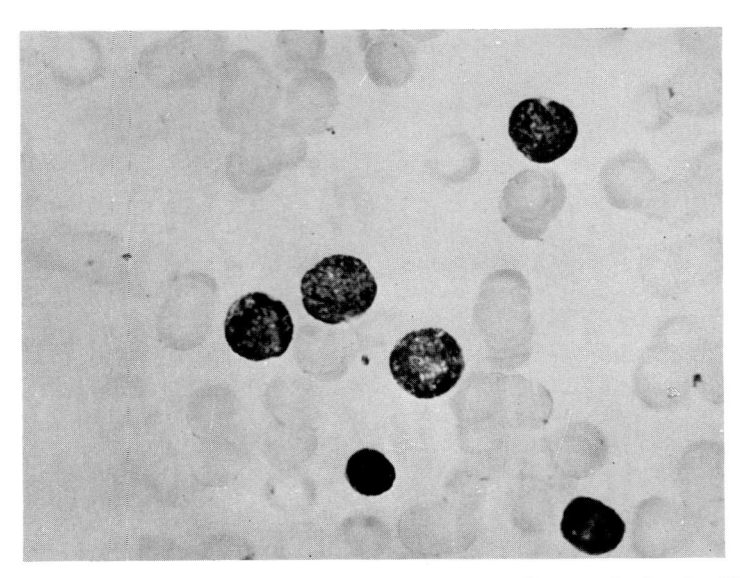

Fig. 68. Photomicrograph from blood smear of a patient with acute leukemia. Note lighter staining and finely granular or stippled appearance of nucleus in lymphoblasts in upper section. Compare with dark staining basichromatin of nuclei of two normal lymphocytes in lower section. (×1200.)

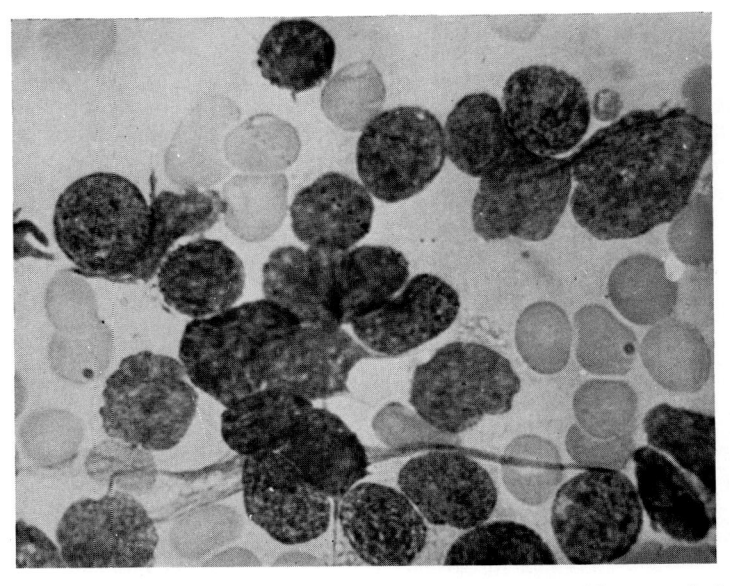

Fig. 69. Photomicrograph of bone marrow smear from a patient with acute leukemia. Note uniform infiltration by lymphoblasts. (×1200.)

acute myelocytic, and chronic myelocytic or myelogenous.

ACUTE MYELOBLASTIC OR PROMYELOCYTIC LEUKEMIA. Acute myeloblastic leukemia is described in the patient in whom myelobasts predominate and constitute from 30 to 60% of the circulating cells.[280] The diagnosis of the myeloblast is based on certain differential characteristics: round or oval nuclei composed of fine chromatin which is not condensed about the edges, several large nucleoli, and deep blue cytoplasm possessing few or no granules. The diagnosis of these immature cells is helped by the presence of later forms possessing granules, characterizing them as promyelocytes. The presence of Auer bodies in these and in most immature cells provides a further clue to the designation of both types as myeloid in origin.

In Chapter 18 the peroxidase reaction is described for differentiating myeloid cells from cells of other series. After blood or bone marrow films are heated with benzidine and hydrogen peroxide, the benzidine is oxidized by the peroxide in the presence of peroxidase. Peroxidase-positive granules are found in promyelocytes, myelocytes, metamyelocytes, neutrophils, eosinophils, monocytes, and promonocytes. Myeloblasts, lymphoblasts, lymphocytes, basophils, and plasma cells are peroxidase negative.[52] Acute myeloblastic leukemia, the most frequent member of the granulocytic group, is a disease in which the predominant cells are myeloblasts or early myelocytes (myelocytes A and B). The terms acute myeloblastic leukemia and acute promyelocytic leukemia are sometimes used interchangeably for this type, because either blast forms or promyelocytes may predominate at one time or another in the same patient. However, in contrast to the myeloblast which is devoid of granules, a few darkly stained granules are found in the promyelocyte. Cases reported as acute granulocytic leukemia probably fit into this category. In some descriptions the cells are designated as being intermediate between myelocytes and promyelocytes,[100] in others as possessing immature nuclei with nucleoli and Auer rods of unusually large size.[80]

Acute promyelocytic leukemia is characterized not only by a predominance of promyelocytes but also by fibrinogenopenia.[128] This deficiency, together with thrombocytopenia and frequent factor V deficiency, accounts for severe bleeding tendency.[80,226] Fibrinogen deficiency is characteristic of this form of leukemia and rare in other forms. Factor V deficiency is a frequent accompaniment but less specific than fibrinogen deficiency. These deficiencies disappear during a remission and reappear in terminal relapse. Infusions of fibrinogen disappear rapidly from the blood in this condition.

ACUTE MYELOCYTIC LEUKEMIA. In patients with acute myelocytic leukemia, the blood smear and especially the bone marrow are characterized by the presence of more mature granules than those of the promyelocytic form. The cells possess numerous granules scattered throughout the somewhat grayish or basophilic cytoplasm. Because of the greater number of granules and the more advanced maturity, this type of cell is often termed myelocyte C, in contrast to less mature myelocytes A and B containing fewer granules, characterizing the promyelocytic form. Acute myelocytic leukemia is differentiated from the chronic myelogenous type not only by the more moderate leukocytosis but also by the narrow range of maturity of the abnormal forms. One of the features of acute myelocytic leukemia is the cytologic resemblance in many of the cells to the monocyte, especially with regard to the nucleus. (See Fig. 70.)

Morphologically typical Gaucher's cells were found in the marrow and liver of a 9½-year-old Caucasian girl with acute leukemia.[281] Gaucher's cells are seen only rarely in childhood leukemia although their occurrence is an established phenomenon in chronic adult myelocytic leukemia. The Gaucher's cells in these circumstances probably represent a "secondary" phenomenon and do not reflect the presence of a second, genetically determined disease. Since granulocytes are the principal source of sphingolipid, the predominance of acute lymphoblastic leukemia in childhood may explain the rarity of Gaucher's cells in children with leukemia. In the present patients the leukemia was acute and probably myelogenous.[281]

CHRONIC MYELOCYTIC (GRANULOCYTIC, MYELOID, OR MYELOGENOUS) LEUKEMIA. Chronic leukemia is infrequent in childhood, being confined to the chronic myelocytic type which accounts for about 2% of all leukemias in this age period. Hyperleukocytosis is common, with segmented and nonsegmented neutrophils constituting 75% of the total. Myelocytes and metamyelocytes are present in increased numbers (Fig. 71). The bone marrow may show

554   BLOOD DISEASES OF INFANCY AND CHILDHOOD

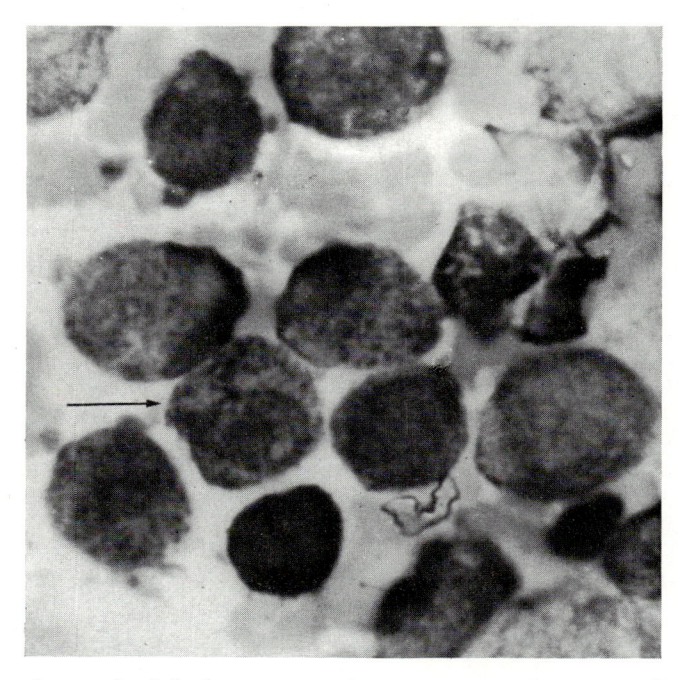

Fig. 70. Photomicrograph of the bone marrow from a patient with acute myelocytic leukemia. The majority of the cells are myelocytes. Arrow points to a promyelocyte containing a nucleolus. (Courtesy Dr. Richard T. Silver, New York, N. Y.)

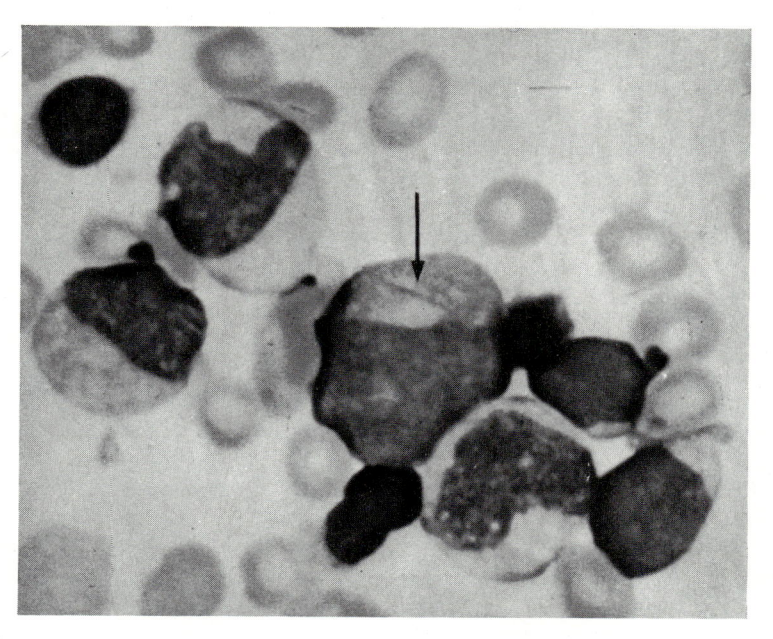

Fig. 71. Photomicrograph of a blood smear from a child 13 years of age with chronic granulocytic leukemia. Note a metamyelocyte, several myelocytes, and a myeloblast. Arrow points to an Auer body in the myeloblast, which also contains an irregular nucleolus. (×1200.) (Courtesy Dr. Julius Rutsky, Pontiac, Mich.)

larger numbers of myelocytes than the peripheral blood, although samples from both areas are characteristically similar. Relatively few myeloblasts or immature myelocytes are found at any time except terminally. Basophils are increased (2 to 10% and higher), and platelet counts are either normal in number or may reach levels of 1 million per cubic millimeter or more. In patients with chronic myelogenous leukemia the neutrophils contain very little alkaline phosphatase, whereas in those with pyogenic infections associated with a leukocytosis or a leukemoid reaction corresponding cells exhibit a great increase in this enzyme.[150,266,267,279] It has been observed that with treatment, cellular leukocyte alkaline phosphatase returns to normal in chronic granulocytic leukemia, although the $Ph^1$ chromosome persists in the marrow cells.[49,274] Auer bodies, rod-shaped structures in the cytoplasm which are peroxidase positive, may be present in the myeloblasts or myelocytes. As the disease progresses, anemia and thrombocytopenia prevail as in patients with the acute leukemias.

Chronic granulocytic leukemia remains one of the less common varieties of leukemia in children. In one series of 570 cases of childhood leukemia, the incidence was 1.2%.[136] In a case of a 12-year-old girl the outstanding feature was the precipitous evolution of a blast crisis within days of her initial presentation. At the end of a brief remission her count rose to 896,000 per cubic millimeter, with 78% blasts.[196] Although several forms of therapy result in temporary clinical and hematologic improvement of patients with chronic granulocytic leukemia, the final phase is characterized by progressive anemia, a rising white blood count, thrombocytopenia, fever, an enlarging liver and spleen, and characteristically a myeloblast crisis at the time of death. In fifty-four adult patients studied by Karanas and Silver[143] the most common heralding characteristics of the onset of the terminal phase were myeloblasts and myelocytes of over 30%, fever of undetermined origin, or both.

The disease is rare in childhood but is often seen in the first months of life as a form of congenital leukemia. In affected infants the cells are as well differentiated as they are in patients with the adult form of the disease, but, in contrast to the prolonged survival in the latter, the course in the infant is short. The older child may survive for a period of several years. Nevertheless, the designation chronic myelocytic leukemia in the young patient refers to the type of blood picture rather than to the length of the survival.

The onset of the disease is particularly difficult to designate in patients with chronic myelocytic leukemia because the symptoms are vague. A routine blood count made because of continued low-grade fever and fatigue frequently calls attention to an underlying hematologic disorder. The marked leukocytosis with a shift of the neutrophils to the left and the presence of a few metamyelocytes and myelocytes suggest a diagnosis of a leukemoid reaction initially. Hepatosplenomegaly and lymphadenopathy are usually marked in patients with this form of leukemia. At the onset these features may be absent except for a palpable spleen which enlarges as the disease progresses. Pain about the hip may become so pronounced that walking is painful. The marked limp which develops early rarely correlates with an abnormal finding in the roentgenogram.

During the chronic phase of chronic myelocytic leukemia a characteristic blast cell crisis emerges. The terminal blast cell leukemic phase may follow the appearance of invasive tissue-destroying lesions composed of blast cells.[99] Busulfan is effective in reducing the number of blast cells to very low levels in patients who have not previously received it.

The spleen may reach an enormous size and relief of discomfort associated with enlargement may prompt consideration of irradiation of this organ. In cases in which thrombocytopenia is marked, this form of therapy is approached with reluctance and on advice of the radiotherapist is usually rejected.

Several authors have noted that the disease occurring in infants and young children differs in certain respects from that of older children in whom it usually resembles chronic granulocytic leukemia of adults.[122,221] Cases of chronic leukemia studied cytogenetically have demonstrated an abnormally small chromosome, probably chromosome 21, which has lost about half of its long arm.[13,200] (See Figs. 72 and 73.) It is now commonly referred to as the Philadelphia ($Ph^1$) chromosome, from the city in which it was discovered. Often it is difficult to decide with absolute certainty whether autosome 21 or 22 is involved, although the former is regarded to be more likely.

Reisman and Trujillo,[221] in cytogenic stud-

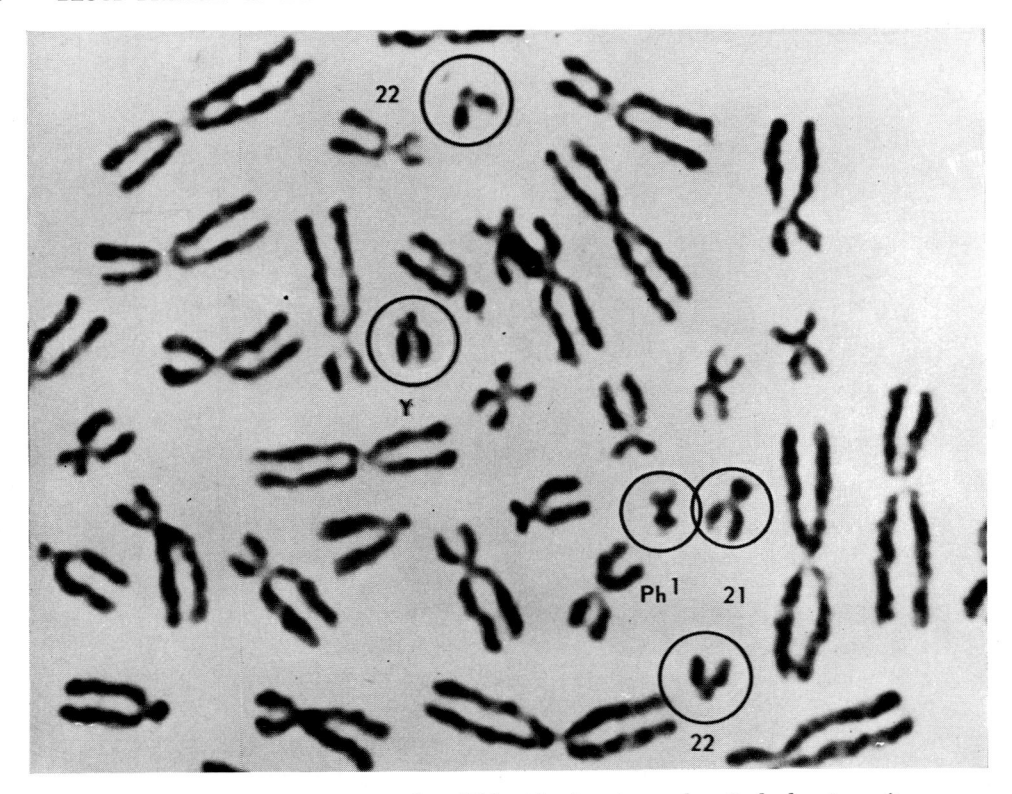

**Fig. 72.** A chromosome preparation of a child with chronic myelocytic leukemia as it appears with a light microscope. The chromosome not seen in normal cells is designated as the Ph[1] chromosome and is near a normal No. 21 chromosome. The Ph[1] chromosome is only about half the size of the smallest normal chromosome, and its constriction is in the middle instead of near the end. The other circled chromosomes are the other members of group G, the smallest group of chromosomes. (Courtesy Dr. Roy D. Schmickel, Rockville, Md.)

ies performed on cells from peripheral blood culture and direct marrow preparations, noted that five children with the adult type of disease demonstrated the Ph[1] chromosome, but none of the four infants (studied within the first 3 years of life) had this abnormal chromosome. Hardisty and co-workers[122] found in four children 8 to 11 years of age that the disease resembled the disease in adults and that the four young children showed the features of the juvenile type. In addition to the absence of Ph[1] chromosome, the juvenile type is characterized by greater lymph node involvement, less marked splenomegaly than the adult type, and the tendency to run a relatively short course. Both types show the hyperleukocytosis with a predominance of granulocytes, an increased number of myelocytes and metamyelocytes in both peripheral blood and bone marrow, and a relatively small number of blasts and immature cells. The total leukocyte count is usually not as high as in the adult type.[122] In contrast to the normal or increased platelet counts in the early stages in the adult type of disease and in children in the older age group, the infantile group presents early thrombocytopenia with hemorrhagic manifestations and decreased or absent megakaryocytes. Response to chemotherapy also differs in the two groups—the infants responding poorly to busulfan and impressively to 6-mercaptopurine, the older children consistently having prolonged remissions with busulfan.[221] The alkaline phosphatase activity of the polymorphonuclear cells is typically reduced in both types.

An exception to the difference in the disease in

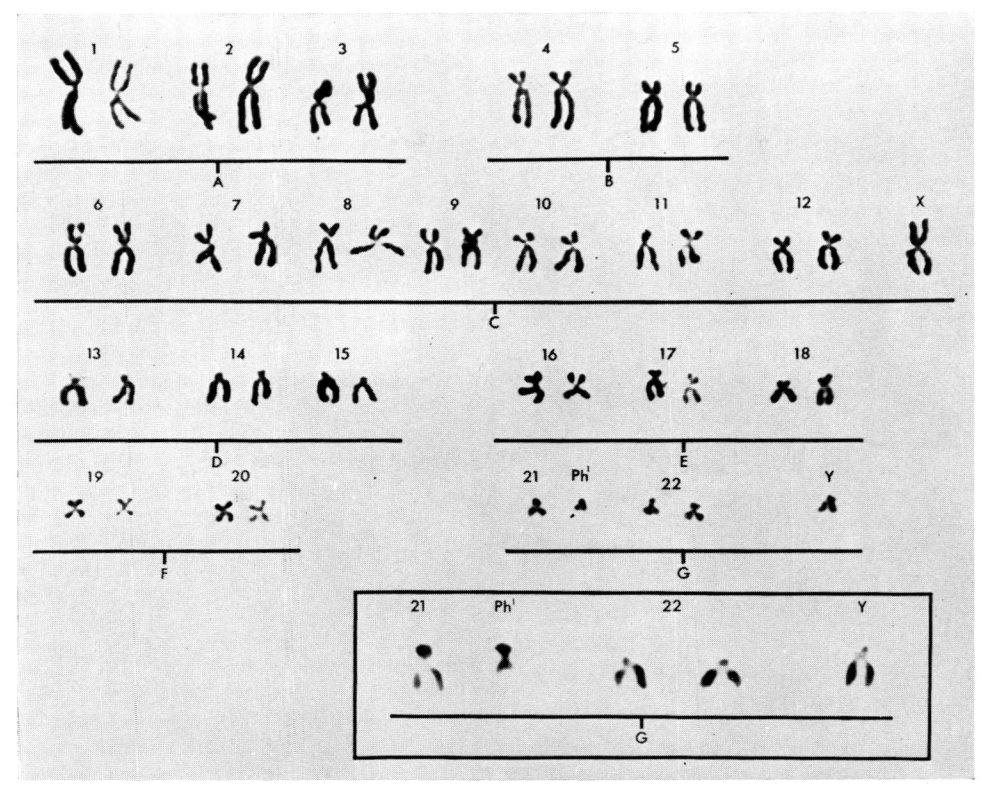

Fig. 73. From a photograph of chromosomes as they appear in Fig. 72, a karyotype can be prepared by grouping chromosomes according to their size and the position of the constriction where the chromatids meet, the *centromere*. The karyotype shows that there is only one instead of the normal two No. 21 chromosomes. Also, an abnormal Ph¹ chromosome is present. From the inset, it can be seen that the Ph¹ chromosome appears to be a No. 21 chromosome after deletion of a portion of its longer arms. (Courtesy Dr. Roy D. Schmickel, Rockville, Md.)

the two age groups is the report[32] of the occurrence of chronic myelogenous leukemia of the adult type in an 8-month-old infant. The fetal hemoglobin levels were about 1%. The Philadelphia chromosome was found in the bone marrow regardless of the stage of the disease; it was also found in the peripheral blood during relapse.

In two infants 16 months and 22 months of age with the juvenile type of granulocytic leukemia, the fetal hemoglobin measured 55 and 49%, respectively.[122] Whereas the fetal hemoglobin averages 40 to 50% in the juvenile type, it averages less than 2 to 7% in the adult type.[122] The continued HbF production after birth may indicate that this type of granulocytic leukemia is congenital in origin, requiring a variable time for the development of its full effect, including also the appearance of the Ph¹ chromosome. An alternative hypothesis is that the juvenile form of chronic granulocytic leukemia is associated with a reversion to a more primitive state of erythropoiesis characterized by reactivation of fetal hemoglobin synthesis.[122]

Acute myelocytic leukemia has been reported in a user of several hallucinogenic drugs, among them LSD.[113] The leukemic leukocytes of the patient contained a Ph¹-like chromosome. Several studies have demonstrated that LSD has been associated with chromosomal abnormalities in cells in vivo and cultured in vitro.[56,84,113] The Ph¹-like chromosome is similar to that commonly associated with chronic myelocytic leukemia but only rarely with acute myelocytic leukemia.

Although the Philadelphia chromosome is most often associated with chronic myeloid leukemia, it has been reported, though rarely, in acute leukemia, myeloid metaplasia, polycythemia vera, atypical myeloproliferative syndrome with marked thrombocytopenia, eosinophilic leukemia, and in apparently healthy descendants of patients with chronic myeloid leukemia.

Miller[177] has found very high (13 to 50%) concentrations of fetal hemoglobin, as is usually found in the juvenile type of chronic granulocytic leukemia or erythroleukemia (Di Guglielmo's syndrome), in three leukemic children: one with acute myeloblastic, another with histiomonocytic leukemia, and a third with acute monomyeloblastic leukemia.[177] HbF was increased in eighteen (55%) of thirty-two other children with leukemia.

Mild to moderate elevation of fetal hemoglobin (HbF) has been noted in many blood disorders, including congenital hypoplastic anemia, constitutional aplastic anemia, juvenile congenital pernicious anemia, paroxysmal nocturnal hemoglobinuria, hereditary persistence of HbF, thalassemia syndromes, and hemoglobinopathies. It is of interest that two of the children in this report with very high HbF had an atypical reticuloendotheliosis syndrome associated with frequent infections, lymphadenopathy, pulmonary infiltration, hepatosplenomegaly, skin rash, and monocytosis and developed overt leukemia 2 to 5 years after the onset of their initial symptoms.

A relationship has been postulated between chronic myelocytic leukemia, polycythemia vera, and essential thrombocytosis, i.e., that all three diseases may be the result of a generalized proliferative disorder of the bone marrow.[73] Although overproduction of one cell dominates the clinical picture of these diseases, increased numbers of granulocytes, erythrocytes, and platelets, respectively, may be found in each of these conditions. Increased granulocyte production and turnover rate were demonstrated in each of these three disorders.[171]

The Ph¹ chromosome has also been identified in the erythroblasts.[55] From this observation it was postulated that a single stem cell serves as a common primordial cell in chronic myeloid leukemia.

*Monocytic leukemia.* Monocytic leukemia is similar to the other types in most respects. The onset may be insidious, with a fatal outcome in a few weeks or months, or it may be sudden, with the disease running its course within a few days. In patients with the latter type of onset the spleen is slightly enlarged, and the liver and lymph nodes may not be palpable. The disease has an age incidence ranging from early infancy to later childhood. The symptoms and physical signs are similar to those of other types of leukemia except that hypertrophied and spongy gums have been described more frequently in patients with the monocytic type.

Two types of monocytic leukemia are described. When the blood picture is marked by the simultaneous presence of both myelocytes and monocytes or immature cells intermediate between myeloblasts or myelocytes and monocytes, the disease is designated as the Naegeli type or myelomonocytic leukemia. When the immature cells resemble monocytes and reticuloendothelial cells, the disease is designated as the Schilling type (Fig. 74). (See Chapter 18.)

Chronic monocytic leukemia is extremely rare in childhood. Only two patients in this category were observed in a series of 900 cases of childhood leukemia.[203] The disease may be difficult to diagnose in the early stage because of predominant megaloblastic blood and bone marrow changes, diverse skin lesions, and spontaneous remissions. However, the finding of varying numbers of cells resembling adult monocytes and their precursors in the peripheral blood and bone marrow should arouse suspicion of the underlying disease. Early in the course of the disease there may be a marked leukocytosis or a leukopenia.

Acute monocytic leukemia has been reported in a case of peripheral monocytosis of 11 years' duration.[216] This 11-year illness differs from preleukemia in being of much greater duration. Many features of a preleukemic condition were manifested, however, including progressive, chronic, normocytic, normochromic anemia, chronic monocytosis, variable chronic neutropenia, and a fulminating terminal recrudescence. Earlier bone marrow examination showed no evidence of acute leukemia.

Three cases have been reported[44] which demonstrate an association between refractory sideroblastic anemia and chronic monocytic leukemia. From the point of view of the anemia the cases are characterized by ineffective erythropoiesis, a hyperplastic erythroid bone marrow showing megaloblastoid changes in numerous ringed erythroblasts, and hypochromic microcytic red cells. An absolute monocytosis with mature but somewhat atypical monocytes appears in the peripheral blood and in the bone marrow. Serum muramidase levels are increased. Those cases seem to be at the benign end of a spectrum of neoplastic diseases involving the monocytic and erythrocytic series simultaneously. At the most malignant

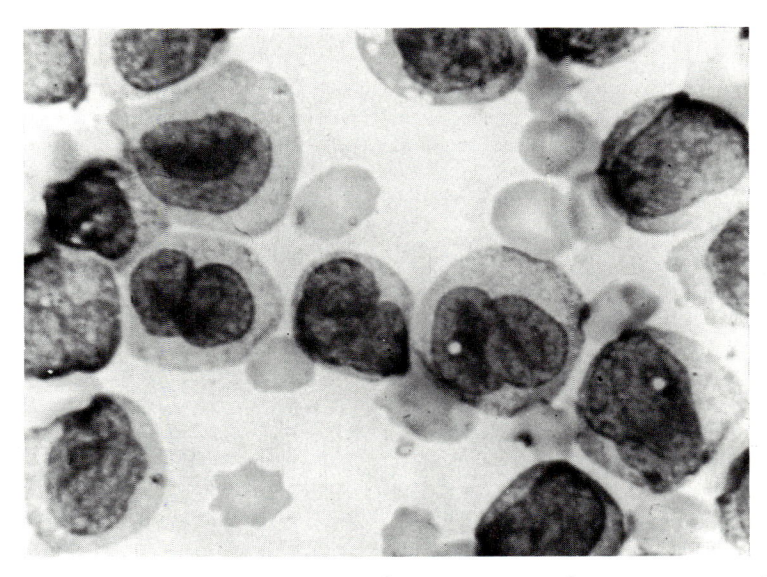

Fig. 74. Photomicrograph of the bone marrow from a patient with acute monocytic leukemia. Note infiltration with increased numbers of mature monocytes, promonocytes, and monoblasts to the exclusion of lymphocytes and myelocytes (Schilling type). All cells, regardless of maturity, possess the characteristic nucleus of the mature monocyte: the nucleus has lacy chromatin, is indented, and is folded on itself, giving a lobulated appearance. Some of the nuclei contain vacuoles. The nucleus of the cell in the lower left corner contains a nucleolus. (×1185.) (Courtesy Dr. Richard T. Silver, New York, N. Y.)

end of this spectrum are the cases in which acute leukemia characterized by a proliferation of erythroblasts and monoblasts develops suddenly without a preleukemic phase and is rapidly fatal.

*Eosinophilic leukemia.* Eosinophilic leukemia is an acute disease of childhood in which the majority of cells in the peripheral blood and tissues are mature eosinophils but in some cases are associated with myeloblasts and myelocytes. Enlargement of the liver, spleen, and lymph nodes, anemia, and thrombocytopenia may not be present until late in the disease. The blood picture may change to that of an acute myeloblastic leukemia, but more often tissue infiltration and the peripheral blood disclose invasion by the adult eosinophil. The slight elevation in the number of myeloblasts occasionally encountered is not sufficient for the diagnosis of acute leukemia.[50,89,110]

The diagnosis of eosinophilic leukemia has been controversial because of the predominance of mature eosinophils and the frequent absence of blast cells.[22] Benvenisti and Ultmann[23] also found that the difficulty in establishing a diagnosis of eosinophilic leukemia is that the majority of reported cases are not associated with a significant number of immature granulocytes. In presenting their cases of eosinophilic leukemia, the following features were accepted: hepatosplenomegaly, lymphadenopathy, and marked persistent eosinophilia, usually accompanied by anemia and thrombocytopenia. In a review of forty-eight cases, blast cells were observed in the peripheral blood of twenty-seven patients, and in eight patients there were over 20% blasts. Of twenty-nine bone marrow examinations, nineteen showed eosinophilic promyelocytes, myelocytes, and metamyelocytes. Eosinophilia ranging from 30 to 80% was found in all cases.

The main nonmalignant disorders that may simulate eosinophilic leukemia are syndromes in the classes of allergic and autoimmune disease such as Löffler's syndrome, pulmonary infiltrate with eosinophilia (P.I.E. syndrome), disseminated eosinophilic collagen disease, and polyarteritis nodosa. Various disorders such as allergic, parasitic, collagen, or malignant diseases that may exhibit intense eosinophilia were excluded by autopsy examination.

Histochemical, phase, and electron microscopic studies have revealed many abnormalities in the leukemic eosinophils: asynchronous nuclear-cytoplasmic maturation, the presence of fibrillar formation in some of the leukemic cells, extensive deposition of glycogen in the cytoplasm, and the demonstration of increased phosphorylase activity.[2]

In a 9-year-old boy with esinophilic leukemia, the leukocytes, which numbered 88,000 per cubic millimeter of blood (80% mature eosinophils), were associated with diffuse parenchymal infiltration of both lungs and intermittent fever. In this patient, steroids (prednisone) produced a temporary regression of lung infiltration and symptomatic relief. Postmortem examination revealed widespread tissue infiltration with mature eosinophils.

**Muramidase (lysozyme) in leukemia.** It is now generally accepted that, within the hematopoietic system, muramidase is limited to the cells of the granulocytic and monocytic series. Previous studies have shown that the major portion of measurable serum muramidase is usually derived from degradation of granulocytes but there is a moderate to increased activity of serum muramidase in patients with acute monocytic leukemia and other forms of monocytosis.

The muramidase activity of serum, urine, and leukocytes was measured in a group of patients with acute and chronic leukemia.[208] The results of these studies indicated that serum muramidase activity is markedly elevated in patients with the monocytic forms of acute leukemia,[193] moderately elevated in the acute and chronic granulocytic forms of leukemia, and reduced or normal in the lymphocytic forms of leukemia. The data suggest that serial measurements of serum muramidase may be of value in determining the efficacy of antileukemic therapy. Enzyme values appear to return to normal when complete remissions are attained, while increased serum activity persists with incomplete marrow remissions. (See Chapter 18 for further comments on muramidase.)

. . .

In terms of clinical severity, stem cell, lymphoblastic, myeloblastic or promyelocytic, myelomonocytic, monocytic, chronic myelocytic, and eosinophilic leukemias are acute leukemias in childhood. Chemotherapy and other modern supportive measures, however, have modified their course and have prolonged life. It should be borne in mind that acute stem cell leukemia is essentially a disease of infancy and childhood, although no age group is spared. In rare instances chronic myelocytic leukemia in children will run a prolonged course simulating that in the adult. Aleukemic leukemia is the designation for leukemia in patients in whom there is either no leukocytosis or a marked reduction in leukocytes but usually with the presence of abnormal cells in the peripheral blood and tissue histology showing the true nature of the disease. In some instances cytologic evidences of leukemia are found only in the bone marrow. Chronic lymphocytic leukemia is the most protracted and benign type of leukemia and occurs invariably in adults.

**Incidence, age distribution, sex, and frequency of types.** Acute leukemia is commonest between 2 and 5 years of age, with the incidence rising from a moderate elevation in the first 2 years of life to a peak in the third and fourth years.[58,65] It has been pointed out that the peak in mortality rates in the age-span between 3 and 4 years results, at least in the United States, as much from a decline in rates in the group under 2 years of age as from an increase at 3 to 4 years.[250] The decline among infants under 1 year of age began in the early 1940's, and with the passage of time affected successively older ages for unknown reasons. Although acute lymphoblastic leukemia predominates in the first 4 to 5 years of life, myelocytic leukemia is the most common form of the chronic disease up to the age of 60 years, after which the lymphocytic type is most frequently encountered. In total numbers chronic myelocytic leukemia and chronic lymphocytic leukemia are more frequent in the groups over 50 years of age.[61,104,164]

In a group of 1,770 children with leukemia treated in eleven pediatric centers by members of Children's Cancer Study Group A,[212a] acute lymphoblastic or undifferentiated leukemia accounted for 78% of all cases; cases of non-acute lymphoblastic leukemia totaled 19% and included acute granulocytic (myeloblastic) leukemia (8.5%), acute monocytic leukemia (8.3%), leukosarcoma (1.8%), and acute erythromyeloid leukemia (0.7%). Chronic granulocytic leukemia and miscellaneous unspecified types comprised only 3% of all cases.

In most series there is a preponderance of males. According to Cooke,[58] there is a gradual increase in the proportion of males to females who have acute leukemia, with the predominance of boys being greater in later childhood than during infancy. In the first year of life more cases are observed in girls than in boys; leukemia is more commonly observed in the male than in the female at all other ages.

Mortality statistics show that there has been a progressive increase in the death rates from leukemia until about 1960. In patients in the youngest age group (0 to 4 years) the rate rose from 2.2 to 5.1 per 100,000 deaths between 1930 and 1949.[61] In one study[72] the incidence in one large hospital from 1932 to 1948 was 0.42% of all admissions to the general pediatric service. Figures showing the changing incidence of leukemia cannot be truly ascertained from hospital admissions alone since there is a tendency for patients with leukemia, especially in the younger age groups, to be concentrated in large hospitals and medical centers. However, the recorded death rate from leukemia at all ages rose steadily in the United States from 1.4 in 1921 to 6.3 per 100,000 in 1953.[240] Later figures[8] give the incidence for males as 6.5 in 1950 to 1952 and 7.5 per 100,000 population in 1960 to 1962. For females the incidence over the same period was 4.6 and 4.8, respectively, per 100,000 population. In recent years a similar increase in all types of leukemia has also been noted in England and Wales.[131] In Scotland an approximate doubling of the incidence of admissions for leukemia to several large hospitals was recorded during the period from 1938 to 1951.[108]

In a paper by Kyle and co-workers[155] dealing with mortality figures cited for leukemia for the United States' white population during the years 1935 through 1964, more than a threefold rise (from approximately 2.4 per 100,000 in 1930 to 7.5 per 100,000 in 1963) was revealed. The reported rise in mortality and the incidence rates for leukemia in recent decades could be interpreted as evidence of a significant increase in leukemogenic environmental agents or an increased exposure to such agents. This increase may be a result of improvement in diagnostic techniques. In very recent years the decline in leukemia mortality may be due to increased awareness and protection against the risk of radiation exposure.[155]

Fraumeni and Miller[97] also found that, in the most recent 5-year period studied (1961-1965), the leukemia rates were for the first time lower than those for the previous period in all age groups from 1 through 74 years. The decline was greatest among children of 1 to 4 years. The reasons were the same as those given previously, namely, lessened exposure to environmental leukemogens and to radiation.

Racial susceptibility may play a role in the incidence of leukemia. Leukemia incidence, for instance, is lower for the American Negro population than for the country's entire population.[104] While this difference may be attributed to better case-finding among white persons, the relatively lower mortality may be due to basic factors relating to disease susceptibility among races. American Indians, for instance, appear to have less leukemia than either Caucasions or Negroes.[253] In a study in England, Lee[158] found that, from 1946 to 1960, a summer peak was noted in the incidence of acute lymphatic leukemia.

*Epidemiology.* Evidence suggesting that cases of leukemia may occur in clusters within communities has been accumulating. Within 6 months we observed three unrelated children under 5 years of age with acute leukemia, living within one-half mile of each other. Intensive investigation, however, revealed no known leukemogenic agent to which the three children had been exposed. This relationship in so many aspects seemed a startling experience and may eventually prove to be more than coincidental. In a study in Buffalo, clusters of two or three cases were found with a frequency of suggestive significance.[214] Between 1957 and 1960, eight cases of leukemia in children 3 to 13 years of age occurred among children in one residential area of Niles, Illinois.[124] Seven of the eight children either attended the community's one parochial elementary school or had older siblings who attended. The eight cases occurred within two separate periods of time and were accompanied by a "rheumatic-like" illness among pupils in the same parochial school. Schwartz and associates[236] found antibodies to a variety of leukemic antigens in the blood of one to three members of the families of all leukemic patients. Positive reactions were noted most often in the mother or a sibling closest in age to the patient with leukemia. The failure to find antibodies in the patient was interpreted as a lack of adequate response to the leukemogenic viruses. Such challenging observations require more extensive experience in other outbreaks of leukemia. At any rate the report of clusters in Buffalo, Niles, and other parts of this country and the world may implicate environmental or infectious factors in the causation of this disease in the human being.

On rare occasions leukemia has been reported in multiple occupants of the same house.[173] Leukemia occurred in four persons associated with a single house in a small town between 1950 and 1962. Three of these persons had acute leukemia and one had chronic granulocytic leukemia progressing to acute leukemia. Radiation survey of the house and its surroundings revealed no abnormalities. Several mechanisms (infectious, physical, or chemical) can be envisioned by which occupants in a given house might predispose to leukemia. Whatever the mechanism of leukemogenesis may be, the association of such leukemia cases with one house is rare.

Of 29,457 death certificates for children under 15 years of age who died of cancer in the United States between 1960 and 1966, the most common neoplasms in order of frequency were leukemia, gliomas, lymphoma, neuroblastoma, Wilms' tumor, bone cancer, rhabdomyosarcoma, and primary liver disease.[182] In this group leukemia was most common—14,240 cases, or 34.55%.

Glass and associates,[105] in a study of leukemia clusters in Los Angeles County, found that a great diversity of epidemiologic tests of hypotheses about leukemogenesis failed to support the concept of an infectious mode of spread. They favor as most promising subjects for such study the persons who are at exceptionally high risk of leukemia, for example, the identical twin of a leukemic child, patients with radiation-treated polycythemia vera, and persons with Bloom's syndrome or Fanconi's aplastic anemia.

Two sets of infant siblings with the juvenile Philadelphia chromosomal negative form of chronic myelocytic leukemia have been reported.[131] Each of the patients developed the disease within a short time of each other. Electron microscopic study of bone marrow and spleens of these children failed to reveal virus particles, and all attempts to isolate virus in cell cultures have been unsuccessful.

*Etiology.* Various physical, chemical, and metabolic agents have been found capable of precipitating or activating the development of leukemia. Infectious agents, trauma,[285] and exposure to drugs and chemicals have appeared to be so closely associated with leukemia as to suggest a causative relationship. Arsenicals, sulfonamides, and benzol poisoning[166] have been prominently mentioned, but evidence is still incomplete. The widespread use of antimicrobial and antibiotic agents in the treatment of patients with infectious disease has led to the impression that they may possess leukemogenic activity, although there has been no proof of this relationship.

The morphologic analogy between the maturation arrest in the bone marrow of patients with pernicious anemia and the blast cells in those with acute leukemia has suggested that leukemia represents a metabolic or deficiency disease, but treatment on this basis has given negative results.[53] In another theory, leukemia is based on disordered hormonal or metabolic functions. In one group of experiments[178] specific substances that produce myeloid and lymphoid proliferation and maturation in animals have been extracted from the urine of patients with leukemia. Data have also been obtained supporting the concept that the failure of cell maturation in patients with leukemia is associated with a loss of factors which inhibit cell proliferation.[67] Leukemia has also been compared to a type of autoimmunization involving the proliferation of one of the white cell-forming tissues in which the response, once begun, is self-replicating and permanent.[76] The stimuli for such leukemogenic activities are ionizing radiation, carcinogenic chemicals, and viruses.

A sufficient number of cases of acute leukemia has occurred in patients taking phenylbutazone (Butazolidin) to prompt inquiring into a cause-and-effect relationship. In a study by Woodliff and Dougan,[284] eight of fifty-five patients with acute leukemia in a registry of leukemia and allied disorders had taken this drug. In five of the eight cases the authors considered that there was a close relationship with the development of leukemia. However, the significance of this high incidence of association awaits the acquisition of more data and an appraisal of the relationship between the clinical condition for which phenylbutazone was given and the incidence of leukemia.

While it is known that acute leukemia appears with regularity in polycythemia vera, a new syndrome has recently been recognized in patients who have had multiple myeloma. Kyle and co-workers[156] have recently reported a rapidly progressive acute myelomonocytic leukemia that developed in four patients who had received prolonged courses of melphalan (phenylalanine mustard), ranging from 30 to 57 months. Since exposure to radiation is a known cause of acute leukemia, it might be expected that the administration of cytotoxic drugs which mimic the effect of radiation might also result in acute leukemia. Kyle and associates[156] point out that melphalan damages deoxyribonucleic acid, as does radiation. It is possible that the prolonged use of an alkylating agent can cause leukemogenesis in man.[130]

*Infections.* The role of infections in the causation of leukemia receives periodic emphasis. Cooke[58] has pointed out that infection frequently antedates the development of acute leukemia in childhood and that the character of the age incidence for leukemia tends to parallel the frequency of acute infections. One of the difficulties in accepting the infectious concept of leukemia, however, has been the well-established observation that in human beings with leukemia, as in experimental animals with leukemia, there is the lack of communicability which characterizes other infectious diseases.

Research on the etiology of leukemia is continuing in many centers, with on-going contributions from the areas of genetics, oncology, and epidemiology. An extensive literature has accumulated on the immunologic defenses against cancer.[126] In recent years the immunologic aspects of acute leukemia have also been under investigation.[126,159] It is postulated that the leukemic cell contains antigens foreign to its host. These are derived either from viruses or by mutation. Attempts to develop host immunity to such antigens have been in progress. Serendipitously, the protective effect of guinea pig serum against leukemia of other species led to the discovery of L-asparaginase as an effective agent in inducing remissions in acute lymphoblastic leukemia. Another approach is the active and passive immunization with specific antigens. B.C.G. has also been found to induce an antileukemic immune reaction.[170]

*Viral etiology.* With the possibility that nonspecific infections conceivably may be causally related to acute leukemia of childhood, a number of studies have focused their attention on a viral etiology for human leukemia. The demonstration by Ellerman and Bang[85] that chicken lymphomatosis could be transmitted by filtered extracts stimulated interest in the causation of leukemia and allied diseases in other species as well as in human beings.

Gross[112] demonstrated a viral etiology for lymphoid leukemias in mice which is noncontagious but is communicated to offspring during embryonal life through either the male or the female parent, resulting in leukemia after a period of latency of one-third to one-half of the life-span of the animal. According to this hypothesis, leukemia develops when the dormant agent is activated any time during the life-span of the mouse. The viral agent thus exists in active form, manifesting malignant capabilities only when challenged by as yet obscure but presumably trigger stimuli such as x-rays, chemicals, infections, or products of endogenous metabolic activities. Also, the virus would not necessarily become activated during the life-span of a single carrier host but would be transmitted from one generation to another in a vertical pattern.

Besides leukemia in mice, transmissible leukemia has been detected in fowl (the first experimental animal), in domestic animals, and in the cow.[82] Since a temporary remission may follow a virus infection, a series of viruses were given to a patient with acute myelogenous leukemia not responding to chemotherapy.[275] An unexpectedly prolonged course, together with decreases in both the number of circulating myeloblasts and size of the spleen and lymph nodes, was repeatedly observed in conjunction with the administration of six different viruses. The predominantly blastic composition of the bone marrow was unchanged during this study.

Schwartz and Schoolman[237] extended these observations to show that cell-free filtrates prepared from the brain of patients who died from acute leukemia are capable of accelerating the development of or inducing this disease in a leukemic strain (AKR) of mice. These studies based on animal experimentation are provocative and provide a basis for explaining many of the features of human leukemia seen in clinical practice. More significant than these laboratory experiments have been two significant observations occurring in man. The first of these is the "lymphoma belt" in Africa,[137] a belt that extends across the waist of the continent and follows a geographic pattern characterized by a minimum temperature of 60° F. (15.6° C.), making it possible for an arthropod vector to survive and transmit the lymphoma or its causative agent to susceptible children. The second phenomenon is the increasing awareness of "leukemia clusters." So far, the only satisfactory explanation of the occurrence of such clusters is that they represent focuses of infection,[124] although the possibility that so-called clusters may represent statistical coincidence cannot be ruled out. The demonstration of virus-like particles in leukocyte preparations of two patients with acute leukemia is also of interest.[5] The direct relationship of leukemia is still to be determined since passenger virus can be present in malignant tissue. The confirmation of the infectious nature of human leukemia, however, awaits the discovery of the virus in man. A detailed comparison between any type of human leukemia, with response of an inbred animal strain, to any leukemogenic virus has yet to be justified.[194,262]

An antibody reaction to extracts of leukemia and Hodgkin's disease tissues of man has been demonstrated by a variety of techniques.[111] The antigenic differences between normal and leukemic tissue extracts may reflect the presence of viruses or alterations caused by them.

The interest surrounding the reports of virus-like particles observed by electron microscopy in the serum of leukemic patients created the impression that viruses were implicated as causative factors of the disease. However, a definitive virus etiology for human cancer or leukemia awaits different virologic techniques than have heretofore been employed.[172] In summary, it appears that, in contrast to avian and murine leukemia which might be induced by virus infection, the viruses that accompany human leukemia have not been found to be etiologic agents. Rather, those that are present are passengers and not disease.[83]

That RNA oncogenic viruses play a role in the etiology of acute leukemia in humans has received considerable support from a number of recent studies.[14a,255a,263a] Gallo and co-workers[98a] identified RNA-dependent DNA polymerase activity in lymphoblasts of patients with leukemia but not in those of normal donors. This important enzyme, analogous to that of RNA tumor viruses, is capable of using an RNA template from mammalian cells to synthesize DNA and may be a mechanism by which viruses insert stable genetic information into a host genome, resulting in the disordered cell differentiation that characterizes human leukemia.

*Heredity.* The agents found to be leukemogenic or to accelerate the onset of leukemia in mice depend upon the genetic constitution of the mouse.[147] In the human being as well, attention has been drawn to the possibility that the genetic constitution may condition susceptibility to leukemia. Many instances have been reported in which leukemia developed simultaneously in several members of the same family or in successive generations. The most striking family history is that reported by Anderson[9] in which five of eight siblings developed leukemia at 5 to 8 years of age. An instance of familial leukemia has been reported in which the disease occurred in a mother and her 5-year-old son, after a heavy exposure to insecticide spray.[151] Acute myelogenous leukemia occurred in the child 8 months after exposure and 5 years after exposure in the mother. Steinberg,[256] in an extensive investigation of the close relation of 249 patients who become ill with acute leukemia before 16 years of age, found no increased incidence of leukemia among the patients' relatives. In another series of 182 cases of leukemia, there were only three instances in close relatives (father and son and two first cousins), suggesting that the environmental rather than the genetic factors determine the onset of leukemia.[42] On the other hand, Heath and Moloney[125] described a family in which five cases of acute leukemia occurred in three consecutive generations over a 60-year period. Each case in this family was probably of a myelocytic variety. They pointed out that the sequence of cases was compatible with the concept of "vertical" viral transmission proposed by Gross[112] for murine leukemia—i.e., the vertical passage of leukemogenic virus from one generation to the next through the germ cells.

The occurrence of leukemia in twin children, especially in identical twins, has been the subject of several reports.[10,59,115] Gunz and Dameshek[115] reported a family in which a man, 53 years of age, died of chronic lymphocytic leukemia 27 years after his father and the father's identical twin died of the same disease, both at the age of 56 years. From a series of seventy-two twin sets selected by the presence of at least one member affected by leukemia in childhood, there were five sets in which both members were affected.[165] In the five the sex was the same; two sets were males and three were females. Although only two sets were thoroughly investigated, it seems probable that all five were monozygous. In two sets of twins the diagnosis was made at the same time and in the others the disease was diagnosed from 4 months to 2 years apart. The onset ranged from 6 months of age to 9½ years. The parallel response to chemotherapy in these twins[283] and the implication of a prenatal or prezygotic origin of childhood leukemia prompted an intensive study of leukemia in twins.[204]

Analysis of large series of cases in any one hospital provides little evidence, however, that heredity is of any importance in human leukemia. On the other hand, in the light of experimental and unequivocal evidence of multiple cases in one family, the hereditary factor cannot be categorically dismissed. Videbaek,[268] for instance, finding a familial incidence of leukemia of about 8% in Denmark as compared with 0.5% in control families, concluded nevertheless that leukemia was a matter of an inherited predisposition rather than of direct chromosomal inheritance.

In a family of New Zealand Maoris of nine children, four and possibly five developed acute lymphocytic leukemia in the space of 5 years. The age of occurrence was from 10 months to 6 years. No major chromosome abnormalities were found in the parents or affected children.[117] This family is one of the extremely few in the literature in which leukemia affected multiple close relatives in the same generation. Such an occurrence probably reflects a highly unusual genetic constellation which differed greatly from that in most individuals with leukemia.

Leukemia has never been known to pass the placental barrier either in the mouse[47] or in the human being. In the experimentally produced disease the leukemic cells are found only on the maternal side of the placenta, the fetal circulation remaining normal. Experience has been universal that leukemic mothers give birth to normal infants, the placenta apparently serving as an effective barrier.[6,26,63]

A probable exception to this observation is the report of a mother with signs and symptoms of leukemia beginning in the seventh month of pregnancy in whom acute lymphocytic leukemia was diagnosed 8 days postpartum and whose infant developed the same disease at 9 months of age.[68] The problem here is one of establishing an absolute relationship between leukemia in the mother and infant because of the lapse of time until the disease was noted. If transplacental passage of the agent occurred late in pregnancy, it is theoretically possible for the disease not to have become manifest until some time after birth.[68]

Leukemia in the newborn is unusual and may be confused with leukemoid reactions complicating mongolism, congenital syphilis, viremia, septicema, toxoplasmosis, hemolytic anemia, thrombocytopenic purpura, erythroblastosis fetalis, and cytomegalic inclusion disease.[51] A case of rapidly progressive acute lymphatic leukemia in a neonate has been described.[51] The onset was marked by purpura on the eighth day, followed by hepatosplenemogaly and pallor. The leukocytosis reached a peak of 1,300,000 cells per cubic millimeter, with 71% lymphoblasts. Microscopic study at autopsy at 7 weeks of age disclosed extensive leukemic infiltration of kidneys, spleen, bone marrow, and lymph nodes. Identical herpes virus–type particles were found in the peripheral blood leukocytes of the mother and child. There were no features in the child to suggest Down's syndrome. Serologic tests in the infant were negative and she had no herpetic lesions.

A high proportion of pregnancies, especially with acute leukemia, terminate in premature labor, abortion, stillbirth, and neonatal death. Congenital malformations have been notably uncommon, however, in the infants, except when potentially teratogenic therapy was used. Several patients with chronic myelocytic leukemia receiving busulfan (Myleran) therapy alone bore normal infants who have continued to develop normally over the years.[223] In one case the child died at 1 month, with infection and anomalies attributable to busulfan. Normal infants were delivered of two other patients with acute leukemia who were treated with corticosteroids and 6-mercaptopurine.[163] Follow-up studies of offspring beyond the newborn period do not indicate that the offspring are at increased risks of developing leukemia.[12] An exhaustive review of the world literature since 1930 on leukemia and pregnancy revealed that twenty-four males and thirty-two females were born alive to mothers suffering from acute leukemia, while thirty-seven males and twenty-eight females occurred among the liveborn offspring of mothers with chronic leukemia.[96] These differences are not statistically significant. A shift in sex ratio together with knowledge that visible chromosome defects occur in leukemia have given further support of the genetic origin of the disease.

On the basis of epidemiological research,

Miller[181] has identified five classes of persons with exceptionally high risk of leukemia. Common to all is a distinctive genetic or cytogenetic characteristic either inherited or acquired. (1) *Identical twins*—at greatest risk thus far known is the child whose identical twin has developed leukemia. The probability is about one in five that he will develop this disease within weeks or months after his twin falls ill.[165] There is no such risk among fraternal twins. (2) *Inherited tendency to chromosomal breakage*—Bloom's syndrome (photosensitive telangiectasia of the face) shows an unusual susceptibility to acute leukemia. This syndrome is marked by excessive chromosomal breakage and rearrangement in cell culture, a trait shared with Fanconi's aplastic anemia and ataxia-telangiectasia, inherited disorders which predispose to acute leukemia. (3) *Acquired chromosomal breaks*—chromosomal breaks can be produced by a variety of agents to which man is exposed. Two of these—ionizing radiation and benzene—have been implicated in human leukemogenesis. Observations on the Japanese survivors of the atomic bombs provide convincing evidence that whole body radiation in sufficient dosage is leukemogenic in man. Studies of patients given radiotherapy for ankylosing spondylitis indicate that partial body exposure may also induce leukemia. In both studies, the frequency of the neoplasm was proportionate to the radiation dose, and the peak incidence occurred about 6 years after exposure. (4) *Extra chromosomes*—an accumulation of reports suggests that Klinefelter's syndrome, in which there is an XXY sex-chromosome complement, predisposes to leukemia. Borges and associates[37] found that four of twenty-five nonmongoloid children with acute leukemia were demonstrated to have cytogenetic variants of prezygotic origins, indicating that the aneuploid cell is more susceptible to malignant change. (5) *Sibs of leukemic children*—it is to be expected that acute leukemia may also aggregate among sibs in families with other heritable leukemia-prone disorders such as Bloom's syndrome, Fanconi's aplastic anemia, and congenital (X-linked) agammaglobulinemia. Although certain viruses alter chromosomes, induce leukemia in experimental animals, and cause human tissue cultures to undergo malignant transformation, no virus has as yet been implicated in the genesis of human leukemia. Epidemiological tests have failed to show that the disease is transmitted from one person to another.

Gibson and co-workers[101] found that the highest risk for leukemia in children 1 to 4 years of age occurred when the following factors were associated in the same individual: irradiation of the mother before conception, in utero irradiation of the child, previous history of reproductive wastage, and early childhood virus disease. The highest risk was for children exposed to all four factors. Irradiation both preconception and in utero is viewed as a triggering agent of a sequence of events that increases the child's risk for leukemia.

**Chromosomes and leukemia.** Short-term cultures of bone marrow and blood have established the normal diploid number of chromosomes as forty-six (euploid). The culture of leukemic blood has demonstrated a variety of abnormal mitoses belonging to leukemic cell lines. In acute forms there is a very high incidence of chromosome abnormalities, consisting of alterations in number and structure. Among the former are aneuploidy (a state in which a chromosome is extra or missing) and polyploidy (multiple complete sets of chromosomes). Structural changes include chromosome deletion and translocation. The abnormalities are extremely variable, but are unique in each case.

It has been postulated that leukemia is the result of autosomal mutation leading to the propagation of an aneuploid stem line. Gunz and Fitzgerald[116] explained the mechanism of genetic change as a disturbance, either inherited or acquired, in an unknown locus, regulating normal cell division leading to chromosomal imbalance. Such changes may in turn enhance alteration in other chromosomes, thus leading to the abnormalities found in acute leukemia. Reisman and co-workers[220,222] observed aneuploidy at the time of leukemic infiltration of the bone marrow, that the modal number of the aneuploid cell lines varied from case to case but appeared to be fixed for each individual, and that it persisted unchanged during prolonged relapse and reemerged in consecutive relapses. During remission the normal number of chromosomes was restored and found to persist, regardless of duration or type of agent used. According to Zuelzer,[286] remission might, therefore, be viewed as the temporary suppression of the mutant in favor of the normal stem line. Relapse after remission would indicate reemergence of a residue of mutant cells.

In one study acute lymphoblastic leukemias as a group showed the highest incidence of aneuploidy (77% versus 12% for nonleukemic controls),[231] but no constant malformation was demonstrated. In contrast to acute leukemias, a constant abnormality has been found in most cases of chronic granulocytic leukemia in which the Ph[1] chromosome can be demonstrated.[13,200] Occasionally, Ph[1] cells have been found in the marrow before the clinical symptoms and hematologic evidence of leukemia were fully developed.[146] This chromosomal abnormality occurs in hematopoietic cells but in no other somatic cells.[116] With the rise and fall of the Ph[1] in chronic granulocytic leukemia, relapses and remissions produced by therapy may be followed.

The problem still remains whether chromosomal changes can be interpreted either as causative or as a part of the changes coincident with the disease. Whether the chromosomal breakage incident to radiation exposure may persist to produce leukemia in some susceptible individuals is still problematic. Thus far, the evidence is that visible changes are not of primary etiologic significance. No consistent pattern of changes is found in acute leukemia in childhood.[132]

**Glossary of chromosomal terminology.** An abbreviated glossary of chromosomal terminology may be helpful in the interpretation of the aberrations of the karyotypes encountered in leukemia.

*chromosomes* tiny, subcellular bundles of DNA which determine all the physical characteristics of an individual from eye color to sex, and control body chemistry as well.

*chromatid* one of the two longitudinal subunits of a chromosome which becomes morphologically (i.e., visibly) distinct at late prophase and metaphase. They separate at anaphase, one sister chromatid passing to each of the daughter cells. A chromosome consists of the two sister chromatids after it duplicates itself during the intermitotic period, before the onset of mitosis.

*chromatid exchange* transposition of a segment of a chromatid, within one, or between two or more, chromosomes, giving rise to a structural change (chromosome mutation).

*chromatid break* a visible discontinuity in a chromatid. Without displacement of the distal segment of the affected chromatid, breaks are difficult to separate from gaps.

*chromatid gap* a discontinuity in a chromatid but with maintenance of alignment and with close approximation of the proximal and distal pieces.

*endoreduplication* chromosome duplication twice in succession without separation of the sister chromatids, represented at metaphase by chromosomes with four rather than two chromatids.

*metaphase* midpoint of mitotic division, with chromosomes aligned on or close to the equatorial plane.

*karyotype* a systematized array of the chromosomes showing their number, size, and shape in a somatic cell, with the implication that this cell is representative of the chromosomes of an individual species; the karyotype of a normal individual shows 46 chromosomes: 22 autosomal pairs and 2 sex chromosomes—XY in a normal male and XX in a normal female.

*autosomes* chromosomes other than sex chromosomes.

*sex chromosomes* X and Y (XX, female; XY, male).

*diploid* the characteristic somatic number of chromosomes in man, 46. Chromosomes are found in pairs. Thus 46 chromosomes of the human karyotype consist of 23 essentially identical pairs. One-half of the diploid number in man is 23 and is designated as the haploid number. Of these, 22 are autosomes or nonsex chromosomes. All body cells contain a member of each pair of chromosomes from one parent and one member from the other parent.

*homologues* chromosomes occurring in usually morphologic indistinguishable pairs; they contain identical sets of loci.

*euploid* having the normal number of chromosomes.

*aneuploid* a deviation from the characteristic chromosome number (a chromosome is extra or missing).

*polyploidy* having multiple sets of chromosomes.

*trisomy* having three chromosomes of a particular pair instead of two (mongoloids are trisomic for chromosome 21).

*deletion* a piece of chromosome breaking off and becoming lost.

*translocation* exchange of segments between chromosomes, producing abnormally long or short chromosomes. Reciprocal translocation happens when two pieces of chromatin not of the same size are broken off from two nonhomologous chromosomes and their positions exchanged. The result is that one chromosome will have too little chromatin and the other too much.

*nondisjunction* during cell division the failing of two chromosomes to separate and pass into each gamete. Instead, both members of a pair pass into the same gamete. Thus, one cell has an extra chromosome and the other has too few. If such cells survive and continue to divide, clinical abnormalities result. Mongoloids, for example, almost always have 47 chromosomes. The extra one is an autosome.

*mosaicism* the presence in somatic tissues within one individual of two or more cell types, differing either in chromosome number or in chromosome morphology.

*Radiation.* In addition to the long-term genetic effects of ionizing radiation,[28,175] there is mounting evidence that this agent is strongly implicated in the causation of leukemia and is a major factor in the steadily increasing death rate from this disease. The evidence for irradiation as a leukemokenic agent in human beings includes the increased incidence of leukemia among radiologists as compared with other physicians,[169] in patients receiving radiation therapy for ankylosing spondylitis,[64] in children who received radiation to the mediastinum for enlarged thymus in infancy,[245,246] and among atomic bomb survivors in Hiroshima and Nagasaki.[94,188,189] Hematologic surveys in Hiroshima indicated that after atomic radiation there was a "latent period" of several years before leukemia was in evidence. Chronic myelogenous leukemia was most common, followed in frequency by acute myelogenous and acute lymphatic types.[187]

Chronic granulocytic (myelogenous) leukemia occurred predominantly in the middle age groups, but it was also seen with unusual frequency in children.[43] After exposure to mixed gamma and neutron radiation, the incidence of leukemia was found to start 1 to 1½ years following irradiation. Maximal risk occurs approximately 4 to 7 years after irradiation. There was a significant increase in proximally exposed survivors in Hiroshima and Nagasaki. Survivors who were under 10 years of age at the time of exposure showed the greatest increase in leukemia following close exposure to the bomb. In the age period up to 19 years there was a striking incidence of acute lymphocytic leukemia. It is of interest that among Japanese survivors who had been exposed in utero no cases of leukemia have been identified to date. High rates of stillbirth, abortion, and neonatal death, however, reduced the size of the group at risk. The studies in Hiroshima and Nagasaki, therefore, established unequivocally that a sufficiently large whole-body exposure to radiation can induce leukemia in man.[43]

It has been postulated that the increased exposure of the population to ionizing radiations employed in medicine and dentistry also contributes to the accelerated death rates from leukemia.[74] There is a possibility that the spontaneous incidence of leukemia may be due to radiation from natural background sources. Quantitative estimates have been made of the probability of developing radiation-induced leukemia in the average person in a population.[162]

It is of interest that age has been shown to be a factor of importance in experimentally induced leukemia. Animals exposed to whole body irradiation before puberty develop a far higher incidence than older animals.[142] Besides causing genetic damage, diagnostic pelvimetry during pregnancy or threatened abortion may occasionally cause leukemia or cancer in the unborn child.[95,258] Gunz, Borthwick, and Rolleston[114] have reported from New Zealand the case of a child who received excessive doses (five heavy exposures) of diagnostic radiation in utero during the third trimester of pregnancy and died of acute granulocytic leukemia at 10 months of age.

In one study mortality rates from leukemia and other cancers were each estimated to be about 40% higher when there was prenatal x-ray exposure than when there was not.[165] The relative risk was greatest at 5 to 7 years of age. On the other hand, the increased risk of childhood malignancy due to fetal radiation during x-ray pelvimetry of the mother has been doubted by others.[66]

Bloom and Tjio[31] have shown that patient body x-irradiation at diagnostic level kilovoltage is capable in some cases of producing chromosome damage in vivo. Five adult patients in whom gastrointestinal tract evaluation was performed had a low rate of structural abnormalities of the chromosomes. In one child with Down's syndrome chromosomal fragments were produced after cardiac catheterization. In five cases with aberrations the effects disappeared within 2 weeks, in another it persisted for 2½ months after irradiation. Chromosome damage has been shown to persist as long as 20 years in some cases in the peripheral leukocytes of patients receiving x-ray therapy[46] for ankylosing spondylitis. Since the mortality from leukemia is increased tenfold among patients treated with x-rays for this disease, it is tempting to link the rise and fall of the cells with unstable abnormalities and the rise in the leukemia to its peak values. More extensive studies are required before it can be concluded that the greater frequency of chromosomal abnormalities among the older spondylitic patients is of necessity related to the higher risk of leukemia among them. Furthermore, there is a vast difference between the transitory chromosomal changes after diagnostic x-ray examinations in children and the level of the x-ray dose in therapy of the older subject with spondylitis.

• • •

In the light of these concepts, it would appear that certain genetic influences acting in conjunction with both identified and as yet unidentified external factors transform normal hematopoietic cells and their precursors into those with an unrestrained and purposeless growth.[260] Exposure to ionizing radiation in the environment, infections, contamination of the atmosphere with chemical pollutants, and marrow-depressing drugs and chemicals may serve as such activating agents.[235] Despite these incriminating data for the carcinogenic effect of radiation, it is not yet possible in man to determine whether or not a threshold dose for the induction of leukemia does or does not exist.[70]

It may be concluded that in the etiology of leukemia radiation undoubtedly plays a part, but it is likely to be a small one.[75] Authenticated cases are known to have followed the administration of moderately large or large quantities of radiation to the whole body or to large parts of the body. Despite statistics to the contrary,[257] no firm evidence exists to show that diagnostic radiology has caused leukemia. There is also nothing to indicate that extremely small quantities of radiation from fallout are leukemogenic.

**Preleukemic stage of leukemia.** Cases of leukemia have been recorded in which a nonleukemic blood disorder of variable duration preceded the onset of acute leukemia.[93] This preliminary period is usually characterized by a deficiency of one or more cellular elements in the peripheral blood resulting in anemia, neutropenia, thrombocytopenia, or combinations thereof. The bone marrow is moderately hyperplastic and may or may not show an arrest in the granulocytic series.[30] In one patient the preleukemic stage extended over a period of 9 years and was punctuated by a remission before the terminal development of myeloblastic leukemia.[277]

The anemia is frequently hemolytic in nature although not always accompanied by an elevated reticulocyte count.[174] In one case in our experience acute stem cell leukemia in a child 4 years old was preceded 2 years earlier by severe iron-deficiency anemia. Neither the blood nor bone marrow showed evidence of immature white blood cell precursors. In the intervening period the child was asymptomatic without changes in the blood status. Another child under our observation who had been seriously ill for many years with recurrent staphylococcal infections, a chronic anemia, and a slightly enlarged spleen developed acute leukemia at 5 years of age. Bone marrow studies 1 year before the development of leukemia showed an entirely normal pattern. In another report[21] an adult presented the features of autoimmune hemolytic anemia and hypersplenism for 18 years and finally developed fulminating leukemia. Still another patient developed aplastic anemia after extensive exposure to benzene. Pancytopenia persisted for a 15 year period and finally emerged as a subacute myelocytic leukemia.[77]

Two other patients followed by us gave evidence of a preleukemic stage of leukemia. One was a child of 2 years who had had a persistent fever for 3 weeks; at termination of the fever a profound anemia was noted. The platelets ranged from 400,000 to 500,000 per cubic millimeter, the white count was normal, and reticulocytes were increased. Bone marrow aspiration revealed erythroid hypoplasia. Iron therapy resulted in marked improvement of the anemia. One month later pancytopenia developed and the bone marrow was heavily infiltrated by stem cells. Another child showed petechiae at 3 months of age, marked thrombocytopenia at 3 years of age, and many normal bone marrow samples during the first 8 years of life. At 8 years of age the peripheral blood revealed increasing numbers of macrocytes for the first time and bone marrow aspiration revealed evidence of the Naegeli type of monocytic leukemia, namely, heavy myelomonocytic infiltration. In this connection, the report of Pretlow[216] is pertinent in that acute leukemia developed after 11 years of peripheral monocytosis.

Other cases have been reported of aplastic anemia followed by acute monocytic leukemia, in one after an interval of 10 months.[168] In another case acute myeloid leukemia followed 7 years of aplastic anemia induced by chloramphenicol.[57] Fanconi's anemia is also known to precede leukemia; a case of acute myelomonocytic leukemia has been reported illustrating this relationship.[81] The term preleukemia can be applied to those cases inasmuch as a prodrome of bone marrow dysfunction existed prior to the clear-cut diagnosis of acute leukemia.[57] These cases fit in with the concept that "any agent capable of producing aplasia of the bone marrow should be considered as potentially leukemogenic."[69]

The possible relationship between autoimmunity and leukemia has previously been postulated.[76] In children, prolonged neutropenia and leukopenia or aplastic anemia may appear to precede acute leukemia, but when this sequence is evaluated further it appears possible that they represent a remission phase in the course of the latter disease. Abnormal cells indicative of leukemia are not found in the blood or bone marrow of patients with these antecedent disorders, and there is no associated splenomegaly or lymphadenopathy. Still to be determined by a more direct approach than circumstantial evidence is the extent to which the initial disorder is involved in the subsequent development of leukemia.

*Leukemia in the newborn period (congenital leukemia).* Congenital leukemia is a rare disease, of which approximately fifty adequately documented cases have been reported.[211,259a] Some infants exhibit signs of leukemia at birth and succumb shortly thereafter. In another group the infant appears normal at birth but develops clinical and hematologic signs later in the newborn period. In the third group the disease is not detected until the third to the sixth week of life,[41] with a suggestive history of a hematologic disturbance dating back to the first weeks of life.

The leukemia is principally myelogenous and is marked by a hyperleukocytosis and a predominance of promyelocytes and myelocytes. Myeloblasts vary from 10 to 80%. The granulocytic leukemia is noted in both the blood and bone marrow.* Anemia is uncommon in the newborn infant but develops soon thereafter, with a rapid progression to pancytopenia. Large numbers of nucleated red blood cells may be present in the peripheral blood, regardless of anemia. Those cases that develop later show anemia when diagnosed. Platelets are reduced in number. Physical signs include hemorrhages of the skin, bleeding from the mucous membranes and umbilical stump, nodular skin infiltration, and enlargement of the liver and spleen.

In the newborn period, leukemia is to be differentiated principally from the leukemoid reaction of sepsis and congenital syphilis, erythroblastosis, folate deficiency,[157] and congenital thrombocytopenic purpura. In patients with a leukemoid reaction, myelocytes, as well as segmented and nonsegmented polynuclear cells, are increased, but myeloblasts are absent. Eventually, the causative agent of the sepsis is discovered by blood culture or by evidences of specific organ involvement with infection. The essential differentiating feature is the extensive infiltration of the nonhematopoietic organs as well as the liver, spleen, and lymph nodes by immature cells of the granulocytic series in infants with leukemia and the absence of such infiltration in patients with a leukemoid reaction. Erythroblastosis, which may also be accompanied by leukocytosis, anemia, and myelocytes in the peripheral blood can be diagnosed by evidences of blood group incompatibility. Although the decreased number of platelets in patients with congenital thrombocytopenia may have to be considered, hepatosplenomegaly is absent and promyelocytes and myelocytes do not appear in the blood smear. It is of interest that, except for the case reported by Cramblett and associates,[68] no other case of congenital leukemia has ever been encountered in a newborn infant whose mother had leukemia during pregnancy. Furthermore, leukemia diagnosed soon after birth must have had an intrauterine origin without affecting the mother.

Treatment of leukemia with current methods (Chapter 23) is ineffective, and the duration of life varies from several days to 2 or 3 months. This rapidly fatal course is in contrast to the prolonged course of chronic myelogenous leukemia in adults and in children beyond infancy.[60]

The presence of associated cardiac, orthopedic, skeletal, and other developmental anomalies in patients with congenital leukemia[25] is analogous to the well-documented combination of leukemia and mongolism.[152,153,176,233] In addition to trisomy 21, other specific congenital anomalies that have been associated with congenital or perinatal leukemia include

---

*See references 25, 71, 144, 145, and 215.

isolated malformations such as absence of radii,[259a] Klippel-Feil syndrome,[259a] patent ductus arteriosus,[259a] atrial and ventricular septal defects,[259a] and the $D_1$ trisomy[231a] and Bonnevie-Ullrich[216a] syndromes. In a 2-week-old male infant with a variant of Ellis-van Creveld syndrome and acute myeloblastic leukemia,[177a] no chromosomal aberration was observed. Leukemia has been reported[259] to be three to twenty times more common in children with mongolism than in the general population. In a survey of 519 sibship histories of leukemic children, mongolism was more common than usual, not only among the leukemic children but also among their sibs.[180,232] One-third of the mongolism-leukemia cases reviewed by Krivit and Good[153] were classified as acute granulocytic leukemia. It is of interest, therefore, that leukocyte alkaline phosphatase values are increased in uncomplicated mongolism, a condition in which patients are trisomic for chromosome 21.[202] In chronic granulocytic leukemia, in which there is a low alkaline phosphatase, there is a deletion of chromosomal material from 21 chromosome ($Ph^1$ chromosome).[200,265] The structural and enzymatic changes in both conditions affecting the same chromosome may be of more than coincidental significance (Chapter 20).

The hypothesis that attributed mongolism to toxic factors of endogenous or exogenous origin, inducing changes in the fetus during the early weeks of pregnancy,[135] requires revision in the light of the newer observations that mongolism is associated with a specific chromosomal pattern. Of the patients with mongolism studied thus far, nearly all have had an extra chromosome (trisomy) of pair 21 (Group 21-22—Denver classification), making a total of 47 chromosomes.[160] Occasional cases have been reported with 46 chromosomes in which there has been a translocation of one of the parts of a chromosome 21 without a trisomy being present. In these cases the main portion of chromosome 21 has attached itself to another chromosome, usually to the chromosome 15 or to some member of the chromosome 13 to 15 (D) group.[39,238] Another abnormality apparently characteristic of mongolism is the reduced number of lymphocytes in the peripheral blood and the presence of polynuclear leukocytes with an increased proportion of cells with an unsegmented nucleus.[185]

Other hematologic peculiarities of Down's syndrome include a shift to the left of the lobe count of granulocytes, a tendency for myeloid leukemia, transient congenital leukemia, labile granulopoiesis, myeloproliferative disorder, and a low HbF at birth. With reference to the latter, Wilson and co-workers[278] found that in twelve infants with Down's syndrome (G trisomy), with one exception, a low HbF and a relatively elevated hemoglobin $A_2$ was present in the first several months of life. These findings are the direct opposite of the hemoglobin changes in D trisomy syndrome.

The increased incidence of leukemia in mongolism[259] has been attributed to the imbalance of genes on the chromosome 21. This imbalance is believed to bring about the mongoloid anatomic anomalies upsetting the humoral coordination of tissue and organ growth during crucial stages of embryonic development. In later life leukopoietic growth regulation may be so erratic as to increase the risk of leukemia.[231]

*Spontaneous remissions.* Complete and spontaneous clinical and hematologic remissions have been observed in some patients, without apparent relation to therapy. They have also occurred in patients on supportive therapy including transfusions and especially following infections. An incidence of spontaneous remissions as high as 10% of cases has been given in one series in children[79] and as low as only 1 in 105 children with transfusions as the sole therapy.[254] Remissions following infections have been described more frequently. Remarkable improvement and complete and dramatic arrest of the disease have been reported in a group of children with acute leukemia following infection caused by streptococcus, staphylococcus, and varicella and by inoculation with the feline panleukopenia virus.[27] Four spontaneous remissions were observed in a young child over a 17-month period on supportive therapy and antibiotics.[16] Characteristic of the majority of cases was an antecedent stage of severe leukopenia, frequently a leukopenic agranulocytic phase, and hypoplasia or aplasia of the marrow associated with anemia. It is of interest that therapeutically induced remissions also demonstrate a hypoplastic phase preceding remission. This transformation to a normal status is usually short-lived, varying from several weeks to a few months, and in one adult reported on complete remission lasted 21 months.[29] Following the remission, however, the disease returns to its original severity, uninfluenced by the temporary reversal to normal.

A series of cases has been compiled with the provocative finding of recoveries from congenital leukemia among children with mongolism.[87,227] Initially the patients' disease was indistinguishable from acute leukemia. The manifestations included hepatosplenomegaly, anemia, thrombocytopenia, purpura, and typical blast cells in the bone marrow and peripheral blood. Five of the seven cases were either granulocytic or myeloblastic, the other two stem cell and monocytic. Recovery occurred spontaneously without any uniformity of treatment by 5½ months (usually within the first 4 months). In three of the seven patients from 3 to 6 years of age, death due to other causes revealed no evidence of leukemia. The authors concluded that whether these cases belong in the category of true leukemia is not so important as the concept that this pathologic process has the capability, even though rare, of undergoing a spontaneous and complete remission. Differentiation from a leukemoid reaction is still, however, of the greatest urgency before it is concluded that leukemia can result in a complete remission.

Other cases have been reported adding further support to the hypothesis of the existence of ineffective regulation of production and maturation of bone marrow elements in association with Down's syndrome.[227] Behrman and colleagues[20] reported a family with three siblings who had mongolism, two of whom presented as newborn infants with thrombocytopenia and a marked derangement in erythropoiesis as well as granulopoiesis. They presented with polycythemia and increased myeloblasts and erythroblasts in the peripheral blood. At postmortem examination, one infant had widespread infiltrates of cells such as may be seen in chronic myelocytic leukemia. Miller and associates[179] reported a patient with Down's syndrome and associated myeloproliferative disease with the unique finding of increased platelet number and size. The hematocrit was 70%, hemoglobin 18.4 gm./100 ml., a white blood count of 230,000/cu. mm., with 80% myeloblasts and a platelet count of 1,200,000/cu. mm. Many platelets were as large as red cells. It was considered that the persistent abnormality did not represent leukemia. Postmortem evidence revealed extramedullary hematopoiesis and not a leukemic infiltration.

During an epidemiologic study of neonatal polycythemia, Weinberger and Oleinick[271] observed nine infants with Down's syndrome among 402 study cases whose hematocrits ranged from 77 to 86%. The time elapsed until cord clamping was not excessive. None of these infants had cyanotic congenital heart disease. In one patient there was a qualitative shift in the form of an abundance of red cell precursors. Quantitatively and qualitatively red cell proliferation in these infants appears analogous to granulocyte and platelet abnormalities previously reported and suggest an extensive congenital defect of the bone marrow function in newborn infants with Down's syndrome.

Wegelius and co-workers reported the case of a newborn monogoloid female infant who showed atypical blast cell infiltration in the bone marrow.[270] At 14 days of age the total white blood count numbered 130,000 per cu. mm., with 91% atypical blast cells. The blood and bone marrow became normal at about 6 weeks of age without any specific antileukemic therapy. At the age of 4 years the child was still healthy and the blood and bone marrow were normal.

On the other hand, an occasional case is encountered in which the blood picture of the newborn demonstrates an immaturity simulating that found in Down's syndrome in the absence of this condition. Gordon[106] reported the case of a newborn infant who on the twelfth day of life demonstrated the clinical and laboratory manifestations of leukemia. Autopsy on the following day revealed the features of myeloid metaplasia but the marrow was not leukemic. The patient's postmortem marrow was not strikingly different from an active or at most reactive newborn marrow. The diagnosis was that of a leukemic-like myeloproliferative disorder in the absence of Down's syndrome.

***Clinical features.*** The clinical features of leukemia combine the constitutional manifestations of the disease, blood deficiencies, particularly thrombocytopenia and anemia, and involvement of organ systems.

*Symptomatology.* The clinical manifestations and course of acute leukemia are strikingly similar and show no differences with respect to the predominating cell type. The onset of this disease is insidious, with localized symptoms obscuring the systemic nature of the disease. Symptomatology often follows a well-defined pattern, and several sets of symptoms are observed. Frequently, the onset is ill defined, with the patient exhibiting pallor, anorexia, irritability, abdominal pain, and malaise. These symptoms may pass unnoticed until diagnosis by blood examination prompts a retrospective review of the history. Other patients have persistent low-grade fever with intermittent periods of moderate or marked temperature elevations which either are unexplained or are attributed to a sore throat. In some the disease is ushered in by high fever and an upper respiratory infection from which the child does not recover as expected with routine treatment. In still others there is the appearance of hemorrhagic manifestations such as bleeding from the gums, epistaxis, and a tendency to bruise. Persistent hemorrhage after a minor operation or after tonsillectomy may be the first evidence of acute leukemia.

More rarely, the onset is abrupt with the clinical picture of an acute infectious disease marked by hyperpyrexia, severe prostration, nausea, vomiting, abdominal pain, anemia, and purpura. In a patient with this type of fulminating disease with a duration of several days, the spleen and lymph nodes may be only slightly or moderately enlarged. Symptoms such as local or generalized pain, limp, and bruising dating from a specific injury are often so definite to permit an exact documentation of the onset of symptoms to the time of a traumatic episode. Migratory bone and joint pains, and at times acute arthritis with signs of local inflammation, pallor, weakness, epistaxis, and an irregular febrile reaction simulate the clinical picture of rheumatic fever. Spontaneous rupture of the spleen is a rare occurrence in patients with acute leukemia and may produce the initial symptomatology of the disease.[282] Initial symptoms and manifestations of the disease may be related to local leukemic infiltration of the central nervous system, kidneys, testes, pericardium, or thyroid rather than to the more commonly occurring hematologic abnormalities.

*Physical findings.* Early in the course of acute leukemia the physical examination may be essentially normal. Sooner or later, the lymph nodes usually enlarge, and the edge of the spleen is palpable on deep inspiration. Lymph node enlargement is most marked in the cervical region but may be conspicuous over the occipital and postauricular areas and elsewhere over the scalp. It is often less pronounced than in patients with chronic leukemia. Involvement of the lymphoid tissue resulting in bilateral painless enlargement of the salivary and lacrimal glands is designated as the Mikulicz syndrome.[129] The liver and spleen may be enormously enlarged, but the spleen may fluctuate in size, especially during treatment, with little accompanying change in the liver. Infarcts and perisplenitis may occur in the spleen and result in such pain and tenderness as to suggest the presence of an abdominal emergency.[263] If a ruptured spleen is suspected by the presence of blood on aspiration, surgical exploration and splenectomy should be promptly performed.

Hemorrhages into the skin consist of petechiae, purpura, and extensive ecchymoses that recede and reappear during the disease. Hemorrhages into eye grounds and in mucous membranes, especially in the mouth and nose, are common. Ulcerations in the buccal mucosa result from leukemic infiltration as well as from hemorrhage.

Swollen, spongy hypertrophied gums, to the extent that the teeth are hidden, which characterizes monocytic leukemia, may also be found in patients with acute stem cell leukemia. Ulcerations may extend from the gums to the tonsils and palate.

Skin involvement is varied. It is either specific with leukemic infiltration or nonspecific with erythema multiform-like papulonecrotic and eczematous lesions. More specific are the small yellow discrete and elevated flat-topped plaques which are either widespread or confined to localized areas on the abdomen and extremities. Infrequently, maculopapular eruptions cover the face initially and spread to the chest and back and eventually to the abdomen and extremities (Figs. 75 and 76). Each lesion may become hemorrhagic and necrotic, and is eventually covered by a grayish membrane. Biopsy reveals extensive leukemic infiltration around blood vessels and adnexa in the epidermis and subcutaneous tissue.

Mediastinal involvement should be suspected in the presence of symptoms of respiratory distress. The kidneys are often greatly enlarged, and glomerulonephritis may precede or accompany the overt blood changes of leukemia.

Radiological studies of a 12-year-old boy with acute lymphocytic leukemia complicated by dysphagia and chest pain showed the presence of filling defects along the distal one-third of the esophagus.[7] A leukemic infiltrate of the esophagus was suspected and radiotherapy to the distal one-third of the esophagus was instituted. Prompt cessation of the chest pain and dysphagia occurred. Involvement of the esophagus in patients with leukemia is a rare complication although gastrointestinal lesions in patients with leukemia are not uncommon.[75]

Priapism has been reported in children with chronic and acute granulocytic leukemia and marked leukocytosis.[109,138,224] Among the various mechanisms proposed for priapism is sludging and mechanical obstruction of the

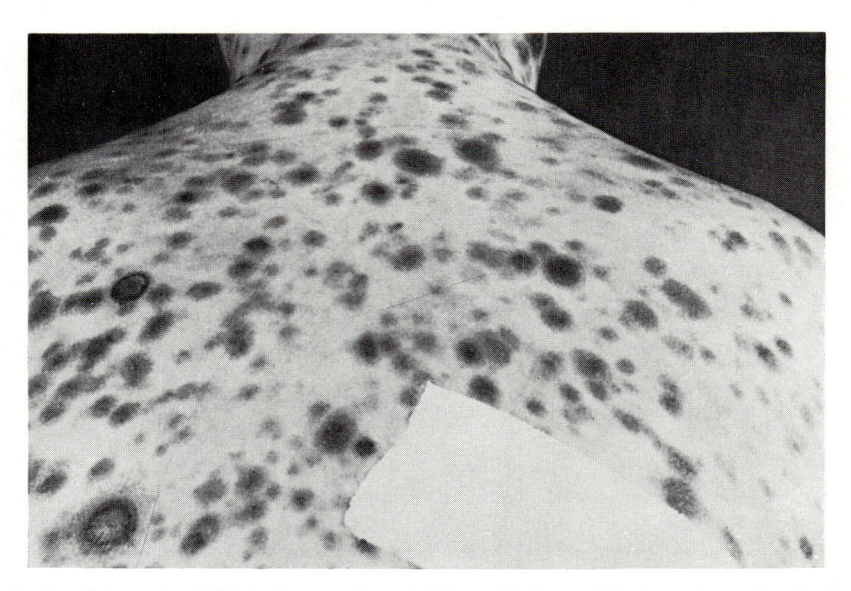

**Fig. 75.** Skin lesions in child with acute lymphoblastic leukemia (leukemia cutis). The lesions, originally discrete, were later confluent and covered the face, trunk, and eventually the entire body. The individual lesions were slightly nodular, erythematous, and purpuric. Many were eventually necrotic.

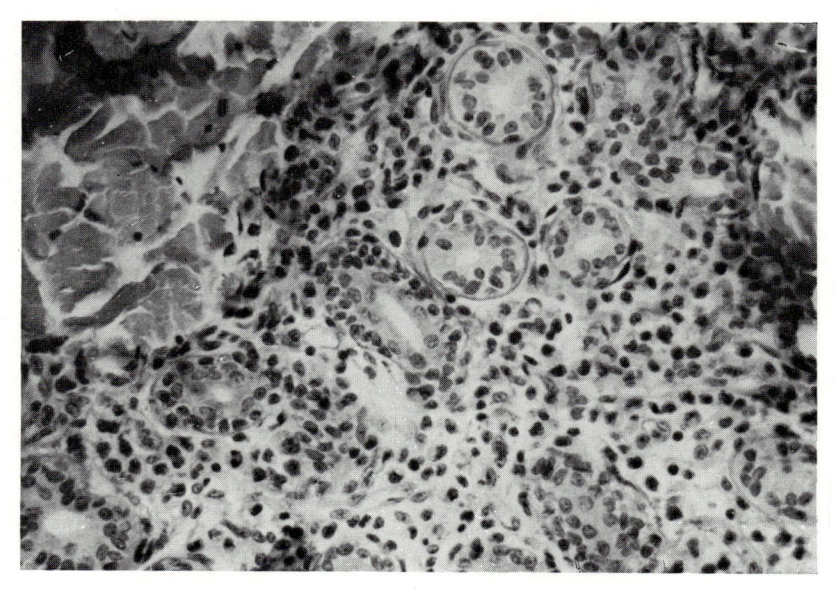

**Fig. 76.** Biopsy of skin lesion from patient shown in Fig. 75. Note leukemic cells densely infiltrating corium about sweat glands. ($\times 435$.)

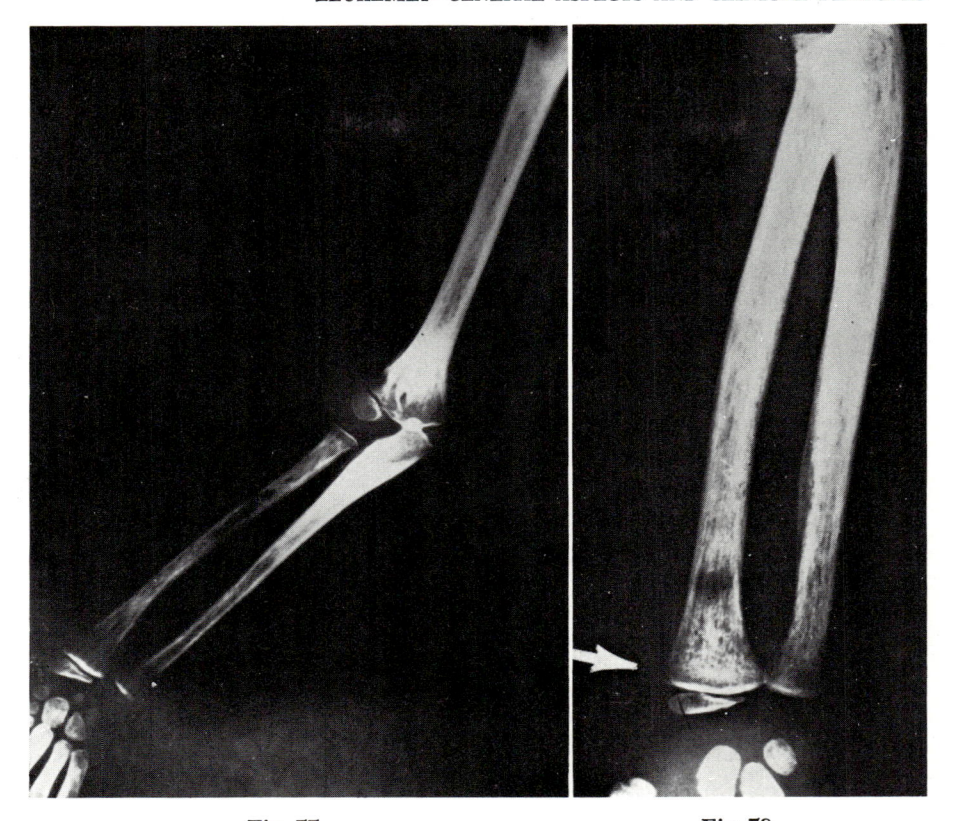

Fig. 77                                                            Fig. 78

Fig. 77. Skeletal lesions of leukemia. Note generalized and local rarefaction and focal areas of bone absorption associated with replacement of bone marrow by leukemic tissue.

Fig. 78. Arrow points to a narrow, deep, transverse zone of rarefaction just proximal to the metaphysis of the long bones, usually most marked in the lower end of the radius. Note also multiple areas of rarefaction in medullary portion of bones.

corpora cavernosa and dorsal veins of the penis by leukemic infiltration[109] or coagulation of the platelet-rich leukemic blood within the corpora cavernosa of the penis. It has been postulated that the association of priapism with chronic granulocytic leukemia rather than acute lymphocytic leukemia in children may be related to the more frequent occurrence of a normal or elevated platelet count and leukocytosis in patients with chronic granulocytic leukemia.

Among the remedies offered in addition to antileukemic therapy is radiation over the spleen which reduces the white blood count and radiation over the penile area.

*Skeletal changes.* The encroachment upon actively functioning marrow by leukoblastic cells within the bony skeleton at a period when nonfunctioning yellow marrow is not yet available accounts for the changes observed by roentgenography in patients with this disease. Skeletal lesions and symptoms are less common in adults, since they possess large amounts of fatty marrow which can be replaced by leukemic cells before osseous changes occur.[3,141,251]

Bone changes consist of transverse bands of diminished density, osteolysis, and periosteal elevation with new bone formation. Most commonly, multiple areas of destruction and production are seen at variable skeletal sites (Fig. 77). The evidence of skeletal lesions varies in different series, being given as 50% in one group[244] and 73% in another.[72]

Bone pain develops with increased intraosseous tension secondary to the proliferation of the leukemic cells. Less frequently, bone pain is caused by infiltration of the synovial membranes of several joints by leukemic cells.[19] These eventually destroy the spongiosa, producing local or diffuse rarefaction. Leukemic cells penetrate the cortex of bone and, extending beyond it, lift up the periosteum which becomes the site of new bone formation. The lifting of the periosteum also results from subperiosteal hemorrhages secondary to thrombocytopenia.

An important diagnostic feature is the marrow translucent zone just proximal to the metaphysis of the shaft of the long bone[18] which is most marked in areas of most rapid growth: the distal femur, tibia, radius, and ulna, in decreasing order of frequency. These zones of diminished density are demonstrated in the radius (Fig. 78). Osteosclerosis occurs least frequently, may be either focal or diffuse, and is secondary to excessive formation of spongiosa.

The changes observed by roentgenographic examination may be summarized as follows: (1) osteoporosis, (2) transverse lines of increased density (growth areas), (3) radiotranslucent bands[18] (metaphyseal and epiphyseal), (4) osteolytic lesions (cortical and medullary), (5) cortical thinning and destruction, (6) leukemic infiltrations and hemorrhage, (7) periosteal lifting and new bone formation, and (8) pathological fractures (Fig. 79).

*Course.* The course of acute leukemia is beset by many complications despite the fact that with chemotherapeutic agents and supportive therapy the patient is free of symptoms for prolonged periods and temporary remissions are induced. The major problems arise from a tendency toward hemorrhage, local or systemic infection, and leukemic infiltration of tissues and organs resulting in disturbances from their increased size and interference with function.

In a 10-year study of 414 patients, the major causes of death in acute leukemia were infection in 70% of patients and hemorrhage in 52%.[127] In 38% there was more than one

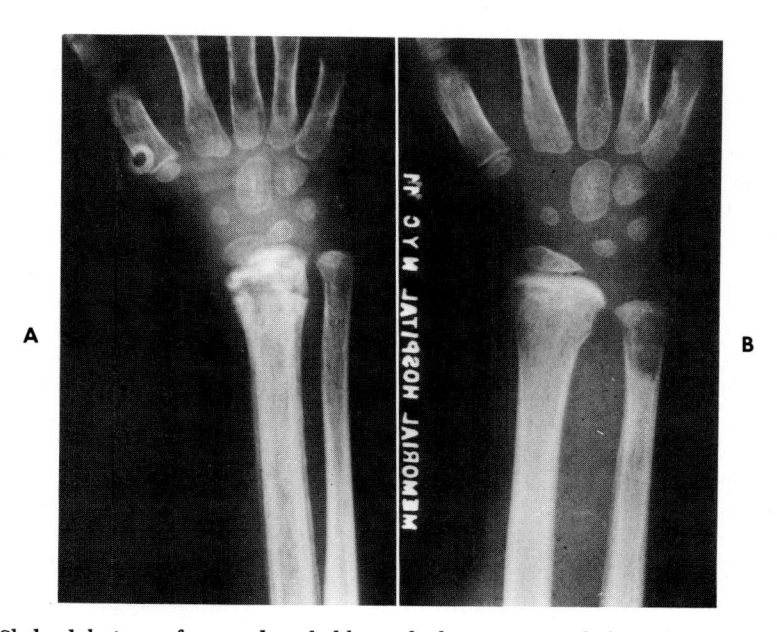

Fig. 79. Skeletal lesions of acute lymphoblastic leukemia. **A,** Pathological fracture of distal radius with marked destruction by diffuse osteolytic involvement of entire radius and periosteal reaction along shaft of radius. **B,** Four months after treatment with 6-mercaptopurine, steroids, and radiation therapy, residual demineralization with slight deformity at area of fracture is present, but otherwise complete restoration. (Courtesy Dr. M. Lois Murphy, New York, N. Y.)

cause of death. A striking finding was the decline in fatal hemorrhage subsequent to the institution of platelet transfusion therapy. While fatal staphylococcal infection declined from 23.5 to 3.1%, fatal infection due to fungi increased from 8.2 to 23.2%.

*Hemorrhage.* The hemorrhagic manifestations of leukemia can usually be accounted for by a reduction in the number of platelets, although bleeding need not necessarily occur with it. Why one patient bleeds and another with comparable thrombocytopenia does not is puzzling. The depletion of platelets has been attributed to the depression of megakaryocytes by replacement of bone marrow by primitive cells. Hypoprothrombinemia and factor V deficiency due to liver damage have been demonstrated in some patients, but there is no consistent relationship with any of these factors.[209] Circulating fibrinolysin resulting in a fibrinogenopenia with massive hemorrhage has also been reported.[62]

The control of bleeding by the adrenal steroid hormones without resulting increase in the number of platelets suggests, however, that vascular dysfunction may result from causes other than thrombocytopenia.

Normal as well as unusually low or high levels of fibrinogen were observed in a group of patients with untreated leukemia.[88] Factor VIII was consistently increased in the active state of the disease and remained elevated in patients in long-term remission. Plasminogen was low in six of twenty-six untreated patients, five of whom died soon after admission. Low factor V levels were observed in two patients with abnormally low fibrinogen concentrations, but occurred also in patients with normal fibrinogen levels. The results in this study showed widely varying changes in parameters of coagulation and fibrinolysis in blood from patients with untreated acute leukemia resulting in normal values with unusually large standard deviations.

Besides skin involvement with petechiae and ecchymoses, serious bleeding can occur in more strategic areas. Intracranial hemorrhage is a frequent terminal complication, especially when the number of circulating abnormal cells is high. For this reason the additional hazard of the hypertensive side effects of steroids must be watched for during treatment. Epistaxis, hematuria, gastrointestinal hemorrhage, and oozing from the gums, ulcerations of the buccal mucous membranes, and interruptions in the mucocutaneous junctions occur frequently, especially in the later stages of the disease. Episodes of severe bleeding occur repeatedly with extreme degrees of thrombocytopenia in both phases of agranulocytosis and leukemic leukocytosis when the bone marrow is heavily infiltrated. Chemotherapeutic agents such as amethopterin (Methotrexate) administered for prolonged periods or in excessive amounts may produce toxic effects such as ulcerations and bleeding in the buccal mucosa and lips and in the gastrointestinal canal. Necrotic lesions are often present in sites of ulcerated and hemorrhagic areas, especially about the mouth.

*Anemia.* Diagnostically, the red cells are both normochromic and normocytic, and anisocytosis, poikilocytosis, and achromia are minimal. Occasionally, large numbers of elliptical and oval cells are present. The crowding out of the normal bone marrow elements and their precursors by leukemic tissue has been offered as a cause of thrombocytopenia, anemia, and agranulocytosis. The mechanism of the anemia cannot be uniformly correlated, however, with the extent of bleeding or erythropoietic failure. Also, the appearance of the bone marrow with regard to the extent of leukemic invasion is often unrelated to the degree of anemia.

The pathogenesis of the anemia is now viewed more as a dynamic process than a crowding out of erythroid elements.[264] It has been demonstrated by cell-tagging techniques[24,45,228] that the anemia of chronic leukemia is due in part to a decreased survival of erythrocytes, perhaps caused by an intrinsic corpuscular defect. A similar increased hemolysis is also an important factor in advanced nonlymphomatous neoplastic disease.[134] When red cell production and red cell destruction were measured simultaneously in patients with leukemia,[273] no single mechanism could be established for the causation of the anemia in every case. There was extreme variability between the degree of red cell survival (normal or short) and adequate or inadequate compensatory red cell production. Autoantibodies appeared to be the cause of hemolysis in some instances but antibody could be found in low titer without any effect on the red cell.[205] Multiple factors, therefore, contribute to the anemia.

Pallor, fatigability, dyspnea on exertion, and listlessness are attributable to the anemia. The increased basal metabolic rate in patients with acute leukemia is responsible for these symptoms as well as for anorexia, weight loss, and irregular fever.

*Relationship of hyperleukocytosis to severity of the disease.* The patients who present themselves with a marked leukocytosis at the onset are much more severely affected, and the disease may run a more fulminant course than in those with leukopenia. When the disease has become stabilized, whether spontaneously or by therapy, and the cells are reduced in numbers, the clinical course is not significantly different from that of patients with a moderate leukocytosis or a leukopenia.

Hardisty and Till[123] have shown that, while patients with acute lymphoblastic leukemia usually respond much better to treatment than those with other cytological types, extensive infiltration of organs at the time of diagnosis, and the presence of large numbers of leukemic cells in the peripheral blood appeared to be adverse prognostic signs. They also found that patients over 3 years of age at diagnosis did better than younger ones, and those without significant thrombocytopenia had a longer course than the remainder.

*Infections and fever.* The increased susceptibility of the patient to infection is attributable to the absence of granulocytes in the peripheral blood. It has been shown also that, in persons with acute leukemia, phagocytosis of *Brucella* organisms by mature neutrophils was not impaired[241] and that the absolute mature neutrophil count when infection develops varies from patient to patient. It is remarkable, however, that children can go for long periods with an agranulocytic blood picture free from infection without the continuous use of antibiotics. Other factors therefore must account for the development of bacterial infections in patients with acute leukemia. The bouts of fever, often with hyperpyrexia, usually are ascribed to infection, but the source is not always discernible. The predominance of negative blood cultures in our experience is probably the result of the immediate use of antibiotic and antimicrobial therapy with the onset of fever. Indeed, with the advent of chemotherapy, the cause of death is often some complication of the disease or its therapy rather than the malignant process itself. In one series the most common infection was septicemia due to gram-negative bacilli.[183] In other reported series *Bacillus proteus* is also included.[210] The majority of organisms isolated are usually the normal flora of the skin and gastrointestinal tract which have become invasive.[243] Impaired antibody formation has long been considered responsible for the increased incidence of infection in leukemia.[242] However, antimetabolites and deficient caloric intake may be factors in the difference in antibody response between the leukemic and control group.[183] Delayed or diminished granulocytic reaction to inflammation may be contributory.[207]

The suppression or alteration of the enteric flora by the intermittent use of antibiotics, as often happens in leukemia, may result in decreased resistance to parenteral infections. It has been demonstrated that the normal flora have a significant influence upon the ability of the host to mobilize leukocytes into an area of injury.[1] It is conceivable that with an altered flora from prolonged antibiotic therapy the protection afforded by leukocytic exudation is no longer available for utilization in areas of leukemic infiltration.

Bodey and co-workers[34] noted that the risk of developing infection increased with prolonged duration of granulocytopenia. The highest fatality rate occurred among patients with persistent severe granulocytopenia. They calculated that a fall in granulocyte level carries a 12% risk of infection, a 60% risk if granulocytopenia persists for 3 weeks, and 100% risk if the level of granulocytes is less than 100 per cu. mm.

Infection contributes to the hemorrhagic tendency, and its control often coincides with subsistence of the bleeding. Localized infection in soft tissues leads to necrotic lesions requiring persistent and assiduous treatment but frequently remaining unhealed. Although usually confined to the oral cavity, monilial infections are particularly troublesome and may become widespread. In one of our patients moniliasis extended to the blood vessels of kidneys and spleen, producing extensive infarcts. Despite conflicting experimental data there is suggestive evidence that the increased incidence of infection and tendency for this complication from ordinarily minor lesions and from organisms of low virulence seen in patients receiving the steroid hormones may be due to a failure of the tissues involved to localize the infection in a normal fashion.[184]

In a series[243] of ninety-two febrile episodes encountered in patients with acute leukemia, fifty-nine appeared to be related to infection. In the remaining thirty-three episodes, bacterial, viral, or fungal infections could not be incriminated as a cause for fever. In this group the most common clinical illnesses associated with the proved infections were pharyngitis, pyelonephritis, and septicemia. The most frequently encountered organisms were *Escherichia coli, Micrococcus pyogens* var. *aureus*, coagulase positive, and *Pseudomonas aeruginosa*. The cause for persistent fever in the patients who had no demonstrable infection remained obscure. Fever in this group of patients occurred only when the leukemia was in relapse. In another series[218] it was pointed out that the drop in the neutrophil count that preceded infection was always accompanied by a relapse in the leukemic process. Individuals who were neutropenic due to drug therapy apparently were not as susceptible to infections as those patients neutropenic with relapse of leukemia. This differentiation cannot always be made since it is unlikely that the seriously involved child would be free from chemotherapy. While marked leukopenia and unexplained and prolonged intermittent fever are often ominous, remissions have followed such an episode. Penicillin, streptomycin, and tetracycline were the common drugs employed.

An outbreak of *Pneumocystis carinii* pneumonia was reported from one hospital in patients treated principally for acute lymphatic leukemia and a lesser number for various neoplastic diseases.[139,206] *Pneumocystis carinii* pneumonitis complicating leukemia has been the subject of many reviews.[190] In sixteen multiple cases reported from the present hospital, pulmonary aspiration was employed for diagnosis and demonstration of the organism by methenamine silver nitrate stain. It was postulated that the emergence of clinical *Pneumocystis* pneumonia in this institution was due to more intensive chemotherapy of patients with malignant disease which in turn may have activated an apparent *P. carinii* infection. Also the intensive use of cancer chemotherapy and radiation in controlling neoplastic disease invariably results in degrees of immunosuppression.

*P. carinii* is considered a protozoan whose complete life cycle is within the alveolus.[15] The suggested treatment after aspiration and diagnosis is a regimen of pentamidine isethionate. The dosage is 4 to 5 mg./kg. of body weight daily for 10 to 14 days, given either intravenously or intramuscularly.[139] The drug regimen may be tapered as clinical improvement or toxicity appears.

Cytomegalovirus pneumonia has also been observed secondary to immunosuppression.[276] Suspicious x-ray findings of the lung were observed although laboratory confirmation was not always obtainable by culture of the virus, complement-fixation antibody titer changes, or observation of the inclusion bodies in the urine. Remarkable clinical improvement was associated with the administration of 5-FUdR (5-fluorodeoxyuridine—a pyrimidine antagonist).

Severe and overwhelming varicella[92] and measles[86] have been reported in leukemia. In varicella, the principal pathologic changes in fatal cases are focal hepatic necrosis and pulmonary hemorrhage, with a lack of inflammatory cells in the visceral lesions.[213] In measles complicating leukemia, giant cell pneumonia with intranuclear inclusions in the alveolar cells is observed.[86,247] In certain individuals with acute leukemia whose natural mechanisms of resistance are depressed,[35] the use of attenuated measles virus employed as a vaccine may prove pathogenic, inducing fatal giant cell pneumonia.[186] A reduction in the amount of steroid to physiologic doses is usually recommended in the event of exposure to measles and its discontinuation suggested in varicella. These decisions are made on an individual basis, depending on the state of leukemia.

In addition to fungal infections, such as moniliasis (*Candida albicans*), a number of unusual organisms have been reported in acute leukemia. Cytomegalic inclusion disease has been found in leukemia and lymphosarcoma, especially in the terminal state.[107] It may be disseminated in the lung, adrenals, and thyroid, probably as a result of decreased host resistance. The virus has been isolated from the urine of children with leukemia and other malignant disease.[120] Death in acute leukemia has also been reported in a child with sepsis due to *Listeria monocytogenes*.[78] Complicating fungous infections such as mucormycosis and aspergillosis, a significant cause of death, are often associated with severe neutropenia.[14]

*Gastrointestinal disturbances.* The vomiting of blood may be caused by persistent oozing from the nasopharyngeal area or from ulcerations in the esophagus and stomach. Severe abdominal pain constitutes one of the most distressing symptoms, and the source may not be obvious, even on postmortem examination. The small punctate hemorrhages in the gastric mucosa, submucosal hemorrhage, enlarged Peyer's patches, infiltration of the mesentery of the small bowel, and marked enlargement of the abdominal lymph nodes could account for the abdominal pain. Ulceration of the leukemic infiltrates in the gastrointestinal tract with multiple perforation has been observed.[90] An intramural hematoma of the small bowel or a polypoid mass in the ileum may provide a basis for intussusception.[91] Acute appendicitis occurring in childhood leukemia does not often have the diagnostic confirmation of a white blood cell count, since serious involvement may be associated with extreme leukopenia with few polynuclear cells.

Acute appendicitis was found in six of twenty-two consecutive necropsies in children with acute leukemia.[140] The pathologic changes in the appendix consisted of extensive infarction and necrosis with minimal exudate. All patients with appendicitis had sepsis due to *Pseudomonas aeruginosa*.

For children under treatment with steroid hormones, gastrointestinal ulceration and perforation are rarely found by the roentgenography or examination of the tissues, but these should not be overlooked. Necrotic ulcerative lesions of the lower rectum are associated with severe and persistent agranulocytosis as well as with monilial infection.

In a series of 148 cases of leukemia, the frequency of gross leukemic lesions in the gastrointestinal tract was 25%.[217] The study emphasized the relatively high incidence of leukemic infiltrates of the gastrointestinal tract with the lesions increasing in frequency from the duodenum to the terminal ileum. The leukemic infiltration of the intestines frequently assumes a polypoid appearance and may affect one segment in the intestinal tract. Nodular lesions of the stomach mucosa and submucosa were also present. There was an increased frequency of monilial lesions with ulcerations and erosions in patients undergoing therapy. Necrotic and hemorrhagic lesions were attributable to antimetabolites, corticosteroids, and leukemic necrosis. A relatively high incidence of surgical complications of the gastrointestinal tract, perforation of the small or large intestine, and agranulocytic abscesses of the bowel and liver were noted. Perforations in different parts of the stomach occurred within a period of ten days in one of our patients who had been on corticosteroid therapy.

Abdominal pain and vomiting may be accompanied by hypercalcemia, probably a manifestation of rapid bone destruction. In a child with acute myelocytic leukemia, the syndrome, presumably due to hypercalcemia, abated when corticosteroids affected a return of the serum calcium to normal.[154]

*Specific organ changes.* The enlargement of superficial lymph nodes may be marked or they may be of normal size.

The liver and spleen are very moderately enlarged and only occasionally reach enormous proportions, usually toward the end of the disease. The size of the spleen fluctuates spontaneously or with treatment; the liver remains more resistant to change. In patients with chronic myeloid leukemia the spleen shows progressive enlargement.

Rarely, the lacrimal and salivary glands in children may be involved in a symmetrical painless enlargement designated as the Mikulicz syndrome.[129]

Infiltration of the heart has been estimated in one-third of patients with leukemia. In most cases the lesions are myocardial and consist only of small interstitial focuses. In our own experience a 13-year-old child, with stem cell leukemia in whom substernal pain was prolonged, died suddenly due to hemopericardium with cardiac tamponade. Rupture of a coronary vessel had occurred following necrosis of its wall, secondary to leukemic infiltration. Clinical, radiologic, and electrocardiographic abnormalities of the heart due to leukemic infiltration have been reported in one series in thirty-four of 143 subjects.[40] In a study of 420 autopsy cases, Roberts and associates[225] found only twenty patients with cardiac symptoms. Of these, nine had chest pain typical of pericarditis. In 69% (288 cases) of the hearts examined at autopsy, hemorrhages or leukemic cell infiltrates or both were found. Diseases of the pericardium (in addition to petechial or leukemic infiltration) occurred in fifty-six patients (13%). A majority of these patients (thirty-nine) had fluid in the pericardial space. Battle and co-workers[17] reported a patient 6 years of age in whom pericarditis was present as the rare initial manifestation of acute leukemia. Symptoms of myocarditis, pericarditis, or heartblock may occur due to leukemic infiltration of the myocardium, pericardium, or the conductive mechanism. This diagnosis should be considered with a picture of heart failure unresponsive to conventional treatment. In one child with acute leukemia intractable cardiac failure was controlled after anterior mediastinal irradiation.[118] Usually, however, heart failure in leukemia is not the result of specific lesions, but of myocardial degeneration resulting from long-continued anemia.[11,148]

Pleural effusion or pneumonia or both may be prominent during the disease. In one patient with eosinophilic leukemia confirmed by postmortem examination, persistent cough and fever were associated with extensive infiltration of both sides of the chest. While pneumonia is common in leukemia, nodular lesions of the lung parenchyma are unusual roentgenographic manifestations. Pathologically, there is noted a variable degree of leukemic invasion of the walls of the alveolar septa, cellular aggregates constituting dense infiltrations compressing the capillaries, and at times the alveoli, focal collections of leukemic cells around or adjoining small bronchioles and blood vessels, and subpleural cellular infiltrations. Usually no specific changes of leukemia are seen on the x-ray film because the leukemic pulmonary infiltrations are mainly of microscopic size.[195] Occasionally, migratory pulmonary infiltrations and miliary lesions resembling Boeck's sarcoid appear. In one series of thirty-three cases with leukemic infiltrations observed at autopsy, only seven had roentgenographically demonstrable disease. This usually consisted of diffuse peribronchial infiltration which was not localized to a specific segment or lobe. Hilar and mediastinal lymphadenopathy and pleural fluid were the most frequent findings.[149] In summary, the lungs are not infrequently involved in leukemia, but clinical symptoms resulting from such involvement are unusual.

The lungs[195] and kidneys[201] are most frequently involved, but the degree of infiltration of these and other organs is not necessarily correlated with the extent of their dysfunction. The kidneys frequently are markedly enlarged by the extensive parenchymal infiltration which is difficult to eradicate. Hemorrhage into the renal parenchyma is usually accompanied by generalized hemorrhagic manifestations.[199] Gross hematuria is common, but in some patients it is confined to the terminal phase, whereas in others it appears at the onset. Uremia is usually associated with very large kidneys. The increase in blood and urinary excretion of uric acid in patients with leukemia[230] results from the disintegration of large numbers of primitive cells with excessive catabolism of nuclear protein. It has been suggested that this factor coupled with the effects of infiltration may seriously interfere with kidney function. It has been stressed that the use of potent chemotherapeutic agents is capable of producing rapid and extensive destruction of blast cells with injurious effects on the kidney. The impairment of kidney function, however, is not a universal occurrence. Some have claimed that renal function in leukemia is not impaired from leukemic infiltration but by dehydration and intrarenal precipitation of uric acid.[103] In patients dying with renal failure sludged urate is demonstrable in the collecting tubules. Urate stones may form, and associated uremia with or without oliguria contributes to mechanical blockade.[36]

In a study conducted in a group of thirty-five children with leukemia, it was concluded that there was no evident impairment of renal function during the course of leukemia despite the presence of gross and microscopic infiltration of the kidney parenchyma at postmortem examination.[103] On the other hand, it has been stressed that impairment of renal function with delayed excretion markedly increases the blood level of antileukemic drugs such as amethopterin, producing severe toxicity.[48] These discordant opinions emphasize the need for individualizing cases of acute leukemia in children, especially with respect to the susceptibility to drug administration.

The impairment of renal function due to uric acid deposits was observed in a 5-year-old child with acute lymphoblastic leukemia and a white blood cell count of 41,000 per cubic millimeter. The urea nitrogen rose to 81 mg. per 100 ml. and uric acid increased to 8.1 mg. per 100 ml. The calcium dropped to 4.4 mg./100 ml. and phosphorus rose to 12.2 mg./100 ml. Signs of tetany were controlled by calcium gluconate given intravenously and normal blood values for electrolytes were restored with hydration.

A syndrome consisting of anorexia, nausea, persistent vomiting, extreme weakness and lethargy has been described in children with acute leukemia.[248] Two of these children developed coma and convulsions. All of the patients had an extreme elevation of the serum uric acid concentration which ranged from 20 to 55 mg./100 ml. The xanthine oxidase inhibitor allopurinol has been shown to be of value in the management of hyperuricemia associated with acute leukemia. The hyperuricemia of leukemia is more amenable to prevention than to treatment. The prompt determination of the serum uric acid when nausea, vomiting, and lethargy appear, and the institution of measures to control hyperuricemia such as the reduction in dosage of chemotherapeutic agents, should prevent the development of this complication.

The testes are infrequently involved in patients with acute leukemia. When affected, they show progressive enlargement with nodular formation due to localized infiltration with leukemic cells.

The central nervous system is frequently involved in its many component structures by hemorrhage, thrombosis, and infiltration by leukemic cells.[191] Central nervous system complications include intracerebral and subarachnoid hemorrhage, meningeal leukemia, and infiltrative lesions of the cranial nerves, spinal cord, and nerve roots. While the cellular infiltrations that extend into the vascular wall are a contributing factor, hemorrhage is due primarily to a deficiency of circulating platelets. Intracranial hemorrhage, which is the most common nervous system complication, is predominantly a late complication of the disease, occurring usually after the leukemia is no longer responsive to chemotherapy.[212]

Hypothalamic and/or pituitary infiltration found at autopsy probably account for hyperphagia and marked obesity demonstrated in some patients, even in periods when steroids are not given. Neurologic signs and symptoms were present in 20 to 25% of the patients in one series. Hemorrhage into the brain sufficiently extensive to be the immediate cause of death occurred in approximately 29%.[272] Subarachnoid hemorrhage is also to be included in nervous system complications.

A 3½-year-old boy with erythromyelocytic leukemia has been reported[229] in whom diabetes insipidus occurred as a complication. Leukemic infiltration of the pituitary stalk was believed to be the etiologic mechanism causing his diabetes insipidus. The extensive perivascular infiltrate of leukemic cells within the pituitary stalk was not present in the hypothalamus and posterior pituitary gland. The authors believe that the pituitary stalk infiltration caused disruption of the normal antidiuretic hormone (ADH) pathway and resulted in the clinical manifestation of diabetes insipidus.

Exophthalmos due to retrobulbar hemorrhage or infiltration of the bones about the orbit is to be differentiated from chloroma, which it closely resembles. Retinal hemorrhages are common and occasionally extensive and may be associated with impaired vision or actual blindness. Pathologic findings consist largely of leukemic infiltrations and hemorrhages in different combinations and of varying intensity.[4] The vascular structures of the eye—the choroid and retinal tissues—are most frequently affected. Hemorrhage occurs most commonly in the retina and may infiltrate into the vitreous body, forming large cloudlike masses of blood. Blood may also rupture into the subretinal space to produce massive retinal detachment. In an 11-month-old infant with monocytic leukemia, blood entered the anterior chamber of one eye with hemorrhage into the cornea (Fig. 80). The iris of the other eye showed patchy new growth, presumably due to leukemic infiltration. Radia-

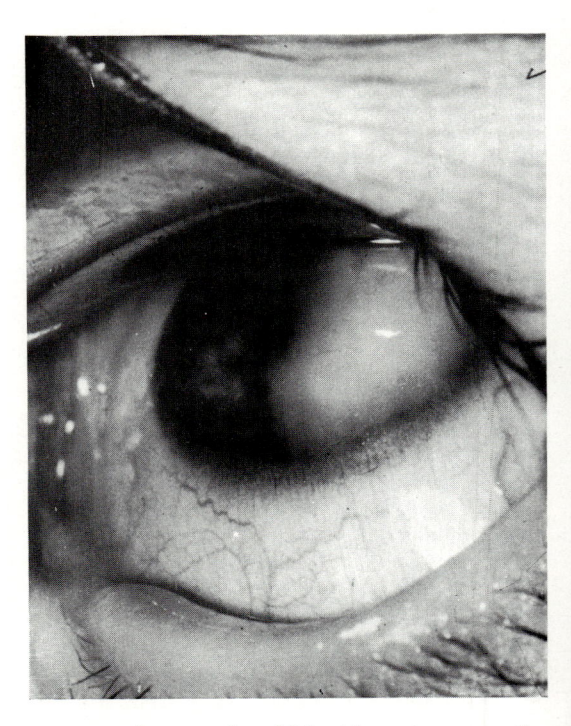

Fig. 80. The eye of a child with acute monocytic leukemia. Note the fluffy white leukemic aggregates, conglomerate and more discrete, occupying part of the anterior chamber.

tion therapy of both eyes resulted in clearing of the affected areas. Although hemorrhages are ordinarily a valuable sign of intracranial bleeding, they may be found in leukemic patients without other signs of nervous system involvement.[272]

The cranial nerves, especially the sixth, seventh, and eighth (Fig. 81), may be infiltrated, and involvement is diagnosed by specific neurologic signs and symptoms.[234]

Increased intracranial pressure is a serious prognostic sign and is due to leukemic infiltration primarily of the meninges and, to a lesser extent, of the cerebral parenchyma. Its pathogenesis has been attributed to infiltration of leukemic cells into the arachnoid, which then interferes with the flow of cerebrospinal fluid in the subarachnoid space and at the base of the brain. The increased fluid pressure produces a symmetric dilation of all four ventricles and hydrocephalus.[191] It may be asymptomatic but is frequently accompanied by severe headache, vomiting, meningismus, papilledema, drowsiness, and coma. The cerebrospinal fluid is clear under increased pressure, the protein and cell count are elevated, and microscopic examination reveals blast forms and a low or normal concentration of sugar. Roentgenograms of the skulls of the younger children show separation of the sutures. It has been suggested[261] that there has been a greater incidence of this complication in patients treated with steroids and chemotherapy than in previously untreated patients. According to this premise, the brain is attacked later than are the other organs so that prolonged survival permits the eventual involvement of the central nervous system. Such agents as 6-mercaptopurine[119] and amethopterin cross the blood-brain barrier in greatly reduced amounts, even though the disease is under control elsewhere. The latter feature should be emphasized, i.e., that intracranial complications frequently occur while the peripheral blood and bone marrow are in a complete hematologic remission.

Leukemic meningitis occasionally simulates the bacterial form with cloudy fluid and decreased sugar content, but examination of the cells reveals its leukemic etiology.[102]

Meningeal leukemia is not an uncommon complication, judging from the incidence noted in various series: twenty-six of 232 cases of childhood leukemia (11%),[212] 150 episodes in fifty-three children of a total of 480 patients,[88] twenty-five of 150 patients (16.7%),[239] and 109 episodes in fifty-nine children with leukemia.[133] Central nervous system involvement has been noted at the onset of leukemia or at any time during its course, when the disease was apparently under good therapeutic control as well as during relapse. Of interest was the observation that this complication occurred less frequently when the disease was under treatment with steroids. While the mean duration of response to 6-mercaptopurine was only 4.1 months, Hyman and co-workers[133] found the median interval from the onset of leukemia to central nervous system involvement was approximately 7 months. These pa-

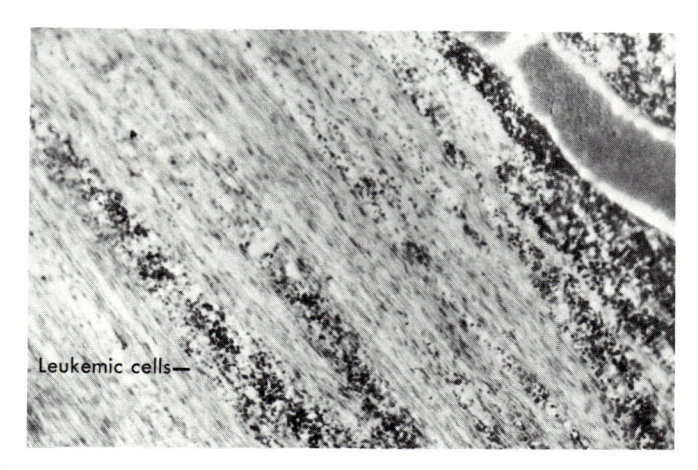

Fig. 81. Leukemic cell infiltration in the eighth cranial nerve in a child with acute lymphoblastic leukemia. (×125.) (Courtesy Dr. Ferdinand La Venuta and Dr. James A. Moore, New York, N. Y.)

tients were already refractory to 6-mercaptopurine, their initial drug, when central nervous system involvement developed. While the opening spinal fluid pressure in these patients is usually elevated (median of 335 mm. of H$_2$O versus a normal of less than 200 mm. H$_2$O), the cerebrospinal fluid findings may exceptionally be normal. In such cases the diagnosis of central nervous system involvement is made on the basis of other signs and symptoms of nervous system irritation.

The central nervous system complications of leukemia have been summarized as follows:[198] paraplegia, monoplegia, and transverse myelitis; hyperphagia with marked obesity in some patients with hypothalamic or pituitary infiltration or both; and cranial nerve infiltration. Infiltration of the meninges as a complication in children with acute leukemia occurs in 30 to 50% in some stage of the disease. Leukemia of the central nervous system usually appeared in patients in hematologic remission. The pressure of the cerebrospinal fluid is sometimes increased to as high as 600 mm. of water. The spinal fluid protein is increased and the concentration of sugar is decreased, being less than half that of the blood sugar. Diabetes insipidus has been reported in a 10-year-old girl with an acute lymphocytic leukemic transformation of a preexisting lymphocytic lymphoma.[167] Physiologic evidence pointed to a direct involvement of the posterior pituitary gland by the malignancy.

Nies and associates[197] claim from a review of their cases that the diagnosis of meningeal leukemia could be established by the presence of ten or more mononuclear cells per cubic millimeter of spinal fluid.

Several methods have been offered for the staining of the spinal fluid cells in meningeal leukemia. One is the use of acidified crystal violet on the counting chamber. The other is the use of Wright's stain and phosphate buffer at pH 7.4, and serum or plasma. The spinal fluid is centrifuged, the supernatant fluid is withdrawn with a pipette, and a small drop of serum or plasma is added to the sediment. The cells are resuspended in the serum and thin cover-slip preparations are drawn. The dried cover-slips are stained with equal parts of Wright's stain and buffer for 5 minutes, washed with distilled water, air dried, and mounted. The presence of nucleoli, nuclear clefts, or lobulation of the nucleus is characteristic of abnormal or immature cells.[249]

**Differential diagnosis.** Usually, leukemia in childhood is diagnosed without difficulty after examination of the peripheral blood and bone marrow. In equivocal cases leukemia must be differentiated from disorders in which overlapping occurs in some aspect of the hematologic picture. The most important feature of the diagnosis of childhood leukemia is the critical evaluation of the clinical picture so that leukemia is suspected and the peripheral blood and bone marrow are examined.

A 25-month-old Negro child presenting with anemia and reticulocytosis was found to have changes of acute undifferentiated leukemia in one iliac marrow aspirate and erythroid hyperplasia in a concomitant from the opposite iliac crest.[219] Within 3 days the previously erythroid marrow became leukemic. These findings suggested that acute leukemia is not necessarily a generalized bone marrow disease at its onset. Diagnostic marrow is more likely to be found if aspiration is directly into an area of bone destruction or reaction. Also in questionable cases with roentgenographic signs of bone involvement, direct aspiration from those sites may have immediate diagnostic import.

*Normal leukocytic changes in infancy and childhood.* Normal leukocytic changes in infancy and childhood may simulate leukemia. The lymphocytic increase in the first years of childhood must be kept in mind so that unnecessary significance is not attached to conditions in which these cells predominate. A mistaken diagnosis of leukemia can be made in young children because of a moderate elevation in the number of white blood cells, a preponderance of lymphocytes, the presence of small or moderately sized cervical nodes, and a palpable spleen. In these children, the white count is at the upper limit of normal, as is the lymphocyte count. Furthermore, the finding of enlarged cervical lymph nodes and careful search of many smears fail to reveal blast cells. The cervical nodes are enlarged from repeated tonsillar infections, and a palpable spleen with a smooth edge is not an uncommon finding in normal young children.

*Idiopathic thrombocytopenic purpura.* Idiopathic thrombocytopenic purpura may be suggested by the appearance of petechiae, purpura, and hemorrhagic manifestations. However, bone marrow aspiration reveals a conspicuous increase of megakaryocytes, whereas they are suppressed in patients with leukemia. In patients with thrombocytopenic purpura severe anemia is absent and the marrow reveals normal granulopoiesis and erythropoiesis in contrast to the anemia and infiltration by immature cells in patients with leukemia.

*Reticuloendotheliosis.* In reticuloendotheliosis in infants not associated with characteristic skin lesions, sudden hematemesis and melena may occur with a diminution in the number of platelets. Bizarre reticuloendothelial cells occasionally may be identified in the bone marrow and skin scrapings[192] as compared with the marked invasion of both the peripheral blood and marrow by abnormal cells in patients with leukemia.

*Aplastic anemia.* The most frequent pancytopenic condition to be confused with leukemia is aplastic anemia. In patients with aplastic anemia the bone marrow shows a progressive decrease in the myeloid elements, nucleated red cells, and megakaryocytes. In leukemia, except in the hypoplastic stage induced by chemotherapy or the infrequent spontaneous remission, the bone marrow and peripheral blood are infiltrated by immature cells.

*Neuroblastoma.* The bone marrow in patients with neuroblastoma of the type referred to as sympathicoblastoma is sometimes sufficiently infiltrated by clusters of undifferentiated cells to suggest leukemia.[54] The confusion is increased in the rare case of neuroblastoma associated with splenomegaly and pancytopenia. Differentiation is especially difficult where groups of cells in the bone marrow are surrounded by discrete cells giving the appearance of stem cells. The identification of pseudorosettes with cells arranged about a central mass of fibrils in patients with neuroblastoma separates the two conditions morphologically. Also, the peripheral blood of patients with neuroblastoma is free from abnormal cells. Other clinical features such as the presence of an abnormal mass with displacement of the kidney and focal areas of calcification are indicative of neuroblastoma. The roentgenogram cannot be employed for differentiation, since leukemia of the skeleton closely resembles metastatic sympathicoblastoma.[121]

*Infectious mononucleosis.* Infectious mononucleosis can be differentiated by the absence of significant anemia, thrombocytopenia, and close examination of the blood smear. Lymphadenopathy and splenomegaly may be slight to moderate, similar to early cases of acute leukemia. Sore throat may be present in patients with both conditions but not to the extent found in those with the pharyngeal type of infectious mononucleosis.

The serum of patients with infectious mononucleosis usually has a high titer of agglutinins for sheep cells. The elevated heterophil antibody titer encountered occasionally in patients with leukemia and other neoplastic diseases can be shown to be normal Forssman antibodies by means of an absorption test (complete absorption by guinea pig kidney).[255]

The atypical mononuclear cell in patients with infectious mononucleosis presents morphologic features distinct from those of the leukemic cell. Although the occasional Downey type III cells may resemble the lymphoblast, the appearance of significant numbers of characteristic atypical cells points to a diagnosis of infectious mononucleosis. In doubtful cases bone marrow aspiration will exclude leukemia, but this is rarely necessary.

*Acute infectious lymphocytosis.* Acute infectious lymphocytosis occurs sporadically as well as in epidemic form and is characterized by a hyperleukocytosis due to an increase in normal small lymphocytes. The mildness of the clinical course, the absence of anemia, thrombocytopenia, and the lack of enlargement of spleen and lymph nodes serve to distinguish this condition from acute leukemia. Bone marrow examination fails to reveal the characteristic cell pattern found in patients with leukemia. The blood picture of patients with acute infectious lymphocytosis, however, may closely resemble that of those with chronic lymphocytic leukemia by the extreme elevation of white cells and the preponderance of small mature lymphocytes. The age incidence of the two diseases is very different, since chronic lymphocytic leukemia is a disease of older persons, rarely seen in those under 40 years of age.

*Rheumatic fever and rheumatoid arthritis.* Leukemic patients with low-grade fever, slight anemia, leukopenia, cardiac murmur, and migratory bone and joint pain simulate the clinical and hematologic pictures in patients with rheumatic fever and rheumatoid arthritis.[3,252] The diagnosis of leukemia is further obscured, for a time at least, by the absence of enlarged lymph nodes and spleen and of a clear-cut blood picture. The presence of polyarthritis with the associated signs of local inflammation provides additional evidence of the possibility of rheumatic disease.[251] Suspicion as to the true nature of the disease should be aroused by the failure of the patient to respond to salicylates and by a favorable response to transfusion. Destructive changes of the skeleton observed by roentgenography exclude rheumatic fever and direct attention to leukemia as the underlying disease. Close examination of the blood smear, including preparations of buffy coat, despite the paucity of white cells, usually reveals an occasional cell which can be identified as being leukemic in origin. Bone marrow aspiration subsequently confirms the diagnosis of acute leukemia.

*Leukemoid reactions.* The differentiation between leukemia and a leukemoid reaction may be difficult with respect to congenital leukemia and sepsis in the newborn infant and cases of chronic myelogenous leukemia in later childhood. Confusion exists particularly when the blood and bone marrow show increased numbers of myelocytes and transitional forms including metamyelocytes and segmented and nonsegmented polynuclear cells. The milder anemia, normal platelet count, and absence of splenomegaly in patients with the leukemoid reaction are contrasted with the severe anemia, thrombocytopenia, and enlarged spleen in those with leukemia. Measurement of the leukocyte alkaline phosphatase activity will aid in the differentiation since the level of this enzyme is increased in leukemoid reactions and is decreased in chronic myelogenous leukemia.[107] In fulminating cases of congenital leukemia the differentiation is often made only at postmortem examination when tissue infiltration with white blood cell precursors reveals the leukemic nature of the disease. In the patient with acute leukemia there is also a gap (hiatus leukemicus) between the myeloblast, lymphoblast, or promyelocyte and the polymorphonuclear neutrophil which is not present in the patient with a leukemoid reaction.

*Australia antigen in leukemia sera.* Reference has been made elsewhere to the presence of an isoprecipitin in the sera of patients with hemophilia (Chapter 7) that reacts with a protein, the Australia antigen. The total absence of this antigen from normal United States subjects and its relatively high frequency in acute leukemia (10%) suggests that its presence may be of diagnostic value in early acute leukemia.[33]

### REFERENCES

1. Abrams, G. D., and Bishop, J. E.: Normal flora and leukocyte mobilization, Arch. Path. 79:213, 1965.
2. Ackerman, G. A.: Eosinophilic leukemia; a morphologic and histochemical study, Blood 24:373, 1964.
3. Aisner, M., and Hoxie, T. B.: Bone and joint pain in leukemia, simulating acute rheumatic fever and subacute bacterial endocarditis, New Eng. J. Med. 238:733, 1948.
4. Allen, R. A., and Straatsma, B. R.: Ocular involvement in leukemia and allied disorders, Arch. Ophthal. 66:490, 1961.
5. Almeida, J. D., Hasselback, R. C., and Ham, A. W.: Virus-like particles in blood of two leukemia patients, Science 142:1487, 1963.
6. Almklov, J. R., and Hatoff, A.: Acute lymphatic leukemia and pregnancy, Amer. J. Dis. Child. 72:202, 1946.
7. Al-Rashid, R. A., and Harned, R. K.: Dysphagia due to leukemic involvement of the esophagus, Amer. J. Dis. Child. 121:75, 1971.
8. American Cancer Society: 1965 Cancer facts and figures, New York, 1965, The Society, p. 11.
9. Anderson, R. C.: Familial leukemia, Amer. J. Dis. Child. 81:313, 1951.
10. Anderson, R. C., and Hermann, H. W.: Leukemia in twin children, J.A.M.A. 158:652, 1955.
11. Aronson, S. F., and Leroy, F.: Electrocardiographic findings in leukemia, Blood 2:356, 1947.
12. Ask-Upmark, E.: Leukemia and pregnancy, Acta Med. Scandinav. 170:635, 1961.
13. Baikie, A. G., Court-Brown, W. M., Buckton, K. E., Harnden, D. G., Jacobs, P. A., and Tough, I. M.: A possible specific chromosome abnormality in chronic myeloid leukaemia, Nature, London 188:1165, 1960.
14. Baker, R. D.: Leukopenia and therapy in leukemia as factors predisposing to fatal mycoses, mucormycosis, aspergilloses and cryptococcosis, Amer. J. Clin. Path. 37:358, 1962.
14a. Baltimore, D.: Viral RNA-dependent DNA polymerase, Nature 226:1209, 1970.
15. Barton, E. G., and Campbell, W. G.: *Pneumocystis carinii* in lungs of rats treated with cortisone acetate; ultrastructural observations relating to the life-cycle, Amer. J. Path. 54:209, 1969.
16. Bassen, F. A., and Kohn, J. L.: Multiple spontaneous remissions in a child with acute leukemia; the occurrence of agranulocytosis and aplastic anemia in acute leukemia and their relationship to remissions, Blood 7:37, 1952.
17. Battle, C. U., Bonfiglio, T. A., and Miller, D. R.: Pericarditis as the initial manifestation of acute leukemia; report of a case, J. Pediat. 75:692, 1969.
18. Baty, J. M., and Vogt, E. C.: Bone changes of leukemia in children, Amer. J. Roentgen. 34:310, 1935.
19. Bedwell, G. A., and Dawson, A. M.: Chronic

myeloid leukemia in a child presenting as acute polyarthritis, Arch. Dis. Child. **29:** 78, 1954.
20. Behrman, R. E., Sigler, A. T., and Patchefsky, A. S.: Abnormal hematopoiesis in 2 of 3 siblings with mongolism, J. Pediat. **68:**569, 1966.
21. Ben-Ishay, D., Freund, M., and Groen, J. J.: A case of autoimmune hemolytic anemia with circulating cold agglutinins presenting for many years as "hypersplenism" and terminating in leukemia, Blood **22:**100, 1963.
22. Bentley, H. P., Jr., Reardon, A. E., Knoedler, J. P., and Krivit, W.: Eosinophilic leukemia; report of a case with review and classification, Amer. J. Med. **30:**310, 1961.
23. Benvenisti, D. S., and Ultmann, J. E.: Eosinophilic leukemia; report of two cases and review of literature, Ann. Intern. Med. **71:** 731, 1969.
24. Berlin, N. I., Lawrence, J. H., and Lee, H. C.: The pathogenesis of the anemia in chronic leukemia; measurement of the life span of the red blood cell with glycine-2C14, J. Lab. Clin. Med. **44:**860, 1954.
25. Bernhard, W. G., Gore, I., and Kilby, R. A.: Congenital leukemia, Blood **6:**990, 1951.
26. Bierman, H. R., Aggeler, P. M., Thelander, H., Kelly, K. H., and Cordes, F. L.: Leukemia and pregnancy; problem in transmission in man, J.A.M.A. **161:**220, 1956.
27. Bierman, H. R., Crile, M., Dod, K. S., Kelly, K. H., Petrakis, N. L., White, L. P., and Shimkin, M. B.: Remissions in leukemia in childhood following acute infectious disease, Cancer **6:**591, 1953.
28. Biological effects of atomic radiation; summary reports from study by National Academy of Sciences, National Research Council, 1956.
29. Birge, R. F., Jenks, A. L., Jr., and Davis, S. K.: Spontaneous remission in acute leukemia; report of a case complicated by eclampsia, J.A.M.A. **140:**589, 1949.
30. Block, M., Jacobson, L. O., and Bethard, W. F.: Preleukemic acute human leukemia, J.A.M.A. **152:**245, 1953.
31. Bloom, A. D., and Tjio, J. H.: In vivo effects of diagnostic x-irradiation on human chromosomes, New Eng. J. Med. **270:**1341, 1964.
32. Bloom, G. E., Gerald, P. S., and Diamond, L. K.: Chronic myelogenous leukemia in an infant; serial cytogenetic and fetal hemoglobin studies, Pediatrics **38:**295, 1966.
33. Blumberg, B. S., Alter, H. J., and Visnich, S.: A "new" antigen in leukemia sera, J.A.M.A. **191:**541, 1965.
34. Bodey, G. P., Buckley, M., Sathe, Y. S., and Freireich, E. J.: Quantitative relationships between circulating leukocytes and infection in patients with acute leukemia, Ann. Intern. Med. **64:**328, 1966.
35. Boggs, D. R.: Inflammatory exudate in human leukemias, Blood **15:**466, 1960.
36. Boggs, D. R., Wintrobe, M. M., and Cartwright, G. E.: The acute leukemias; analysis of 332 cases and review of the literature, Medicine **41:**163, 1963.
37. Borges, W. H., Nicklas, J. W., and Hamm, C. W.: Prezygotic determinants in acute leukemia, J. Pediat. **70:**180, 1967.
38. Brakman, P., Snyder, J., Henderson, E. S., and Astrup, T.: Blood coagulation and fibrinolysis in acute leukemia, Brit. J. Haemat. **18:** 135, 1970.
39. Breg, W. R., Miller, O. J., and Schmickel, R. D.: Chromosomal translocations in patients with mongolism and in their normal relatives, New Eng. J. Med. **266:**845, 1962.
40. Bregani, P., and Perrotta, P.: Il cuore nelle leucemie (Aspetti clinici ed elettrocardiografici), Folia cardiol. **19:**193, 1960.
41. Brescia, M. A., Santora, E., and Sarnatora, V. F.: Congenital leukemia, J. Pediat. **55:** 35, 1959.
42. Bridges, J. M., and Nelson, M. G.: Familial leukaemia, Acta haemat. **26:**246, 1961.
43. Brill, A. B., Tomonaga, M., and Heyssel, R. M.: Leukemia in man following exposure to radiation, Ann. Intern. Med. **50:**590 (and supp.), 1962.
44. Broun, G. O.: Chronic erythromonocytic leukemia, Amer. J. Med. **47:**785, 1969.
45. Brown, G. M., Elliott, S. M., and Young, W. A.: Haemolytic factor in anaemias of lymphatic leukaemia, J. Clin. Invest. **30:**130, 1951.
46. Buckton, K. E., Jacobs, P. S., Court-Brown, W. M., and Doll, R.: Study of chromosomal damage persisting after x-ray therapy for ankylosing spondylitis, Lancet **2:**676, 1962.
47. Burchenal, J. H.: Experimental studies on the relation of pregnancy to leukemia, Amer. J. Cancer **39:**309, 1940.
48. Burchenal, J. H., Murphy, M. L., and Tan, C. T. C.: Review article, treatment of acute leukemia, Pediatrics **18:**643, 1956.
49. Carbone, P. P., Whang, J., Frei, E., III, and Tjio, J. H.: Cytogenetic studies in patients with chronic myelogenous leukemia (CML) undergoing intensive treatment, Blood **24:** 833, 1964.
50. Carmel, W. J., Minno, A. M., and Cook, W. L., Jr.: Eosinophilic leukemia with report of a case, Arch. Intern. Med. **87:**280, 1951.
51. Carper, S. M., O'Donnell, W. M., and Monroe, J. H.: Neonatal leukemia; detection of herpes virus in the mother and child, Amer. J. Dis. Child. **115:**61, 1968.

52. Cartwright, G. E.: Diagnostic laboratory hematology, ed. 4, New York, 1968, Grune & Stratton, Inc., p. 169.
53. Castle, W. B., Meyer, O., and Chew, W. B.: Negative results of treatment of chronic myelogenous leukemia as a deficiency disease, Proc. Soc. Exp. Biol. Med. 32:660, 1935.
54. Christenson, W. N., Ultmann, J. E., and Mohos, S. C.: Disseminated neuroblastoma in an adult presenting the picture of thrombocytopenic purpura, Blood 11:273, 1956.
55. Clein, G. P., and Flemans, R. J.: Involvement of the erythroid series in blastic crisis of chronic myeloid leukaemia; further evidence for the presence of Philadelphia chromosome in erythroctyes, Brit. J. Haemat. 12:754, 1966.
56. Cohen, M. M., Hirschhorn, K., and Frosch, W. A.: In vivo and in vitro chromosomal damage induced by LSD-25, New Eng. J. Med. 277:1043, 1967.
57. Cohen, T., and Creger, W. P.: Acute myeloid leukemia following seven years of aplastic anemia induced by chloramphenicol, Amer. J. Med. 43:762, 1967.
58. Cooke, J. V.: The incidence of acute leukemia in children, J.A.M.A. 119:547, 1942.
59. Cooke, J. V.: Acute leukemia in twins, J.A.M.A. 152:1028, 1953.
60. Cooke, J. V.: Chronic myelogenous leukemia in children, J. Pediat. 42:537, 1953.
61. Cooke, J. V.: The occurrence of leukemia, Blood 9:340, 1954.
62. Cooperberg, A. A., and Neiman, G. M. A.: Fibrinogenopenia and fibrinolysis in acute myelogenous leukemia, Ann. Intern. Med. 42:706, 1955.
63. Coopland, A. T., Friesen, W. J., and Galbraith, P. A.: Acute leukemia in pregnancy, Amer. J. Obstet. Gynec. 105:1288, 1969.
64. Court-Brown, W. M., and Abbatt, J. D.: The incidence of leukaemia in ankylosing spondylitis treated with x-rays, Lancet 1:1283, 1955.
65. Court-Brown, W. M., and Doll, R.: Leukaemia in childhood and young adult life; trends in mortality in relation to aetiology, Brit. M. J.: 1:981, 1961.
66. Court-Brown, W. M., Doll, R., and Hill, A. B.: Incidence of leukaemia after exposure to diagnostic radiation in utero, Brit. M. J. 2: 1539, 1960.
67. Craddock, C. G.: The physiology of granulocytic cells in normal and leukemic states, Amer. J. Med. 28:711, 1960.
68. Cramblett, H. G., Friedman, J. L., and Najjar, S.: Leukemia in an infant born of a mother with leukemia, New Eng. J. Med. 259:727, 1958.
69. Cronkite, E. P.: Evidence for radiation and chemicals as leukemogenic agents, Arch. Environ. Health 3:297, 1961.
70. Cronkite, E. P., Moloney, W., and Bond, V. P.: Radiation leukemogenesis, Amer. J. Med. 28:673, 1960.
71. Cross, F. S.: Congenital leukemia; report of two cases, J. Pediat. 24:191, 1944.
72. Dale, J. H., Jr.: Leucemia in childhood; a clinical and roentgenographic study of seventy-two cases, J. Pediat. 34:421, 1949.
73. Dameshek, W.: Some speculations on the myeloproliferative syndromes, Blood 6:372, 1951.
74. Dameshek, W., and Gunz, F .W.: Diagnostic and therapeutic x-ray exposure and leukemia, J.A.M.A. 163:838, 1957.
75. Dameshek, W., and Gunz, F.: Leukemia, ed. 2, New York, 1964, Grune & Stratton, Inc.
76. Dameshek, W., and Schwartz, R. S.: Leukemia and auto-immunization; some possible relationships, Blood 14:1151, 1959.
77. DeGowin, R. L.: Benzene exposure and aplastic anemia followed by leukemia 15 years later, J.A.M.A. 185:112, 1963.
78. Delta, B. G., and Pinkel, D.: Listeriosis complicating acute leukemia; report of a case, J. Pediat. 60:191, 1962.
79. Diamond, L. K., and Luhby, L. A.: The pattern of "spontaneous" remissions in leukemia in childhood; a review of 26 remissions in 300 cases, Amer. J. Med. 10:236, 1951.
80. Didisheim, P., Trombold, J. S., Vandervoot, R., and Mibashan, R. S.: Acute promyelocytic leukemia with fibrinogen and factor V deficiencies, Blood 23:717, 1964.
81. Dosik, H., Hsu, L. Y., Todaro, G. J., Lee, S. L., Hirschhorn, K., Selirio, E. S., and Alki, A. A.: Leukemia in Fanconi's anemia; cytogenetic and tumor virus susceptibility studies, Blood 36:341, 1970.
82. Editorial: Virus and leukemia, Lancet 1: 1259, 1964.
83. Editorial: Viruses and leukemia, Lancet 2: 442, 1968.
84. Egozcue, J., Irwin, S., and Maruffo, C. A.: Chromosomal damage in LSD users, J.A.M.A. 204:214, 1968.
85. Ellerman, V., and Bang, O.: Experimentelle Leukamie bei Huhner, Zentralbl. Bakt. 46: 595, 1908.
86. Enders, J. F., McCarthy, K., Mitus, A., and Cheatham, W. J.: Isolation of measles virus at autopsy in cases of giant cell pneumonia without rash, New Eng. J. Med. 261:875, 1959.
87. Engel, R. R., Hammond, G. D., Eitzman, D. V., Pearson, H., and Krivit, W.: Transient congenital leukemia in 7 infants with mongolism, J. Pediat. 65:303, 1964.
88. Evans, A. E., D'Angio, G. J., and Mitus, A.:

Central nervous system complications of children with acute leukemia; an evaluation of treatment methods, J. Pediat. 64:94, 1964.
89. Evans, T. S., and Nesbit, R. R.: Eosinophilic leukemia; report of case with autopsy confirmation; review of literature, Blood 4:603, 1949.
90. Everett, C. R., Haggard, M. E., and Levin, W. C.: Extensive leukemic infiltration of the gastrointestinal tract during apparent remission in acute leukemia, Blood 22:92, 1963.
91. Feldman, B. H., and Schulaner, F. A.: Intussusception as a cause of death in acute leukemia; report of a case, J. Pediat. 63:463, 1963.
92. Finkel, K. C.: Mortality from varicella in children receiving adrenocorticosteroids and adrenocorticotrophin, Pediatrics 28:436, 1961.
93. Firkin, B., and Moore, C. V.: Clinical manifestations of leukemia; recent contributions, Amer. J. Med. 28:764, 1960.
94. Folley, J. H., Borges, W., and Yamawaki, T.: Incidence of leukemia in survivors of the atomic bomb in Hiroshima and Nagasaki, Japan, Amer. J. Med. 13:311, 1952.
95. Ford, D. D., Paterson, J. C. S., and Trsuting, W. L.: Fetal exposure to diagnostic x-rays and leukemia and other malignant diseases in childhood, J. Nat. Cancer Inst. 22:1093, 1959.
96. Fraumeni, J. F., Jr.: Sex ratio of children born of leukemic mothers, Pediatrics 33:587, 1964.
97. Fraumeni, J. F., Jr., and Miller, R. W.: Leukemia mortality; downturn rates in the United States, Science 155:1126, 1967.
98. Furth, F.: Recent studies on the etiology and nature of leukemia, Blood 6:964, 1957.
98a. Gallo, R. C., Yang, S. S., and Ting, R. C.: RNA dependent DNA polymerase of human acute leukemic cells, Nature 228:927, 1970.
99. Galton, D. A. G.: Chemotherapy of chronic myelocytic leukemia, Seminars Hemat. 6:323, 1969.
100. Ghitis, J.: Acute promyelocytic leukemia, Blood 21:237, 1963.
101. Gibson, R. W., Bross, I. D. J., Gruham, S., Lilienfeld, A. M., Schuman, L. M., Levin, M. L., and Dowd, J. E.: Leukemia in children exposed to multiple risk factors, New Eng. J. Med. 279:906, 1968.
102. Gilbert, E. F., and Rice, E. C.: Neurologic manifestations of leukemia; report of three cases simulating acute bacterial meningitis, Pediatrics 19:801, 1957.
103. Gilbert, E. F., Rice, E. C., and Lechaux, P. A.: Renal function in children with leukemia, Amer. J. Dis. Child. 93:150, 1957.
104. Gilliam, A. G.: Age, sex, and race selection at death from leukemia and lymphomas, Blood 8:693, 1953.
105. Glass, A. G., Hill, H. A., and Miller, R. W.: Significance of leukemia clusters, J. Pediat. 73:101, 1968.
106. Gordon, H. W.: Myeloid metaplasia masquerading as neonatal leukemia, Amer. J. Dis. Child. 118:932, 1969.
107. Gottmann, A. W., and Beatty, E. C., Jr.: Cytomegalic inclusion disease in children with leukemia or lymphosarcoma, Amer. J. Dis. Child. 104:180, 1962.
108. Gould, W. R., Innes, J., and Robson, H. N.: Survey of 647 cases of leukemia, Brit. M. J. 1:585, 1953.
109. Graw, R. G., Jr., Skeel, R. T., and Carbone, P. P.: Priapism in a child with chronic granulocytic leukemia, J. Pediat. 74:788, 1969.
110. Gray, J. D., and Shaw, S.: Eosinophilic leukaemic and familial eosinophilia; two illustrative cases, Lancet 2:1131, 1949.
111. Greenspan, I., Brown, E. R., and Schwartz, S. O.: Immunological specific antigens in leukemic tissues, Blood 21:717, 1963.
112. Gross, L.: Is leukemia caused by a transmissible virus? A working hypothesis, Blood 9:557, 1954.
113. Grossbard, L., Rosen, D., McGolvray, E., de Capoa, A., Miller, O., and Bank, A.: Acute leukemia with Ph¹-like chromosome in an LSD user, J.A.M.A. 205:791, 1968.
114. Gunz, F. W., Borthwick, R. A., and Rolleston, G. L.: Acute leukaemia in an infant following excessive intrauterine irradiation, Lancet 2:190, 1958.
115. Gunz, F., and Dameshek, W.: Chronic lymphocytic leukemia in a family, including twin brothers and a son, J.A.M.A. 164:1323, 1957.
116. Gunz, F. W., and Fitzgerald, P. H.: Chromosomes and leukemia, Blood 23:394, 1964.
117. Gunz, F. W., Fitzgerald, P. H., Crossen, P. E., MacKenzie, I. S., Powles, C. P., and Jensen, G. R.: Multiple cases of leukemia in a sibship, Blood 27:482, 1966.
118. Haddy, T. B.: Cardiac irradiation in childhood leukemia, Amer. J. Dis. Child. 108:559, 1964.
119. Hamilton, L., and Elion, G. B.: The fate of 6-mercaptopurine in man, Ann. N. Y. Acad. Sci. 60:304, 1954.
120. Hanshaw, J. B., and Weller, T. H.: Urinary excretion of cytomegaloviruses by children with generalized neoplastic disease; correlations with clinical and histopathologic observations, J. Pediat. 58:305, 1961.
121. Hansman, C. F., and Girdany, B. R.: The roentgenographic findings associated with neuroblastoma, J. Pediat. 51,621, 1957.

122. Hardisty, R. M., Speed, D. E., and Till, M.: Granulocytic leukaemia in childhood, Brit. J. Haemat. 10:551, 1964.
123. Hardisty, R. M., and Till, M. M.: Acute leukaemia 1959-64; factors affecting prognosis, Arch. Dis. Child. 43:107, 1968.
124. Heath, C. W., Jr., and Hasterlik, R. J.: Leukemia among children in a suburban community, Amer. J. Med. 34:796, 1963.
125. Heath, C. W., Jr., and Moloney, W. C.: Familial leukemia, five cases of acute leukemia in three generations, New Eng. J. Med. 272:882, 1965.
126. Hellstrom, K. E., and Hellstrom, I.: Immunologic defense against cancer, Hosp. Pract. 5:45, 1970.
127. Hersh, E. M., Bodey, G. P., Nies, B. A., and Freireich, E. J.: Causes of death in acute leukemia: a ten-year study of 414 patients from 1954-1963, J.A.M.A. 193:105, 1965.
128. Hillestead, L. K.: Acute promyelocytic leukemia, Acta Med. Scandinav. 159:189, 1957.
129. Hird, A. J.: Mikulicz's syndrome, Brit. M. J. 2:416, 1949.
130. Holland, J. F.: Epidemic acute leukemia, New Eng. J. Med. 283:1165, 1970.
131. Holton, C. P., and Johnson, W. W.: Chronic myelocytic leukemia in infant siblings, J. Pediat. 72:377, 1968.
132. Hungerford, D. A.: Chromosome studies in human leukemia. I. Acute leukemia in children, J. Nat. Cancer Inst. 27:983, 1961.
133. Hyman, C. B., Bogle, J. M., Brubaker, C. A., Williams, K., and Hammond, G. D.: Central nervous system involvement by leukemia in children. I. Relationship to systemic leukemia and description of clinical and laboratory manifestations, Blood 25:1, 1965.
134. Hyman, G. A.: Studies on anemia of disseminated malignant neoplastic disease; the hemolytic factor, Blood 9:911, 1954.
135. Ingalls, T. H.: Etiology of mongolism; epidemiologic and teratologic mechanism, Amer. J. Dis. Child. 94:147, 1947.
136. Iverson, T.: Leukaemia in infancy and childhood; a material of 570 Danish cases, Acta Paediat. Scand. 167(supp.):1, 1966.
137. Jacobs, P. A., Tough, I. M., and Wright, D. H.: Cytogenetic studies in Burkitt's lymphoma, Lancet 2:1144, 1963.
138. Jaffe, N., and Kim, B. S.: Priapism in acute granulocytic leukemia, Amer. J. Dis. Child. 118:619, 1969.
139. Johnson, H. D., and Johnson, W. W.: *Pneumocystis carinii* pneumonia in children with cancer; diagnosis and treatment, J.A.M.A. 214:1067, 1970.
140. Johnson, W., and Borella, L.: Acute appendicitis in childhood leukemia, J. Pediat. 67:595, 1965.
141. Kalayjian, B. S., Herbut, P. A., and Erf, L. A.: The bone changes of leukemia in children, Radiology 47:223, 1946.
142. Kaplan, H. S.: On the etiology and pathogenesis of the leukemias; a review, Cancer Res. 14:535, 1954.
143. Karanas, A., and Silver, R. T.: Characteristics of the terminal phase of chronic granulocytic leukemia, Blood 32:445, 1968.
144. Keith, H. M.: Chronic myelogenous leukemia in infancy; report of a case, Amer. J. Dis. Child. 69:366, 1945.
145. Kelsey, W. M., and Anderson, D. H.: Congenital leukemia, Amer. J. Dis. Child. 58:1268, 1939.
146. Kemp, N. H., Stafford, J. L., and Tanner, R.: Aetiology of leukaemias, Lancet 2:95, 1963.
147. Kirchbaum, A.: Recent studies in experimental mammalian leukemia, Yale J. Biol. Med. 17:163, 1944-1945.
148. Kirshbaum, I. D., and Preuss, F. S.: Leukemia; clinical and pathologic study of 123 fatal cases in a series of 14,400 necropsies, Arch. Intern. Med. 71:777, 1943.
149. Klatte, E. C., Yardley, J., Smith, E. B., Rohn, R., and Campbell, J. A.: The pulmonary manifestations and complications of leukemia, Amer. J. Roentgen. 89:589, 1963.
150. Koler, R. D., Seamon, A. J., Osgood, E. E., and Vanbellinghen, P.: Myeloproliferative diseases, diagnostic value of the leukocyte alkaline phosphatase test, Amer. J. Clin. Path. 30:295, 1958.
151. Kolmeier, K. H., and Bayrd, E. D.: Familial leukemia; report of incidence and review of the literature, Proc. Staff Meet. Mayo Clinic 38:523, 1963.
152. Krivit, W., and Good, R. A.: The simultaneous occurrence of leukemia and mongolism; report of 4 cases, Amer. J. Dis. Child. 91:218, 1956.
153. Krivit, W., and Good, R. A.: Simultaneous occurrence of mongolism and leukemia; report of a nationwide survey, Amer. J. Dis. Child. 94:289, 1957.
154. Kronfield, S. T., and Reynolds, T. B.: Leukemia and hypercalcemia; report of a case and review of the literature, New Eng. J. Med. 271:399, 1964.
155. Kyle, R., Nobrega, F. T., Kurland, L. T., and Elveback, L. R.: The 30-year trend of leukemia in Olmstead County, Minnesota, 1935 through 1964, Mayo Clin. Proc. 43:342, 1968.
156. Kyle, R. A., Pierre, R. V., and Bayrd, E. D.: Multiple myeloma and acute myelomonocytic leukemia, New Eng. J. Med. 283:1121, 1970.
157. Lahey, M. E., Beier, F. R., and Wilson, J. F.: Leukemia in Down's syndrome, J. Pediat. 63:189, 1963.

158. Lee, J. A. H.: Seasonal variation in the incidence of the clinical onset of leukaemia, Path. Microbiol. 27:772, 1964.
159. Lee, S. L.: Leukemia; immunologic approaches to therapy, N. Y. State J. Med. 70:2982, 1970.
160. Lejeune, J., Gautier, M., and Turpin, R.: Étude des chromosomes somatiques de neuf enfants mongoliens, Compt. rend. Acad. sc. 248:1721, 1959.
161. Leonard, B. J., and Wilkinson, J. F.: The acute leukemias. In Wilkinson, J. F., editor: Modern trends in blood diseases, New York, 1955, Paul B. Hoeber, Inc.
162. Lewis, E. B.: Leukemia and ionizing radiation, Science 125:963, 1957.
163. Lloyd, H. O.: Acute leukemia complicated by pregnancy, J.A.M.A. 178:1140, 1961.
164. MacMahon, B., and Clark, D.: Incidence of common forms of human leukemia, Blood 11:871, 1956.
165. MacMahon, B., and Levy, M. A.: Prenatal origin of childhood leukemia; evidence from twins, New Eng. J. Med. 270:1082, 1964.
166. Mallory, T. B., Gall, E. O., and Brickley, W. J.: Chronic exposure to benzene (benzol); pathologic results, Indust. Hyg. Toxicol. 21:355, 1939.
167. Malter, I. J., Gross, S., and Teree, T. M.: Diabetes insipidus complicating acute lymphocytic leukemia, Amer. J. Dis. Child. 117:228, 1969.
168. Manganaro, J. S.: Aplastic anemia preceding acute myeloblastic (histiocytic) leukemia, J.A.M.A. 173:1559, 1960.
169. March, H. C.: Leukemia in radiologists in 20-year-period, Amer. J. Med. Sci. 220:282, 1950.
170. Mathé, G., Amiel, J. L., Schwarzenberg, L., Schneider, M., Cahan, A., Schlumberger, J. R., Hayatt, M., and DeVassal, F.: Acute immunotherapy for acute lymphoblastic leukemia, Lancet 1:697, 1969.
171. Mauer, A. M., and Jarrold, J.: Granulocyte kinetic studies in patients with proliferative disorders of the bone marrow, Blood 22:125, 1963.
172. McAllister, R. M.: On the role of viruses in human cancer, J. Pediat. 69:175, 1966.
173. McPhedran, P., and Heath, C. W., Jr.: Multiple cases of leukemia associated with one house, J.A.M.A. 209:2021, 1969.
174. Meachen, G. C., and Weisberger, A. S.: Early atypical manifestations of leukemia, Arch. Intern. Med. 41:780, 1954.
175. Medical Research Council: Hazards to man of nuclear and allied radiations, London, 1956, Her Majesty's Stationery Office.
176. Merrit, D. H., and Harris, J. S.: Mongolism and acute leukemia, Amer. J. Dis. Child. 92:41, 1956.
177. Miller, D. R.: Raised foetal haemoglobin in childhood leukaemia, Brit. J. Haemat. 17:103, 1969.
177a. Miller, D. R., Newstead, G. J., and Young, L. W.: Perinatal leukemia with a possible variant of the Ellis-van Creveld syndrome, J. Pediat. 74:300, 1969.
178. Miller, F. R., and Turner, D. L.: The action of specific stimulators on the hematopoietic system, Amer. J. Med. Sci. 206:146, 1943.
179. Miller, J., McC., Sherrill, J. G., and Hathaway, W. E.: Thrombocythemia in the myeloproliferative disorder of Down's syndrome, Pediatrics 40:847, 1967.
180. Miller, R. W.: Down's syndrome (mongolism), other congenital malformations and cancers among the sibs of leukemic children, New Eng. J. Med. 268:393, 1963.
181. Miller, R. W.: Persons with exceptionally high risk of leukemia, Cancer Res. 27:2420, 1967.
182. Miller, R. W.: Fifty-two forms of childhood cancers; United States mortality experience, 1960-1966, J. Pediat. 75:685, 1969.
183. Miller, S. P., and Shanbrom, E.: Infectious syndromes of leukemias and lymphomas, Amer. J. Med. Sci. 246:240, 1963.
184. Mills, L. C., Boylston, B. F., Greene, S. A., and Moyer, J. H.: Septic arthritis as a complication of orally given steroid therapy, J.A.M.A. 164:1310, 1957.
185. Mittwoch, U.: The leukocyte count in children with mongolism, J. Ment. Sci. 104:457, 1958.
186. Mitus, A., Holloway, A., Evans, A. E., and Enders, J. F.: Attenuated measles vaccine in children with acute leukemia, Amer. J. Dis. Child. 103:413, 1962.
187. Moloney, W. C.: Leukemia in survivors of atomic bombing, New Eng. J. Med. 253:88, 1955.
188. Moloney, W. C., and Kastenbaum, M. A.: Leukemogenic effects of ionizing radiation on atomic bomb survivors in Hiroshima City, Science 121:308, 1955.
189. Moloney, W. C., and Lange, R. D.: Leukemia in atomic bomb survivors; observations on early phases of leukemia, Blood 9:663, 1954.
190. Moore, D. L., Carnehan, C. E., Mills, S. D., and Burgert, E. O., Jr.: *Pneumocystis carinii* pneumonitis complicating leukemia, Mayo Clin. Proc. 44:162, 1969.
191. Moore, E. W., Thomas, L. B., Shaw, R. K., and Freireich, E. J.: The central nervous system in acute leukemia, Arch. Intern. Med. 105:451, 1960.
192. Moore, T. D.: A simple technique for the

diagnosis of nonlipid histiocytosis, Pediatrics 19:438, 1957.
193. Muggia, F. M., Heinemann, H. O., Farhangi, M., and Osserman, E. F.: Lysozymuria and renal tubular dysfunction in monocytic and myelomonocytic leukemia, Amer. J. Med. 47:351, 1969.
194. Murphy, W. H., Furtado, D., and Plata, E.: Possible association between leukemia in children and virus-like agents, J.A.M.A. 191:110, 1965.
195. Nathan, D. J., and Sanders, M.: Manifestation of acute leukemia in the parenchyma of the lung, New Eng. J. Med. 252:797, 1955.
196. Neerhout, R. C.: Chronic granulocytic leukemia; early blast crisis simulating acute leukemia, Amer. J. Dis. Child. 115:66, 1968.
197. Nies, B. A., Thomas, L. B., and Freireich, E. J.: Meningeal leukemia; a follow-up study, Cancer 18:546, 1965.
198. Nievi, R. L., Burgert, E. O., Jr., and Groover, R. V.: Central nervous system complications of leukemia; a review, Mayo Clin. Proc. 43:70, 1968.
199. Norris, H. J., and Wiener, J.: The renal lesions in leukemia, Amer. J. Med. Sci. 241:512, 1961.
200. Nowell, P. C., and Hungerford, D. A.: A minute chromosome in human chronic granulocytic leukemia, Science 132:1497, 1960.
201. Oehme, J., Janssen, W., and Hagitte, C.: Leukamie im Kindesalter; Beiträge zur Morphologie, klinik Pathophysiologie und Therapie, Leipzig, 1958, Georg Thieme Verlag.
202. O'Sullivan, M. A., and Pryles, C. V.: A comparison of leukocyte alkaline phosphatase determinations in 200 patients with mongolism and in 200 "familial" controls, New Eng. J. Med. 268:1168, 1963.
203. Pearson, H. A., and Diamond, L. K.: Chronic monocytic leukemia in childhood, J. Pediat. 53:259, 1958.
204. Pearson, H. A., Grello, F. W., and Cone, T. E., Jr.: Leukemia in identical twins, New Eng. J. Med. 268:1151, 1963.
205. Pengelly, C. D. R., and Wilkinson, J. F.: The frequency and mechanism of haemolysis in the leukaemias, reticuloses and myeloproliferative diseases, Brit. J. Haemat. 8:343, 1962.
206. Perera, D. R., Western, K. A., Johnson, H. D., Johnson, W. W., Schultz, M. G., and Akers, P. V.: *Pneumocystis carinii* pneumonia in a hospital for children; epidemiologic aspects, J.A.M.A. 214:1074, 1970.
207. Perillie, P. E., and Finch, S. C.: The local exudative cellular response to leukemia, J. Clin. Invest. 39:1353, 1960.
208. Perillie, P. E., Kaplan, S. S., Lefkowitz, E., Rogoway, W., and Finch, S. C.: Studies of muramidase (lysozyme) in leukemia, J.A.M.A. 203:79, 1968.
209. Perry, S.: Coagulation defects in leukemia, J. Lab. Clin. Med. 50:229, 1957.
210. Pierce, M. I.: The acute leukemias of childhood, Ped. Clin. N. Amer. 4:447, 1957.
211. Pierce, M. I.: Leukemia in the newborn infant, J. Pediat. 54:691, 1959.
212. Pierce, M. I.: Neurologic complications in acute leukemia in children, Ped. Clin. N. Amer. 9:425, 1962.
212a. Pierce, M. I., Borges, W. H., Heyn, R. M., Wolff, J. A., and Gilbert, E. S.: Epidemiological factors and survival experience in 1,770 children with acute leukemia, Cancer 23:1296, 1969.
213. Pinkel, D.: Chickenpox and leukemia, J. Pediat. 58:729, 1961.
214. Pinkel, D., and Nefzeger, D.: Some epidemiological features of childhood leukemia in the Buffalo, New York, area, Cancer 12:351, 1959.
215. Poncher, H. G., Weir, H. F., and Limarzi, L. R.: Chronic myelogenous leukemia in early infancy; case report, J. Pediat. 21:73, 1942.
216. Pretlow, T. G.: Chronic monocytic dyscrasia culminating in acute leukemia, Amer. J. Med. 46:130, 1969.
216a. Pridie, G., and Dumitriscu-Pirvu, D.: Laucemie acuta sindrom Bonnevie-Ullrich la un non rascat, Pediatria 10:345, 1961.
217. Prolla, J. C., and Kirsner, J. B.: The gastrointestinal lesions and complications of the leukemias, Ann. Intern. Med. 61:1084, 1964.
218. Raab, S. O., Hoeprich, P. D., Wintrobe, M. M., and Cartwright, G. E.: The clinical significance of fever in acute leukemia, Blood 16:1609, 1960.
219. Raney, R. B., and McMillan, C. W.: Simultaneous disparity of bone marrow specimens in acute leukemia, Amer. J. Dis. Child. 117:548, 1969.
220. Reisman, L. E., Mitani, M., and Zuelzer, W. W.: Chromosome studies in leukemia. I. Evidence for the origin of leukemic stem lines from aneuploid mutants, New Eng. J. Med. 270:591, 1964.
221. Reisman, L. E., and Trujillo, J. M.: Chronic granulocytic leukemia of childhood, J. Pediat. 62:710, 1963.
222. Reisman, L. E., and Zuelzer, W. W.: Serial chromosome studies in acute leukemia (abstract), Blood 22:818, 1963.
223. Reyes, G. R., and Perez, R. T.: Leukemia and pregnancy: observation of a case treated with busulfan (Myleran), Blood 18:764, 1961.
224. Ritz, N. D., and Purfar, M.: Chronic myeloid

leukemia with priapism in eight-year-old child, New York J. Med. **64**:553, 1964.
225. Roberts, W. C., Bodey, G. P., and Wertlake, P. T.: The heart in acute leukemia; a study of 420 autopsy cases, Amer. J. Cardiol. **21**: 388, 1968.
226. Rosenthal, L. L.: Acute promyelocytic leukemia associated with hypofibrinogenemia, Blood **21**:495, 1963.
227. Ross, J. D., Maloney, W. C., and Desforges, J. F.: Ineffective regulation of granulopoiesis masquerading as congenital leukemia in a mongoloid child, J. Pediat. **63**:1, 1963.
228. Ross, J. F., Crockett, C. L., Jr., and Emerson, C. P.: Mechanism of anemia in leukemia and malignant lymphoma, J. Clin. Invest. **30**:668, 1951.
229. Roy, S., III, and Johnson, W. W.: Diabetes insipidus in a child with erythromyelocytic leukemia, Amer. J. Dis. Child. **119**:82, 1970.
230. Sandberg, A. A., Cartwright, G. E., and Wintrobe, M. M.: Studies on leukemia; uric acid excretion, Blood **11**:154, 1956.
231. Sandberg, A. A., Ishihara, T., Miwa, T., and Hauschka, T. S.: The in vivo chromosome constitution of marrow from 34 human leukemias and 60 nonleukemic controls, Cancer Res. **21**:(Part I) 678, 1961.
231a. Schade, H., Schoeller, L., and Schultze, K. W. D.: D-trisomie (Patau) mit kongenitaler myeloischer Leukaemie, Med. Welt. **50**:2690, 1962.
232. Schuman, L. M., Ager, E. A., Wallace, H. M., Rosenfeld, A. B., and Collen, W. H.: An epidemiological study of childhood leukemia, J. Chron. Dis. **18**:113, 1965.
233. Schunk, G. J., and Lehman, W. L.: Mongolism and congenital leukemia, J.A.M.A. **155**: 250, 1954.
234. Schwab, R. S., and Weiss, S.: The neurologic aspect of leukemia, Amer. J. Med. Sci. **189**: 766, 1935.
235. Schwartz, E. E., and Lipton, E. E.: Factors influencing the incidence of leukemia; special consideration of the role of ionizing radiation, Blood **13**:845, 1958.
236. Schwartz, S. O., Greenspan, I., and Brown, E. R.: Leukemic cluster in Niles. III. Immunologic data in families of leukemic patients and others, J.A.M.A. **186**:106, 1963.
237. Schwartz, S. O., and Schoolman, H. M.: The etiology of leukemia; the status of the virus as causative agent; a review, Blood **14**:279, 1959.
238. Sergovich, F. R., Valentine, G. H., Carr, D. H., and Soltan, H. C.: Mongolism (Down's syndrome) with atypical clinical and cytogenic features, J. Pediat. **65**:197, 1964.
239. Shaw, R. K., Moore, E. W., Freireich E. J., and Thomas, L. B.: Meningeal leukemia; a syndrome resulting from increased intracranial pressure in patients with acute leukemia, Neurology **10**:823, 1960.
240. Shimkin, M. B.: Mortality from leukemia and lymphoma in the United States, Sixth International Congress of the International Society of Hematology, Boston, 1956.
241. Silver, R. T., Beal, G. A., Schneiderman, M. A., and McCullough, N. B.: The role of the mature neutrophil in bacterial infections in acute leukemia, Blood **12**:814, 1957.
242. Silver, R. T., Utz, J. P., Fahey, J., and Frei, E., III: Antibody response in patients with acute leukemia, J. Lab. Clin. Med. **56**: 634, 1960.
243. Silver, R. T., Utz, J. P., Frei, E., and McCullough, N. B.: Fever, infection and host remission in acute leukemia, Amer. J. Med. **24**:25, 1958.
244. Silverman, F. N.: The skeletal lesions in leukemia, Amer. J. Roentgen. **59**:819, 1948.
245. Simpson, C. L., and Hempelmann, L. H.: Association of tumors and roentgen-ray treatment of thorax in infancy, Cancer **10**: 42, 1957.
246. Simpson, C. L., Hempelmann, L. H., and Fuller, L. M.: Neoplasia in children treated with x-rays in infancy for thymic enlargement, Radiology **64**:840, 1954.
247. Simpson, C. L., and Pinkel, D.: Pathology in leukemia complicated by fatal measles, Pediatrics **21**:436, 1958.
248. Sinks, L. F., Newton, W. A., Jr., Nagi, N. A., and Stevenson, T. D.: A syndrome associated with extreme hyperuricemia in leukemia, J. Pediat. **68**:578, 1966.
249. Skeel, R. T., Yankee, R. A., and Henderson, E. S.: Two simple methods for rapid detection of malignant cells in spinal fluid, J.A.M.A. **205**:863, 1968.
250. Slocum, G. J. C., and MacMahon, B.: Changes in mortality rates in the first five years of life, New Eng. J. Med. **268**:922, 1963.
251. Smith, C. H.: Leukopenic myeloid leukemia associated with arthritis, Amer. J. Dis. Child. **45**:123, 1933.
252. Smith, C. H.: Leucemia in childhood with onset simulating rheumatic disease, J. Pediat. **7**:390, 1935.
253. Smith, R. L.: Recorded and expected mortality among the Indians of the United States with special reference to cancer, J. Nat. Cancer Inst. **18**:385, 1957.
254. Southam, C. M., Craver, L. F., Dargeon, H. W., and Burchenal, J. H.: Study of natural history of acute leukemia, with special reference to duration of disease and occurrence of remissions, Cancer **9**:39, 1951.

255. Southam, C. M., Goldsmith, Y., and Burchenal, J. H.: Heterophile antibodies and antigens in neoplastic diseases, Cancer 4:1036, 1951.
255a. Siegelman, S., Burny, A., Das, M. R., Keydar, J., Schlom, J., Travnicek, M., and Watson, K.: DNA-directed DNA polymerase activity in oncogenic RNA viruses, Nature 227:1029, 1970.
256. Steinberg, A. G.: The genetics of acute leukemia in children, Cancer 13:985, 1960.
257. Stewart, A., Pennybacker, W., and Barber, R.: Adult leukaemias and diagnostic x-rays, Brit. M. J. 2:882, 1962.
258. Stewart, A., Webb, J., Giles, D., and Hewitt, D.: Malignant disease in childhood and diagnostic irradiation in utero, Lancet 2:447, 1956.
259. Stewart, A., Webb, J., and Hewitt, D.: A survey of childhood malignancies, Brit. M. J. 1:1495, 1958.
259a. Stransky, E.: Perinatal leukemia, Acta Paediat. Acad. Sc. Hungaricae 8:121, 1967.
260. Sturgis, C. C.: Some aspects of the leukemia problem, J.A.M.A. 150:1551, 1952.
261. Sullivan, M. P.: Intracranial complication of leukemia in children, Pediatrics 20:757, 1957.
262. Syverton, J. T., and Ross, J. D.: The virus theory of leukemia, Amer. J. Med. 28:683, 1960.
263. Tartaglia, A. P., Scharfman, W. B., and Propp, S.: Splenic rupture in leukemia, New Eng. J. Med. 267:31, 1962.
263a. Temin, H. M., and Mizutani, S.: RNA-dependent DNA polymerase in virions of Rous sarcoma virus, Nature 226:1211, 1970.
264. Troup, S. B., Swisher, S. N., and Young, L. E.: The anemia of leukemia, Amer. J. Med. 28:751, 1960.
265. Trubowitz, S., Kirkman, D., and Masek, B.: The leukocyte alkaline phosphatase in mongolism, Lancet 2:486, 1962.
266. Valentine, W. N.: The metabolism of the leukemic leukocyte, Amer. J. Med. 28:699, 1960.
267. Valentine, W. N., and Beck, W. S.: Biochemical studies on leucocytes; phosphatase activity in health, leucocytosis and myelocytic leucemia, J. Lab. Clin. Med. 38:39, 1951.
268. Videbaek, A.: Heredity in human leukemia and its relation to cancer, London, 1947, H. K. Lewis & Co., Ltd.
269. Virchow, R.: Weisses Blut und Miltztumoren, Med. Zeitung, Berlin 15:157, 163, 167, 1846 (erste); 16:9, 15, 1847 (zweiter).
270. Wegelius, R., Väänänen, I., and Koskelai, S-L.: Down's syndrome and transient leukaemia-like disease in a newborn, Acta Paediat. Scand. 56:301, 1967.
271. Weinberger, M. M., and Oleinick, A.: Congenital marrow dysfunction in Down's syndrome, J. Pediat. 77:273, 1970.
272. Wells, C. E., and Silver, R. T.: The neurologic manifestations of the acute leukemias; a clinical study, Ann. Intern. Med. 46:439, 1957.
273. Wetherley-Mein, G., Epstein, I. S., Foster, W. D., and Grimes, A. J.: Mechanisms of anaemia in leukaemia, Brit. J. Haemat. 4:281, 1958.
274. Whang, J., Frei, E., III, Tjio, J. H., Carbone, P. P., and Brecher, G.: The distribution of the Philadelphia chromosome in patients with chronic myelogenous leukemia, Blood 22:664, 1963.
275. Wheelock, E. F., and Dingle, J. H.: Observations of the repeated administration of viruses to a patient with acute leukemia; a preliminary report, New Eng. J. Med. 271:645, 1964.
276. Wilbur, J. R., Sutow, W. W., Sullivan, M. P., and Mumford, D. M.: Treatment of acute leukemia in children; in leukemia-lymphoma, Chicago, 1970, Year Book Medical Publishers, Inc., p. 347.
277. Williams, M. J.: Myeloblastic leukemia preceded by prolonged hematologic disorder, Blood 10:502, 1955.
278. Wilson, M. G., Schroeder, W. A., Graves, D. A., and Kach, V. D.: Postnatal change of hemoglobin F and $A_2$ in infants with Down's syndrome (G trisomy), Pediatrics 42:349, 1968.
279. Wiltshaw, E., and Moloney, W. C.: Histochemical and biochemical studies on leukocyte alkaline phosphatase activity, Blood 10:1120, 1955.
280. Wintrobe, M. M.: Clinical hematology, ed. 5, Philadelphia, 1961, Lea & Febiger.
281. Witzleben, C. L., Drake, W. L., Jr., Sammay, J., and Mohabbat, O. M.: Gaucher's cells in acute leukemia of childhood, J. Pediat. 76:129, 1970.
282. Wolfson, I. N., Groce, E. J., and Fite, F. K: Acute leukemia with rupture of the spleen as the initial symptom, New Eng. J. Med. 251:735, 1954.
283. Wolman, I. J.: Parallel responses to therapy in identical twin infants with concordant leukemia, J. Pediat. 60:91, 1962.
284. Woodliff, H. J., and Dougan, L.: Acute leukaemia associated with phenylbutazone treatment, Brit. M. J. 1:744, 1964.
285. Yaguda, A., and Rosenthal, N.: The relation of trauma to leukemia, Amer. J. Clin. Path. 9:311, 1939.
286. Zuelzer, W. W.: Implications of the long term survival in acute stem cell leukemia in childhood treated with composite cyclic therapy, Blood 24:477, 1964.

# 23 LEUKEMIA—TREATMENT

The aim of therapy in patients with leukemia is the eradication of the leukemic process in the blood and tissues and the restoration of hematopoiesis to normal. No curative agent or method has as yet been discovered which permanently controls the disease. Although it is invariably fatal, substantial gains have been made in achieving remission and in prolonging life, especially in patients with acute leukemia of childhood.

Based on concepts derived from studies of leukemia in animals, it has been reasoned that a single leukemic cell may double and redouble and finally produce fatal disease.[117] The goal of treatment is a 100% kill of leukemic cells. The lethal number of leukemic cells in the patient with a diagnosis of acute leukemia is estimated at approximately one trillion ($10^{12}$). A patient can be in "complete remission," that is, blood and bone marrow apparently normal and all signs and symptoms of disease absent, and still have a leukemic cell count of one billion ($10^9$). With intensive courses of drug combinations, the leukemic cell populations in patients with acute lymphatic leukemia is approximately one million ($10^6$). At this time the patient has no sign of disease. In the absence of a method of measuring the number of leukemic cells required for their complete destruction, the duration of maintenance of remission without drug therapy is an index of the number of leukemic cells persisting at the end of treatment. The goal of modern therapy of leukemia has been succinctly summarized as follows: "The reduction in leukemic cells from one trillion ($10^{12}$) to zero, with the best results achieved to date is with intensive courses of drug combinations and with optimal supportive care, including transfusions of platelets and antibiotic therapy."[177]

*Treatment.* The principal therapeutic agents in current use in childhood leukemia are as follows:

A. Antileukemic chemotherapeutic agents
  1. Antimetabolites
     a. Folic acid antagonists
        (1) Amethopterin (methotrexate)
     b. Purine antagonists
        (1) 6-mercaptopurine (Purinethol)
        (2) 6-thioguanine
     c. Pyrimidine antagonist
        (1) Cytosine arabinoside (Cytosar)
     d. Enzyme producing nutritional deficiency
        (1) L-asparaginase
B. Cytotoxic agents
  1. Radiation therapy
  2. Busulfan (Mylaren)
  3. Cyclophosphamide (Cytoxan)
  4. Vincristine sulfate (Oncovin)
  5. Daunorubicin (Daunomycin); adriamycin (an antibiotic which inhibits DNA synthesis)
  6. Nitrosureas (BCNU or 1,3 bis-(2-chloroethyl)-1-nitrosurea)
C. Immunotherapy
  1. ACTH
  2. Cortisone, hydrocortisone, prednisone, prednisolone
  3. Triamcinolone, methylprednisolone, dexamethasone
D. Hormones
E. Supportive therapy
  1. Transfusions—packed cells, platelets, leukocytes
  2. Antibiotics
  3. Protective environment
  4. Allopurinol
F. Bone marrow transplantation

Skillful management depends upon the judicial selection of these agents for administration alone or in combination. Antileukemic therapy may be classified as specific and nonspecific. In the specific group reliance is placed mainly upon the adrenal corticosteroids, such as prednisone (or prednisolone and like compounds); the folic acid antagonist amethopterin (methotrexate); the purine antagonist 6-mercaptopurine (6-MP); the alkaloid vincristine; and the alkylating agent cyclophosphamide (Cytoxan). Busulfan (Mylaren) and x-ray therapy are employed to a lesser extent. Supportive or nonspecific therapy in the form of transfusions of blood derivatives and antibiotics are directed, respectively, toward correction of the anemia and bleeding tendencies and treatment of infection.

*Chemotherapeutic agents—antimetabolites.*[96] The antimetabolites include the folic acid antagonist amethopterin and the purine antagonist 6-mercaptopurine. Cytosine arabinoside is a pyrimidine antagonist.

*Principle of the antagonist (analogues, antimetabolite).* The use of a number of drugs in the therapy of leukemia is based on their ability to inhibit one or more of the steps in nucleic acid biosynthesis. It has been well established that structurally related compounds may be biologically antagonistic. Antimetabolites in use in the treatment of leukemia are compounds in which the chemical structure differs only slightly from a vitamin, an amino acid, or a precursor of nucleic acid. These substances are so closely related chemically that they replace the metabolite in its particular enzyme system. Thus, folic acid analogues combine with folic acid systems because of their similar chemical structure. In view of the structure not being the same as that of the metabolite, the reaction ceases, and the enzyme system and, in this case, the utilization of folic acid is blocked.[157,158] For example, synthetic analogues of many vitamins which inhibit the growth of organisms have been prepared. Woods[156] originally observed that the bacteriostatic action of sulfanilamide was reversed by the chemically related para-aminobenzoic acid. These observations led also to the concept that the analogues exhibit their effects by producing signs of deficiency of the metabolite which they resemble structurally.

The advent of potent antimetabolites which affect the synthesis of nucleic acid has focused considerable interest on its structure. The nucleic acids are composed of relatively simple primary units: phosphate, the sugars ribose or deoxyribose, the purines, and the pyrimidines. The building materials involved in purine synthesis are glycine, carbon dioxide, ammonia, and certain one-carbon compounds such as formate. Folic acid is quite generally involved in one-carbon unit metabolism, and it appears to be specifically concerned with the synthesis of the purines. It is assumed that by virtue of this fact the antifolic acid compounds exert their growth inhibitory action. Thus, nucleic acid synthesis might be interfered with by the use of folic acid antagonist which blocks one-carbon unit incorporation or by the use of purine or pyrimidine analogues (to block interconversion reactions and incorporation).[102]

*Folic acid antagonists:* Folic acid (PGA), a vitamin which occurs in nature and which is also synthesized, consists of pteridine, para-aminobenzoic acid, and glutamic acid. Since it is essential for the growth of erythroid and myeloid cells of the bone marrow, megaloblastosis results when it is deficient. In addition to its specific action upon megaloblastic marrow, folic acid exerts many other nutritional effects and participates in specific metabolic functions frequently in conjunction with vitamin $B_{12}$. Of basic importance is the fact that folic acid is essential for the growth of certain types of leukemic cells and, with its derivatives, plays an essential role in the biosynthesis of nucleic acid. Leukocytes of patients with leukemia contain higher levels of folic acid than do leukocytes from normal individuals.[140] The more immature the cell the higher the level, so that proliferating tissues are therefore more susceptible to antifols.[110] It is now appreciated that the main action of antifols is their ability to combine with the enzyme folic acid reductase which normally reduces folic acid to tetrahydrofolic acid prior to its conversion to citrovorum factor.[43,63] Citrovorum factor (folinic acid, Leucovorin) is a derivative of and probably the active form of folic acid. Conversion of folic acid to the citrovorum factor is enhanced in vivo and in vitro by ascorbic acid. Citrovorum factor is necessary for the incorporation of one-carbon groups into bases of nucleic acid and nucleic acid biosynthesis is, therefore, impaired by the administration of methotrexate.[63] The essential rise in folic acid reductase activity during treatment of patients with methotrexate may be one of the factors associated with drug resistance.[110]

Certain compounds biologically antagonistic to folic acid have the property of inhibiting cell growth. The folic acid antagonists that have been more widely used are Aminopterin and amethopterin (methotrexate). Both involve a change in the folic acid molecule by the addition of an amino group in the 4-position of the pteridine ring. The administration of either of these antagonists in controlled doses prevents the utilization of folic acid. Normal as well as leukemic tissues are affected by these agents, but the development of rapidly growing immature cells is impaired more than that of the mature slowly growing cells. The body therefore is placed in a state of folic acid deficiency insufficient to injure normal cells.[20]

The analogues Aminopterin (4-aminopteroylglutamic acid) and amethopterin (4-amino-$N^{10}$-methylpteroylglutamic acid) appear to exert their antimetabolic effect by blocking the conversion of folic acid to citrovorum factor itself. These folic acid derivatives enter into the synthesis of purines and pyrimidines, and in blocking the activity of purines and pyrimidines, nucleic acid formation is reduced and cell growth is retarded.

In many instances it seems likely that the leukemic cells rapidly acquire resistance to the folic acid and other antagonists. Thus, experience has shown that eventually all patients ultimately become resistant to these compounds, but the mechanism by which this is accomplished is not definitely established.[44]

AMINOPTERIN. The chemotherapeutic agent Aminopterin was among the first of the analogues of folic acid to be employed successfully in the treatment of patients with acute leukemia.[37,133] Although substantial improvement and complete remissions have been obtained with this drug, clinical experiences have demonstrated the superiority of amethopterin. The latter possesses a much wider margin of safety and therefore is less prone to produce toxicity from the dosages used than is Aminopterin.

METHOTREXATE (AMETHOPTERIN). The dosage of amethopterin ranges from 1.25 to 5 mg. given orally once daily. The usual dose is 1.25 mg. for very small children and 2.5 mg. daily for children over 2 years of age. At this dosage, treatment can be carried out for prolonged periods without toxic effects. In some patients 5 mg. is required to obtain a remission, but at this level evidences of toxicity frequently appear. (In some schedules 5 mg. daily is the prescribed dosage for children over 10 years of age.) Intravenous methotrexate, 3 mg. per kilogram every 2 weeks in combination with prednisone, has also been successful in inducing remission. The drug is rapidly absorbed, and constant supervision is necessary to avoid serious complications. Intermittent therapy is sometimes useful in children, particularly those susceptible to toxic reactions. One such schedule for remission maintenance includes 30 mg. per square meter twice weekly, orally or intramuscularly.

A remission following the administration of folic acid antagonists generally takes 3 to 8 weeks, although satisfactory responses have been obtained within 10 days to 2 weeks. Remissions with methotrexate have been maintained for periods of several months to 1 year and longer by skillful management by either continuous or intermittent therapy. Good clinical and hematologic remissions may be expected in 30 to 50% of patients[20] with complete remissions in 20 to 30%. Others have been able to induce complete remission in 21% of affected children with this drug.[47] Following a remission, therapy is usually continued on a dosage adjusted to maintain a normal blood and bone marrow status without signs of toxicity. During treatment the bone marrow should be examined at 4- to 8-week intervals to detect early signs of relapse which may precede clinical and peripheral blood changes. Unless the number of leukemic cells in the bone marrow is very low, relapses can occur quite rapidly. Occasionally, enlargement of the spleen, lymphocytosis, granulocytopenia, or thrombocytopenia may herald a relapse. Repeated remissions may be obtained with amethopterin, but each successive one is usually of shorter duration and more difficult to produce. It is of interest that children can be maintained on amethopterin for prolonged periods in relatively good health with the bone marrow and blood showing partial relapse.

TOXIC EFFECTS. The initial symptoms of toxicity are loss of appetite and abdominal pains. The areas involved are the buccal mucous membrane, gastrointestinal tract, and bone marrow. Small shallow ulcers which are painful and which interfere with feedings may appear on the buccal mucosa of the lips and the cheeks and on the tongue. At this point the dosage should be reduced or the drug discontinued; otherwise serious ulceration of the gastrointestinal canal with massive hemorrhages develops. Erythematous and hemorrhagic rashes of the scalp, face, neck, and trunk, nausea, anorexia, diarrhea, epistaxis, and alopecia are other signs of toxicity. These manifestations, including bone marrow hypoplasia or aplasia, usually ascribed to toxic effects of the drug may represent part of the leukemic process itself.

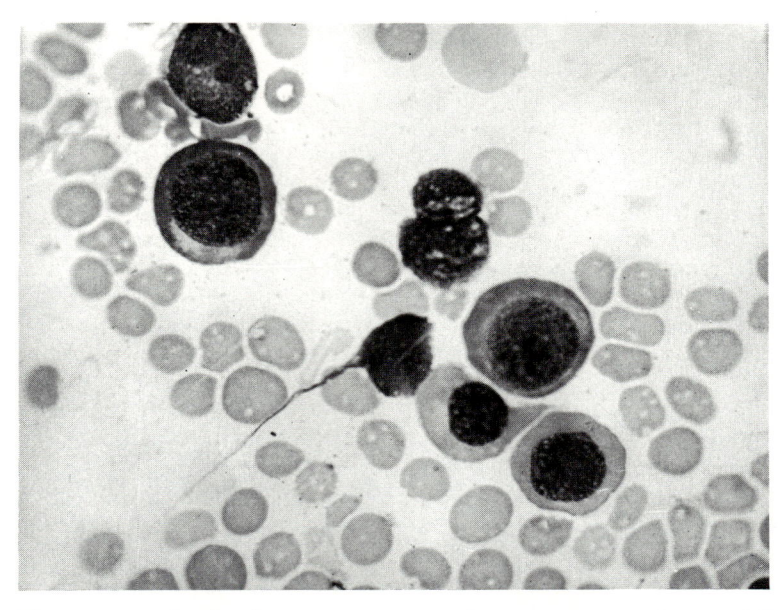

**Fig. 82.** Photomicrograph of a bone marrow smear from a patient with stem cell leukemia. Megaloblasts appeared while the patient was on antifolic therapy (methotrexate). (×960.)

Ulceration of the lips and buccal mucous membranes often subsides with elimination of the drug. For stubborn involvement, mycostatin, xylocaine (Lidocaine), glyoxide, or other local remedies are sometimes necessary.

A megaloblastic transformation of the bone marrow and peripheral macrocytosis represent true folic acid deficiency (Fig. 82). The bone marrow may show varying degrees of injury with respect to the red and white blood cell elements and the megakarocytes. Ultimately, an aplastic bone marrow results with pancytopenia and bleeding unless the drug is withdrawn. With prolonged administration reversibility is more difficult to obtain.

Usually the megaloblastic bone marrow encountered with methotrexate therapy is associated with few leukemic cells and persistent anemia. Under circumstances of pancytopenia, therapy had best be stopped and transfusions given to correct the anemia. Methotrexate may be resumed when the pancytopenic state subsides. Although folinic acid prevents the toxic effects of folic acid antagonist, it also interferes with their antileukemic action.[20]

In the event of a hypoplastic marrow due to therapy with cytotoxic drugs, a trial of androgens has been suggested to stimulate regeneration.[29] Antileukemic therapy is later reinstituted. This treatment awaits further trial.

A severe but self-limited respiratory illness characterized by fever, dyspnea, cyanosis, and bilateral pulmonary infiltrates developed in seven consecutive patients with acute lymphoblastic leukemia who received intermittent therapy with methotrexate, while in clinical and hematologic remission of the leukemia. No infectious agent could be identified, and a moderate blood eosinophil count accompanied the illness in five of the seven patients. Lung biopsy performed on one patient revealed an allergic type of granulomatous reaction. It is suggested but not proved that the pulmonary disease represented an adverse reaction to methotrexate therapy. Two patients received methotrexate by intramuscular injection, the other patients were given methotrexate by mouth. The pulmonary disorder appeared 12 to 100 days after the initiation of methotrexate therapy, at which time the leukemia in all seven patients was in complete remission. Administration of methotrexate was continued throughout the pulmonary illness in five patients, interrupted for 9 days in one patient, and discontinued in one patient.[22]

Severe bone pain, osteoporosis, and pathological fractures have been attributed to long-term methotrexate therapy.[119] Discontinuation of the drug resulted in resolution of the clinical and radiographic abnormalities which were confused with local leukemic infiltrates, which failed to respond to radiation therapy. Prolonged therapy has also resulted in hepatic fibrosis.[72]

*Purine antagonist—6-mercaptopurine (Purinethol).* This analogue of the nucleic acid constituent adenine and the physiologic purine base hypoxanthine, 6-mercaptopurine,[76] has been found particularly effective in the treatment of acute leukemia in children. Its activity in leukemias which are resistant to the antifols is indicative of an antipurine rather than an antifolic acid mode of action. The drug interferes with the formation of purines and their subsequent incorporation into nucleic acid, whereas the folic acid antagonists interfere with the de novo synthesis of purines and pyrimidines involved in nucleic acid formation.

DOSAGE. The usual initial dose of 6-mercaptopurine is 2.5 mg. per kilogram of body weight to the nearest 12.5 mg. given once daily. The approximate dose is 50 mg. in an average 5-year-old child, and in children of all ages the range is from 25 to 150 mg. daily. The drug has a specific leukopenic effect which is manifested in 7 to 10 days after administration, although maximal benefits require 3 to 8 weeks of treatment. As with amethopterin, 6-mercaptopurine may be increased above the stated dosage when the response is inadequate, especially in the later stages of the disease.

The drug is discontinued temporarily at the first evidence of a precipitous drop in the white blood cell count, especially in patients with marked leukocytosis, since a continued drop often follows the cessation of therapy. When the leukocyte count rises or becomes stabilized for several days, with counts ranging from 1,000 to 1,500 granulocytes per cubic millimeter, treatment is reinstituted. The same program is followed with elevated but more moderate initial white blood cell counts. Periodic bone marrow aspiration is useful in determining to what extent the peripheral leukopenia is associated with leukemic infiltration. If the bone marrow is still heavily involved, treatment can be resumed provided the blood count does not fall below 1,000 white blood cells per cubic millimeter. From this level the white blood cell count usually rises again within a few days. A rapid decrease in the white blood cells in patients with hyperleukocytosis occasionally results in hyperuricemia and impaired renal function, which may be obviated with xanthine oxidase inhibitor, allopurinol. When this drug is used in combination with 6-mercaptopurine, the dose of the latter should be reduced by three-fourths.

A suitable maintenance dose should be established, depending upon the character of the response in the initial treatment. As with amethopterin, 6-mercaptopurine may be given continuously or intermittently following a remission. Relapses usually occur within 4 to 6 weeks after treatment is stopped. Good clinical and hematologic remissions were observed in 47% of patients in one series of eighty-seven children.[20] In another series[47] the drug induced complete remissions in 27% of forty-three children. The drug produces remissions in children with acute leukemia who have been previously untreated and in those in whom the disease has become resistant to amethopterin and the steroid hormones. Clinical improvement with reduction in size of the liver, spleen, and lymph nodes accompanies the return to normal of the bone marrow and peripheral blood. 6-Mercaptopurine is rapidly metabolized, disappearing from the plasma almost completely in 24 hours. Only in a dosage higher than that usually prescribed does the drug pass the blood-brain barrier in appreciable amounts.[64]

TOXIC EFFECTS. The chief toxic manifestations are hematologic, with marked leukopenia and bone marrow aplasia. The drug is less toxic to the mucosa of the gastrointestinal tract than are the folic acid antagonists. Mouth lesions, nausea, vomiting, anorexia, and mild diarrhea occur exceptionally. The development of nausea and an enlarging, tender liver may herald a toxic hepatitis.[100] Bile stasis, a pronounced disruption of the normal hepatic architecture, and a loss of hepatic cords are seen. The acute hepatitis and intrahepatic blockage clear when the drug is stopped.[21]

*6-Mercaptopurine combined with azaserine:* The combination of 6-mercaptopurine and azaserine has been subjected to clinical trial in the treatment of patients with acute leukemia following the demonstration of its synergistic therapeutic effect in experimental animals. Azaserine, an analogue of serine which also blocks nucleic acid synthesis, is given orally in a dosage of approximately 2.5 mg. per kilogram of body weight. Ulceration of the tongue and buccal mucosa is an indication for temporary withdrawal of this drug alone. It is later resumed at a lower dosage of 1.25 mg. per kilogram of body weight together with the full dose of 6-mercaptopurine. In one series[20] complete remissions were obtained with an average duration of 6 months, thus delaying the resistance to 6-

mercaptopurine alone on the average of about 2 months. In another and more extensive study[73] the duration of the remissions obtained with the combined therapy was not significantly longer than when 6-mercaptopurine was used alone.

DON, a tumor-inhibitory antibiotic related to azaserine, is also a glutamine antagonist. It has little therapeutic value in human leukemia of itself, but like azaserine it may have a synergistic effect with 6-mercaptopurine but not consistently so.

*Cytotoxic agents.* The principle cytotoxic agents used in the treatment of childhood leukemia are radiation therapy and the drugs cyclophosphamide, vincristine, and busulfan (Myleran).

*Radiation therapy.* Roentgen-ray irradiation finds a place in the treatment of acute leukemia in childhood. It is effective in relieving pressure symptoms and pain due to enlargement of infiltrated organs and localized leukemic masses. It is an excellent adjuvant in relieving severe headache in patients with acute leukemia and in intractable bone and joint pain and disability in those with any type of leukemia, especially in the infrequent chronic myelocytic form in children. In patients with chronic myelocytic leukemia, especially, it reduces the leukocyte count and the number of immature forms. The technique of treatment is highly specialized and requires a consideration of the advantages of local versus generalized irradiation. As with the specific drugs, treatment needs to be carefully controlled by regular hematologic examinations so as to avoid pancytopenia and aplastic bone marrow.

Ten children with acute leukemia were treated with local radiation therapy following bone marrow remission.[129] Although local infiltrates in the liver and kidney seemed to have been eliminated, the ultimate outcome in regard to relapse and survival remained unchanged. Despite these negative findings, radiation to the skull and spine supplements combination drug therapy in some schedules.

Prophylactic irradiation to the skull and vertebral axis early in remission has significantly decreased the incidence of central nervous system leukemia which occurs in approximately 50% of children with acute lymphoblastic leukemia.[114]

*Busulfan (Myleran)—use in patients with chronic myelocytic leukemia.* The search for a less toxic analogue of nitrogen mustard led to the discovery of a sulfonic acid ester, busulfan. This drug has been found to be invaluable in the treatment of chronic myelocytic leukemia,[16,54,61,95] and of little or no value in other types of leukemia. It has largely replaced irradiation by x-ray and the mitotic inhibitors urethan (ethyl carbamate) and demecolcin (a derivative of colchicine) previously used in treatment of this type of leukemia.

Kyle and associates[93] have reported a number of cases in which hyperpigmentation of the skin, severe weakness, fatigue, anorexia, nausea, and weight loss developed after long-term busulfan therapy for leukemia. In those cases it was difficult to distinguish the clinical syndrome from true Addison's disease, but the diagnosis could not be substantiated by laboratory tests alone. While the etiology is obscure, it does not seem unreasonable to assume that busulfan inactivates sulfhydryl groups in the skin, thus removing an inhibitor of tyrosinase and accelerating the formation of melanin.

MODE OF ACTION. Busulfan is myelotoxic and depresses normal and abnormal myeloid tissue. It tends to act selectively on granulocytes, but in large doses platelets, red cells, and lymphocytes are also depressed. Reduction in the leukocyte count is the prominent feature and may be achieved in 10 to 14 days or delayed for 3 or 4 weeks. The remission is accompanied by the correction of the anemia, a reduction or even a disappearance of the immature myeloid cells from the blood, a decrease in the cellularity of the bone marrow, a diminution in the size of the liver and spleen, and pronounced subjective improvement. Large daily doses may produce thrombocytopenia and serious bone marrow depression. Toxic side effects are confined to the bone marrow, and little, if any, other discomfort is encountered. Prolonged remissions lasting 6 to 12 months have been reported in adults. Busulfan has been found to be superior to 6-mercaptopurine for the overall control of chronic granulocytic leukemia.[81] It may reduce the granulocyte count somewhat more slowly than does 6-mercaptopurine, but the effect is more prolonged.

DOSAGE. Busulfan is available in 2 mg. tablets. The usual dosage is 4 mg. daily until a maximum hematologic and clinical improvement is obtained. Administration of the drug is continued until the white blood cell count drops to just below 10,000 per cubic millimeter.[154] Occasionally, 6 mg. per day is required to attain a remission. However, the amount given must be individualized, especially in children, for a precipitous decrease in the leukocyte count may develop, necessitating withdrawal of the drug until the white blood cell count is stabilized. The need for maintenance therapy is still debatable. A small dose, adjusted to the particular patient, may be given to prevent elevation or further reduction in the white blood cell count. Some resume therapy when there is a substantial rise in the leukocyte count (to 50,000 per cubic millimeter).[154]

In chronic myelocytic leukemia, stem cell differentiation is overbalanced toward granulopoiesis and sometimes to platelet proliferation, homeostasis is defective, and the abnormal cell line enlarges until the total granulocyte mass is 10 to 150 times the normal.[58] Cytotoxic agents reduce the greatly expanded total granulocyte mass, the spleen size is diminished, the absolute and relative counts of blast cells, of promyelocytes, myelocytes, and metamyelocytes fall, the hemoglobin concentration rises, the blood picture returns to normal, and the myeloid pattern in the bone marrow approaches normal. Busulfan has proved to be as effective as radiotherapy both in shrinking the spleen and maintaining a state of regression for long periods.

The acute blast cell crisis erupts during the chronic phase of the disease, accompanied by lytic lesions in various portions of the skeleton, often by enlargement of the spleen and lymphadenopathy. Busulfan is effective in reducing the blast cells but where this agent is ineffective dibromomannitol, hydroxyurea, vincristine, methotrexate, or steroids alone or in various combinations are effective. Dibromomannitol acts as an alkylating agent and may restore control when busulfan has lost its effect. Marrow hypoplasia may result from overdose of busulfan and other chemotherapeutic agents.

*Cyclophosphamide (Cytoxan).* This alkylating agent has proved of significant benefit in lymphomas and leukemia.[134] The drug is inactive in vitro but is activated in vivo to cytostatic and alkylating metabolites by an oxidation process in liver microsomes and thus differs considerably from alkylating nitrogen mustards which require no prior activation.[10] Neoplastic cells contain an elevated concentration of phosphatases and phosphamidases, enzymes active in the breakdown of cyclophosphamide.

It has a lesser destructive effect on megakaryocytes or platelets or both for the equivalent leukopenic or anticancer effects produced by other agents. Remissions with this drug have been obtained in up to 35% of adequately treated cases.[94] In another series of forty-four children a complete remission was achieved in 18% and a partial remission in another 11%.[39] Almost all patients who showed significant improvement did so in 7 to 14 days. Blasts often disappeared from the blood in 3 to 7 days.[39] In this group of children with leukemia complete remissions were independent of antecedent or concomitant steroid therapy and persisted from 3 to 15 months.

This alkylating agent, as others, functions by inactivating DNA. Cyclophosphamide may be administered by the oral or intravenous route—approximately 3 mg. per kilogram of body weight orally daily until the white blood cell count is reduced to a level of 2,000 per cubic millimeter. From this point the white blood cell count may drop steadily. The drug is resumed when the count returns above these levels. Beneficial results have also been obtained by giving the drug intravenously at a dose of 5 to 15 mg. per kilogram administered once a week.

Side effects are few—occasional alopecia, nausea, leukopenia, and vomiting. Chemical cystitis is due to the presence in the bladder of irritating breakdown products of the agent. Forcing fluids before the administration of the drug prevents its occurrence. Hydration is also effective if cystitis occurs after treatment. An increased number of Döhle bodies (cytoplasmic inclusions) has been reported during cyclophosphamide therapy.[77]

*Vincristine (Oncovin).* This is one of a series of alkaloids obtained from a common flowering herb, the periwinkle plant. This antineoplastic agent falls into the group of antimitotic agents. Despite differences in structure, colchicine and vincristine have similar effects in cell division. Remission rates up to 50% have been reported in acute lymphocytic leukemia.[104] In one series nine of thirteen patients with advanced refractory acute leukemia achieved a complete remission with vincristine which was maintained from 2 weeks to over 3 months.[85] With a remission following vincristine one of the previous antimetabolite drugs is reinstituted. In many clinics vincristine is employed as a starting drug to induce a remission. In addition to its use in acute lymphocytic leukemia and in malignant tumors (Hodgkin's disease, lymphosarcoma, and reticulum cell sarcoma), vincristine has been found valuable in acute and chronic myeloid and monocytic leukemia.[97]

Vincristine is obtained as a white powder, 1 mg. per vial, and is readily dissolved in 10 ml. of isotonic saline solution to give a concentration of 0.1 mg. per milliliter. It is administered intravenously at weekly intervals, either directly or through an infusion tubing. The usual dosage is 0.05 to 0.075 mg. per kilogram or 1.5 to 2.0 mg. per square meter per week for 6 weeks. With counts below 1,000 the drug is reevaluated in terms of bone marrow findings. The most frequent and severe toxic manifestations relate to the neuromuscular system. These consist of paresthesias, usually involving the periphery of the extremities, ataxia, difficulties in grasping and performing delicate movements, depression of deep tendon reflexes, foot drop, and facial weakness. Other side effects are leukopenia, abdominal pain, constipation, face, jaw, or throat pain, dysphagia, and alopecia. Erythropoiesis is disordered and the peripheral blood of patients treated with vincristine reveals anisocytosis, poikilocytosis, basophilic stippling, and normoblastemia.[106a] Hyponatremia is a rare complication of therapy.[14a]

Radioactive phosphorus ($^{32}$P) and nitrogen mustard and its derivatives such as triethylene melamine (TEM), although effective in patients with chronic leukemias, have not been found to be particularly valuable in those with acute leukemias.

A number of other agents, including the fluorinated pyrimidines (FudR), 5-fluorouracil (FUJ), and 6-azauracil (6AzU), have been investigated, but striking benefits have not been observed in acute leukemia.[84] FUJ and FudR, which inhibit thymidylate synthetase, an enzyme required in the synthesis of thymidylic acid producing a thymidine deficiency, have had extensive trials against cancer in man with varying results. 6AzU prevents uridylic acid formation by inhibiting orotidylate synthetase. Incomplete responses were observed in patients with leukemia. By these mechanisms the cell is rendered deficient in essential materials necessary for growth.

Methyglyoxal-bis-guanylhydrazone (methyl GAG) has been known to produce a remission in acute myelocytic leukemia in a child.[94]

*More recent antileukemic therapuetic agents. Daunorubicin* (daunomycin, rabidomycin) is an antibiotic derived from *Streptomyces ceruleorubidus,* which inhibits DNA and RNA synthesis. It is equally effective against acute myeloblastic and acute lymphoblastic leukemia. The dose is a variable one. According to one schedule the dose is 2 mg./kg. given daily intravenously for a total quantity no greater than 30 mg./kg. A remission is usually induced in 1 month with a duration of 1 to 5 months. Up to 40 to 50% of patients have responded with a complete remission, but response is related to duration of disease and previous chemotherapy.

The drug has not been effective in preventing or treating meningeal leukemia. Daunomycin is more effective when used in combination with prednisone or with prednisone plus vincristine, in the latter case given once per week only.[70] Major toxicity is myelosuppression, cardiotoxicity, gastrointestinal disturbances, fever, and alopecia.

*Adriamycin* is an antitumor antibiotic, similar in structure and mechanism of action to daunomycin.[30a] Early clinical trials with this compound, the 1-4 hydroxy analogue of daunomycin, have demonstrated activity against acute leukemias in children and adults and certain solid tumors including carcinomas and lymphosarcomas.[8a,155a] Dose and schedules are still to be established, but most studies have employed a total dose range of 60 to 90 mg. per square meter. Toxicity includes alopecia, nausea and vomiting, mucositis, myelosuppression, phlebitis, and cardiac toxicity.[102a] Electrocardiographic changes including premature ventricular contractions and ST-T wave changes appear to be dose-related. Deaths related to congestive heart failure have been reported.[102a] Further clinical trials will be required to establish the antitumor specificity of this agent.

*Cytosine arabinoside* (Cytarabine, ara-c) is the only pyrimidine antimetabolite. Its antileukemic action is primarily due to its ability to inhibit DNA synthesis by inhibiting the availability of deoxycytidylic acid.[70]

The dosage is 3 to 5 mg./kg. or 100 mg./square meter given daily intravenously for 10 days. The drug is rapidly deactivated in the blood and quickly becomes ineffective. Slow continuous infusion in moderate doses allows the drug to achieve increased destruction of leukemic cells. The drug is effective in inducing a remission in about 2 to 3 weeks in 18 to 25% of cases of acute lymphocytic leukemia and in 30 to 50% of cases of acute myelocytic leukemia when combined with thioguanine. Remissions are short—7 to 8 weeks to 4 months. Cytosine arabinoside has been particularly effective in the treatment of adults with acute granulocytic leukemia. Its value in the treatment of children with acute lymphocytic leukemia has not yet been completely evaluated.[152]

Major toxicity of cytosine arabinoside is myelosuppression, mild hepatic dysfunction, nausea, and vomiting.

*L-asparaginase* induces asparagine deficiency in sensitive malignant cells. Most mammalian cells can make their own asparagine, an essential amino acid, even if deprived of an external supply in the blood and extracellular fluid because they possess an enzyme asparagine synthetase. Others lack this enzyme. If treated with L-asparaginase, asparagine is destroyed in their environment and, unable to synthesize their own asparagine, they die of malnutrition. The antitumor activity of the enzyme presumably is due to inhibition of protein synthesis in tumor cells that require an exogenous source of asparagine, that is, cells that contain no asparagine synthetase activity. Cells containing adequate asparagine synthetase activity would be resistant to L-asparaginase activity. Research in this area was developed from the identification of L-asparaginase as the moiety responsible for the antitumor activity of guinea pig serum.[11,12]

Dosage varies from 50 to 2,000 units/kg./day intravenously for 28 days. The average required to induce a remission varied from 21 to 28 days. The response rate in patients with acute lymphocytic leukemia with a complete remission was 50 to 60% and 25 to 30% in acute myelocytic leukemia. The mean duration of remission in acute lymphocytic leukemia was 60 days. The duration of remission appeared to be independent of the dose.

L-asparaginase has proved to be among the most effective preparations for inducing remission in acute lymphocytic leukemia and occasionally in acute myelocytic leukemia as well.[11] Leukemic cell populations appear to develop resistance rapidly to asparaginase activity.[70]

TOXICITY. Nausea, vomiting, weight loss, fever, anemia, liver dysfunction, central nervous system toxicity, hypofibrinogenemia, elevated blood urea nitrogen, hypersensitivity reactions, pancreatitis, and pericarditis have been reported by a number of investigators.[152] When a hypersensitivity reaction occurs during desensitization (following a positive skin test), treatment is terminated when there is a threat of anaphylaxis. In a group of children refractory to conventional antileukemic agents, L-asparaginase was administered intravenously by two dosage schedules—one group by daily injections and the second in weekly injections of a larger dose. Toxicity appeared to be greater when L-asparaginase was administered daily rather than weekly.[116]

L-asparaginase differs fundamentally from all other chemotherapeutic agents that are used in the treatment of neoplastic disease in man in that its action is based on a specific metabolic defect of cancer cells. Kidd[87] had originally observed that certain lymphomas of the mouse and rat were suppressed by treatment with guinea pig serum. Later the inhibitory factor was shown by Broome[11] to be L-asparaginase, and this was confirmed by several groups.

*Immunotherapy.* Another avenue of exploration is concerned with immunological studies of cancer and leukemia. Extensive electron microscopic and immunological studies on animal leukemia and solid tumors have demonstrated an extraordinary similarity of viruses involved in the origin of these disorders in animals of various species.[32] Mathé and associates[98] investigated the efficacy of immune reactions in the control of human leukemia. The demonstration of virus-specific new antigens in murine leukemia induced by a virus and similar findings in the cells of human leukemia prompted the application of active immunotherapy procedures. One direction of research was nonspecific immunotherapy to stimulate the immune defenses, the other was specific, consisting of vaccination by the tumor cells themselves.

A nonspecific immunotherapy with B.C.G. was chosen. The other was vaccination from a part of allogenic leukemic "lymphoblasts" pretreated with formalin or irradiated in vitro. Whereas all in the control group treated with chemotherapy alone relapsed, eight out of twenty patients treated by immunotherapy without further chemotherapy had prolonged remissions. Three types of immunotherapy were tested—B.C.G., irradiated leukemic cells, and a combination of both. The leukemic cells that were injected came from pooled cells taken from patients with acute lymphoblastic leukemia but excluding the patient's own leukemic cells.

The drawbacks[152] in attempting immunotherapy are possible immunologic enhancement of tumor growth, the risk of inducing autoimmune reactions, and the possibility that undetected carcinogenic viruses may be transmitted.

*Hormones.* The hormones that have been used in the treatment of leukemia in childhood include ACTH, cortisone, hydrocortisone, prednisone, prednisolone, triamcinolone, methylprednisolone, and dexamethasone. Of these, prednisone and prednisolone are now in most common use usually in combination with one or more chemotherapeutic agents for inducing a remission.

*Hematologic response in normal subjects:* The blood response to the administration of ACTH in human subjects with unimpaired adrenal function is well known—within 4 hours of the intramuscular injection of 25 mg. of ACTH, there is an increase in circulating neutrophils and a decrease in lymphocytes and eosinophils.[75] The involution of lymphoid tissue and dissolution of lymphocytes previously reported with the adrenocortical hormones[38] provided a basis for clinical trial of these hormones in human beings with leukemia. The mechanisms by which neutrophilia, eosinopenia, and lymphocytopenia are produced are not entirely understood, nor has the mode of action in leukemia found a satisfactory explanation. The inhibition of incorporation of a structural analogue of thymidine ([131]I-labeled iodeoxyuridine) into DNA by cortisone may implicate the latter directly or indirectly in nucleotide metabolism.[57]

*Role in treatment of leukemia:* Corticotrophin (ACTH) and the adrenocortical steroids (cortisone, hydrocortisone, prednisone, and prednisolone) have proved particularly effective in the treatment of acute leukemia in childhood. In contrast to the folic acid antagonists and 6-mercaptopurine, which require 3 to 8 weeks to produce a satisfactory response, these hormones act rapidly. When serious bleeding occurs and the patient's condition is otherwise precarious, the hormones are the treatment of choice.

Rapid and dramatic improvement has been brought about by these hormones in critically ill patients with acute stem cell (lymphoblastic) leukemia within several days of treatment, and complete remission has been noted in 3 to 4 weeks. Satisfactory clinical and hematologic remissions occur with the initial use of adrenal corticosteroids in 50 to 75% of children with acute leukemia.[49,108,111,120] The response in patients with acute myeloblastic and monoblastic leukemia is much less favorable.

In the first weeks of successful hormone therapy there is a disappearance of fever, a return of appetite, greater activity, a subsidence of bone and joint pain, a lessening of hemorrhagic manifestations, and a regression of enlarged lymph nodes and spleen. Within 1 week the white blood cell count decreases, the blast cells decrease in the blood and bone marrow, and the reticulocyte count rises. Platelets increase in number after the first week, and hemoglobin levels rise. Bone marrow hypoplasia is not infrequently observed during the second week of treatment. Erythroblastic and granulocytic cells make their appearance, and in many patients a complete remission is achieved by the third to fourth week of treatment. Remission is relatively short and in most patients extends from 3 weeks to 3 months, but it occasionally extends from 6 to 9 months without further treatment. Successive remissions are less frequent, incomplete, and of shorter duration.

*Types and dosage:* No definite dosage can be stated for hormonal therapy since the speed of response and signs of hypercorticism which limit its use are subject to individual variation. The following schedule serves as a guide to treatment and is based upon dosages in current use. In order to provide sustained hormonal effects, the total daily dosage must be divided.

ACTH. ACTH is administered in 25 mg. doses by continuous intravenous drip in a glucose infusion over an 8- to 12-hour period. Rarely is more than one treatment given daily. Intramuscular injection of an aqueous preparation, or preferably the gel, of 60 to 80 units daily is given in two divided doses to children under 4 years of age, and 80 to 120 units is given to older children.[111] ACTH is rapidly absorbed following intravenous or intramuscular injection. ACTH has been superseded by prednisone and prednisolone, the corticosteroids of choice.

CORTISONE. Cortisone is administered orally in a total daily dosage of 100 to 200 mg. It is given in divided doses at 6-hour intervals. It has been largely replaced by hydrocortisone.

HYDROCORTISONE. Hydrocortisone (compound F) can be given orally, intravenously,* or intramuscularly, depending upon the urgency of treatment. It produces maximal physiologic effects when given by continuous intravenous drip. Be-

---

*Hydrocortisone succinate (Solu-Cortef), which contains 100 mg. of hydrocortisone in each vial, is particularly suitable for intravenous use, especially in emergency situations when high levels of hydrocortisone are needed immediately.

cause its effects are terminated rapidly when intravenous administration is stopped, it is necessary to supplement it with the oral or intramuscular preparation. The intravenous dosage is 100 mg. daily. Total oral dosage is 60 to 80 mg. in younger children and 80 to 120 mg. in older children. Hydrocortisone is given at 6-hour intervals in four divided doses.

PREDNISONE AND PREDNISOLONE. Prednisone and prednisolone in combination with vincristine or 6-mercaptopurine or methotrexate serve at present as common drugs in the initiation of treatment. ACTH and hydrocortisone used originally at the onset of the disease now are rarely, if ever, used as primary therapy. Prednisone and prednisolone possess the advantage of rapid onset of action and prompt therapeutic effects. These hormones are available in 5 mg. tablets and are given at 6- or 8-hour intervals. In young children the tablets are crushed in stewed fruit or apple sauce.

These compounds are produced by subtle modification in chemical structure of cortisone and hydrocortisone, respectively. Thus endowed with a potency three to five times greater than that of the parent compounds, they possess relatively marked decreases in electrolyte side effects. In moderate dosage (approximately 2 mg. per kilogram or 60 mg. per square meter per day) therapy is not complicated by sodium retention and excessive potassium excretion which occur with the older corticosteroid agents. Although these precautions, therefore, do not apply to prednisone and prednisolone in average therapeutic doses, hypopotassemia, sodium retention, and elevated blood pressure may occur when massive or excessive amounts are given over prolonged periods, and appropriate measures must be taken to obviate these side effects.

Remission was induced with prednisone in 330 children with acute leukemia.[155] Complete remission occurred in 40% and good partial remission occurred in 34% of patients. Complete bone marrow remission occurred in 63%. Remission was maintained without treatment for a median duration of 58 days. Infants under 1 year of age with initially high white cell counts and those with a diagnosis of acute granulocytic leukemia responded less favorably than the other children. Dosage of the drug was 2.0 mg./kg. to the nearest 1.25 mg. daily by mouth in three divided doses every 8 hours. Bone marrow aspirations were performed 28 and 42 days after the start of therapy.

The following milligram equivalents differentiate the glucocorticosteroids: dexamethasone (Deronil, Decadron), 0.75 mg.; methylprednisolone (Medrol), triamcinolone (Aristocort, Kenacort), 4 mg.; prednisone and prednisolone, 5 mg.; hydrocortisone, 20 mg.; and cortisone, 25 mg. It is claimed that products like dexamethasone, methylprednisolone, and triamcinoline require smaller dosage and produce a lesser incidence of side effects. The 4 mg. tablet of Artistocort, Kenacort, and Medrol corresponds to the 5 mg. tablet of prednisone so that if trial is contemplated, the dosage should be adjusted on the basis of four-fifths of Meticorten. One 0.75 mg. tablet of Decadron or Deronil replaces 4 mg. of methylprednisolone or triamcinolone or 5 mg. of prednisone or prednisolone.

Despite the effectiveness of prednisone in inducing a remission when used alone, the plan of current therapy is to achieve rapid control of the disease and restoration of normal bone marrow function. While each of the antileukemic agents in general use is capable of inducing a clinical and hematological remission, experience has shown that the combined use of certain of these drugs results in a higher incidence of induction remission. An effective combination commonly used is prednisone 2 mg./kg./day in four divided doses, and 6-mercaptopurine, 2.5 mg./kg. as a single daily dose, or prednisone in the same dosage orally, and vincristine, 0.05 mg./kg./day given weekly intravenously. One may expect with either combination a remission in acute lymphocytic leukemia of approximately 90% of children in 3 to 4 weeks. The success of this initial treatment is documented by the reappearance of normal blood and bone marrow constituents as well as clinical improvement.

Cross-resistance between the hormones and folic acid antagonists or purine antagonists does not occur so that a patient who has become resistant to any of these agents may still be expected to respond to the others.

*Massive hormone therapy.* Remissions have been reported in adults and, to a lesser extent, in children with acute leukemia of various types morphologically differentiated and undifferentiated following massive doses of prednisone and prednisolone. Dosages of 1 gm. daily (occasionally higher) have been recommended until satisfactory improvement is obtained with a variable toxicity.[74,120] Experience has shown that large individual doses of prednisone and other steroids have not proved more effective in acute lymphocytic leukemia.[70] The reports of the use of 250 to 1,000 mg. per day of prednisone and other steroids to patients with acute myelocytic leukemia showed no greater effectiveness than the 10 to 20% response rate observed in those patients receiving a more conventional dose.

*Toxic and side effects.* Serious toxic and side effects indicative of hypercorticism develop with prolonged and excessive administration. They consist of acneiform eruption, hirsutism, and increased deposition of fat in various parts of the body, giving the "moon face" and the "buffalo hump" effect on the back of the neck. Edema, osteoporosis, glycosuria, and elevated blood sugar, a tendency toward infections, gastric ulcer, myopathy, and clinical, chemical, and electrocardiographic evidences of hypokalemia represent other diverse effects. Encephalopathy and cerebral hemorrhage in patients with severe thrombocytopenia also necessitate a reduction or withdrawal of hormone therapy (Plate 3). Severe hypertension, however, is a rare complication in childhood. Patients whose dosage of corticosteroids is being tapered may develop signs and symptoms of increased intracranial pressure and pseudo-tumor cerebri. As with other chemotherapeutic agents, the rapid destruction of white cells may lead to severe azotemia. Pancreatitis may also be associated with steroid administration and was found in 16% of leukemic children at autopsy.[108]

*Exposure to chickenpox.* The severe and often fatal nature of chickenpox occurring during the course of acute leukemia has been generally observed. Histologic study in fatal cases reveals focal hepatic necrosis and pulmonary hemorrhage and edema.[112] The lack of inflammatory cells in the visceral pox lesion reflects a deficiency in the cellular response to chickenpox. Fulminating infection has been noted in other conditions in which the patient is receiving steroids, but notably in leukemia.[42] The serious nature of chickenpox complicating acute leukemia may be due to impairment of the immune mechanism in leukemia itself or to the drugs used in its treatment. The adrenal steroids, 6-mercaptopurine and methotrexate, all tend to depress host resistance. There is some clinical evidence that large doses of pooled gamma globulin may exert some beneficial effect,[112] but control studies are necessary to substantiate its value. The dosage of gamma globulin used in the modification of chickenpox in family contacts[124] has also been extended on an empirical basis to patients with leukemia. All steroids are withdrawn and gamma globulin is administered in a dosage of 0.6 to 1.2 ml. per kilogram of body weight. Because of the increased quantity in the older child, it may be given in three divided doses at 24-hour intervals. It should be emphasized that more extended trial is needed to substantiate its therapeutic value.

Others[5] have emphasized, however, that the prognosis is not always serious with this complication and that the outcome probably depends largely on the stage of the leukemic process. For patients in remission they claim the risk is negligible; for those in relapse the disease is more serious, but the outcome can still be favorable. On the other hand, we have observed exceptions to this classification and the development of varicella in children in remission must still be looked on with the greatest apprehension.

*Adjuvant treatment with the adrenocortical steroids.* With prednisone and comparable compounds sodium retention is not significant; excessive potassium loss is easily controlled by having the patient take potassium chloride syrup or foods rich in potassium such as orange juice, tomato juice, grapefruit, or bananas. Patients treated with intravenous hydrocortisone should be maintained on a low-salt diet with additional potassium chloride. Sodium and potassium determinations should be carried out initially and repeated only for clinical indications.

*Remissions—criteria.* Therapeutic responses are classified as either complete or partial, depending upon the extent to which the bone marrow, peripheral blood, and organ involvement revert to normal. In accordance with the established standards of the Leukemia Chemotherapy Cooperative Study Group A[25,73] a complete remission includes the following criteria. In the bone marrow there are reductions in the number of blasts to less than 5% with lymphocytes and blasts to less than 40% and essentially normal-appearing granulopoiesis, erythropoiesis, and thrombopoiesis. In the peripheral blood there are return to and maintenance for more than 1 month of hemoglobin greater than 11 gm. per 100 ml. for children

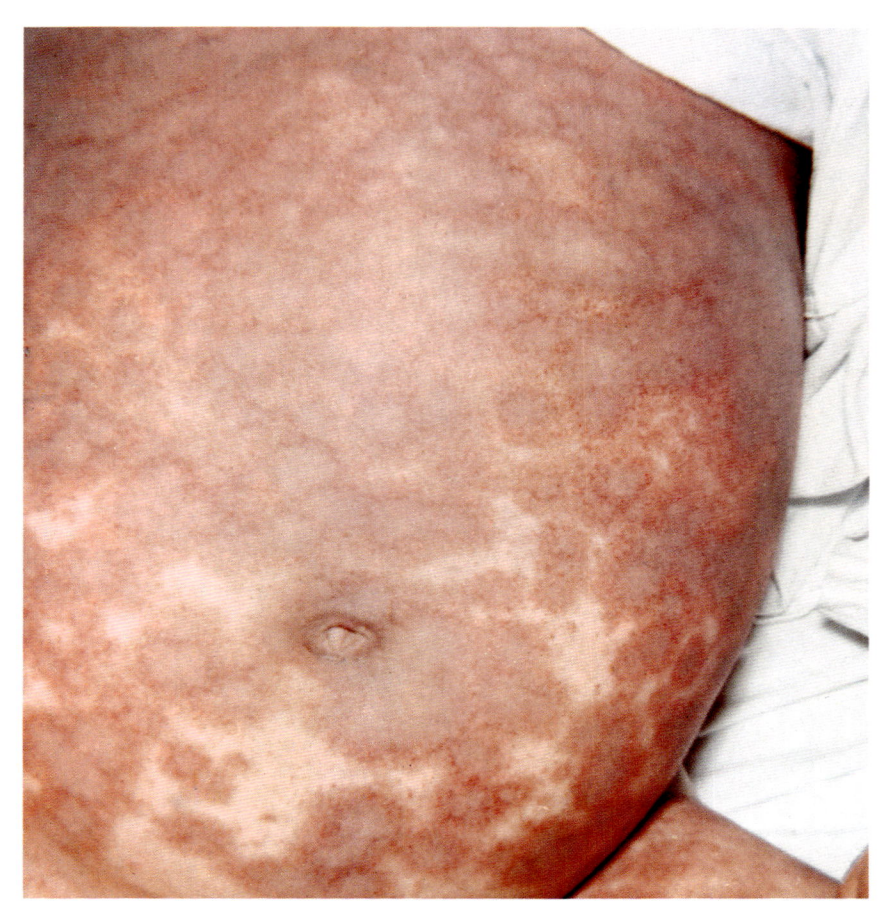

**Plate 3.** Diffuse hemorrhagic measles in child with leukemia while under treatment with prednisone and 6-mercaptopurine. The extensive hemorrhagic eruption noted on the abdomen was typical of the eruption covering the entire body and mucous membranes. Chemotherapy was discontinued. The thrombocytopenia was treated by the daily administration of two units of concentrated platelets. Remission followed subsidence of the measles.

under 15 years of age or 10 gm. for infants under 2 years of age, granulocyte levels in excess of 1,500 per cubic millimeter, platelet counts greater than 100,000 per cubic millimeter, and an absence of leukemic cells in the blood smear. Clinically, signs ascribable to leukemia should be absent. Criteria of a partial remission and a relapse involve increasing clinical and hematologic evidences of leukemic infiltration. In general, these criteria differ only in minor aspects from the criteria published by other cancer chemotherapy study groups.[146]

With satisfactory hematologic and clinical improvement, the patient should return to complete health and activity, appetite should be normal, and no overt toxic effects of drug therapy should be manifested.

***Detailed program of treatment.*** With the diagnosis of leukemia the following factors require consideration: choice of chemotherapeutic agent in relation to type of leukemia, choice of a drug with which to initiate treatment, the need for blood transfusions and other supportive therapy, and the question of hospitalization and of psychologic factors, especially with relation to the parents.

*Choice of chemotherapeutic agent in relation to type of leukemia.* Experience has demonstrated that significant differences in the therapeutic effects of various chemotherapeutic agents depend upon the type of leukemia diagnosed. Following are the chemotherapeutic agents of choice in the treatment of various types of leukemia.

*Acute stem cell (lymphoblastic) leukemia*
1. Adrenocortical steroids
2. Amethopterin (Methotrexate)
3. 6-Mercaptopurine (Purinethol)
4. Cyclophosphamide (Cytoxan)
5. Vincristine sulfate (Oncovin)
6. Daunomycin
7. Cytosine arabinoside
8. L-asparaginase

*Eosinophilic leukemia*
1. Adrenocortical steroids
2. 6-Mercaptopurine (Purinethol) (less effective)

*Acute myeloblastic, promyelocytic, and myelocytic and monocytic leukemia*
1. Adrenocortical steroids
2. 6-Mercaptopurine (Purinethol)
3. 6-Thioguanine
4. Amethopterin (Methotrexate)
5. Cytosine arabinoside
6. Daunomycin
7. Vincristine sulfate (Oncovin)
8. Cyclophosphamide (Cytoxan)

*Chronic myelocytic leukemia*
1. Busulfan (Myleran)

The acute stem cell (lymphoblastic) leukemia responds to the adrenocortical steroids, amethopterin, 6-mercaptopurine, vincristine, cyclophosphamide, and the newer drugs cytosine arabinoside, daunomycin, and L-asparaginase. Eosinophilic leukemia responds principally to the adrenocortical steroids and less favorably to 6-mercaptopurine. Acute myeloblastic, promyelocytic, and myelocytic and monocytic leukemias respond poorly to the adrenocortical steroids and better to combinations of 6-mercaptopurine, or 6-thioguanine and cytosine arabinoside. Other useful agents used either alone or in combination include vincristine, methotrexate, daunomycin, cytoxan, and steroids. Chronic myelocytic leukemia responds to busulfan. Although these recommendations are more or less specific, it is frequently necessary to deviate from them to introduce another drug when the response is greatly delayed. The antimetabolites may have to be pushed, however, to the point of inducing severe leukopenia before deciding on their ineffectiveness. To accomplish this the dosage may have to be increased, with a close watch for toxicity. At present busulfan appears to be the drug of choice in the treatment of chronic myelocytic leukemia.

With the exception of the adrenocortical steroids, the antileukemic agents enumerated are capable of injuring the bone marrow. The fact that myelotoxicity, responsible for bone marrow aplasia, is also destructive to leukemic cells suggests that, for an agent to be of value therapeutically, it must also have myelotoxic properties.[26] This fact must be kept in mind in prolonged treatment with a chemotherapeutic agent and emphasizes the need for periodic bone marrow examinations.

Occasionally, early in treatment the antimetabolites produce signs of toxicity of sufficient severity to warrant withdrawal of the drug. These signs consist of anorexia, listlessness, fever, extreme leukopenia, and increased bleeding from the gums and other areas. In such an event the adrenocortical steroids and fresh whole blood, packed cells, or platelets

Table 28. Selected chemotherapeutic agents for the treatment of leukemia*

| Drug | Available as | Dose† | Toxicity — Requiring temporary interruption of therapy | Toxicity — Other | Usual time to induce remission | Patients responding with complete or partial remission | Usual duration of remission | Comment |
|---|---|---|---|---|---|---|---|---|
| 6-Mercaptopurine (Purinethol) (purine analogue) | 50 mg. tablets | 2.5 mg./kg./day | Rare at recommended doses; at higher doses same as for methotrexate | Increased pigmentation of skin | 1–2 mo. | 50% | 4 mo. | |
| Methotrexate (amethopterin) (folic acid antagonist) | 2.5 mg. tablets | 2.5 mg./day or 30 mg./M² twice weekly | Oral ulcers, diarrhea, marrow depression, dermatitis, hepatitis and pulmonary fibrosis | Alopecia, increased pigmentation of skin, anorexia | 1–2 mo. | 30% | 7 mo. | Doses to 5 mg./day may be used in older children; dose reduction to 1.25 mg./day may be necessary in others to avoid toxicity |
| | 50 mg. ampules for dilution with distilled water to concentrations of 2.5 mg./ml. | 2.5–5 mg./kg. I.V. every 7–14 days | | | | | | Because of better tolerance of higher dose, I.V. route may be tried in patients who have relapsed on, or failed to respond to, or become toxic to, oral doses |
| | 5 mg. ampules; dissolved in 2–5 ml. of distilled water | Intrathecally 0.25–0.5 mg./kg. every 3–5 days | | | | | | Oral or I.V. methotrexate temporarily suspended while intrathecal methotrexate is given; may be restarted 3–5 days after last intrathecal dose |

| | | | | | | |
|---|---|---|---|---|---|---|
| Prednisone (hormone) | 5 mg. tablets | 2 mg./kg./day divided in three equal doses; dose may be reduced to 1 mg./kg. if side effects severe | Hypertension, cerebral edema, gastric ulcers | Cushinoid facies, osteoporosis, acne, mild edema | ½–1½ mo. | 70% | 1½ mo. Principal use to induce remissions in combination with vincristine, 6-mercaptopurine, or methotrexate |
| Cyclophosphamide (Cytoxan) (alkylating agent) | 50 mg. tablets<br><br>100 and 200 mg. amps.; dilute in sterile H$_2$O to concentration of 10 mg./ml. | 2–3 mg./kg./day orally in one dose<br><br>15–20 mg./kg. I.V. weekly | Hemorrhagic cystitis, stomatitis, vomiting, diarrhea, dermatitis, and leukopenia or other marrow depression | Alopecia | ½–2 mo. | 35% | 6 mo. (?) Dose may be raised to 5 mg./kg./day orally or 5 to 15 mg./kg. I.V. weekly, if not responding after 2–3 wk. at lower dose; maintain adequate fluid intake; sometimes must maintain W.B.C. count as low as 2,000 in order to obtain desired effects |
| Vincristine (Oncovin) (alkaloid agent) | 1 and 5 mg. amps. for I.V. use; dilute to concentration of 1 mg./ml. with saline, water, or glucose | 0.05–0.075 mg./kg. or 1–2 mg./M² weekly for 6 weeks | More frequent with higher doses or longer courses; peripheral neuritis, weakness, fever, severe constipation, marrow depression | Alopecia, mild constipation, sleeplessness | ½–1 mo. | Approximately 50% | 2 mo. (?) Because of serious side effects, main usefulness may be in inducing remissions; dose continued until remission obtained or until toxic effects preclude further use, another drug then substituted for maintenance |

\*Based on Murphy, M. L.: In Gellis, S. S., and Kagan, B. M., editors: Current pediatric therapy, Philadelphia, 1964, W. B. Saunders Co.
†Consult text for variation in dosage of drugs listed above as well as the newer drugs: daunomycin, cytosine arabinoside, and L-asparaginase.

are valuable in tiding the patient over the period until the specific therapy is reinstituted.

Although the beneficial effects of corticosteroid therapy in the treatment of lymphocytic leukemia have been well established, the value of these drugs in the treatment of acute granulocytic leukemia remains questionable.[89] Corticosteroid therapy frequently causes marked leukocytosis and clinical deterioration in adults with acute granulocytic leukemia or chronic granulocytic leukemia in blast crisis. This noxious response to corticosteroids was not observed in prepubertal patients or in the aged.

Despite this possible shortcoming, the steroids serve as useful chemotherapeutic agents at some phase in the course of all types of leukemia in childhood.

*Programs of drug therapy in acute leukemia (stem cell, lymphoblastic).* The approach to chemotherapy in acute leukemia may be divided broadly into two categories—the induction of remission and the maintenance of remission. The induction of remission is a simpler matter than maintenance.

The current treatment of acute leukemia has been influenced by several factors, among which are the advent of newer chemotherapeutic agents, a clearer understanding of the kinetics of leukemic cell growth, and the fact that chemotherapeutic "cure" is now a realistic goal. Burchenal[18] has gathered more than 100 individuals from the world's experience, many of whom, now without evident disease in excess of 10 years, have experienced a prolonged remission or who might be considered cured.

The target of treatment based on animal studies is the total destruction of leukemic cells (from all tissues of the body), whether in the stem cell or proliferating cell pool, while the differentiated cell pool of malignant cells will be eliminated through senescence. It is hoped, as shown experimentally, that the thorough destruction of replicating leukemic cells will result from the combined use of several drugs if necessary.[128] As stated by Henderson,[70] "the aim of the chemotherapist must be to effect the greatest possible ultimate reduction of the leukemic cell population consistent with conservation of that amount of normal cells requisite for survival." In treatment it cannot be overemphasized that the side-effects of a particular mode of therapy must be assessed in evaluating its relative success. "The price that the patient must pay in terms of painful procedures, length of hospitalization, and life-threatening side effects must be weighed against the long term success achieved by that therapy."[152]

It is advisable from the outset for treatment to be planned as a cooperative venture between the patient's own physician and an investigational center in leukemia therapy located in a university hospital or a research institution.[78] The reasons are many—the increased number of antileukemic agents available, the variety and complexity of programs offered for treatment, their control by detailed hematologic procedures, vigilance in detailing side-effects, as well as the management of hemorrhage and infection.

The ideal treatment of acute leukemia, regardless of the type, is directed toward the complete eradication of the malignant process rather than its temporary suppression. The objective is to produce remissions of maximum duration. Many programs of treatment are under current investigation; yet, surprisingly, patients with unusually prolonged remissions have been reported from many sources with varied schedules. As a basic principle, agents that produce complete remissions with initial treatment also improve survival. It is therefore important to choose for initial chemotherapy the agent or agents that experience has demonstrated to be most effective. With the combination of prednisone and 6-mercaptopurine, or with vincristine and prednisone, complete remission rates in excess of 80% have been achieved.[45,48]

Skipper and associates[182] have shown in experimental mouse leukemia that a single leukemic cell will eventually cause death. The difficulties of achieving complete eradication in man are shown by questionable results when four drugs are combined ("VAMP").[29] It has also been observed that leukemic cells persist in extramedullary leukemic infiltrates (kidney, liver, testes, bowel, lung, central nervous system, and lymph nodes) during bone marrow remission.[107]

The principal therapeutic agents in current use in acute stem cell leukemia are amethopterin (methotrexate), 6-mercaptopurine, cyclophosphamide (Cytoxan), vincristine, and the adrenocortical steroids. Daunomycin, cytosine arabinoside, and L-asparaginase are recent additions to the antileukemic agents. Of these, main reliance is placed initially on prednisone (or other prednisone-like adrenocortical steroids), in combination with either vincristine, 6-mercaptopurine, or methotrexate. Formerly, the practice was to prescribe each drug in turn as resistance developed to the previous one. Methotrexate and 6-mercaptopurine alone produced longer remissions than the adrenocortical steroids but generally required 3 to 8 weeks for a maximal response.

With the adrenocortical steroids, remissions occur within 1 to 3 weeks but are shorter than with the antimetabolites. In the era before combined therapy (such as prednisone and 6-mercaptopurine) remissions of 7 and 8 months occasionally occurred following the initial use of prednisone alone. A plan formerly adopted was to introduce 6-mercaptopurine or methotrexate in full dosage just as soon as the initial remission with the adrenocortical hormones was reached.

In combined studies it was observed that when prednisone alone was used for remission induction for subsequent 6-mercaptopurine maintenance, 57% of patients entered complete remission as compared with 82% when prednisone was combined with 6-mercaptopurine.[48] However, when only 6-mercaptopurine was used to induce remission and the complete remission rate was 27%, the median duration of remission was only 18 weeks.[47] It was clear in these studies, too, that patients who do not achieve complete remission with initial treatment have a significantly shorter survival.

The steroids are employed to control bleeding manifestations at any time during the disease, regardless of the drug in current use. In the gravely ill child with other than stem cell or undifferentiated leukemia, usually the granulocytic and monocytic types, the hormones are nevertheless administered. These agents are supplemented by supportive treatment until the immediate emergency is over, when the specific drug may be given.

Since the white blood cell count frequently undergoes a precipitous drop with steroids, it is necessary to modify the dosage to avoid too-rapid dissolution of white blood cells leading to hyperuricemia and kidney impairment. Cases of hyperleukocytosis are carefully controlled by blood uric acid and urea nitrogen determinations. Instead of the standard dose of prednisone of 2 mg. per kilogram per day, it is usually advisable to give one-half the dose for the first day or two, until the state of kidney function is established. It is not uncommon to observe patients with leukopenic peripheral blood in whom the bone marrow reveals marked hyperplasia and dissolution of the leukemic cells. In one such case marked elevation of serum uric acid occurred. In cases with high leukocyte counts the need for lowered dosage in the first 24 to 48 hours is even more important, unless the patient is critically ill.

The excretion of large amounts of uric acid following antileukemic therapy may be explained by the destruction of white cells releasing large amounts of nucleoprotein which is degraded to uric acid. Another source of uric acid is from the accumulation of nucleic acid purines that ordinarily would have gone into leukemic cells, but whose production is inhibited by chemotherapeutic agents.[126] In a 13-year-old child with acute lymphoblastic leukemia, marked leukocytosis and extreme hyperuricemia, acute renal failure, and severe gouty arthritis developed under treatment with 6-mercaptopurine.[150] The hot, red, swollen, exquisitely tender joints responded dramatically to colchicine. The acute gouty arthritis may possibly also have been a reflection of a familial gouty diathesis.

A syndrome consisting of anorexia, nausea, persistent vomiting, extreme weakness, and lethargy has been described in children with acute leukemia when serum uric acid concentrations rose to 20 to 55 mg./100 ml.[131]

Since uric acid nephropathy is the most common cause of renal failure in leukemia,[46] prevention or prompt therapy is an essential part of leukemic chemotherapy. Successful prophylaxis depends on effective urinary alkalinization or a brisk urine flow in order to attain maximal solubility of uric acid. A regimen has been suggested which includes the administration of acetazolamide (Diamox), sodium bicarbonate, and intravenous hydration.[121] In the majority of patients with leukemia the clinical condition is fairly good, and the white blood cells range from a leukopenia to a moderate leukocytosis. The best results, however, depend upon early detection of the disease and control of its progress as vigorously as possible with antileukemic therapy.

With the advent of allopurinol, hyperuricemia has been more effectively controlled. This drug, an isomer of hypoxanthine, is capable of inhibiting xanthine oxidase, the enzyme responsible for the oxidation of hypoxanthine to xanthine to uric acid. This drug has been used in the treatment or prevention of hyperurecemia in children with various neoplastic diseases in whom severe uremia was present or in whom it might have been expected as a result of antineoplastic therapy. It was found a useful agent in the treatment or prevention of uric acid nephropathy in children with leukemia, the uric acid being derived from the degradation of nucleic acid purines.

In the group of children studied[90] allopurinol (Zyloprim), which is supplied as 100 mg. scored tablets, was given orally in total daily doses of approximately 10 mg. per kilogram divided into three or four doses.

It is impossible to set forth absolute criteria for the administration of antileukemic therapy except in the seriously ill child in whom the adrenocortical steriod therapy is mandatory. The individual response is so varied with each class of compounds that judgment must be exercised in the replacement of one drug by another and in relation to dosage.

In our clinic at one time we had initiated treatment with predisone only. A remission was predictable with this agent in at least 70% of patients with acute stem cell leukemia within 3 to 4 weeks of treatment. This was succeeded by continuing prednisone with daily oral doses of 6-mercaptopurine. At the present time the induction phase is carried out with a combination of daily oral treatment with prednisone and weekly intravenous injections of vincristine.

Another method[13] is to give daily oral prednisone (2 mg. per kilogram per day) and intermittent intravenous methotrexate (3 mg. per kilogram every 14 days). This combination was used as initial therapy for fourteen children with acute lymphocytic or acute undifferentiated leukemia. Complete or partial remissions were achieved in eight of fourteen patients by day 14 and in all patients by day 28. Toxicity attributable to methotrexate was noted in only one patient, who developed mild ulcerations of the buccal mucosa.

Increased success in achieving induction remission appears to have been accomplished with the use of drugs in combination. Krivit and associates[91] have described an 80% induction remission with prednisone plus methotrexate and an 86% remission with prednisone plus 6-mercaptopurine. Other investigators have reported bone marrow remission in approximately 90% or more of patients receiving combination of prednisone and vincristine,[56] prednisone and 6-mercaptopurine,[127] prednisone and methotrexate,[13] and multiple drug combinations such as prednisone, vincristine, and daunomycin.[99]

Another important observation has been the demonstration that the use of prednisone and vincristine can successfully reinduce remissions two to four times or more.[152]

*Cyclic use of chemotherapeutic agents.* One of the methods aimed to effect a more thorough suppression of the leukemic process is to rotate the metabolites for relatively short periods. This approach is based on the hypothesis that resistance to one or the other drug might be postponed by the sequential use of the chemotherapeutic agents. Based on the need for the continued inhibition of folic acid reductase which converts folic acid to its active form, tetrahydrofolic acid, Welch[147] recommended the introduction of a second drug immediately after a remission. Resistant leukemic (stem) cells would be exposed and hopefully eliminated by the second drug. Cyclic therapy is directed toward preventing hematologic and clinical relapse by successfully eliminating neoplastic cells that have become resistant or have re-emerged in spite of the drug in current use. The program has been subjected to many individual variations. Zuelzer,[159,160] for instance, initiated treatment of acute lymphoblastic (stem cell) leukemia with prednisone combined with 6-mercaptopurine. After 3 months, methotrexate replaced 6-mercaptopurine, steroids meanwhile having been eliminated. Methotrexate and 6-mercaptopurine were interchanged at 3-month intervals.

In this as in any program before a chemotherapeutic agent is introduced, antibiotics and transfusions are given as required. Prednisone is then given in a dosage of 2 mg. per kilogram daily in divided doses, except in cases of excessive leukocytosis, in which case the dose is reduced to prevent uric acid accumulation. Critically ill patients receive hydrocortisone intravenously instead of oral prednisone. From the start, all patients able to tolerate oral medication receive 6-mercaptopurine in a single dose of 2.5 mg. per kilogram, irrespective of the white blood cell count. Steroid therapy is continued simultaneously for 1 full month, after which the dose is reduced by one-half on alternate days and discontinued after 1 week's time. 6-Mercaptopurine is continued for 3 months. Only when anemia supervenes is the dose temporarily reduced but not for moderate leukopenia and neutropenia. After 3 months methotrexate is substituted for 6-mercaptopurine and is given in a total single dose daily of 1.25 to 5 mg., depending on the size of the patient. (In some programs[160] the dose of methotrexate for patients less than 2 years of age is 1.25 mg. per day; for patients 2 to 10 years of age, 2.5 mg. per day; and for patients over 10 years, 5 mg. per day.)

With toxicity the drug is temporarily discontinued. If a deficiency state attended by megaloblastosis seems to require it, transfusions or steroids or both are given in addition. At the end of 3 months of therapy with methotrexate, 6-mercaptopurine is resumed, and the two antimetabolites are thus alternated at regular intervals. This regimen is maintained indefinitely until a relapse occurs. This is marked by falling hemoglobin levels, thrombocytopenia, severe neutropenia, the reappearance of "blast" cells in the blood, and clinically by fatigability, pain, fever, loss of appetite, and increasing size of the spleen or lymph nodes or both. When this complication develops, the bone marrow is examined; otherwise the aspiration is carried out at the end of each cycle.

With relapse, steroid therapy is resumed in full dosage for about 1 month and the metabolite currently in use is replaced by its alternate. If remission is induced, the drug is continued; otherwise as relapse progresses, other agents (cyclophosphamide or vincristine) are substituted. Brubaker and associates[14] rotating prednisone (2.2 mg. per kilogram), methotrexate (0.2 mg. per kilogram per day), and 6-mercaptopurine (2.5 mg. per kilogram per day) for 6-week cycles, achieved a mean duration of clinical control of approximately 17 months in 135 patients. In twenty-four of his patients, the disease was controlled for 2 years or more; in nine, for 3 years or more; and in six, for 4 to more than 7 years. Zuelzer[159] noted that the duration of the initial remission was generally a decisive factor for determining longevity. Of 175 patients surviving at least 1 month after diagnosis, the percentage survival ranged from 17 months (50%) to 45 months (10%) and the mean survival of expired patients was 17.7 months. Six patients were alive in uninterrupted remission from 4 to 9 years after diagnosis. Patients with white blood counts initially below 20,000 cells per cubic millimeter had twice the mean survival of those above this value.

An adult has been reported with a 7-year remission with massive doses of corticosteroids.[28] The patient had received 1,000 mg. of prednisone daily over a period of several weeks, followed by a short course of 6-mercaptopurine.

These treatment schedules apply to acute stem cell (undifferentiated) leukemia, but do not apply to granulocytic, monomyelogenous, and monocytic leukemia. Stem cell leukemia reaches a peak between the ages of 3 and 4 years. The incidences of other types are not as rigidly confined by age.

Additional trials of cyclic drug regimens for acute childhood leukemia have been recently reported. In one study,[23] after induction with vincristine and prednisolone cases were randomly allocated to cyclic and noncyclic regimens in each of which vincristine, 6-mercaptopurine, cyclophosphamide, and methotrexate were given in sequence. The results analyzing the various measurements of mortality and morbidity have shown a remarkable absence of difference between the cyclic and noncyclic groups. The survival time of both series was on the order of 2 years.

In another group, after initial induction with oral prednisone and 6-mercaptopurine or vincristine, cyclic therapy consisted of rotating oral 6-mercaptopurine, methotrexate, and cyclophosphamide.[153] Relapses were treated with prednisolone and weekly intravenous vincristine. Thereafter cyclic therapy was reinstituted, resulting in a median survival from diagnosis of over 82 weeks (19 months).

Ninety-four children with acute leukemia were treated with sequential drug therapy.[127] Remission was induced with prednisone and 6-mercaptopurine in some and in others with cyclophosphamide and vincristine. For maintenance, 6-mercaptopurine and methotrexate were used. The remission rates were 94% for cases of acute lymphoblastic leukemia and 57% for acute myeloblastic leukemia. The median survival of patients was 17 months with acute lymphoblastic leukemia and 8 months with acute myeloblastic leukemia. The study indicated that sequential therapy offers results equal to those of cyclic drug therapy.

*Miscellaneous schedules.* The selection and scheduling of these drug combinations includes the following principles: "to take maximum advantage of the antileukemic capability of each drug, to utilize the drugs with different mechanisms of action and to combine drugs which have different types of major toxicity."[152] Some of the combinations employed have been VAMP[50] (vincristine, amethopterin, 6-mercaptopurine, and prednisone) and POMP[68] (prednisone, Oncovin, methotrexate, and Purinethol). In another series[47] methotrexate and 6-mercaptopurine, each alone and in combination, were studied for remission rates. For children with acute lymphoblastic (stem cell) leukemia, combination therapy resulted in a remission rate of 59%, 47% for 6-mercaptopurine alone, and 29% for methotrexate. The median duration of complete remission (4 to 5 months) for the three treatments was not different. There were no differences between the three treatment programs in regard to survival. The median survival from the onset of therapy to death was 9 months. There was no evidence that prior treatment with one of the metabolites altered response to the other antimetabolites.

The assumption that early use of steroids interferes with its subsequent effectiveness is not borne out by experience. Second and third remissions can be induced by steroids; the more readily, the greater the time interval since the last administration. There is also no advantage in withholding steroids until antimetabolites become ineffective since an excellent response is realized late in the course, when steroids are combined once more with an antimetabolite to which the patient appears to be resistant.

In still another schedule[7] all untreated patients with lymphoblastic leukemia, irrespective of age, receive 40 mg. of prednisone per day for 6 weeks or longer if their blood values have not returned to normal or are improving. When normal values are attained, 6-mercaptopurine (2.5 mg. per kilogram daily) is prescribed and prednisone tapered off and stopped. The drug is maintained at this dosage except for interruption necessitated by toxicity or until the patient is clearly relapsing. With relapse, 6-mercaptopurine is stopped and prednisone is given as before. When improved from the second course of prednisone, 1.25 to 5 mg. of methotrexate is given daily, depending on age and size of the patient, as maintenance therapy in the same fashion as 6-mercaptopurine had been given. If the second trial of prednisone therapy proves of no benefit, remission is attempted with methotrexate. With relapse from the second remission, prednisone is tried again, followed by any current drug that appears to hold promise (cyclophosphamide or vincristine).[7]

Another method of dealing with patients in relapse while receiving oral therapy is to administer methotrexate intravenously.[109] Metrotrexate for parenteral use is dissolved in sterile water for injection and given intravenously over a 2- to 3-minute period. The drug is given in a dose of 3 mg. per kilogram every 2 weeks. Each 50 mg. vial is reconstituted with 20 ml. of water for injection. In one series a new remission was obtained in ten of twelve patients who had relapsed or failed to respond to standard courses of 6-mercaptopurine or methotrexate given orally. No side effects were observed except occasional vomiting and severe leukopenia. The intravenous use of methotrexate is contraindicated in the face of renal impairment.

*Current program of treatment in stem cell (lymphoblastic) leukemia.* Before the emphasis was placed on "total" therapy with the combined use of several chemotherapeutic agents, the patient with acute lymphoblastic leukemia was treated with prednisone or prednisolone exclusively. These steroids were gradually withdrawn when the bone marrow returned to normal. Following cessation of therapy, the bone marrow was reexamined at 2- to 4-week intervals. In our experience maintenance therapy with small doses of prednisone given daily or intermittently has not prolonged the remission. Many others have claimed complete or partial remissions in more than 90% of cases of acute leukemia treated with adrenal hormones alone and complete remissions in 50%. Vietti and co-workers[146] noted that the remission rates with prednisone (2.2 mg. per kilogram per day, ranging from 20 mg. to 60 mg. daily) in forty-six children with untreated disease and in forty-one children in relapse for the second time were 59% and 46%, respectively. Hyman and associates[83] found the median time necessary to produce a full bone marrow remission with steroids was 29 days. The particular advantage of these agents is their rapidity of action in comparison with other forms of chemotherapy. Steroid-induced remissions are relatively short, averaging 3 months in duration. Another advantage of the steroids is their nonspecific hemostatic effect, and they are frequently used in the severe thrombocytopenic periods of relapsing leukemia.[94]

When prednisone is employed as the only

drug for inducing remission, 6-mercaptopurine is begun when the blood and bone marrow return to normal. This is given normally in a dose of 2.5 mg./kg. body weight as maintenance therapy and prednisone is gradually reduced and discontinued at the end of 10 to 14 days.

The variety of programs advocated by different workers may be so bewildering that a choice is often difficult. In stem cell leukemia in young children, however, prednisone and the antimetabolites usually exert a predictable depressant and lytic effect of variable duration upon the proliferation of leukemic tissue.

The plan that is currently being followed in our clinic for patients with stem cell leukemia is to initiate treatment with prednisone and vincristine for 6 weeks.[45] When a remission is established and confirmed by bone marrow examination, prednisone is tapered over a 2-week period and discontinued. In an effort to further reduce the leukemic cell burden, "consolidation" therapy with intravenous methotrexate is given during the next 8 weeks. At this time, the bone marrow is reexamined and, if remission persists, "maintenance" therapy with oral methotrexate, 30 mg. per square meter twice weekly, is given. Once each month "reinducer" doses of vincristine with oral prednisone for 1 week are administered.[80]

With relapse there are several alternatives—the reintroduction of prednisone and vincristine or the use of prednisone and either 6-mercaptopurine, cyclophosphamide, or cytosine arabinoside. With the establishment of remission, 6-mercaptopurine would be the drug of choice for maintenance therapy. Nagao and co-workers[105] found that methotrexate given intravenously at 2-week intervals in doses of 3 to 6 mg./kg. appears to be an effective form of maintenance therapy for acute childhood leukemia. They report that prolonged remission periods are achieved with minimal risk of drug toxicity. Brubaker and colleagues[14] reported that daily oral prednisone (2 mg./kg./day) and intermittent intravenous methotrexate (3 mg./kg. every 14 days) used as initial therapy in children with acute lymphoblastic leukemia gave complete or partial remissions in every case. Toxicity attributed to methotrexate was noted in only one patient, who developed mild ulcerations of the buccal mucosa.

*Prolonged complete remissions.* With the use of methotrexate, 6-mercaptopurine, corticosteroids, and vincristine in various dosages and combinations, as initial clinical remission can be assured in 80 to 90% of patients with acute lymphoblastic leukemia. The median life-span from the day of diagnosis prior to the availability of effective chemotherapy was 3 to 4 months, as compared to the current median life-span of 18 to 24 months.

Krivit and co-workers[92] investigated the need for continuing or discontinuing chemotherapy to maintain a prolonged complete remission in acute leukemia in childhood. Fifteen children whose disease had been in total control for 2¾ to 3⅓ years had been divided into two groups—one a "continuous," the other "no therapy" group. No significant difference was found between these two groups during the ensuing 2 years. Disadvantages of chemotherapy include evidence of hepatic toxicity and immunosuppression.

A variation of this regimen is treatment with vincristine and prednisone which is followed by 5-day parenteral intensive courses of methotrexate for a period of 8 additional months.[79] After every third course of methotrexate, another inducer course of vincristine and prednisone is given. Seventy-five percent of these children are alive at 24 months, with the projected probability that 25% will survive 5 years or more.

That aggressive therapy results in improved prognosis with prolonged remissions without continuous therapy has been the experience of clinics with large numbers of children with leukemia under treatment, perhaps to justify the statement that "it is possible that acute lymphocytic leukemia has a 15% cure rate and that this may increase shortly."[113]

In a national survey Burchenal and Murphy found seventy-one patients who survived longer than 5 years,[19] and by 1968[18] there were 157 patients with acute leukemia who had survived 5 years or more from the diagnosis of their disease. Of 127 children, eighty-seven were living and were with no evidence of disease, and forty had died or were living with signs of leukemia. Burchenal's recommendation was that in the patient with acute leukemia who is living over 7 years after diagnosis of disease and who has had no evidence of leukemia for the past 4 years it should be reasonably safe to discontinue treatment on the assumption that all leukemic cells had been eradicated. In this connection, the case reported by Feldman and Tan[38] is pertinent. The patient with acute leukemia diagnosed at 2½ years of age relapsed and finally died 16 months after an initial remission which lasted 11 years. During the period of remission the patient had been treated with methotrexate and 6-mercaptopurine cycled monthly. The explanation for the relapse after the long period of remission was either the emergence of leukemic cells resistant to methotrexate and 6-mercaptopurine or that these drugs suppress host defenses to a point where they are unable to prevent reinduction of the disease. Thus maintenance chemotherapy must be considered as a possible threat as well as a potential advantage in maintaining remissions.

In one program describing "total" therapy of acute lymphoblastic leukemia, vincristine and prednisone were used for induction. This was followed by an intensive short-term high-dosage course of treatment with methotrexate, mercaptopurine, and cyclophosphamide given in sequence prior to radiotherapy to the entire craniospinal axis and a continuous combined maintenance regimen with methotrexate, mercaptopurine, cyclophosphamide, and vincristine simultaneously. The median duration of complete remission in twenty-seven of thirty-one children with acute lymphoblastic leukemia who had previously been untreated was 78 weeks, the median duration of over-all remission was 95 weeks, and the median survival time was 135 weeks. Six patients (22% without therapy for 6 months or longer) survived in continuous complete remission for an average of 153 weeks (3 years). Radiotherapy with the dosage used did not influence the subsequent development of central nervous system leukemia.

**Treatment of acute myeloblastic leukemia.** Induction of complete remission in acute myeloblastic, monomyeloblastic, and monocytic leukemia in childhood has been far less successful than in acute lymphoblastic leukemia. Complete remission rates of 20%, 40%, and 70% have been achieved with combination of 6-mercaptopurine and methotrexate,[47] 6-mercaptopurine and methyl GAG (methylglyoxal-bis-guanylhydrazone),[8] and vincristine, prednisone, 6-mercaptopurine, and methotrexate.[69] Other treatment programs have utilized cytosine arabinoside in combination with thioguanine[55] or with cyclophosphamide and vincristine,[135] in which remission rates of approximately 50% have been obtained. Cytosine arabinoside or daunomycin alone have produced similar remission rates.[70] The limiting factor in the treatment of acute myeloblastic leukemia has been severe and often life-threatening myelotoxicity produced by these agents. Protected environments and massive platelet, red cell, and leukocyte replacement therapy are often necessary adjuvant therapy which is best carried on in a specialized center. There appears to be a correlation between duration of remission and survival in acute myeloblastic leukemia and, as expected survival is longer in patients responding to treatment.[69]

*Supportive therapy.* Transfusions and antibiotics are the methods of supportive therapy chiefly relied upon in patients with leukemia.

*Transfusions:* Blood is administered to combat anemia and to control hemorrhage. There is also evidence that the action of blood may not be confined solely to its capacity for raising hemoglobin but that it may also be responsible for an occasional remission. This rare phenomenon noted after ordinary transfusions has led to the hypothesis that normal blood contains an antileukemic substance. More directly, it has been shown that fresh blood rather than stored blood was effective in producing a decline in the total number of leukocytes without, however, modifying the differential count.[148]

The hemoglobin value at which a transfusion is indicated varies with the associated signs and symptoms present in the patient. Although the requirements for raising hemoglobin levels to correct anemia can be met by the administration of packed cells, whole blood is often more desirable because thrombocytopenia is commonly present, especially during chemotherapy. Fresh whole blood obtained in siliconized equipment or platelet concentrates derived from such a sample has proved remarkably effective in the control of hemorrhage.

For overwhelming and persistent hemorrhage from the nose, mouth, and gastrointestinal canal we have found that a routine of continuous treatment with whole blood and its products is beneficial. Fresh blood collected in a plastic bag is given until the hemoglobin level is normal. This is followed at once by platelet concentrates also obtained by plastic bag technique and given daily until evidence of bleeding has ceased. By assiduous application of this program of intensive and continuous therapy, bleeding is usually controlled.

It should be remembered that patients receiving multiple transfusions of whole blood may occasionally develop thrombocytopenia due to the formation of antibodies against platelets.

Concentrated platelets in patients with severe bleeding have proved effective in producing temporary hemostasis,[88] but in an emergency they are usually difficult to prepare. With adequate dosage, the platelet count in acute leukemia returns to preinfusion levels within 24 hours but occasionally remains elevated for 48 to 96 hours.[1]

The infusion of platelet concentrates[31] prepared as a by-product of ordinary blood banking by means of plastic bag systems increases the number of circulating platelets in leukemia patients who are thrombocytopenic. Given in adequate dosage (the minimum is usually platelets separated from 2 pints, or 1 liter, of fresh blood), overt bleeding in the form of epistaxis and hematuria is usually controlled, but melena subsides less readily. It has been estimated that each unit of platelet concentrate will increase the platelet count 12,000 per cu. mm. per square meter of surface area.

As has already been stated, corticosteroids have been shown to increase capillary resistance[122,123] so that these hormones are useful adjuncts in the control of bleeding. It has been shown, however, that ecchymoses may occur in patients undergoing prolonged steroid therapy.[30,136] The administration of ascorbic acid (200 to 300 mg. daily) has therefore been recommended as supplementary treatment.[137]

Bleeding from accessible areas is occasionally controlled by the local application of thromboplastin, Gelfoam, or packs, or packs saturated with a mixture of thrombin and Adrenalin or neosynephrine.

Unless there is associated hemorrhage, transfusions are not required until hemoglobin levels decrease to 7 or 8 gm. per 100 ml. The dosage of whole blood, packed cells, and plasma for the different age groups are listed in Chapter 7.

*Antibiotics:* The policy of giving broad-spectrum antibiotics routinely whenever adrenocortical steroids are administered is open to question. Prolonged administration of the steroids is known to inhibit the inflammatory process with the result that serious infection can develop without the usual clinical signs and symptoms. Advocates of this policy also cite the fact that the leukemic patient is prone to develop infections as a result of the depletion of myeloid elements in the blood and bone marrow.

The difficulties with routine use of antibiotics with the steroids and the antimetabolites are the possibility of eventual resistance of specific pathogenic organisms and the development of widespread and fulminating monilial infection. A more realistic approach is to administer antibiotics when infection is present. This is often manifested in the initial stages of the disease and at varying periods subsequently.

When sepsis is suspected, the choice of an effective antibiotic depends upon bacteriologic methods. It is not always possible, however, to isolate the causative organism in order to determine its susceptibility to antibiotics by in vitro tests.[130]

In the presence of persistent and markedly elevated temperatures late in the course of the disease, when blood cultures are negative and the focus of infection is obscure, definitive antibiotic therapy is difficult to prescribe. It is a temptation to regard the fever as unrelated to an infectious process and due to a product of proliferating leukemic tissues. Terminally, the febrile period is nearly always refractory to anti-infectious agents.[118] In one series 32% of the febrile episodes were associated with major hemorrhage, which was usually accompanied by infection.[130]

For control of infection in patients with leukemia the following program has been useful. Until cultures are available: (1) methicillin—150-200mg./kg./day, intravenously, in divided doses given every 4 hours (for staphylococci, streptococci, and pneumococci); (2) ampicillin—200 mg./kg./day, intravenously in divided doses given every 4 to 6 hours (some gram-negative organisms, some *E. coli,* most *Proteus mirabilis,* streptococci, and pneumococci); (3) gentamycin—3 mg./kg./day given in divided doses every 6 hours, intravenously (most gram-negative organisms including *Pseudomonas* and *Proteus* species); (4) carbenecillin may be used for treatment of *Pseudomonas* infections or for other infections with gram-negative organisms when other agents are not effective. There is some evidence of synergism of carbenecillin and gentamycin so that both may be given in serious *Pseudomonas* infections.

Despite its theoretic advantages, the routine use of gamma globulin failed to demonstrate its effectiveness as adjunctive therapy against infections occurring in patients with acute leukemia.[6] In this study, sodium methicillin and colistin were employed to provide coverage for both the control group and those receiving gamma globulin.

Fungal infections such as moniliasis (*Candida albicans*) are treated with antifungal antibiotics such as nystatin (Mycostatin). In general, it is undesirable to give oral antibiotics in serious infections. For serious involvement amphotericin B may be useful and should be given intravenously, never intrathecally.[143]

*Hospitalization.* Except for the most seriously ill patients, for whom hospitalization is urgent, the average patient with leukemia can be managed on an ambulatory basis. For patients especially with a hyperleukocytosis, hospitalization is necessary because a precipitous drop in the white blood cell count frequently occurs soon after treatment is instituted, necessitating adjustment of dosage.

Whether the leukemic child with even the mildest form of the disease should be treated from the first on an ambulatory program is debatable. In our experience an introductory period of hospitalization for about 1 week or 10 days at the time of the diagnosis has proved extremely useful, regardless of the chemotherapeutic agents that are chosen and the degree of severity of the disease. It permits a more adequate compilation of data, including roentgenographic studies, on the basis of which a program of treatment is planned.

When the antimetabolites are introduced initially, severe myelotoxic effects may be manifested within the first 2 weeks of treatment in sensitive patients. Hospitalization during this period offers an opportunity for institution of adjuvant treatment, especially in patients with prolonged bleeding. Following this hospitalization, however, ambulatory treatment is desirable unless serious clinical and hematologic relapses develop.

*Emotional support.* The medical management of the child with leukemia requires special medical competence but providing emotional support for the patient and his family invariably is more demanding of and challenging to the physician's skills. The initial interview at which time the diagnosis is presented to the parents, as well as all subsequent discussions, should be frank, open, and honest. Frequent interviews with the attending physician will be required to acquaint parents with miscellaneous details concerning the nature of the disease and its management which they are anxious to ascertain. Considering the excellent remission rates and improved survival in acute lymphoblastic leukemia, a cautiously optimistic approach is warranted but speculative, omniscient predictions of survival times and the creation of false hope should be assiduously avoided.

Parental support requires an understanding of and an ability to deal positively with the initial reactions of shock, guilt, denial, hostility, and anger that frequently occur. The patterns of adjustment and adoptive mechanisms developed by parents or "coping behavior" will protect parents from overwhelming stress and permit them to function more effectively in providing their child with as normal a life as possible.[51]

Green[60] has outlined a number of important principles of management of children with fatal illnesses and includes the competence and availability of the physician, continuity and personalization of care, and preparation for required medical procedures. The problem of what to tell the child about his disease has led to the recent appreciation that all children should be permitted to have an active role,[86] ask questions, and maintain lines of communication between their parents and physician about their illness. Discussions about the disease and its treatment will depend upon the age and maturity of the child, but it has been suggested that the child who is totally cut off from any meaningful discussion concerning his disease may have anxieties and develop feelings of hopelessness and guilt.[145]

Total emotional support requires an understanding of the impact of the disease on other family members, including siblings and grandparents. Recent studies have emphasized the relatively high incidence of emotional disturbances during the course or following the death of a child with leukemia.[4] Preparing families for the death of a child[52] or anticipatory grieving may decrease the sudden, overwhelming sense of loss that occurs in parents who were unwilling or unable to accept the implications of the diagnosis. Interviews with parents after the death of a child may be extremely valuable in clarifying unanswered questions.

A team approach beginning at the time of diagnosis is extremely important. The enlistment of the combined resources of medical, nursing, medical social service, and community personnel will improve the quality and continuity of care.

Finally, the problems and reactions of the physician himself should not be overlooked. Emotional overinvolvement may compromise medical management and decision-making on the one hand, whereas repulsion by death and the impulse to retreat from the dying child on the other hand may deny the child and his family vital emotional support. The physician who treats children with leukemia, and whose aim is to provide optimal total care, must find a compromise between these extremes.[125]

*Bone marrow transplantation.*[27,40,65,141] The demonstration that several species of animals given lethal doses of irradiation will recover after the infusion of normal bone marrow prompted trial of this procedure in human beings. Leukemia particularly has been the object of energetic clinical experimentation.

It is of great interest that marrow injected intravenously seeks out the denuded marrow spaces and repopulates them. Theoretically, total body irradiation destroys the immunologic defenses so that heterotransplants of normal human bone marrow material might conceivably generate normal blood elements. The results thus far have been uniformly unsuccessful, although questionable transient improvement has been cited.[2] The collecting and storing of human marrow from living persons or cadavers for subsequent injection present formidable problems which are now in the process of solution. The successful transplantation of human bone marrow would offer long-sought-for help in the treatment of patients with aplastic anemia, leukemia, and disseminated neoplastic disease.

In summarizing the results of bone marrow transplantation, Ferrebee and Thomas[41] concluded that this procedure was experimental at present and only rarely useful to patients. Even with the transplantation of isogenic marrow (from an identical but normal twin) recurrences of leukemia have been discouragingly rapid in irradiated subjects. Either the leukemic cells are not eradicated by the amounts of radiation and drugs that are administered, or the agent of the disease finds itself resistant and equally able to infect the isogenic marrow that has been engrafted. The use of allogenic marrow (cells from donors with a different genetic background than the recipient) requires preliminary heavy radiation to render the recipient's marrow aplastic with the further risk of a serious or fatal wasting syndrome.

A number of attempts to utilize allogenic marrow grafts in patients with marrow failure or leukemia followed the demonstration of a transient marrow graft in a leukemic patient and the treatment of victims of an irradiation accident. Failure of recent attempts have been due to graft-versus-host disease or unsuccessful engraftment. Buckner and co-workers[15] believe that transplantation failures were caused for a variety of reasons. Donors had not been selected on the basis of histocompatibility testing, or patients were terminal at the time of transplantation, or isoimmunization against transplantation antigens had been induced by multiple prior transfusions. With recent advances in sophisticated histocompatibility testing and immunosuppressive therapy, more successful bone marrow transplants are to be expected. It had been hoped that allogenic bone marrow grafts might act as a powerful weapon by the action of the graft against the leukemic cells and perhaps against the leukemia virus.

In another case, an 8-year-old boy with acute lymphoblastic leukemia, no longer responsive to conventional chemotherapy after 2 years, was successfully grafted with bone marrow from his HL-A genotypically identical 10-year-old sister.[58] Except for the occurrence of a possible graft-versus-host reaction and a documented cytomegalovirus infection, the patient remained clinically well until full return of his leukemia 91 days after the transplant. This case also demonstrated that bone marrow transplantation can be accomplished between HL-A identical siblings even though the recipient may have been previously sensitized to other HL-A antigens by earlier transfusions. A regimen of immunosuppression using intravenous cyclophosphamide (180 mg./kg. given in four divided daily doses) after a stimulating dose of leukocytes from the donor was employed. Methotrexate was given after the donor bone marrow infusion to combat the possible graft-versus-host reaction. It is of interest that there was a slow disappearance of the marker chromosomes from the patient's marrow as leukemia recurred and that circulating female lymphocytes persisted in the patient's peripheral blood as late as 114 days following the graft.

During the past few years, the main transplantation antigen system of man—the HL-A system—has been identified. Therefore it was surprising that a graft-versus-host reaction ranging from mild to severe was observed in three of seven patients with acute lymphoblastic leukemia who had had an allogenic bone marrow engraftment from their HL-A antigen identical siblings.[59] Two patients died as a direct result of this complication of marrow transplantation. No definitive explanation could be given for the graft-versus-host reaction except that another transplantation system may be presumed to exist. It appears, therefore, for the success of clinical bone marrow transplantation, that more information is needed for specific tolerance and immunological enhancement.[34]

The successful outcome of bone marrow failure with bone marrow transplants from an identical twin carries the hope that this procedure will eventually be equally useful in leukemia. This possibility was also suggested in a group O child with acute lymphoblastic leukemia in whom 56% of the red cells were group AB, 6 weeks after he received white cell–rich plasma from a group AB donor with chronic myelogenous leukemia.[9] It was postulated that erythroid precursors or undifferentiated multipotential stem cells contained in the blood of the AB donor were successfully grafted to an O recipient whose immunologic mechanisms were temporarily impaired. The graft that produced AB cells was rejected 48 hours after the AB transfusion. It was also conceived that the $Ph^1$ chromosome present in chronic myeloid leukemia involves common precursor cells,[149] since both platelets and white cells rose after the transfusion.

The treatment of leukemia by extracorporeal irradiation has been successful in reducing the level of circulating leukemic lymphocytes. Whether or not this method will prove of value in childhood leukemia, especially in the leukopenic patients, awaits further study.[142]

**Laboratory determinations.** In the patient who is hospitalized, daily peripheral blood counts are important to determine the effect on the leukocyte count and leukemic cells; platelet and reticulocyte counts may be done periodically. The bone marrow is examined at the outset and again at the end of the initial induction period. Subsequently, peripheral blood counts may be carried out at weekly or biweekly intervals. Bone marrow examinations are required if suspicious signs of relapse develop, if marked leukopenia is noted in the peripheral blood, or if the patient's condition deteriorates so that a change in therapy is contemplated. Patients treated according to cooperative protocol studies require periodic bone marrow examinations. Not infrequently, bone marrow relapse is evident in the absence of abnormal physical and hematologic findings. Early diagnosis of relapse and prompt initiation of reinduction therapy will often obviate hospitalization.

Blood urea nitrogen and uric acid estimations are necessary in the event of a precipitous fall in the white blood cell count with signs of obstructive uremia. Liver function tests, including serum glutamic oxalacetic and glutamic pyruvic transaminases, and alkaline phosphatase are useful in patients being treated with potentially hepatotoxic agents.

*Treatment of nervous system involvement.* Nervous system involvement has been noted with increasing frequency in children whose lives have been prolonged with chemotherapy.[24,103] Frequently, neurologic symptoms occur while the peripheral blood and bone marrow are in remission. Vomiting, papilledema, separation of the cranial sutures, headache, stiff neck, and pleocytosis (lymphoblasts) point to leukemic infiltration of meningeal and nerve tissues. Some children may present with hyperphagia, weight gain, cranial nerve palsies, and drowsiness.[82] Irradiation to the brain or vertebral column to supplement chemotherapy has often been effective in relieving symptoms and in decreasing the cells in the spinal fluid.

Combined radiation and intrathecal chemotherapy are necessary in those cases in which there is not only involvement of the spinal meninges but also of nerve roots. Spinal involvement is suggested by complaints of leg and low back pain, refusal to walk, and, at times, fecal incontinence. In such circumstances indicating leukemic infiltration of the lumbosacral plexus, x-ray therapy to the lower spine is indicated.[138] When meningeal leukemia is combined with a peripheral seventh nerve paralysis, the treatment of choice is intrathecal methotrexate combined with radiation therapy, the portal being designed to include the extracranial and intraosseous course of the facial nerve.[35] Steroid hormones in the usual or increased dosage have also been useful. Another property of prednisone is that it is the only commonly used antileukemic drug to enter the cerebrospinal fluid in therapeutically significant quantity following oral or parenteral administration. It is often effective in controlling meningeal leukemic infiltrates.[70]

Methotrexate and 6-mercaptopurine in the doses used to control systemic leukemia do not pass the blood-brain barrier in quantities sufficient to control disease in the meninges and central nervous system. Because of this poor penetration into the cerebrospinal fluid, methotrexate (amethopterin) should be given intrathecally.[151] The dose is either 0.25 mg. per kilogram of body weight every second to third day or 0.5 mg. per kilogram every fourth to fifth day, with an additional dose after the spinal cell count has returned to normal.[103] The dose is given in 5 ml. of saline solution through a lumbar puncture at the level of the fourth and fifth lumbar vertebrae. Usually, three doses suffice, but more may be required depending on the spinal fluid response. During intrathecal therapy oral amethopterin (methotrexate) is discontinued.

Radiation therapy has often been proposed for the treatment of meningeal leukemia. This modality was investigated by Sullivan and co-workers[138] with and without intrathecal methotrexate. They found that injecting intrathecal methotrexate 0.5 mg./kg. every 2 to 3 days until the spinal fluid mononuclear cell count decreased to 10 cu. mm. or less produced spinal fluid remission in 78% of fifty-one children experiencing their first episode of CNS leukemia. Radiation of the entire cerebrospinal axis using a tumor dose of 1,000 rads resulted in a spinal fluid remission rate of 92%. A combination therapy of two injections of methotrexate preceding radiation of the entire cerebrospinal axis (750 to 1,000 rads tumor dose for children in marrow remission and 250 to 500 rads tumor dose for children in marrow relapse) and one injection of methotrexate intrathecally following radiation resulted in spinal fluid remission in 100% of the evaluable children in the treatment group. Symptomatic remissions occurred in 94% of the children. The duration of remission, however, was similar to that obtained with conventional intermittent methotrexate therapy.

The program of therapy varies in different clinics. Hyman and co-workers,[82] in an extensive experience, have found the need for administering one to seven courses of treatment in central nervous system leukemia. Each course consists of 0.2 mg. parenteral methotrexate per kilogram of body weight injected intrathecally every other day for four doses. At the time of each injection the spinal fluid pressure, white blood cell count, protein, and sugar are determined. If the cerebrospinal fluid findings are abnormal at the time of the fourth injection, a fifth lumbar puncture is performed 1 week later. If the spinal fluid is still abnormal, a second course of four injections is given. Patients receiving oral methotrexate do not receive oral therapy on the day the medication is given intrathecally, although other antimetabolites are continued unless intolerance or toxicity develops. They found also that intrathecal methotrexate may still be effective therapy for central nervous system leukemia in patients whose systemic disease was initially sensitive but later developed resistance to oral methotrexate. Symptoms of central nervous system leukemia may respond to lumbar puncture without the injection of methotrexate, but the abnormal centrospinal fluid findings were not significantly altered.

In a 9-year study of 205 patients with acute stem cell leukemia, Haghbin and Zuelzer[62] found sixty-one with central nervous system involvement. Treatment intrathecally with Aminopterin in a dosage of 0.1 mg. per kilogram of body weight for two to seven treatments was effective in controlling symptoms and decreasing the spinal fluid cell numbers.

The incidence of symptomatic CNS leukemia was studied in 209 children, all of whom were entered in a cooperative study during 1963-64 and received the same chemotherapeutic agents.[36] The overall incidence was 51% and the median time for occurrence of the first episode was 9 months. The incidence was 56% in patients with acute lymphoblastic leukemia and 25% in those with other forms of leukemia. It was concluded that the increasing survival of children with leukemia is the chief cause for the increased incidence of CNS leukemia. Most of the chemical agents used in the treatment of leukemia appear in the spinal fluid in insignificant concentrations. Corticosteroids, however, cross the blood-brain barrier and these are sometimes used in the treatment of CNS leukemia. It has been suggested that persistence of leukemic cells in the CNS provide a source of cells to reseed the marrow and possibly precipitate a hematologic relapse. Hence the reason for studies employing "sanctuary" therapy such as intrathecal medications, irradiation to the head and spine, or a combination of the two.

Another study showed that central nervous system involvement in leukemia occurred more frequently and more rapidly in patients who presented with elevated peripheral white blood cell counts. CNS infiltration not suspected clinically was identified by spinal fluid examination. However, intrathecal methotrexate administered prophylactically at the time of initial diagnosis of leukemia did not prevent or decrease the frequency of occurence of CNS infiltration. It was thought that it did delay the onset of CNS involvement in patients with elevated white blood cell counts.

The use of larger doses (2,400 R) of prophylactic radiation therapy to the cranium and cerebrospinal axis after the induction of remission has significantly reduced the incidence of CNS leukemia.[114] Controlled studies are now being mounted in an effort to determine optimal dose and treatment schedules.

*Results of treatment—prognosis for survival.* The beneficial effects of treatment may be measured by a comparison of the duration of life in the prehormonal era and in the posthormonal and chemotherapeutic era. In an analysis of cases[144] for the period in which no treatment was available, 50% of the children with acute leukemia given supportive therapy not including antibiotics expired within a period of approximately 4 months after the onset of the first definite symptoms. The middle two-thirds of patients survived from approximately 2 to 8 months and 10% for as long as 11 months. In a smaller series[111] 80% treated with transfusions alone survived less than 6 months. In another untreated group comprised of children and adults with acute leukemia, the figure of 50% survival at 4 months is given.[66]

In contrast to these groups is the effect on longevity of treatment with the antimetabolites, ACTH, and the adrenocortical hormones. With this program of treatment 25% still succumb within the first 6 months, although a small number survive beyond 2 years.[111] The increased survival in patients with the lymphoblastic type of leukemia that is prevalent in childhood has been emphasized, especially in those patients with counts below 10,000 per cubic millimeter.[67] The results of treatment have been summarized as follows[103]: for patients treated before folic acid antagonists were used the 50% survival time was 4 to 5 months as compared with 9.2 months when folic acid antagonists and/or adrenocortical steroids were used and 12.5 months since 6-mercaptopurine has been added.[103] Study of 300 patients with acute leukemia revealed that complete remissions became fewer with advancing age, both for all forms of leukemia taken together and more particularly for lymphoblastic leukemia.[3] In the latter, 75% of remissions occurred in children under 9 years of age, 50% from 9 to 20 years, and 35% thereafter. Equally impressive is the striking clinical improvement in most patients that accompanies the hematologic remission induced by the newer therapy.

In one protocol treatment consisted of vincristine and prednisone followed by 5-day parenteral intensive courses of methotrexate for a period of 8 additional months.[79] After every third course of methotrexate, another inducer course of vincristine and prednisone was added. Seventy-five percent of these children are alive at 24 months with a projected possibility that perhaps 25% will survive 5 years or more.

The National Cancer Institute reported that thirty-five children with acute leukemia treated intermittently with a high-dose, four-drug combination have had a median survival (survival of 50% of the group) of about 3 years. This represents twice the length of time anticipated 5 years previously when therapy was less intensive.[106] Together with the results cited by Burchenal[17] that sixteen children in his series have lived for 12 years or more with no leukemic relapse, this information provides hope for the eventual control of this disease.

Recent studies employing multiple agents with or without CNS irradiation produced median survivals of 33 and 35 months.[71,114] In the latter study, six of the twenty-six patients were alive 5 years after the diagnosis was made. Thus, considering the advances since 1948, it does not seem unreasonable to assume that larger numbers of patients with acute lymphoblastic leukemia will have prolonged survival.

## REFERENCES

1. Alvarado, J., Djerassi, I., and Farber, S.: Transfusion of fresh concentrated platelets to children with acute leukemia, J. Pediat. 67: 13, 1965.
2. Atkinson, J. B., Mahoney, F. J., Schwartz, I. R., and Hesch, J. A.: Therapy of acute leukemia by whole-body irradiation and bone marrow transplantation from an identical normal twin, Blood 14:228, 1959.
3. Bernard, J., and Boiron, M.: Etude de la rémission complete des leucémies aiguës, Bull. World Health Organ. 26:563, 1962.
4. Binger, C. M., Ablin, A. R., Feuerstein, R. C., Kushner, J. H., Zoger, S., and Mikkelsen, C.: Childhood leukemia; emotional impact

on patient and family, New Eng. J. Med. 280:414, 1969.
5. Bodey, G., McKelvey, E., and Karon, M.: Chickenpox in leukemic patients—factors in prognosis, Pediatrics 34:562, 1964.
6. Bodey, G. P., Nies, B. A., Mohberg, N. R., and Freireich, E. J.: Use of gamma globluin in infections in acute leukemia patients, J.A.M.A. 190:1099, 1964.
7. Boggs, D. R., Wintrobe, M. M., and Cartwright, G. E.: The acute leukemias, Medicine 41:163, 1962.
8. Boiron, M., Jacquillat, C., Weil, M., and Bernard, J.: Combination of methylglyoxal-bis-(guanyldrazone) [NSC 329446][1] and 6-mercaptopurine [NSC 755][2] in acute granulocytic leukemia, Cancer Chemother. Rep. 45:69, 1965.
8a. Bonadonna, G., Monfardini, S., De Lena, M., and Fossati-Bellani, F.: Clinical evaluation of adriamycin, a new antitumor antibiotic, Brit. Med. J. 2:503, 1969.
9. Bronson, W. R., McGinniss, M. H., and Morse, E. E.: Hematopoietic graft detected by a change in ABO group, Blood 23:239, 1964.
10. Brock, N., and Hohorst, H. J.: Metabolism of cyclophosphamide, Cancer 20:900, 1967.
11. Broome, J. D.: Evidence that the L-asparaginase activity of guinea pig serum is responsible for its antilymphoma effects, Nature 191:114, 1961.
12. Broome, J. D.: Studies on the mechanism of tumor inhibition by L-asparaginase. Effects of the enzyme on asparagine levels in the blood, normal tissues, and 6C3HED lymphomas of mice; differences in asparagine formation and utilization in asparaginase-sensitive and -resistant lymphoma cells, J. Exp. Med. 127:1055, 1968.
13. Brubaker, C. A., Gilchrist, G. S., Hammond, G. D., Hyman, C. B., Shore, N. A., and Williams, K. O.: Induction of remission in acute leukemia with prednisone and intravenous methotrexate, J. Pediat. 73:623, 1968.
14. Brubaker, C. A., Wheeler, H. E., Sonley, M. J., Hyman, C. B., Williams, K. O., and Hammond, D.: Cyclic chemotherapy for acute leukemia in children, Blood 22:820, 1963.
15. Buckner, C. D., Epstein, R. B., Rudolph, R. H., Clift, R. A., Storb, R., and Thomas, E. D.: Allogeneic marrow engraftment following whole body irradiation in a patient with leukemia, Blood 35:741, 1970.
16. Burchenal, J. H.: The treatment of leukemia, Bull. N. Y. Acad. Med. 30:429, 1954.
17. Burchenal, J. H.: Formal discussion; long-term survival in Burkitt's tumor and in acute leukemia, Cancer Res. 27:2616, 1967.
18. Burchenal, J. H.: Long-term survivors in acute leukemia and Burkitt's tumor, Cancer 21:595, 1968.
19. Burchenal, J. H., and Murphy, M. L.: Long-term survivors in acute leukemia, Cancer Res. 25:1491, 1965.
20. Burchenal, J. H., Murphy, M. L., and Tan, C. T. C.: Review article; the treatment of acute leukemia, Pediatrics 18:643, 1956.
21. Clark, P. A., Hsia, Y. E., and Huntsman, R. G.: Toxic complications of treatment with 6-mercaptopurine; 2 cases with hepatic necrosis and intestinal ulceration, Brit. M. J. 1:393, 1960.
22. Clarysse, A. M., Cathey, W. J., Cartwright, G. E., and Wintrobe, M. M.: Pulmonary disease complicating intermittent therapy with methotrexate, J.A.M.A. 209:1861, 1969.
23. Colebatch, J. H., Balkie, A. G., Clark, A. C. L., Jones, D. L., Lee, C. W. G., Lewis, I. C., and Newman, N. M.: Cyclic drug regimen for acute childhood leukaemia, Lancet 1:313, 1968.
24. Cramblett, H. G.: Recognition and treatment of intracranial manifestations of leukemia, Amer. J. Dis. Child. 97:805, 1959.
25. Criteria used for evaluation of clinical status of acute leukemia (9/15/63), Cancer Chemotherap. Rep. 42:27, 1964.
26. Dameshek, W.: The outlook for the eventual control of leukemia, New Eng. J. Med. 250:131, 1954.
27. Dameshek, W.: Bone marrow transplantation; a present-day challenge, Blood 12:321, 1957.
28. Dameshek, W., and Mitus, W. J.: Seven year remission in an adult with acute leukemia, New Eng. J. Med. 268:870, 1963.
29. Dameshek, W., Necheles, T. F., Finkel, H. E., and Allen, D. M.: Therapy of acute leukemia, 1965 (editorial), Blood 26:220, 1965.
30. Denko, C. W., and Schroeder, L. R.: Ecchymotic skin lesions in patients receiving prednisone, J.A.M.A. 164:41, 1957.
30a. Di Marco, A., Gaetani, M., and Scarpinato, B.: Adriamycin (NSC-123127): a new antibiotic with antitumor activity, Cancer Chemother. Rep. 53:33, 1969.
31. Djerassi, I., Farber, S., and Evans, A. E.: Transfusions of fresh platelet concentrates to patients with secondary thrombocytopenia, New Eng. J. Med. 268:221, 1963.
32. Dmochowski, L.: Current status of the relationship of viruses to leukemia, lymphoma and solid tumors in leukemia-lymphoma, Chicago, 1970, Year Book Medical Publishers, Inc., p. 37.
33. Dougherty, T. F., and White, A.: Role of pituitary adrenotropic hormone in regula-

tion of lymphocytes and other cellular elements of blood, Endocrinology 35:1, 1944.
34. Editorial: Bone marrow transplantation; unexpected results, Lancet 1:26, 1971.
35. Evans, A. F., D'Angio, G. J., and Mitus, A.: Central nervous system complication of children with acute leukemia; an evaluation of treatment methods, J. Pediat. 64:94, 1964.
36. Evans, A. F., Gilbert, E. S., and Zandstra, R.: The increasing incidence of central nervous system leukemia in children (Children's Cancer Study Group A), Cancer 26:404, 1970.
37. Farber, S., Diamond, L. K., Mercer, R. D., Sylvester, R. F., Jr., and Wolff, J. A.: Temporary remissions in acute leukemia in children produced by folic acid antagonist, 4-aminopteroyl–glutamic acid (Aminopterin), New Eng. J. Med. 238:787, 1948.
38. Feldman, F., and Tan, C. V.: Acute leukemia—relapse after a prolonged remission, J. Pediat. 76:926, 1970.
39. Fernbach, D. J., Sutow, W. W., Thurman, W. G., and Vietti, T. J.: Clinical evaluation of cyclophosphamide; a new agent for the treatment of children with acute leukemia, J.A.M.A. 182:30, 1962.
40. Ferrebee, J. W., Atkins, L., Lochte, H. L., Jr., McFarland, R. B. Jones, A. R., Dammin, G. J., and Thomas, E. D.: The collection, storage and preparation of viable cadaver marrow for intravenous use, Blood 14:140, 1959.
41. Ferrebee, J. W., and Thomas, E. D.: Present status of bone marrow transplantation, Ped. Clin. N. Amer. 9:851, 1962.
41a. Fine, R. N., Clarke, R. R., and Shore, N. A.: Hyponatremia and vincristine therapy, Amer. J. Dis. Child. 112:256, 1966.
42. Finkel, K. G.: Mortality from varicella in children receiving adrenocorticosteroids and adrenocorticotropin, Pediatrics 28:436, 1961.
43. Fischer, G. A.: Increased levels of folic acid reductase as a mechanism of resistance to amethopterin in leukemic cells, Biochem. Pharmacol. 7:75, 1961.
44. Fountain, J. R.: The chemotherapy of acute leukemia; a review of its present status, Edinburgh M. J. 61:69, 1954.
45. Frei, E., III.: Chemotherapy of acute leukemia, C.A. 14:252, 1964.
46. Frei, E., III, Bentzel, C., Roselbach, R., and Block, J.: Renal complications of neoplastic disease, J. Chron. Dis. 16:757, 1963.
47. Frei, E., III, and others: Studies of sequential and combination antimetabolite therapy in acute leukemia; 6-mercaptopurine and methotrexate, Blood 18:431, 1961.
48. Frei, E., III, and others: The effectiveness of combinations of antileukemic agents in inducing and maintaining remission in children with acute leukemia, Blood 26:642, 1965.
49. Freireich E. J., and Frei, E., III: Recent advances in acute leukemia. In Moore, C. V., and Brown, E. B., editors: Progress in hematology, vol. IV, New York, 1964, Grune & Stratton, Inc.
50. Freireich, E. J., Karon, M., and Frei, E., III: Quadruple combination therapy (VAMP) for acute lymphocytic leukemia in childhood (abstract), Proc. Amer. Ass. Cancer Res. 5:20, 1964.
51. Friedman, S. B.: Care of the family of the child with cancer, Pediatrics 40 (Part II): 498, 1967.
52. Friedman, S. B., Chodoff, P., Mason, J. W., and Hamburg, D. A.: Behavioral observation on parents anticipating the death of a child, Pediatrics 32:610, 1963.
53. Galton, D. A. G.: Chemotherapy of chronic myelocytic leukemia, Seminars Hemat. 6:323, 1969.
54. Galton, D. A. G., and Till, M.: Myleran in chronic granulocyte leukemia, Lancet 1:425, 1955.
55. Gee, T. S., Yu, K-P., and Clarkson, B. D.: Treatment of adult acute leukemia with arabinosylcytosine and thioguanine, Cancer 23:1019, 1969.
56. George, P., Hernandez, K., Hustu, H. O., Borella, L., Holton, C. P., and Pinkel, D.: A study of "total therapy" of acute lymphocytic leukemia in children, J. Pediat. 72:399, 1968.
57. Gitlin, D., Commerford, L., and Hughes, W. L.: Inhibition of the incorporation of iododeoxyuridine into DNA by cortisone, Society for Pediatrics Research, paper No. 10, 30th annual meeting, May 3 and 4, 1960, Swampscott, Mass.
58. Graw, R. G., Jr., Brown, J. A., Yankee, R. A., Leventhal, B. G., Whang-Peng, J., Rogentine, G. N., and Henderson, E. S.: Transplantation of HL-A identical allogenic bone marrow to a patient with acute lymphoblastic leukemia, Blood 36:736, 1970.
59. Graw, R. G., Jr., Herzig, G. P., Rogentine, G. N., Jr., Yankee, R. A., Leventhal, B., Whang-Peng, J., Halterman, R. H., Krüger, G., Bernard, C., and Henderson, E. S.: Graft-versus-host reaction complicating HL-A matched bone marrow transplantation, Lancet 2:1053, 1970.
60. Green, M.: Care of the dying child, Pediatrics 40(Part II):492, 1967.
61. Haddow, A., and Timmis, G. M.: Myleran in chronic myeloid leukemia, Lancet 1:207, 1953.
62. Haghbin, M., and Zuelzer, W. W.: A long-

term study of cerebrospinal leukemia, J. Pediat. 67:23, 1965.
63. Hall, T. C.: Chemotherapy of cancer, New Eng. J. Med. 266:238, 1962.
64. Hamilton, L., and Elion, G. B.: The fate of 6-mercaptopurine in man, Ann. N. Y. Acad. Sci. 60:304, 1954.
65. Haurani, F. I., Repplinger, E., and Tocantins, L. M.: Attempts at transplantation of human bone marrow in patients with acute leukemia and other marrow depletion disorders, Amer. J. Med. 28:794, 1960.
66. Haut, A., Altman, S. J., Cartwright, G. E., and Wintrobe, M. M.: The influence of chemotherapy on survival in acute leukemia, Blood 10:875, 1955.
67. Haut, A., Altman, S. J., Wintrobe, M. M., and Cartwright, G. E.: The influence of chemotherapy on survival in acute leukemia, comparison of cases treated during 1954 to 1957 with those treated during 1947 to 1954, Blood 14:828, 1959.
68. Henderson, E. S.: Combination chemotherapy of acute lymphocytic leukemia of childhood, Cancer Res. 27:2570, 1967.
69. Henderson, E. S.: Treatment of acute leukemia (editorial), Ann. Intern. Med. 69:628, 1968.
70. Henderson, E. S.: Treatment of acute leukemia, Seminars Hemat. 6:271, 1969.
71. Henderson, E. S., and Samaha, R. J.: Evidence that drugs in multiple combinations have materially advanced the treatment of human malignancies, Cancer Res. 29:2272, 1969.
72. Hersh, E., Wong, V. G., Henderson, E. S., and Freireich, E. J.: Hepatoxic effects of methotrexate, Cancer 19:600, 1966.
73. Heyn, R. M., Brubaker, C. A., Burchenal, J. H., Cramblett, H. G., and Wolff, J. A.: The comparison of 6-mercaptopurine with the combination of 6-mercaptopurine and azaserine in the treatment of acute leukemia in children; results of a cooperative study, Blood 15:350, 1960.
74. Hill, J. M., Marshall, G. J., and Falco, D. J.: Massive predisone and prednisolone therapy in leukemia and lymphomas in the adult, J. Amer. Geriat. Soc. 4:627, 1956.
75. Hills, A. G., Forsham, P. H., and Finch, C. A.: Changes in the circulatory leukocytes induced by administration of pituitary adrenocorticotrophic hormone (ACTH) in man, Blood 3:755, 1948.
76. Hitchings, G. H., and Elion, G. B.: The chemistry and biochemistry of purine analogues, Ann. N. Y. Acad. Sci. 60:195, 1954.
77. Hoga, T., and Laszlo, J.: Döhle bodies and other granulocytic alterations during chemotherapy with cyclophosphamide, Blood 20:668, 1962.
78. Holland, J. F.: Who should treat leukemia? J.A.M.A. 209:1511, 1969.
79. Holland, J. F.: Hopes for tomorrow become realities of today; therapy and prognosis in acute lymphocytic leukemia of childhood, Pediatrics 45:191, 1970.
80. Holland, J. F., and Glidewell, O.: Induction, consolidation, intensification, reinduction and maintenance chemotherapy of acute lymphocytic leukemia, Abstracts, XII Congress Int. Soc. Hemat. 1968, p. 9.
81. Huguley, C. M., Jr., and others: Comparison of 6-mercaptopurine and busulfan in chronic granulocytic leukemia, Blood 21:89, 1963.
82. Hyman, C. B., Bogle, J. M., Brubacker, C. A., Williams, K., and Hammond, G. D.: Central nervous system involvement by leukemia in children. II. Therapy with intrathecal methotrexate, Blood 25:13, 1965.
83. Hyman, C. B., Borda, E., Brubaker, C. A., Hammond, G. D., and Sturgeon, P.: Prednisone in childhood leukemia, Pediatrics 24:1005, 1961.
84. Karnofsky, D. A., and Clarkson, B. D.: Cellular effects of anticancer drugs, Ann. Rev. Pharmacol. 3:357, 1963.
85. Karon, M. R., Freireich, E. J., and Frei, E., III: A preliminary report on vincristine sulfate; a new active agent for the treatment of acute leukemia, Pediatrics 30:791, 1962.
86. Karon, M., and Vernick, J.: An approach to the emotional support of fatally ill children, Clin. Pediat. 7:274, 1968.
87. Kidd, J. G.: Regression of transplanted lymphomas induced in vivo by means of normal guinea-pig serum. I. Course of transplanted cancers of varying kinds in mice and rats given guinea pig sera, horse sera or rabbit sera, J. Exp. Med. 98:565, 1953.
88. Klein, E., Toch, R., Farber, S., Freeman, G., and Fiorentino, R.: Hemostasis in thrombocytopenic bleeding following infusion of stored, frozen platelets, Blood 11:693, 1956.
89. Knospe, W. H., and Conrad, M. E., Jr.: The danger of corticosteroids in acute granulocytic leukemia, Med. Clin. N. Amer. 50:1653, 1966.
90. Krakoff, I. H., and Murphy, M. L.: Hyperuricemia in neoplastic disease in children; prevention with allopurinol, a xanthine oxidase inhibitor, Pediatrics 41:52, 1968.
91. Krivit, W., Brubaker, C. A., Hartman, J., Murphy, M. L., Pierce, M., and Thatcher, L. G.: Induction of remission in acute leukemia of childhood by combination of prednisone and either 6-mercaptopurine or methotrexate, J. Pediat. 68:965, 1966.

92. Krivit, W., Gilchrist, G., and Beatty, E. C., Jr.: The need for chemotherapy after prolonged complete remission in acute leukemia of chilhood, J. Pediat. 76:138, 1970.
93. Kyles, R. A., Schwartz, R. S., Oliner, H. L., and Dameshek, W.: A syndrome resembling adrenal cortical insufficiency associated with long term busulfan (Myleran) therapy, Blood 18:497, 1961.
94. Leikin, S. L.: Leukemia—current concepts in therapy, Ped. Clin. N. Amer. 9:753, 1962.
95. Louis, J., Limarzi, L. R., and Best, W. R.: Treatment of chronic granulocytic leukemia with Myleran, Arch. Intern. Med. 97:299, 1956.
96. Mandel, H. G.: The physiological disposition of some anticancer agents, Pharmacol. Rev. 11:743, 1959.
97. Martin, J., and Compston, N.: Vincristine sulphate in the treatment of lymphoma and leukemia, Lancet 2:1080, 1963.
98. Mathé, G., Amiel, J. L., Schwarzenberg, L., Schneider, M., Cattan, A., Schlumberger, J. R., Hayat, M., and de Vassal, F.: Active immunotherapy for acute lymphoblastic leukaemia, Lancet 1:697, 1969.
99. Mathé, G., Hayat, M., Schwarzenberg, L., Schneider, M., Cattan, A., Schlumberger, J. R., and Jasmin, C.: Acute lymphoblastic leukemia treated with a combination of prednisone, Vincristine and Rubidomycin; value of pathogen-free rooms, Lancet 2:380, 1967.
100. McIlvanie, S. K., and MacCarthy, J. D.: Hepatitis in association with prolonged 6-mercaptopurine therapy, Blood 14:80, 1959.
101. Melhorn, D. K., Gross, S., Fisher, B. J., and Newman, A. J.: Studies on the use of "prophylactic" intrathecal amethopterin in childhood leukemia, Blood 36:55, 1970.
102. Mercaptopurine and nucleic acid synthesis, Nutrit. Rev. 13:247, 1955.
102a. Middleman, E., Luce, J., and Frei, E. III: Clinical trials with adriamycin, Cancer 28:844, 1971.
103. Murphy, M. L.: Leukemia and lymphoma in children, Ped. Clin. N. Amer. 6:611, 1959.
104. Murphy, M. L.: Acute leukemia. In Gellis, S. S., and Kagen, B. M., editors: Current pediatric therapy, Philadelphia, 1964, W. B. Saunders Co., p. 275.
105. Nagao, T., Lampkin, B. C., and Warren, A. M.: Maintenance therapy in acute childhood leukemia, J. Pediat. 76:134, 1970.
106. National Advisory Cancer Council: Progress against cancer, 1970, p. 8.
106a. Nesbit, M. E., Jr., and Lowman, J. T.: Hematopoiesis and serum iron changes following vincristine sulfate, Blood 34:633, 1969.
107. Nies, B. A., Bodey, G. P., Thomas, L. B., Brecher, G., and Freireich, E. J.: The persistence of extramedullary leukemic infiltrates during bone marrow remission of acute leukemia, Blood 26:133, 1965.
108. Oppenheimer, E. G., and Boitnott, J. K.: Pancreatitis in children following adrenal corticosteroid therapy, Bull. Johns Hopkins Hosp. 107:297, 1961.
109. Perrin, J. C. S., Mauer, A. M., and Sterling, T. D.: Intravenous methotrexate (Amethopterin) therapy in the treatment of acute leukemia, Pediatrics 31:833, 1963.
110. Perry, S.: Biochemistry of the white blood cell, J.A.M.A. 190:918, 1964.
111. Pierce, M. I.: The acute leukemias of childhood, Ped. Clin. N. Amer. 4:497, 1957.
112. Pinkel, D.: Chickenpox and leukemia, J. Pediat. 58:729, 1961.
113. Pinkel, D.: Prognosis of childhood leukemia, Pediatrics 44:619, 1969.
114. Pinkel, D.: Five year follow-up of childhood leukemia, J.A.M.A. 216:648, 1971.
115. Pinkel, D. P., Simone, J. V., Hustu, H. O., and Aur, R. J.: "Total therapy" of childhood acute lymphocytic leukemia, Proc. Soc. Ped. Res. 1971, Atlantic City, p. 70.
116. Pratt, C. B., Simone, J. V., Zee, P., Aur, R. J. A., and Johnson, W. W.: Comparison of daily versus weekly L-asparaginase for the treatment of childhood acute leukemia, J. Pediat. 77:474, 1970.
117. Progress against Cancer—A report by the National Advisory Cancer Council, 1969, p. 35, published by U. S. Department of Health, Education and Welfare.
118. Raab, S. A., Hoeprich, P. D., Wintrobe, M. M., and Cartwright, G. E.: The clinical significance of fever in acute leukemia, Blood 16:1609, 1960.
119. Ragab, A. A., Frech, R. S., and Vietti, T. J.: Osteoporotic fractures secondary to methotrexate therapy of acute leukemia in remission, Cancer 25:580, 1970.
120. Ranney, H. M., and Gellhorn, A.: The effect of massive prednisone and prednisolone therapy on acute leukemia and malignant lymphomas, Amer. J. Med. 22:405, 1957.
121. Rieselbach, R. E., Bentzel, C. J., Cotlove, E., Frei, E., III, and Freireich, E. J.: Uric acid excretion and renal function in the acute hyperuricemia of leukemia; pathogenesis and therapy of uric acid nephropathy, Amer. J. Med. 37:872, 1964.
122. Robson, H. N., and Duthie, J. J. R.: Capillary resistance and adrenocortical activity, Brit. M. J. 2:971, 1950.
123. Robson, H. N., and Duthie, J. J. R.: Further observations on capillary resistance and ad-

renocortical activity, Brit. M. J. 1:994, 1952.
124. Ross, A. H.: Modification of chickenpox in family contacts by administration of gamma globulin, New Eng. J. Med. 267:369, 1962.
125. Rothenberg, M. B.: Reactions of those who treat children with cancer, Pediatrics 40 (Part II):507, 1967.
126. Sandberg, A. A., Cartwright, G. E., and Wintrobe, M. M.: Studies on leukemia, Blood 11:154, 1956.
127. Saunders, E. F., Kauder, E., and Mauer, A. M.: Sequential therapy of acute leukemia in childhood, J. Pediat. 70:632, 1967.
128. Saunders, E. F., and Mauer, A. M.: Reentry of nondividing leukemic cells into a proliferative phase in acute childhood leukemia, J. Clin. Invest. 48:1299, 1969.
129. Sharp, H. L., Nesbit, M. E., D'Angio, G. J., and Krivit, W.: Addition of local radiation after bone marrow remission in acute leukemia in children, Cancer 20:1403, 1967.
130. Silver, R. T.: Infectious fever and host resistance in neoplastic disease, J. Chron. Dis. 16:677, 1963.
131. Sinks, L. F., Newton, W. A., Jr., Nagi, N. A., and Stevenson, T. D.: A syndrome associated with extreme hyperuricemia in leukemia, J. Pediat. 68:578, 1966.
132. Skipper, H. E., Schabel, F. M., Jr., and Wilcox W. S.: Experimental evaluation of potential anticancer agents. XIII. On the criteria and kinetics associated with "curability" of experimental leukemia, Cancer Chemotherapy Rep. 35:3, 1964.
133. Smith, C. H., and Bell, W. R.: Aminopterin in treatment of leukemia in children; serial aspirations of bone marrow as a guide to management and appraisal of treatment, Amer. J. Dis. Child. 79:1031, 1950.
134. Solomon, J., Alexander, M. J., and Steinfeld, J. L.: Cyclophosphamide; a clinical study, J.A.M.A. 183:165, 1963.
135. Sonley, M. J., Nesbit, M. E., Samuels, L., Thatcher, L. G., Karon, M., and Hammond, G. D.: Cytosine arabincside, cyclophosphamide and vincristine in children with acute myelogenous leukemia, Proc. Am. Soc. Hemat. 1970, San Juan, p. 104.
136. Stefanini, M.: Ecchymoses following prednisone therapy, J.A.M.A. 164:1383, 1957.
137. Stefanini, M., and Martino, N. B.: Use of prednisone in the management of some hemorrhagic states, New Eng. J. Med. 254:313, 1956.
138. Sullivan, M. P.: Leukemic infiltration of meninges and spinal nerve roots, Pediatrics 32:63, 1963.
139. Sullivan, M. P., Vietti, T. J., Fernbach, D. J., Griffith, K. M., Haddy, T. B., and Watkins, W. L.: Clinical investigations in the treatment of meningeal leukemia; radiation therapy regimens vs. conventional intrathecal methotrexate, Blood 34:301, 1969.
140. Swenseid, M. E., Bethell, F. H., and Bird, O. D.: Concentration of folic acid in leukocytes, Cancer Res. 9:441, 1963.
141. Thomas, E. D., Lochte, H. L., Jr., and Ferrebee, J. W.: Irradiation of the entire body and marrow transplantation; some observations and comments, Blood 14:1, 1959.
142. Thomas, E. D., Epstein, R. B., Eschbach, J. W., Jr., Prager, D., Buckner, C. D., and Marsaglia, G.: Treatment of leukemia by extracorporeal irradiation, New Eng. J. Med. 273:6, 1965.
143. Tilley, R. F.: Present status of antifungal antibiotics, Ped. Clin. N. Amer. 9:377, 1962.
144. Tivey, H.: Prognosis for survival in leukemias of childhood; review of literature and proposal of simple method of reporting survival data for these diseases, Pediatrics 10:48, 1952.
145. Vernick J., and Karon, M.: Who's afraid of death on a leukemia ward? Amer. J. Dis. Child. 109:393, 1965.
146. Vietti, T. J., Sullivan, M. P., Berry, D. H., Haddy, T. B., Haggard, M. E., and Blattner, R. J.: The response of acute childhood leukemia to an initial and a second course of prednisone, J. Pediat. 66:18, 1965.
147. Welch, A. D.: The mechanism of action of folic and antagonists, Proceedings of the Third Annual Meeting of the American Society of Hematology, Montreal, 1960.
148. Wetherley-Mein, G., and Cottone, D. G.: Fresh blood transfusion in leukemia, Brit. J. Haemat. 2:25, 1956.
149. Whang, J., Frei, E., III, Tjio, J. H., Carbone, P. P., and Brecher, G.: The distribution of the Philadelphia chromosome in patients with chronic myelogenous leukemia, Blood 22:664, 1963.
150. Whitaker, J. A., Shaheedy, M., Baum, J., James, J., and Flume, J. B.: Gout in childhood leukemia; report of a case and concepts of etiology, J. Pediat. 63:961, 1963.
151. Whiteside, J. A., Philips, F. S., Dargeon, H. W., and Burchenal, J. H.: Intrathecal methotrexate therapy in children with neurological manifestations of acute leukemia, Arch. Intern. Med. 101:279, 1958.
152. Wilbur, J. R., Sutow, W. W., Sullivan, M. P., and Mumford, D. M.: Treatment for acute leukemia in children, Chicago, 1970, Year Book Medical Publishers, Inc.
153. Willoughby, M. L. N., and Laurie, H. C.: Cyclic chemotherapy in childhood acute leukaemia, Arch. Dis. Child. 43:187, 1968.

154. Wintrobe, M. M.: Clinical hematology, ed. 5, Philadelpha, 1961, Lea & Febiger.
155. Wolff, J. A., Brubaker, C. A., Murphy, M. L.: Pierie, M. I., and Severo, N.: Prednisone therapy of acute childhood leukemia; prognosis and duration of response in 330 treated patients, J. Pediat. **70**:626, 1967.
155a. Wollner, N., Tan, C., Ghavimi, F., Rosen, G., Tefft, M., and Murphy, M. L.: Adriamycin in childhood leukemia and solid tumors, Proc. 62nd Ann. Amer. Ass. Cancer Res., April 8-10, 1971, Chicago.
156. Woods, D. D.: Relation of p-aminobenzoic acid to mechanism of action of sulphanilamide, Brit. J. Exp. Path. **21**:74, 1940.
157. Woolley, D. W.: A study of antimetabolites, New York, 1952, John Wiley & Sons, Inc.
158. Woolley, D. W.: Antimetabolites, Science **129**:615, 1959.
159. Zuelzer, W. W.: Implications of long-term survival in acute stem cell leukemia of childhood treated with composite cyclic therapy, Blood **24**:477, 1964.
160. Zuelzer, W. W., and Flatz, G.: Acute childhood leukemia; a ten-year study, Amer. J. Dis. Child. **100**:866, 1960.

# 24 LEUKEMIA—ALLIED DISORDERS

There are a number of conditions of a leukemic nature that occur infrequently which resemble the more common forms clinically and are characterized by an abnormal cell of an unusual type. Also allied to this unusual group of leukemias are the solid leukocytic neoplasms such as chloroma and the lymphomas in which the process is aleukemic in a few sites at the onset but which, as it becomes generalized, may simulate the typical blood and bone marrow picture of leukemia.

**Infrequent types of leukemia.** Among the unusual types of leukemia and extremely uncommon in children are the mast cell, basophilic, and plasma cell leukemias.

*Mast cell leukemia.* Mast cells which have been shown to produce the characteristic skin lesions in urticara pigmentosa can occasionally infiltrate many viscera and supporting tissues. Ellis[42] described the involvement of the skin, bone marrow, mesenteric lymph nodes, spleen, and liver in a 1-year-old infant. Bone marrow involvement is reflected in the roentgenogram by marked thickening and increased density especially of the frontal bone of the skull and coarsening of the trabeculations and thinning of the cortices in the small and large tubular bones.[103] Conditions in which there is splenic involvement with a generalized visceral distribution of cells, hepatosplenomegaly, the appearance of mast cells in the peripheral blood, anemia, and at times thrombocytopenia have been classified as mast cell leukemia.[41,48,141] The difficulty of separating the mast cell from the blood basophil is reflected in the patient in whom tissue and marrow mastocytosis is associated with blood basophilia.[4] The differentiation between the tissue mast cell and basophilic leukocyte is described elsewhere (Chapter 18).

*Basophilic leukemia.* Increased numbers of basophilic cells have been described in the course of chronic myelocytic leukemia. In one instance of acute leukemia in a 5-month-old infant, mature basophilic leukocytes and myelocytes predominated.[34] In another case in a young adult mature basophilic cells characterized the blood smear but were not associated with immature forms.[53]

*Plasma cell leukemia.* Cases of leukemia have been described in which plasma cells appeared in large numbers in the peripheral blood accompanied by anemia and leukocytosis. These cells were found to have diffusely infiltrated the spleen, liver, lymph nodes, and bone marrow rather than to have aggregated as nodular masses as they do in multiple myeloma.[85,89] Hyperglobinemia and occasionally Bence Jones proteinuria can sometimes be present.[89] These cases are often difficult to differentiate from multiple myeloma, which may also be accompanied by substantial numbers of plasma cells in the peripheral blood.[119]

Multiple myeloma is primarily a disease of later life and occurs rarely in childhood.[25] In a 7½-year-old Negro male with multiple myeloma, severe epistaxis was the presenting symptom. Pancytopenia was present, and the bone marrow showed typical myeloma cells.[99] Serum gamma globulin was greatly elevated (32.5%).

The typical myeloma cells are moderately large (15 to 25$\mu$), usually oval, with a large nucleus and abnormally large and prominent nucleoli. The chromatin is not as coarse as in the plasma cell, and the wheelspoke arrangement is absent. The cytoplasm is basophilic and bright blue, not blue-green as in the plasma cell. Acidophilic inclusions (Russell bodies) may be present.

A bizarre type of plasma cell has been found in the bone marrow of multiple myeloma which is designated as the "grape cell" because the cytoplasm contains multiple globular bodies apparently adherent to each other.[130] They have a gray-blue stain and are differentiated from Russell bodies, which have an affinity for the red or eosin stain.

Cases of multiple myeloma should be further differentiated from plasmacytosis and hypergammaglobulinemia. Transient marked plasmacytosis of the bone marrow and hypergammaglobulinemia have been observed in a 12-year-old girl with acute leukemia and may have been the manifestation of a reaction to penicillin.[131]

**Bone marrow replacement and leukoerythroblastosis.** Space-occupying lesions of the bone marrow resulting from infiltration with foreign cells or an overgrowth of fibrous or bony tissue are associated with a heterogeneous group of diseases. This process results in a chronic progressive anemia, a low or occasionally greatly elevated leukocyte count, and the presence of varying numbers of immature myeloid and erythroid cells in the peripheral blood.[98] These conditions are accompanied by marked enlargement of the spleen and liver in which blood cells are produced, which normally originate in the bone marrow. The resulting blood disorders have been described under the title of myelophthisic or leukoerythroblastic anemia, and since anemia need not necessarily be present the blood response may be termed leukoerythroblastosis.

Leukoerythroblastosis is characterized by the presence of immature leukocytes of the myeloid series in the peripheral blood and nucleated red cells out of proportion to the degree of anemia. It may be provoked by invasion of the bone marrow by malignant cells of organs likely to metastasize to the bones, usually carcinomas. Children with lymphosarcoma and Hodgkin's disease may develop this type of blood response. The abnormal blood picture results from irritation or stimulation of normal adjacent marrow into excessive myeloid and erythropoietic activity.

**Myelofibrosis.** The syndrome of myelofibrosis is a myeloproliferative process involving the bone marrow, accompanied by extramedullary hemopoiesis and splenic enlargement. It occurs less frequently in children than in adults. The process may be either focal or generalized or primary or secondary and is of varying grades of severity. Myelosclerosis is characterized by increased production of fibrous (myelofibrosis) and bony tissue (osteosclerosis). Fibrosis and osteosclerosis of the marrow occur as a primary and idiopathic disease and in connection with such conditions as polycythemia in the course of the disease and in the "spent" phase, leukemia, Hodgkin's disease, Gaucher's disease, xanthomatosis, tuberculosis, infections caused by chemical or physical agents, and renal rickets.[44] A diverse terminology has been applied to the syndrome, such as myeloid metaplasia of the spleen, leukoerythroblastic anemia, osteosclerosis, agnogenic myeloid metaplasia of the spleen, and erythroleukemia (Di Guglielmo's syndrome).

Theories regarding pathogenesis include necrobiosis (due to the toxic action of radioactive phosphorus, radium, benzene, or other agents) or primary bone marrow failure, with myeloid metaplasia as a compensatory process. A current theory classifies myelofibrosis in the group of myeloproliferative disorders.[40] Depending on the phase of the disease or the form it takes in a particular patient, the myeloproliferative disorder may take the form of polycythemia vera, myelogenous leukemia, erythroleukemia of Di Guglielmo, or myelofibrosis. Although a myelostimulatory factor has been heretofore postulated, there is now evidence from a study of Hiroshima victims to implicate ionizing irradiation as a causative factor in cases of myelofibrosis.[2]

Agnogenic myeloid metaplasia is currently regarded as part of the myeloproliferative disorders.[91] Frequently it is impossible to distinguish agnogenic myeloid metaplasia from chronic myelocytic leukemia during life. A number of cases of myeloid metaplasia terminate in acute leukemia.

Myelofibrosis is associated with slight to marked leukocytosis, a leukemoid reaction with early granulocytes, myelocytes, and occasionally myeloblasts, variation in red cell morphology with normoblasts and teardrop-shaped erythrocytes,[16,73] anisocytosis, poikilocytosis, variable platelet levels, circulating megakaryocytic fragments, and tissue megakaryocytosis.[12] The hemoglobin level is usually low but may be normal. Aspiration of a hypocellular bone marrow and difficulty in obtaining marrow at aspiration because of hardness of the bone indicate the presence of fibrous or other pathologic tissue. Dry taps are frequently encountered in attempts to aspirate the marrow.[143] Bone marrow biopsy, which is frequently necessary, reveals patchy myelofibrosis, hyperplastic focuses of myelopoiesis, and often increased numbers of megakaryocytes. Roentgenographic examination reveals changes suggestive of osteosclerosis in variable parts of the skeleton such as the ribs, pelvis, spine, and femora. As the disease progresses, the liver and spleen enlarge and anemia develops. Evidence of increased hemolysis is indicated by fecal urobilinogen, reticulocytosis, and red cell survival studies.[69]

Although fibrosis of the bone marrow with extramedullary hematopoiesis usually occurs in adults, such cases have been reported in pediatric patients. The findings in the latter also consist of fibrosis of the bone marrow, hepatosplenomegaly with immature granulocytic and erythrocytic elements in the peripheral blood, and a predominance of megakaryocytes in the spleen and bone marrow.[104] A typical case has been reported in a 7½-month-old infant.[113]

Treatment consists of transfusions and splenectomy when blood requirements are excessive. Despite the apparent need for the spleen as a source of extramedullary hematopoiesis, splenectomy has often been effective when the hemolytic component accompanies its enlargement.[12,52] Preliminary treatment with adrenocorticosteroids has been employed to determine whether it will stimulate red cell production, decrease the rate of hemolysis, or both.[12] Testosterone has been found of considerable value in adults. With prolonged treatment, increased hemoglobin, reticulocytosis, a hypercellular marrow, and reduced transfusion requirements have been reported.[68] Splenectomy is not undertaken until full evaluation is made, especially for the presence of islands of red cells and megakaryocytes in the bone marrow and possibly in the liver. The prognosis is interrelated with the underlying disease.

*Familial myeloproliferative disease.* A severe myeloproliferative disorder with clinical and laboratory findings suggesting chronic or subacute myelogenous leukemia has been observed in nine children who were related as first or second cousins.[102] The disease is characterized by an early onset, marked splenomegaly, hepatosplenomegaly, leukocytosis (25,000 to 100,000 per cubic millimeter) with immature granulocytes, anemia, and thrombocytopenia. Bone marrow examination revealed marked granulocytic (blasts and promyelocytes) and slight erythroid hyperplasia, a cell distribution similar to that of certain forms of myelogenous leukemia. An important differential feature is that the liver and spleen show evidence of extramedullary hematopoiesis without leukemic infiltration. The Ph$^1$ chromosome usually observed in older children with chronic myelogenous leukemia is apparently not present in the peripheral blood. The normal levels of fetal hemoglobin also distinguish these cases from those with juvenile chronic myelogenous leukemia. In contrast to a high leukocyte alkaline phosphatase level found in most of the myeloproliferative disorders and in a leukemoid reaction, a very low level was found in four children with the disease and in eighteen of twenty related but asymptomatic members in three generations of the kindred. Early death occurred in three and chronic symptoms in six patients. Antileukemic therapy was without value. Two of the latter children recovered completely during adolescence after 10 to 12 years of illness.

*Osteopetrosis (marble-bone disease, Albers-Schönberg disease).* Osteopetrosis (Fig. 83) is a rare disease characterized by increased thickening and density of the cortical and spongy portions of the entire osseous system.[81] The onset is usually in fetal life, less often in later childhood. The bones are rigid and brittle, and there is a tendency for spontaneous fractures and slipping of the epiphyses to occur. The individual bones, including those of the skull, appear opaque, heavy, and lacking in finer structure, and in the roentgenogram normal markings are obliterated. Hydrocephalus is not uncommon in infancy. The disease follows a strong familial and hereditary pattern.[83] It has been attributed to a failure of resorption of the calcified cartilaginous matrix during endochondral bone formation or to the influence of an unknown agent which damages the bone-forming blastema.[149]

The clinical picture includes anemia, splenomegaly, enlargement of the liver, and body deformities. Recurrent purulent abscesses and lymphadenitis occur later in the disease. Anemia is common but not invariable and is associated with a leukoerythroblastic response. Normoblasts and myeloid cells appear in the peripheral blood, in some patients resembling myeloid leukemia (Fig. 84). Thrombocytopenia may be marked and associated with massive hemorrhage. Transfusions are given as required. While the anemia has been attributed to encroachment of space reserved for blood formation in the bone marrow, there has been increasing evidence that a hemolytic process was also in progress (anemia, reticulocytosis).[49,122,151] The absence of haptoglobin and the short life-span of the red cells labeled with radioactive chromium confirm the evi-

632  BLOOD DISEASES OF INFANCY AND CHILDHOOD

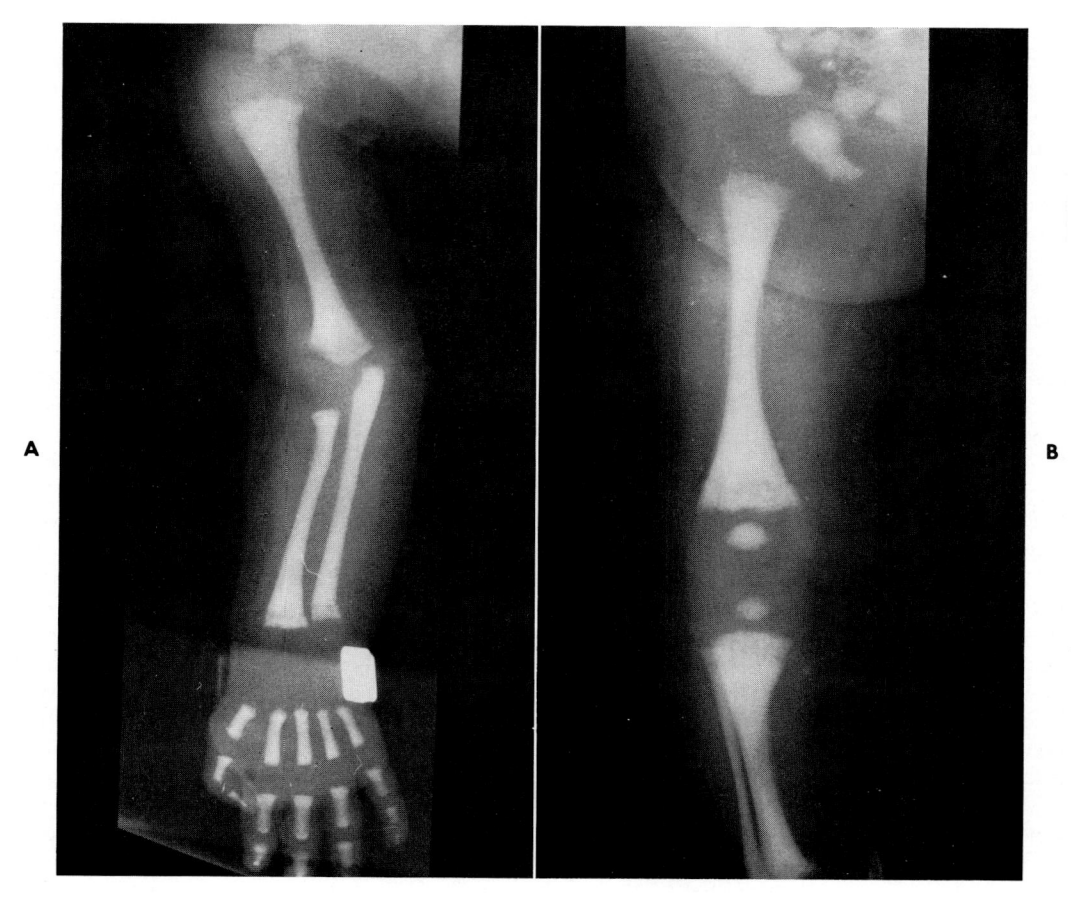

Fig. 83. Osteopetrosis in a 3-month-old infant showing marked generalized sclerosis of the long bones. **A**, Upper extremity. **B**, Lower extremity.

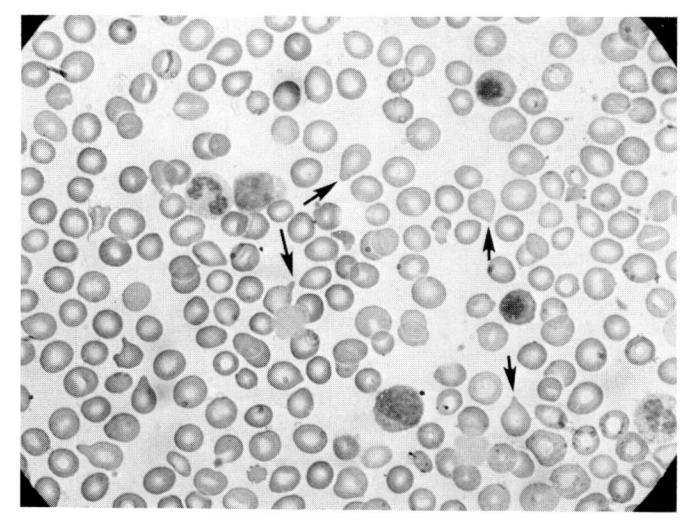

Fig. 84. Peripheral blood film from a patient with osteopetrosis showing normoblasts, a myelocyte, tailed poikilocytes (arrows), and erythrocyte fragmentation.

dences for increased blood destruction.[49] Accordingly, splenectomy has been recommended in cases in which a shortened red cell survival has been demonstrated. In such instances the anemia is ascribed to an extracorpuscular hemolytic process, in all probability due to hypersplenism. Splenectomy relieves the anemia in selected cases, often prolonging the red cell life-span. In all instances thrombocytopenia was improved.

On the basis that osteopetrosis was due to a primary biochemical abnormality resulting from an overabsorption of calcium from the diet, a child with this disease was placed on a strict calcium-depleting regimen.[28] He showed a great spurt in growth and had less dense bone which showed signs of remodeling. In this case red cell studies showed that most of the active marrow was in the liver and spleen and that most of the red cell destruction occurred in the spleen. After splenectomy, the red cell life-span markedly increased and corticosteroid therapy could be eliminated.

Johnston and co-workers[62] have reviewed the literature in this disease, dividing the cases into clinically benign, a dominantly inherited form, and a malignant recessive form. In the severe group optic atrophy and hepatomegaly were common and the acid phosphatase usually elevated. Patients in the dominantly inherited group are asymptomatic and the diagnosis is made by x-ray alone. The most frequent complaint is easy fracturing of bones. A few develop osteomyelitis, and a small number develop cranial nerve palsies, probably due to compression of the nerves in the bony foramina.

A syndrome of facial palsy associated with roentgenographic evidence of osteopetrosis affecting the long bones, pelvis, spine, and skull has been described in several members of the same family and in several generations.[144] This form is benign and is associated with hepatosplenomegaly or abnormalities of the blood. Bony encroachment of the seventh nerve is responsible for the palsy.

*Extramedullary megakaryocytosis and acute megakaryocytic leukemia.* Hyperplasia of the bone marrow with respect to myeloid, erythroid, and megakaryocytic cells has been described in which the megakaryocytes predominate.[27] The term megakaryocytosis, in contrast to the term leukocytosis, applies to an increased number of megakaryocytes in any tissue, intramedullary or extramedullary, usually the latter. Megakaryocytes appear with an aleukemic or subleukemic blood picture, often with chronic myelogenous leukemia, with megakaryocytosis in the hematopoietic tissues, or with myelosclerosis.[115] Extramedullary megakaryocytosis is less efficient in the formation of platelets than is the bone marrow and accounts for the discrepancy between the platelet count and the number of megakaryocytes in the metaplastic organs.[115] Whether the condition can be categorized as megakaryocytic leukemia in the absence of invasion of these cells into the blood stream is still controversial.[82]

*Thrombocythemia.* Megakaryocytic hyperplasia of the bone marrow with markedly increased platelet counts (thrombocythemia) is regarded as a proliferative disorder of the bone marrow. Primary[94] and secondary types have been recognized. Secondary thrombocythemia occurs in association with an underlying condition such as carcinoma, regional ileitis, ulcerative colitis, myelogenous leukemia, polycythemia, and Hodgkin's disease and following splenectomy. It has also been described as an idiopathic disease with prolonged bleeding time, venous thromboses, splenomegaly, spontaneous hemorrhage, and a normal coagulation time. The cause of the hemorrhage and prolonged bleeding time is not known.[45] Abnormal platelet function has been detected in essential thrombocythemia and is associated with decreased platelet aggregation with ADP, absent response to epinephrine, decreased serotonin uptake, but normal platelet factor III activity.[129]

Primary thrombocytosis with platelet counts varying from 900,000 to 5 million per cubic millimeter was observed in an 8-year-old child with myocardial infarction and multiple thromboses.[128] Although the platelet count remained elevated (1.3 million per cubic millimeter), there was no recurrence of the thrombotic phenomenon in an 8-year follow-up. Hepatosplenomegaly, which was present early in the course, had disappeared when the child was seen at the age of 14 years. Electrocardiographic abnormalities resulting from myocardial infarction receded. This syndrome with idiopathic elevations of blood platelets is contrasted with secondary thrombocytosis in which platelets are increased in association with acute infections, Boeck's sarcoidosis, hemorrhage, cancer, chronic leukemia, and polycythemia vera and in postsplenectomy states.

***Erythremic myelosis (Di Guglielmo's disease).*** Erythremic myelosis is a rare disease described by Di Guglielmo,[32] characterized by erythropoietic hyperplasia within the bone marrow and extramedullary sites. Irregular remittent fever, splenomegaly proportionally greater than hepatomegaly, thrombocytopenia, granulopenia, and anemia are associated with enormous numbers of erythroblasts in the peripheral blood which are basophilic, multinucleated, or otherwise atypical.[78] Both the bone marrow and the peripheral blood show overcrowding with erythroid elements which become progressively immature. This neoplastic disorder affecting erythropoietic tissue is analogous in its cellular specificity to involvement of myeloid cells in leukemia.

Anemia results from failure of release of cells from the bone marrow as well as from hemolysis. Survival of patients' $^{51}$Cr-tagged red cells is shortened.[120] Cases have been reported in patients in younger age groups[43,84,142] as well as in adults. In contrast to hemolytic anemia which it resembles, the reticulocyte count is low and remains so. The disease occurs as a short and acute form of several months' duration or a chronic and prolonged form lasting up to 2 years. Transfusions, splenectomy, and steroids have been employed in treatment, but the disease is ultimately fatal with hemorrhagic manifestations.

A strongly positive periodic acid–Schiff (PAS) reaction (for glycogen and mucopolysaccharides) occurs in many of the erythroblasts from the bone marrow and blood of patients with Di Guglielmo's disease.[5,101] A strongly positive reaction also occurs in many erythroblasts of patients with iron-deficiency anemia and thalassemia major. Erythroblasts are uniformly negative in the bone marrow of normal persons and in that of patients with pernicious anemia, nutritional macrocytic anemia, aplastic anemia, and polycythemia.

Erythroleukemia is a condition in which hyperplasia of erythroblastic and leukoblastic tissues are combined. The peripheral blood and bone marrow reveal an admixture of myeloblasts and immature erythroblasts.[54] According to another concept, erythremic myelosis may eventually emerge as leukemia, particularly when life is prolonged by intensive transfusion therapy.[22] In one such patient the anemia was characterized by intensive erythroblastemia, marrow erythroblastosis, and a hemorrhagic state. At death the patient was found to have changes characteristic of acute granulocytic leukemia.[33]

Erythroleukemia has been designated as cases in which pure erythroid neoplasia is present—erythremic myelosis or Di Guglielmo's disease—is present together with an additional leukoblastic component. In a report of three children with this disorder,[38] the criteria for diagnosis were anemia, granulocytopenia, thrombocytopenia, presence of nucleated red cells, megaloblasts or blast cells in the peripheral blood, and bone marrow examination showing crowding with megaloblastic erythroid elements and Auer bodies in granulocytic precursors. Myeloblasts in increased numbers were not essential for the diagnosis. One of the children revealed a missing C chromosome, with only 45 chromosomes in the bone marrow. The benign type reverted to normal during remission.

Dameshek[21] conceived of this condition as one of the members of the group of conditions called the "myeloproliferative syndrome." He defined the Di Guglielmo syndrome as a "self-perpetuating myeloproliferative disorder of undetermined origin characterized by progressive anemia, striking erythroblastic hyperplasia of the bone marrow and of megaloblastic, megaloblastoid, or normoblastic types; and often in the course of years, of increasing numbers of myeloblasts." Eventually sufficient myeloblasts are present to justify the diagnosis of erythroleukemia and later of myeloblastic leukemia. It can be thought of as a highly variable myeloproliferative disorder in which erythremic myelosis, erythroleukemia, and myeloblastic leukemia may all appear either in sequence or conjointly so that classification is difficult.

Additional criteria of the Di Guglielmo syndrome include hyperferremia both in the blood serum and in the marrow, large numbers of erythroblasts with iron granules (sideroblasts), large amounts of iron in the mitochondria of sideroblasts leading to a picture of "ringed" sideroblasts, ineffective erythropoiesis, "heme" diversion, and frequently a low blood granulocyte alkaline phosphatase, increased fetal hemoglobin, and decreased hemoglobin A$_2$.[55]

***Chloroma and chloroleukemia.*** In rare cases of acute leukemia in children and young adults, there are coexisting localized tumor masses found in close relationship to the periosteum of the bones of the face, ribs, sternum or vertebrae, and less commonly in the viscera. Chloromas may occasionally produce central or peripheral neurologic disturbance. Compression of the spinal cord from invasion of the spinal canal may produce varying patterns of motor and sensory defects.[77] These tumors are referred to as chromas because of a pale greenish color on the cut surface that fades rapidly on exposure to light and air but reappears on addition of hydrogen peroxide. The nature of the pigment causing the green color is still controversial, with theories involving white blood cells and hemoglobin derivatives. A green pigment has been isolated with a high peroxidase activity closely resembling verdoperoxidase, an enzyme perhaps elaborated by the primitive cells.[114] These tumors consist of primitive white blood cells, usually myeloblasts, less commonly myelocytes and monocytes. Clinically, the classic case of chloroma is characterized by an orbital tumor, frequently causing exophthalmos and proptosis, lymphadenopathy, and a rapid progressing anemia associated with acute myelogenous and monocytic leukemia.[110] A congenital case has been reported in a 13-day-old infant.[88]

*Neoplasms of lymphoid tissue (malignant lymphomas).* The malignant lymphomas include Hodgkin's disease and lymphosarcoma. In this classification are included diverse conditions of unknown etiology arising from lymphoid tissues. The cellular constituents found in the lymph nodes and lymph follicles form the basis of specific conditions—i.e., lymphoblast, lymphocyte, reticulum cell, and plasma cell. Single cells alone may be involved, or the histologic patterns may be more complex, with the presence of nodules or granulomatous lesions of several cell types. Exact diagnosis depends upon the identification of distinctive cells or a group of cells. It is often impossible to distinguish between these disorders without access to complete clinical data, multiple laboratory aids such as roentgenograms, bone and lymph node biopsy, bone marrow aspiration, and blood studies. Even with these facilities diagnosis is often difficult and depends upon clinical and laboratory changes during the course of the disease. Transitions are known to occur from one histologic type of neoplasm to another, and several different microscopic patterns are often present in the same patient and same lymph nodes.[20]

A causal relationship between longstanding hyperthyroidism and lymphoma is suggested but not proved. In one study[137] six patients were presented who, subsequent to long-standing hyperthyroidism, developed a lymphoma (one lymphoblastic lymphosarcoma, one Hodgkin's disease, one giant follicular lymphoma, and three lymphocytic lymphosarcoma or leukemia). Such an association may gain support from the experimental evidence that hyperthyroidism stimulates lymphoid structures and promotes tumor growth in animals and hypothyroidism inhibits lymphoid structures. In man, also, hyperthyroidism is frequently associated with lymphoid hyperplasia manifested by lymphocytosis, lymph node enlargement, and splenomegaly. Thyroidectomy results in a reversal of the lymphatic response. These observations indicate that long-standing hyperthyroidism should be considered in differential diagnosis in any lymphoma-like state.

Approximately 30% of patients with malignant lymphoma have hypogammaglobulinemia, some even have agammaglobulinemia.[95] In these cases the hypogammaglobulinemia has been considered secondary to the lymphoma on the assumption that replacement of normal lymphoid tissue by malignant cells reduces the number of gamma globulin–producing cells. Whether malignancy may be due to failure of the body to destroy abnormal mutant cells (the agammaglobulinemic patient, especially, is unable to destroy them), whether he is unable to resist infection, including the viral agent of leukemia, or whether a thymic abnormality is involved are still unknown. Two cases of children with congenital agammaglobulinemia who at 4 years of age developed malignant lymphoma have been reported, one with the blood picture of acute lymphoblastic leukemia.[95] An increased incidence of lymphoma has been reported in other immunological deficiency syndromes, including ataxia-telangiectasia,[97] Wiskott-Aldrich syndrome[135] and sex-linked agammaglobulinemia.[46]

*Hodgkin's disease.* Hodgkin's disease is characterized by a painless and progressive enlargement of the superficial and deep lymph nodes and often of other lymphoid structures of the body and of the spleen. It is protean in its manifestations and, during its course, can resemble both tumor and infections.[86] As in patients with lymphosarcoma, the first evidence of Hodgkin's disease may be detected in the form of a mediastinal mass in the chest observed by roentgenographic examination.[19] However, in contrast to lymphosarcoma, in which symmetrical areas are attacked, in the

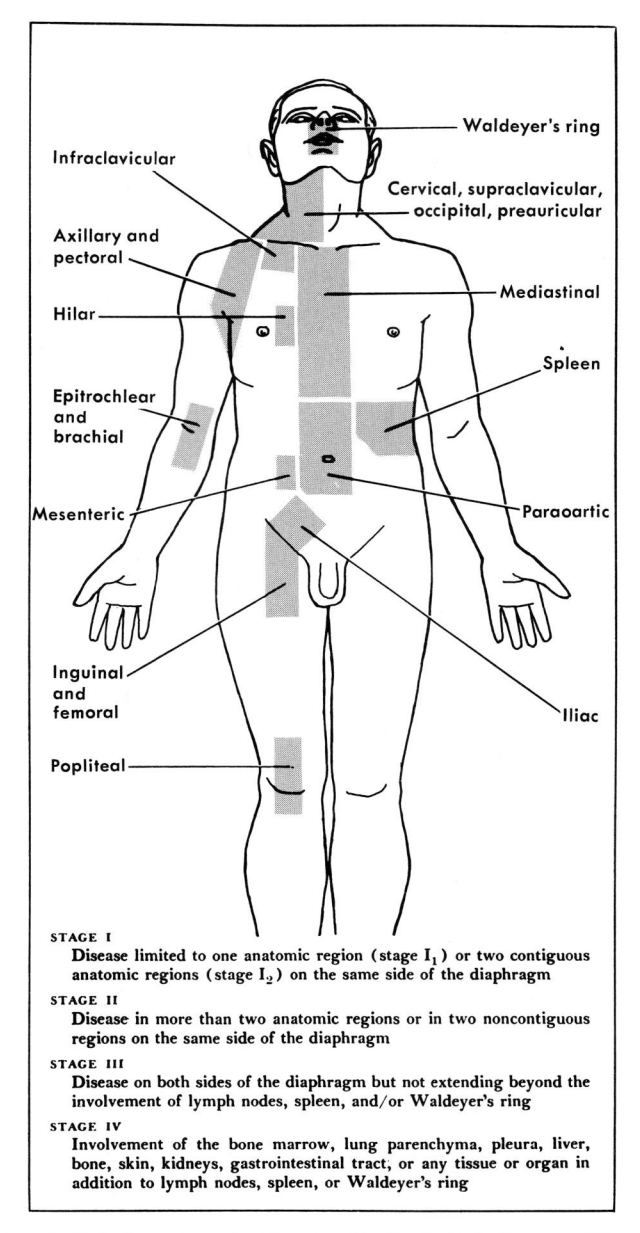

**STAGE I**
Disease limited to one anatomic region (stage $I_1$) or two contiguous anatomic regions (stage $I_2$) on the same side of the diaphragm

**STAGE II**
Disease in more than two anatomic regions or in two noncontiguous regions on the same side of the diaphragm

**STAGE III**
Disease on both sides of the diaphragm but not extending beyond the involvement of lymph nodes, spleen, and/or Waldeyer's ring

**STAGE IV**
Involvement of the bone marrow, lung parenchyma, pleura, liver, bone, skin, kidneys, gastrointestinal tract, or any tissue or organ in addition to lymph nodes, spleen, or Waldeyer's ring

Fig. 85. International clinical staging classification for Hodgkin's disease. (From Kaplan, H. S., and Rosenberg, S. A.: The cure of malignant lymphomas, Hospital Practice 3:31, 1968.)

early stages of Hodgkin's disease the pathology is usually unilateral.

Hodgkin's disease formerly was classified as paragranuloma, granuloma, or sarcoma. The paragranuloma involves chiefly lymph nodes in which the normal architecture may or may not be altered. The granuloma type represents the classic form of the disease in which there is a gradual loss of normal architecture of the lymph nodes and replacement by pleomorphic cellular tissue. Hodgkin's sarcoma represents the most invasive and destructive form of the disease in which cells larger than lymphocytes predominate, normal architecture of the nodes is destroyed, and necrosis is present.[31] Lukes and Butler[76] have provided a revised pathologic classification of Hodgkin's disease. In order of progressive malignancy: lymphocyte predominance (paragranuloma); nodular sclerosis and mixed cellularity (granuloma); and lymphocyte depletion (sarcoma). In the fourth type of lymphocyte depletion the stroma shows a paucity of lymphocytes and may result from diffuse fibrosis or from widespread proliferation of Reed-Sternberg cells.[36]

Symptoms include loss of weight and appetite, weakness, fever, cough, and dyspnea. In a majority of patients the disease progresses through a latent period which is often protracted and during which nodes enlarge without symptoms. This period is followed by one of further progressions and generalization during which symptoms of varying severity appear with cachexia as a terminal symptom.[39] Fatigue, anorexia, loss of weight, and intermittent fever (Pel-Ebstein) herald or accompany the disease. The spleen is enlarged in about 60 to 70% of patients with advanced disease.[80]

The incidence of jaundice varies widely— from 3 to 8%. In a series of 875 cases 13% had jaundice.[72] Common causes of jaundice in autopsy cases include liver involvement, hemolytic anemia, extrahepatic bile duct obstruction due to tumor, and hepatitis.

Accurate clinical staging is important for optimal therapy. An international clinical staging classification for Hodgkin's disease is diagrammed in Fig. 85.

The causative agent is unknown, although viral and bacterial, especially tuberculous, etiologies have been suggested but not fully established. Inflammatory and neoplastic theories have also been advanced but unproved. The disease affects males more often than females, with a predominance in the ratio of 3 to 1. It is most common in adults between 20 and 40 years of age and comparatively rare in children, in whom it occurs between 4 and 12 years of age and even earlier.[37]

The nodes involved in order of prevalence are the cervical, axillary, inguinal, mediastinal, and mesenteric nodes. The cervical nodes are involved in 50 to 75% of all patients. The nodes are usually discrete, and the capsule is rarely infiltrated. The essential histologic features of Hodgkin's disease are the Reed-Sternberg cells, pleomorphism of the cellular tissue, the presence of eosinophils, and fibrosis.[3] The pathologic changes vary from patient to patient and in different areas in the same patient.

The diagnosis is based on the distinctive histopathologic alteration in an involved area. The microscopic picture is characterized by a proliferation of the large reticuloendothelial cells replacing the lymphoid tissue and the presence of giant cells derived from the reticulum cells. The latter are the nucleated and multinucleated Reed-Sternberg cells, the pathognomonic cell and essential diagnostic feature of Hodgkin's disease. The large nucleus of the Reed-Sternberg cell has a well-defined membrane with many folds and outcroppings.[124] Nucleoli are especially prominent. The diagnostic lesions consist of eosinophils, lymphocytes, endothelial cells, Reed-Sternberg cells, myelocytes, and megakaryocytes. Eosinophils may be especially prominent. Mixed osteolytic and osteoblastic lesions are noted in at least 15% of cases of Hodgkin's disease.[79]

It has been stated that the histologic components associated with Reed-Sternberg cells are a reflection of the state of the host and relate to the immunologic abnormalities of Hodgkin's disease.[75] The belief that lymphocytes play a primary role in immunity is supported by the realization that when there is a lymphocytic and/or histiocytic proliferation, Reed-Sternberg cells are rare, the disease is quiescent, and median survivals are prolonged. According to this hypothesis, the stage of the disease, the rate of progression, and the length of time the patient survives are determined by the state of the host rather than by the effectiveness of therapy.

In the later stages the usual structure of the lymph nodes disappears and is gradually replaced by fibrous tissue. From the initial manifestation of Hodgkin's disease as a painless swelling of one or more groups of superficial nodes, the disease progresses. Mechanical pressure of the enlarging nodes produces local clinical manifestations, such as dyspnea from tracheal and mediastinal involvement. The disease may become actively invasive, however, extending beyond the confines of the lymph nodes to involve the spleen, liver, bones, lungs, and, to a lesser extent, other organs, including the central nervous system. Radiation results in increased fibrosis and matting together of the nodes.

Reed-Sternberg cells have been found in the bone marrow biopsies or aspirations in Hodgkin's disease but the yield has been low. In the case reported by Willerson and associates,[145] the patient presented with pancytopenia. A smear of the bone marrow treated with Wright's stain revealed numerous giant cells, eosinophilic myelocytes, and reticulum cells. Binucleate cells with large nucleoli had the appearance of classical Reed-Sternberg cells. In this case the disease was apparently confined to the bone marrow. Autopsy yielded only small lymph nodes which on sectioning had normal architecture.

They also commented that in the early stages of the disease the cervical lymph nodes are most commonly involved (60 to 80%). The next most frequently involved are axillary (6 to 20%), inguinal (6 to 12%), and mediastinal lymph nodes (6 to 11%). The spleen is involved in 80% of cases and the liver in more than 50%. There have been few reports of organ involvement limited to the spleen or spleen and bone marrow. There is also a report that while Reed-Sternberg cells are generally considered essential to the diagnosis of Hodgkin's disease they may be found in Burkitt lymphoma.[146]

Although the disease was considered uniformly fatal, the period of survival has been extended in recent years. The average survival time following diagnosis is 2 to 3 years, but in individual cases it varies from a few months to 10 to 15 years or more. In others, the condition may be chronic and benign, extending to more than 20 years. Possible and even probable cures are anticipated with modern treatment.[123] Prior to 1950, the 5-year survival period following diagnosis and treatment in most of the large series reported was given as under 20%. Another survey showed a 5-year survival of over 30%.[121] Despite the limitations of histopathologic evidence as a prognosticator,[111] in one series a relationship could be shown between such a classification and survival. Three hundred eighty-eight cases of Hodgkin's disease among white male soldiers during World War II were histopathologically differentiated into paragranuloma (35), granuloma (308), sarcoma (5) and unspecified types (40).[14] A follow-up period of 17 years showed 8.4% of the men with granuloma and 28.6% of those with paragranuloma still alive. All five men with Hodgkin's sarcoma were dead within a year. The long survival of patients with granuloma and paragranuloma suggest that Hodgkin's disease may not be invariably fatal.

Smithers[125] suggested that Hodgkin's disease is one progressive myeloblastic disorder, from lymphocytic predominance through mixed cellularity to lymphocytic depletion, in which host resistance may develop; when this occurs the process is represented histologically by a nodular-sclerosis and clinically by a tendency for the disease to be arrested in Stage II. The histological appearances which determine the diagnosis vary considerably. However, if Reed-Sternberg cells are seen by the pathologist in the relevant cellular and architectural environment, they are accepted as confirmation of the diagnosis of Hodgkin's disease. The diagnosis, though suspected clinically, is thus made histologically. Reed-Sternberg cells, however, have occasionally been found in infectious mononucleosis, recurrent Burkitt's lymphoma, and treated lymphosarcoma.

According to Lukes and Butler,[76] several definite conclusions appear to be indicated from evaluating the significance of the histologic features and clinical stages in Hodgkin's disease. Lymphocytic and histiocytic proliferation was associated predominantly with Stage I disease and with prolonged median survivals. The lymphocytic depletion types represented histologically by diffuse fibrosis and the predominant Reed-Sternberg cell proliferation in the reticular type are usually observed in Stage III disease, with rapidly progressive disease of brief duration.

*Lymphosarcoma.* The term lymphosarcoma has been used to include all primary malignant tumors of lymphoid origin except Hodgkin's disease and has been subdivided into giant follicular lymphosarcoma, reticulum cell sarcoma, and lymphosarcoma.[106] In its restricted terminology the predominant cell in lymphosarcoma corresponds to the small mature lymphocyte so that the condition is often termed small cell lymphosarcoma. In the reticulum cell sarcoma the typical cell is the reticulum cell which is more than one and one-half times the size of the mature lymphocyte. Reticulum cell sarcoma mimics lymphosarcoma and is regarded as its most undifferentiated type. Lymphosarcoma and reticulum cell sarcoma can be discussed together from the clinical, pathologic, and therapeutic standpoints, although the latter is generally more highly malignant and invasive and metastasizes even more readily than the lymphosarcoma.[31]

Lymphosarcoma occurs with greater frequency in adults than in children but in sufficient numbers in the latter to prompt a review of its clinical and hematologic aspects. In a series of 583 children with malignant tumors treated at the Memorial Center, twenty-seven (5%) had lymphosarcoma.[24] The malignant neoplasms comprising this group are often difficult to classify, but orientation is facilitated by considering the clinical features together with an interpretation of the specific cellular components. In addition to lymphocytic and reticulum cell forms arising from the periphery and germinal center of the lymph follicle, respectively, lymphoblastic and mixed lymphocytic and reticulum cell types have been described.

Lymphosarcoma occurs infrequently within the first month of life as well as throughout childhood. Any lymph node or lymphoid structure may be the primary site. All sites have been reported, the lymphoid tissue of the adenoids and the tonsils or the thymus, the gastrointestinal tract, and lymph nodes of the cervical, mediastinal, and retroperitoneal areas are common sites. Occasionally the multiple organs and nodes are involved when the patient presents. In contrast to Hodgkin's disease, localized lymphosarcoma is usually not characterized by systemic manifestations. The frequency with which lymphosarcoma and reticulum cell sarcoma invade and replace the bone marrow and convert to a leukemic process has been increasing with each reported series and is as high as 60%.

These tumors of the lymphosarcoma group originate within and outside the lymph nodes in the many anatomic regions in which lymphoid tissue is present. Expansion of these areas by overgrowth of malignant cells results in destruction of the normal architecture of lymphoid tissue and infiltration of surrounding tissues. The disease therefore may be limited initially to a single locus or to a region or may be generalized with constitutional symptoms and signs.[30]

Symptoms and signs originate in the area of primary involvement or from the areas invaded by direct extension from affected lymph nodes. The eyes, nervous system, skin, thymus, gastrointestinal tract, and cervical, mediastinal, mesenteric, and retroperitoneal nodes serve as primary sites. The anterior mediastinum is frequently involved.

In an appreciable number of patients lymphoblastic leukemia develops during the course of lymphosarcoma, either following roentgen irradiation or occurring spontaneously, regardless of the site involved. Of a group of forty-two children with small cell lymphosarcoma, nine, or 21.4% showed a transition into leukemia.[106] In another composite series of lymphosarcoma the overall leukemic transformation was 29.8% (sixty-two of 208 cases).[63] An average of 2.4 months elapsed from the time of diagnosis of lymphosarcoma to the manifestations of frank leukemia. This conversion to leukemia was more likely with lymphosarcoma of the small cell type (81.9%). To this association with a leukemia component the term leukosarcoma has been applied.

The actual time relationship to the development of leukemia is not always apparent, for examination of the blood smear may reveal a small percentage of abnormal cells at any stage of the disease. These cells, however, may represent tumor cells rather than actual lymphoblasts. Attempts have been made to differentiate between the typical lymphoblast of stem cell leukemia and the lymphosarcoma cell reaching the bloodstream by invasion from the primary focus. One of the main features of the lymphosarcoma cell is the coarsely reticular and more deeply staining chromatin as compared with the leptochromatic or more lightly staining nucleus of the lymphoblast. A distinctive feature of the lymphosarcoma cell[57] is the nucleolus, which stands out as a sky-blue round area surrounded by a deep blue-black rim of chromatin. In the course of lymphosarcoma, the bone marrow may become heavily infiltrated with lymphosarcoma cells without their appearance in the bloodstream. It may be that death ensues before the peripheral blood is invaded.

We have seen a patient in whom this process appeared to have been reversed. In an 11-year-old child with anemia, thrombocytopenia, and splenomegaly, the bone marrow and, to a lesser extent, the peripheral blood were heavily infiltrated with blast cells. On the basis of a diagnosis of lymphoblastic leukemia, steroids were administered, and a complete remission was obtained which persisted for 15 months. At this time the onset of abdominal pain led to the discovery of a retroperitoneal lymphosarcoma. Radiotherapy produced a prompt resolution of the mass. One month after the beginning of this treatment, leukemic cells were again found in the blood and bone marrow. The initial leukemic cells may have represented metastasis from a quiescent focus of lymphosarcoma which later became reactivated.

Massive enlargements of the mediastinum causing circulatory or respiratory distress which precede the blood picture of acute leukemia have been reported in children.

Whether the mass is of thymic origin exclusively or associated with mediastinal lymph nodes is not certain. In these patients irradiation with the roentgen ray produces marked relief from the shortness of breath. The mediastinal tumor disappears completely and permanently within a few days, although patients have been known to succumb later to acute leukemia.[17] Roentgen therapy as a factor in precipitating the leukemic phase may have been overemphasized.[7]

The records of 113 patients dying of documented reticulum cell sarcoma revealed six persons whose course terminated with symptoms resembling those of acute leukemia.[150] Their course was characterized by weakness, pallor, petechiae, hemorrhages, and hepatosplenomegaly. The blood showed anemia, leukocytosis (20,000 to 80,000 per cu.mm.), and thrombocytopenia. Differential count in the blood and bone marrow revealed a high percentage of immature cells (35 to 96%). They were identified as reticulum cells in three patients, as myeloblasts in two, and as monocytoid granulocytes in one. Systemic infection or hemorrhage occurred within 2 months of one leukemic blood picture. Therapy with 6-mercaptopurine, adrenocortical steroids, or both gave no benefit. On the other hand, others regard monocytic leukemia as the leukemic counterpart of reticulum cell sarcoma.[23] Not all reticulum cell sarcomas have a leukemic phase; many remain localized in tissues.

*Chronic lymphadenopathy simulating malignant lymphomas.* A symptom complex has been described as "lymphadenopathy simulating lymphoma"[10] with the following features: onset of disease between 1 month and 2 years of age, hepatosplenomegaly, significant generalized lymphadenopathy with a decrease in node size during infections, fever, variable lymph node histological changes, hypercellular bone marrow with occasional blast cells, deviations in immunologic status with various manifestations of autoimmune disease, altered responses to immunosuppressive drugs, and chronic disease. Organomegaly decreased during periods of spontaneous remission or following therapy. Two patients required splenectomy, one for hemolytic anemia and the other for pancytopenia. Thrombocytopenic purpura was present in three patients. Many aspects of this disorder suggest an immunological disease. Zuelzer and co-workers[152] have reported cases of chronic lymphadenopathy with intermittent hemolytic anemia associated with the presence of cytomegalic virus in cells of lymph nodes and other tissues at the time of active hemolysis. This virus could not be demonstrated in the patients reported. The symptom complex described simulated malignant lymphoma but in prolonged follow-up no evidence of malignancy has developed.

FOLLICULAR LYMPHOSARCOMA (GIANT FOLLICULAR LYMPHOBLASTOMA, BRILL-SYMMERS DISEASE). This type of lymphosarcoma involves the lymph nodes, spleen, and other lymphoid tissues and is characterized by a prominance of the follicular structure. Clinically, it consists of generalized lymphadenopathy, splenomegaly, delayed appearance of anemia, tendency toward pleural and peritoneal effusions, bone involvement, and unilateral exophthalmos. Hyperplasia of lymph follicles and malpighian bodies with an increase in these elements numerically and in size is a striking feature. As the disease progresses, follicular hypertrophy and hyperplasia are replaced by lymphosarcoma, lymphocytic leukemia, or rarely Hodgkin's disease.[109] The disease is of long duration and is remarkably sensitive to x-ray therapy, more so than any other form of lymphoma. This is particularly true in the earlier phase but less so in the later malignant phases.

*Burkitt's tumor.* Burkitt's tumor is a lymphoma of childhood of which one of the more characteristic features is involvement of one or more quadrants of the jaw by a rapidly growing osteolytic tumor. Tumors may also be found in the salivary glands, thyroid, heart, liver, kidneys, adrenals, retroperitoneum, gonads, and long bones. Histologically, this tumor is a lymphoma with a uniform pattern of sheets of immature lymphoid cells interspersed with nonmalignant histiocytes that often assume a clear or vacuolated form, giving the tumor a characteristic "starry sky" appearance.[92] Alkylating agents and antimetabolites have resulted in complete remission and prolonged survival. Terminal lymphoblastic leukemia may occur.[13] This tumor has its highest incidence in areas were the rainfall is greater than 20 inches per annum and the mean temperature above 60° F.[9] It is particularly prevalent in children in Kenya and Uganda. These climatic conditions are the most favorable to certain arthropods that may carry a causative virus.[58] Cases have also been reported in the United States,[15,35] England,[147] Brazil, and New Guinea.[148]

*Blood changes in the lymphoma group.* The degree of anemia and the white blood cell and platelet levels show great variations in patients with the malignant lymphomas. In patients with the early stages of lymphosarcoma and in those with follicular lymphoblastoma, the anemia may be absent or slight but eventually progresses. In patients with Hodgkin's disease the anemia usually is normochromic, and normocytic. Various mechanisms may be involved in producing the anemia. Prior to the advent of the Coombs test and techniques to determine red cell survival, the anemia in patients with this group of diseases and in those with leukemia was ascribed to crowding out of the marrow by pathologic cells.

On the basis of immunologic studies the mechanism of hemolysis in many of these patients has now been shown not to differ significantly from that of patients with idiopathic autoimmune hemolytic anemia.[108] Anemia, reticulocytosis, spherocytosis, bilirubinemia of the direct type, and a positive Coombs test are conspicuous. In a small number of patients autoimmune antibodies are not detected, and the signs of hemolysis are slight or absent. In the latter the anemia is normochromic, there are no abnormalities in the red cell morphology, and transfusion requirements are occasionally increased.[140] In patients with either type, red cell survival is decreased. Steroids act favorably in patients with autoimmune hemolytic anemia, but there is no response in those with the contrasting type.

In another study[47] no shortening of the lifespan was apparent until the hemoglobin level dropped below 7.5 gm. per 100 ml., and inadequate erythropoiesis was a major cause of anemia in patients with a negative Coombs test.

The leukocyte count in patients with Hodgkin's disease may be normal, low, or moderately increased. Leukopenia is uncommon, however, and lymphocytosis is rare.[71] The white blood cell count in this disease usually ranges from 10,000 to 15,000 per cubic millimeter but may reach levels of 30,000 per cubic millimeter or more. The higher counts usually accompany the late stages of the disease. The differential count reveals a tendency toward polymorphonuclear predominance ranging from 85 to 90%. Monocytosis, eosinophilia, and lymphocytopenia characterize the peripheral blood of the patient with Hodgkin's disease.

Extreme degrees of eosinophilia are infrequent. Aisenberg[1] pointed out that in the patient with advanced Hodgkin's disease a depression of the peripheral lymphocyte count is regularly observed and antibody formation is depressed as well. He drew a parallel between the Hodgkin's patient in this phase and the "Swiss" form of agammaglobinemia, a disease characterized by lymphocytopenia, thymic hypoplasia, frequent bacterial and fungal infections, and early death.

The white blood cell count in patients with lymphosarcoma and follicular lymphoblastoma may be normal, or there may be relative or absolute lymphocytosis. Tumor cells of lymphosarcoma may be found in the blood smear. Both lymphosarcoma and follicular lymphoma may be associated with lymphocytic leukemia during the progression of each disease. Hematogones have been found[109] in increased numbers in the peripheral blood of patients with follicular lymphoblastoma. These are cells smaller than lymphocytes with nuclei composed of dense chromatin and almost devoid of cytoplasm so that the cells give the appearance of naked nuclei. An indentation or a horizontal crack through the cell may be seen. Leukemoid blood pictures have been observed occasionally in all members of the lymphoma group.

The platelet count in patients with Hodgkin's disease is usually normal. Markedly increased numbers of platelets and bizarre forms occasionally present reflect the excessive numbers of megakaryocytes in the bone marrow. The platelet count in patients with lymphomas other than Hodgkin's disease is usually normal or occasionally reduced. Thrombocytopenia in patients with lymphomas including those with Hodgkin's disease may represent the effects of a pathologically involved spleen exerting a hypersplenic effect.

Abnormal and primitive reticulum cells with morphologic features of Reed-Sternberg cells have been described in the peripheral blood of a patient with Hodgkin's disease.[74] In a study of 135 patients,[8] it was observed that 37% of those suffering from Hodgkin's disease exhibit abnormal cells in the leukocyte concentrates of the peripheral blood during the course of their illness. Typical Reed-Sternberg cells were found in 18.5% of patients and were present only in the advanced stages of generalized Hodgkin's disease. These observations suggest the hematogenous metastasis of Hodgkin's disease. Typical L.E. cells have infrequently been reported in both lymphosarcoma and Hodgkin's disease.[56]

*Bone marrow changes.* It has been stated[18] that bone marrow aspiration is of greatest diagnostic value in patients with lymphosarcoma in whom abnormal lymphocytic tumor cell infiltrates may be found. In patients with Hodgkin's disease, myeloid and megakaryocytic hyperplasia is common. In patients with this disease reticulum cells, plasma cells, polymorphonuclear leukocytes, and lymphocytes are increased, and in many, eosinophils are conspicuous. In rare cases cells resembling Reed-Sternberg cells are found in bone marrow aspiration.[6,139] They must be distinguished from the neighboring megakaryocytes which they resemble. The cells appear as hypertrophied reticulum cells with one or several very large blue nucleoli; in other cells a large number of nuclei are grouped together, forming a giant cell. The presence of giant nucleoli which stain pale to deep blue with Romanowsky stains serves as a distinguishing feature from megakaryocytes, in which the nucleoli are small and inconspicuous and present only in the youngest cells.[139] In a recent case in a boy 15 years of age, these abnormal cells as well as a marked increase of eosinophils were found in the bone marrow. The chief complaint was abdominal pain and marked loss of weight. The lymph nodes were not enlarged, and the spleen was only slightly increased in size.

Lymphosarcoma and reticulum cell sarcoma can be identified more frequently in bone marrow specimens.

*Treatment.* The malignant lymphomas may be considered as a group with regard to the general principles of treatment. Lymphosarcoma and Hodgkin's disease require special consideration since they figure more prominently in pediatric practice. Surgery, roentgen-ray irradiation, and chemotherapy, together with supportive treatment (including transfusions and antibiotics), constitute the agents of direct attack upon these diseases.

As a guide to treatment, the lymphomas, and more particularly Hodgkin's disease, have been classified according to the following stages.[90,93,96,112] The classification divides Hodgkin's disease into four stages on the basis of anatomic distribution of the sites of involvement. According to Kaplan,[64] these stages embrace the following: Stage I refers to disease limited to one anatomic region or to two contiguous anatomic regions on the same side of the diaphragm. The disease is designated Stage II when involved lymphatic structures are present in more than two anatomic regions or in two noncontiguous regions on the same side of the diaphragm. Stage III disease is still limited to the lymphatic structures—that is, to lymph nodes, thymus gland, spleen and Waldeyer's ring—but is present on both sides of the diaphragm. Stage IV is a heterogeneous one because there is involvement of bone marrow, lung parencyma, pleura, liver, bone, skin, kidneys, gastrointestinal tract, or a tissue or organ in addition to lymph nodes, spleen, or Waldeyer's ring. All states are subclassified as A or B, indicating the absence or presence, respectively, of systemic manifestations which include fever, night sweats, and pruritis.

Proper staging requires a careful history and physical examination, complete blood counts, urinalysis, radiograms of the chest, skeletal survey, bone marrow aspiration and biopsy, liver function tests, and lower extremities lymphangiography. Lymphangiography is recommended for all Stage I and II cases since intravenous pyelography detects only a small fraction of Hodgkin's disease involving the retroperitoneal nodes. It now appears that laparotomy as well should be part of the initial diagnostic investigations. Laparotomy, splenectomy, liver biopsy, and para-aortic lymph node biopsy have proved to be valuable supplements to the diagnostic evaluation of selected patients with Hodgkin's disease. The precise delineation of intra-abdominal sites of involvement permits the use of extended field megavoltage radiation therapy with curative intent.[50] There is some suggestion that splenectomized patients tolerate subsequent chemotherapy better than comparable patients who retain their spleen.[51]

Splenectomy provides an opportunity to examine the spleen very carefully for evidence of Hodgkin's disease.[51] It is of interest that, of twelve patients with palpable spleens, only eight had identifiable Hodgkin's disease; yet eighteen of the fifty-six patients whose spleens were thought preoperatively to be normal had splenic Hodgkin's disease by histology. The lymphangiogram was also evaluated, and in six of the twenty patients with positive studies, biopsy failed to confirm the lymphographic reading; conversely, seven of the twenty-four patients whose para-aortic nodes were negative by lymphography had positive biopsies.

Early, aggressive treatment of Hodgkin's disease has been shown to lead to a higher survival rate. This is an imperative reason for trying to establish the diagnosis as soon as possible. The choice and intensity of therapy depend upon whether the disease is strictly localized or is widespread. Surgical excision has been recommended in the few patients in whom the lesion is confined to a single accessible focus and in whom complete examination, including roentgenograms of the chest, skeleton, and gastrointestinal tract, reveals no other involvement.[19] Excisions are followed postoperatively by roentgen-ray irradiation.

Roentgen-ray therapy, however, represents the most effective and dependable suppressive agent, especially for localized lesions,[30] and has been regarded as the sheet anchor of treatment. It is claimed that there is no doubt that radiotherapy is the correct primary treatment for Stages I and II disease, that as many as 80% of such patients may survive 10 years, and that a proportion of patients are probably cured.[51] There is even the belief "that if a patient has survived for five years after the initial course of treatment without evidence of relapse, there is probably a greater than 95 percent chance that permanent cure has been attained."[64]

Initially roentgen-ray therapy is often used alone or in conjunction with chemotherapy, especially when patients are no longer responsive to roentgen irradiation alone. Karnofsky[65,67] regards radiation therapy as the most effective treatment, even for localized Hodgkin's disease, with prophylactic irradiation of adjacent lymph node–bearing areas. Fairly extensive so-called eradicative doses of radiation should be administered to the involved nodes. The area to be irradiated must be left to the radiotherapist. Jenkin and co-workers[61] report twenty-five children with Hodgkin's disease treated mainly by irradiation. The 5-year survival was 33%, dropping to 24% at 10 years. Others claim the superiority of surgery in Stage I Hodgkin's disease and are concerned with the late effects of irradiation in the large dosage needed for obliteration in the younger patient.[123]

Chemotherapeutic agents are of value in Stages III and IV and can produce temporary but complete remission in 50% of patients and partial remission in 25%. The drugs used in this category are vinblastine, vincristine, cytoxan, nitrogen mustard, or chlorambucil and prednisone. More recently procarbazine has been employed as an antineoplastic agent in Hodgkin's disease.[26] In recent trials treatment with combined chemotherapy has achieved a higher rate of remission than has the use of any single agent.[29,138]

In lymphosarcoma in childhood roentgen-ray therapy constitutes the mainstay of treatment. In mediastinal lesions with symptoms of respiratory obstruction, radiation should be administered cautiously. Treatment is known to precipitate transient enlargement of nodes with aggravation of respiratory distress. While nitrogen mustard (mechlorethamine) may have little lasting benefit,[106] cyclophosphamide (Cytoxan), another alkylating drug, is currently the agent of choice in generalized involvement. The plan of therapy with this drug is similar to that in leukemia. Adrenocorticosteroids or amethopterin (methotrexate) may be used when no further response is obtained with cyclophosphamide. It is still to be determined whether the polyfunctional alkylating agents or other agents given systemically at tolerated dosages can be expected to permanently control the course of Hodgkin's disease.[65]

Lymphangiography and inferior venacavagrams[70,116] have been shown to be more effective and reliable in demonstrating femoral, inguinal, iliac, and retroperitoneal node involvement by lymphoma than physical examination. Direct palpation of lymph nodes may give a misleading impression of the extent of neoplastic involvement. Intravenous pyelograms have also been shown to be less reliable than the other procedures. By the newer techniques, lymphosarcoma and reticulum cell sarcoma have rarely been found to be localized at the time the patient presents himself to the physician. Many patients who initially present as clinical Stages I and II, Hodgkin's disease, are shown to have retroperitoneal involvement. Those patients, with no evidence of disease below the diaphragm, seem to be potentially curable. In localized Hodgkin's disease the need for alkylating agents in addition to irradiation has been questioned. Prophylactic radiotherapy (aggressive radiotherapy of the diseased area and all contiguous node-bearing areas) may be inadequate in lymphosarcoma and reticulum cell sarcoma since they do not disseminate by direct extension to adjacent groups as in the case in Hodgkin's disease.[70] In Hodgkin's disease, in which lymphangiograms reveal retroperitoneal involvement in cases previously diagnosed as Stage I, more aggressive therapy than surgical removal is necessary.

Nitrogen mustard and its derivatives possess the ability to arrest mitosis and owe their effectiveness to their toxicity for all cells but more so to bone marrow, lymphoid, and reticuloendothelial tissues. With these compounds improvement sets in within a few days with subsidence of fever and shrinkage of lymph nodes and spleen and persists from periods of a month to a year or longer. Nausea, vomiting, and depression of the bone marrow with pancytopenia are likely to result from use of these compounds. Leukopenia, thrombocytopenia, and anemia may become marked within a few days to a week following treatment and persist from 3 to 5 weeks. Rigid attention, therefore, should be given to blood studies before and after treatment, especially with regard to leukopenia and thrombocytopenia. This caution is particularly applicable when successive courses of nitrogen mustard ($HN_2$) are contemplated. In general it is inadvisable to employ this form of treatment when the white blood cell count is below 3,500 per cubic millimeter.[132]

$HN_2$ (nitrogen mustard), the principal member of this group of drugs, is given intravenously in a total dosage of 0.4 mg. per kilogram of body weight. It may be divided in a fractional dosage of 0.1 mg. per kilogram in 4 consecutive days when there is evidence of abnormal depression of the bone marrow and widespread disease. The calculated dose is injected into an intravenous infusion of physiologic saline solution or 5% glucose in water.

TEM (triethylene melamine), a compound with nitrogen mustard activity, has the advantage of oral administration permitting ambulatory treatment. The dosage is 0.12 mg. per kilogram orally. A single course consists of 10 mg., divided into 2.5 mg. doses daily for 4 days.[90] The restoration to normal white blood cell and platelet counts is a prerequisite for repetition of treatment.

Chlorambucil (Leukeran), another nitrogen mustard derivative, is available in 2 and 4 mg. tablets. It is given orally in a dosage of 0.2 mg. per kilogram of body weight. With proper adjustment of dosage chlorambucil has been found as effective as other alkylating agents in the treatment of patients with Hodgkin's disease, lymphosarcoma, chronic lymphocytic leukemia, and also chronic myelocytic leukemia.[87] To achieve maximum results, the drug is given to the point of early bone marrow depression. Close observation of the hemoglobin level, white blood cell count, and platelet level is mandatory. Chlorambucil is given initially in a dosage of 0.1 mg. per kilogram when the bone marrow function has been previously impaired by radiation or chemotherapy. Cyclophosphamide (Cytoxan), also related to the nitrogen mustards, is a potent cytotoxic agent. This compound possesses the alkylating groups of nitrogen mustard attached to a cyclic phosphorus compound. Its special advantage is that it is activated only when the alkyl groups are released by phosphamidase activity which is high in many malignant tumors. It is useful not only in leukemia, but also especially in soft tissue malignancies in children, such as the lymphomas.[93,127] Significant benefit has been obtained with giant follicular lymphoma, Hodgkin's disease, lymphosarcoma, and reticulum cell sarcoma. Cyclophosphamide, an inactive transport form of an alkylating agent that requires in vivo activation, may be given by oral, intramuscular, and intravenous routes. The oral dosage is 2.5 mg. per kilogram of body weight in one oral dose daily or 5 to 15 mg. per kilogram intravenously and repeated at weekly intervals, observing the white blood cell count. As soon as leukopenic levels of 2,000 to 2,500 per cubic millimeter are reached, the drug is discontinued, as the white blood cells may continue to fall.

In a study of twenty-four children with disseminated neuroblastoma, the incidence of response to cyclophosphamide was superior to that with any other chemotherapeutic agent.[136] Seven of ten children showing favorable responses had neuroblastoma cells in the bone marrow that disappeared from the marrow during therapy. Improvement in the disease may be observed as early as 21 days. These children received cyclophosphamide in doses of 5 mg. per kilogram of body weight given intravenously each day for 10 days, depending on the white blood cell count. Therapy was continued orally at a maintenance level of 2.5 mg. per kilogram per day. Significant leukopenia (white blood cell count of 2,500 per cubic millimeter or less), gastrointestinal symptoms, hyperpigmentation, alopecia, and cystitis may occur in varying degree.

Cyclophosphamide was administered concurrently with vincristine sulfate to nine consecutive children (3 weeks to 11 years of age) with unresectable neuroblastma.[60] Objective tumor regression was observed in all nine children and complete remission in seven. Two of the nine patients expired within 1 year of diagnosis. The remaining seven continued to respond after 12 months. These results compare with a median survival of 6 months in a larger series of thirty-one patients, 75% of whom had expired by 1 year from the time of diagnosis. In the combined therapy group vincristine sulfate was administered intravenously on the first day and was repeated every 2 weeks in dosages of 1.5 mg. per square meter of body surface. Cyclophosphamide was injected intravenously on the eighth day and from then on every 2 weeks in dosages of 300 mg. per square meter of body surface. The duration of chemotherapy was 2 to 12 months. The findings indicate that some unresectable neuroblastomas will respond to chemotherapy alone or chemotherapy followed by radiation therapy to an extent that allows complete surgical removal.

PROCARBAZINE.[26] This agent has recently been used in patients with widespread Hodgkin's disease resistant to vinca alkaloids and alkylating agents. All responses (in thirteen out of twenty-two patients) were clinically evident 3 weeks after therapy was begun. Four complete and nine partial remissions were achieved, ranging from 4 to more than 40 weeks in duration, with a mean duration of 10 weeks. Procarbazine hydrochloride therapy was initiated in this series at daily doses of 50 to 100 mg. in an attempt to avoid early nausea and vomiting. Within 1 to 2 weeks drug dosage was increased to 200 mg. daily and continued until antineoplastic effects or drug toxicity was observed. The drug was discontinued if relapse could not be reversed by dosages producing leukopenia (3,000/cu.mm.) in several weeks. Central nervous system manifestations of depression and lassitude were complications, but the major limitations of the drug were leukopenia and thrombocytopenia. The drug is known to inhibit the biosynthesis of DNA and RNA.

VINCRISTINE. Vincristine, an alkaloid of the periwinkle plant, has been successfully used in the treatment of inoperable malignant solid tumors. It is related to colchicine and, as a mitotic inhibitor, blocks cell division in metaphase without interfering with DNA replication or premitotic events.[66] In one group of nineteen children,[59] tumor regression was observed in two of three children with Hodgkin's disease, three of seven with neuroblastoma, two with Wilms' tumor, and one each with lymphosarcoma and neurofibrosarcoma, Ewing's sarcoma, malignant teratoma, and retinoblastoma. One child with localized inoperable neuroblastoma responded to vincristine therapy, followed by ionizing radiation to such an extent that the localized tumor could be excised completely. Comparable results have been obtained in other series.[11,117,134] The drug is given intravenously in single weekly doses, ranging from 0.03 to 0.075 mg. per kilogram, watching the white blood count for evidences of marked leukopenia (below 1,000 per cubic millimeter). Small daily priming doses (0.02 mg. per kilogram) are sometimes recommended but are not generally used to treat lymphomas or Hodgkin's disease.[134] Side effects of vincristine are alopecia, gastritis, esophagitis, and neurotoxicity such as paresthesias, loss of deep tendon reflexes, peripheral neuritis, and severe constipation with ileus.

COMBINATION THERAPY. Recent investigations have indicated that the use of several chemotherapeutic agents simultaneously in generalized Hodgkin's disease and lymphosarcoma have increased the rate of remission. The National Cancer Institute[29] employed combination chemotherapy in previously untreated patients with Stage III and IV Hodgkin's disease. Patients received six 2-week cycles of drugs administered over a period of 6 months, each cycle consisting of vincristine, 1.4 mg. per square meter, and nitrogen mustard, 6 mg. per square meter on days 1 and 8; procarbazine, 100 mg. per square meter orally for 14 days of each cycle; and prednisone, 40 mg. per square meter orally for each day of cycles 1 and 4. In the forty-three patients treated, the response rate was 100% and the complete remission rate was 81%. The median duration of remission was 19 months. Similar chemotherapy programs for lymphocytic lymphoma and reticulum cell sarcoma have been effective in inducing remission and prolonging the duration of unmaintained remission.[118] In refractory cases combined therapy has been used, consisting of actinomycin D, $10 \mu g$ per kilogram of body weight, and 5 mg. of cyclophosphamide per kilogram, each given intravenously, and 2.5 to 5 mg. of methotrexate given orally. This combined therapy is given daily for 7 to 14 days. The hemoglobin, white blood cell count, and platelet count are determined before treatment and then every other day. If the platelet count falls from normal to 100,000 to 150,000 per cubic millimeter, all three drugs should be discontinued and counts then followed twice a week for the first week and weekly until returned to normal. In patients with lymphoma, blood urea nitrogen and uric acid should be obtained before therapy and once or twice a week during therapy. Toxic reactions such as mouth ulcers, nausea, vomiting, abdominal pain, and other side reactions of each drug should be evaluated before therapy is stopped. Responses have been seen in patients with metastatic Ewing's sarcoma, embryonal rhabdomyosarcoma, neuroblastoma, and lymphoma.

In lymphoma, actinomycin D has also been used in combination with cyclophosphamide only—the former in a dose of 15 $\mu$g per kilogram and the latter, 5 mg. per kilogram given intravenously every second or third day, each for five doses.[93]

TREATMENT OF A TYPICAL CASE OF LYMPHOSARCOMA. The low 5-year survival rate of lymphosarcoma necessitates the use of energetic methods of treatment.[93] For a localized and surgically accessible lesion, radical excision is indicated, followed by roentgen therapy to the tumor site and contiguous node regions. Chemotherapy is then instituted for the reasons already stated. In cases in which the disease is already widespread, surgery is indicated for diagnosis and perhaps exploration, followed by radiation therapy. Available agents designed to destroy or inhibit tumor growth have now increased in numbers and choice of the ideal drug or combination may be difficult.

In a typical case of a child with lymphosarcoma situated in a peripheral lymph node in whom substantial numbers of neoplastic cells were found in the bone marrow, management was as follows. Following biopsy to establish the diagnosis, nitrogen mustard ($HN_2$) was prescribed in a dosage of 0.4 mg. per kilogram given intravenously as a single-dose course (fractional doses of 0.2 mg. per kilogram on each of 3 days may be given as an alternative method). A course of roentgen-ray therapy was immediately begun. On its termination, chlorambucil was given in a daily dosage of 0.2 mg. per kilogram of body weight for a period of 3 to 4 weeks, depending on bone marrow depression. As an alternative drug, cyclophosphamide (Cytoxan) may be given in a daily oral dose of 2 to 5 mg. per kilogram. As soon as leukopenic levels are reached (below 2,000 white blood cells per cubic millimeter), the drug is discontinued. The drug is reintroduced with the return of higher white blood cell counts.

The adrenocortical steroids known to cause lympholysis are useful when the disease is generalized and constitutional symptoms are present. They also are important accessory therapeutic agents with the development of an acquired hemolytic anemia. When the disease has become generalized, therapy of acute lymphoblastic leukemia, as outlined in Chapter 23, should be employed.

Hemolytic anemia may be so severe and splenomegaly so marked in patients with lymphosarcoma that splenectomy may be required in spite of continued transfusion and steroid administration to achieve stability of the hemoglobin level.

As with leukemia, effective therapeutic agents in Hodgkin's disease and lymphosarcoma can produce excessive rapid breakdown of nucleoprotein. A large increase in uric acid excretion during the early days of treatment of a patient with lymphosarcoma is often indicative of a responsive tumor. With continued treatment, obstructive uric acid nephropathy or uropathy may supervene.[100] Allopurinol, a xanthine oxidase inhibitor, should be used to prevent these hazardous complications. The usual dose in children is 100 to 300 mg. per day.

*Prognosis.* With the combination of therapeutic agents the duration of life of patients with the lymphomas can be extended to many years. Survivals of 3 and 5 years and longer have been reported, during which time the patient appeared in good health.[106] In children the course is shorter and the disease more aggressive than in adults. Despite periods of remission, recurrences are invariable, and inevitably a fatal outcome ensues.

The gravity of lymphosarcoma is reflected in a series of twenty-nine children, in whom 60% with lymphosarcoma died within 44 weeks of onset of symptoms.[133] Jones and Klingberg[63] in a composite series of 213 children with lymphosarcoma (omitting Hodgkin's disease and giant cell follicular lymphosarcoma), which included forty-three cases of their own, found an increased incidence of the disease between 3 to 5 years of age. Of the entire group only 9.3% were survivors of 5 years. Fifty percent were alive at the end of 6 months and 10% at the end of 15 months. Leukemic transformation in this series occurred in 29.8% of cases.

In a series of 1,269 patients with lymphosarcoma of all ages, the median survival was 7.5 months for children up to 15 years of age as compared with that of the adults (16 to 92 years), 27.7 months.[105,107] Five-year survival for children was 17.4% and for adults 29%. In another series[93] 18% is given as a 5-year survival and 8% at 10 years for lymphocytic lymphosarcoma. This compares with 30% for 5 years in Hodgkin's disease and 17% at 10 years; 100% survival for 5 years in follicular lymphoblastoma and 40% in 10 years. For reticulum cell sarcoma the 5-year survival was 16%, 8% at 10 years.

# REFERENCES

1. Aisenberg, A. C.: Lymphocytopenia in Hodgkin's disease, Blood 25:1037, 1965.
2. Anderson, R. E., Hoshino, T., and Yamamoto, R.: Myelofibrosis with myeloid metaplasia in survivors of atomic bomb in Hiroshima, Ann. Intern. Med. 60:1, 1964.
3. Anderson, W. A. D.: Synopsis of pathology, ed. 8, St. Louis, 1971, The C. V. Mosby Co.
4. Asboe-Hansen, G., and Kaalund-Jorgensen, O.: Systemic mast cell disease involving skin, liver, bone marrow and blood associated with disseminated xanthomata, Acta Haemat. 16:273, 1956.
5. Baldini, M., Fudenberg, H. H., Fukutake, K., and Dameshek, W.: The anemia of the Di Guglielmo syndrome, Blood 14:344, 1959.
6. Bayrd, E. D., Paulson, G. S., and Hargraves, M. M.: Hodgkin's specific cells in bone marrow aspiration; a brief review and report of two cases, Blood 9:46, 1954.
7. Bogart, F. B.: Leukosarcoma, Amer. J. Roentgen. 55:743, 1946.
8. Bouroncle, B. A.: Sternberg-Reed cells in the peripheral blood of patients with Hodgkin's disease, Blood 27:544, 1966.
9. Burkitt, D.: Determining climatic limitations of children's cancer common in Africa, Brit. J. Med. 2:1019, 1962.
10. Canale, V. C., and Smith, C. H.: Chronic lymphadenopathy simulating malignant lymphoma, J. Pediat. 70:891, 1967.
11. Carbone, P. P., Bono, V., Frei, E., III, and Brindley, C. D.: Clinical studies with vincristine, Blood 21:640, 1963.
12. Cartwright, G. E., Finch, C. A., Loeb, V., Jr., Moore, C. V., Singer, K., and Dameshek, W.: Panels in therapy; splenectomy in myeloid metaplasia with myelosclerosis, Blood 10:550, 1955.
13. Clift, R. A., Wright, D. H., and Clifford, P.: Leukemia in Burkitt's lymphoma, Blood 22:243, 1963.
14. Cohen, B. M., Smetana, H. F., and Miller, R. W.: Hodgkin's disease; long survival in a study of 388 World War II Army cases, Cancer 17:856, 1964.
15. Cohen, M. H., Bennett, J. M., Berard, C. W., Ziegler, J. L., Vogel, C. L., Sheagren, J. N., and Carbone, P. P.: Burkitt's tumor in the United States, Cancer 23:1259, 1969.
16. Cook, J. E., Franklin, J. W., Hamilton, H. E., and Fowler, W. M.: Syndrome of myelofibrosis, Arch. Intern. Med. 91:704, 1953.
17. Cooke, J. V.: Mediastinal tumor in acute leukemia; a clinical and roentgenologic study, Amer. J. Dis. Child. 44:1153, 1932.
18. Cooper, T., and Watkins, C. H.: An evaluation of sternal aspiration as an aid in diagnoses of the malignant lymphomata, Blood 4:534, 1949.
19. Craver, L. F.: Some aspects of the treatment of Hodgkin's disease, Cancer 7:927, 1954.
20. Custer, R. P., and Bernhard, W. G.: The interrelationship of Hodgkin's disease and other lymphatic tumors, Amer. J. Med. Sci. 216:625, 1948.
21. Dameshek, W.: The Di Guglielmo syndrome revisited, Blood 34:567, 1969.
22. Dameshek, W., and Baldini, M.: The Di Guglielmo syndrome (editorial), Blood 13:192, 1958.
23. Dameshek, W., and Gunz, F.: Leukemia, ed. 2, New York, 1964, Grune & Stratton, Inc., pp. 24-26.
24. Dargeon, H. W.: Lymphosarcoma in childhood. In Levine, S. Z., editor: Advances in pediatrics, Chicago, 1953, Year Book Medical Publishers, Inc.
25. Dargeon, H. W.: Tumors of childhood, New York, 1960, Paul B. Hoeber, Inc.
26. DeConti, R. C.: Procarbazine in the management of late Hodgkin's disease, J.A.M.A. 215:927, 1971.
27. De La Fuente, V.: Megakaryocytic reaction localized in the bone marrow, Arch. Intern. Med. 78:387, 1946.
28. Dent, C. E., Smellie, J. M., and Watson, L.: Studies in osteopetrosis, Arch. Dis. Child. 40:7, 1965.
29. DeVita, V. T., Serpick, A., and Carbone, P. P.: Combination chemotherapy of advanced Hodgkin's disease, Proc. Amer. Ass. Cancer Res. 10:19, 1969.
30. Diamond, H. D.: The natural history and management of lymphosarcoma, Med. Clin. N. Amer. 40:721, 1956.
31. Diamond, H. D.: The medical management of cancer, New York, 1958, Grune & Stratton, Inc.
32. Di Guglielmo, G.: Les maladies érythémiques, Rev. hémat. 1:355, 1946.
33. Discombe, G., and Nickol, K.: Myelosis involving the granulocytic and erythrocytic systems, J. Clin. Path. 7:211, 1954.
34. Doan, C. A., and Reinhart, H. L.: The basophil granulocyte, basophilcytosis and myeloid leukemia, basophil and "mixed granule" types; and experimental clinical and pathological study, with the report of a new syndrome, Amer. J. Clin. Path. 11:1, 1941.
35. Dorfman, R. F.: Diagnosis of Burkitt's tumor in the United States, Cancer 21:563, 1968.
36. Dorfman, R., and Reinhard, E.: Hodgkin's disease, J.A.M.A. 208:325, 1969.
37. Douglas, D. M., and Claireaux, A. E.:

Hodgkin's disease in childhood, Arch. Dis. Child. 28:222, 1953.
38. Dyment, P. G., Melnyk, K. J., and Brubaker, C. A.: A cytomegalic study of acute erythroleukemia in children, Blood 32:997, 1968.
39. Editorial: Hodgkin's disease, J.A.M.A. 139:380, 1949.
40. Editorial: Myelofibrosis (panmyelosis) in Hiroshima, J.A.M.A. 189:767, 1964.
41. Efrati, P., Klajman, A., and Spitz, H.: Mast cell leukemia? Malignant mastocytosis with leukemia-like manifestations, Blood 12:869, 1957.
42. Ellis, J. M.: Urticaria pigmentosa; report of case with autopsy, Arch. Path. 48:426, 1949.
43. Emery, J. L.: Erythraemic myelosis in a girl aged 13 years, J. Path. Bact. 63:395, 1951.
44. Erf, L. A., and Herbut, P. A.: Primary and secondary myelofibrosis; clinical and pathological study of thirteen cases of fibrosis of the bone marrow, Ann. Intern. Med. 21:862, 1944.
45. Fanger, H., Cella, L. J., Jr., and Litchman, H.: Thrombocythemia; report of three cases and review of literature, New Eng. J. Med. 250:456, 1954.
46. Fraumeni, J. F., Jr., and Miller, R. W.: Epidemiology of human leukemia; recent observations, J. Nat. Cancer Inst. 38:593, 1967.
47. Freymann, J. G., Burrell, S. B., and Marler, E. A.: Role of hemolysis in anemia secondary to chronic lymphocytic leukemia and certain malignant lymphomas, New Eng. J. Med. 259:847, 1958.
48. Friedman, B. I., Will, J. J., Freiman, D. G., and Braunstein, H.: Tissue mast cell leukemia, Blood 8:70, 1958.
49. Gamsu, H., Lorber, J., and Rendle-Short, J.: Haemolytic anaemia in osteopetrosis; a report of two cases, Arch. Dis. Child. 36:494, 1961.
50. Gladstein, E., Guernsey, J. M., Rosenberg, S. A., and Kaplan, H. S.: The value of laparotomy and splenectomy in the staging of Hodgkin's disease, Cancer 24:709, 1969.
51. Goldman, J. M.: Laparotomy for staging of Hodgkin's disease, Lancet 1:125, 1971.
52. Green, T. W., Conley, C. L., Ashburn, L. L., and Peters, H. R.: Splenectomy for myeloid metaplasia of the spleen, New Eng. J. Med. 248:211, 1953.
53. Groat, W. A., Wyatt, T. C., Zimmer, S. M., and Field, R. E.: Acute basophilic leukemia, Amer. J. Med. Sci. 191:457, 1936.
54. Hedenstrom, G., and Soderstrom, M.: Di Guglielmo's disease; comments on a case of erythroleucemic myelosis, Acta Paediat. 43:78, 1954.
55. Horton, B. F., Chernoff, A. I., and Meadows, R. W.: The hemoglobin profile and erythroleukemia, Cancer 26:904, 1970.
56. Howqua, J., and MacKay, I. R.: L.E. cells in lymphoma, Blood 22:191, 1963.
57. Isaacs, R.: Lymphosarcoma cell leukemia, Ann. Intern. Med. 11:657,1937.
58. Jacobs, P. A., Tough, I. M., and Wright, D. H.: Cytogenetic studies in Burkitt's lymphoma, Lancet 2:1144, 1963.
59. James, D. H., Jr., and George, P.: Vincristine in children with malignant solid tumors, J. Pediat. 64:534, 1964.
60. James, D. H., Jr., Hustu, O., Wrenn, E. L., and Pinkel, D.: Combination chemotherapy of childhood neuroblastoma, J.A.M.A. 194:123, 1965.
61. Jenkin, R. D. T., Peters, M. V., and Darte, J. M. M.: Hodgkin's disease in children, Amer. J. Roentgen. 100:222, 1967.
62. Johnston, C. C., Jr., Lavy, N., Lord, T., Vellios, F., Merritt, A. D., and Deiss, W. P., Jr.: Osteopetrosis; a clinical genetic, metabolic and morphologic study of the dominantly inherited benign form, Medicine 47:149, 1968.
63. Jones, B., and Klingberg, W. G.: Lymphosarcoma in children; a report of 43 cases and a review of the literature, J. Pediat. 63:11, 1963.
64. Kaplan, H. S.: Clinical evaluation and radiotherapeutic management of Hodgkin's disease and the malignant lymphomas, New Eng. J. Med. 278:892, 1968.
65. Karnofsky, D. A.: Hodgkin's disease; chemotherapy, J.A.M.A. 191:30, 1965.
66. Karnofsky, D. A., and Clarkson, D. D.: Cellular effects of anticancer drugs, Ann. Rev. Pharmacol. 3:357, 1963.
67. Karnofsky, D. A., Miller, D. G., and Phillips, R. F.: Role of chemotherapy in the management of early Hodgkin's disease, Amer. J. Roentgen. 90:968, 1963.
68. Kennedy, B. J.: Effect of androgenic hormone in myelofibrosis, J.A.M.A. 182:116, 1962.
69. Korst, D. R., Clatanoff, D. V., and Schilling, R. F.: On myelofibrosis, Arch. Intern. Med. 97:169, 1956.
70. Lee, B. J., Nelson, J. H., and Schwartz, G.: Evaluation of lymphangiography, inferior venacavography and intravenous pyelography in the clinical staging and management of Hodgkin's disease and lymphosarcoma, New Eng. J. Med. 271:327, 1964.
71. Levinson, B., Walter, B. A., Wintrobe, M. M., and Cartwright, G. E.: A clinical study

of Hodgkin's disease, Arch. Intern. Med. **99**:519, 1957.
72. Levitan, R., Diamond, H. D., and Craver, L. F.: Jaundice in Hodgkin's disease, Amer. J. Med. **30**:99, 1961.
73. Lineman, J. W., and Bethell, F. H.: Angogenic myeloid metaplasia; its natural history and present day management, Amer. J. Med. **22**:107, 1957.
74. Ludman, H., and Spear, P. W.: Reed-Sternberg cells in the peripheral blood; report of a case of Hodgkin's disease, Blood **12**:189, 1957.
75. Lukes, R. J.: Hodgkin's disease; prognosis and relationship of histologic features to clinical stage, J.A.M.A. **190**:914, 1964.
76. Lukes, R. J., and Butler, S. S.: The pathology and nomenclature of Hodgkin's disease, Cancer Res. **26**(Part I):1063, 1966.
77. Lusher, J. M.: Chloroma as a presenting feature of acute leukemia, Amer. J. Dis. Child. **108**:62, 1964.
78. Mackenzie, I., and Stephenson, A. G.: A case of erythremic myelosis (Di Guglielmo's anemia), Blood **7**:927, 1952.
79. McAlister, W.: Hodgkin's disease; clinicopathologic conference, Amer. J. Med. **40**:414, 1966.
80. McCausland, D. J. M.: Hodgkin's disease in children, Arch. Dis. Child. **16**:59, 1941.
81. McCune, D. J., and Bradley, C.: Osteopetrosis (marble bones) in an infant, Amer. J. Dis. Child. **48**:949, 1934.
82. McDonald, J. B., and Hamrick, J. G.: Acute megakaryocytic leukemia, Arch. Intern. Med. **81**:73, 1948.
83. McPeak, C. N.: Osteopetrosis; report of eight cases occurring in three generations of one family, Amer. J. Roentgen. **36**:816, 1936.
84. Menten, M. L., and Gaffney, P. C.: Immature cell erythremia, Amer. J. Dis. Child. **80**:982, 1950.
85. Meyer, L. M., Halpern, J., and Ogden, F. N.: Acute plasma cell leukemia, Ann Intern. Med. **22**:585, 1945.
86. Meyer, O. O.: Treatment of Hodgkin's disease, J.A.M.A. **161**:1484, 1956.
87. Miller, D. G., Diamond, H. D., and Craver, L. F.: The clinical use of chlorambucil; a critical study, New Eng. J. Med. **261**:525, 1959.
88. Morrison, M.: Congenital leukemia with chloromas, Amer. J. Dis. Child. **58**:332, 1939.
89. Moss, W. T., and Ackerman, L. V.: Plasma cell leukemia, Blood **1**:396, 1946.
90. Murphy, M. L.: Leukemia and lymphoma in children, Ped. Clin. N. Amer. **6**:611, 1959.
91. Nakai, G. S., Craddock, C. G., and Figueroa, W. G.: Agnogenic myeloid metaplasia; a survey of twenty-nine cases and a review of the literature, Ann. Intern. Med. **57**:419, 1962.
92. O'Conor, G. T., and Davies, J. N. P.: Malignant tumors in African children: with special reference to malignant lymphoma, J. Pediat. **56**:526, 1960.
93. Origenes, M. L., Jr., Need, D. J., and Hartmann, J. R.: Treatment of the malignant lymphomas in children, Ped. Clin. N. Amer. **9**:769, 1962.
94. Ozer, F. L., Truax, W. E., Miesch, D. C., and Levin, W. C.: Primary hemorrhagic thrombocytopenia, Amer. J. Med. **28**:807, 1960.
95. Page, A. R., Hansen, A. E., and Good, R. A.: Occurrence of leukemia and lymphoma in patients with agammaglobulinemia, Blood **21**:197, 1963.
96. Peters, M. V.: Hodgkin's disease; radiation therapy, J.A.M.A. **191**:28, 1965.
97. Peterson, R. D. A., Kelly, W. O., and Good, R. A.: Ataxia-telangiectasia; its association with a defective thymus, immunological deficiency disease and malignancy, Lancet **1**: 1189, 1964.
98. Pisciotta, A. V.: Clinical and pathologic effects of space-occupying lesions of the bone marrow, Amer. J. Clin. Path. **20**:915, 1950.
99. Porter, F. S.: Multiple myeloma in a child, J. Pediat. **62**:602, 1963.
100. Primikirios, N., Stutzman, L., and Sandberg, A. A.: Uric acid excretion in patients with malignant lymphomas, Blood **17**:701, 1961.
101. Quaglino, D., and Hayhoe, F. G. J.: Periodic-acid-Schiff positivity in erythroblasts with special reference to Di Guglielmo's disease, Brit. J. Haemat. **6**:26, 1960.
102. Randell, D. L., Reiquam, C. W., Githens, J. H., and Robinson, A.: Familial myeloproliferative disease; a new syndrome closely simulating myelogenous leukemia in childhood, Amer. J. Dis. Child. **110**:479, 1965.
103. Rider, T. L., Stein, A. A., and Abbuhl, J. W.: Generalized mast cell disease and urticaria pigmentosa, Pediatrics **19**:1023, 1957.
104. Rosenberg, H. S., and Taylor, F. M.: The myeloproliferative syndrome in children, J. Pediat. **52**:407, 1958.
105. Rosenberg, S. A., Diamond, H. D., and Craver, L. F.: Lymphosarcoma; the effects of therapy and survival of 1,269 patients in a review of 30 years' experience, Ann. Intern. Med. **53**:877, 1960.
106. Rosenberg, S. A., Diamond, H. D., Dargeon, H. W., and Craver, L. F.: Lymphosarcoma in childhood, New Eng. J. Med. **259**:505, 1958.

107. Rosenberg, S. A., Diamond, H. D., Jaslowitz, B., and Craver, L. F.: Lymphosarcoma in childhood; a review of 1,239 cases, Medicine **40**:31, 1961.
108. Rosenthal, M. C., Pisciotta, A. V., Komninos, Z. D., Goldenberg, H., and Dameshek, W.: The auto-immune hemolytic anemia of malignant lymphocytic disease, Blood **10**:197, 1955.
109. Rosenthal, N., Dreskin, O. H., Vural, I. L., and Zak, F. G.: The significance of hematogones in blood, bone marrow and lymph node aspiration in giant follicular lymphoblastoma, Acta Haemat. **8**:368, 1952.
110. Ross, R. R.: Chloroma and chloroleukemia, Amer. J. Med. **18**:671, 1955.
111. Rubin, P.: Hodgkin's disease, J.A.M.A. **190**:910, 1964.
112. Rubin, P.: Hodgkin's disease; comment, J.A.M.A. **190**:917, 1964.
113. Say, B., and Berkel, I.: Idiopathic myelofibrosis in an infant, J. Pediat. **64**:580, 1964.
114. Schultz, J., Shay, T. L., and Gruenstein, M.: Chemistry of experimental chloroma. I. Porphyrins and peroxidases, Cancer Res. **14**:157, 1954.
115. Schwarz, E.: Extramedullary megakaryocytosis in chronic myelosis, Amer. J. Clin. Path. **24**:629, 1954.
116. Schwarz, G.: Hodgkin's disease; the role of lymphangiography, J.A.M.A. **190**:912, 1964.
117. Selawry, O. S., and Hananian, J.: Vincristine treatment of cancer in children, J.A.M.A. **183**:741, 1963.
118. Serpick, A. A., Lowenbraun, S., and DeVita, V. T.: Combination chemotherapy of lymphosarcoma and reticulum cell sarcoma, Proc. Amer. Ass. Cancer Res. **10**:78, 1969.
119. Sharnoff, J. G., Belsky, H., and Melton, J.: Plasma cell leukemia or multiple myeloma with osteosclerosis, Amer. J. Med. **17**:582, 1954.
120. Sheets, R. F., Drevets, C. C., and Hamilton, H. E.: Erythroleukemia (Di Guglielmo syndrome); a report of clinical observations and experimental studies in seven patients, Arch. Intern. Med. **111**:295, 1963.
121. Shimkin, M. B.: Hodgkin's disease; effectiveness of treatment in control, J.A.M.A. **190**:916, 1964.
122. Sjolin, S.: Studies on osteopetrosis. II. Investigation concerning the nature of the anaemia, Acta Paediat. **48**:529, 1959.
123. Slaughter, D. P.: Hodgkin's disease; radical surgery, J.A.M.A. **191**:26, 1965.
124. Smetana, A. F., and Cohen, B. M.: Mortality in relation to histologic type in Hodgkin's disease, Blood **11**:211, 1956.
125. Smithers, D. W.: Hodgkin's disease; one entity or two? Lancet **2**:1285, 1970.
126. Sohn, D., Valensi, Q., and Miller, S. P.: Neurologic manifestations of Hodgkin's disease; intracerebral Hodgkin's granuloma, Arch. Neurol. **17**:429, 1967.
127. Solomon, J., Alexander, M. J., and Steinfel, J. L.: Cyclophosphamide, J.A.M.A. **183**:165, 1963.
128. Spach, M. A., Howell, D. A., and Harris, J. S.: Myocardial infarction with multiple thromboses in a child with primary thrombocytosis, Pediatrics **31**:268, 1963.
129. Spaet, T. H., Lejnieks, I., Gaynor, E., and Goldstein, M. L.: Defective platelets in essential thrombocythemia, Arch. Intern. Med. **124**:135, 1969.
130. Stich, M. H., Swiller, A. I., and Morrison, M.: The "grape cell" of multiple myeloma, Amer. J. Clin. Path. **25**:601, 1955.
131. Stickler, G. B., and Pinkel, D.: Plasmacytosis in bone marrow and hypergammaglobulinemia in acute leukemia, Pediatrics **22**:659, 1958.
132. Sturgis, C. C.: Hematology, ed. 2, Springfield, Ill., 1955, Charles C Thomas, Publisher.
133. Sullivan, M. P.: Leukemia transformation in lymphosarcoma in childhood, Pediatrics **29**:589, 1962.
134. Sutow, W. W., Thurman, W. G., and Wendmiller, J.: Vincristine (Leurocristine) sulfate in the treatment of children with metastatic Wilms' tumor, Pediatrics **32**:880, 1963.
135. ten Bensel, R. W., Stadlan, E. M., and Krivit, W.: The development of malignancy in the course of the Aldrich syndrome, J. Pediat. **68**:761, 1966.
136. Thurman, W. G., Fernbach, D. J., Sullivan, M. P., and the Writing Committee of the Pediatric Division of the Southwest Cancer Chemotherapy Study Group: Cyclophosphamide therapy in childhood neuroblastoma, New Eng. J. Med. **270**:1336, 1964.
137. Ultmann, J. E., Hyman, G. A., and Calder, B.: Occurrence of lymphoma in patients with longstanding hyperthyroidism, Blood **21**:282, 1963.
138. Ultmann, J. E., and Nixon, D. D.: The therapy of lymphoma, Seminars Hemat. **6**:376, 1969.
139. Varadi, S.: Hodgkin's disease; specific findings in sternal puncture material, Brit. J. Haemat. **1**:184, 1955.
140. Wasserman, L. R., Stats, D., Schwartz, L., and Fudenberg, H.: Symptomatic and hemopathic hemolytic anemia, Amer. J. Med. **18**:961, 1955.
141. Waters, W. J., and Lacson, P. S.: Mast cell

leukemia presenting as urticaria pigmentosa; report of a case, Pediatrics 19:1033, 1957.
142. Wegelius, R., and Peltonen, T.: Erythraemic myelosis (Di Guglielmo) in an infant, Acta Paediat. 43:280, 1954.
143. Weisberger, A. S.: The significance of "dry tap" bone marrow aspirations, Amer. J. Med. Sci. 229:63, 1955.
144. Welford, N. T.: Facial paralysis associated with osteopetrosis (marble bones); report of a case of the syndrome occurring in five generations of the same family, J. Pediat. 55:67, 1959.
145. Willerson, D., Becker, C. E., Boushey, H., Kimball, R. S., and Kass, C.: Hodgkin's disease exclusively with bone marrow involvement, J.A.M.A. 214:2197, 1970.
146. Wright, D. H.: Reed-Sternberg-like cells in recurrent Burkitt lymphoma, Lancet 1:1052, 1970.
147. Wright, D. H.: Burkitt's tumor in England—a comparison with childhood lymphosarcoma, Int. J. Cancer 1:503, 1966.
148. Wright, D. H.: Burkitt's tumor and childhood lymphosarcoma, Clin. Pediat. 6:116, 1967.
149. Zawisch, C.: Marble bone disease; a study of osteogenesis, Arch. Path. 43:55, 1947.
150. Zeffren, J. L., and Ultmann, J. E.: Reticulum cell sarcoma terminating in acute leukemia, Blood 15:277, 1960.
151. Zetterström, R.: Osteopetrosis (marble bone disease); clinical and pathological review, Mod. Prob. Pädiat. 3:488, 1957.
152. Zuelzer, W. W., Mastrangelo, R., Stulberg, C. S., Poulik, M. D., Page, R. H., and Thompson, R. I.: Autoimmune hemolytic anemia; natural history and viral-immunologic interactions in childhood, Amer. J. Med. 49:80, 1970.

# 25 DISORDERS OF THE SPLEEN AND THE RETICULOENDOTHELIAL SYSTEM

*Role of the spleen in blood disorders.* The spleen plays an essential part in the pathogenesis of so many blood disorders that a review of its structure and function serves as a frame of reference for appraising deviations from the normal.

*Structure of the spleen.* The spleen is structurally organized to perform its main physiologic functions of blood formation, sequestration and destruction of blood cells, principally the erythrocytic series, and protection against infection. It possesses a smooth muscle capsule and trabeculae permitting its contraction, a vascular system with connecting sinusoids allowing withdrawal of cells from the circulation, a lymphoid system (malpighian corpuscles) corresponding to similar tissue elsewhere in the body, and a rich supply of reticuloendothelial tissue.[42] Elements of the reticuloendothelial system are either scattered through the pulp or line the vascular and lymphatic sinusoids. Whether free or fixed, these cells exert a phagocytic action. Mesenchymal cells and lymphoid tissue serve as a source of monocytes and lymphocytes. The sequestration of blood into pulp spaces and venous sinuses exposes bacteria and particulate matter to phagocytosis by the reticuloendothelial tissue and at the same time promotes the stasis and destruction of red blood cells.

The spleen is the largest mass of lymphatic tissue in the body, but, unlike other similar collections of this tissue, it is integrally associated with the bloodstream.[97] Splenic tissue fills the spaces between the capsule and trabeculae and is composed of white pulp and red pulp. The white pulp is made up of diffuse and nodular or cylindrical masses of lymphoid tissue (malpighian bodies), forming a sheath about small arterial branches. The red pulp consists of venous sinuses, while the tissue filling the spaces between them contains the splenic cords. The splenic artery subdivides into arterioles and capillaries, the majority terminating in venous sinuses. The veins of the spleen begin as networks of venous sinuses. The sinuses are lined by long narrow cells, and fixed macrophages, which are identical in properties with those in surrounding splenic cords. The precise manner of the connection of arterioles and venules in the spleen is still controversial. The closed circulation theory[52] presupposes that the blood in the spleen follows endothelial-lined pathways throughout so that arterial capillaries communicate directly with venous sinuses without initial sidetracking through the splenic cords. According to the open circulation theory, the arterial capillaries pour their blood directly into the pulp cords, and it then filters into venous sinuses. The exact manner of connection of arterioles and venules in the spleen, therefore, still awaits clarification.

It is now known that the sinus wall is a fenestrated membrane perforated by numerous slits through which the sinuses communicate with the surrounding pulp cords. Through a system of sphincters it is possible for the red cells to be sequestered in the venous sinuses for considerable periods of time, during which the plasma filters through the slits in the sinus wall into the cords.[19] Inspissated blood is eventually discharged from the sinuses into veins, but during the process of deplasmatization the entrapped red corpuscles are made more spheroidal, their membrane weakened and thus rendered susceptible to hemolysis in the trauma of the circulation.

*Normal functions of the spleen.* The normal functions of the spleen include the production, storage, and destruction of blood and protection against infection.

*Blood production.* The spleen is one of the principal sites of blood formation from the second to the fifth month of fetal life. After passing through the hemocytoblast stage, mesenchymal cells in the fifth month give rise to erythroblasts. After the fifth month red cell production diminishes and is absent by the sixth month.[33] Lymphocytes are produced in the spleen mainly in the white pulp (lymphatic tissue, malpighian bodies). According to the unitarian theory, monocytes are derived from lymphocytes upon migrating into the red pulp. In stress situations such as hemorrhage, hemolysis, and leukoblastic infiltration in infants and children, fetal blood foci are reactivated with the resumption of hematopoiesis. This function by which the spleen, liver, and lymph nodes revert to their fetal function of hematopoiesis is known as extramedullary hematopoiesis and applies equally to the production of red blood cells, granulocytes, and platelets. The relationship of the spleen to blood formation is further confirmed by the observation that in adult mice recovery of blood-forming tissues after total irradiation is accelerated by previously shielding the surgically exteriorized spleen with lead.[73]

Splenic control of normal maturation of the red cell surface is indicated by the loss of stickiness of the reticulocytes during maturation, the loss of reticulum, and shrinkage of diameter and volume due to loss of water.[33] This function is lost after splenectomy. Evidence of splenic control over the bone marrow is also suggested by the peripheral blood changes occurring after splenectomy—i.e., prompt increase in the number of white blood cells, platelets, nucleated red cells, and target cells, tendency toward thinness of the red cells, decreased osmotic fragility, and appearance of siderocytes, Heinz bodies, and red cells containing nuclear fragments (Howell-Jolly bodies).[149] On the other hand, erythrocytes containing Heinz bodies are removed and destroyed primarily in the spleen.[135] In a study in which such damaged cells were injected intravenously, the rate of their disappearance was slower in splenectomized patients than in control subjects.[3]

The "culling" function of the spleen describes the ability of this organ to scrutinize passing cells and to remove from the circulation those which do not meet certain minimum requirements.[33] The "pitting" function refers to its ability to remove a solid particle from the cytoplasm of a red cell without destroying the cell itself.[33] The increase in normoblasts following splenectomy may be due to the loss of an organ which is able to remove the nucleus of these red cells. While the spleen may remove nucleated red cells from the circulation, some, at least, are normally pitted and returned to the circulation. The "pitting" function may extend to siderin granules and other intraerythrocytic inclusions.

*Postsplenectomy thrombocytosis.* In any patient who has undergone splenectomy the number of platelets may rise excessively. While hemorrhagic and thromboembolic complications have been reported with postsplenectomy thrombocytosis in adults,[67] these have not occurred in our patients or in the experience of others dealing with splenectomized children.[38] Accordingly, the need for instituting anticoagulant therapy is minimal.

*Blood storage.* Although the spleen serves as a reservoir of red blood cells in the dog, cat, and horse, evidence indicates that blood reservoirs of this nature do not exist in man.[46,123] In the average-sized adult the spleen holds 20 to 30 ml. of red blood cells.[33] During the passage through the spleen even normal red blood cells are rendered more fragile, and a mild degree of spherocytosis is attained. It has been estimated that of the 120-day life cycle of the human red blood cell, about 2 days are spent in the spleen.[33] However, in patients with pathologic conditions, significant withdrawal of red blood cells from the circulation may take place, producing sudden severe anemia.[108]

In many enlarged spleens a stasis compartment exists in which blood slowly exchanges with the main arteriovenous stream. This "pool" of closely packed cells is especially prominent in conditions with splenomegaly.[165] During repeated circuits through this compartment, the red cells become progressively more susceptible to splenic destruction. In patients with red cell abnormalities splenic pooling is greater in relation to spleen size than in those patients in whom normal cells are circulating. In sickle cell anemia in young children sudden pooling of the blood into the spleen results in increased size of the organ, accompanied by severe anemia (Chapter 16).

It has been demonstrated that circulation of $^{51}$Cr-labeled red cells is slowed in patients with splenomegaly, leading to increased erythrostasis.[64] Whereas in normal subjects labeled red cell mixing in the spleen is completed within less than 1 minute, in patients with splenomegaly complete red cell mixing may require 45 minutes. The resulting erythrostasis may be associated with destruction of red cells within the spleen or the movement of altered cells through the circulation. The detention of red cells in an enlarged spleen and their resulting spheroidicity may account for transient hemolytic anemias encountered in a variety of systemic infections such as bacterial endocarditis, infectious hepatitis, infectious mononucleosis, etc.[76]

*Blood destruction.* Through the reticuloendothelial system the spleen removes worn out and fragmented cells and red cells sensitized by agglutination, resulting in degradation of hemoglobin and formation of bile pigment. That abnormally shaped red cells are trapped and destroyed by the normal spleen is illustrated by the fate of the spherocytes in patients with hereditary spherocytosis.

The activity of the enzymes of the red cell gradually diminishes[8]; the aging cell grows thinner,[150] becomes brittle and mechanically fragile,[158] and, hence, more susceptible to fragmentation. The fragments of the old red cells are finally destroyed in the spleen. ATP is a known determinant of erythrocyte deformability, i.e., the ability of the erythrocyte to traverse the restrictive passages of the microcirculation of the spleen and other reticuloendothelial structures.[179a] The intracellular content of ATP decreases with aging, and a significant difference in the concentration of ATP between young and old erythrocytes has been detected.[124a] Thus, with ATP depletion, spheroidicity and membrane rigidity increase, deformability decreases, and erythrocyte fragmentation occurs, leading to splenic entrapment and destruction of aged erythrocytes.[82a]

*Protection against infection.* It has been pointed out that the spleen with its abundant content of macrophages, plasma cells, and lymphocytes is strategically located in the direct stream of the circulating blood for effective phagocytosis and antibody production.[108] The extent to which the spleen participates in antibody response is estimated by comparing the normal with the splenectomized animal and human being after the injection of microorganisms and other antigens. It has been shown that in the rabbit abolition of antibody formation by roentgen rays may be prevented by shielding the surgically mobilized spleen.[74] A comparison of the antibody response to different types of agents in the splenectomized and nonsplenectomized animals and human beings has led to divergent results.\* These differences may be due to the need for intravenous[138,139] rather than subcutaneous[140] injections to demonstrate the depression of antibody response following splenectomy. There is satisfactory evidence that filtration of organisms or other particulate material takes place from the bloodstream by the local phagocytic action of the macrophages in the spleen. Evidence for such a protective mechanism is suggested by experiments[17] in which intravenously injected bacteria cleared from the blood were recovered in the macrophages of the reticuloendothelial tissues of the liver and spleen. Trapping of organisms by removal mechanisms of the liver and spleen have been demonstrated for staphylococci and *Escherichia coli.*[129,130]

Properdin, a natural serum protein which (in association with magnesium and complement) is involved in the destruction of selected bacteria and viruses, has been found to be in lower concentration in splenectomized persons than in normal persons.[23]

Several studies have recently reemphasized the fact that under certain circumstances the splenectomized child may show increased susceptibility to infection, particularly in the form of septicemia and meningitis.[69,154,155] The least susceptible is the child who has sustained a traumatic rupture of the spleen. An increased incidence, 10% or more, is found in children with portal hypertension and thalassemia major. The splenectomized infant is most susceptible, with an incidence of infection of 20%.[69] The basis of this increased susceptibility is not known. Perhaps it is due to removal of a substantial part of the reticuloendothelial system lodged in the spleen, or to the fact that this organ provides an important site of antibody synthesis.[59] Recently Shinefield and associates[147] found that splenectomized mice are strikingly susceptible to *Diplococcus pneumoniae* type 6. By using small numbers of organisms in contrast to previous investigators who had experimented with large numbers, they were able to show that earlier and increased death rates were observed in splenectomized mice, that diminished resistance persisted for a prolonged period after splenectomy, and that factors other than a deficiency of blood clearance of these organisms by the spleen were responsible for increased susceptibility.

Since serious infections occur most frequently in the first 2 years after splenectomy, oral therapy with antibiotics, usually penicillin, has been prescribed as a continuous prophylactic measure during this period. Although

---

\*See references 104, 120, 127, 138-140, and 153.

the incidence of postsplenectomy infection is avowedly small in comparison with the ever-increasing number of splenectomies, close supervision of the splenectomized child is necessary for several years postoperatively until further information is obtained. Such patients should receive immediate and energetic treatment in the event of sudden and severe illness.[153]

It has been suggested that the high transferrin level appearing after splenectomy supports the concept of an immunologic function for this protein in addition to iron-binding capacity.[144] In another report,[99] three children following splenectomy developed septicemia and disseminated intravascular coagulation, and a fourth patient with congenital asplenia had a similar course. *Diplococcus pneumoniae* was isolated from the blood of three patients. Only one of the four patients survived.

Later confirmatory studies[39,49] have further documented the hazard of overwhelming infection following splenectomy. There should be little remaining doubt that splenectomy in the child is associated with a significant risk of severe infection. These data have emphasized the risk of infection following splenectomy in infants and in all age groups in which there was a serious primary disease. The risk has been well summarized in an earlier publication,[69] that there were on record at least four isolated cases in which septicemia or meningitis occurred in children over 1 year of age following splenectomy for traumatic rupture of the spleen, that the risk of such infection after hereditary spherocytosis (2.3%) or after splenectomy for thrombocytopenic purpura (4.8%) was higher, and that the risk was much higher for thalassemia and portal hypertension.

*Splenic aspiration.*[25,177] Splenic aspiration serves as an aid in hematologic examinations in patients with undiagnosed splenomegaly to determine the nature of the abnormal cell responsible for the condition. It has been helpful in the diagnosis of lymphoma, myeloid metaplasia, kala-azar, and Gaucher's disease, especially when these conditions are suspected and bone marrow aspiration has been negative or inconclusive. Aspiration of the spleen also permits observations on its pathophysiology in patients with the hemolytic disorders and in those with hypersplenic syndromes. Cooperation of the patient is essential in carrying out this procedure because of the danger of excessive hemorrhage. It is, therefore, contraindicated in patients with a hemorrhagic tendency.

***Adrenaline test in diagnosis of hypersplenic syndromes.*** The adrenaline test has been employed to confirm the diagnosis of various hypersplenic syndromes with a depletion of one or more cells in the peripheral blood.[43] Epinephrine is said to prompt the mobilization of sequestered cells into the peripheral blood. In one investigation,[24] it was shown that this test provided only indirect corroborative evidence of the functional status of the blood-forming tissues. In splenomegalic conditions, for instance, there was no correlation between the degree of splenic contraction and the degree of hematopoietic response.

It should be remembered that, after entering the blood from the bone marrow, the neutrophil does not always stay in the circulation but may transiently marginate along vessel walls.[79] These two aggregations of the blood neutrophil population are about equal in size and in constant equilibrium. Epinephrine effects a redistribution of granulocytes of the blood by causing a shift from the "marginal" to the "circulatory" compartment. To cells mobilized in this way are supplemented those cells sequestered in the spleen. The object of this test is to determine the nature of the cell elements sequestered in the spleen. The results are not always constant.

As a clue to bone marrow contents and to demonstrate the adequacy of the granulocyte reserves from patients with hematologic disorders, the use of bacterial endotoxin (Pyrexal),[95,162] or etiocholanolone,[60] or the Rebuck skin-window[125] is more reliable (see Chapters 18 and 19).

***Indications for splenectomy.*** Splenectomy is most successful in patients with hereditary spherocytosis and, to a lesser extent, in those with thrombocytopenic purpura. By removing an inhibitory or destructive influence in patients with secondary hypersplenism, it frequently restores the blood count to normal either in part or completely. As mentioned elsewhere (Chapter 16), in patients with severe Cooley's anemia, the beneficial effects of splenectomy result in the elimination of a hemolytic factor and in a material decrease in transfusion requirements. With respect to the following conditions, splenectomy is discussed in connection with management of the individual disorders.

1. Hemolytic disorders
   a. Hereditary spherocytosis
   b. Acquired hemolytic anemia
   c. In selected cases
      (1) Thalassemia major (Cooley's anemia)
      (2) Sickle cell anemia
      (3) Certain nonspherocytic hemolytic anemias
2. Hypersplenic syndromes
   a. Without splenomegaly
      (1) Chronic idiopathic thrombocytopenic purpura
   b. With splenomegaly
      (1) Banti's syndrome
      (2) Splenic neutropenia
      (3) Splenic hematopenia
      (4) Gaucher's disease
      (5) Other lipid storage diseases
3. Miscellaneous
   a. Rupture of spleen
   b. Cysts
   c. Tumors (i.e., lymphosarcoma and follicular lymphoblastoma)
   d. Selected cases of hypoplastic anemia (including pure red cell anemia)

## DISORDERS OF THE SPLEEN
*Splenomegaly*

In Chapter 15 it was stated that splenomegaly is associated more commonly with the hemolytic than with other anemias. In young children with anemia of comparable severity, the spleen is more likely to be enlarged in those with severe Cooley's anemia than in those with sickle cell anemia or hereditary spherocytosis. The enlarged spleen in the patient with sickle cell anemia becomes progressively smaller and more fibrotic as the patient gets older. In interpreting the pathologic significance of an enlarged spleen, it is important to remember that the spleen may be palpable in normal infants and children and at times does not recede in size until puberty. At birth the weight of the spleen is approximately 10 gm.; at 1 year of age, approximately 30 gm.; at 6 years of age, about 55 gm.; at puberty, approximately 95 gm.; and in the adult, about 155 gm.[176] It is estimated that spleens must be enlarged two and one-half to three times the normal size to be palpable. As is shown in the following list, splenomegaly accompanies both hematologic and nonhematologic disorders.

1. Blood dyscrasias
   a. Hemolytic anemias
      (1) Acquired hemolytic anemia
      (2) Hereditary spherocytosis
      (3) Severe Cooley's anemia
      (4) Sickle cell anemia
      (5) Many of the hemoglobinopathies
      (6) Nonspherocytic hemolytic anemia
   b. Leukemia
2. Infiltrative
   a. Lipid
      (1) Gaucher's disease
      (2) Niemann-Pick disease
      (3) Neurovisceral lipidosis
   b. Nonlipid
      (1) Letterer-Siwe disease (nonlipid reticuloendotheliosis)
   c. Amyloidosis
   d. Mucopolysaccharidosis
3. Vascular
   a. Chronic congestive splenomegaly (Banti's syndrome)
   b. Chronic passive congestion
4. Infectious
   a. Acute
      (1) Septicemias
      (2) *Salmonella* infections
      (3) Brucellosis
      (4) Infectious mononucleosis
   b. Chronic
      (1) Malaria
      (2) Kala-azar
      (3) Trypanosomiasis and other parasitic infections
   c. Subacute bacterial endocarditis
   d. Tuberculosis
   e. Sarcoidosis
   f. Syphilis
5. Neoplasms and cysts
   a. Lymphosarcoma
   b. Hodgkin's disease
   c. Follicular lymphoma
   d. Reticulum cell sarcoma
   e. Hemangioma and lymphangioma
   f. Dermoids
6. Miscellaneous
   a. Lupus erythematosus
   b. Rheumatoid arthritis

In a group of 2,200 entering college students 2.86% had palpable spleens.[100] Of the sixty-three students studied, approximately 30% persisted with this finding for at least 3 years after the initial detection. The finding of a palpable spleen could not be explained on the basis of body habitus or infectious mononucleosis or other blood dyscrasias.

The soft edge of the spleen tip can be palpated in many normal children and even in young adults.

*Hypersplenism*

The spleen exerts a regulatory influence on the control of blood formation and in the delivery of cellular elements from the bone marrow. This function is greatly exaggerated when the spleen becomes hyperactive, a condition that is termed hypersplenism and implies an exaggeration of inhibitory and destructive activities of the spleen. Hypersplenism represents a functional and not an anatomic change. Inherent in this concept is the reduction of one or more cellular elements in the peripheral blood with compensatory hyperplasia in the bone marrow of the corresponding cells, the presence of an enlarged spleen, and the expectation that the peripheral blood picture will return to normal, or nearly normal, by splenectomy. The blood disturbances dependent upon hypersplenism have been attributed to either selective sequestration and increased destruction of formed cell elements in the enlarged spleen[43] or to an inhibitory influence upon a normal or hyperactive bone marrow by a hormonal mechanism.[35,36] By inhibitory action it is understood that the growth and maturation of various cells are prevented, or else their delivery from the marrow to the blood is blocked. There is increasing evidence favoring the concept of hypersplenic sequestration, but it does not exclude the possibility that other splenic mechanisms may cause cytopenic diseases. In reviewing the data on which the two concepts of hypersplenism are based, Crosby[34] concludes that "although the evidence in favor of inhibitory hypersplenism is fragile and loopholed, there is still reason to suspect the existence of splenic humoral factors." In either case, whether by increased destruction or inhibition, the removal of an abnormally functioning spleen has been shown to restore normal blood levels with varying degrees of success. Hypersplenism, therefore, is associated with neutropenia, thrombocytopenia, or anemia either singly or in combination, by splenomegaly and a normal or hypercellular marrow.

Hypersplenism may be primary when there is no obvious cause for the depletion of blood cell types as there is in patients with splenic neutropenia, splenic panhematopenia, or pancytopenia, and idiopathic thrombocytopenic purpura. It is secondary in patients with splenomegaly in combination with well-defined disorders such as Banti's syndrome, Hodgkin's disease, chronic leukemia, Gaucher's disease, lymphosarcoma, or Boeck's sarcoid. Splenectomy frequently restores a normal peripheral blood picture without affecting the underlying disorder.

Experimental hypersplenism has been produced by a variety of methods. The most consistent of these is the intraperitoneal injection into rats of macromolecular inert polymers such as methyl cellulose.[118] Splenomegaly of up to eight times its normal weight can be produced by this method in the rat. The histology of such spleens reveals packing of splenic phagocytes with methyl cellulose particles and congestion of the pulp with blood. The rats develop anemia, leukopenia, and thrombocytopenia with hyperplastic bone marrow. The spleen, liver, and kidneys are infiltrated with "storage cell" macrophages. The administration of methyl cellulose to previously splenectomized rats produced similar histologic lesions but failed to produce the hematologic abnormalities. In experimental hypersplenism of this type a humoral factor is responsible for the thrombopenia which is eliminated in the urine. When such urine is given to normal rats, it is responsible for the thrombopenia and partially for the anemia.[119]

In the differential diagnosis of liver enlargement, one can take advantage of the presence of fetoprotein. Normally this alpha fetoprotein becomes detectable in early fetal life at about 6 to 8 weeks of gestation. It reaches its peak serum concentration of 150 to 300 mg./100 ml. at about 12 to 20 weeks, followed by a subsequent decline. In the event of hepatocellular carcinoma there is a resynthesis of fetoprotein. Its presence in hepatoblastoma is of diagnostic importance.[9,54]

## Congenital absence of the spleen

Agenesis of the spleen usually occurs in combination with malformation of the heart, commonly atrioventricular communis, and partial transposition of the abdominal viscera.[21,122,124] Rarely is there an absence of an associated anomaly.[72,109,110] In either case a presumptive diagnosis of agenesis of the spleen can be made from the peripheral blood by the presence of normoblastemia and Howell-Jolly bodies and Heinz bodies in the erythrocytes. The diagnostic value of Heinz bodies (particles of denatured hemoglobin) has been emphasized by their presence in 10% of the red cells in the peripheral blood of mature newborn infants with agenesis of the spleen.[56]

Hereditary splenic hypoplasia has been described in three siblings in whom the use of radioactive scanning techniques helped to establish the diagnosis.[80]

## Primary splenic neutropenia

Varying degrees of leukopenia and granulocytopenia accompany most conditions with splenomegaly in the form of a secondary hypersplenism. Primary splenic neutropenia,[181] however, consists strictly of neutropenia, with normal erythrocytes and platelets, often a palpable spleen, but without evidence of an underlying disease. Primary splenic neutropenia is a rare disease in childhood and should be differentiated from chronic or periodic neutropenia. The symptoms and signs in both conditions overlap. There are frequent bouts of fever, sore throat, ulcerative lesions of the gums, mouth, tonsils, vulva, and vagina. The leukocyte count varies between 1,000 and 3,000 per cubic millimeter with granulocytes varying from 0 to 20%.[35] In the typical patient, symptoms are completely relieved by splenectomy.

## Felty's syndrome

Felty's syndrome occurs in adults. It consists of neutropenia, splenomegaly, and chronic rheumatoid arthritis and usually responds to splenectomy.[132]

## Primary splenic panhematopenia

Although primary splenic panhematopenia occurs frequently in children with splenomegaly as a manifestation of secondary hypersplenism, the primary disease is rare. The case of a 14-year-old girl with the primary disease was described by Doan and Wright[43] with complaints of weakness, pallor, unexplained fever, skin disorders, and anorexia, accompanied by pancytopenia, a hyperplastic marrow, a slightly palpable nontender spleen, and no adenopathy. Splenectomy was followed by a hematologic as well as clinical recovery. As contrasted with aplastic anemia in which pancytopenia also exists, the bone marrow in patients with primary splenic panhematopenia is hyperplastic, and each cellular element is present in normal or increased numbers.

• • •

A few of the better-known disorders in infancy and childhood, nonleukemic or neoplastic in origin, are associated with a greatly enlarged spleen. Outstanding examples are chronic congestive splenomegaly (Banti's syndrome) and Letterer-Siwe disease, Gaucher's disease, and Niemann-Pick disease. The latter are diseases of the reticuloendothelial system.

## Chronic congestive splenomegaly (Banti's syndrome, portal hypertension, splenic anemia)

Chronic congestive splenomegaly is characterized by enlargement of the spleen, progressive anemia, leukopenia, often thrombocytopenia, gastrointestinal hemorrhage due to portal hypertension, and, in later stages, cirrhosis of the liver and ascites.

**Etiology and pathogenesis.** As originally described by Banti in 1894,[13] the disease progresses in three stages. The first is that of splenic enlargement and increasing anemia; the second, enlargement of the liver and jaundice; and, terminally, cirrhosis of the liver, gastrointestinal hemorrhage, and ascites. The sequence according to this concept is initiated by a toxin, elaborated by an enlarged spleen that acts locally, and is also carried to the liver and other tissues and organs. The causative agent, being lodged primarily in the arteriole of the malpighian corpuscle, produces a thickening of the surrounding reticulum while maintaining a glandlike structure. Banti designated this pathologic picture as "fibroadenie." It has since been shown[101] that "fibroadenie" was indeed a peripheral fibrosis representing a nonspecific manifestation of passive congestion and end result of hemorrhage around the splenic arterioles. More recently, the concept of Banti's disease has been changed from a homogeneous entity originating in the spleen to one of congestion and enlargement of the spleen resulting from high portal venous pressure.[180] Congestive splenomegaly has, therefore, replaced the term Banti's disease.

The veins that form the portal system are the portal, the superior and inferior mesenteric, and the splenic veins and their tributaries. The portal vein itself is formed by the union of the superior mesenteric and splenic veins. Unlike other veins the portal vein ends like an artery, breaking up into numerous small channels which ultimately terminate in capillaries in the substance of the liver. The portal vein has no valves and carries about three-fourths of the circulation of the liver, whereas the hepatic artery carries oxygen and supplies the other fourth of the circulation.[4] Both vessels have a common outlet in the hepatic vein which empties into the inferior vena cava. It is important to bear in mind that back pressure in the valveless portal system does not possess the anatomic barriers found in the peripheral veins.[179]

The location of the obstruction in the portal system determines the type of portal hypertension. If obstruction is within the liver, it is classified as intraphepatic; if outside the liver parenchyma, it is classified as extrahepatic. Normally, the venous pressure in the portal system ranges from 140 to 220 mm. of saline solution or from 60 to 140 mm. of water.[179] In the adult the portal pressure is normally below 225 mm. of water so that readings above 250 mm. can be regarded as abnormally high.[63]

The commonest cause of portal obstruction is cirrhosis of the liver resulting from congenital diseases, infiltrations, hepatitis, schistosomiasis, Wilson's disease, and neoplasms. Fibrocystic disease of the pancreas is one of the more important causes of biliary cirrhosis and portal hypertension in childhood. It stems from mechanical obstruction of the bile ductules by inspissated secretions.[41] Cirrhosis of the liver, which accounts for 70% of cases of portal hypertension in the adult, is rare in children. In children extrahepatic lesions are the more common and are due to congenital malformations such as congenital stenosis or atresia, aneurysm of the splenic artery, and distortions of the portal vein extending into the liver. Other causes are thrombosis resulting from thrombophlebitis caused by omphalitis or generalized infection in early life involving splenic or portal veins or both, cavernomatous transformation of the portal vein, hepatic fibrosis secondary to irradiation in Wilms' tumor, and compression from pancreatic fibrosis and tumors, especially of the pancreas.

Extrahepatic portal vein obstruction and portal hypertension may result from umbilical vein catheterization in the course of exchange transfusion.[116,146] To avoid the potential hazard of portal vein thrombosis as a consequence of catheterization, it has been recommended that fluids should not be administered parenterally via an indwelling umbilical vein catheter, that catheters should not be left in the umbilical vein between exchange transfusions, and if clinical evidence of umbilical sepsis exists or difficulty is encountered during insertion of the catheter, another site for catheterization should be chosen.[116]

*Collateral circulation.* In the patient with chronic portal hypertension a collateral circulation which tends to lower the pressure in the portal system develops between the portal and systemic veins. These collaterals are located at the lower end of the esophagus and the upper end of the stomach, in the umbilicus, and in the rectum. Collateral vascular channels are sometimes seen in the abdominal wall. Of the greatest clinical significance are the collateral routes beneath the mucous membranes at the cardioesophageal junction which give rise to esophageal varices. The latter are thin walled and are likely to rupture when exposed to trauma, resulting in massive and at times fatal hemorrhage. The hemorrhoidal varices represent connections between the portal system and systemic veins through the middle hemorrhoidal vessels and constitute a souce of hemorrrhage.[179] Although it is known that bleeding from ruptured esophageal varices can occasionally occur in the absence of associated portal hypertension, patients with a high portal venous pressure and massive bleeding from esophageal varices have been described in whom neither intrahepatic nor extrahepatic portal vein obstruction was found.[163] Esophageal varices have been observed also in patients with extensive intrahepatic Hodgkin's disease.[86]

*Pathology.* The long-standing back pressure on the venous sinuses of the spleen eventually results in hemorrhage, with fibrotic and regenerative changes within this organ resulting in a characteristic fibrotic spleen.[180] The pathologic histology of the spleen has been described as consisting of periarterial hemorrhages developing into areas of periarterial fibrosis, siderotic nodules, and dilated venous sinuses with thickening of the reticulum of the wall, giving a collagen-staining reaction.[101]

*Clinical features.* The onset is insidious, usually with an unexplained enlargement of the spleen. The most common manifestations are fatigability, pallor, splenomegaly, hematemesis, or melena. Portal hypertension should be suspected in children of any age, even in the first year of life, when hematemesis or melena is associated with an enlarged spleen. In an infant who had had melena and hematemesis from 3 months of age, splenoportography at 14 months revealed anomalies of the portal system. In patients with fully developed chronic congestive splenomegaly, the liver is palpable and the spleen is massive, and in over one-half of the patients hematemesis has occurred. Less often, hemorrhoids are a source of bleeding. The bulk of these features are attributable to the rupture of varices in strategic locations. Epistaxis and early bruising are noted in a small number of patients.

*Laboratory data.* Normochromic and hypochromic anemia and leukopenia, with or without thrombocytopenia, are usually noted. With increasing size of the spleen, marked reduction in the number of leukocytes occurs, ranging usually between 1,500 and 4,000 white blood cells per cubic millimeter, with a predominance of lymphocytes. Leukocytosis accompanies severe hemorrhage, and when blood loss is repeated, a hypochromic microcytic anemia results. In the presence of portal cirrhosis the red blood cell survival may be shortened and indirect serum bilirubin may be elevated.[7] The mechanism postulated for hemolysis is a high portal venous pressure and probably a major degree of congestive splenomegaly with red cell stasis. Macrocytosis,[183] target cells, teardrop poikilocytes, and an increase in the mean corpuscular hemoglobin value have been noted in patients with long-standing disease and cirrhosis of the liver.[133] In patients with marked thrombocytopenia, prolonged bleeding time and occasionally increased bruising follows, but this association is inconstant. The coagulation time is usually normal. The bone marrow reveals either a normal pattern, despite leukopenia and anemia, or a hyperplasia involving megakaryocytes and myeloid and erythroid elements.

*Diagnosis.* The combination of massive enlargement of the spleen, a palpable liver, and pancytopenia often presents a difficult diagnostic problem. A history of hematemesis or melena is, of course, highly suggestive of portal hypersplenism. After barium is swallowed esophageal varices are visualized in only about 40% of patients.[37] Esophagoscopy with the flexible esophagoscope is utilized to visualize varices at the site of the lesion. In patients suspected to have chronic congestive splenomegaly, the use of percutaneous splenoportal venography has been helpful in diagnosis. With this method roentgenographic visualization of the portal vein and its branches is achieved by percutaneous intrasplenic injection of contrast material.[51] Percutaneous arteriography of the celiac axis may aid diagnosis by delineating during the arterial phase abnormalities of the hepatic circulation, during the venous phase the condition of the splenic and portal veins and the presence of esophageal varices.

Before a definite diagnosis can be made, other conditions associated with splenomegaly, leukopenia, and pancytopenia must be eliminated. These include Gaucher's disease, Niemann-Pick disease, nonlipid reticuloendotheliosis (Letterer-Siwe disease), and infiltrations of the bone marrow with leukemic or neoplastic cells.

*Course and prognosis.* The course depends upon the degree and site of obstruction and the effectiveness of a remedial operation in relieving the excessive portal venous pressure and retarding liver damage. The control of gastrointestinal hemorrhage from ruptured varices and eradication of the obstruction are important factors in projecting the outcome. The presence of ascites and persistent anorexia are of serious prognostic import.

The site of portal venous obstruction is the most significant single factor in the management and prognosis of patients with portal hypertension in childhood. Intrahepatic portal obstruction carries a much poorer outlook than extrahepatic obstruction because of the serious and progressive nature of the primary hepatic disease. Posthepatic obstruction of the hepatic veins rarely leads to the development of esophageal varices and bleeding.[166]

*Treatment.* Adequate treatment depends upon the discovery of the site and nature of the portal obstruction. Extrahepatic portal hypertension may be differentiated from that which is secondary to liver cirrhosis[70] and is suggested by the following: a history of omphalitis or severe bacterial infection during early infancy which is followed by an uneventful course until signs of portal hypertension appear; an essentially negative and benign history prior to the onset of signs of portal hypertension, such as hematemesis and/or splenomegaly; an absence of jaundice or other signs of liver disease prior to the onset of symptoms; and normal liver function tests. In contrast, portal hypertension secondary to cirrhosis of the liver is suggested by positive liver function tests, evidence of a previous history of jaundice or liver enlargement, hepatomegaly, and tenderness of the liver which is prominent. Hepatic enlargement, ascites, and other evidences of liver failure tend to appear prior to portal hypertension.

Newer techniques have led to an elucidation of the factors concerned with the pathogenesis of portal hypertension and the possible identification of the site of obstruction. Appraisal of liver function, manometric measurement of portal pressures, and the use of portal venography and celiac axis arteriography contribute to the accuracy of diagnosis and facilitate surgical intervention for decompression of the portal area.[143] In portal venography, the portal venous system is rendered opaque by contrast medium and then visualized by serial roentgen studies. At present percutaneous splenoportography is in common use and provides important data with regard to size and conformation of the vessels and thus aids in the selection of the optimal type of shunt.[185]

Splenorenal, mesocaval, and portacaval anastomoses are the three types of shunts in common use, and the choice of one of these depends largely upon the patency and caliber of the vessels available for the procedure. Splenectomy might be considered preferable in children with moderate or marked enlargement of the spleen, especially when pancytopenia exists. Although blood values would be restored to normal or nearly normal, it is now realized that once the spleen is removed the splenic vein is no longer available for anastomosis should it later become necessary. Splenectomy without a venovenous shunt is indicated only in patients with lesions obstructing the splenic hilum.[136] The prognosis is best in those children with a normal liver and with obstruction located in the splenic vein.

Splenectomy with a splenorenal shunt is usually recommended in patients with marked splenomegaly, hypersplenism, large caliber splenic veins, or an obliterated portal vein resulting from cavernomatous transformation or aplasia of the portal vein. A portacaval shunt is advocated with small caliber splenic veins or cirrhosis of the liver. Because of the progressive nature of the disease and the likelihood that a fair percentage of splenorenal shunts will tend to close spontaneously, there has been a tendency to decompress the portal system by an immediate portacaval shunt, especially in the small child. Should the latter procedure eventually prove ineffective, the now larger splenic vein will be available for anastomosis.

In general, the most effective relief of portal hypertension in children with intrahepatic obstruction is obtained from portacaval anastomosis, a procedure normally successful in children over the age of 5 years.[166] For children with extrahepatic portal obstruction the most effective remedy is to bypass the obstruction by means of a portal-system venous shunt. Since the portal vein is usually occluded by the obstructive process, a splenorenal or mesocaval shunt may be used. The former procedure has rarely been found successful under 10 years of age.[166] When a shunt is inadvisable or impossible and control of bleeding cannot otherwise be achieved, the mesocaval shunt devised by Marion and Clatworthy[26,171] may prove useful. This shunt is worthwhile in patients whose portal and splenic veins have been rendered useless for shunting. The mesocaval shunt represents an anastomosis of the proximal end of the divided inferior vena cava into the root or side of the superior mesenteric vein in an end-to-side fashion. There is no definite way, unfortunately, to visualize the superior mesenteric vein preoperatively to determine its patency. Celiac and superior mesenteric arteriograms may be utilized to demonstrate the venous phase of the superior mesenteric vein, but this method is not sufficiently trustworthy.

It is of interest that a salutory effect on the hematologic features of hypersplenism has been observed after a portacaval shunt, with a reversal of the pancytopenia and without splenectomy.[47] Once portal hypertension is relieved, esophagogastric varices recede, the hazard of hemorrhage diminishes, and the spleen shrinks in size.[172,175] Transthoracic ligation and endoscopic injection of esophageal varices have also proved of value for the temporary control of esophageal bleeding.

Anemia due to hemorrhage responds to iron therapy. Blood transfusions are given for values of 8 gm. per 100 ml. or less, but the hemoglobin concentration need not be elevated to maximal levels. Esophageal bleeding remains a constant source of concern, and methods for its control by tamponade with esophageal balloons have proved of questionable value.

## DISEASES OF THE RETICULOENDOTHELIAL SYSTEM

The reticuloendothelioses constitute a group of disorders of unknown etiology, having in common hyperplasia of cellular elements of the reticuloendothelial system. Reticulum cells and histiocytes undergo proliferation principally in the spleen, liver, bone marrow, lymph nodes, and, to some extent, in other tissues and organs. These disorders have been subject to varied classifications but are now separated on the basis of presence or absence of distinctive intracellular lipids. Gaucher's disease and Niemann-Pick disease are the prominent members of the storage disease group, and Letterer-Siwe disease (nonlipid reticuloendotheliosis), Hand-Schüller-Christian disease, and eosinophilic granuloma constitute the inflammatory group. The difficulty of classification is exemplified by Hand-Schüller-Christian disease in which the proliferating histiocytes initially contain very little cholesterol but later accumulate enough to give the appearance of foam cells.

## Gaucher's disease

Gaucher's disease is an uncommon hereditary metabolic disorder characterized by the storage of kerasin and other cerebrosides in the reticuloendothelial system. It has been most often observed in Jewish families, but cases have been described in many nationalities over the world. The disease occurs as an acute infantile type and a chronic or adult type. Gaucher[57] first described this entity in 1882, regarding it as a primary epithelioma of the spleen.

*Pathology and pathogenesis.* At least three substances have been isolated from tissues containing Gaucher cells: a galactocerebroside

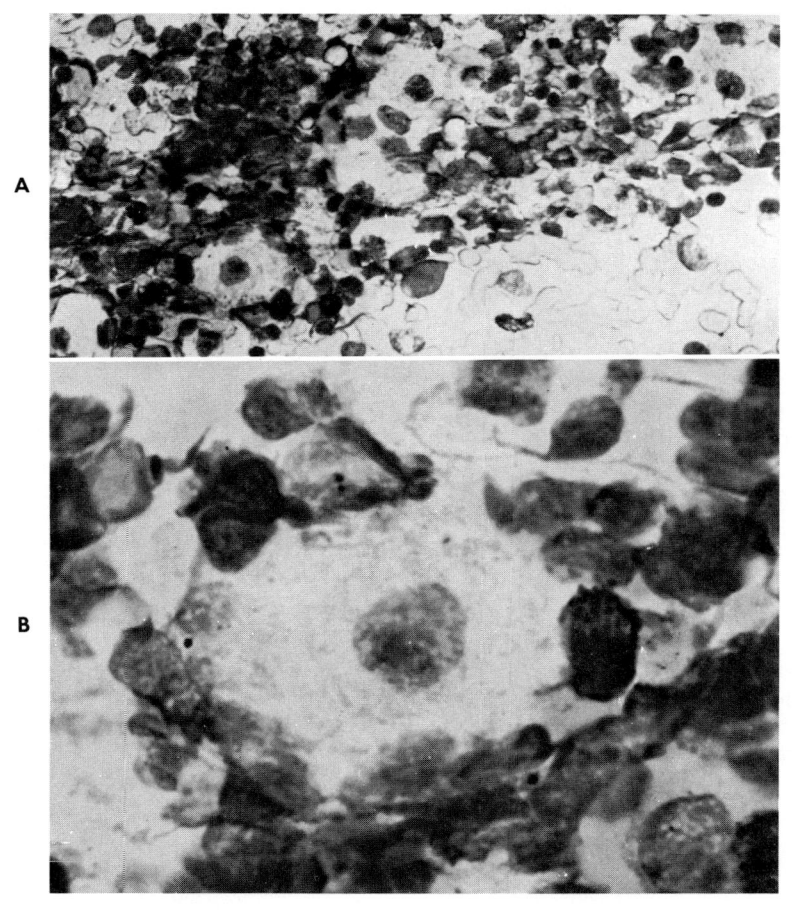

Fig. 86. **A**, Photomicrograph of nest of Gaucher cells in smear of bone marrow. (×900.) **B**, A single Gaucher cell from the smear shown in **A**. Note crinkled, fibrillar appearance of cytoplasm and relatively small, slightly eccentric nucleus. (×1500.)

(kerasin), a glucocerebroside, and a water-soluble glycolipid polycerebroside.[167,168] The pathogenesis of the disease has not been fully established. It has been ascribed to a primary disturbance of intermediary lipid metabolism causing an elevation of cerebrosides in the serum with later storage in reticuloendothelial cells or to a primary disturbance in the reticulum cells causing increased synthesis and storage of cerebrosides.[161] It has been postulated that the site of the biochemical error in most patients with the disease is at the conversion of the glucocerebroside to the galactocerebroside so that the abnormal glucose form accumulates.[157] Postmortem examination reveals Gaucher cells in the spleen, liver, lymph nodes, bone marrow, lungs, and other organs (Fig. 86). The disease is diagnosed by the demonstration of these cells in areas where they proliferate, the most accessible of which is the bone marrow. Splenic puncture also serves as a useful means of demonstrating the source of Gaucher cells. These cells are large and distinctive, 20 to 80$\mu$ in diameter, round or oval, and possess one or more small dense nuclei eccentrically located. The cytoplasm has an opaque wrinkled tissue paper appearance due to the presence of fine wavy fibrils running parallel to the long axis of the cell. The cytoplasm occupies the major part of the Gaucher cell and stains slightly gray or bluish. It exhibits an intense periodic acid–Schiff reaction for glycogen and a positive reaction for acid phosphatase.[52] Electron microscopy indicates that the cytoplasmic striations, pathognomonic of the Gaucher cell, correspond to tubule-containing bodies. Mitochondria could be identified within such bodies. These round or ovoid bodies may be derived from transformations of the mitochondria.[52]

**Clinical features.** The clinical features of the acute infantile and chronic forms of Gaucher's disease are discussed separately.

*Acute infantile form.* The infant may appear normal at birth and for the first weeks and months of life but soon undergoes mental and physical retardation and deterioration. Splenomegaly followed by enlargement of the liver contribute to prominence of the abdomen, which is further exaggerated by wasting of the extremities. Severe neurologic symptoms and signs characterize the infantile form of the disease. Generalized hypertonia, opisthotonus and rigidity, dysphagia, laryngeal spasm, cyanosis, severe cough due in part to pulmonary infiltration with Gaucher cells,[128] and fever dominate the clinical picture. Death follows before the age of 2 years.[1,58] The cerebral changes observed at postmortem examination indicate chronic disease of the ganglion cells progressing to sclerosis and complete destruction. Rarely, typical Gaucher cells are found in the intracerebral vascular spaces.[169]

Lipid analysis of liver and spleen in young patients reveals a consistent increase in the level of water-insoluble glycolipid (cerebroside). Acid phosphatase is increased in these tissues. The elevations of cerebroside and acid phosphatase usually found are not of the magnitude characteristic of childhood patients with the chronic disease. Alteration in the metabolism of certain large neurons results in an accumulation of glycolipid within their cytoplasm which is then apparently followed by cell death and neuronophagia. A patchy loss of nerve cells is especially marked in layers three and five of cortex, as well as a prominence of microglia and Gaucher cells in the same location.[12] Neuronophagia is a conspicuous finding in the nuclei of the basal ganglia and brainstem. In contrast it is rare in Tay-Sachs, Hurler's, and Niemann-Pick diseases.

*Chronic form.* The chronic form has an insidious onset (starting in childhood or at any age thereafter), most commonly with splenomegaly followed soon after by liver enlargement. Lymphadenopathy is not a conspicuous feature. The skin reveals a yellow or patchy brown pigmentation which is particularly prominent on exposed parts of the body—face, neck, hands, and legs. Pingueculae of the conjunctiva are rare in children and common in adults. They consist of a brownish yellow wedge-shaped thickening of the subconjunctival tissue with bases situated close to the corneal margins and apices pointed to the inner and outer canthi. Infiltration with Gaucher cells causes pulmonary and bone involvement. Pulmonary infiltration is infrequent in the chronic form although common in the acute form of the disease. Pain in the legs, occasionally accompanied by swelling of adjacent joints, is due to bony infiltration by Gaucher cells. The roentgenogram shows diffuse or localized destructive and productive changes often producing a characteristic deformity in the lower femora. This consists of a widening

664  BLOOD DISEASES OF INFANCY AND CHILDHOOD

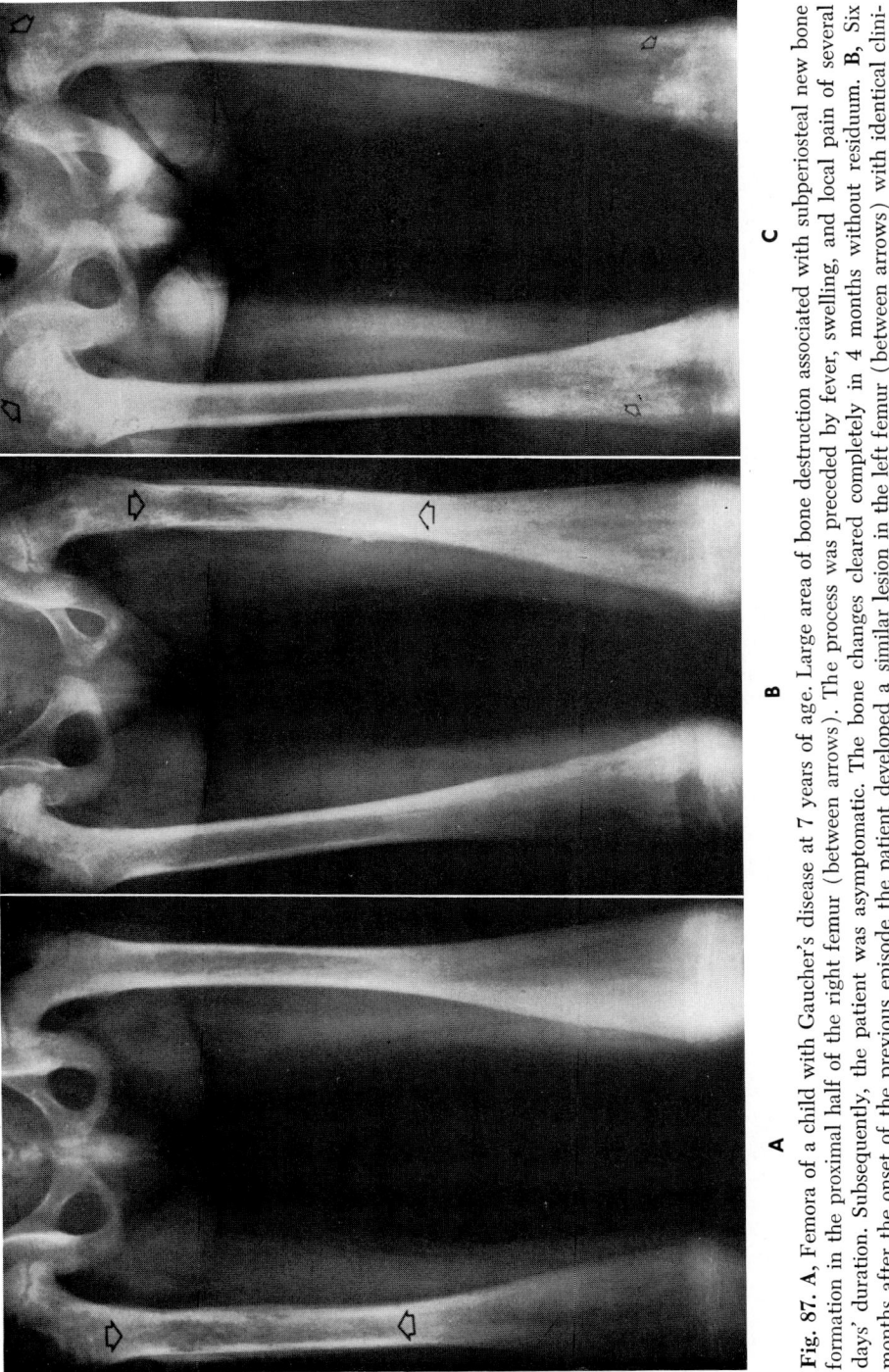

Fig. 87. *A*, Femora of a child with Gaucher's disease at 7 years of age. Large area of bone destruction associated with subperiosteal new bone formation in the proximal half of the right femur (between arrows). The process was preceded by fever, swelling, and local pain of several days' duration. Subsequently, the patient was asymptomatic. The bone changes cleared completely in 4 months without residuum. *B*, Six months after the onset of the previous episode the patient developed a similar lesion in the left femur (between arrows) with identical clinical history, findings, course, and duration. *C*, Seven months later; complete clearing of the destructive process in the left femur. Note undertubulation of the distal segment of the femoral shafts (Erlenmeyer flask appearance) characteristic of Gaucher's disease (arrows). Note also in *B* and *C* signs (more marked in *C*) of aseptic necrosis of the femoral heads and necks (arrows)—not uncommon complications of Gaucher's disease. Radiolucent defects in distal femoral metaphysis presumably due to infiltration of bone by Gaucher cells.

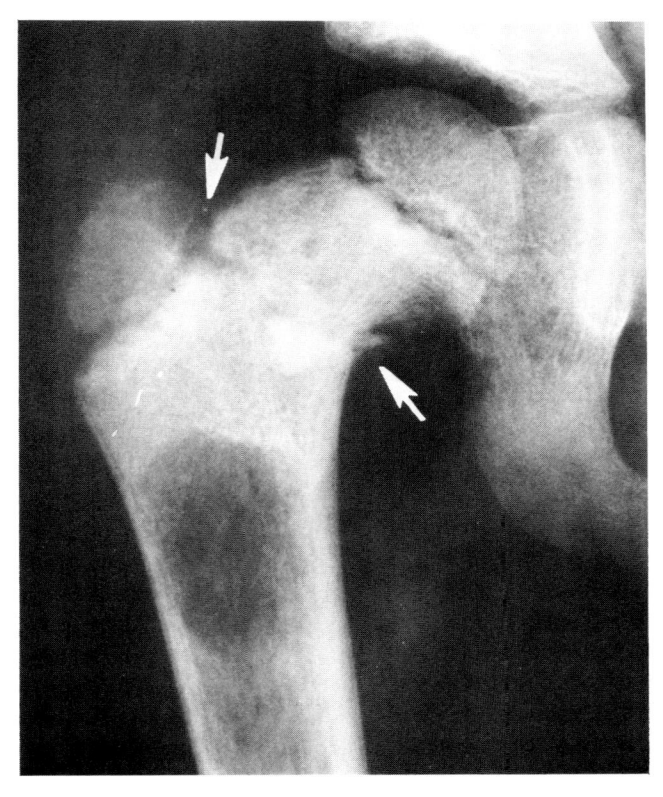

Fig. 88. Pathologic fracture of right hip in a 9-year-old girl with Gaucher's disease of 4 years' duration. Fracture and mild subluxation of right femoral neck indicated by arrows.

of the lower halves and thinning and flaring of the cortices, giving a trumpet or an Erlenmeyer flask appearance.[126] This feature is reminiscent of the swollen appearance in similar areas in patients with severe Cooley's anemia. Pathologic fractures due to marked osteoporosis and replacement by Gaucher cells may occur.[65] (See Figs. 87 and 88.)

In some cases osteosclerosis is a major feature of the disease. New bone may be laid down around and between areas of bone destruction, or it may be found along the inner aspect of the cortex in the affected areas.[107] A periosteal reaction is produced by elevation of the periosteum by Gaucher cells, resulting in new bone formation.[160] The clinical picture of osteomyelitis may be simulated. Gaucher's disease may also exhibit the roentgenographic features of Legg-Perthes disease.[44] Proliferation of Gaucher cells in the femoral heads, leading to their subsequent collapse, creates a picture indistinguishable from aseptic necrosis.[107,164] Gaucher cell infiltration of the vertebrae may lead to their collapse.

The clinical differentiation between osteomyelitis and the condition produced by extensive infiltration of the bone marrow by Gaucher cells may be extremely difficult. It has been emphasized that an intractable sinus may result when patients with Gaucher's disease are subjected to operation under the mistaken diagnosis of osteomyelitis.[160] The difficulties of diagnosing bone infection are illustrated in the following case: Splenectomy was performed in a 4½-year-old child with Gaucher's disease because of increasing splenomegaly and hypersplenism. At the age of 6 years persistent pain over each thigh was associated in sequence with fever. As the clinical picture regressed, x-ray findings revealed destruction of bony trabeculae and thinning of cortices. (Fig. 87). Antibiotics were administered during the febrile period and the child recovered. Soon thereafter bilateral aseptic necrosis of the femoral heads was noted, presumably caused by Gaucher cell infiltrates. Most recently the patient complained of severe pain in the groin accompanied by a temperature reaching 102° to 106° F. Within a few weeks destructive changes in the left ilium were noted. A large quantity of purulent fluid was eventually aspirated from this area which grew out *Salmonella derby*. The infection came under control with appropriate antibiotic therapy. Whether the earlier episodes of bone pain over the femur were due to osteomyelitis or to compression by Gaucher cell infiltrates has still not been determined.

**Blood.** The anemia is usually of a mild or moderate normochromic and normocytic type. Leukopenia with relative lymphocytosis and slight to marked thrombocytopenia may be present. Thrombocytopenia with hemorrhage may be sufficiently severe to require splenectomy. The complete pancytopenic blood picture of hypersplenic disorders may ultimately develop. Serum lipid and cholesterol levels are normal. With phenylphosphate substrate the serum acid phosphatase level is elevated in Gaucher's disease, perhaps by spillage from tissue accumulations.[31,50] Gaucher cells have been found very infrequently in smears of the peripheral blood. They should be sought along the edges of the slide. In one case in which this finding was reported, a leukoerythroblastic reaction was observed many years after splenectomy.[186]

**Heredity.** The disease has been noted in siblings, in a parent and child both with the full clinical picture of Gaucher's disease,[71] and in asymptomatic parents of typically affected children.[62,159] In this respect the parent can be regarded as a carrier. The mode of inheritance varies with different groups, the majority of cases being caused by an autosomal recessive gene.[71] Zoltnick and Groen[186] in an analysis of cases of Gaucher's disease found that the disease tends to become more severe in successive generations. The authors noted that not a single patient with Gaucher's disease was born of a father or mother with manifest disease, indicating that death in utero results from the severe metabolic disturbance. They concluded that "patients with manifest Gaucher's disease can at least be freed from worry about their offspring." The patients can expect either healthy children or none at all. More extensive observations are required in confirmation of this principle.

**Course and treatment.** There is no cure for Gaucher's disease, and in children beyond infancy the disease may either progress or remain chronic. Pregnancy does not aggravate the course of Gaucher's disease, nor is there any effect on the fetus.[68] The lives of those who survive to adolescence are prolonged for many years. Most adults die of intercurrent diseases rather than of Gaucher's disease. Steroids are sometimes of value in relieving bone pains and joint swelling without altering the progress of the disease. Splenectomy is usually effective in relieving the development of a massive spleen and in reversing the severe pancytopenia.[102] Acceleration of bone involvement due to splenectomy has been a controversial issue since the spleen is the main storage place for glucocerebrosides. However, based on wide experience, the theory that splenectomy hastens the onset of bone lesions finds no support from most writers on this subject.[126] Splenectomy induces improvement in symptoms, particularly if there are signs of hypersplenism such as bleeding from thrombocytopenia. Occasionally, massive enlargement of the liver follows splenectomy. In these cases microscopic examination reveals diffuse infiltration by Gaucher cells, some arranged in tumorlike nodules.

Cases of hepatosplenomegaly have been described in which abnormal cells, probably of reticuloendothelial origin, containing large blue cytoplasmic granules have been found in bone marrow and other organs[94,141] Cells similar to those initially described by Sawitsky and co-workers[141] have been observed in the bone marrow by Silverstein and colleagues[148] in a Negro girl who had been followed from the age of 16 months until her death at 10 years of age. This disorder, termed the syndrome of the "sea-blue histiocyte," is characterized by the presence of this destructive, blue, granulated histiocyte and an associated splenomegaly. Clinically patients with the disease may have a relatively benign course, with mild purpura secondary to thrombocytopenia or may have progressive hepatic cirrhosis, hepatic failure, and death. Two biochemical events appear to accompany this disease: storage of specific phospholipids and glycosphingolipids; and abnormal urinary excretion and perhaps hepatic storage of mucopolysaccharide-type substances. All patients had numerous sea-blue histiocytes in aspirated specimens of bone marrow demonstrated by either Wright's or Giemsa stain. This histiocyte is a large cell, up to $20\mu$ in diameter, containing a varying number of blue-staining granules. The cells are differentiated from those of Gaucher's disease, Niemann-Pick disease, and other storage diseases.

Two siblings 10 and 12 years of age with the sea-blue histiocyte syndrome have been reported.[77] The 10-year-old child had an enlarged spleen, and chest x-ray showed diffuse nodular densities in both lung fields with bilateral hilar adenopathy. He had varying degrees of hypersplenism as manifested by mild anemia, leukopenia, and thrombocytopenia. Bone marrow aspiration showed numerous large histiocytes whose cytoplasm contained varying numbers of granules staining light-blue with Wright's or May-Grunewald-Giemsa stain. A 12-year-old sister had bone marrow containing numerous "sea-blue histiocytes" identical in number and morphology to those found in the patient's bone marrow. Her spleen was not palpable. It was postulated that this is a hereditary disorder of lipid metabolism transmitted as an autosomal recessive trait.

Objection has been made that the "sea-blue histiocyte" is not a specific cell. Kattlove and associates[78] regard this cell as a normal reticuloendothelial cell that contains partially digested cells which become apparent when there is increased destruction of blood or bone marrow cells. They believe that the inclusions are the remnants of partially phagocytosed cells and are responsible for the appearance of these histiocytes on light microscopy.

### Niemann-Pick disease

Niemann-Pick disease is a rare heredofamilial disease, resembling in its clinical features the infantile type of Gaucher's disease. It is characterized by the widespread storage of lipids, mainly sphingomyelin, in the reticuloendothelial system, the nervous system, and some other tissues.

*Clinical features.* The onset may date from birth or may occur after the first 6 months of life. Progressive physical and mental deterioration is accompanied by massive and equal enlargement of the liver and spleen. In contrast, in patients with Gaucher's disease the spleen is larger than the liver. A brownish yellow pigmentation occurs, especially in the parts exposed to light. In an appreciable number of patients estimated as high as 60%,[169] a cherry-red spot appears in the macula corresponding to that seen in patients with amaurotic familial idiocy (Tay-Sachs disease). Nervous system involvement is manifested by spasticity, blindness, and deafness; the patient finally lapses into a state of apathy and idiocy. With the patient profoundly emaciated, death usually occurs before the third year of life. Although the bone marrow is infiltrated with foam cells, survival is not sufficiently prolonged for changes to be conspicuously apparent on x-ray examination.

Chronic forms of the disease are described extending to adolescence,[30,53,92] and in cases reported in two brothers death occurred at 29 and 33 years of age, respectively.[161] In patients who have survived beyond infancy extensive pulmonary infiltrations are observed on roentgenographic examination. In a 19-year-old boy under observation from early childhood with the typical Niemann-Pick cells in the bone marrow, marked hepatosplenomegaly, and pulmonary infiltration, normal mental and physical growth took place.

*Pathology and pathogenesis.* The striking features at autopsy are involvement of the liver, spleen, lungs, bone marrow, and lymph nodes and the replacement of reticular cells and histiocytes by the foam or Niemann-Pick cells. The nervous system is almost invariably affected. Degenerative changes take place in the ganglion cells. The large neurons are distended or ballooned with loss of their usual triangular or pyramidal shape. Usually, there are lipid deposits in the ganglion and neurolgia cells.[169] Often, there is a paucity of nerve cells as if many had disintegrated.[30]

The storage material in the foam cells which accumulates in the viscera of patients with Niemann-Pick disease consists largely of phospholipids, chiefly lecithin and sphingomyelin. These foam cells which characterize the disease are readily available for examination by bone marrow aspiration. These are large, more or less rounded, occasionally oval or polyhedral cells averaging 15 to 90$\mu$ in diameter[30] and containing one or two nuclei often eccentrically placed with loosely arranged chromatin material. The abundant cytoplasm is filled with highly refractile lipid droplets giving a web-like, honeycombed, or foamy appearance. Unlike the Gaucher cells, the foam cells of the disease are readily detected in the counting chamber and can be separated from the megakaryocytes[121] (Fig. 89). Electron microscopy revealed in one case that the lipid inclusions were made up of lamellated multiple membranes.[92]

Assays of sphingolipid-cleaving enzymes in the leukocytes of patients with lipidosis are of diagnostic value and have provided much useful information concerning the abnormal lipid metabolism in these diseases. Decreased activ-

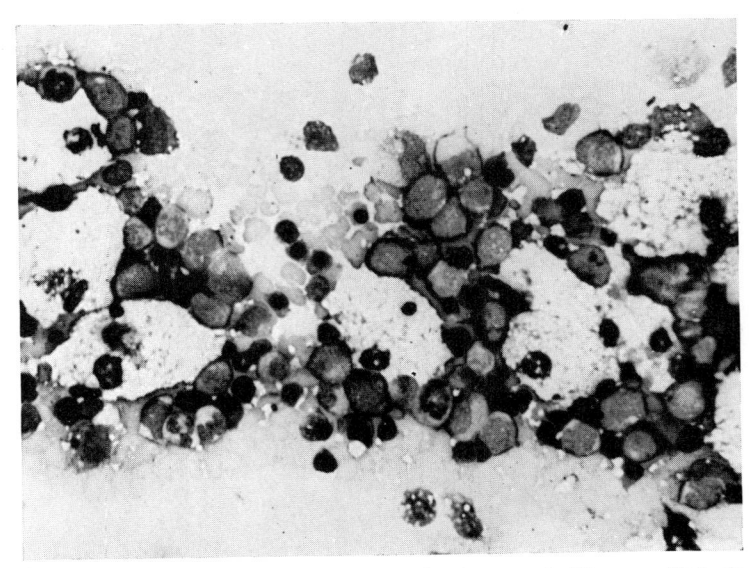

**Fig. 89.** Photomicrograph of bone marrow smear of patient with Niemann-Pick disease. Note group of typical cells—their large size, relatively small, round, or oval nucleus, and foam droplets giving a honeycomb appearance of cytoplasm.

ity of glucocerebrosidase and sphingomyelinase has been correlated with Gaucher's disease and Niemann-Pick disease, respectively.[156] The spleen and skin fibroblasts also demonstrate these enzymatic lesions.[20]

*Blood.* Vacuoles appear in the cytoplasm of the circulating lymphocytes and monocytes, but no definite histochemical studies on such cells are known. The vacuoles are discrete, unstained, and round and vary in number from 1 or 2 to 15 or 20.[30]

In the older patient anisocytosis and poikilocytosis with many oval cells are noted. A mild or moderate microcytic anemia is found. White blood cells vary between slight leukocytosis and moderate leukopenia. Blood cholesterol either is not increased or is slightly elevated.

*Heredity.* There is a striking predilection for Jews which is more marked than in Gaucher's disease. The occurrence among siblings is well known. Tay-Sachs disease has been noted among relatives of patients with Niemann-Pick disease.

*Treatment.* There is no effective treatment. Splenectomy has been carried out, but except for the relief of anemia and mild evidences of hypersplenism this procedure has not altered the course of the disease.[30]

### Generalized gangliosidosis

In patients with generalized gangliosidosis[85] ($GM_1$ gangliosidosis, familial neurovisceral lipidosis, pseudo-Hurler disease, Hurler variant, Tay-Sachs disease with visceral involvement), abnormal, gargoyle-like facies, macroglossia, peripheral edema, hepatosplenomegaly, and, infrequently, cherry-red spots in the macula have been described. The clinical and radiological features resemble Hurler's disease. Vacuoles in the lymphocytes and monocytes, Reilly bodies in the polymorphonuclear leukocytes, and foam cells in the bone marrow are prominent hematologic characteristics. Pathologically, there is lipid histiocytosis of the reticuloendothelial system, neural lipidosis, and ballooning of the glomerular epithelium. The metabolic abnormality, present in the brain, liver, skin, leukocytes, and other tissues, is due to a deficiency of $\beta$-galactosidase, with progressive accumulation of ganglioside.[113] Death usually occurs before the second or third year of life.

### Wolman's disease

Wolman's disease or "primary familial xanthomatosis with involvement and calcification of the adrenals" was originally described in

Israeli children[182] and has been reported in children from New Zealand,[6] Austria,[40] and the United States.[32] Clinically patients have failure to thrive, gastrointestinal complaints, and hepatosplenomegaly. Death usually occurs by 2 to 4 months of age. Vacuolated lymphocytes in the peripheral blood and foam cells in the bone marrow, similar to those seen in Neimann-Pick disease, have been described. Markedly increased amounts of structurally normal cholesterol have been identified in the liver, spleen, and, to a lesser extent, brain of these patients, suggesting that the biochemical defect may be an abnormality in the regulation of the rate of production or disposal of cholesterol.[134]

## Letterer-Siwe disease, Hand-Schüller-Christian disease, and eosinophilic granuloma (histiocytosis X)

There is considerable evidence that these three syndromes are members of a closely related group of disorders in which underlying pathology is an inflammatory histiocytosis. Each has distinctive clinicopathologic features which are currently regarded as different expressions of the same basic disorder.[75] Of these, Letterer-Siwe disease is acute and malignant, eosinophilic granuloma is the most benign, and Hand-Schüller-Christian disease occupies an intermediate position. Overlapping occurs to the extent that some histologic changes will be found in each entity that are similar to those of the other two.[10]

A generic term, histiocytosis X, was suggested by Lichtenstein[87,88] to embrace these diseases since all three share the common origin of inflammatory histiocytosis. The difficulties of separating these entities on either a clinical or histopathologic basis have frequently been emphasized. Oberman[112] regards the assessment of the rapidity of progression of the disease as the most accurate guide to the ultimate outcome. Consequently, those patients in whom the disease at the onset is localized to the bone have a less aggressive form of the disease than those in whom there is multiple system involvement initially (visceral and soft tissue lesions and generalized maculopapular eruption). In reticuloendotheliosis in children, excluding those patients who had only solitary bone lesions, a composite study indicates that one-third die of the disease.[84] This fatality rate must be considered only as an approximation since periods of apparent complete remission may be followed by widespread dissemination after a lapse of many months or even years.

In 1969 Lieberman and co-workers[89] analyzed eighty-two cases of histiocytosis X and concluded that there was no justification for the current theory that eosinophilic granuloma of bone, Hand-Schüller-Christian disease, and Letterer-Siwe disease represent component parts of a single nosologic entity. They concluded that eosinophilic granuloma of bone is a benign disorder but may in the multifocal form be responsible for considerable morbidity and that the Hand-Schüller-Chirstian triad is nonspecific: foam cells were of no help in diagnosis and are usually found in areas of nonspecific reaction. They felt that Letterer-Siwe disease is a clinical term which has been used to characterize various malignant histiocytic lymphomas and occasional infectious processes. In summary, they state that the term histiocytosis X is unnecessary and may lead to therapeutic errors. As for therapy, they suggested simple biopsy and/or curettage for management of unifocal eosinophilic granuloma supplemented by radiation therapy, and systemic therapy for the multifocal form. Systemic agents such as vinca alkaloids and steroids in addition to transfusions and antimicrobial therapy were recommended.

## Letterer-Siwe disease (nonlipid reticuloendotheliosis)

Letterer-Siwe disease is an acute rarely familial disease appearing before the age of 2 years, with a rapidly fatal course within weeks or months of the onset.[2,151,152,174] The etiology is unknown. Often the disease is ushered in as an acute infection; at times there is no relation to infection. Irritability, malaise, diarrhea, and development of a skin eruption which may date from birth are early features. A hemorrhagic tendency manifested by petechiae and purpura combines with a yellow, scaly, greasy, seborrheic eruption that is accentuated over the scalp and trunk.[66,90,170] A purulent otitis media, hepatosplenomegaly, moderately enlarged and tender lymph nodes, abdominal enlargement, and fever characterize the disease in the infant. Bronchitis and bronchopneumonia are common. Circular areas of rarefaction in the calvaria and cystlike defects in the lower ends of the femora and upper ends of the tibiae have been described.[27] Pulmonary involvement due to histiocytic infiltration appears on the roentgenogram as diffuse irregularly nodular involvement. Progression

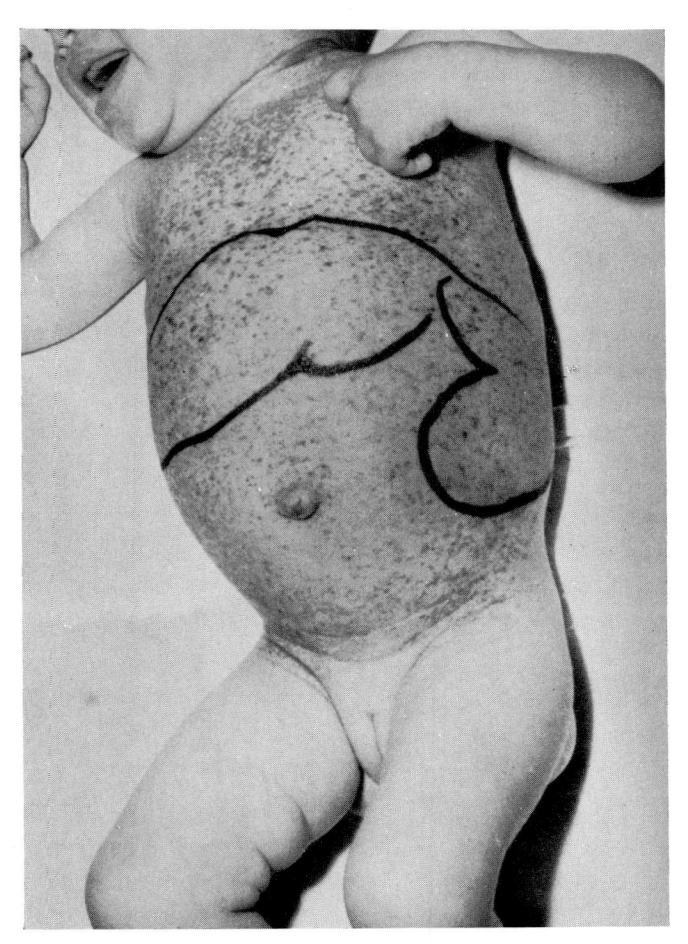

Fig. 90. Child of about 6 months of age with typical Letterer-Siwe disease. Note diffuse seborrheic eruption over the body in combination with petechiae and purpura. The enlarged liver and spleen are outlined. (Courtesy Dr. Philip Lanzkowsky, New York, N. Y.)

to multiple lung cysts has been described.[81] A familial occurrence has been described.[131] In two such siblings the most outstanding features were anemia, thrombocytopenia, hepatosplenomegaly, and the presence of histiocytes in the reticuloendothelial system at autopsy. Of two other siblings[142] one showed central nervous system involvement with extensive histiocytic infiltration of brain and leptomeninges, while the other had much less extensive meningeal involvement. Reticuloendotheliosis has been described in a full-term infant who died shortly before the onset of labor. Whatever etiologic factors were involved in the development of this disease, the case demonstrated that these may be active in utero.[5] (See Fig. 90.)

*Pathology.* The spleen, liver, lymph nodes, skin, lungs, and bone marrow are heavily infiltrated by sheets of histiocytes, granulomatous nodules, and multinucleated giant cells. There is no lipid storage except in occasional patients in whom there are foam cells containing cholesterol. The rapid course of the disease precludes progression to the histologic picture of Hand-Schüller-Christian disease.

*Diagnosis.* A hemorrhagic tendency, eczematoid eruption, enlargement of the liver, spleen, and lymph nodes, roentgenographic evidence of bony defects, and progressive anemia in a young infant are highly suggestive of Letterer-Siwe disease. The characteristic eruption is not invariable in the infant, nor does it appear in the older child, in which case diag-

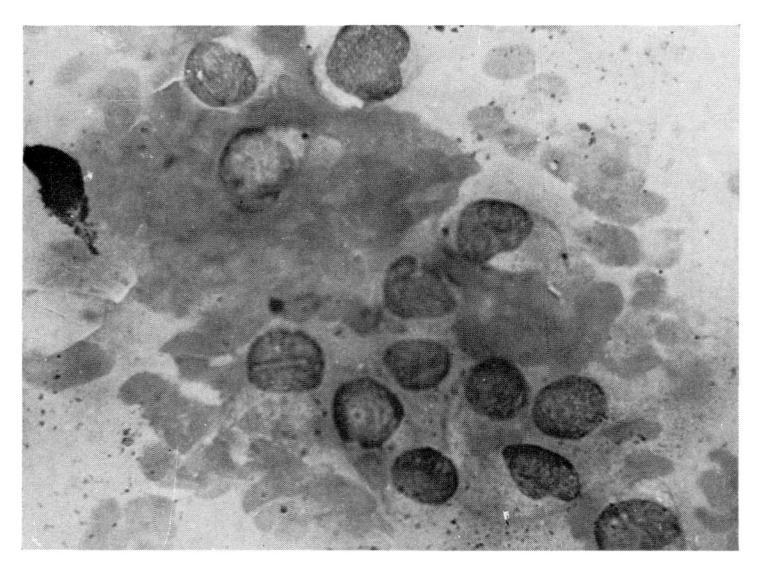

Fig. 91. Touch preparation from the skin lesions of a 20-month-old patient with nonlipid histiocytosis (Letterer-Siwe disease). The large mononuclear cells resemble those seen in affected lymph nodes. (×725.) (From Moore, T. D.: A simple technique for the diagnosis of nonlipid histiocytosis, Pediatrics 19:438, 1957.)

nosis depends upon roentgenographic findings and the pathologic evidence of a generalized hyperplasia of histiocytes. Biopsy of skin or lymph nodes reveals evidence of proliferating histiocytes and occasional foam cells.

Bone marrow aspiration often demonstrates increased numbers of histiocytes. These are irregularly round, oval, or polyhedral cells with protoplasmic projections containing ingested particles, red blood cells, and leukocytes. The nucleus is round, oval, or kidney shaped and is usually eccentrically placed.[66] It should be remembered that occasional phagocytic histiocytes of this type are seen in bone marrow smears of patients with many pathologic states. Skin scrapings show cells similar to the proliferating reticulum cells in the lymph nodes, spleen, liver, and bone marrow and serve as a diagnostic aid.[106] (See Fig. 91.)

*Blood.* Severe and progressive anemia is a prominent feature. The red cells are normochromic and normocytic and the white blood cell count ranges from leukopenic to moderate leukocytosis, with lymphocytosis or a normal differential count. Hemohistiocytes have been identified in the peripheral blood.[115] Despite the hemorrhagic nature of the disease, the platelets may be normal or only slightly decreased in numbers. Occasionally, there is marked thrombocytopenia. Pancytopenia and a hyperplastic bone marrow are occasionally noted. The etiology of the hematologic changes is by no means clear. A hemolytic mechanism has been considered on the basis of persistent reticulocytosis, nucleated red cells in the peripheral smears, slightly elevated serum bilirubin, and erythroid hyperplasia of the bone marrow.[90]

*Treatment and course.* Supportive therapy, transfusions, radiation, and antibiotics[18] have been employed. Improvement with steroids[15] has been reported, but this form of therapy awaits further trial. The disease is usually fatal in infants. Three patients with proved Letterer-Siwe syndrome were treated with gratifying results with vinblastine sulfate.[16] Treatment with large doses of steroids alternating with antifolic acid compounds[55] has given good responses, but relapse is a constant possibility. The chronic case in the older patient may represent a transitional form between Letterer-Siwe disease and Hand-Schüller-Christian disease.

A patient diagnosed as having Letterer-Siwe disease has been reported[96] presenting a hemorrhagic skin rash, thrombocytopenia, and a clotting profile indicative of intravascular coagulation. These abnormalities appeared to respond quickly to heparin. She continued to improve following the administration of prednisone and cyclophosphamide. The liver and spleen regressed although still palpable and the hemoglobin and platelets have maintained satisfactory levels, although she has been intermittently leukopenic.

### Hand-Schüller-Christian disease

Hand-Schüller-Christian disease is a constitutional disorder of metabolism characterized by a classic triad consisting of defects of membranous bones, exophthalmos, and diabetes insipidus. These features and associated phenomena result from the localized accumulation of histiocytes containing cholesterol and its esters, giving the appearance of foam cells (xanthomas).

**Clinical features.** The onset is insidious, occurring most often in children before the age of 7 years and often after an infection. The disease is ushered in by varied signs and symptoms indicative of underlying accumulations of histiocytes and foam cells. Ulceration of the mouth, loose teeth, swollen gums, dwarfism, yellow to brownish colored plaques and nodules of the skin, and chronic otitis media with mastoid involvement are characteristic findings.[137,169] Papular eczematoid lesions, which resemble the dermatitis of Letterer-Siwe disease, start on the scalp and spread over the face and trunk. Xanthomatous lesions are uncommon. When present, they consist of pinpoint to pea-sized nodules from the deeper layer of the skin and are covered by normal epidermis.[137]

Lesions in the calvaria are part of a generalized skeletal disease and consist of numerous "punched-out" areas of bone, resulting in defects of irregular size and producing a "geographic pattern." The defects are filled by a yellow granulomatous tissue originating in the dura or periosteum. Although the skull defects are most prominent, the facial bones, pelvis, ribs, scapula, and spine may be subject to granulomatous formation giving rise to localized areas of bone destruction which can be visualized on roentgenograms.[173] Pathologic fractures result from cysts in the long bones and punched-out areas. Diabetes insipidus is due to xanthomatous involvement of the region of the hypophysis and base of the brain. Exophthalmos follows destruction of the orbit and replacement by abnormal tissues. Visceral involvement leads to serious complications. Brain involvement is unusual. Infiltration of the lungs, suggesting the picture of pneumoconiosis on the roentgenogram, leads ultimately to marked fibrosis, cor pulmonale, and right heart failure. Involvement of the liver, spleen, and lymph nodes is less common than involvement of other systems, although it may be a predominant feature.[10] Growth and sexual development are retarded.

**Pathology.** On microscopic examination the most notable histologic feature is the presence of foam cells lodged in different tissues giving a yellow coloration. The fully developed foam cell is large, pale, round or ovoid, and 20 to 40μ in diameter, having abundant cytoplasm and one or two small nuclei. In the fresh state it is loaded with small droplets of fatlike material.[137] Biopsies show a hyperplasia of histiocytic foam cells or an admixture with granulomatous tissues rich in eosinophils. This close pathologic relationship is confirmed by cases demonstrating the transition from eosinophilic granuloma to Hand-Schüller-Christian disease.[45,91,173]

**Diagnosis.** Although membranous bone defects, exophthalmos, and diabetes insipidus are the cardinal features of Hand-Schüller-Christian disease, they are not always present together, especially in the initial stages. In one series they were present in combination in only three of twenty-nine patients.[10] Examination of a single biopsy specimen does not permit unequivocal classification of any given case. In such a case, the diagnosis and subsequent course must be deferred until the disease becomes generalized. With an incomplete picture there may be confusion with isolated bone cysts, multiple myeloma, Ewing's sarcoma, and metastatic neuroblastoma. Usually, there is no anemia; if it does occur, it is mild. A severe progressive anemia is indicative of serious involvement of blood-forming organs. Serum cholesterol is normal.

**Course.** The course is chronic and protracted, but spontaneous remissions occur. When the onset is early in life, the course is more likely to be severe than when it comes later. Visceral and neurologic lesions presage a fulminating course.[137] Of the series of twenty-nine cases cited previously, the mortality was 13%.[10] The prognosis is always doubtful, and a true estimate still awaits the results of more extensive experience with modern therapy.

*Treatment.* Roentgen-ray therapy results in definite improvement, being limited to the lesion toward which it is directed.[10] In soft tissue masses and enlarged lymph nodes a response is obtained within 2 to 3 weeks, and in bone defects a response is obtained after 3 to 4 months. It is the quickest available method for healing bone lesions and for relieving exophthalmos.[103] Steroid therapy, intravenous nitrogen mustard, and the antifols, such as amethopterin, are useful adjuvants. While adrenocorticoid therapy is capable of reversing all the skeletal and visceral manifestations, its overall effectiveness is still equivocal and difficult to assess.[11] Vinblastine sulfate (Velban) has been recommended as an extremely effective agent in treatment of this disorder.[29] Polydypsia and polyuria of diabetes insipidus are easily controlled by injection or insufflation of Pitressin.[103]

## Eosinophilic granuloma

Eosinophilic granuloma, the main feature being the presence of single or multiple skeletal lesions,[14,117] is regarded as the most benign member of the reticuloendothelial group.[61,75] It occurs predominantly in infants, children, and young adults. Any bone in the body may be involved, but there appears to be a predilection for the bones of the skull, vertebrae, extremities, and pelvis. Visceral involvement is rare. There is no hepatosplenomegaly or lymph node enlargement. Usually, there is little or no systemic evidence of illness. Symptoms, when present, are referable to the local lesion and consist of mild fever, local pains, swelling, and redness. The foci of destruction, as well as demarcated areas of rarefaction, are represented in the roentgenograms. Expansion of the lesions in the medullary cavity of the long bones results in erosion of the cortex and spontaneous fractures. In other instances cyst formation in the long bones is associated with regional cortical thickening.[22] The bony defects showing a punched-out appearance are similar to those of Hand-Schüller-Christian disease. Pulmonary nodular infiltrations of eosinophilic granuloma may coexist with[178] and without[83,98] associated skeletal lesions.

Histologically, the lesions consist of granulomatous inflammatory collections interspersed among which are polymorphonuclear leukocytes and accumulations of eosinophilic leukocytes. Multinuclear giant cells and foam cells occasionally are present. The number of eosinophilic leukocytes in the peripheral blood is usually not increased. Transitional forms between Hand-Schüller-Christian disease and eosinophilic granuloma occur. The lesions respond well to surgical excision or simple curettage performed at the time of biopsy. Roentgen ray therapy is also effective. Spontaneous cures have been observed. The prognosis is favorable but must be guarded because of the possibility of skeletal lesions appearing elsewhere.

## Histiocytic medullary reticulosis

Histiocytic medullary reticulosis[145] is a rare disorder originally described by Scott and Robb-Smith in 1939. The clinical picture is characterized by a fulminant illness with fever, wasting, pancytopenia, lymphadenopathy, hepatosplenomegaly, and death in a matter of weeks to a few months. In the terminal stages there is profound leukopenia, anemia, purpura, and jaundice. The disease occurs mainly in adults but has been observed in children. The pathologic histology was described as showing a progressive and "at times neoplastic" cellular hyperplasia throughout the lymphoreticular tissues, associated with active histiocytic phagocytosis (Fig. 92). Pathologists sometimes encounter giant cells which are difficult to differentiate from Reed-Sternberg cells of Hodgkin's disease.

Two siblings were reported[93] also diagnosed as having histiocytic medullary reticulosis in whom Letterer-Siwe disease had been suspected. The first child died at the age of 3 months, the second child born about a year later died in the first year of life, about 8 months after the onset of the illness. Autopsy findings in both cases were characterized by hyperplasia of histiocytic cells, erythrophagocytosis, and infiltration of lymphocytes and histiocytes in almost every organ. In the older infant the leptomeninges were heavily infiltrated with lymphocytes and histiocytes, some of the latter containing erythroctyes.

At The New York Hospital a 10-year-old male child was admitted with respiratory distress following an upper respiratory infection. He had lost 28 pounds in 1 month and at this time had bloody diarrhea. He was pale, and had massive lymphadenopathy in the neck and a firm mass at the angle of the right jaw. Chest x-ray revealed a superior mediastinal mass and hilar lymphadenopathy. The

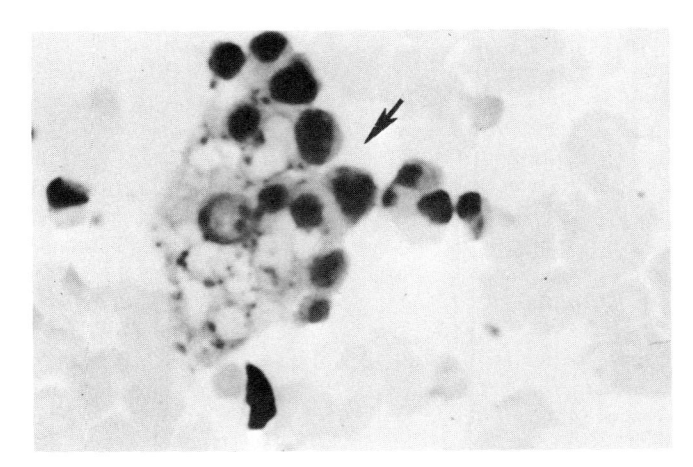

**Fig. 92.** Histiocytic medullary reticulosis. Bone marrow aspirate from a 10-year-old male who presented with fever and adenopathy showed erythroid hyperplasia and marked erythrophagocytosis.

liver was palpable up to 4 to 5 cm. in the midclavicular line but there were no other abdominal masses and the spleen was not palpable. Hemoglobin was 8.8 gm. per 100 ml., hematocrit 26%, and platelets 60,000/cu.mm. The WBC was 10,200/cu.mm., with 80% polynuclear forms. There were no abnormal leukocytes. Bone marrow revealed erythroid hyperplasia with erythrophagocytosis. Lymph node biopsy was consistent with histiocytic medullary reticulosis. Radiation, prednisone, and cyclophosphamide produced only a very short response. Death occurred 4 months after the diagnosis. Autopsy confirmed the diagnosis of histiocytic medullary reticulosis with involvement of lymph nodes, bone marrow, kidneys, liver, spleen, esophagus, stomach, colon, adrenals, lungs, leptomeninges, and conjunctiva.

The diagnosis of histiocytic medullary reticulosis was established during life by bone marrow examination in a 45-year-old Caucasian man with bone pain and anemia.[184] Results of electron microscopy of the neoplastic histiocytes and ferrokinetic studies supported the hypothesis that the anemia in patients with this disorder was due to the unavailability of iron stores resulting from excessive erythrophagocytosis.

Another example of this disease but presenting a leukemic blood picture has been reported by Clarke and Dawson[28] in a 17-year-old boy. After an initial response to prednisone therapy a relapse occurred with a protein-losing enteropathy. Autopsy revealed the characteristic changes of histiocytic medullary reticulosis with the characteristic marked infiltration with histiocytic erythrophagocytic cells. The terminal enteropathy was interpreted as histiocytic infiltration of the lamina propria of the small intestine.

Other conditions have also been described that do not exactly fit into any of the three forms of histiocytosis X. One of these has been described as familial, generalized, lymphohistiocytic infiltrative disease, which is to be differentiated from Letterer-Siwe disease and the Chediak-Higashi syndrome.[111]

Concurrence of a familial malignant reticuloendotheliosis in a complete sibship of five girls has been reported.[105] Twelve cases of familial reticuloendotheliosis with eosinophilia have been documented in six sibships of a large family containing many consanguineous matings.[114] These syndromes have been uniformly fatal and etiologic agents have escaped identification.

## REFERENCES

1. Aballi, A. J., and Kato, R.: Gaucher's disease in early infancy: review of the literature and a report of a case with neurological symptoms, J. Pediat. 13:364, 1938.
2. Abt, A. F., and Denenholz, E. J.: Letterer-Siwe's disease splenohepatomegaly associated with wide-spread hyperplasia of non-lipid-storing macrophages; discussion of the so-called reticuloendothelioses, Amer. J. Dis. Child. 51:499, 1936.
3. Acevedo, G., and Mauer, A. M.: The capacity for the removal of erythrocytes containing Heinz-bodies in premature infants and patients following splenectomy, J. Pediat. 63:61, 1963.
4. Ackerman, L. V.: Surgical pathology, ed. 4, St. Louis, 1968, The C. V. Mosby Co.
5. Ahnquist, G., and Holyoke, J. B.: Congenital Letterer-Siwe disease (reticuloendothe-

liosis) in a term stillborn infant, J. Pediat. **57**:897, 1960.
6. Alexander, S.: Niemann-Pick's disease showing calcification in the adrenal glands, New Zealand Med. J. **45**:43, 1946.
7. Allen, F. A., Carr, M. H., and Klotz, A. P.: Decreased red blood cell-survival time in patients with portal cirrhosis; correlation of laboratory and clinical findings, J.A.M.A. **164**:955, 1957.
8. Allison, A. C., and Burn, G. P.: Enzyme activity as a function of age in the human erythrocyte, Brit. J. Haemat. **1**:291, 1955.
9. Alpert, M. E., and Seeler, R. A.: Alpha fetoprotein in embryonal hepatoblastoma, J. Pediat. **77**:1058, 1970.
10. Avery, M. E., McAfee, J. G., and Guild, H. G.: The course and prognosis of reticuloendotheliosis (eosinophilic granuloma, Schüller-Christian disease and Letterer-Siwe disease); a study of forty cases, Amer. J. Med. **22**:636, 1957.
11. Avioli, L. U., Laserohn, J. T., and Lopresti, J. M.: Histiocytosis X (Schüller-Christian disease); a clinico-pathological survey review of ten patients and the results of prednisone therapy, Medicine **42**:119, 1963.
12. Banker, B. Q., Miller, J. Q., and Crocker, A. C.: The neurological disorder in infantile Gaucher's disease, Tr. Am. Neurol. A. **86**:43, 1961.
13. Banti, G.: La splenomegalia con cirrose del fegato, Sperimentale (sez biol.) **48**:407, 1894.
14. Bass, M. H.: Solitary eosinophilic granuloma of bone, Amer. J. Dis. Child. **61**:1254, 1941.
15. Bass, M. H., Sapin, S. O., and Hodes, H. L.: Use of cortisone and corticotropin (ACTH) in treatment of reticuloendotheliosis in children, Amer. J. Dis. Child. **85**:393, 1953.
16. Beier, F. R., Thatcher, L. G., and Lahey, M. E.: Treatment of reticuloendotheliosis with vinblastine sulfate, J. Pediat. **63**:1087, 1963.
17. Bennett, I. L., Jr., and Beeson, P. B.: Bacteremia; a consideration of some experimental and clinical aspects, Yale J. Biol. Med. **26**:241, 1954.
18. Bierman, H. R., Lanman, J. T., Dod, K. S., Kelly, K. H., Miller, E. R., and Shimkin, M. B.: The ameliorative effect of antibiotics on nonlipid reticuloendotheliosis (Letterer-Siwe disease) in identical twins, J. Pediat. **40**:269, 1952.
19. Bjorkman, S. E.: The splenic circulation with special reference to the function of the spleen sinus wall, Acta Med. Scandinav., supp. 191, 1947.
20. Brady, R. O.: Genetics and the sphingolipidosis, Med. Clin. N. Amer. **53**:827, 1969.
21. Bush, J. A., and Ainger, L. E.: Congenital absence of spleen with congenital heart disease, Pediatrics **15**:93, 1955.
22. Caffey, J.: Pediatric x-ray diagnosis, Chicago, 1956, Year Book Medical Publishers, Inc.
23. Carlisle, H. N., and Saslaw, S.: Properdin levels in splenectomized persons, Proc. Soc. Exp. Biol. Med. **102**:150, 1959.
24. Chatterjea, J. B., Dameshek, W., and Stefanini, M.: The adrenalin (epinephrin) test as applied to hematologic disorders, Blood **8**:211, 1953.
25. Chatterjea, J. B., Mesa Arrau, C., and Dameshek, W.: Splenic puncture, Brit. M. J. **1**:987, 1952.
26. Child, C. G., III: The liver and portal hypertension. In Dunphy, J. E., consulting editor: Major problems in clinical surgery, Volume 1, Philadelphia, 1964, W. B. Saunders Co.
27. Claireaux, A. E., and Lewis, I. C.: Reticuloendothelial granuloma; a review with a report of a case of Letterer-Siwe disease, Arch. Dis. Child. **24**:142, 1950.
28. Clarke, B. S., and Dawson, P. J.: Histiocytic medullary reticulosis presenting with a leukemic blood picture, Amer. J. Med. **45**:314, 1969.
29. Cole, D. R., and Pingitore, N. E.: Hand-Schüller-Christian disease, New York State Med. J. **70**:2346, 1970.
30. Crocker, A. C., and Farber, S.: Niemann-Pick disease; a review of eighteen patients, Medicine **37**:1, 1958.
31. Crocker, A. C., and Landing, B. H.: Phosphatase studies in Gaucher's disease, Metabolism **9**:341, 1960.
32. Crocker, A. C., Vawter, G. F., Neuhauser, E. B. O., and Rosowsky, A.: Wolman's disease; three new patients with a recently described lysidosis, Pediatrics **35**:627, 1965.
33. Crosby, W. H.: Normal functions of the spleen relative to red blood cells; a review, Blood **14**:399, 1959.
34. Crosby, W. H.: Is hypersplenism a dead issue? Blood **20**:94, 1962.
35. Dameshek, W.: Hypersplenism, Bull. N. Y. Acad. Med. **31**:113, 1955.
36. Dameshek, W., and Estren, S.: Hypersplenism, Med. Clin. N. Amer. **34**:1271, 1950.
37. De Gruchy, G. C.: Clinical haematology in medical practice, ed. 2, Springfield, Ill., 1964, Charles C Thomas, Publisher.
38. Diamond, L. K.: Indications for splenectomy in childhood, Amer. J. Surg. **39**:400, 1938.
39. Diamond, L. K.: Splenectomy in childhood and the hazard of overwhelming infection, Pediatrics **43**:886, 1969.
40. Dienet, G., and Hamperl, H.: Lipoid spleno-

hepatomegalie (typus Niemann-Pick), Wien. Klin. wschr. **40**:1432, 1927.
41. Di Sant'Agnese, P. A., and Blanc, W. A.: A distinctive type of biliary cirrhosis of the liver associated with disease of the pancreas; recognition through signs of portal hypertension, Pediatrics **18**:387, 1956.
42. Doan, C. A.: The spleen and reticuloendothelial system. In Sodeman, W. A., editor: Pathologic physiology, Philadelphia, 1956, W. B. Saunders Co., chap. 29, p. 852.
43. Doan, C. A., and Wright, C. S.: Primary congenital and secondarily acquired splenic panhematopenia, Blood **1**:10, 1946.
44. Draznin, S. Z., and Singer, K.: Legg-Perthes disease; a syndrome of many etiologies with clinical and roentgenographic findings in a case of Gaucher's disease, Amer. J. Roentgen. **60**:490, 1948.
45. Dumermuth, G.: Reticulogranulomatose: Zwei Fälle von Eosinophileim Granulom mit Übergang in Hand-Schüller-Christiansche Krankheit, Helvet. Paediat. Acta **13**:15, 1958.
46. Ebert, R. V., and Stead, E. A., Jr.: Demonstration that in normal man no reserves of blood are mobilized by exercise, epinephrine and hemorrhage, Amer. J. Med. Sci. **201**:655, 1941.
47. Ekman, C. A.: Portal hypertension; diagnosis and surgical treatment, Acta Chir. Scandinav. (supp. 222) **1**:143, 1957.
48. Ellis, E. F., and Smith, R. T.: The role of the spleen in immunity; with special reference to the post-splenectomy problem in infants, Pediatrics **37**:111, 1966.
49. Erickson, W. D., Burgert, E. O., Jr., and Lynn, H. B.: The hazards of infection following splenectomy in children, Amer. J. Dis. Child. **116**:1, 1968.
50. Estborn, B., and Hillborg, P. O.: On the increased serum acid phosphatase in Gaucher's disease, Scandinav. J. Clin. Lab. Invest. **12**:504, 1960.
51. Figley, M. M.: Splenoportography; some advantages and disadvantages, Amer. J. Roentgen. **80**:313, 1958.
52. Fisher, E. R., and Reidbord, H.: Gaucher's disease; pathogenetic considerations based on electron microscopic and histochemical observations, Amer. J. Path. **41**:679, 1962.
53. Forsythe, W. I., McKeown, E. F., and Neill, D. W.: Three cases of Niemann-Pick's disease in children, Arch. Dis. Child. **34**:406, 1959.
54. Fraumeni, J. F., Jr., Rosen, P. J., Hall, E. W., Barth, R. F., Shapiro, S. R., and O'Conner, J. F.: Hepatoblastoma in infant sisters, Cancer **24**:1086, 1969.
55. Freud, P.: Treatment of reticuloendothelioses; use of corticosteroids and anti-folic acid compounds, J.A.M.A. **175**:82, 1961.
56. Gasser, C., and Willi, H.: Spontane Innenköperbildung bei Milzagenesie, Helvet. Paediat. Acta **7**:369, 1952.
57. Gaucher, E.: De l'épithelima primitif de la rate, Theśe de Paris, 1882.
58. Geddes, A. K., and Moore, S.: Acute (infantile) Gaucher's disease, J. Pediat. **43**:61, 1953.
59. Gitlin, D., Rosen, F. S., and Janeway, C. A.: Undue susceptibility to infection, Ped. Clin. N. Amer. **9**:405, 1962.
60. Godwin, H. A., Zimmerman, T. S., Kimball, H. R., Wolff, S. M., and Perry, S.: The effect of etiocholanolone on the entry of granulocytes into the peripheral blood, Blood **31**:461, 1968.
61. Green, W. T., and Farber, S.: "Eosinophilic or solitary granuloma" of bone, J. Bone Joint Surg. **24**:499, 1942.
62. Groen, J.: The hereditary mechanism of Gaucher's disease, Blood **2**:1328, 1948.
63. Gross, R. E.: The surgery of infancy and childhood; its principles and techniques, Philadelphia, 1953, W. B. Saunders Co.
64. Harris, I. M., McAlister, J. M., and Prankerd, T. A. J.: Splenomegaly and the circulating red cell, Brit. J. Haemat. **4**:97, 1958.
65. Harrison, W. E., Jr., and Louis, H. S.: Osseous Gaucher's disease in early childhood; report of a case with extensive bone changes and pathological fractures with splenomegaly, J.A.M.A **187**:107, 1964.
66. Harvard, E., Rather, L. J., and Farber, H. K.: Nonlipoid reticuloendotheliosis (Letterer-Siwe's disease), Pediatrics **2**:474, 1950.
67. Hayes, D. M., Spurr, C. L., Hutaff, R. J., and Sheets, J. A.: Postsplenectomy thrombocytosis, Ann. Intern. Med. **58**:259, 1963.
68. Hoja, W. A.: Gaucher's disease in pregnancy, Amer. J. Obstet. Gynec. **79**:286, 1960.
69. Horan, M., and Colebatch, J. H.: Relation between splenectomy and subsequent infection, Arch. Dis. Child. **37**:398, 1962.
70. Hsia, D. Y-Y., and Gellis, S. S.: Portal hypertension in infants and children, Amer. J. Dis. Child. **90**:290, 1955.
71. Hsia, D. Y-Y., Naylor, J., and Bigler, J. A.: Gaucher's disease; report of two cases in father and son and review of the literature, New Eng. J. Med. **261**:164, 1959.
72. Ivemark, B. I.: Implications of agenesis of the spleen on the pathogenesis of cono-truncus anomalies in childhood, Acta Paediat. (supp. 104) **44**:1, 1955.
73. Jacobson, L. O., Marks, E. K., Gaston, E. O., Simons, E. L., and Robson, M. J.: Modifica-

tion of radiation, Bull. N. Y. Acad. Med. **30**: 675, 1954.
74. Jacobson, L. O., Robson, M. E., Marks, E. K., and Goldman, M. C.: The effect of x-radiation on antibody formation, J. Lab. Clin. Med. **34**:1612, 1949.
75. Jaffe, H. L., and Lichtenstein, L.: Eosinophilic granuloma of the bone; a condition affecting one, several or many bones, but apparently limited to the skeleton and representing the mildest clinical expression of the peculiar inflammatory histiocytosis also underlying Letterer-Siwe disease and Schüller-Christian disease, Arch. Path. **37**:99, 1944.
76. Jandl, J. H., Jacob, H. S., and Daland, G. E.: Hypersplenism due to infection; a study of 5 cases manifesting hemolytic anemia, New Eng. J. Med. **264**:1063, 1961.
77. Jones, B., Gilbert, E. F., Zugibe, F. T., and Thompson, H.: Sea-blue histiocyte disease in siblings, Lancet **2**:73, 1970.
78. Kattlove, H. E., Gaynor, E., Spivack, M., and Gottfried, E. L.: Sea-blue indigestion, New Eng. J. Med. **282**:630, 1970.
79. Kauder, E., and Mauer, A. M.: Neutropenias of childhood, J. Pediat. **69**:147, 1966.
80. Kevy, S. V., Tefft, M., Vawter, G. F., and Rosen, F. S.: Hereditary splenic hypoplasia, Pediatrics **42**:752, 1968.
81. Keats, T. E., and Crane, J. F.: Cystic changes of the lungs in histiocytosis, Amer. J. Dis. Child. **88**:764, 1954.
82. Knisely, M. H.: Microscopic observations of the circulatory system of living unstimulated mammalian spleens, Anat. Rec. **65**:23, 131, 1936.
82a. La Celle, P. L., and Weed, R. I.: The contribution of normal and pathological erythrocytes to blood rheology. In Brown, E. B., and Moore, C. V., editors: Progress in hematology, vol. VII, New York, 1971, Grune & Stratton, Inc.
83. Lackey, R. W., Leaver, F. Y., and Fatinacci, C. J.: Eosinophilic granuloma of the lung, Radiology **59**:504, 1952.
84. Lahey, M. E.: Prognosis of reticuloendotheliosis in children, J. Pediat. **60**:664, 1962.
85. Landing, B. H., Silverman, F. N., Craig, J. M., Jacoby, M. D., Lahey, M. E., and Chadwick, D. L.: Familial neurovisceral lipidosis, Amer. J. Dis. Child. **108**:503, 1964.
86. Levitan, R., Diamond, H. D., and Craver, L. F.: Esophageal varices in Hodgkin's disease involving the liver, Amer. J. Med. **27**:137, 1959.
87. Lichtenstein, L.: Histiocytosis X, Arch. Path. **56**:84, 1953.
88. Lichtenstein, L.: Histiocytosis X (eosinophilic granuloma of the bone, Letterer-Siwe disease and Schüller-Christian disease); further observations of pathological and clinical importance, J. Bone Joint Surg. **46**:76, 1964.
89. Lieberman, P. H., Jones, C. R., Dargeon, H. W. K., and Begg, C. F.: A reappraisal of eosinophilic granuloma of bone, Hand-Schüller-Christian syndrome and Letterer-Siwe syndrome, Medicine **48**:375, 1969.
90. Lipton, E. L.: Hemolytic and pancytopenic syndrome associated with Letterer-Siwe disease, Pediatrics **14**:533, 1954.
91. Love, F. M., and Fashena, G. J.: Eosinophilic granuloma of the bone and Hand-Schüller-Christian disease, J. Pediat. **32**:46, 1948.
92. Lynn, R., and Terry, R. D.: Lipid histochemistry and electron microscopy in adult Niemann-Pick disease, Amer. J. Med. **37**:987, 1964.
93. MacMahon, H. E., Bedizel, M., and Elks, C. A.: Familial erythrophagocytic lymphohistiocytosis, Pediatrics **32**:868, 1963.
94. Malinin, T. I.: Unidentified reticuloendothelial cell storage disease, Blood **17**:675, 1961.
95. Marsh, J. C., and Perry, S.: The granulocyte response to endotoxin in patients with hematologic disorders, Blood **23**:581, 1964.
96. Mauger, D. C.: Letterer-Siwe's disease (acute disseminated histiocytosis X); a case complicated by disseminated intravascular coagulation responding to heparin therapy, Pediatrics **47**:435, 1971.
97. Maximow, A. A., and Bloom, W.: A text book of histology, ed. 6, Philadelphia, 1953, W. B. Saunders Co.
98. Mazzitello, W. F.: Eosinophilic granuloma of the lung, New Eng. J. Med. **250**:804, 1954.
99. McCracken, G. H., and Dickerman, J. D.: Septicemia and disseminated intravascular coagulation; occurrence in four asplenic children, Amer. J. Dis. Child. **118**:431, 1969.
100. McIntyre, O. R., and Ebaugh, F. G.: Palpable spleens in college freshmen, Ann. Intern. Med. **66**:301, 1967.
101. McMichael, J.: Pathology of hepatolienal fibrosis, J. Path. Bact. **39**:481, 1934.
102. Medoff, A. S., and Bayrd, E. D.: Gaucher's disease in 29 cases; hematologic complications and effects of splenectomy, Ann. Intern. Med. **40**:481, 1954.
103. Mermann, A. C., and Dargeon, H. W.: The management of certain nonlipid reticuloendotheliosis; 28 cases treated over a 22-year period, Cancer **8**:112, 1955.
104. Meyerson, R. M., Stout, R., and Havens, W. P.: Production of antibody by splenectomized persons, Amer. J. Med. Sci. **234**:297, 1957.

105. Miller, D. R.: Familial reticuloendotheliosis; concurrence of disease in five siblings, Pediatrics **38**:986, 1966.
106. Moore, T. D.: A simple technique for the diagnosis of nonlipid histiocytosis, Pediatrics **19**:438, 1957.
107. Moseley, J. E.: Bone changes in hematologic disorders, New York, 1963, Grune & Stratton, Inc.
108. Motulsky, A. G., Casserd, F., Giblett, E. R., Broun, G. O., Jr., and Finch, C. A.: Anemia and the spleen, New Eng. J. Med. **259**:1164, 1958.
109. Muir, C. S.: Splenic agenesis and multilobulate spleen, Arch. Dis. Child. **34**:431, 1959.
110. Murphy, J. W., and Mitchell, W. A.: Congenital absence of the spleen, Pediatrics **20**:253, 1957.
111. Nelson, P., Santamaria, A., Olson, R. L., and Mayak, N. C.: Generalized lymphohistiocytic infiltration; a familial disease not previously described and different from Letterer-Siwe disease and Chediak-Higashi syndrome, Pediatrics **27**:931, 1961.
112. Oberman, H. A.: Idiopathic histiocytosis; a clinicopathologic study of 40 cases and review of the literature on eosinophilic granuloma of bone, Hand-Schüller-Christian disease and Letterer-Siwe disease, Pediatrics **28**:307, 1961.
113. Okada, S., and O'Brien, J. S.: Generalized gangliosidosis; beta galactosidase deficiency, Science **160**:1002, 1968.
114. Omenn, G. S.: Familial reticuloendotheliosis with eosinophilia, New Eng. J. Med. **273**:427, 1965.
115. Orchard, N. P.: Letterer-Siwe's syndrome; report of a case with unusual peripheral blood changes, Arch. Dis. Child. **25**:151, 1950.
116. Oski, F. A., Allen, D. M., and Diamond, L. K.: Portal hypertension; a complication of umbilical vein catheterization, Pediatrics **31**:297, 1963.
117. Otani, S., and Ehrlich, J. C.: Solitary granuloma of bone simulating primary neoplasm, Amer. J. Path. **16**:479, 1940.
118. Palmer, J. G., Eichwald, E. J., Cartwright, G. E., and Wintrobe, M. M.: The experimental production of splenomegaly, anemia and leukopenia in albino rats, Blood **8**:72, 1953.
119. Perez-Tamayo, R., Mora, J., and Montfort, J.: Humoral factor(s) in experimental hypersplenism, Blood **16**:1145, 1960.
120. Perla, D., and Marmorston, J.: The spleen and resistance, Baltimore, 1935, Williams & Wilkins Co.
121. Pick, L.: Niemann-Pick disease and other forms of so-called xanthomatosis, Amer. J. Med. Sci. **185**:601, 1933.
122. Polhemus, D. W., and Schafer, W. B.: Absent spleen syndrome; hematologic findings as an aid to diagnosis, Pediatrics **24**:254, 1959.
123. Prankerd, T. A. J.: The spleen and anaemia, Brit. J. Med. **2**:517, 1963.
124. Putschar, W. G. J., and Manion, W. C.: Congenital absence of the spleen and associated anomalies, Amer. J. Clin. Path. **26**:429, 1956.
124a. Ramot, B., Brok, F., and Ben-Bassat, I.: Alterations in the metabolism of human erythrocytes with aging, Plenary Session Papers, XII Cong. Int. Soc. Hematol., New York, 1968.
125. Rebuck, J. W., and Crowley, J. H.: A method for studying leukocyte functions in vivo, Ann. N. Y. Acad. Sci. **59**:757, 1955.
126. Reich, C., Seife, M., and Kessler, B. J.: Gaucher's disease; a review and discussion of 20 cases, Medicine **30**:1, 1951.
127. Robinson, T. W., and Sturgeon, P.: Postsplenectomy infection in infants and children, Pediatrics **25**:941, 1960.
128. Rodgers, C. L., and Jackson, S. H.: Acute infantile Gaucher's disease, Pediatrics **7**:53, 1951.
129. Rogers, D. E.: Studies on bacteremia; mechanisms relating to the persistence of bacteremia in rabbits following the intravenous injection of staphylococci, J. Exp. Med. **103**:713, 1956.
130. Rogers, D. E., and Melly, M. A.: Studies on bacteremia; the blood stream clearance of *Escherichia coli* in rabbits, J. Exp. Med. **105**:113, 1957.
131. Rogers, D. L., and Benson, T. E.: Familial Letterer-Siwe disease, J. Pediat. **60**:550, 1962.
132. Rogers, H. M., and Langley, F. H.: Neutropenia associated with splenomegaly and atrophic arthritis (Felty's syndrome); report of a case in which splenectomy was performed, Ann. Intern. Med. **32**:745, 1950.
133. Rosenberg, D. H.: Macrocytic anemia in liver disease, particularly cirrhosis, Amer. J. Med. Sci. **192**:86, 1936.
134. Rosowsky, A., Crocker, A. C., Tritis, D. H., and Modest, E. J.: Gas-liquid chromatographic analysis of the tissue sterol fraction in Wolman's disease and related lipidosis, Biophys. Acta **98**:617, 1965.
135. Rothberg, H., Corallo, L. A., and Crosby, W. H.: Observations on Heinz bodies in normal and splenectomized rabbits, Blood **14**:1180, 1959.
136. Rousselot, L. M.: The present status of sur-

gery for portal hypertension, Amer. J. Med. 16:874, 1954.
137. Rowland, R. S.: Constitutional disturbances of lipid metabolism and the reticuloendothelial system, constitutional disturbances of the lipid metabolism. In McQuarrie, I., and Kelley, V. C., editors: Brennemann's practice of pediatrics, Hagerstown, Md., W. F. Prior Co., Inc., vol. 3, chap. 23, p. 15.
138. Rowley, D. A.: The effect of splenectomy on the formation of circulating antibody in the adult male albino rat, J. Immunol. 64:289, 1950.
139. Rowley, D. A.: The formation of circulating antibody in the splenectomized human being following intravenous injection of heterologous erythrocytes, J. Immunol. 65:515, 1950.
140. Saslow, S., Bouroncle, B. A., Wall, R. L., and Doan, C. A.: Studies on the antibody response in splenectomized persons, New Eng. J. Med. 261:120, 1959.
141. Sawitsky, A., Hyman, G. A., and Hyman, J. B.: An unidentified reticuloendothelial cell in bone marrow and spleen, Blood 9:977, 1954.
142. Schoeck, V. W., Peterson, R. D. A., and Good, R. A.: Familial occurrence of Letterer-Siwe disease, Pediatrics 32:1055, 1963.
143. Schuckmell, N., Grove, W. J., and Remenchik, A. P.: The diagnosis of operable portal obstruction in children, Amer. J. Dis. Child. 90:692, 1955.
144. Schumacher, J. J.: Serum immunoglobulins and transferrin levels after childhood splenectomy, Arch. Dis. Child. 45:114, 1970.
145. Scott, R. B., and Robb-Smith, A. H. T.: Histiocytic medullary reticulosis, Lancet 2:194, 1939.
146. Shaldon, S., and Sherlock, S.: Obstruction to the extra-hepatic portal circulation in childhood, Lancet 1:63, 1962.
147. Shinefield, H. R., Kaye, D., and Eichenwald, H. F.: The effect of splenectomy on the mortality of mice inoculated with *Diplococcus pneumoniae*, J. Pediat. 65:1104, 1964.
148. Silverstein, M. N., Ellefson, R. D., and Ahern, E. J.: The syndrome of the sea-blue histiocyte, New Eng. J. Med. 228:1, 1970.
149. Singer, K., Miller, E. B., and Dameshek, W.: Hematologic changes following splenectomy in man with particular reference to target cells, hemolytic index and lysolecithin, Amer. J. Med. Sci. 202:171, 1941.
150. Singer, K., and Weisz, L.: The life cycle of the erythrocyte after splenectomy and the problems of splenic hemolysis and target cell formation, Amer. J. Med. Sci. 210:301, 1945.
151. Siwe, S. A.: Die Reticuloendotheliose—ein neues Krankheitsbild unter den Hepatosplenomegalien, Ztschr. Kinderh. 55:212, 1933.
152. Siwe, S.: The reticulo-endothelioses in children. In Levine, S. Z., editor: Advances in pediatrics, vol. 4, New York, 1949, Interscience Publishers, Inc., p. 117.
153. Smith, C. H., Erlandson, M. E., Schulman, I., and Stern, G.: Hazard of severe infections in splenectomized infants and children, Amer. J. Med. 22:390, 1957.
154. Smith, C. H., Erlandson, M. E., Stern, G., and Hilgartner, M. W.: Postsplenectomy infection in Cooley's anemia; an appraisal of the problems in this and other blood disorders, with a consideration of prophylaxis, New Eng. J. Med. 266:737, 1962.
155. Smith, C. H., Erlandson, M. E., Stern, G., and Hilgartner, M. W.: Postsplenectomy infection in Cooley's anemia, Ann. N. Y. Acad. Sci. 119:748, 1964.
156. Snyder, R. A., and Brady, R. O.: The use of white cells as a source of diagnostic material for lipid storage diseases, Clin. Chem. Acta 25:331, 1969.
157. Stein, M., and Gardner, L. J.: Acute infantile Gaucher's disease, Pediatrics 27:491, 1961.
158. Stewart, W. B., Stewart, J. M., Izzo, M. J., and Young, L. E.: Age as affecting the osmotic and mechanical fragility of dog erythrocytes tagged with radioactive iron, J. Exp. Med. 91:147, 1950.
159. Stransky, E., and Conchu, T. L.: Heredity in the infantile type of Gaucher's disease, Ann. Paediat. 177:319, 1951.
160. Strickland, B.: Skeletal manifestations of Gaucher's disease with some unusual findings, Brit. J. Radiol. 31:246, 1958.
161. Thannhauser, S. J.: Lipoidoses: diseases of the cellular lipid metabolism, ed. 2, New York, 1950, Oxford University Press.
162. Thatcher, L. G., and Smith, N. J.: Granulocyte responses of children to bacterial endotoxin, J. Pediat. 62:484, 1963.
163. Tisdale, W. A., Klatskin, G., and Glenn, W. W. L.: Portal hypertension and bleeding esophageal varices, their occurrence in the absence of both intrahepatic and extrahepatic obstruction of the portal vein, New Eng. J. Med. 261:209, 1959.
164. Todd, R., and Keidan, S. E.: Changes in the head of the femur in children suffering from Gaucher's disease, J. Bone Joint Surg. 34-B:454, 1952.
165. Toghill, P. J.: Red-cell pooling in enlarged spleens, Brit. J. Haemat. 10:347, 1964.
166. Trusler, G. A., Morris, F. R., and Mustard, W. T.: Portal hypertension in childhood, Surgery 52:664, 1962.

167. Uzman, L. L.: The lipoprotein of Gaucher's disease, Arch. Path. **51**:329, 1951.
168. Uzman, L. L.: Polycerebrosides in Gaucher's disease, Arch. Path. **55**:181, 1953.
169. van Creveld, S.: The lipoidoses. In Levine, S. Z., editor: Advances in pediatrics, vol. 6, Chicago, 1953, Year Book Medical Publishers, Inc., p. 190.
170. Varga, C., Richter, M. N., and De Sanctis, A. G.: Systemic aleukemia reticuloendotheliosis (Letterer-Siwe's disease), Amer. J. Dis. Child. **75**:376, 1948.
171. Vorhees, A. B., Jr., and Blaksmore, A. H.: Clinical experience with superior mesenteric vein, inferior vena cava shunt in the treatment of portal hypertension, Surgery **51**:35, 1962.
172. Walker, R. M., Shaldon, C., and Vowles, K. D. J.: Late results of portacaval anastamoses, Lancet **2**:727, 1961.
173. Wallace, W. S.: Reticuloendotheliosis; Hand-Schüller-Christian disease and the rare manifestations, Amer. J. Roentgen. **62**:189, 1949.
174. Wallgren, A.: Systemic reticuloendothelial granuloma nonlipid reticuloendotheliosis and Schüller-Christian disease, Amer. J. Dis. Child. **60**:471, 1940.
175. Wantz, G. E., and Payne, M. A.: Experience with portacaval shunt for portacaval hypertension, New Eng. J. Med. **265**:721, 1961.
176. Watson, E. H., and Lowrey, G. H.: Growth and development of children, Chicago, 1951, Year Book Medical Publishers, Inc.
177. Watson, R. J., Shapiro, H. D., Ellison, R. R., and Lichtman, H. C.: Splenic aspiration in clinical and experimental hematology, Blood **10**:259, 1955.
178. Weinstein, A., Francis, H. C., and Sprofkin, B. F.: Eosinophilic granuloma of bone; report of a case with multiple lesions of bone and pulmonary infiltration, Arch. Intern. Med. **79**:176, 1947.
179. Welch, C. S.: Portal hypertension, New Eng. J. Med. **243**:598, 1950.
179a. Wennberg, E., and Weiss, L.: The structure of the spleen and hemolysis, Ann. Rev. Med. **20**:29, 1969.
180. Whipple, A. O.: Problems of portal hypertension in relation to hepatosplenopathies, Ann. Surg. **122**:449, 1945.
181. Wiseman, B. K., and Doan, C. A.: Primary splenic neutropenia; a newly recognized syndrome, closely related to congenital hemolytic icterus and essential thrombocytopenic purpura, Ann. Intern. Med. **16**:1097, 1942.
182. Wolman, M., Sterle, V. V., Gatt, S., and Frenkel, M.: Primary familial xanthomatosis with involvement and calcification of the adrenals, Pediatrics **28**:742, 1961.
183. Wright, D. O.: Macrocytic anemia in Banti's disease, Ann. Intern. Med. **8**:814, 1935.
184. Zawadzki, Z. A., Pena, C. E., and Fisher, E. R.: Histiocytic medullary reticulosis; case report with electron microscopic study, Acta Haemat. **42**:50, 1969.
185. Zeid, S. S., Felson, B., and Schiff, L.: Percutaneous splenoportal venography, with additional comments on transhepatic venography, Ann. Intern. Med. **52**:782, 1960.
186. Zlotnick, A., and Groen, J. J.: Observations on a patient with Gaucher's disease, Amer. J. Med. **30**:637, 1961.

# 26 BLOOD COAGULATION

An abnormal tendency to bleed is the most obvious indication of a disturbance of hemostasis. Such an event calls for an investigation of possible defects in one or more of the components which normally maintain hemostasis. A description of these factors and their interaction will be reviewed as a background to discussion of the hemorrhagic disorders.

The arrest of hemorrhage is a complex process involving vascular integrity, platelets, and a group of specific circulating proteins which are active in blood coagulation. The sequence from the initial response to skin and blood vessel injury to the formation of a clot requires the proper functioning and coordination of a series of vascular and clotting mechanisms. These are so closely integrated that it has been stated that a single abnormality of one of the hemostatic mechanisms does not necessarily result in bleeding if all the others are normal.[353]

## NORMAL HEMOSTATIC MECHANISMS

*Role of vascular factors.* When a vessel is injured sufficiently to permit the escape of blood, an immediate reflex contraction occurs. In the smallest venules and capillaries hemostasis is accomplished by direct adhesions of endothelial surfaces.[84] Since the media of veins contain less muscle than those of arteries, vasoconstriction is less marked. Venous hemostasis depends mainly on the accumulation of platelets at the edges of the vessel wall which eventually occludes the vessel. In the small arteries and arterioles, vasoconstriction permits adherence and subsequent clumping of platelets by contracting the smooth muscle. The formation of large amorphous hyaline clumps derived from the platelets (viscous metamorphosis) seals off the injured area. Contraction of the vessel is reinforced by this aggregation of platelets and by the release of a powerful vasoconstrictor, serotonin (5-hydroxytryptamine).[401,405] The difficulties in defining the platelet clumps morphologically has led to the use of various terms such as platelet aggregation, agglutination, clumping, and fusion,[339] in addition to the older term viscous metamorphosis. The newer terms perhaps more accurately describe initial platelet changes than does viscous metamorphosis,[403] which refers to subsequent changes in which an irreversible structural alteration in platelets occurs, resulting in their fusion and loss of identity.

In the small arteries the platelet mass is reinforced by fibrin resulting from blood coagulation during vasoconstriction. Platelets and precipitated fibrin threads form a hemostatic plug which fills the lumen of the vessel. The clot subsequently retracts and is partially digested and organized, and the vessel is recanalized. Hemorrhage from a larger artery is controlled with difficulty until the blood pressure drops sufficiently within the vessel for a blood clot to form. Extravascular factors such as subcutaneous tissue, muscle, bone, and skin contribute to the arrest of the hemorrhage by presenting a firm surface so that the local accumulation of blood compresses the affected blood vessel. Ascorbic acid is regarded as a necessary factor for the synthesis of intercellular cement substance in the capillaries that unites the individual endothelial cells—hence its use in ill-defined bleeding syndromes due to increased vascular fragility. Spontaneous bleeding occurs with loss or changes in the cement substance. The continuity of capillaries is further strengthened by the adherence of platelets to this substance. Vitamin P is apparently also involved in some unknown manner in maintaining capillary permeability, but its administration therapeutically (rutin, hesperidin, and bioflavinoids) has been disappointing.

*Role of platelets.* While the size of the injured vessel and its ability to contract, and the ability of supporting tissues to limit blood loss are important factors in hemostasis, the cessation of bleeding is ultimately due to platelet function. The collagen of injured vessels initiates many phases of hemostasis. When a vessel is injured sufficiently to expose the subendothelial basement membrane or connective tissue, a chain of events is set in motion in the flowing blood that results in thrombus formation. The collagen of injured vessels initiates many of the phases of hemostasis. Platelets accumulate at the point of injury by adhesion and aggregation to the exposed collagen that has become denuded in the process of injury[346] and in doing so many of the phases of hemostasis are initiated. Following trauma, the walls of the damaged vessel with denuded collagen adhere together spontaneously or by pressure. When platelets adhere to collagen they undergo profound changes including degranulation and release adenosine tri- and diphosphate, which induce platelet aggregation. It is this aggregation that is responsible for the platelet plug.[396] The phospholipid procoagulant, platelet factor III (PF3) is released by platelets in the hemostatic plug. An important consequence of platelet plug formation is precipitation of the chain reaction leading to blood coagulation. At the same time or shortly after the platelet aggregation, Hageman factor (factor XII), presumably activated by collagen, interacts with factor XI (PTA) to form the contact product and thereby initiates the intrinsic pathway of blood coagulation.[395] The same product, thromboplastin, formed in the first phase of clotting may be formed in the extravascular compartment through the activation of factor X (Stuart-Prower factor) in the presence of factor VII to form extrinsic thromboplastin. The activated factor X requires factor V and phospholipid for full activity. The blood platelets form a mass or plug which initially halts the loss of blood and subsequently interact with protein coagulants to provide more permanent hemostasis through clot formation.

*The blood platelet.* Platelets normally are small, granular, disk-shaped, nonnucleated bodies measuring 2 to $5\mu$ in diameter. In patients with disease they may vary in size from fine particles to masses of agranular cytoplasm about twice the size of the normal platelet. Platelets arise by budding from the cytoplasm of megakaryocytes in the bone marrow. When labeled with $^{32}$DFP a linear relationship was found between time and platelet-bound reactivity, suggesting a life-span of normal platelets of 8 to 9 days.[212] Transfused platelets labeled with $^{51}$Cr in normal recipients had a survival period of 9 to 11 days.[1] By means of volume measurements, it has been estimated that 3,000 to 4,000 platelets are produced from a single megakaryocyte.[234] In the earlier forms of megakaryocytes, the megakaryoblast and promegakaryocyte, the cytoplasm stains deep blue, is nongranular, and shows no evidence of platelet formation. These primitive cells are increased in numbers in patients with thrombocytopenic purpura. In the mature megakaryocyte the cytoplasm is abundant and basophilic and contains numerous azurophilic granules. Masses of mature platelets often adhere to the periphery of the cells. The nuclei are large and are joined together in an irregularly lobulated ring. By means of fluorescent technique, the common antigenic structure in human platelets and megakaryocytes can be demonstrated, supporting the hypothesis that platelets are derived from megakaryocytes.[380]

The presence of megakaryocytes in the lung has long been known, as well as the fact that infections and other conditions that stimulate megakaryocytopoiesis are associated with increased numbers of pulmonary megakaryocytes. Evidence has been presented[196] which indicates that megakaryocytes present in the lungs do not originate there, although once present in this site they are evidently able to deliver platelets to the blood. Megakaryocytes have been shown to be transported from elsewhere in the body, especially from areas rich in bone marrow (e.g., lower vena cava blood), and are carried to the lungs in the venous blood to be filtered by the pulmonary capillaries. It has also been noted that surgery is a potent stimulus to megakaryocyte production and that the numbers of megakaryocytes found in the lung postoperatively are significantly increased.

Megakaryocytes arise from mononuclear precursors.[151] The number of nuclei doubles with each mitosis. In normal bone marrow about 65% of megakaryocytes contain eight diploid nuclei, 25% have sixteen nuclei, and 10% have four nuclei. According to Harker,[151] the cell accumulates cytoplasm in direct proportion to the number of nuclei formed during nuclear proliferation. After maturation is completed the mass of preformed platelets is apparently delivered to the circulation through an opening in the cell's outer shell. About two-thirds of the platelets are found in the general circulation; the remainder are pooled in the spleen. With splenomegaly an increased proportion of platelets is pooled in the spleen, resulting in a decreased concentration of platelets in the general circulation.[151] According to Harker,[151,452] megakaryocyte size is a clinically useful indicator of thrombopoietic stimulation because of the inverse relation normally observed between the circulating platelet count and megakaryocyte size.

Megakaryocytes have been demonstrated in central venous blood of patients undergoing cardiac catheterization.[195] It has been calculated that from 20 to 50% of the mature megakaryocyte population enters the blood and ultimately reaches the lungs and that 7 to 17% of the body platelets are released in the pulmonary capillaries. It was further postulated that during periods of great platelet demand, immature megakaryocytes are forced from the bone marrow and that an even greater percentage of the body's platelet release may take place in the lungs.

Many properties and activities associated with coagulation and hemostasis have been identified with platelet function. Some of these have been mentioned in connection with vascular factors. Platelets tend to adhere to injured blood vessels, check the formation of petechiae and extravasations of blood in spontaneous hemorrhage, promote clot retraction, and enhance vasoconstriction. It has been demonstrated that the platelet is a highly adsorptive structure and that many of the factors are merely carried on or are adherent to their surface.[281] Thus, three major functions of platelets are known: maintenance of the vascular endothelium, participation in blood coagulation, and transport of various chemical substances. The plasma accelerator globulin (labile factor), for instance, which functions in blood coagulation, is adsorbed by the platelet.[170] There is considerable evidence in favor of the theory that many of the platelet factors, and perhaps vascular factors, are adsorbed onto its surface from the plasma.[15] According to this concept the platelet is a sponge, adsorbing coagulation and perhaps vascular factors on its surface and carrying them through the circulation to the site of vessel wall injury. Among the factors adsorbed on the surface are prothrombin, AHG (factor VIII), PTC (factor IX), Stuart-Power factor (factor X), PTA (factor XI), fibrin stabilizing factor (factor XIII), labile factor (factor V), stable factor (factor VII), fibrinogen, and antifibrinolysin. In addition to liberating a vasoconstrictor substance, platelets contribute a number of factors to coagulation. Platelets accelerate the conversion of prothrombin to thrombin (platelet factor 1), accelerate the conversion of fibrinogen to fibrin (platelet factor 2), participate in the formation of thromboplastin (platelet factor 3), and neutralize the action of heparin (platelet factor 4). An example of the relation of platelet factors to coagulation is observed in patients with severe thrombocytopenia in whom the marked reduction of platelets (less than 20% of normal) retards prothrombin conversion to thrombin and is responsible for poor clot retraction.[378]

It is of interest that the most important, if not the only, functions of the platelets under physiologic conditions appear to be those concerned with blood coagulation and hemostasis.[32] Apart from these disturbances, severe thrombocytopenia or functional platelet defects do not seem to be associated with other physiologic changes which can be related to the decrease or dysfunction of platelets per se. (See p. 741 for discussion of platelet adhesiveness.)

The sequence of steps of platelet function in relation to hemostasis has been summarized as follows: adhesion, release action, and aggregation.[30] Platelet aggregation is the property of platelets to stick to one another and platelet adhesiveness the property of platelets to adhere to a foreign or damaged surface. Platelets adhere to damaged endothelium, to other damaged cells, and to collagen. Adenosine diphosphate (ADP) encourages adhesion, adenosine monophosphate (AMP) and adenosine triphosphate (ATP) inhibit it.

ADP released from platelets by the action of collagen does not originate from platelet ATP but is preformed in the platelets themselves.[233] Serious damage to a vessel wall is likely to expose collagen to which platelets adhere in vivo. ADP is subsequently released, thus favoring platelet aggregation and the formation of the platelet plug, which in small blood vessels will ensure hemostasis. Release of thrombin in turn activates the clotting process and a firm clot closes the vessel. Collagen-induced platelet aggregation is thought to be mediated by a release of ADP from the platelets. Contact of platelets with collagen results in important biochemical and morphologic changes in the platelet.

In considering possible sites of defects in platelet function, one would include the platelet membrane with its intrinsic stickiness; the platelet alpha granules with their release action liberating nucleotides and hydrolytic enzymes; thrombosthenin, the contractile protein of platelets; and defects of energy metabolism.

An important consequence of the interaction of thrombin and platelets is platelet contraction. This process is mediated by the contractile protein thrombosthenin which represents about 15% of platelet protein. Platelet contraction is to be distinguished from clot retraction, which probably results from the contraction of platelet pseudopods which are attached to fibrin strands.[234]

The platelet factor participating in thromboplastin generation (factor 3) is a phospholipid.[378] Numerous phosphatides, among them brain[40] and soybean cephalins,[330] have been substituted for platelets in a variety of test systems to measure thromboplastin formation.

Platelets are the source of a large part of the acid phosphatase in normal serum, the enzyme being liberated from the platelets during clotting.[406] Serum prepared from platelet-poor (high spun) plasma contains much less acid phosphatase than serum prepared from clotted whole blood, the difference resulting from enzyme contributed by the platelets. The content of acid phosphatase in platelet-free plasma has been employed in the differentiation of types of purpura.

Platelets may be considered small cytoplasmic structures, containing a small amount of ribonucleic acid (RNA) but no deoxyribonucleic acid (DNA). They contain large amounts of adenosine triphosphate (ATP) and, on the basis of total protein in the cell, more than 150 times that in red cells. The metabolism of platelets is, therefore, high compared with the metabolism of other cells. Platelets contain the full complement of enzymes required for glycolysis, the pentose-phosphate and citric-acid cycles, cellular respiration, and the splitting of ATP and transaminase.[179] ATP plays an important role in clot retraction, glucose is utilized, and lactic acid is produced during this process. Clot retraction is inversely proportional to the fibrinogen content and red cell mass.

Whether platelets contain their own fibrinogen or utilize what is adsorbed at the surface from plasma has been a subject of study. Many authors point out that the addition of pure thrombin to washed platelets leads to platelet clumping and viscous metamorphosis followed by a coagulum that is very similar to fibrin. The properties of platelet fibrinogen and its role in thrombosis were further defined by Johnson and McKenna.[189] A mild bleeding tendency in a young man was attributed to a deficiency of platelet fibrinogen. The authors indicate that platelet fibrinogen is involved in the reaction of thrombin with platelets and suggest that platelet fibrinogen may be essential for normal hemostasis.[189]

Fibrinogen has been clearly established as a platelet component. It is known to be firmly adsorbed to the platelet surface and is not removed by multiple washing. There seems little doubt that retractable fibrinogen is immunologically identical to plasma fibrinogen. The detection of extractable fibrinogen in the platelets of the hypofibrinogenemic patients when it was possible to be reasonably certain that all adsorbed fibrinogen was removed gives strong support for an intracellular fraction.[82] Intraplatelet fibrinogen may be derived from the megakaryocyte.

Nachman[254] demonstrated a thromboclottable protein immunologically identical to fibrinogen within the platelet and concluded that fibrinogen forms an intricate part of the internal platelet structure as well as being adsorbed on the platelet membrane. Plasminogen and fibrinogen were described in platelets, and the fibrinogen appears to be part of the intracellular structure.

Contrast media used in roentgenographic studies have been found to depress blood coagulation factors, presumably by binding with globulin.[354]

**Blood coagulation mechanism.** In the classical coagulation theory of Morawitz,[252a] thromboplastin originates from two sources, the tissues and the platelets (Fig. 93). When tissues are injured, preformed thromboplastin (thrombokinase) is liberated which, in the presence of calcium, converts prothrombin to thrombin. Acting as an enzyme, thrombin then converts fibrinogen to fibrin. These studies provided a basis for subsequent investigations dealing with coagulation.

It is now known that platelets contain no preformed thromboplastin but that they do interact with plasma factors to form plasma thromboplastin (intrinsic prothrombinase). In the presence of calcium, plasma thromboplastin converts prothrombin to thrombin without the aid of accessory factors. In contrast, tissue extract (incomplete thromboplastin) performs the same function but only after it has been activated by specific factors in the blood. This form of thromboplastin is termed extrinsic prothrombinase. Plasma (intrinsic) thromboplastin evolved during the coagulation of normal blood is, therefore, differentiated from the extrinsic thromboplastin formed by the reaction of tissue extracts with other factors. The intrinsic and extrinsic mechanisms operate concur-

## PLASMA THROMBOPLASTIN SYSTEM

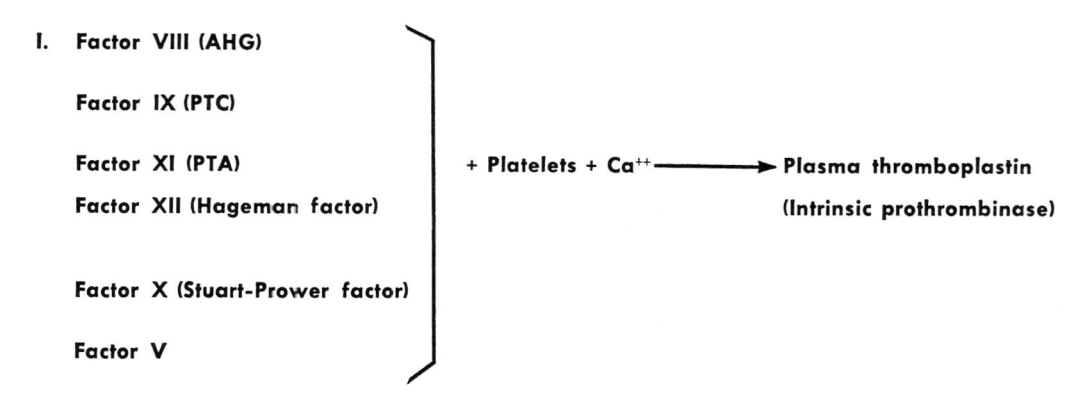

I.  Factor VIII (AHG)

    Factor IX (PTC)

    Factor XI (PTA)

    Factor XII (Hageman factor)     + Platelets + $Ca^{++}$ ⟶ Plasma thromboplastin (Intrinsic prothrombinase)

    Factor X (Stuart-Prower factor)

    Factor V

II. Plasma thromboplastin + $Ca^{++}$ + Prothrombin ⟶ Thrombin

III. Thrombin + Fibrinogen ⟶ Fibrin

## TISSUE THROMBOPLASTIN SYSTEM

I.  Tissue extract

    +

    Factor V

    +

    Factor VII     ⟶ Tissue thromboplastin (Extrinsic prothrombinase)

    +

    Factor X

    +

    $Ca^{++}$

II. Tissue thromboplastin (Extrinsic prothrombinase)     + $Ca^{++}$ + Prothrombin ⟶ Thrombin

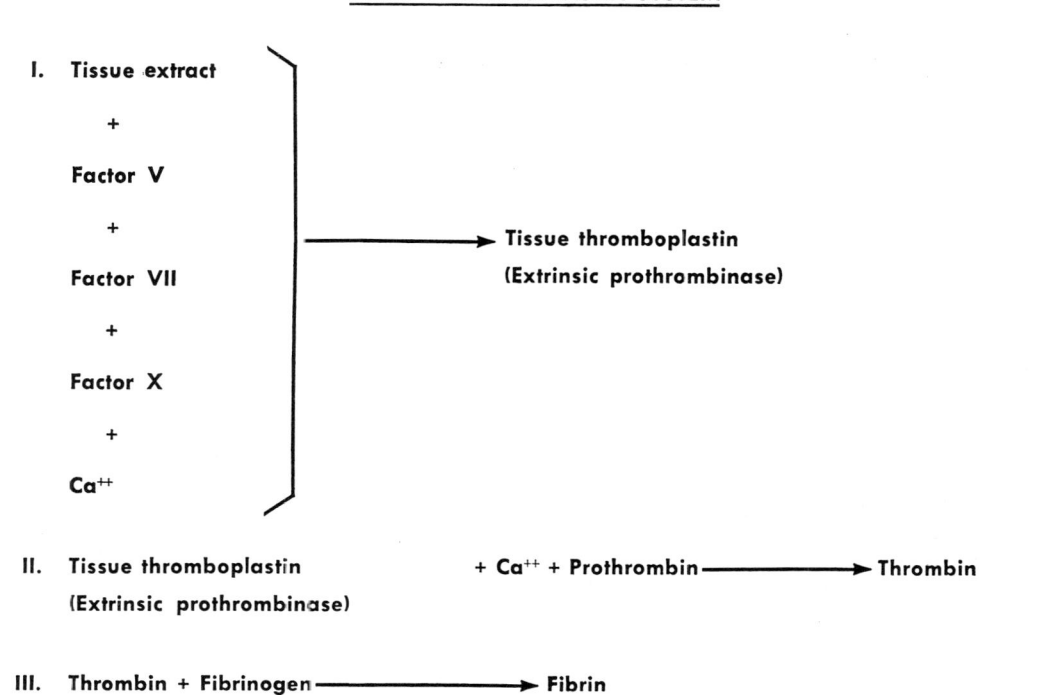

III. Thrombin + Fibrinogen ⟶ Fibrin

Fig. 93. Schematic outline of the coagulation mechanism.

| EXTRINSIC SYSTEM | | INTRINSIC SYSTEM |
|---|---|---|
| (Measured by one-stage prothrombin time) | | (Measured by thromboplastin generation test) |
| Tissue extract | | Factor VIII |
| | | Factor IX |
| | | Factor XI |
| | | Factor XII |
| | | Platelets |
| Factor VII | | ///////// |
| Factor V | | Factor V |
| Factor X | | Factor X |
| Calcium | | Calcium |

Extrinsic prothrombinase → Thrombin ← Intrinsic prothrombinase

Prothrombin → Thrombin

Fibrinogen → Fibrin

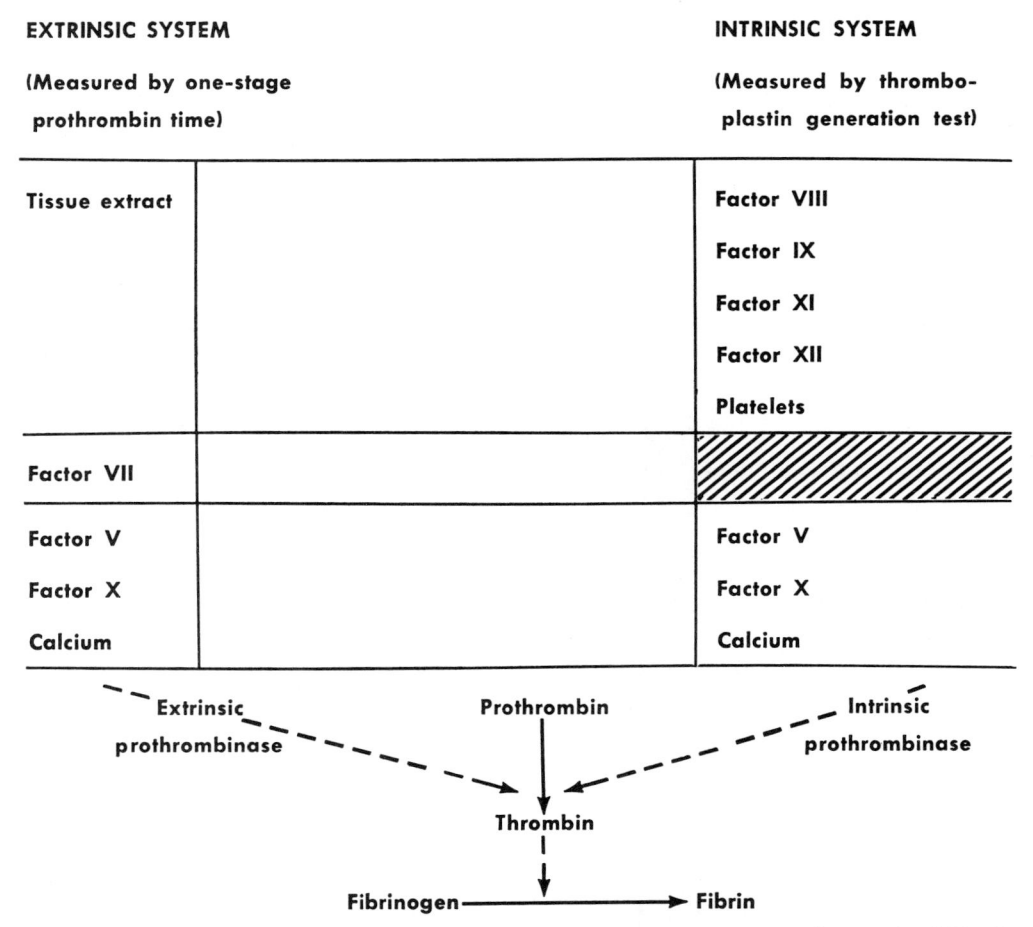

Fig. 94. The modern scheme of blood coagulation. (From Hougie, C.: Fundamentals of blood coagulation in clinical medicine, New York, 1963, McGraw-Hill Book Co.)

rently, the latter being more immediately mobilized for hemostasis in injured areas.

The concept of extrinsic and intrinsic thromboplastin forming systems envisions two pathways of thromboplastin formation, each culminating in a potent substance called prothrombinase (Fig. 94).[132] In vivo, both mechanisms must be intact for normal hemostasis. Extrinsic prothrombinase is formed in seconds in contrast to the minutes required for the formation of the intrinsic prothrombinase. The two types of prothrombinase are approximately of equal potency. The extrinsic system is important when the clotting of blood follows tissue damage, whereas the intrinsic system is more important in the absence of such damage. Both extrinsic and intrinsic mechanisms must be intact in vivo to ensure normal hemostasis.

A deficiency of the factors essential to intrinsic prothrombinase formation is detected by the thromboplastin generation test, while a deficiency of those factors essential for extrinsic thromboplastin is revealed by the one-stage Quick prothrombin time.

*Coagulation factors.* Coagulation of blood free from tissue juice has been arbitrarily divided into three stages: the elaboration of plasma thromboplastin, the conversion of prothrombin to thrombin, and the interaction of thrombin with fibrinogen to form the fibrin clot. These main stages are assisted by accelerating and inhibitory mechanisms. The precise mode of action of several of the factors and their relative importance in each phase of coagulation are still being elucidated and in many ways are still controversial.

**Table 29.** Blood-clotting factors

| Coagulation factors | Descriptive names (synonyms and abbreviations) |
|---|---|
| Factor I | Fibrinogen |
| Factor II | Prothrombin |
| Factor III | Thromboplastin, prothrombinase, tissue thromboplastin |
| Factor IV | Calcium |
| Factor V | Ac-globulin, proaccelerin, labile factor |
| Factor VII | Proconvertin, serum prothrombin conversion accelerator (SPCA), stable factor |
| Factor VIII | Antihemophilic globulin (AHG), antihemophilic factor (AHF) |
| Factor IX | Plasma thromboplastin component (PTC), Christmas factor |
| Factor X | Stuart-Prower factor |
| Factor XI | Plasma thromboplastin antecedent (PTA) |
| Factor XII | Hageman factor (HF) |
| Factor XIII | Fibrin-stabilizing factor (FSF) |

Many of the coagulation factors in plasma and serum to be discussed are described under numerous synonyms and abbreviations, some of which are given in Table 29.[400]

PHASE 1. The first phase of blood coagulation is concerned with the elaboration of plasma thromboplastin free from tissue juice. Contact with a foreign surface and injury to a blood vessel initiate coagulation by the disintegration of platelets and the release of a lipoid thromboplastic factor. Many cofactors react with platelets. Several cofactors may be regarded as ones of major importance in coagulation: antihemophilic globulin (factor VIII, AHG),[364] plasma thromboplastin component (factor IX, PTC),[18,51,331] plasma thromboplastin antecedent (factor XI, PTA),[321,322] factor V (labile factor), and factor X (Stuart-Prower factor).* Another participating factor is factor XII (Hageman factor).[308,314] Calcium is essential. These soluble plasma-clotting factors, with the exception of fibrinogen, are present in small amounts. Nevertheless, for the synthesis of active intrinsic thromboplastin, it is obligatory that they be available in adequate concentration.

The importance of factor XI (PTA) in coagulation has been previously questioned.[55] It had been considered by many to represent an association of factor VIII (AHG) and factor IX (PTC) deficiencies. Its status as a separate entity is now well established. In our experience a substantial decrease of factor XI results in a hemophilia-like clinical picture similar in many respects to factor VIII and factor IX deficiencies.

In patients with factor XII (Hageman factor) deficiency[308] coagulation time is prolonged, but affected persons have no symptoms and have been operated upon without excessive bleeding. The clot-promoting effect of glass upon normal human plasma requires the presence of the Hageman factor.[313] This factor, a surface activation factor, probably aids in the initiation of the clotting process. A 9-year-old boy with a deficiency of the Hageman factor was completely free of hemorrhagic symptoms despite a prolonged clotting time.[205] In a 13-year-old white girl in whom factor XII (Hageman factor) deficiency was discovered at the time of routine coagulation screening tests, no bleeding was observed at the time of tonsillectomy and adenoidectomy.[9] The content of factor XII (Hageman factor) may be low in many infants during the newborn period. Unlike factor VII, factor X (Stuart-Prower factor) and factor IX (plasma thromboplastin component, PTC), which do not reach normal levels until 6 weeks of age or more, the concentration of Hageman factor is normal by 10 to 14 days of life.[205] It is likely that the earliest events in plasma thromboplastin (intrinsic prothrombinase) formation involve activation of factor XII (Hageman factor) by "contact" and subsequent reaction with factor XI (plasma thromboplastin antecedent),[311] forming an early intermediate product.[347] While the two factors are difficult to separate from one another, pa-

---
*See references 101, 140, 181, 334, and 365.

tients who lack factor XI (plasma thromboplastin antecedent) show clinical bleeding and those with factor XII deficiency (Hageman factor) are free of symptoms and show no bleeding tendency. Blood of such common fowl as the chicken, turkey, goose, pigeon, and duck lacks factor XII (Hageman factor) and can be used as a convenient substitute for factor XII (Hageman factor)–deficient human plasma or serum. Simplified methods based on the recalcification clotting time of oxalated plasma have also been described for the laboratory detection of a deficiency in factor XII (Hageman factor).[277] The partial thromboplastin time can also be used for the detection of this factor (see p. 739).

Factor X (Stuart-Prower factor) is necessary for both the first and second phases of blood coagulation. It is utilized for the production of thromboplastin as well as for the conversion of prothrombin to thrombin. A deficiency of factor X (Stuart-Prower factor) retards the thromboplastin generation test and prolongs the prothrombin time. This factor is gradually assuming increasing clinical importance with the observation that it may be deficient in congenital and acquired liver disease and in hemorrhagic disease of the newborn infant.[334]

Factor VIII (antihemophilic globulin) is associated with the globulin of the fibrinogen fraction of the plasma protein. It is labile when stored and is completely utilized in the process of clotting, whereas factor IX (PTC) and factor XI (PTA) are stable when stored and are not consumed in this process. These properties are of practical importance in laboratory testing and in the selection of therapeutic agents. Factor XI (PTA) is said to deteriorate as fast as factor V in banked blood.

There is evidence that factor VIII (plasma antihemophilic globulin) increases with age, at least from the range of 15 to 70 years.[288] The rate of increase is approximately 0.7 to 0.8% a year. Between the ages of 40 and 50 years, for instance, factor VIII (AHG) concentrations range between 60 and 190%. Both parents appear to make roughly equal and significant contributions to the concentrations of antihemophilic globulin of their children. The range in males was between 75 and 195% and in females, 50 to 160%. The best donors for treatment of patients with hemophilia would, therefore, be the older male population in whom the AHG level is greatest.[87]

Increased AHG (factor VIII) levels have also been observed in a variety of stressful situations, i.e., during febrile states, after surgery, after strenuous exercise, and after infusions of Adrenalin. It also occurs in pathologic states, often in association with acute stress, i.e., thrombocytopenia, x-irradiation, thyrotoxicosis, coronary artery disease, pancreatitis, and some malignancies. It has also been claimed that in the acutely stressful situation, the spleen plays an important role in increasing the level of factor VIII (AHG), whereas in chronic pathologic conditions only the inverse variation of factor VIII (AHG) and platelets appears significant.[219] Hypothyroidism is associated with subnormal levels of AHG (factor VIII), while hyperthyroidism is characterized by specific elevation of activity of this factor.[341]

Data obtained in dogs with hemophilia placed in cross-circulation with normal or splenectomized dogs indicate that the spleen is an important organ for the maintenance of AHG (factor VIII) under stress and that it serves as a site for its formation and storage.[72]

The levels of a number of coagulation factors are raised in posttraumatic and postpartum periods.[96] This increase applies not only to factor VIII (AHG) but also to factor IX (PTC), factor X (Stuart-Prower factor), and fibrinogen.

Coagulation by either the intrinsic or extrinsic systems involves a stepwise sequence of reactions in which the precursors of proteolytic enzymes—zymogens—are activated and in turn act on the subsequent zymogen in "cascade" or "waterfall sequence."[97]

Each clotting factor must, therefore, circulate either as a precursor or as a specific molecule which reacts only with another factor that circulates as a precursor.[327] This concept is in accord with the principle that the protein-clotting factors interact in pairs in which one factor behaves like an enzyme and the other like a substrate.[97] Through this interaction the various clotting factors are converted in succession to active enzymes which eventually bring about the conversion of prothrombin to thrombin. The enzyme thrombin converts fibrinogen to fibrin (Fig. 95).

Accordingly, the Hageman factor (factor XII) is activated by contact with glass, with collagen, or with some fatty acid such as ellagic acid. It forms a complex with PTA (factor XI), which activates PTC (factor IX),[327] the second enzyme of the intrinsic pathway. When activated it complexes with AHF (factor VIII) and phospholipid in plasma[231] to activate Stuart-Prower factor (factor X), the third enzyme. This complexes with platelet factor 3 (phospholipoprotein) and factor V to split prothrombin, the fourth enzyme of the sequence, becoming thrombin. The latter acts on fibrinogen to release two peptides (A and B) and forms fibrin monomers. The monomer polymerizes to urea-soluble fibrin. A fifth enzyme, factor XIII (fibrin stabilizing factor), is activated perhaps also by collagen, and is a transaminase. It causes peptide linkages between the amine of lysine residues and the COOH groups of glutamic acid. As a result, urea-insoluble fibrin is formed.

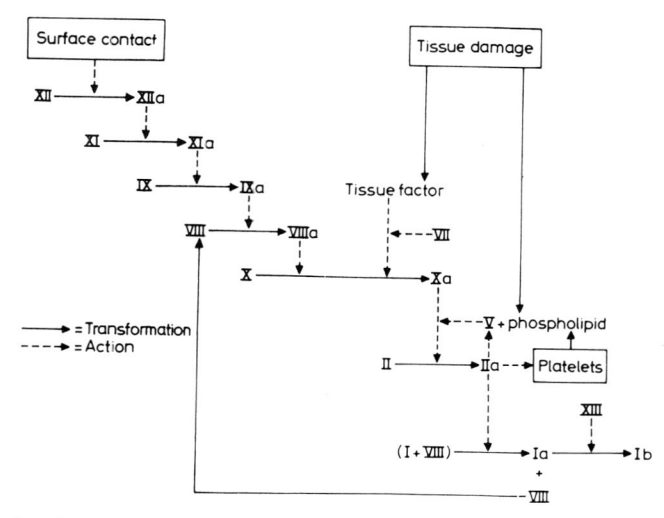

Fig. 95. A cascade scheme of blood coagulation based on existing evidence and showing autocatalytic effects of thrombin. Thrombin, IIa; fibrin, Ia. (From Macfarlane, R. G.: The basis of the cascade hypothesis of blood clotting, Thromb. Diath. Hemorrh. 15:591, 1966.)

As for the extrinsic pathway, the tissue factor can be split into a protein moiety and phospholipid.[258] The latter is analogous to platelet factor 3, though there is different specificity of phospholipids in the two systems. At any rate, the protein activates factor VII, which is probably a zymogen. The complex of tissue factor protein–active factor VII is an enzyme which, like the PTA-AHF complex of the intrinsic systems, activates factor X. The latter then makes use of the phospholipid already present in the tissue factor and adds factor V to form a complex which converts prothrombin to thrombin.

PHASE 2. The second phase of blood coagulation is concerned with the conversion of prothrombin to thrombin. In this process intrinsic thromboplastin generated in the first phase reacts with prothrombin and calcium to form thrombin. Tissue juice liberated by trauma reacts with the accessory factors (factor V, factor VII, and calcium) to form an extrinsic thromboplastin or prothrombinase.[146,178,275] The interaction of these two substances is conceived as follows: active plasma thromboplastin and calcium initially convert prothrombin to thrombin slowly in small amounts. At this point prothrombinase formed in the presence of calcium increases the velocity of the prothrombin conversion and is responsible for the rapid phase of thrombin formation.[275] Factor V and factor VII, once activated, are referred to as the accelerators of prothrombin conversion. They are not precursors of thrombin but are accelerators which influence the speed at which thrombin is formed in the presence of tissue extracts.[55]

Although no authentic case of hemorrhagic disease due to a deficiency of calcium has been reported, calcium appears to play a role in the first two phases of coagulation. This activity takes place in its diffusible ionized form. The anticoagulant effect of citrate is mediated through suppression of calcium ionization, whereas in the case of oxalate, free calcium is precipiated.

Prothrombin is a glycoprotein that is stable when stored and utilized in excess of 25% during the coagulation process. A sufficient intake of vitamin K is necessary for normal synthesis of prothrombin, provided liver function is normal.

Factor V deteriorates in oxalated plasma and therefore is referred to as the labile factor. It is also called ac-globulin and proaccelerin. Factor VII is also known as stable factor, proconvertin, and serum prothrombin conversion accelerator (SPCA).

Factor V is consumed during clotting; stable factor it not. A deficiency in either factor V, factor VII, or Stuart-Power factor results in a hemorrhagic state due to decreased formation of extrinsic prothrombinase, with subsequent inadequate thrombin formation. Factor V and Stuart-Power factor (factor X) are also necessary for the formation of intrinsic thromboplastin in the first phase of coagulation. Factor VII is not necessary for thromboplastin generation in coagulating blood, in contrast to the Stuart-Prower factor (factor X), or for conversion of prothrombin to thrombin by the intrinsic or plasma thromboplastin.[19] Factor VII represents one of the factors that is involved in the reaction with tissue extract to form extrinsic thromboplastin which directly activates prothrombin.

In the sequence of blood clotting it has become clear that the final reaction, the conversion of fibrinogen to fibrin by thrombin, must result from a series of preliminary reactions. The final reaction involves the conversion of precursor to an activated form.[327] As each factor is activated by the product of the preceding reaction, coagulation proceeds. Thus, an activated form of PTC (PTC'), which incorporates the properties of both native PTC and activated PTA (PTA'), has already been identified.

PHASE 3. In the final phase of coagulation fibrinogen is converted to fibrin through the action of thrombin liberated in phase 2. Fibrinogen, with a molecular weight of 350,000, is an unstable soluble protein formed in the liver. In the plasma, fibrinogen reaches a concentration of 250 to 400 mg. per 100 ml. The final step, clot retraction, appears to be controlled by intact platelets. Disorders characterized by inadequate fibrin formation include congenital afibrinogenemia and congenital and acquired hypofibrinogenemia.

Thrombin, the proteolytic enzyme which results from the series of reactions of either the intrinsic or extrinsic coagulation systems, acts on fibrinogen with great selectivity. Four arginyl-glycine bonds are split, liberating two pairs of peptides (A and B), roughly 3% of the fibrinogen molecule. Once the A and B peptides are removed the molecule becomes fibrin. It has now the ability to undergo further chemical and physical changes on the pathway to clotting.[135] The residual fibrin monomer now polymerizes rapidly to form long thin strands of fibrin which are soluble in 6M urea. (A monomer is a subunit of fibrin that is formed by the action of thrombin on fibrinogen and that polymerizes spontaneously to form fibrin.[340]) An enzyme, fibrinase (fibrin stabilizing factor, FSF, factor XIII), now creates peptide links between five amine groups of one fibrin strand and the free acid groups of a neighboring fibrin chain.

In the presence of factor XIII, adjacent fibrin monomers join through chemical bonds, stabilizing the clot. The insoluble fibrin strands later contract through the action of the platelet protein, thrombasthenin, into the firm fibrin clot. Dissolution of the clot with recanalization of the vessel and restoration of the free flow of blood is accomplished through the action of the fibrinolytic system (see p. 723).

*Fibrin-stabilizing factor.* Laki and Lorand[207,223] observed that "fibrin clots," formed by the addition of calcium and thrombin to purified fibrinogen solutions, were readily soluble in 5M urea and 1% monochloracetic acid, while "plasma clots," formed by the recalcification of oxalated plasma, were insoluble in these solvents. Hence, a factor present in plasma was responsible for rendering the fibrin clots insoluble. This factor is known as the fibrin-stabilizing factor (FSF), Laki-Lorand factor, or fibrinase. Its presence, however, is responsible for the formation of a fibrin structure that is insoluble in hydrogen bond–breaking solvents. It has received the designation of factor XIII and has been defined as a substance in plasma or serum which, when present during the thrombin-fibrinogen reaction, leads to the formation of a fibrin that is insoluble in urea. The lack of factor XIII does not cause any change in the ultrastructure of the fibrin meshwork. After treatment with urea solution, however, the cross striation of fibrin fibers found in the patient's blood disappears within a short time. The insoluble clot produced in normal blood undergoes no alteration in urea solution.[363]

Congenital[116] and acquired deficiency of the fibrin-stabilizing factor cause hemorrhagic symptoms similar to mild and moderate grades of hemophilia. Blood samples taken from twenty adults, sixty-eight infants, and sixty-seven children revealed a FSF activity in cord blood only 36% of the normal adult level. From the fifth month to the fourth year of life, values were similar to the neonatal period. A persistent rise in FSF content begins in the fifth year and reaches adult levels at about the eighth year of life.[204] In confirmation of these findings are three infants with bleeding from the umbilical cord due to FSF (factor XIII) deficiency. Bleeding was stopped by blood transfusion.[224] The healing of wounds is less satisfactory with deficiency of FSF. The bleeding time, platelet count, and routine coagulation tests are normal. The defect is diagnosed by demonstrating that the patient's blood clot dissolves in solutions of urea or monochloracetic acid. It may also be detected if a clot formed in the patient's recalcified plasma is soluble in a 5M urea solution when left at room temperature for 24 hours.

Fresh blood or fresh plasma should be used when replacement is necessary. In a survey of plasma FSF assays of 322 patient's, ninety-five patients were found to have plasma with markedly or moderately diminished FSF activity.[269] Notable in the group were patients with severe cirrhosis, tumor metastases to the liver, and acute granulocytic leukemia.

In a 12-year-old boy with a congenital deficiency of fibrin-stabilizing factor the symptomatology consisted of prolonged umbilical hemorrhage, ecchymoses, hematomas, cerebromeningeal hemorhages, and posttrauamtic hemarthroses. The usual coagulation tests were all within normal limits. A brother died of cerebral hemorrhage and a sister was suspected of a tendency to bleed.[86]

A boy 5½ years of age with many bleeding episodes dating from circumcision at 24 hours of age was found to be deficient in factor XIII (FSF).[67] In vivo survival studies after transfusion with fresh frozen plasma indicated a half-life of factor XIII of 5 to 7 days. The concentration of factor XIII was determined as approximately 50 to 76% in the newborn infant with a rapid rise to adult levels within 1 month, which remained so with only normal variations. Factor XIII levels in the parents and siblings were significantly lower than in twenty normal individuals, suggesting an autosomal recessive inheritance of Factor XIII deficiency.

Britten,[73] in a review of previous cases of factor XIII deficiency, contributed an additional report of a child of 3 years who bled initially after circumcision. He points out that the urea solubility test is highly specific. Once it has been shown that the patient's fibrin is soluble in 5M urea, the diagnosis of factor XIII deficiency is almost certain and few alternatives need be considered.

In another case report,[141] a 13-year-old boy had a congenital factor XIII deficiency and history of serious bleeding dating back to the neonatal period. He was successfully treated with monthly infusions of a single unit of plasma obtained from a maternal aunt with the same blood type as the patient.

Congenital severe deficiency of factor XIII has been reported in three siblings, two girls and one boy, from a family of fourteen children.[145] Recurrent hematamesis which occurred in one of the siblings had heretofore not been reported. A mild deficiency of factor XII (Hageman factor) coexisted in two of these patients and in two other members of the family. The factor XIII deficiency characteristically was manifest at the time of the separation of the cord with the development of umbilical hemorrhage. Intracranial hemorrhage was frequently observed and hemarthrosis was not uncommon, as previously thought. Fibrinogen infusions (probably by factor XII contamination), fresh frozen plasma, and blood transfusions were effective in controlling the bleeding of factor XIII deficiency in these cases. Severe factor XII deficiency usually causes no bleeding tendency.

*Dynamics of coagulation.* Blood clotting should be thought of as a dynamic process moving in the direction of fibrin formation. It should be emphasized that the sequence of events outlined here in three distinct phases is based upon in vitro studies. They serve a convenient and useful purpose in the clinical and laboratory approach to the patient with a hemorrhagic disorder. Blood coagulation in vivo probably does not occur in such sharply demarcated series of steps but in a slow initial phase and a succeeding accelerated one.

As soon as a small amount of thrombin is formed, platelets begin to be further aggregated. This leads to the formation of thromboplastin, which in turn converts prothrombin to thrombin. From this point, the generation of thrombin takes place with increasing velocity, reaching explosive force. The rapid phase has been referred to as a chain reaction or an autocatalytic mechanism and assures the presence of enough thrombin[250] at the site of injury. The initial slow phase parallels the period from the aggregation of platelets to the formation of small amounts of thrombin. The succeeding accelerated phase extends from steps involving the rapid evolution of thrombin to the conversion of fibrinogen to fibrin. Thrombin thus represents the key substance in the chain reaction of blood coagulation. These changes correspond roughly to blood coagulation in a test tube in which the blood remains fluid for several minutes (slow phase) and then clots solidly in a short fraction of time (accelerated phase).

*Natural inhibitors of coagulation.* With the forces favoring coagulability of the blood, there are corresponding opposing physiologic inhibitors and anticoagulants that maintain its fluidity. Maintaining the continuity of the vascular endothelium constitutes one of the most important factors preventing the formation of thromboplastin. In vivo the formation of thrombin is counteracted by natural inhibitors such as antithrombin and heparin. The latter is extracted from the liver and is also present in the granules of the mast cells. The adsorption of thrombin by fibrin may also be regarded as a neutralizer of thrombin.

The reticuloendothelial system has been assigned an important role in clearing the bloodstream of particulate intermediates of clotting and of partially polymerized thrombin. In addition, the liver is capable of rapidly removing activated factors IX (PTC') and XI (PTA') from the circulation.[106]

## DISORDERS DUE TO A DEFICIENCY OF FACTORS REQUIRED FOR THROMBOPLASTIN FORMATION (PHASE 1 OF COAGULATION)

*General consideration of the hemophilias.* Until studies demonstrated its manifold nature, the term hemophilia was applied to a single disorder—a deficiency of the antihemophilic globulin factor VIII (AHG), known to be essential for clotting and hemostasis. The discovery of the additional thromboplastin precursors, plasma thromboplastin component factor IX (PTC) and factor XI (plasma thromboplastin antecedent, PTA), led to the realization that hemophilia was not an isolated condition but a group of entities with a similar symptomatology.[53] The pathogenesis of each of the three members could then be attributed to a congenital inability to produce a specific thromboplastin precursor. As in patients with classic hemophilia, those with other hemophilias also demonstrate a bleeding tendency from childhood and give a history of other bleeders in the family. From the standpoint of management and specific therapy the separation of the hemophilias has proved to be necessary.

In due course, methods were developed for the differentiation of each type of defect within the hemophilia group. An extension of these and other techniques revealed also that many cases of clotting disorders which had heretofore been classified as hemophilia were due to deficiencies in other phases of coagulation, principally in the prothrombin complex. In all types and grades of hemophilia, the platelet count, bleeding time, clot retraction, prothrombin time, and fibrinogen concentrations are normal.

A feature of major importance in the diagnosis of hemophilia is the variation in its severity. The mild form of the disease is most deceptive since its manifestations emerge suddenly and unexpectedly after surgical procedures, especially dental extraction or tonsillectomy. The degree of clinical severity in mildly affected patients is correlated inversely with the percentage of antihemophilic globulin in the plasma.

Hemophilioid diseases refer rather loosely to all deficiencies of the coagulation factors resembling classic hemophilia due to factor VIII (AHG) deficiency, Christmas disease due to plasma thromboplastin component (PTC, factor IX) deficiency, plasma thromboplastin antecedent (PTA, factor XI) deficiency, Stuart-Prower (factor X) deficiency, and deficiencies of prothrombin, labile factor (factor V), stable factor (factor II), and fibrinogen. The hemophilioid states are differentiated from the purpuras on clinical grounds and laboratory tests. Whereas bleeding is often intramuscular and deep hematomas occur in the former, bleeding in the latter is usually cutaneous and characterized by mucosal petechiae and/or ecchymoses.[179] In the hemophilioid states the bleeding time is always normal and usually prolonged in the purpuras.

### Classic hemophilia (hemophilia A, factor VIII [AHG] deficiency)

*Hereditary aspects.* Classic hemophilia is a severe congenital disorder consisting of a hereditary defect in blood thromboplastin formation due to a congenital deficiency of antihemophilic globulin.[200] The plasma AHG in severe hemophilia ranges from less than 1 to 3%.[72] The condition is inherited as a sex-linked recessive mendelian trait with transmission to affected males by asymptomatic carrier females who possess a normal content of antihemophilic globulin. The daughter of an affected male is capable of transmitting the trait to half of her sons who will have the disease and half of her daughters who will be carriers. Hemophilic carriers as a group show significantly lower than normal plasma antihemophilic globulin concentrations, but a considerable overlap with the normal range may exist.[42,265,286] Abnormal results with available tests for blood coagulation were obtained in a substantial number of carriers with hemophilia A (AHG deficiency) and hemophilia B (PTC deficiency).[108] In rare instances, classic hemophilia occurs in the female as a product of the marriage between a hemophilic male and a carrier female.[244] In other cases severe hemophilia due to factor VIII (AHG) deficiency occurred in females (verified by chromosomal studies) who were the product of a carrier female and a nonhemophilic father.[100] Possibly, a spontaneous mutation produced a hemophilic gene on the chromosome inherited from the father.[243] Lusher and co-workers[227] described a case of antihemophilic globulin (factor VIII) deficiency with abnormal bleeding tendency in a 14-month-old Negro female with a negative family history and also reviewed recently reported cases in the female.

The plasma concentration of factor VIII (AHG) in mothers at delivery is abnormally high (135% as compared with 97.5% in the normal control groups).[96] Pregnancy may increase the mean concentration of factor VIII by as much as 50%.[291] This high level may be connected with the fact that the fibrinogen concentration is raised in pregnant women, the two factors being closely associated. The AHG level of normal babies bears no relation to that of the mother at parturition, falling within the normal adult range. Factor VIII (AHG) does not readily cross the placental barrier, but babies born with genetically controlled deficiency of this factor may be expected to manifest the deficiency from birth. Pregnancy has been referred to as a "hypercoagulable" state, characterized by an increase in the factors participating in the formation of intrinsic thromboplastin and in the conversion of prothrombin to thrombin.[279] Factor IX (PTC) is also increased in pregnancy.[312]

Classic hemophilia occurs sporadically in children without a previous family history in about 25 to 30% of patients, either because the disease has gone unrecognized or because it is the end result of a mutation, with the de novo appearance of either hemophilic males or female carriers.[55]

Strauss[356] has shown that sporadic cases constitute approximately a third of all cases of hemophilia A and one-fifth of cases of hemophilia B. These cases have been ascribed to mutations or ignorance of family history. In the families he studied, sporadic occurrence was strikingly associated with severe disease. It was speculated that sporadic cases were due to gene mutation or to transmission of the gene through several generations of female carriers without known expression in males. From determinations for factor VIII levels and the high proportions of noncarriers among maternal grandmothers as compared with the carriers in mothers, he concluded that the hemophilic gene in the sporadic cases arose by recent mutation. In these studies, Strauss[356] designated severe hemophilia A as cases in which factor VIII level was less than 0.5%, nonsevere as those in which it ranged between 1 and 35%.

Classic hemophilia (factor VIII deficiency) comprises about 80% of the heritable coagulation disorders. In Minneapolis the relative incidence of hemophilia A (factor VIII deficiency), hemophilia B (factor IX deficiency, Christmas disease), and PTA deficiency (factor XI deficiency) was 45:6:4, in New York City it was 32:6:2.[126] Of 267 patients with hemophilia syndromes seen at Manchester Royal Infirmary, 84.1% had classic hemophilia (factor VIII deficiency) and 15.9% had Christmas disease (factor IX deficiency).[394]

It has been demonstrated that about 5 to 10% of patients with hemophilia A[183] and B[182] make factors VIII and IX molecules that completely neutralize their respective antibodies but which are without clotting activity. While the majority of patients with hemophilia A and B fail to synthesize their respective factor VIII and IX, variants of each have been described in which a nonfunctional but antigenically cross-reacting AHF-like protein inactivates an anticoagulant to either AHF or factor IX. Conceivably this polymorphism of hemophilia A and B represents a heterogenous group with different genetic mechanisms.

This polymorphism has not yet been found in von Willebrand's disease, in which AHF synthesis apparently occurs with transfusion of normal plasma, hemophilic plasma, or serum.

An immunological assay using rabbit antiserum against crude human factor VIII has been used to quantitate factor VIII protein or cross-reacting material in the plasma of patients (or relatives of patients) with hemophilia.[41] Three types of hemophilia were distinguished, ranging from one in which there is no biological activity and no factor VIII-like protein to one with low levels of factor VIII activity and associated with normal amounts of factor VIII-like protein.

Three patients with Christmas disease have been reported[102] whose plasma was shown to have a prolonged one-stage prothrombin time with ox brain thromboplastin. These patients were found to have an inhibitor for the reaction between factor X, factor VII, and ox brain extract. The abnormal constituent responsible for this inhibitor appears to be factor IX which is functionally inactive but antigenically indistinguishable from normal factor IX. Christmas disease might, therefore, be classified into two types: (1) hemophilia B+ (Christmas disease+) for the defect observed in the three patients who have an abnormal reaction to ox brain and whose blood contains a protein antigenically indistinguisable from factor IX; and (2) hemophilia B− (Christmas disease−), or classic Christmas disease, in which factor IX is absent.

Although most clotting factors are known to be made in the liver, there is evidence that the spleen is capable of synthesizing factor VIII. The spleen appears to be capable of either storing or releasing factor VIII or of effecting release of factor VIII from some other site.[220,268] It is believed that approximately three-fifths of circulating factor VIII is synthesized in the liver, one-fifth in the spleen, and lesser amounts in the thymus and bone marrow.[267] Human splenic transplants in critical hemophilia cases are under consideration.

*Clinical aspects.* The disease is characterized by recurrent episodes of bleeding from various parts of the body, occurring either spontaneously or following slight injury. The tendency toward prolonged hemorrhage is observed in the first days of life either from the umbilical cord, which is rare, or from circumcision, which is common. The bleeding from the latter source may be trivial or moderate or may require transfusion because of its persistence. Hemorrhage occurs almost invariably in the first year of life with the onset of walking, commonly following injuries of the nose and mouth, especially lacerations of the lips, tongue, frenulum of the upper lip, and gums. Excessive bleeding during inoculations or during eruption or loss of deciduous teeth suggests hemophilia.

Petechiae are rare. Subcutaneous and intramuscular hemorrhages are common. A significant amount of blood may be lost into the large muscles such as those of the thighs and gluteal regions. A person with hemophilia may bleed from the mucous membranes, into the pleural or peritoneal cavities, the gastrointestinal tract, solid viscera, or central nervous system. Hematuria is common and often persistent but responds to vigorous therapy. Epistaxis is uncommon in childhood. Hemorrhage into the retroperitoneal region, into the mesentery, and into the iliopsoas may simulate acute appendicitis. Abdominal pain presents complex problems in differential diagnosis. More often, the signs and symptoms are due to bleeding into the intestinal wall and peritoneal cavity than to inflammation, although mild leukocytosis can be present in either case.

In general, petechiae and mucous membrane and intracranial hemorrhage are common in thrombocytopenia and thrombocytopathia, whereas hematuria and hemarthrosis are common in deficiencies of coagulation factors. Epistaxis is most common in thrombocytopenia and less frequent in hemophilia, although there are many exceptions.

In addition to blood loss, tissue hemorrhages may cause serious pressure effects. Hematomas in strategic areas such as those in the extremities may obstruct circulation. Bleeding into the tissues of the mouth, neck, and thorax may seriously interfere with respiration, producing asphyxia.

Spontaneous hemorrhages frequently are cyclic with short episodes recurring at approximately 3- to 8-week intervals, despite the constancy of the deficiency. With equal deficiency of antihemophilic globulin, children show variations in clinical severity.

Bleeding after circumcision in one newborn infant with hemophilia and no bleeding in another with equally severe hemophilia must be due to the amount of tissue juices expressed during the procedure. The cord blood from a newborn infant with classic hemophilia was found to be devoid of antihemophilic globulin,[109] indicating the lack of passage of a plasma factor from the mother.

Moderate to marked elevations of factor VIII (antihemophilic factor, AHF) have been observed in normal subjects following a variety of stimuli: strenuous exercise, epinephrine infusions, fever induction, intravascular hemolysis, during pregnancy, hyperthyroidism, hemolytic anemias, and recently in sickle-cell anemia.[13] Contrary to other opinons, the administration of corticosteroids had no effect on factor VIII levels in hemophilic and nonhemophilic subjects.[81]

*Hemarthrosis.* The most characteristic site of hemorrhage is the joint cavities, usually of the ankles, knees, and especially the elbows. The shoulders, wrists, and hips may also be involved. Acute hemarthroses occur suddenly with severe pain, swelling, heat, tenderness, and limitation of motion. Although early hemorrhages are readily absorbed, the recurrence of bleeding eventually leads to extensive damage and thickening of synovial membranes, destruction of articular surfaces, and erosion of bone, with chronic inflammatory lesions, contractures, and permanent crippling.

*Management.* Treatment of the patient with severe hemophilia requires detailed attention to many aspects of the disease. As an initial step it is essential to determine whether the deficiency is due to the AHG factor or PTC factor and to assay the degree of deficiency by laboratory tests. The parents must be informed of the physical and emotional adjustments that will have to be made by both the patient and the family. Of major importance is the recognition of the special aptitudes of the child so that necessary training will be given for a protected occupation in adult life.

The individual management of the patient with hemophilia entails a knowledge of treatment of local bleeding sites and acute internal bleeding episodes, of preparation before dental extraction, minor operations, emergency surgery, and of orthopedic care.

*Treatment of bleeding.* Treatment of bleeding consists of local measures and transfusions of whole blood or fresh frozen or lyophilized plasma.

*Local measures.* Treatment consists of the application of a suitable coagulant and local pressure at the bleeding site. For open wounds, powdered thrombin and local packing with absorbable packs, such as a fibrin foam, oxidized cellulose (Oxygel or Surgicel), or gelatin sponge (Gelfoam) saturated in a solution of topical thrombin and Adrenalin followed by firm pressure, are valuable hemostatic devices. When it is not possible to apply digital pressure to an accessible bleeding site, a useful procedure is to spray a mixture of Adrenalin and thrombin on the local area after it has been freed of excess clot.[98] Thrombin is not to be given intravenously. Cauterization is always contraindicated. Suturing a wound should be avoided since it may provoke more serious local bleeding and tissue necrosis. Local measures are not a substitute for transfusion or replacement therapy, especially if the bleeding is located in a potentially dangerous area.

*Transfusion of whole blood or plasma.* For the patient who has suffered extensive blood loss, immediate transfusion with whole blood or packed cells is necessary. Fresh whole blood is preferable if available. In many patients it is unnecessary to bring the hemoglobin level to maximum concentrations; levels of 10 to 11 gm. per 100 ml. are adequate. Short of severe anemia, the basic objective in treatment of the patient in the acute phase or in preparation before a surgical procedure to prevent bleeding is to inject into the circulation a sufficient amount of antihemophilic globulin to raise its concentration to a level which will assure effective hemostasis.[112] In Christmas (PTC) disease the same objective is sought.

USE OF PLASMA—FRESH FROZEN AND LYOPHILIZED. Transfusion of type-specific fresh frozen plasma cryoprecipitate (see p. 701) is the treatment of choice. Many clinics, however, regard the matching of plasma as an unnecessary precaution. A whole blood transfusion is given if the patient is anemic. A knowledge of the properties of plasma is important: factor VIII (AHG) is labile, its life-span in the circulation is 12 to 24 hours, and its half-life is 4 to 6 hours, so that 50% of the initial level will remain after 4 hours, 25% after 8 hours, etc.

Fresh plasma that is withdrawn a few hours after collection of blood, frozen rapidly at $-20°$ C., and stored in a frozen state maintains its activity for variable periods of time. According to one estimate, fresh frozen plasma kept at $-20°$ C. loses roughly one-half its strength in 1 month, after which time the remaining factor VIII tends to be stable.[280] According to another study,[289] up to one-half of the donor's factor VIII is lost during centrifugation for separation of the plasma; the half-life of the remainder in the wet frozen state is about 16 weeks. In contrast, factor VIII activity in bank blood and plasma shows progressive deterioration, with about 30 to 60% of the initial factor VIII remaining after 3 weeks' storage.[280]

The plasma from freshly collected blood may be lyophilized and reconstituted with saline solution before use. Factor VIII in lyophilized plasma is also remarkably stable for as long as 1 year. One commercial preparation of frozen lyophilized plasma (Antihemophilic Plasma) contains factor VIII levels averaging 72% of fresh normal plasma.[289] This preparation is of value in traveling and in areas where fresh frozen plasma is not readily available.

Studies in our laboratory have confirmed the findings of Brinkhous and coworkers[74] with regard to the factor VIII concentration required for hemostasis in patients with hemophilia. They found that the minimum hemostatic level of factor VIII may be as low as 5% of normal, although some data suggested that it might be 15 to 20% of normal or higher. A constant level of factor VIII between 10 and 20% is realized by administering plasma in a dose of 10 ml. per kilogram of body weight initially and 5 ml. per kilogram every hour.[332] It has been frequently observed that active hemorrhage will persist in patients with hemophilia after inadequate amounts of plasma or blood are given, although the clotting time becomes normal.

Brinkhous[72] has emphasized that the plan for transfusion therapy (fresh frozen plasma) consists of an initial large priming transfusion, approximately 1% of body weight, followed by smaller transfusion maintenance at frequent intervals. With the initial transfusion, the level of AHG (factor VIII) is rapidly elevated in the circulating plasma in direct proportion to the amount administered. The rapid disappearance of factor VIII from the plasma results particularly from distribution to the empty extravascular compartment as well as from utilization. Transfusions are prescribed for maintenance in a volume of approximately 0.5% of the body weight. If given within 4 to 6 hours after the primary transfusion, the level of factor VIII is raised to approximately the level reached with the primary transfusion. The decrease is now less rapid and reflects chiefly the consumption of factor VIII. Careful scrutiny for the development of an inhibitor, pulmonary edema, and hypervolemia is necessary when large amounts of fresh frozen plasma are required.

The accompanying schedules provide guides for treatment of hemorrhage in patients with various clinical conditions and for preparation of patients for surgical procedures. Amounts in excess of those given in the schedules may be necessary, because the plasma factor VIII values of normal persons vary widely—in one estimate ranging from about 60 to 175% of the mean.[52] In treatment of patients with hemophilia the initial dose of plasma should be injected fairly rapidly (within a period of 45 minutes to 1 hour) in order to supply the bleeding area with adequate amounts of factor VIII to control hemostasis. It should be remembered that within 1 hour after exposure to room temperature, 50% of factor VIII activity disappears.

Occasionally, vigorous treatment over a prolonged period with plasma will lead to progressive edema and abdominal pain without cessation of bleeding from such sites as an extracted tooth or from the kidneys. To overcome this "refractoriness" we have found it expedient, in emergency, to stop plasma infusions while maintaining local hemostasis. After a rest period, transfusions with packed cells, whole blood, or plasma are reinstituted, depending upon the hemoglobin level.

Quick[295] has classified hemophilic patients into several groups on the basis of their concentration of factor VIII. The most severe group has a level below 0.1% and a clotting time of 40 minutes or more; a second group has a concentration of 0.5% and a clotting time of 18 to 30 minutes; and in a third group the level ranges from 1 to 5%. In the last group the clotting time is only slightly prolonged, the bleeding tendency is mild, and hemarthrosis is uncommon. It can, however, be fatal after trauma or surgery.

Biggs and Macfarlane[54] classified severely affected patients with spontaneous bleeding as having less than 1% of factor VIII, mildly affected patients as having more than 5%, and the variably affected group as having between 0 and 5%. Concerning treatment, they state that all patients requiring transfusions had less than 30% of factor VIII, that if the factor VIII level can be raised to between 15 and 30% postoperative bleeding will be less excessive, and that if the factor VIII level can be raised to more than 30% postoperative bleeding may be prevented. Brinkhous[71] pointed out that injected factor VIII is quickly redistributed between vascular and extravascular compartments. Once equilibrium is established between these compartments the rate of loss of factor VIII from the plasma may then be an indication of its biologic half-life.

The maintenance of adequate and continuous concentrations of factor VIII is especially important in patients with deep tissue hemorrhages in whom important structures may be involved. Such situations are encountered in the preparation for and during emergency surgery, especially of an abdominal nature, and in patients with central nervous system bleeding. Fatalities in patients with hemophilia are often due to ill-advised surgery. Hemorrhage into the tissues of the tongue and throat require active treatment with plasma and prompt pharyngeal or laryngeal intubation to prevent fatal asphyxia.[229] Hemothorax usually occurs spontaneously and produces serious respiratory and cardiac embarrassment. Aspiration is usually urgent and should be preceded by the rapid administration of fresh frozen plasma in adequate quantities.

Repeated infusions of plasma or concentrates carry the hazard of a refractory state due to the development of circulating anti-

This therapy schedule, as proposed, is ideal therapy which is presented as a guide for treatment of the patient with hemophilia. It is recognized that such therapy is not always possible and that the ultimate decision must lie with the physician treating the patient.

### Therapy schedules

*In emergency and major surgery* (for all deficiencies if concentrates are not available)

A priming dose of type specific fresh frozen plasma, 20 ml. per kilogram of body weight, is given 30 minutes before the procedure. If the procedure is longer than 1 hour, an additional 5 ml. per kilogram is given. Blood is replaced during the procedure as necessary.

After surgery, 5 ml. of fresh frozen plasma per kilogram is given every 4 hours for 48 hours, is extended to 6 to 8 hours for an additional 48 to 72 hours, and then 10 ml. per kilogram is given every 12 hours for 72 hours.

Therapy for 7 days should be sufficient or until all sutures are removed if the surgical procedure is minimal.

If the operation is major (abdominal, thoracic, or orthopedic, or if drains have been left in a cavity), it is usually wise to maintain a minimum of 50% of the adult normal values for the deficient factor for at least 8 to 10 days and 30% for an additional 4 days. Such levels are difficult to obtain by using the foregoing regimen because of problems associated with giving such large volumes of plasma. Adequate levels are easier to achieve with less hazard for the patient with the use of concentrates. For the patients with AHF (factor VIII) deficiency or von Willebrand's disease, cryoprecipitate or one of the more highly purified concentrates is the product of choice. The von Willebrand factor is present in cryoprecipitate and the other less concentrated products.

When cryoprecipitate is used the amount of AHF present is variable, depending on the amount present in the donor and the precipitation process, since each pack is extracted from single donations of whole blood. The AHF present can be assumed to be between 80 and 100 Standard AHF Units. (One Standard AHF unit is that amount of AHF found in 1 ml. of pooled fresh normal plasma, assumed to be 100%.) The therapy suggested is based on this assumption.

When major surgery is contemplated, give 4 packs of cryoprecipitate (each bag cryoprecipitate 80 to 100 AHF units) per 10 kilograms body weight 30 minutes before the procedure and again in 6 hours. Give 4 packs cryoprecipitate per 10 kilograms daily, thereafter for 8 to 10 days, then 3 packs for an additional 4 days. A minimum of 50% AHF should be maintained with this regimen for the 8- and 10-day period and a minimum of 30% for the last 4 days.

The high purity concentrates of AHF are available in smaller volumes, greater purity, and known content per cubic centimeter. The amount to be used may be calculated according to the formula of Abildgaard and co-workers,[11] as follows:

AHF units required=body weight (in kg.) $\times$ 0.5 $\times$ desired AHF increase (in percentage of normal)

For example:

400 AHF units are required for a 20 kg. boy $\times$ 0.5 (constant) to raise his AHF to 40%

A minimum of 50% of adult normal should be maintained for 8 to 10 days and then 30% for an additional 3 to 4 days.

### Bleeding into hazardous areas

Any head injury in a patient with severe AHF or PTC deficiency, irrespective of degree of symptomatology, should be treated as though bleeding existed. Although brain tissue has a high concentration of thromboplastin, it should not be relied upon to control all silent bleeding.

Fresh frozen plasma is given initially at 20 ml. per kilogram of body weight, and is followed by 5 ml. per kilogram every 4 to 6 hours for 48 hours for bleeding into hazardous areas such as the brain or retropharyngeal areas.

Therapy is tapered to every 8 to 12 hours and continued thereafter for 3 to 4 days or longer if deemed necessary.

When cryoprecipitate or the high purity concentrates are used, a minimum of 50% AHF should be maintained for 48 hours, then tapered to 30% for an additional 48 hours, and longer if deemed necessary. These levels may be accomplished by giving 5 packs of cryoprecipitate per 10 kilograms daily, tapered to 3 packs per 10 kilograms daily.

*Continued.*

*Dental extractions*

Fresh frozen plasma, 20 ml. per kilogram, is given 30 minutes before the extraction, followed by 5 ml. per kilogram every 4 to 6 hours for 6 days. Cryoprecipitate and the concentrates should be used to achieve a minimum of 40% adult normal AHF level for 6 days.

*Hemarthrosis*

Fresh frozen plasma, 20 ml. per kilogram body weight, is given initially, followed by 5 ml. per kilogram in 4 to 6 hours; 10 ml. per kilogram is repeated in 12 hours if pain persists.

Cryoprecipitate given at 3 packs per 10 kilogram body weight in one dose should give good hemostasis for 24 hours. This should be accompanied by prednisolone, 2 mg. per kilogram body weight per day, for 3 days to decrease the inflammation, and immobilization with ice for 24 hours. Passive exercise may be begun at 24 hours and active exercise at 48 hours.

If concentrates are used, a dose should be given to achieve 75 to 80% adult normal levels of AHF. With normal decay some hemostatic control may be present for at least 24 hours. Joints are aspirated in our clinic when swelling appears to be extensive and the swelling has been so great that blood supply of the joint is compromised.

*Muscle hemorrhage*

Fresh frozen plasma is given, 10 ml. per kilogram body weight, or cryoprecipitate, 1 to 2 packs per 10 kilogram body weight, with rest, ice, and Ace bandage. Passive exercise should begin at 24 hours and full ambulation at 48 hours.

*Genitourinary bleeding*

*For moderate bleeding* (most common), prednisolone is administered in a dosage of 1 to 2 mg. per kilogram and bed rest prescribed for 48 hours. If bleeding persists beyond 48 hours, plasma or cryoprecipitate is administered as for severe bleeding, and prednisolone is continued.

*For severe bleeding,* 20 ml. of fresh frozen plasma per kilogram of body weight is given, followed by 5 ml. per kilogram every 4 to 6 hours for 3 days, then tapered to 5 ml. per kilogram every 12 hours for 2 days. Prednisolone is continued simultaneously. Packed red cells should be given for anemia. Should bleeding persist, one course of therapy may be repeated.

When cryoprecipitate or a concentrate is used, a minimum of 40% adult normal levels of AHF should be maintained for 3 days, followed by 20% for 2 additional days.

*Mucous membrane bleeding*

In the young infant bleeding from the mucous membranes of the mouth or the frenulum is difficult to control unless a minimum level of 50% adult normal is achieved. This can be achieved best on an inpatient basis. The patient should be sedated, restrained, and maintained on intravenous therapy and should be given nothing by mouth for at least 48 hours.

Fresh frozen plasma therapy is begun at 20 ml. per kilogram of body weight, followed by 5 ml. per kilogram every 4 to 6 hours for 5 days. Cryoprecipitate or concentrate should be given to achieve the minimum level of 50% adult normal AHF level.

After 48 hours, clear liquids may be given orally by small spoon, with attention not to dislodge the clot. If a large friable mushroom-shaped clot forms through a small seepage of blood, it is sometimes of value to remove the clot and restore therapy with 10 ml. of fresh frozen plasma per kilogram body weight (if this has been the therapeutic dose). Should the infant dislodge the clot before complete healing has taken place, plasma therapy must be instituted with the original amounts.

When cryoprecipitate or concentrates are used the high values achieved at all times usually remove the possibility of these complications and allow treatment on an outpatient basis, with therapy daily for 6 days. Cryoprecipitate can be given at 4 packs per 10 kilograms of body weight daily.

*Gastrointestinal bleeding*

Fresh frozen plasma, 20 ml. per kilogram of weight, followed by 5 ml. per kilogram every 4 to 6 hours for 24 to 48 hours, will usually suffice; therapy may be continued longer if necessary. Concentrates should achieve 40% minimum level for the same period of time.

**Supplementary therapy schedule**

1. Hematoma:

   *Factor VIII deficiency*
   | | | |
   |---|---|---|
   | Fresh frozen plasma | (FFP) | 10 ml./kg. |
   | Cryoprecipitate | (Cryo) | 2 packs/10 kg. |
   | Factor VIII concentrate | | 20 units/kg. |

   *Factor IX deficiency*
   | | | |
   |---|---|---|
   | Factor VIII deficient plasma | | 10 ml./kg. |
   | Factor IX concentrate | (Konȳne) | 10 units/kg. |

2. Hemarthrosis:

   *Factor VIII deficiency*
   Fresh frozen plasma (FFP) 20 ml./kg. immediately followed by 5 ml./kg. in 4 to 6 hours
   Cryoprecipitate (Cryo) 3 to 4 packs/ 10 kg.
   Factor VIII concentrate 25 to 30 units/kg.; repeat if necessary, or factor VIII    40 units/kg. stat once
   Prenisolone  2 mg./kg./day for 3 days (not to exceed 40 mg./day)
   (May be used as an adjuvant to replacement therapy.)

   *Factor IX deficiency*
   Factor VIII deficient plasma   20 ml./kg.   10 ml./lb.
   Factor IX concentrate (Konȳne)   30 units/kg.

   Should joint swelling become excessive or should the skin become shiny, an orthopedist should be consulted and the joint should be aspirated either just before or as the replacement material is given. If orthopedic problem persists for longer than 1 week, the patient should be referred for orthopedic rehabilitation.

3. Hematuria:

   Prednisolone 2 mg./kg./day for 2 days with bed rest has been found useful as preliminary therapy; if no improvement, start on replacement therapy

   *Factor VIII deficiency*
   FFP 20 ml./kg., followed by 5 ml./kg. every 4 to 6 hours for 5 days
   Cryo 4 packs/10 kg. for 5 days

   *Factor IX deficiency*
   Factor VIII deficient plasma 20 ml./kg. followed by 10 ml./kg. every 8 hours for 5 days
   Factor IX concentrate (Konȳne) 40 units/kg./day for 5 days

4. Mucous membrane bleeding and dental extractions:

   *Factor VIII deficiency*
   Dental extractions should only be done in major center under laboratory control with the patient admitted to hospital; mucous membrane bleeding can be controlled with daily visits to the outpatient department for transfusions
   FFP 20 ml./kg. immediately followed by 5 ml./kg. every 4 to 6 hours for 5 days; cryo 5 packs/10 kg./day for 5 days (this may be given in divided dose twice daily if desired)
   Factor VIII concentrate 40 units/kg. for 5 days
   *Factor IX deficiency*
   Factor VIII deficient plasma 20 ml./kg. followed by 10 ml./kg. every 8 hours for 5 days
   Factor IX concentrate (Konȳne) 40 units/kg./day for 5 days

   Epsilon amino caproic acid    70 mg./kg. immediately before the procedure, followed by 40 mg./kg. every 4 hours is a usual adjuvant for dental extractions (for Factor VIII and IX deficiencies)

*Continued.*

**Supplementary therapy schedule—cont'd**

5. Hazardous areas (retropharyngeal, CNS, floor of the mouth):

   *Factor VIII deficiency*
   FFP 20 ml./kg. immediately followed by 5 ml./kg. every 4 to 6 hours for 48 hours; cryo 5 packs/10 kg.
   Factor VIII concentrate 40 units/kg. stat

   *Factor IX deficiency*
   Factor VIII deficient plasma 20 ml./kg. immediately followed by 10 ml./kg. every 8 hours for 48 hours.
   Factor IX concentrate (Konȳne) 40 units/kg./day

   Patients should be given an initial dose and then transferred to a major center, where length of therapy depends on the severity of bleeding and danger of the hemorrhage.

6. Surgery:  Should only be done in major centers

   Prior to surgery
   
   *Factors VIII and IX deficiency*
   Concentrates to achieve 100% correction to be given 30 minutes before procedure

   Maintain 50% correction for 4 days and 30% until all sutures are removed. All patients should have a preliminary screening procedure done for the presence of inhibitors. The test should be performed according to the method of Biggs and Bidwell.[48] The patient should be given a test dose of the material to be used for replacement therapy to determine maximal effect and half-life in the patient at that time.

---

coagulants.[319] The deficient factor introduced in this fashion acts as a foreign protein inducing antibody formation. The inhibitor present in the blood of some patients with circulating anticoagulants is a gamma globulin antibody[120,359] which destroys antihemophilic globulin.[48] Management of the refractory state is unsatisfactory and depends on the actual inhibitor level present at the time. Large amounts of factor VIII concentrates can be used to achieve hemostasis within the 5- to 7-day period during which the anticoagulant is present at minimal levels. When these are ineffective in overcoming the presence of a potent inhibitor, other forms of treatment are available such as corticosteroids and immunosuppressive agents. In life-threatening situations in enclosed soft tissue bleeding areas repeated exchange transfusions with fresh blood may prove effective.[226,357]

Biggs and Bidwell[48] have described a method of determining the presence of inhibitor by mixing AHG (factor VIII) and diluted inhibitory plasma, incubating at 37° C., and removing samples after measured intervals and testing for AHG content. As a control, AHG is similarly incubated with diluted hemophilic plasma.

More important in prophylaxis is the protection of the infant and young child against trauma by carefully selecting toys, padding the crib, removing potential sources of injury from furniture when the child begins to walk, and supervising play activities. With advancing age and greater understanding, accidents are decreased.

*Use of concentrates of factor VIII (AHF, AHG).* Concentrates from animal and human sources have been prepared which are under constant investigation for purification and concentration.[172]

The introduction of factor VIII concentrates has led to changes in the management of major bleeding episodes in hemophilia and other bleeding disorders. The advantage of concentrates which are prepared from plasma over the plasma itself is the elimination of the vascular overload from an excessive infusion of protein. The danger of circulatory overload arises not so much from the volume of fluids infused but rather from the osmotic load of infused proteins. The large amounts of albumin and other proteins present in plasma have interfered with raising the level of factor VIII without compromising the circulation.

The use of concentrates permits higher concentrations of factor VIII than previously achieved with the use of plasma alone and the possibility of lengthening the interval between administrations, so as to sustain these levels for longer periods of time. Frequently single doses of factor VIII concentrates have replaced the need for repeated infusions of plasma to maintain hemostatic levels of AHF.

Many of these concentrates are still in preparation and those that are in manufacture are not available in all parts of the world. Hence reliance on fresh frozen plasma or cryoprecipitate is essential, as well as knowledge of adequate dosage.

A unit of antihemophilic factor is defined as the activity present in 1 ml. of average normal pooled plasma less than an hour old.

The clinical manifestations of hemophilia A due to a deficiency of factor VIII and of hemophilia B due to a deficiency of factor IX are similar with respect to chronic and recurring invalidism caused by spontaneous hemarthrosis, spontaneous or easy and extensive bruising, difficulty in controlling hemorrhage after dental extraction, or hematuria. The condition in either disease may be very mild and the patient unaware of it until trauma or surgery causes severe loss of blood. The frequency of administration of the particular product to replace the deficiency either of factor VIII or of factor IX will depend on the half-life of their respective deficient factors. The half-life of factor VIII is short; its life-span in the circulation is 12 to 24 hours, and its half-life is from 4 to 6 hours. The half-life of factor IX ranges from 8 to 20 hours. The maintenance of adequate levels of factor VIII and factor IX depends on the knowledge of these differences.

*Cryoprecipitate.* The cryoprecipitate method of Pool and her associates[290] was based on the observation that when frozen plasma is thawed in the cold, most of the factor VIII remains in the cold-insoluble precipitate and provides a simple means of preparation of potent antihemophilic globulin concentrates suitable for introduction as a routine blood-banking procedure.[77]

Cryoprecipitate is prepared from blood, as soon after collection as possible but no more than 6 hours after donation. After cold (4° C.) centrifugation, the fresh plasma is frozen in a deep freeze at −65° C. or colder, or in a dry ice-alcohol mixture. It may remain frozen for several months, but usually within the week after collection it is thawed at 1 to 6° C. in a refrigerator. As soon as thawing is completed (18 to 24 hours) the plasma pack is centrifuged at 4° C. for 20 minutes at 1,600g. All but 10 to 15 ml. of the supernate is removed. The cryoprecipitate remains behind on the walls of the pack, and this material with remaining plasma is refrozen and stored for up to 1 year at below −20° C.[77,92]

Under ideal conditions, the average pack of cryoprecipitate will contain 125 to 150 units of factor VIII; when prepared routinely in a blood bank, however, the average factor VIII content is best calculated at 100 units per pack.

As is true for all AHF containing materials, 40 units/kg. will give a 30-minute posttransfusion level of 100%. The dose to be administered can be thus calculated and will depend upon the level of AHF desired.

If, for hemarthroses, a level of 60 to 100% is achieved (by administering 24 to 32 units/kg. AHF; ¼ to ⅓ pack/kg.), repeat therapy is rarely necessary. For surgical procedures a level of 80 to 100% should be maintained from just prior to operation through the third or fourth postoperative day, followed by therapy which maintains the AHF level at 40 to 50% for an additional 6 to 8 days.

For von Willebrand's disease essentially the same dosage schedule is recommended; however, since patients with this disorder may be stimulated by cryoprecipitate administration to produce their own AHF, therapy in surgical patients should be initiated 24 hours prior to operation.

Cryoprecipitate is also the treatment of choice for factor XIII (FSF) deficiency. A single dose of 1 to 2 packs per 10 kg. is recommended. The precipitate contains only minimal amounts of fibrinogen, but does contain isohemagglutinins. It is thus recommended that type-specific or AB plasma be used as a source of this material.

*Courtland antihemophilic factor (human).*\* This substance is a stable dried concentrate of antihemophilic factor (factor VIII, AHF, AHG) and an excellent product for surgical proce-

---

\*Manufactured by Courtland Scientific Products, Los Angeles, California.

dures and major bleeds in the therapy of hemophilia A. It is a lyophilized product and is reconstituted with 30 ml. of sterile water. It should be administered with a filter immediately after reconstitution. Factor VIII half-life is 8 to 12 hours. Before surgical procedures enough of the product is given to achieve 100% correction. Levels of factor VIII of over 50% are to be maintained for 5 days and then at over 30% until all sutures are removed. The dosage for hemarthrosis is 25 to 30 units per kilogram. Since this product is prepared from freshly pooled plasma, viral hepatitis may be a frequent complication. Also, while the blood group isoagglutinins are not present in significant amounts, with extensive correction of patients who are not either type O or $A_2$, hemolytic anemia can be prevented by the addition of A and/or B specific soluble blood group substance. (Blood group substance SSBGS, Pfizer, is recommended.)

*Hemofil (antihemophilic factor [human]) method four.** This substance is prepared from fresh normal plasma. It supplies six or more times higher potency AHF than cryoprecipitates or previous glycine preparations with relatively smaller amounts of fibrinogen and other protein and is therefore of value in long-term therapy. The factor VIII half-life with this preparation is 10 hours. Recovery in vivo is 80 to 90%. The product comes as a lyophilized material and is reconstituted with 10 ml. of sterile water. It should be given immediately after reconstitution. Dosage is calculated according to need. One unit gives approximately 2% rise in factor VIII. Since the concentrate is prepared from large pools of fresh human plasma it may contain the causative agents of viral hepatitis. The preparation contains trace amounts of blood groups A and B isohemagglutinins. When large volumes are given to individuals who are not either type O or $A_2$, the addition of A and/or B specific soluble blood group substance is recommended, as for the Courtland antihemophilic factor.

*Cohn's fraction 1.* Concentrated AHG is made from human blood (specifically from Cohn's fraction 1 as starting material) and, when reconstituted for use, is usually three to five times more concentrated than the original plasma.[264] The resulting fraction, designated 1-0, which is rarely used today, contains 86 to 90% of the original fibrinogen and 100% of AHG. It has been reported effective in controlling bleeding.[60,264] Human AHG is being prepared in limited quantities, endeavoring to obtain more concentrated material from smaller quantities of blood.

A concentrate marketed as Fibrinogen (human)* has an AHG content four times that of fresh frozen plasma. This material has great value, particularly for the pediatric patient, but its use is limited because of cost and availability. Side effects of hemolysis, clumping of red cells, and a falsely positive Coombs test may be encountered after the administration of amounts that give levels greater than 1,000 mg. of fibrinogen per 100 ml. of blood. Each gram contains an AHG activity equivalent to approximately 75 to 100 ml. of plasma not more than 18 hours old. Fibrinogen (human) can be given in amounts sufficient to raise AHG activity to within 30 to 60% of normal. This product has already been found useful for replacement therapy in patients with classic hemophilia (factor VIII deficiency).[361]

*Concentrates from animal serums.* Potent concentrates of AHG from human or animal sources (bovine or pig globulin[44,45]) have been successfully employed. Both cows and pigs have a considerably higher concentration of factor VIII in their blood than is found in man, making this product more available. Because it is a foreign protein, AHG derived from animal sources is potentially antigenic and carries the hazard of anaphylactic reactions.[55] A crude animal (porcine) factor VIII has been further purified and was successfully employed during an appendectomy of a severe hemophiliac.[247] Animal factor VIII can only be given in one bleeding episode and in desperate situations, because its repetition may lead to serious reactions.

Human factor VIII preparations are less potent than animal preparations. The purification factor of the best human preparations is only 25 and compares unfavorably with a purification factor of 400 for the best bovine preparations.[179] Human preparations are, however, preferable to animal preparations, despite their lesser potency. Since they are derived from fresh frozen plasma, the supply of human material is necessarily restricted.

A home transfusion program has been reported

---

*Manufactured by the Hyland Laboratories, Costa Mesa, California.

*Manufactured by Merck Sharp & Dohme, West Point, Pennsylvania.

for treatment of patients with classic hemophilia (hemophilia A).[302] For joint or soft tissue hemorrhage cryoprecipitate is injected in a dose of 10 to 20 units per kilogram of body weight. The member of the family who most frequently performed the infusion (venipuncture) was the mother. This procedure is carried out after consultation of the hemophiliac patient's family with the supervising physician. Thus far this program appears eminently successful. It has been pointed out that hemophiliac patients are often better judges of a bleeding episode than the physician and are able to decide the indications for treatment.

*Use of corticosteroids.* Corticosteroids have been effectively used to control bleeding due to thrombocytopenia, without actually increasing platelet numbers. The improvement in vascular resistance has been related to changes in the concentration of mucopolysaccharides at the level of the vessel wall.[369] In oral surgery it seems to minimize the tendency toward unwarranted postoperative hemorrhage and provide a firmer clot at the extraction site.[353] In various clinics the use of the corticosteroids has been extended to the adjuvant treatment of hemarthrosis and genitourinary bleeding. The dosage of prednisone, or a comparable compound, is 1 to 2 mg. per kilogram of body weight daily, in four divided doses.

*Epsilon-aminocaproic acid (Amicar).* A search for a synthetic inhibitor of plasmin, the enzyme causing clot lysis (fibrinolysin), led to the discovery of epsilon-aminocaproic acid (EACA).[362] This substance inhibits the enzymatic process involved in plasminogen activation by urokinase, streptokinase, or blood activator. The peculiar property of epsilon-aminocaproic acid of inhibiting the enzyme dissolving clots has been applied to the treatment of hemophilia. It has been postulated that the patient with hemophilia has difficulty in forming clots but dissolves them once they have been formed. It is also possible that in a hemorrhagic episode activation of the clot-dissolving process may be accelerated. While this drug does not replace the deficient factor VIII (antihemophilic globulin) in the hemophiliac, the slowing down of clot dissolution, once it has been formed, has already proved beneficial in dental bleeding. While EACA is of value in the prophylaxis of spontaneous bleeding in the hemophiliac[6] and has contributed to the cessation of hematuria in a young adult,[31] there are reports of intrarenal obstruction as a probable complication of this therapy.[83,164]

In a group of thirty-one dental extractions performed on eleven hemophiliac patients, EACA was administered (12 to 40 gm. daily by mouth in syrup or tablet form) preoperatively and postoperatively, in conjunction with careful packing of the socket and protection of the extraction area.[315] Transfusions of blood and antihemophilic globulin or plasma were found unnecessary.

It is to be emphasized that this drug (EACA) has been designed basically for use when hemorrhage results from an overactivity of the fibrinolytic system. Its application in hemophilia is directed toward inhibiting clot lysis.

This product will be discussed further in a subsequent section of this chapter on fibrinolysis.

At one time peanuts were regarded as an effective agent in suppressing the bleeding tendency in hemophilia,[66] acting through an inhibitory effect on clot dissolution.[29] In recent years there has been little mention of their therapeutic usefulness in controlling hemostasis.

*Treatment of hematuria.* It has been stated that no type of bleeding in hemophilia is as likely to be overtreated as much as hematuria, since a surprisingly small amount of blood in the urine may make it appear almost pure blood.[296] In our experience hematuria can be controlled within 48 hours by complete bed rest and prednisone (1 to 2 mg. per kilogram).[167] If bleeding continues beyond this period, fresh frozen plasma or factor VIII concentrates are given as outlined previously, while continuing the use of prednisone. If microscopic hematuria is not cleared to approximately 50 to 100 red blood cells per high-power field with this regimen, throat and urine cultures are taken to rule out other causes of hematuria. A local lesion rather than a hemophilic state may be responsible for the hematuria. If hematuria persists, the patient is not re-treated, but is watched carefully before a complete urologic investigation is made. Epsilon-aminocaproic acid (EACA) has been recommended in hematuria but is still undergoing trial.[31] Intrarenal obstruction has been reported with the use of this drug.[351] It is probable that this complication occurs in hemophilia regardless of EACA therapy.[164]

***Dental extractions.*** When loose deciduous teeth are being removed, hemostasis is relatively simple. When permanent teeth are extracted, the socket is packed with an absorbable thromboplastin and one loose, holding suture is inserted. The patient is maintained on intravenous fluids with nothing by mouth for 48 hours, after which time clear fluids are given by spoon. Extraction of more than two molars or three incisors at one time is not recommended. Fresh frozen plasma or factor VIII concentrates are administered as outlined previously. Prednisone (1 to 2 mg. per kilogram) is begun 12 hours before the procedure and continued through the period of plasma therapy. The administration of epsilon-aminocaproic acid has been recommended but is still under trial.[315]

***Treatment of hemarthroses.*** Hemarthroses are particularly troublesome and tend to recur. Acute joint bleeding is to be treated promptly and vigorously for 3 to 4 days with plasma or factor VIII concentrates, as suggested in the schedules for treatment. Reassurance, analgesics, plasma therapy, bed rest, and elevation with slight flexion of the joint surrounded by ice packs constitute initial treatment (plastic ice bags should be kept immediately available in the refrigerator). An elastic compression bandage is useful. Following arrest of hemorrhage, orthopedic supervision is necessary for conserving maximum function and preventing deformities.

It is now known that any amount of blood in a joint may lead to prolonged arthritic changes. Hence orthopedic supervision and prompt administration of fresh frozen plasma or a factor VIII concentrate in adequate dosage is necessary. Repeated hemorrhage into a joint is eventually associated with deterioration of the synovium and accumulation of excessive fluid containing proteolytic enzymes.

With the control of bleeding, cautious active motion within painless areas and massage are instituted until the former range of movement is obtained.[95] Active motion favors absorption of residual blood and prevents contracture of capsular and pericapsular tissues.[103] Slow ambulation with passive exercises is begun at 48 hours. Aspiration of the joint cavity may relieve the symptoms in an occasional patient, especially when the skin is under tension over a very large, painful, and distended joint that has not responded to immobilization and analgesics. Aspiration must be done under coverage with adequate amounts of plasma or factor VIII concentrate, since needling of a hemophilic joint may precipitate fresh bleeding. More extensive experience is needed to evaluate aspirations, since the proponents of both forms of management claim equally good results. With the use of fresh frozen plasma or factor VIII concentrate, immobilization, and early ambulation, there has been less permanent joint deformity, regardless of aspiration.

There has been renewed interest in the surgical treatment of hemarthrosis.[118] Aspiration of the joint cavity has been recommended[57] if there is evidence of accumulation of an appreciable amount of fluid. Factor VIII concentrate or fresh frozen plasma is given *after* the aspiration with the assurance that the joint was immobilized. Others[384] give cryoprecipitate in the dose of 1 unit (i.e., the amount obtained from one unit of blood) per 10 kg. body weight, or factor VIII concentrate (10 to 20 units per kg.) to cover possible bleeding *after* aspiration. By these procedures the period of immobilization is reduced in aspirated patients with the aim of preventing serious permanent damage to the joint.

Experience in our clinic has demonstrated the value of prednisone or prednisolone 2 mg./kg./day (not to exceed 40 mg./day, in divided doses) in reducing pain. It is given for 3 to 5 days after joint bleeding has been controlled by fresh frozen plasma or factor VIII concentrates. In patients with milder hemarthroses, steroid may be given without the use of plasma. If synovitis is a complication, corticosteroids are extended for a longer period. Occasional use of salicylates in ordinary doses is permissible, but for prolonged use a substitute analgesic is preferable. Where a joint has been repeatedly affected, rehabilitation with traction, casts, and braces is necessary.[192]

For muscle hemorrhage fresh frozen plasma is given, 10 ml. per kilogram of body weight, or a factor VIII concentrate, 20 units per kilogram of body weight, with rest, ice packing, and ambulation in 24 to 48 hours. Repeated therapy is usually not necessary for the usual hematoma. Steroid therapy to decrease inflammation is usually not required. However, severe muscle bleeding will require repeated doses of plasma, 5 ml. per kilogram of body weight every 4 to 6 hours, or a factor VIII concentrate, 10 units per kilogram of body weight, following the initial dose until bleeding is controlled.

With the use of factor VIII concentrates it is now possible to provide the entire therapeutic AHF replacement in a single infusion instead of repeated infusions of plasma in order to maintain hemostatic levels of AHF over a 48-hour period.[173] Single doses of 20 to 30 units of AHF per kilogram of body weight were given and this treatment was sufficient to produce a postinfusion AHF level of about 50%. Advantages of the single dose regimen include fewer venipunctures, ease of administration, less need for hospitalization and greater patient acceptance. In another report,[199] splinting and immobilization with acute hemarthrosis could be further eliminated by a single infusion of 25 units of AHF per kilogram and a short-term course of corticosteroids. The total dose of prednisone consisted of 1 mg. per pound of body weight per day in two divided doses for 3 days, with a limit of 80 mg. per day followed by half the initial dose for the next 2 days. In the control group of those not receiving prednisone a considerable number needed additional replacement for complete return of joint function. The investigators felt that immobilization and splinting tended to weaken the surrounding muscle structure thereby increasing the amount of physical therapy and the time needed before ambulation and complete return of function were possible.

The knees of a group of hemophilia patients requiring orthopedic care were aspirated to relieve pressure from acute or chronic hemarthrosis.[27] The acid phosphatase was markedly elevated in the joint fluid from hemophilic patients and higher than that found in the fluid from patients with rheumatoid arthritis. The rationale for treatment of acute and chronic hemarthrosis is based upon the hypothesis of active enzymatic destruction of cartilage. Treatment consists of replacement therapy with factor VIII concentrates, frequent joint aspirations, corticosteroids, and active physiotherapy.

*Mild hemophilia.* One of the significant observations made concerning hemophilia as a result of correlating clinical manifestations with laboratory findings is the variation in its severity. On the basis of assay it appears that severely affected persons often have no measurable amounts of antihemophilic globulin in the plasma, or they may range up to 3%.[72] In the most mildly affected patients it ranges from 5 to 20% and in a smaller number it is less than 5%.[54] In general, AHG levels above 5% occur in mildly affected patients.[54] Under strain of the hemostatic mechanism, such as occurs postoperatively, occasionally a seemingly well person with an AHG value between 30 and 45% may suffer from transient bleeding. It has been stated that each person appears to have a constant and characteristic level of this clotting factor.[73] It should again be emphasized that patients with mild deficiencies may not manifest hemorrhage until they sustain a sizable injury or after such common surgical procedures as tonsillectomy or dental extraction.

In a group of mild hemophiliacs in whom the venous clotting time was normal and the thromboplastin generation test impaired, surgical bleeding after tonsillectomy or tooth extraction was the most frequent symptom. Usually the first episode was delayed or ignored until adolescence or adult life. Hemarthrosis or hematuria were far less frequent than in severe cases. The concentration of factor VIII (AHG) in mild hemophilia A (classic) ranged from 8 to 37% and factor IX (PTC) in hemophilia B (Christmas disease), from 9 to 58%.[17] A mild deficiency of factor VIII, affecting both males and females, was reported in which a vascular abnormality had been excluded.[63] The condition was thought to be transmitted as an intermediate dominant or represented a quantitative variant of hemophilia A.

*Diagnosis.* An abnormal bleeding tendency, particularly hemarthroses, dating from infancy, occurring also in other members of the family, and being limited to male members with evidence of sex-linked inheritance suggests hemophilia. In patients with severe grades of hemophilia the marked prolongation of whole blood clotting time is a characteristic feature. In patients with mild types of disease the coagulation time may be slightly prolonged or even normal since as little as 1% of AHG is sufficient to produce a normal clotting time. The prothrombin consumption test and the thromboplastin generation tests are more sensitive tests of an AHG deficiency with amounts below 5% and 20%, respectively, in the plasma.

The thromboplastin generation test, by identifying the deficient factor, will separate hemophilia B due to PTC defect from classic hemophilia which it closely resembles clinically. In the type of pseudohemophilia (von Willebrand's disease) in which there is a combined vascular defect and AHG deficiency, epistaxis and a prolonged bleeding time characterize the former defect and hemarthrosis and a normal bleeding time, the latter.

Mixing tests provide simple diagnostic leads. The three types of plasma correct unrelated hemophilias but not those with the corresponding defect.

*Roentgenographic findings.* In the early stages of hemophilia x-ray findings are nonspecific and consist of swelling and distention of the joint. Skeletal lesions result from bleeding directly into the bones or from secondary changes in the bones due to hemorrhages into adjacent joints.[80] Hemorrhages into the spongiosa of the shafts and epiphyses produce cystic areas of rarefaction. Juxtaarticular cysts, irregular in size and distribution, are an outstanding feature seen on the roentgenogram of the patient with moderate hemophilic anthropathy.[192] (See Fig. 96.)

Marginal bony defects of the epiphyses and erosions of joint margins are noted. In the joints incomplete resorption of blood and retained blood clots result in deformities, disability, and, infrequently, ankylosis. Repeated hemorrhages into joint spaces may lead to accelerated maturation and hypertrophy of the adjacent epiphyses, probably resulting from local hyperemia[80] (Fig. 97.) With limitation of motion, generalized decalcification is noted in the bones adjacent to the affected joint.

*Prognosis.* Deaths from exsanguination following surgical procedures or severe trauma have become less common with the judicious administration of fresh plasma or blood. The protection offered the infant and young child obscures the true nature of the disease which becomes apparent as the child grows older and is exposed to trauma of various kinds. Hemarthrosis, resulting from frequently repeated hemorrhages, eventually results in crippling and disability. It has been stated that the best laboratory guide to prognosis is the determination of the blood concentrations of AHG. Patients with no detectable AHG are usually severely affected, and those with more than 5% are almost invariably mildly affected.[54]

## Von Willebrand's disease (pseudohemophilia, vascular hemophilia)

Von Willebrand's disease is a hereditary hemorrhagic diathesis characterized by a moderate to severe factor VIII (AHG) deficiency combined with a capillary defect, causing prolonged bleeding time.* It was first described[383] by von Willebrand, who observed the condition in several kindreds living in the islands of Åland in the Gulf of Bothnia off the coast of Finland where it is present in high frequency. Von Willebrand originally designated the disease as pseudohemophilia.

The claim that Minot had described a similar condition a few years earlier prompted Quick[297] to suggest that it be designated as the Minot-von Willebrand syndrome.

The main features consist of a markedly prolonged bleeding time, normal clotting time, normal platelet count, normal clot retraction, and occurrence in both males and females. In recent years it has been observed that the platelets in this disease are nonadhesive in vivo. The prolonged bleeding time may be related to a failure of platelets to adhere to the vessel wall, resulting in a delay in platelet plug formation.[65] With the growing interest and confirmation of the defect in platelet adhesiveness, many have felt that this feature should be included in the definition of this disease. (See p. 741 for platelet adhesiveness.) In a considerable number of these patients blood vessel abnormalities have been demonstrated. The morphologic vascular abnormalities consist of coiled, tortuous capillaries in the nail beds and in the venules of the bulbar conjunctivae. These abnormal nail-bed capillaries fail to contract normally after puncture.

Although severe intracranial hemorrhage can occur, the most common symptom in either group of patients, regardless of associated factor VIII deficiency, is severe and spontaneous epistaxis. Also common to both groups is bleeding from the tongue, gums, and teeth following extraction or loss of deciduous teeth. Excessive bruising on slight trauma is also present. The outstanding laboratory finding is a prolonged bleeding time. The clotting time, prothrombin time, platelet count, and clot retraction are normal. The capillary fragility is only occasionally abnormal. The results, however, obtained with all the tests for integrity of the vascular wall suggest that hemostasis is abnormal in von Willebrand's disease.[35] The tourniquet test may give equivocal results, although some have noted positive capillary fragility in

---

*See references 20, 94, 210, 238, 332, 333, 343, and 372.

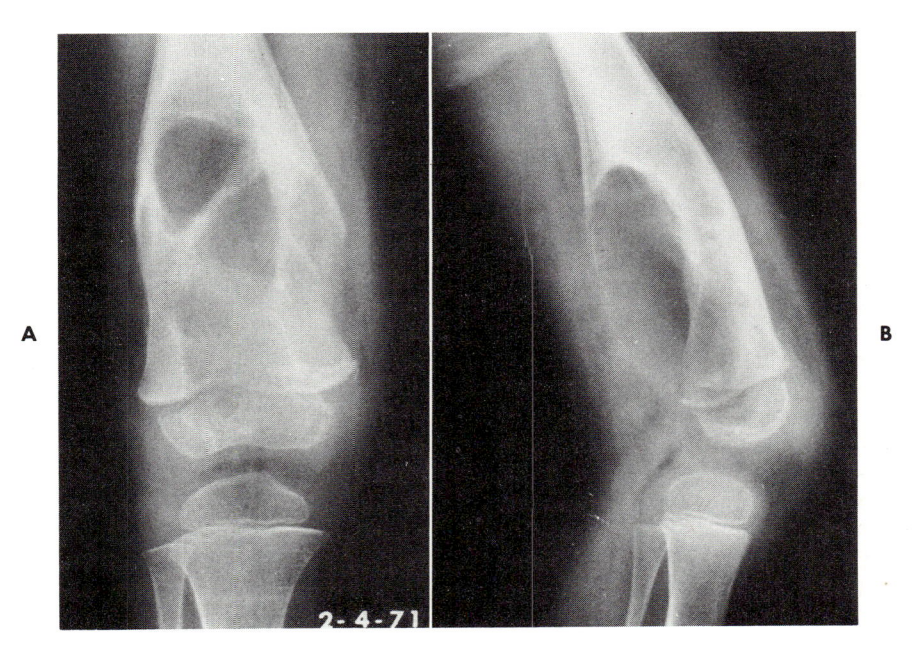

Fig. 96. Cystic changes of femur on AP view, **A**, and posterior extension of tumor mass on lateral view, **B**, in a 1½-year-old patient with severe factor VIII deficiency. (Courtesy Dr. Margaret W. Hilgartner, New York, N. Y.)

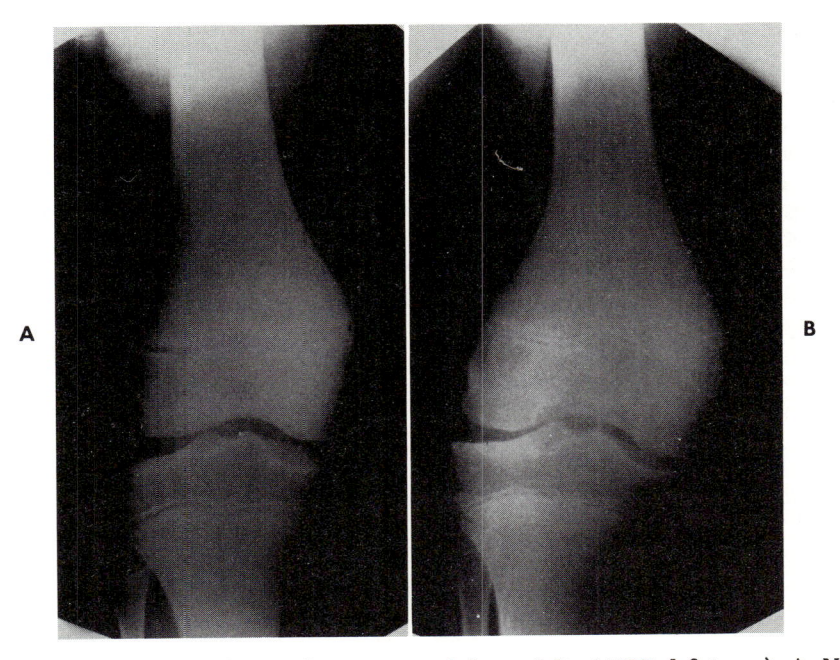

Fig. 97. Roentgenograms of knees of a patient with hemophilia (AHG deficiency). **A**, Normal epiphyses of right knee. **B**, Note hypertrophy of epiphysis of femur and tibia of left knee due to local hyperemia from recurrent hemarthrosis.

the majority of their patients.[260] The coagulation abnormality, deficiency of AHG, if severe enough, may be reflected in the impaired prothrombin consumption and defective thromboplastin generation tests. The amount of antihemophilic globulin is in excess of that found in patients with mild hemophilia. In one study[263] factor VIII deficiency ranged between 30 and 60% of normal. Others found levels to range from 1 to 60% of the mean normal level.[179]

The presence of severe epistaxis, which characterizes vascular hemophilia, separates this disease from mild hemophilia in which the bleeding time is normal. The disease is familial, occurs in both sexes, is probably hereditary, and is transmitted as a simple dominant. Administration of fresh plasma corrects the coagulation defect and has proved of value in treatment before and after dental extraction. Splenectomy is definitely contraindicated. Vitamin P, vitamin C, rutin, and steroids have proved ineffective in controlling epistaxis and other manifestations of the abnormal vascular component.

A source of error in the diagnosis of von Willebrand's disease is to confuse it with mild hemophilia A, since factor VIII deficiency is common to both. A prolonged bleeding time has been relied on for differentiating von Willebrand's disease from hemophilia A. However, milder cases of von Willebrand's disease often have a normal bleeding time. While inherited in an autosomal pattern, it manifests variable expressivity and like hemophilia may appear as a sporadic case. In the absence of a characteristic type of inheritance, von Willebrand's disease can be diagnosed by a diminished adhesiveness of platelets.[358]

While von Willebrand's disease is well established as a hereditary disease, it has been reported as an acquired disease. Findings characteristic of von Willebrand's disease were observed in a 14-year-old boy in the course of lupus erythematosus.[342] The findings of von Willebrand's disease disappeared following corticosteroid therapy of his lupus erythematosus.

Biggs[47] classifies the bleeding in von Willeband's disease into the spontaneous type responsible for the persistent ooze producing epistaxis, bleeding from the gums, gastrointestinal bleeding, and menorrhagia. This type is due primarily to the long bleeding time. The second type of bleeding follows trauma, can probably be related to the low blood concentration of factor VIII, and is essentially hemophilic. The control of traumatic bleeding is related more to the factor VIII concentration than to the bleeding time.

Menorrhagia is a frequent and disabling complication in women. Nilsson and Blombäck[262] reported severe menstrual bleeding in fifteen of twenty-seven mildly affected women. It is of interest that twenty-two had borne children and only eight had experienced abnormal bleeding during and after delivery. The beneficial effect of pregnancy may be ascribed to reported increases of factor VIII occurring spontaneously by the time of delivery.[262] It is of interest that one case report of a patient with von Willebrand's disease during pregnancy showed a spontaneous correction of the prolonged bleeding time and an increase in the level of AHG (factor VIII). After delivery the deviation in AHG and bleeding time returned.[375]

The fact that transfusion of normal plasma[333] or a plasma fraction[263,376] occasionally corrects the bleeding time as well as the coagulation time suggests the possibility that vascular dysfunction may result from a deficiency of a plasma vascular factor required for normal vasoconstriction which is different from AHG (factor VIII). The vascular factor that is distinct from AHG is present in normal and fresh hemophilia A plasma and decreased in von Willebrand's disease.[61,260,263] In still another group an abnormality of platelets is an added feature.[59,304] A reduction in the plasma concentration of antihemophilic globulin was observed in the members of four families suffering from von Willebrand's disease.[287] Such persons were clinically affected.

Reinvestigation of the original patients of von Willebrand still living in the Åland islands revealed not only the hereditary element, but also the dual defect of increased bleeding due to a deficient plasma factor and a coexisting low content of AHG.[61] No defect of the platelets was found. The increased capillary bleeding time could be corrected by a plasma factor, fraction 1-0 (prepared from Cohn's fraction 1 containing 86 to 90% of fibrinogen and 100% of AHG). Here, too, the effect on bleeding time was equally good whether the fraction had been prepared from plasma with a high or low platelet count. In addition, the concentrate fraction 1-0 is equally effective in controlling bleeding in those with von Willebrand's disease and in patients with classic hemophilia, both of whom require replacement of factor VIII.

The coagulation defect of von Willebrand's disease differs from that of hemophilia not only in its mode of inheritance (autosomal dominant in the former, sex-linked recessive in the latter), but also in its response to transfusion. An apparent paradox exists in the correction of AHG deficiency in von Willebrand's disease. In classic hemophilia, following the injection of fresh frozen plasma, the AHG concentration rises abruptly but not to levels above those anticipated. Following the rise there is a rapid decrease, with an estimated circulation half-time of 4 hours or less. Cornu and associates[88,213] have demonstrated that in cases of von Willebrand's disease in which a decreased level of factor VIII exists, the injection of fresh frozen plasma is followed by the expected rise in factor VIII. Subsequently, however, instead of an expected drop of factor VIII, as in classic hemophilia, there is a continued rise which is sustained 24 hours after the administration of the plasma. A similar response has been demonstrated with the transfusions of hemophilic blood and normal serum,[88] both devoid of factor VIII. Several theories have been advanced to explain this unexpected response. One is that an AHG-stimulating or AHG-mobilizing factor is present in the plasma or serum to explain the sustained increase in plasma AHG in von Willebrand's disease.[58] Another is that AHG (factor VIII) deficiency in hemophilia is related to a genetically controlled abnormality late in the cellular processes involved in factor VIII synthesis, while in von Willebrand's disease it is related to another factor that functions earlier in this series of reactions.[213] While the enzymatic defect in the synthesis of factor VIII is different in the two diseases, the final outcome is the same. In classic hemophilia there appears to be an accumulation of nonutilized precursor material from which the patient with von Willebrand's disease can synthesize factor VIII.[88] A study of the nature of the substance stimulating the production of factor VIII in von Willebrand's disease appears to be concentrated in the fibrinogen fraction of plasma.[58]

Immunological studies have been reported from two laboratories[354a,400a] in which rabbit antibody to highly purified human factor VIII was used to test for the presence or absence of factor VIII activity in the plasma of patients with classic hemophilia and von Willebrand's disease. Factor VIII activity was detected immunologically in both the serum and plasma of normal individuals and of patients with factor VIII deficiency. However, serums and plasmas from patients with von Willebrand's disease showed little or no factor VIII activity, suggesting that von Willebrand's disease is a disorder in which a true deficiency of factor VIII exists. It remains to be determined whether classic hemophilia is due to a structurally abnormal, nonfunctional factor VIII or to an inhibitor, but these studies differentiate the two disorders.

The decreased AHG values observed in many patients with von Willebrand's disease indicates that the regulation of plasma AHG is controlled by at least two genes, one of which is on the X-chromosome and abnormal in classic hemophilia, the other on an autosomal chromosome, abnormal in von Willebrand's disease.[388] In many patients plasma transfusion produces not only progressive increase in AHG activity but also corrects the abnormal adhesiveness in platelets in this disease. Weiss[388] has pointed out the great variability of this disease. He defines the term "classic von Willebrand's disease" as an inherited autosomal bleeding disorder in which the dual defects of a prolonged bleeding time and a decrease in AHG occur together. To these criteria abnormal platelet adhesiveness (Salzman test) gives added corroboration of the diagnosis.

In neither hemophiila A nor in von Willebrand's disease has it been definitely established whether a functionally defective AHG-like protein is synthesized or whether there is a simple deficiency of AHG.[12] This problem has a particular bearing in von Willebrand's disease since AHG is apparently synthesized after transfusion of normal plasma, hemophilic plasma, or serum. Abildgaard and colleagues[12] conclude that the diagnosis of von Willebrand's disease ordinarily can be confirmed by measurement (1) of the bleeding time by an appropriate method and (2) of the factor VIII level. The Ivy or modified Ivy bleeding time is more likely to be abnormal than the Duke bleeding time, but both tests are useful. Tests of platelet adhesiveness are of interest but not necessary for the diagnosis of von Willebrand's disease.

### Christmas disease (factor IX deficiency, hemophilia B, plasma thromboplastin component deficiency, PTC deficiency)

Plasma thromboplastin component deficiency,[18,51,331] often designated as Christmas disease,\* is a hemophilia-like disease due to a deficiency of factor IX (plasma thromboplastin component, PTC), one of the necessary thromboplastin precursors. It is inherited as a sex-linked recessive and therefore is confined to males and transmitted by a carrier female as is classic hemophilia. As in patients with factor VIII (AHG) deficiency there is no family history in about 25 to 30% of the patients.

---

\*After a 5-year-old boy named Christmas who was among the first patients in whom this condition was diagnosed.[51]

Cases of hemophilia B due to factor IX deficiency have been reported in a female,[360] as have been cases of hemophilia A. The case of hemophilia B in a girl was the product of a marriage between a hemophilic father and a probable carrier mother who were first cousins.

An 11-year-old girl has been reported[211] who had a bleeding diathesis and was believed to be a symptomatic carrier of Christmas disease. The factor IX level was 5% and she presented with a hemarthrosis. Christmas disease was documented in the family.

**Clinical and laboratory features.** Factor IX (PTC) deficiency constitutes about 15% of all hemophilias and is clinically indistinguishable from classic hemophilia. There are approximately four cases of factor VIII deficiency (hemophilia A) for every one of factor IX (PTC) deficiency. It also exists as a mild disease. The proportion of mild cases that is not detected seems to be higher in factor IX deficiency than in hemophilia A (factor VIII deficiency). Hemarthroses are common. The clotting time is prolonged (normal in patients with the mild form of the disease), and prothrombin consumption is abnormal (due to inadequate thromboplastin formation), but the actual defect is diagnosed by the thromboplastin generation test (located in the serum component as contrasted with the plasma component in patients with classic hemophilia). In newborn infants with hemorrhagic disease and in patients with liver disease, factor IX (PTC) deficiency is often found in combination[62] with prothrombin and stable factor (factor VII) deficiencies. An assay of the factor IX (PTC) demonstrated that a 30% concentration of the factor is sufficient to protect against ordinary everyday stresses and as much as 60% is needed to stop bleeding from major wounds. These figures correspond to 5 to 10% and 30 to 40% factor VIII (AHG), respectively, under the same conditions in patients with classic hemophilia. In one series, 16% of carriers of AHG (factor VIII) deficiency and 37% of carriers of PTC (factor IX) had abnormally low levels of the respective deficient factor.[214] While acquired deficiencies of AHG are rare and are usually associated with circulating inhibitors, acquired deficiencies of PTC are quite common and occur in conjunction with liver disease, vitamin K deficiency, and Dicumarol therapy.

**Treatment.** The general principles of treatment for Christmas disease are the same as those for classic hemophilia (factor VIII deficiency). Experience has shown that fresh frozen plasma is effective in the patient with Christmas disease and that he must be treated with this material as vigorously as the patient with factor VIII deficiency. Comparable amounts are given as in hemophilia A. Fresh frozen plasma is given 4 to 6 hours apart and later every 6 to 8 hours, depending on the site and severity of the bleeding. More frequent intervals are required at the outset in an effort to replenish the body pools with factor IX. As a general rule, traumatic bleeding may be difficult to control, even with fresh frozen plasma and concentrated preparations of factor IX made from human blood which have been hemostatically effective.[49,56] Christmas disease as well as hemophilia A (factor VIII deficiency) may be refractory to treatment due to inhibitors and circulatory antagonists,[217] probably as a result of repeated transfusions of whole blood and plasma. Here, too, concentrated factor IX preparations have been recommended, since hemostasis may be difficult to overcome with blood and plasma transfusions. Details of management in relation to dental extraction, preparation for surgery, and treatment of hemarthroses are similar to those for patients with classic hemophilia.

Another product that has been used is the plasma from which factor VIII has been removed—known as factor VIII–poor plasma. In recent years a new clotting factor concentrate known as Konȳne has become available containing factors II, VII, IX, and X.[171]

Cutter Laboratories, which supplies Konȳne, provides the following specifications:

Factor IX Complex (Konȳne) is a stable dried purified plasma fraction comprising coagulation factors II (prothrombin), VII, IX, and X with a minimal amount of total protein. It is intended for use in the treatment of congenital factor IX deficiency (hemophilia B), congenital factor VII deficiency, congenital factor X deficiency, and in other bleeding disorders resulting from an acquired deficiency of factors II, VII, IX, and X. Each bottle of Konȳne contains 500 units of factor IX, as well as amounts of factors II, VII, and X roughly proportionate to their respective levels in average fresh plasma. One unit of factor IX (or II, or VII, or X) is equivalent to the activity found in 1 ml. of average fresh plasma. Therefore, a 500-unit bottle of Konȳne is equivalent to at least two packages of fresh frozen plasma. One thousand units of Konyne (equivalent to 1 liter of fresh frozen plasma) can be administered in a volume of only 40 ml. containing 1 gm. of protein. Each bottle contains, in general: prothrombin, 500 units; factor VII, 750 units; factor IX 500 units; and factor X 600 units. It comes lyophilized and is reconstituted with 20 ml. sterile water and should be given slowly immediately after reconstitution. The half-life is 8 to 20 hours. Usually 1 unit/kg. will give a rise of 1.5%. For hemarthrosis 25 to 30 units/kg. in one dose is suggested. Levels for other sites of bleeding are the same as the dosage for factor VIII deficiency. Anti-A and anti-B agglutinins are in the range of 1:32 or below. This is considered a clinically insignificant level and the product may be safely used without typing or cross-matching. For prolonged use the same precautions are necessary as for the factor VIII concentrates.

Factor IX complex (human) or Proplex* is a dried preparation of factors II, VII, IX, and X. It is prepared from pooled human plasma and may be used for the treatment of factor IX deficiency (PTC deficiency, hemophilia B), rarer congenital deficiencies of factors II, VII, and X, and clotting factor deficiencies induced by overdoses of coumarin-type drugs. The amount of Proplex required for normal hemostasis depends on the degree of factor deficiency, the area of hemorrhage, and the desired hemostasis level of the deficient factor. Dosage can be calculated according to the following formula,[132b] or in the same manner as Konyne.

Units Proplex required = 0.3 × body weight (kg.) × desired increase (% of "normal")

*Hemophilia prophylaxis.* In a discussion of hemophilia prophylaxis[117] it was emphasized that the feasability of prophylaxis depends on the plasma clotting factor level required for reasonable protection and on the frequency of infusions necessary to maintain that level. Frequent hemorrhages are the rule in patients with severe hemophilia with less than 1% of the average normal activity of factors VIII or IX, whereas hemophiliacs with 4 or 5% activity rarely bleed without provocation. This suggests the value of a regimen of periodic infusions to maintain even these minimal levels.

---

*Manufactured by the Hyland Laboratories, Division of Travenol Laboratories, Inc., Costa Mesa, California.

Of basic importance is the knowledge of the biologic half-life of a clotting factor in order to provide a low but useful activity level in the patient suffering from the specific deficiency. Factor XIII (fibrin-stabilizing factor) has a half-life of about 6 days. Hemorrhage has been prevented in a severely deficient patient with a plasma transfusion every 5 to 6 weeks.[76] The biologic half-life of factor IX is about 31 hours, and weekly infusions of factor IX concentrate almost eliminates severe hemorrhages in patients with this deficiency.[171] In classic hemophilia, infused factor VIII disappears according to its biologic half-life of about 10 hours. Increased levels of factor VIII to maintain the hemophilic patient necessitate infusions every day or every other day. In patients with a deficiency of factor VIII due to von Willebrand's disease, the factor VIII present in the plasma is augmented by the induction of new factor VIII production. A weekly prophylactic plasma infusion may be sufficient for this disorder. A fundamental problem of prophylaxis is the cost involved when frequent administrations of the concentrate are necessary as in classic hemophilia.

*Plasma thromboplastin antecedent deficiency (factor XI deficiency, PTA deficiency, hemophilia C)*

Plasma thromboplastin antecedent deficiency is due to a deficiency of factor XI (PTA), which is required for thromboplastin formation and occurs as an inherited abnormality.[321,322] In contrast to classic hemophilia and factor IX (PTC) deficiency, this form of hemophilia manifests no sex linkage. Sporadic cases are observed as is true of the other hemophilias described.

*Clinical and laboratory features.* Factor XI (PTA) deficiency is inherited as an incompletely recessive trait since the severe defect—major PTA deficiency—results from a homozygous state with respect to PTA, while minor PTA deficiency results from the heterozygous state.[306] In the severely PTA-deficient patient factor XI is present at 3 to 20% of normal activity, the mild PTA-deficient patient has factor XI to the extent of 33 to 65%, and normal persons, greater than 67%. The patient with the severe defect has more serious and more frequent hemorrhages, whereas patients with minor PTA deficiency rarely bleed from surgery. Minor PTA deficiency is found in parents and children of subjects with major PTA deficiency.

The hemorrhagic tendency is usually milder than in patients with factor VIII (AHG) and factor IX (PTC) deficiencies. Spontaneous hemorrhage is rare but may occur as in a patient reported with cerebral hemorrhage.[162] Bleeding is usually related to trauma. Because of the infrequency of spontaneous bleeding and the relative mildness of the bleeding, factor XI (PTA) deficiency often escapes detection. As in patients with the other types of hemophilia, excessive bleeding may follow minor injuries and surgical procedures, usually dental extraction and tonsillectomy. Easy bruising and, occasionally, spontaneous epistaxis have been noted, but hemarthroses are uncommon.

Usually, the whole blood clotting time is normal or only slightly prolonged, and except in the most mildly affected patients prothrombin consumption is abnormal. The deficiency of factor XI (PTA) is detected by the thromboplastin generation test (abnormality in both the serum and plasma component as contrasted with the plasma component alone in AHG deficiency and serum component alone in PTC deficiency).

During pregnancy, fibrinogen, prothrombin, factor VII, and factor IX have been reported to be significantly increased. Recent work suggests that factors VIII and XII may also be increased while the platelet count, bleeding time, tourniquet test, and factor V concentrations are normal.[179] The levels of factor XI (PTA) during the last trimester of pregnancy, on the other hand, fall below those of the normal adult. Neonatal levels are significantly lower than the maternal levels at term and rise gradually so that in 60 days (at times, not until 9 months) normal adult levels are achieved.[168] Vitamin K does not alter the levels within the first 5 days of life and has no effect on accelerating the rate of increase to adult levels. PTA (factor XI) appears to be formed in the liver and probably does not cross the placenta from the mother to infant.[168] It is probably produced in amounts proportional to the maturity of the liver.

Two children with congenital cardiac lesions, one acyanotic with a patent ductus arteriosus and the other cyanotic with a malformation including pulmonary stenosis, exhibited PTA deficiency. Following surgery, with adequate preparation with plasma, the PTA content improved in both children.[165]

Three newborn infants with symptoms of hemorrhagic disease of the neonatal period were found to be deficient in PTA (factor XI).[168] The bleeding symptoms were not controlled by administration of vitamin K. The findings in these infants suggested that decreased activity of PTA in the newborn infant may be responsible for bleeding symptoms similar to those associated with hemorrhagic disease of the newborn infant, but it cannot be prevented by administration of vitamin K. In cases of serious hemorrhage administration of fresh frozen plasma or blood may be necessary.

*Treatment.* Contrary to previous views, there is mounting evidence that factor XI (PTA) deteriorates rapidly in banked blood. For that reason fresh blood or plasma is given in amounts approximating those used in the treatment of factor VIII (AHG) and factor IX (PTC) deficiency. This applies to treatment of the acute bleeding emergency as well as to preparation for surgical procedures.

Several cases have been reported of combination of PTA with other defects in hemostasis. Factor XI deficiency was reported in association with factor VIII (AHG) deficiency and increased vascular fragility.[282] In another case factor XI deficiency occurred with a vascular defect in a girl 15 years of age who showed extensive purpura over both lower extremities and arms.[127] An unusual case of PTA (factor XI) deficiency has been described in which a prolonged bleeding time was attributed to a defect in platelet adhesiveness.[393] The administration of normal platelets rather than fresh plasma corrected the prolonged bleeding time and indicated that the deficiency in PTA (factor XI) was not the cause of this prolonged bleeding.

In order to test for deficiencies of factor XI (PTA), plasma may be artificially depleted of this factor.[176] This is done by adding diatomaceous silica (Filter-Cel, Celite) to plasma which permits the activation and exhaustion of factor XI. This reagent now serves as a means of assay of factor XI and gives results comparable to those obtained with naturally deficient plasma.

# DISORDERS DUE TO A DEFICIENCY OF FACTORS REQUIRED FOR CONVERSION OF PROTHROMBIN TO THROMBIN (PHASE 2 OF COAGULATION)

*General considerations.* Disturbances in the second stage of coagulation result in a deficient formation of thrombin. Both intrinsic (plasma) and extrinsic (tissue) thromboplastin activate the conversion of prothrombin to thrombin in the presence of calcium so that both mechanisms play an important part in hemostasis. It has already been stated that the formation of extrinsic thromboplastin depends upon the interaction of tissue extract and factors V, VII, and X. The deficiency of these factors as well as of prothrombin is most conveniently determined in the laboratory in connection with the second stage of coagulation. The prothrombin complex, therefore, consists of prothrombin and factor V (labile factor), factor VII (stable factor), and factor X (Stuart-Prower factor). Each deficiency will be included in this discussion of phase 2 coagulation, although factors V and X are also involved in the first phase of coagulation with plasma thromboplastin formation. Deficiencies of the factors of the prothrombin complex may be congenital in origin or may be acquired in various disease states. Members of the prothrombin complex are synthesized in the liver so that deficiency of one or all of the factors is found in patients with liver disease. Combined deficiencies of the four components are most commonly found in patients with parenchymal liver disease such as infectious hepatitis and cirrhosis.

*Vitamin K–dependent clotting factors.* Four of the various factors made in the liver are vitamin K dependent. Prothrombin, factor VII (stable factor), factor X (Stuart-Prower factor), and factor IX (Christmas factor, PTC) require vitamin K for synthesis. Factor V (labile factor), factor XI (PTA), and fibrinogen are also made in the liver but are not vitamin K dependent.[345] The vitamin K–dependent clotting factors behave in a like manner during health and disease. These four clotting factors are collectively referred to as the vitamin K–dependent clotting factors, less correctly as the prothrombin complex. The four clotting factors are decreased with Dicumarol administration, vitamin K deficiency, malabsorption, and obstructive jaundice.[218] Their concentration is low at birth and may decrease even further during the first days of life, resulting in hemorrhagic disease of the newborn infant.

*Vitamin K deficiency*

Vitamin K is a dietary principle required for the normal clotting time of blood. In chicks fed fat-free diets Dam and associates[93] observed the development of hemorrhages in various tissues and noted further that is was associated with a longer clotting time of the blood. It was soon determined that the delay in clotting resulting from this deficiency could be corrected by feeding the chicks substances containing an active principle, vitamin K. Prothrombin is synthesized by the liver from vitamin K, but the mechanism by which synthesis is achieved is still unknown. Deficiencies of vitamin K, regardless of cause, are now known to result in a simultaneous depletion of prothrombin and factors VII, IX, and X. The administration of vitamin K corrects deficiencies of these four factors.

Hypoprothrombinemia combined with a deficiency of factors VII, IX, and X occurs in various states in which vitamin K is reduced. Since natural vitamin K is fat soluble, bile is required for its absorption. A deficiency is very likely to occur whenever bile is prevented from entering the intestinal tract as occurs in patients with biliary obstruction and in those with hepatic disease due to toxic and infectious agents since the reactions of vitamin K in prothrombin synthesis are impaired. Deficiencies occur in the presence of faulty intestinal absorption such as occurs in patients with celiac disease, diarrhea, gastrointestinal malformation, and steatorrheas. Green vegetables and products of intestinal bacteria are among the richest sources of vitamin K. Hypoprothrombinemia due to a deficient intake of this vitamin is rare, because prothrombin is capable of being elaborated from the small amounts of this vitamin commonly found in foods and also produced by the intestinal flora. In newborn infants, hypoprothrombinemia occurs in the first days of life until the normal intestinal bacterial flora become established.

It has been pointed out that hemorrhagic manifestations are the exception rather than the rule in vitamin K deficiency,[179] but a tendency to excessive bleeding at surgery will always be present, unless the deficiency is corrected. In vitamin K deficiency the lesions are purpuric (superficial) rather than hemophilioid (deep and intramuscular) in type. The petechial hemorrhages are not as serious as in moderately severe cases of thrombocytopenic purpura. Hemarthroses do not occur. Oozing from surgical wounds is common, and bleeding from the gums or gastrointestinal tract is not unusual.[179] In hemorrhagic disease of the newborn infant, melena is more common and other bleeding manifestations are less common.

While it was formerly believed that vitamin K was concerned with the synthesis of prothrombin alone, it is now known that it is also essential for the synthesis of factors VII, IX, and X. The coumarin-like anticoagulants inhibit the synthesis of these four factors, but their action is reversed by vitamin K. The dicoumarin group has a complex effect on the clotting mechanism, acting as anticoagulants by interfering with the hepatic synthesis of the vitmain K–dependent clotting factors. An early fall is found in factor VII, a later decrease in factors IX and X, and, usually, a less important fall in the prothrombin level.[55] A marked reduction in prothrombin usually occurs only with a gross overdosage. Because of the passage of dicoumarin into breast milk, mothers receiving the drug should not nurse during the period of anticoagulant therapy. By far the most useful test for the detection of vitamin K deficiency is the one-stage prothrombin time test. If this is normal, a deficiency of vitamin K is excluded, while a prolongation indicates presumptive evidence of a deficiency.

Bishydroxycoumarin (Dicumarol) was demonstrated in the circulation of an infant born of a mother receiving anticoagulant treatment for thrombophlebitis.[323] The half-time disappearance of the drug in both mother and infant was 51 hours. Prothrombin and factors VII, IX, and X reduced by the administration of coumarin anticoagulant drugs are further influenced by the variable reduction of these clotting factors observed in cord blood and in the immediate postnatal period due to immaturity of liver function, inadequate formation and absorption of vitamin K, and its abnormal utilization. Factor V is not seriously reduced.

It seems quite clear that factors II (prothrombin), VII, IX (plasma thromboplastin component), and X (Stuart-Prower factor) are synthesized in the liver. These four factors are vitamin K dependent and are commonly deficient in severe liver disease. There is suggestive evidence that the liver is the principal, perhaps the only, site of factor I (fibrinogen) synthesis. Increased fibrinolytic activity of the blood is present in patients suffering from cirrhosis of the liver.[215]

It will be recognized that the administration of oral anticoagulant drugs during pregnancy carries the risk of fetal and neonatal bleeding. The results of Mountain and co-workers[253] suggest that the anticonvulsant drugs, especially barbiturates, when given to the mother during pregnancy, decrease the levels of the vitamin K–dependent clotting factors in the infant during the early neonatal period.

Treatment of the mother with vitamin $K_1$ will prevent the coagulation defect in the neonate. The administration of vitamin $K_1$ controls bleeding in the neonate and may also be used to prevent bleeding in infants born to mothers treated with anticonvulsant drugs.

*Congenital deficiencies.* Congenital deficiencies represent coagulation disorders resulting from isolated deficiencies of one of the factors of the prothrombin complex. The bleeding manifestations are similar to those observed in patients with disorders in which multiple deficiencies exist and will be described later. In the congenital deficiencies (prothrombin, factors V, VII, and X) vitamin K treatment is uniformly unsuccessful.

*Idiopathic (congenital) hypoprothrombinemia.* Congenital prothrombin deficiencies are rare, but authentic cases of failure to synthesize this protein have been reported. There may be a family history of idiopathic hypoprothrombinemia, with hemorrhages appearing in childhood and bleeding from mucous surfaces and into skin and tissues. Since the majority of patients with hypoprothrombinemia usually possess associated deficiencies, it is important to rule out factor V (labile) and factor VII (stable factor) involvement, especially the latter,[299] before the diagnosis of true hypoprothrombinemia is justified.

### Congenital deficiency of factor V (parahemophilia, Owren's disease, labile factor deficiency)

Originally described by Owren[274,275] and since by others,[21] factor V deficiency is detected by a prolonged one-stage prothrombin time with undiluted plasma, which is corrected when the patient's plasma is mixed with deprothrombinized (barium sulfate–absorbed) normal human plasma. The coagulation time of whole blood is prolonged, and the bleeding time may be prolonged or normal. In patients with factor V or factor VIII deficiencies, bleeding is usually from the mucous membranes and skin. In both conditions the bleeding tendency dates from infancy but may not be manifested until later in childhood after trauma or a surgical procedure, such as tonsillectomy. Many newborn infants have low levels of factor V during the first 2 days of life which rise toward normal by the sixth day.[184] A syndrome of congenital factor V deficiency with syndactylism has been reported. In this family with normal parents five of seven siblings had syndactylism and a bleeding tendency. In three of the children a deficiency of factor V in the plasma was demonstrated.[104]

Factor V deficiency is a familial disease affecting both sexes and is transmitted as an incompletely dominant gene.[273] It has also been suggested[198] that the plasma of the homozygous patient is almost entirely lacking in factor V and the patient is a bleeder. However, the heterozygous person has only a partial deficiency and is usually not a bleeder. The disease may be of variable intensity. The only treatment of known value is transfusion with *fresh* normal blood or plasma, because of the lability of the factor. The abnormality is not affected by vitamin K. Acquired factor V deficiency occurs in persons with a variety of clinical conditions, usually in association with prothrombin deficiency since both factors are affected simultaneously after surgical operations, and in the presence of liver disease, leukemia, malignancies, pernicious anemia, and abruptio placentae. A combined deficiency of factor V and factor VIII (AHG) has been reported in two sisters and in a child of a first cousin marriage.[191] The clinical severity of the condition was remarkably slight in the three cases, although each had less than 10% factor V and less than 20% factor VIII. Factor V deficiency has been reported in patients with hemorrhagic scarlet fever (purpura fulminans).[201]

Fresh frozen plasma was effective in maintaining hemostasis in factor V deficiency as long as the levels of this factor remained above 25%.[385] The mean biologic half-life of factor V in transfused frozen fresh plasma is 36 hours.

### Congenital factor VII deficiency (stable factor deficiency, proconvertin deficiency, congenital hypoconvertinemia)

Isolated stable factor deficiency has been reported,* but its incidence is relatively rare. Recent reviews have compiled the cases of isolated congenital factor VII deficiency.[235,272] Affected patients give a history of excessive bleeding dating from early life.[33] Hemorrhagic phenomena are seen in patients with factor VII concentrations of approximately 10% or less

---

*See references 22, 110, 202, 249, and 303.

of normal.[19] Bruising, petechiae, marked epistaxis, menorrhagia, hematuria, hemarthrosis, melena, hematomas, and often bleeding after dental extraction are common phenomena in this group. Spontaneous hemorrhages have been described in the central nervous system, especially subarachnoid bleeding. The disease is familial and transmitted by an autosomal "intermediate" gene which produces severe deficiency in the homozygote and partial deficiency in the heterozygote.[143] The gene for factor VII is, therefore, neither completely dominant nor recessive. A decreased activity of factor VII may be found in relatives of patients who show greatly decreased amounts of this factor. In one family intracranial hemorrhage was the cause of death of the father and the siblings.[275] Three general ranges of plasma factor VII have been differentiated in the families of the propositus: normal (75 to 200%), reduced or intermediate (25 to 75%), and low (0 to 25%). The bleeders probably are homozygous for the abnormal gene. The "carrier" often has a reduced level of clotting factor. However, some carriers have normal levels and can be identified only if they have a severely affected offspring.[235]

As is true of factors V and X, deficiency of factor VII lengthens the prothrombin time. The one-stage plasma prothrombin time of Quick is prolonged and is corrected by the addition of serum (fresh or stored) which contains factor VII but is not corrected by prothrombin-free plasma (barium sulfate treated). The bleeding and whole blood clotting time may be normal or prolonged. Clotting time is normal in the presence of small amounts of factor VII but is prolonged in its complete absence. Acquired factor VII deficiency occurs in patients with many pathologic conditions, probably always with some prothrombin defect (such as are caused by dicoumarin and Tromexan therapy).

The half-life of factor VII is short (35 to 300 minutes). Despite its well-known stability in vitro, factor VII is extremely labile in vivo. Treatment consists of the transfusion of banked blood or plasma. Multiple transfusions are usually necessary. There is sometimes the need for a therapeutic regimen like that required by classic hemophilia, i.e., calculated infusions of blood plasma.[272] Sufficient plasma to produce a factor VII level of 10 to 20% at the time of major surgery and in each of several days postoperatively will assure normal hemostasis.[235] Vitamin K is ineffective since it will not correct a congenital defect in which the inability of the end organ, the liver, to synthesize factor VII exists.

*Bleeding in the newborn.* In orientation to diagnosis of the newborn who is bleeding, the origin of the blood must be determined. A careful maternal and family history is essential. The site of the origin of blood in the gastrointestinal tract may be maternal and swallowed by the infant at the time of delivery or it may come from the infant itself and represent true hemorrhage. The alkali denaturation test described by Apt and Downey (see Chapter 1) may be applied to the vomitus or stool and will differentiate between the mother's blood containing adult hemoglobin and the infant's blood which is predominantly fetal hemoglobin.

*Maternal history.* This should include all infections during pregnancy which may cause a hematologic abnormality in the infant predisposing to hemorrhage such as cytomegalic inclusion disease, toxoplasmosis, syphilis, and any viral infection such as rubella, coxsackie B, or herpes simplex. Other illnesses in the mother which may be transmitted to the infant and present before pregnancy include lupus erythematosus, malignancies such as leukemia, Hodgkin's disease, malignant melanoma, and thrombocytopenic purpura. Drug ingestion either for illnesses listed above or for other complaints of pregnancy is important information. The drugs most commonly known to cause difficulty are the thiazides, quinine, antimalarials, sulfonamides, dicumarol, barbiturates, salicylates, and anticonvulsants. The family history must be scrutinized for "hemophilia," commonly factor VIII, IX, XI, and von Willebrand's disease, and for other rare congenital disorders such as factor XIII deficiency from either maternal or paternal families.

*Physical examination.* The infant should be examined carefully for the site of bleeding, the type of bleeding, whether the lesions are local or generalized, and whether there is oozing from puncture sites. Hemorrhagic disease of the newborn usually presents with bleeding from the gastrointestinal tract or oozing from circumcision or cord. Hemophilia presents with subcutaneous hematomas or cephalhematomas; massive hematomas usually occur with birth trauma; petechiae on the face occur with cord wrapped around the neck or generalized petechiae with platelet anomaly or systemic disease such as cytomegalic inclusion disease. Note color of the skin for icterus or for other signs of sepsis or for organomegaly, particularly liver and spleen, as evidence of systemic disease which might affect the clotting mechanism.

*Laboratory tests.* The basic laboratory tests which may help to determine the extent of bleeding in the infant should begin with a complete blood count including platelet count. The screening tests for the plasmatic factors of the clotting mechanism should include the activated partial thromboplastin time, the Quick prothrombin time, one tube clotting time to be used for observation of clot retraction, and whenever possible a fibrinogen determination and a euglobulin clot lysis time. If the platelets are present in normal numbers and there are no petechiae on physical examination, findings against platelet dysfunction, then a deficiency of the clotting factors should be investigated.

With the aid of the prothrombin time, and the partial thromboplastin time, it is possible to determine deficiencies of the vitamin K–dependent factors or deficiencies of factors VIII, IX, or XI or von Willebrand's disease. With Quick prothrombin time the range for the newborn is 16 to 18 seconds with a normal control of 11 to 12 seconds. The neonatal values return to normal in approximately 1 week. The prothrombin time tests for all of the factors in the second and third stage of the clotting process, namely factors II, V, and X, as well as factor VII and fibrinogen.

The activated partial thromboplastin time (PTT) screens for the presence of all the factors in the intravascular system—I, II, V, VIII, IX, X, XI, and XII—excluding only factor VII. The normal newborn because of the physiologic deficiencies already noted may have a value of 60 to 80 seconds compared with the normal adult value of 36 to 46 seconds. The value for the neonate should fall to the normal range within a week.

In the male infants the common sex-linked recessive deficiencies of factors VIII and IX should be considered first and for female infants the autosomal deficiencies of factor XI and von Willebrand's disease first. If the partial thromboplastin time remains prolonged and the prothrombin time remains long there has been no effect from vitamin K and the rare congenital defects of factor II, V, VII, and X should be considered and appropriate assays performed. Should both the partial thromboplastin time and prothrombin time be relatively normal for the age, a factor XIII deficiency should be considered and the retracted clot observed for friability as well as a qualitative assay for factor XIII be done using monochloracetic acid.

## Hemorrhagic disease of the newborn infant (hypoprothrombinemia in the newborn infant)

Hemorrhagic disease of the newborn infant is a self-limited hemorrhagic disorder, occurring usually between the first and fifth day after birth, caused by a marked deficiency of the vitamin K–dependent clotting factors—i.e., prothrombin and factors VII, IX (PTC), and X (Stuart-Prower factor).*

The disease does not occur during the first 24 hours after birth or later than the fifth day after birth. The one-stage prothrombin time, which is normal at birth, is increased between the first and fifth day due to a fall in the concentration of the vitamin K–dependent clotting factors. After the fifth day the prothrombin time may revert to normal in spite of decreased prothrombin and factor VII levels, a circumstance that may be due to a gross excess of factor V occurring at birth.[179]

The lack of full development of all coagulation factors at birth is shown in Table 30.

The deficiency of the vitamin K–dependent factors is more pronounced in the premature infant than in the full-term baby; and the return to normal takes place more slowly. Premature infants show somewhat more severe alterations of the factor VII complex (factors VII and X) and in the first-stage thromboplastin generation than is sometimes found in the full-term infant.[5] Aballi and deLamerens[5] describe derangement of the first stage of coagulation (thromboplastin generation), which may be due to a deficiency of factors IX and X as well as the deficiency of the other vitamin K–dependent factors, in the newborn infant. Hemorrhagic disease of the newborn infant, however, is caused primarily by the deficiency of the factors in the latter group. To what extent coincidental thromboplastin generation disorders are contribu-

*See references 3, 4, 75, 221, and 334.

Table 30. Coagulation factors in normal full-term newborn

|  | Cord | 3 days | 14 days |
|---|---|---|---|
| Factor I | 250 mg. % | | |
| Factor II | 24-54% | 5-12% | 80% |
| Factor V | 100% | | 70-120% |
| Factor VII | 29-43% | 15-25% | 70-100% |
| Factor VIII | 70-120% | | 70-120% |
| Factor IX | 20-80% | | 40-80% |
| Factor X | 21-54% | | 60-80% |
| Factor XI | 10-60% | 13-85% | 23-79% |
| Factor XII | | 25-100% | 100% |
| Factor XIII | 40-50% | | 100% |

tory requires further study. A secondary type of hemorrhagic disease has also been described unresponsive to vitamin K in which factor V is often very low and thrombocytopenia occasionally occurs,[5] and which is not as clearly attributable to a deficiency of the usual vitamin K–dependent factors and may simulate the manifestations of disseminated intravascular coagulation.

Immaturity of the liver enzyme systems in the newborn with relatively slow maturation is a well-known fact which finds its counterpart in decreased synthesis of the clotting proteins. All of the clotting proteins with the exception of factor VIII are manufactured in the liver. The levels of factors II, VII, IX, X, XII, and XIII are low in cord blood with a fall to even lower levels at 3 days of age and a subsequent rise to normal adult values within 2 weeks for most of the factors but with a lag period of as long as 9 months for factors IX and XI.

There are other factors that are reduced in the normal infant in addition to those involved in the initial stages of coagulation (factors XII, XI, and IX) and the vitamin K–dependent factors (II, VII, IX, and X). These are the "Fletcher factor," low in the newborn infant,[155] and the existence of "fetal fibrinogen."[397] The thrombin time which measures the conversion of fibrinogen to fibrin which is moderately prolonged in the normal newborn infant for the first few days of life may be due to the "fetal fibrinogen" and perhaps to the increased fibrin split products.[154]

Several factors contribute to the genesis of physiologic deficiency of vitamin K–dependent clotting factors: the bacteria-free nature of the newborn infant's intestinal tract which prevents vitamin K synthesis until intestinal flora are established with food ingestion, liver immaturity, a lack of reserve supply of the vitamin, and, in some cases, a depletion of vitamin K in the mother due to poor dietary intake, poor absorption, and impaired utilization due to liver dysfunction.

Although vitamin K may cross the placenta, absolute values in the infant are dependent on the mother's ingestion, diet, or therapeutic supplements and may vary a good deal. Should large amounts of this vitamin cross the placenta to allow for synthesis of the clotting proteins, maintenance of that supply is cut off at delivery and the infant must wait until his gut becomes colonized with organisms which may produce a vitamin K of questionable value or until he ingests sufficient amounts of milk to give the necessary 8 µg of vitamin K per kg. per day. This vitamin is necessary for the synthesis of factor II (prothrombin), VII, IX, and X.

Concentrations of 20 to 25% of vitamin K–dependent clotting factors are critical values below which a potential hemorrhagic state exists. Values of 5% and lower occur in infants with hemorrhagic disease. In the majority of patients, bleeding occurs spontaneously during the period when the concentration of vitamin K–dependent clotting factors is sharply reduced. The incidence of hemorrhagic disease of the newborn infant is given variously as about 1 in 200 to 400 births, but it appears much less commonly at present, perhaps due to the widespread use of vitamin K.

A deficiency of factor IX (PTC), active in the first phase of coagulation, occurs in combination with prothrombin and factor VII deficiencies in the newborn period.[2,241,373,377] Factor IX deficiency follows the pattern of the prothrombin complex in the first weeks of life, with its most marked decrease about the third day of life and spontaneous increases thereafter. Aballi and co-workers[2] observed marked improvement in factor IX concentration by administering vitamin K to full-term infants but saw an inadequate response in the premature infant. Because of the slowness with which prothrombin, factor VII, and factor IX return to nonhemorrhagic levels in the premature infant and because of the inadequacy of vitamin K therapy, it may be safer to defer circumcision for a period of 3 to 4 weeks.

*Clinical and laboratory features.* Bleeding is rarely massive, consisting of persistent oozing from the umbilical cord and mucous surfaces, hematemesis, hematuria, gastrointestinal and vaginal bleeding, petechiae, ecchymoses, and, infrequently, spontaneous central nervous system and meningeal hemorrhage. Serious hemorrhage can occur from minor trauma. Circumcision may result in slow and continued bleeding.[85] There is suggestive evidence that the factor IX deficiency is especially responsible for the prolonged coagulation time and the tendency to bleed encountered in patients with this disease.[3]

The platelet count is normal, and anemia is proportional to blood loss. In addition to prolonged prothrombin time, prolonged coagulation and bleeding times occasionally occur but are not necessary for the diagnosis. The one-stage prothrombin time is prolonged and is often more than twice that of the normal control. As would be expected, factor IX (PTC), which is one of the vitamin K–dependent factors, may also be sufficiently depressed to interfere with thromboplastin generation and produce abnormal first-stage tests.[5] The presence of an associated vascular lesion is suggested by the prolonged bleeding time, rarely positive tourniquet test, and evidence of skin hemorrhages.

*Differential diagnosis.* The stools of many infants are benzidine positive, indicating the presence of blood. A markedly prolonged prothrombin time differentiates hemorrhagic disease of the newborn infant from blood derived from maternal sources such as blood swallowed at birth or while nursing from fissured nipples. In a grossly bloody stool this test is helpful, but the identification of the source of blood in regard to its maternal or fetal nature is even more specific.

The application of the alkali denaturation test distinguishes between maternal blood (adult type) and infant's blood (fetal type), the latter being more resistant to denaturation with alkali than adult hemoglobin.[26] Anticoagulant therapy in the mother may provoke serious bleeding in the fetus and newborn infant.[139] Conditions other than the hypoprothrombinemias deserve consideration in the differential diagnosis. Disorders of thromboplastin formation and afibrinogenemia can be eliminated by appropriate tests. Oozing from the umbilical cord occurs in infants with hemorrhagic disease but is unusual in those with hemophilia. Infants with congenital thrombocytopenic purpura, congenital syphilis, bacteremia, and hemorrhagic manifestations of erythroblastosis fetalis also present clinical bleeding in the first days of life. Petechiae of the face, head, and neck may occur without any marked depletion of platelets and are due to a local or regional increase in venous pressure or are a result of a temporary compression of superficial veins.[121]

*Treatment.* The discovery of vitamin K by Dam[93] and of its relationship to prothrombin formation led to its use in pregnant women before delivery and in the infant at birth to prevent hypoprothrombinemia. Doubt has been thrown on the value of vitamin K in the prevention[157] and management[124] of hemorrhagic disease of the newborn infant. In the premature infant especially, the shortage of vitamin K is not so important as the inadequate synthesis of the clotting factors (vitamin K–dependent group) caused by immaturity of the liver. Occasionally, prothrombin levels have been raised by vitamin K given to the mother or infant, but this did not reduce the incidence of the disease. There is ample evidence, however, that the administration of vitamin K to the newborn infant arrests the fall of the vitamin K–dependent clotting factors although normal levels may not be achieved.[113] In another series, vitamin K administration corrected all the clotting defects (factors VII, IX, and X deficiencies and hypoprothrombinemia) associated with hemorrhagic disease of the newborn infant.[3,4] Until a more effective means of controlling hemorrhagic disease of the newborn infant, with its potentially serious clinical manifestations, becomes available, vitamin K therapy still remains the agent of choice for prophylaxis and treatment.

*Vitamin K.* The large number of vitamin K preparations may be classified as those containing oil-soluble vitamin K and the synthetic analogues, many of which are water soluble. One of the very effective natural vitamin K products, $K_1$, phytonadione (Konakion, Mephyton), can be given intramuscularly, intravenously, or as a tablet for oral use. Two synthetic water-soluble vitamin K preparations which are in common use are menadiol sodium bisulphate (Hykinone) and menadiol sodium diphosphate (Synkavite). They are available for oral use and subcutaneous, intramuscular, and intravenous injection.

Excessive doses of vitamin K are to be avoided because of their known hemolytic action and tendency to cause hyperbilirubinemia, especially in the premature infant. It has, therefore, been recommended by the Council on Drugs of the American Medical Association[111] that, as an equivalent of 1 mg. of synthetic vitamin $K_1$, menadione is adequate to prevent hemorrhagic disease of the newborn infant.

The natural $K_1$ vitamins act more rapidly than the synthetic preparations and raise plasma prothrombin to therapeutic levels within 2 to 4 hours. Phytonadione is of special value in threatening or actual hemorrhage. Prophylaxis of hemorrhagic disease of the newborn infant is achieved by the use of phytonadione (Mephyton) or other natural or synthetic vitamin K (menadione) by giving the mother daily doses of 2 to 4 mg. orally for 1 week before delivery or parenteral injection of an equivalent dose of one of the water-soluble preparations several hours before delivery. For the infant at birth phytonadione is effective when given intramuscularly in a 1 to 2 mg. dose. The water-soluble forms of vitamin K (Hykinone, Synkavite) are, however, completely adequate in the presence of vitamin K–deficiency states.

In our own institution vitamin $K_1$ (phytonadione) is administered intramuscularly to all premature or full-term newborn infants in the delivery room in a dosage not exceeding 1 mg. Phytonadione prevents a neonatal decline in blood levels of the vitamin K–dependent coagulation factors (prothrombin, factors VII, IX and X) when given immediately following birth.

In some areas, vitamin K is given only to poorly nourished groups in which breast feeding is widely practiced.[240] Others have found that as much as 20 mg. of phytonadione given to the mother 4 to 24 hours before delivery serves as a practical prophylactic measure in preventing hemorrhage in the newborn infant, without danger of kernicterus.[386] On the other hand, some have maintained that no specific dose or route of administration of vitamin K could be designated for the woman in labor that would provide effective and safe prophylaxis for the infant. For this reason it has been recommended that vitamin K prophylaxis (parenteral dose of 0.5 to 1 mg. of vitamin $K_1$ or an oral dose of 1 to 2 mg.) be administered to the infant after birth rather than prenatally through administration to the mother.[317]

The danger of hyperbilirubinemia in the infant from excessive dosage of vitamin K given to the mother has been noted.[225] The parenteral administration of 72 mg. of a vitamin K analogue (menadione sodium bisulfate, Hykinone) during labor resulted in bilirubin levels in the newborn premature infant ranging from 21 to 47 mg. per 100 ml. with neurologic sequelae in two patients.

Transfusions of blood or plasma are given to replenish prothrombin, factor VII (stable factor), factor X (Stuart-Prower factor), and factor IX (PTC factor) and in severely affected patients to combat anemia and shock.

Specifically, the dose of 1 mg. of phytonadione may be repeated at once should hematemesis, melena, or ecchymoses occur. The time lag before vitamin K will have its maximum effect is 4 hours. If bleeding has been sufficient to cause anemia, fresh whole blood at 20 ml. per kilogram may then be given for hemostasis. When bleeding persists in the face of therapy, more complete investigation should be undertaken to establish a congenital defect or to document an unusually low PTA (factor XI) level which is unaffected by phytonadione.

Although external bleeding can be controlled, internal bleeding results in an appreciable mortality (estimated at 70%).

### Factor X deficiency (Stuart-Prower factor deficiency)

The Stuart-Prower factor[101,181,334] functions in the formation of both intrinsic and extrinsic thromboplastin. Deficiencies of the factor have been found in patients with liver disease, in newborn infants with hemorrhagic disease, and in patients receiving coumarin compounds.[140] The deficiency is transmitted as an incompletely recessive autosomal character. In the heterozygote this factor is reduced on an average of 36% and causes mild bleeding. The homozygote has a moderately severe hemorrhagic disorder manifested by epistaxis, hematomas, and hemarthrosis. A deficiency of Stuart-Prower factor is an important part of the clotting defect of premature[334] and full-term infants.[4] Treatment with fresh blood or plasma is desirable.

The clinical features of this disease are not strikingly different from those of factor V or factor VII deficiencies. Only when critical levels of 5% are reached does overt bleeding occur.[276] Rabiner and Kretchmer[301] presented evidence suggesting that the two activities of the Stuart-Prower factor (factor X)—i.e., the production of both extrinsic and intrinsic thromboplastin—may vary independently. They studied a boy with a marked deficiency of the factor in both phases; his father had a marked deficiency in the first phase and a moderate deficiency in the second, whereas his sister had a moderate deficiency in the first phase only.

In patients on long-term anticoagulant therapy the most frequent cause of bleeding is a severe depression of factor X.[276] In factor X deficiency the whole blood clotting time and prothrombin consumption may be abnormal. Patients who have active bleeding show a long one-stage prothrombin time using brain thromboplastin or Russell's viper venom and lecithin. The serum of such patients gives poor results in the thromboplastin generation test.[179] One of the clotting activities of rabbit brain thromboplastin is involved in the activation of factor X.[259]

A 7-year-old Negro who had been active and in good health suffered a severe hemorrhagic disease with a single acquired defect in coagulation factor X.[37] No cause for deficiency could be found. He improved spontaneously and was completely healthy 6 months later.

### Factor XII deficiency (Hageman factor deficiency)

The Hageman factor deficiency has been shown to result from the homozygous state of an autosomal recessive characteristic.[314] This factor participates in the early stages of coagulation. Present in an inactive form in normal blood, it is activated by contact with a foreign surface and in turn activates factor XI (PTA), thereby initiating thromboplastin formation. Blood deficiency in this factor shows prolonged clotting time, poor prothrombin consumption, and decreased thromboplastin formation. Despite abnormality of in vitro coagulation, individuals deficient in this factor do not ordinarily manifest hemorrhagic tendencies although a few had menorrhagia or mild bleeding after surgical procedures, childbirth, or injury.[309]

On March 24, 1968, Mr. John Hageman, the index patient with Hageman trait, died unexpectedly 12 days after sustaining fractures of the left ischium and ilium. The cause of death was pulmonary embolism.[307] Neither he nor his family had had a bleeding tendency. He had not bled excessively after tonsillectomy, dental extraction, or injuries. In a glass tube Mr. Hageman's blood had a prolonged clotting time, yet he had had no bleeding diathesis. The Hageman factor apparently inert in circulating blood is "activated" upon contact with glass or similar substances. Once activated, Hageman factor initiates the reactions described as the intrinsic pathway of blood coagulation by changing plasma thromboplastin antecedent (PTA, factor XI) to its active form.

It is worthwhile to recall that the Hageman trait is the inherited deficiency of a specific plasma protein, Hageman factor (factor XII). The trait is inherited in an autosomal recessive manner. One gene locus responsible for the synthesis of Hageman factor could be the short arm of chromosome 6.[99]

The kinins,[197,326] a group of polypeptides with potent biologic activities, are capable of influencing smooth-muscle contraction and increasing blood flow. Microvascular permeability, among other properties, shows a relationship to the Hageman factor. It had been suggested that the activation of the Hageman factor might be an essential step for the activation of a kinin permeability factor.[237]

### Multiple defects

*Capillary and single coagulation factor deficiency.* Von Willebrand's disease (vascular hemophilia) represents a dual hemostatic disorder in which a capillary defect responsible for clinical bleeding is combined with a factor VIII (AHG) deficiency. The vascular defect alone is responsible for an increased bleeding time and often a positive tourniquet test. Capillary disorders have also been found to coexist with either labile or stable factor deficiencies (factors V and VII, respectively), with congenital afibrinogenemia, and with double factor deficiencies.[372] A case of factor XI deficiency has been described in association with a prolonged bleeding time. The failure to correct the prolonged bleeding time with fresh plasma demonstrated that factor XI deficiency was not the cause of the vascular defect.[393]

*Multiple factor deficiencies.* A combined deficiency of factor VIII (AHG) and factor IX (PTC)[169] and of congenital factor V with factor VIII (AHG) deficiency has also been described.[185,336] In another case a hemorrhagic diathesis was described in a young adult with symptoms dating from childhood which were found to be due to deficiencies of factors VIII, IX, and XI.[25] Some of his family members showed a mild disorder of coagulation due to a partial deficiency of one or more factors.

## DISORDERS DUE TO A DEFICIENCY OF FIBRINOGEN (PHASE 3 OF COAGULATION)

A deficiency of fibrinogen is a rare coagulation defect resulting in a profound disturbance of the blood-clotting mechanism. The complete deficiency is congenital, whereas conditions with reduced amounts of fibrinogen (hypofibrinogenemia or fibrinogenopenia) are either congenital or acquired.

Immunochemical methods employing specific antifibrinogen serums have demonstrated that liver parenchymal cells normally contain small amounts of fibrinogen.[34] Only a few parenchymal cells appear to be actively engaged in synthesis. On stimulation, liver parenchymal cells produce and store large quantities of fibrinogen. Neutrophilic leukocytes contain fibrin or fibrinogen breakdown products which have been phagocytized by these blood cells.

The relationship between fibrinogen and platelet structure has been the subject of considerable controversy. Two groups of investigators have debated whether fibrinogen is present in the inner structure or on the surface of platelets. It has been thought that certain adsorbed plasma proteins on the platelet membrane, particularly fibrinogen, play an important role in platelet physiology. When fluorescent-labeled antifibrinogen serum and enzyme-treated platelets were used, evidence was provided that fibrinogen is part of the platelet structure rather than being bound to its surface with physical interaction.[137] Fibrinogen was also present in the cytoplasm of the megakaryocyte. In another study part of the total platelet fibrinogen was localized in the intracellular granule to form an integral part of the interior structure of the platelet.[255] (More on platelet fibrinogen on p. 684, earlier in this chapter.)

### Congenital afibrinogenemia

Congenital afibrinogenemia is marked by a complete, or practically complete, and permanent absence of fibrinogen from the blood resulting in a hemorrhagic syndrome resembling hemophilia, except that it affects either sex.[292] The patient is frequently the offspring of a consanguineous marriage. An incomplete recessive or semidominant inheritance[257] is postulated since low fibrinogen levels are occasionally found in the parents of affected children.[128]

Bleeding is manifest from birth, with excessive oozing from the umbilical cord or from the navel on separation of the cord and after circumcision. Persistent bleeding follows trauma, surgical procedures, and the loss of deciduous teeth. Excessive bruising and epistaxis are common. In contrast to hemophilia, hemarthroses are rare.[216] Joint disability does not result, even in this circumstance, probably due to a lack of fibrin formation. Except for the absence of fibrinogen, the other phases of clotting are normal. Despite incoagulable blood, long intervals with freedom from hemorrhage are common,[23] and the condition is usually associated with only a minor degree of disability.

### Congenital hypofibrinogenemia

Reduced fibrinogen levels may be present in parents of children with afibrinogenemia in whom bleeding is absent or in patients with "constitutional fibrinogenemia" in whom there is a tendency toward abnormal bleeding.

### Acquired fibrinogen deficiency

Acquired fibrinogen deficiencies have been noted in patients with many conditions such as severe liver disease, bone marrow involvement with invasion by leukemic or tumor cells, polycythemia vera, malignancies, tuberculosis, shock, burns, transfusion reactions,[90] and obstetric complications.

**Dysfibrinogenemias.** The term dysfibrinogenemia includes the more descriptive terms hypo- and hyperfibrinogenemia. The term parafibrinogenemia has been employed[38] to designate the presence of fibrinogens not normally encountered in human plasma. The latter refers to congenital variants of human fibrinogen. Mild hemorrhage as well as recurrent thrombosis may be presenting symptoms in patients with abnormal fibrinogen but alterations of the coagulation mechanism due to the presence of abnormal fibrinogen have been described in the absence of such symptoms. Beck[38] suggests that the presence of an abnormal fibrinogen should be suspected under the following circumstances: familial hypofibrinogenemia, prolonged thrombin clotting time, formation of friable clots without evidence of acquired hypofibrinogenemia or activated fibrinolysis, anticoagulant activity interfering with clotting of normal fibrinogen by thombin, and abnormal fibrin stabilization.

An abnormal fibrinogen was reported by Beck and co-workers[39] in a 29-year-old woman with a mild hemorrhagic diathesis. The abnormal fibrinogen represented a dysfibrinogenemia rather than a hypofibrinogenemia. Investigation revealed the presence of a similar abnormal fibrinogen in all three daughters of the proposita, whereas the two sons had normally clottable fibrinogen. The disorder appears to be transmitted by a dominant gene. The abnormal fibrinogen does not interfere with clotting of normal fibrinogen. It can be distinguished from normal fibrinogen by differences in migration in immunoelectrophoresis.

Forman and associates[122] described eight individuals of both sexes who had a defect in the fibrinogen molecule. The disorder seems to lie in the aggregation of soluble fibrin to form a visible clot after the splitting off of fibrinopeptide from fibrinogen by thrombin. It is still questionable whether the existence of an abnormal fibrinogen is a biological handicap. These variations in the fibrinogen molecule are analogous to the hemoglobinopathies.

### Hypofibrinogenemia and other coagulation defects in patients with congenital heart disease: open-heart surgery

A potential hemorrhagic diathesis in congenital cyanotic heart disease has been described.[153] Marked impairment of clot retraction is due to a combination of thrombocytopenia and low blood fibrinogen in the presence of a high hematocrit. The slight to moderate prolongation of prothrombin time is not a cause of the hemorrhagic disorder. Although these abnormal findings were present in patients in all age groups, postoperative hemorrhage was chiefly a problem in adults and adolescents. Children, however, with evidence of marked impairment revealed by hematologic tests underwent operation without hemorrhage. In adults with polycythemia vera, as well as in patients with secondary polycythemia of congenital heart disease, the hemorrhagic tendency is attributed in large measure to fibrinogenopenia. The treatment preoperatively in emergency situations in patients with polycythemia is liberal venesection together with the return of normal plasma to the patient.[353]

Other abnormalities in hemostasis also occur in heart disease. In cyanotic heart disease thrombocytopenia[153,381] has long been recognized, and on occasion it has been indicated as a cause of hemorrhage following thoracotomy for heart surgery.[278] In one set of observations, thrombocytopenia was extremely rare unless the hematocrit was greater than 65% and/or the oxygen saturation was less than 70%. Age exerted an influence for, despite these criteria, the incidence of thrombocytopenia in infants under 1 year of age was only 10%, whereas it approached 60% in children over 1 year.[278] The observation that there was no correlation between the degree of operative hemorrhage (non-pump cardiac surgery) and the platelet count per se was of clinical importance. With a similar degree of extreme thrombocytopenia, significant operative hemorrhage occurred only in patients over 6 years of age.

In another study[328] it was noted that in patients undergoing cardiac surgery with extracorporeal circulation, the lowest platelet counts were reached at the second postoperative day. Recovery to preoperative levels required 7 to 8 days. Both donor and patient's platelets were damaged by passage through the pump oxygenator. In this series no bleeding episodes were due to thrombocytopenia per se (even with levels of less than 60,000 per cubic millimeter, the clinical bleeding range). Multiple minor coagulation defects unrelated to thrombocytopenia, such as fibrinolysis, might potentiate bleeding.

Another defect found prior to cardiac surgery was increased capillary fragility noted in fourteen of 200 children. Three children with this hemostatic defect died with massive hemorrhage during surgery or immediately after the operation. Increased fibrinolytic activity occurred less commonly in this series.[344]

Another feature noted after cardiac surgery was thrombocytopenia after the administration of heparin. It is doubtful, however, if the high dosages of heparin are a primary cause of the bleeding tendency.[138] Further findings resulting from extracorporeal circulation include the increased plasma hemoglobin concentration during the cardiac bypass, probably resulting from trauma to whole blood. The decrease in fibrinogen and increase in fibrinolytic activity are probably due to intravascular clotting. Thrombocytopenia, prolonged bleeding time, poor clot retraction, and prolonged prothrombin time last several days.[131]

In a group of 145 children with congenital heart disease some degree of hemostatic deficiency was frequently found prior to surgery. Marked deviations with postoperative hemorrhage were more common in interventricular septal defect with pulmonary hypertension and tetralogy of Fallot. The most common hemostatic disorders fell into two categories: circulating fibrinolysins and a group consisting of thrombocytopenia, increased bleeding time, and increased capillary fragility. In the latter group, steroid therapy has been found of value.[261]

Incoagulability of the blood as a result of hypofibrinogenemia is a well-known complication of several obstetric conditions; amniotic fluid infusion (embolism), premature separation of the placenta, and prolonged retention of a dead fetus. One of the explanations for the deficiency in fibrinogen is that a thromboplastin-like material associated with these complications gains access to the maternal circulation, resulting in fibrinogen consumption. Another theory is that as fibrin is formed intravascularly it is destroyed by a fibrinolysin released as a result of shock.[209] In this condition intravascular coagulation results in a conversion of all or most of the circulating fibrinogen to fibrin, the latter being laid down either diffusely in the vascular system or in the retroperitoneal clot. However, as both these tissues are rich in lytic activator, some cases also show violent fibrinolytic activity in the blood. In obstetric defibrination it is generally believed that fibrinolysis follows intravascular fibrin formation and that fibrinolysis is seldom the cause per se.[338]

Hypofibrinogenemia has been encountered among the sensitized mothers of severely ill and stillborn infants in the course of erythroblastosis. It has been pointed out that the threat of developing afibrinogenemia in these patients may necessitate early delivery.[379]

### Fibrinolysis (fibrinolytic purpura)

The fibrinolytic process is one in which the living organism dissolves blood clots and disposes of fibrin.[28] This is effected through a complex enzymatic system. The activation of enzymes capable of destroying fibrin occurs acutely in patients with trauma, hemorrhagic shock, extensive burns, transfusion reactions, and obstetric accidents and, chronically, in those with leukemia, liver disease, and disseminated carcinoma.

Fibrinolysis accounts for recanalization of a blood vessel after hemostasis has been completed. Disruption of the hemostatic mechanism in patients with carcinoma or after extensive surgery with severe bleeding manifestations (fibrinolytic purpura) results from enzymatic digestion of fibrin clot, fibrinogen, and other proteins involved in blood coagulation.[352] In patients with hemorrhage following abruptio placentae and after surgery for cirrhosis of the liver the primary causative factor of afibrinogenemia may be fibrinolysis.[283]

Once a clot lodges in a blood vessel, activator enters from the endothelium causing clot lysis and reestablishes a patent circulation. The enzyme causing clot lysis, plasmin (fibrinolysin), is derived from an inactive precursor, plasminogen (profibrinolysin). Fibrinolysis depends upon the liberation into the circulation of tissue "kinases" or activators which activate the inert plasminogen to the active proteolytic enzyme, plasmin. Natural inhibitors of plasmin are present in the blood which may protect against the inappropriate action of this enzyme. High titers of antiplasmin and antiplasminogen activity have been reported in two patients; one of these was an infant with purpura fulminans.[256]

High concentrations of fibrinokinase or tissue activators[28] are present in the arteries, adrenals, prostate, thyroid, lymph nodes, lungs, and ovary and small amounts in other organs. Blood also is normally capable of forming an activator. Streptokinase, an extracellular filtrate of hemolytic streptococci, and urokinase[325] prepared from urine are both activators of plasminogen. Plasmin has a wide spectrum of proteolytic activity; not only does it attack fibrin but also other blood proteins such as fibrinogen, factors V, VIII, and XII, and prothrombin.

The equilibrium normally produced by the activators and inhibitors which prevent the generation of abnormal fibrinolytic activity may be disrupted temporarily by a number of abnormal states. Surgical trauma, for instance, can produce significant but transient increase in fibrinolytic activity in anesthetized patients.[284]

Epsilon-aminocaproic acid (Amicar), a potent synthetic antifibrinolytic agent, may be used as a part of the total treatment of the patient with life-threatening hemorrhage associated with excessive proteolysis due to increased plasminogen (profibrinolysin) activation.[89] This product was discussed in an earlier section in connection with the treatment of hemophilia and its complications (p. 703). It is a monoaminocarboxylic acid that is a competitive inhibitor of plasminogen activators and also of plasmin (fibrinolysin), to a lesser degree. It, therefore, prevents the formation of excessive plasmin that is responsible for the destruction of fibrinogen, fibrin, and other clotting elements. This substance has been shown to reduce postoperative bleeding in conditions associated with hyperfibrinolytic hemorrhage of open-heart surgery, in surgical and nonsurgical bleeding of the urinary tract such as hematomas occurring in hemophilia, and in severe fibrinolysis of abruptio placentae. Since this agent is contraindicated in thrombotic phenomena, the need for a fibrinolytic inhibitor must be clearly defined.

Aminocaproic acid may be administered by intravenous or oral route. Because the drug is excreted by the kidney, decreased renal function will result in higher plasma concentrations so that lower than usual doses may control hematuria.

Aminocaproic acid in a dosage of 70 mg. per kilogram of body weight is given in divided doses within the first hour. The initial dose is administered either orally or by slow intravenous infusion. Doses of 15 mg. per kilogram of body weight are given each hour for the next 8 hours, or until the bleeding has stopped. After 8 hours of continuous therapy a reevaluation of the patient's status is made. When given intravenously, isotonic sodium chloride, 5% dextrose, or Ringer's solution may be used to dilute the aminocaproic acid. The total dose should not exceed 4.5 gm. in any 24-hour period. If the response is poor, fibrinogen may be given in doses up to 4 gm. intravenously. Plasma (10 ml. per kilogram) and prednisone, (1 to 2 mg. per kilogram) given each day may also help to control bleeding.

Plasminogen activator comes from the endothelial cells of the microcirculation. Activators or kinases (specific for plasminogen activators) convert plasminogen to plasmin by opening a specific arginyl-valine bond in plasminogen and exposing the active enzyme center of plasmin.[340] Proteolysis of fibrinogen in the primary fibrinolytic disorders and of fibrin deposited in the microcirculation in the consumption coagulopathies result in degradation or split products which possess anticoagulant properties. They inhibit thrombin action, fibrin polymerization, thromboplastin generation, and platelet aggregation. As these split products accumulate in the plasma they produce a severe hemorrhagic diathesis.

Plasminogen levels at delivery are about one-tenth that of the normal adult and increase rapidly to a low normal level at about 7 months of age. Antiplasmin, on the other hand, is present in the newborn in values comparable to the normal adult.

Fibrin/fibrinogen degradation products have been found in the sera of healthy infants and children of all ages (10.0 ± 4.3 $\mu$g/ml.).[370] These levels are significantly greater than those in adults, but the reasons for this are unknown (Fig. 98).

Fibrinolysis has been defined as a means "whereby the body rids itself of a superfluous scaffolding contrived in order to facilitate repair."[350]

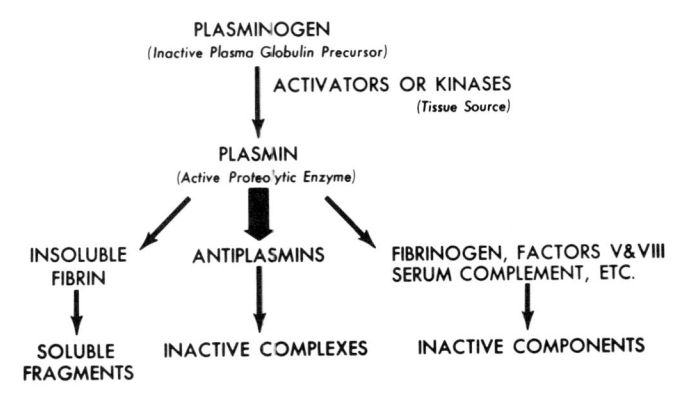

```
                    PLASMINOGEN
            (Inactive Plasma Globulin Precursor)
                           │
                           ▼
                 ACTIVATORS OR KINASES
                      (Tissue Source)
                           │
                           ▼
                        PLASMIN
                (Active Proteolytic Enzyme)
              ╱            │            ╲
            ╱              ▼              ╲
    INSOLUBLE        ANTIPLASMINS      FIBRINOGEN, FACTORS V & VIII
     FIBRIN                             SERUM COMPLEMENT, ETC.
        │                │                      │
        ▼                ▼                      ▼
     SOLUBLE      INACTIVE COMPLEXES      INACTIVE COMPONENTS
    FRAGMENTS
```

Fig. 98. Components of human fibrinolytic enzyme system (plasminogen-plasmin system) and nature of actions. (From Fibrinolytic agents by Sol Sherry, in "Disease-a-Month." Copyright 1969. Year Book Medical Publishers, Inc. Used by permission of Year Book Medical Publishers.)

Physiologic mechanisms are available for the dissolution of fibrin since blood clots are not permanent structures, thereby keeping circulatory pathways patent and efficient. With the discovery of a fibrinolytic agent produced by strains of hemolytic streptococci,[366] mammalian blood, heretofore examined for its coagulative properties, began to be intensively investigated for fibrinolytic mechanisms. While fibrin formation and destruction may occur coincidentally under physiologic conditions, fibrinolysis may be accelerated under pathologic conditions and is attributed to circulating fibrinolytic agents.

### Laboratory findings in fibrinogen deficiencies

In complete afibrinogenemia the whole blood is incoagulable. The absence of fibrinogen is confirmed by the failure of citrated blood or plasma to clot when thrombin is added and by the absence of a precipitate when the plasma is heated to 56° C.[55] If the plasma remains clear, afibrinogenemia exists, since fibrinogen precipitates at about this temperature.

The blood of patients with hemophilia shows a normal one-stage prothrombin time. Hence, if the whole blood clotting time is prolonged and the Quick one-stage prothrombin time shows no clotting or a very incomplete clot, total or partial afibrinogenemia should be suspected.[55] It has been estimated that if the prothrombin time of a given plasma sample is normal its fibrinogen level must be in excess of 100 mg./100 ml.[23]

In hypofibrinogenemia, the clotting time may be normal or slightly prolonged, depending upon the content of fibrinogen. With reduced fibrinogen levels clotting occurs promptly, and retraction of the clot results in a relatively large volume of erythrocytes over which is suspended a very small mass. Eventually, the clot becomes detached and drops into the erythrocyte suspension, by which it is obscured.

### Treatment of the fibrinogen deficiencies

The normal concentration of fibrinogen in the blood is 180 to 400 mg. per 100 ml. Only in the event of a hemorrhagic episode is treatment necessary, and this consists of the administration of blood, plasma, and concentrated fibrinogen (Cohn fraction 1). Approximately 0.2 to 0.3 gm. of fibrinogen is present in 100 ml. of plasma and about 0.7 to 0.9 gm. in 1 pint of whole blood. Cryoprecipitate is an excellent source of fibrinogen since each pack of cryoprecipitate contains approximately 300 mg. of fibrinogen. Concentrated human fibrinogen preparations are now in good supply and constitute the first choice of treatment. In contrast to the labile antihemophilic globulin, fibrinogen remains stable when stored. In critical situations in which severe and persistent bleeding is associated with marked fibrinogen depletion, substantial amounts of human fibrinogen may be given (up to 4 gm. intravenously in children). It must be cautioned, however, that the use of fibrinogen carries a definite hazard of hepatitis.

A critical blood level of 80 mg. of fibrinogen per 100 ml. is required for effective hemostasis, and treatment should be directed toward achieving, at least, this concentration. Gitlin and Borges[134] determined immunochemically that one-half of administered fibrinogen disappeared from the circulation in the first 48 hours. After the first 2 days, the fibrinogen follows a logarithmic decay curve with a half-life of 4 days, indicating that the fundamental defect in these patients is a failure to synthesize adequate amounts of fibrinogen. Fibrinogen labeled with radioactive iodine, $^{131}I$, shows a mean half-life of 5.1 days (range 4.1 to 6 days).[144] A dose of 100 mg. of fibrinogen per kilogram of body weight raises the fibrinogen concentration of a patient with afibrinogenemia to approximately 200 mg. per 100 ml.[329] With the use of plasma, the fibrinogen component may remain in the circulation for as long as 4 days, and with concentrated fibrinogen it may remain twice as long.[150]

In patients with acute fibrinolysis, treatment is urgent and consists of prompt administration of whole blood, plasma, and concentrated fibrinogen (fraction 1). Use of ACTH and the steroid hormones has been suggested as a means of increasing antifibrinolysin activity[353] and controlling bleeding. Epsilon-aminocaproic acid (Amicar) is an effective inhibitor of fibrinolysis. Its use in inhibiting plasminogen activators in a variety of clinical conditions has been referred to previously. Essential to the diagnosis of increased fibrinolysis and the use of aminocaproic acid is the demonstration of increased plasmin and/or plasminogen activator levels in the patient.

In a 16-year-old girl with congenital afibrinogenemia and rheumatic valvular disease an antifibrinogen antibody developed during repeated infusions of human plasma fibrinogen fraction I.[105] The appearance of this antibody was associated with severe infusion reactions and skin hypersensitivity to fibrinogen.

# CIRCULATING ANTICOAGULANTS

*Naturally occurring anticoagulants.* The fluidity of the circulating blood depends upon the integrity of vascular endothelium and the presence of the natural anticoagulants, plasma antithrombin, heparin, and a postulated antithromboplastin.

Antithromboplastin has been described as a lipid inhibitor, an excess of which has been held accountable for hemophilia.[367,368] It has been shown, for instance, that contact of hemophilic plasma with asbestos or glass will normalize its clotting by adsorption of the inhibitor. On the other hand, transfusion of hemophilic plasma treated by removal of the inhibitor in this manner or by extraction with ether still demonstrates a deficiency of AHG in in vivo experiments.[71] Nevertheless, the presence of an inhibitor in hemophilic plasma cannot be discounted. Proof of the presence of circulating anticoagulant as an intrinsic feature of the hemophilic defect within the circulation awaits further corroborative evidences.[46]

*Acquired anticoagulants.* The majority of acquired inhibitors prevents the formation of thromboplastin, either as a complication of hemophilia or causing a hemorrhagic diathesis resembling hemophilia.[177] The best defined blood-clotting inhibitors are those which appear in the blood of the patient with hemophilia following repeated transfusions. This has been ascribed to an immunologic response to the antihemophilic globulin in blood or plasma. These inhibitors are apparently specific for factor VIII and are capable of inducing a transient hemophilic state when injected into dogs.[318] Similar inhibitors of plasma thromboplastin component (PTC) have also been described.[217]

Acquired hemophilia-like disease based on circulating anticoagulants has also been recorded after pregnancy. In one case the anticoagulant was detected in the patient's child during the first 2½ months of life, indicating its transplacental transfer.[125] Circulating anticoagulants have appeared in previously healthy male and female patients or in connection with an associated illness, notably lupus erythematosus, periarteritis nodosa, rheumatoid arthritis, tuberculosis, and glomerulonephritis.

Circulating anticoagulants directed against the first stage of coagulation have appeared in patients who do not have congenital hemophilia.[174] They occur frequently in women in the third and fourth decades with an onset several weeks to a year after parturition and in elderly persons with autoimmune manifestations or without etiologic association. Hemorrhagic disease due to a rise in blood heparin or substances with heparin-like activity has appeared after treatment with physical or chemical reagents such as nitrogen mustard and after exposure to ionizing radiation and probably explains the decreased coagulability of the blood in patients with anaphylaxis.

The presence of a circulating anticoagulant

contributes to the diagnosis of lupus erythematosus. This abnormality may disappear fairly rapidly during steroid therapy.[242] In one patient with this disease severe bleeding was associated with hypoprothrombinemia plus an anticoagulant active against formed blood and tissue prothrombinase.[305]

This anticoagulant is also directed against the activated form of factor X (Stuart-Prower) or the clotting reactions immediately following factor X activation.[70] The circulating anticoagulants in lupus erythematosus have also been found to interfere with the conversion of prothrombin to thrombin.[179] However, patients with lupus erythematosus often develop thrombocytopenia and the occurrence of hemorrhages is more likely due to this cause than to an anticoagulant.[179]

Multiple changes in blood coagulation occur in the course of a number of systemic disorders, in contrast to those congenital defects of hemostasis in which a single clotting factor is deficient. These changes have been summarized by Spaet[345] as follows:

1. *Parenchymal liver disease.* Those factors that are depressed or synthesized by the liver are the prothrombin group consisting of prothrombin, factors VII, IX (PTC), and X (Stuart-Prower factor) and the group consisting of fibrinogen and factor V. The most critical finding that distinguishes the liver group from vitamin K deficiency is the reduction of factor V in the former. Administration of vitamin K to patients with damaged livers will be ineffective and may cause further prolongation of the prothrombin time.

2. *Vitamin K deficiency.* The body's vitamin K stores may be depleted or they may be inhibited by metabolic antagonists such as the coumarin drugs and, more rarely, by salicylates. In any case, a selective depression of the prothrombin group of clotting factors takes place—i.e., prothrombin and factors VII, IX (PTC), and X (Stuart-Prower factor). Since the daily requirement of vitamin K is on the order of 0.5 $\mu$g per kilogram, a few milligrams parenterally of either fat- or water-soluble compounds are sufficient to restore normal clotting to the patient with a simple deficiency.

**Disseminated intravascular coagulation (DIC, defibrination syndrome, consumption coagulopathy).** The terminology of this syndrome has varied with each investigator's approach to its pathophysiology. The varied designations may be used interchangeably but they have in common the consumption of fibrinogen, labile clotting factors, and platelets.

For that reason DIC is also designated as the defibrination syndrome or consumption coagulopathy; there are proponents for each of these designations.[86,245]

In the normal coagulation process a sequential interaction of certain coagulation factors and platelet phospholipid results in fibrin formation. In the clotting of blood in vitro, platelets, prothrombin (factor II), factor V, factor VIII, and fibrinogen (factor I) are consumed, and these factors are lacking in the serum. In the process of intravascular coagulation a similar consumption of factors occurs.[7] In many cases factor XIII is also absent or reduced.[246] A hemorrhagic state follows associated with widespread deposition of fibrin in small blood vessels resulting in local tissue necrosis.

In the patient the clotting process is activated by a variety of stimuli. The etiologic agents and triggering mechanisms include: release of thromboplastic material and bacterial endotoxins, anoxia, sepsis, a generalized Shwartzman reaction, malignant disease especially if accompanied by bone metastasis, leukemia, snakebite, giant hemangiomata, and purpura fulminans (Table 31). Disseminated intravascular coagulation has in recent years been held accountable for a wide variety of diseases or at least for some of their prominent pathophysiologic aspects. It has been described in the newborn period in association with the respiratory distress syndrome,[156] in fatal disseminated herpes simplex virus infection,[248] in septicemia following splenectomy and in patients with congenital asplenia,[239] in the hemolytic-uremic syndrome, and in thrombotic thrombocytopenic purpura.

Once the precipitating event becomes operative, intravascular coagulation occurs and the circulating plasma is depleted of prothrombin, platelets, factors V and VIII, and fibrinogen. The fibrin formed may produce occlusive thrombi in the microvasculature. Widespread vascular injury produces a direct consumption of platelets by damaged endothelium.[151] Bleeding depends upon the extent of depletion of coagulation factors.

Intravascular clots, once formed and lodged in a blood vessel, initiate local fibrinolytic activity. Digestion of fibrin by plasmin or other enzymes produces split products which are released into the general circulation.[246] In the defibrination syndrome described by Merskey

**Table 31.** Conditions in children in which intravascular coagulation may occur as a complication or an intermediary mechanism of pathogenesis*

Infections
   Parasitic (malaria)
   Mycotic
   Bacterial
   Rickettsial
   Viral
Disorders of the newborn period
   Intrauterine infections
   Maternal toxemia or abruptio placenta
   Idiopathic respiratory distress syndrome
Leukemia and other malignancies
Intravascular hemolysis
Giant hemangioma
Purpura fulminans
Hemolytic-uremic syndrome (?)
Thrombotic thrombocytopenic purpura(?)
Hemorrhagic shock
Trauma
Burns
Postoperative states
Snakebite
Cirrhosis
Amyloidosis

*From Abildgaard, C. F.: Recognition and treatment of intravascular coagulation, J. Pediat. 74:163-176, 1969.

**Table 32.** Laboratory tests useful in the detection of intravascular coagulation*

Rapidly available screening tests
   Observation of whole blood clot
   Platelet count (or evaluation of blood smear)
   Fibrinogen (semiquantitative)
      Heat precipitation method
      Fibrinogen titer
      Fi test (Hyland Laboratories)
   Thrombin time
   Prothrombin time
   Partial thromboplastin time
   Protamine precipitation
Quantitative measurements
   Factor V assay
   Factor VIII assay
   Fibrinogen
   Euglobulin clot lysis time
   Fibrin split products

*From Abildgaard, C. F.: Recognition and treatment of intravascular coagulation, J. Pediat. 74: 163-176, 1969.

and associates,[246] studies of fibrinolytic parameters revealed low plasminogen levels and almost invariable presence of abnormal amounts of fibrinolytic split products in the serum, indicating excessive fibrinolysis. It can be assumed that, in disseminated intravascular coagulation once a clot lodges in a blood vessel, activator of the plasminogen enters from the endothelium, causing clot lysis, and reestablishes a patent circulation. The system is so effective that frequently when such patients come to autopsy no thrombi are found. In such cases only the evidence of lysis, such as fibrin split products remain to offer testimony to the original DIC.

The laboratory diagnosis of intravascular coagulation depends upon the demonstration of the depletion of plasma factors consumed in the clotting process—factors V and VIII, prothrombin, and fibrinogen—reduced levels of blood platelets, and increased levels of fibrinolytic split products. Because of the changing nature of the course of disseminated intravascular coagulation the laboratory findings may not reflect equal degrees of depletion. The fibrinogen level for instance may be elevated at some stage of the disease (Table 32).

A bizarre blood picture characterized by distorted and fragmented cells described as triangular, helmet, and burr cells accompanies many of the syndromes associated with disseminated intravascular coagulation.[68,79] It was suggested that mechanical intravascular events were responsible for erythrocyte damage similar to hemolysis from prosthetic heart valves. More specifically the hemolytic anemia occurring in these conditions results from injury to red blood cells buffeting intravascular fibrin strands, comparable to the events taking place in microangiopathic hemolytic anemia. (See discussion of hemolytic-uremic syndrome in Chapter 27.) These distorted cells are not pathognomonic for disorders associated with disseminated intravascular coagulation, but they are suggestive and prompt the need for further investigation.

Treatment is of a dual nature. Primary consideration is given to the investigation of the condition or disease which triggered intravascular coagulation for which supportive and specific therapy may be required. The second is the use of a suitable anticoagulant after appropriate screening tests have established the extent of the coagulation coagulopathy. In time the effects of intravascular coagulation dominate the clinical picture.

In acute episodes heparin is the drug of choice and is given intravenously in a dosage of 1 to 1.5 mg. per kilogram of body weight initially. The larger dose is usually required for the premature infant with the respiratory distress syndrome, the smaller dose for older children. The subsequent amounts of heparin are controlled by determining the clotting time before each succeeding dose, to maintain the whole blood clotting time at 20 to 30 minutes. With this method of control the dosage after the initial administration is approximately 1 mg. per kilogram every 4 hours for the infant with the respiratory distress syndrome and half this dosage for the older child. The drug in any case is best given by intravenous drip. When successful, heparin appears to arrest the defibrination process and leads to the restoration of the depressed clotting factors. To neutralize the heparin in the patient's plasma, protamine is administered intravenously in a dose of 5 to 8 mg./kg. for 24 hours.

The presence of intravascular coagulation and favorable response to heparin have been reported in the therapy of purpura fulminans,[24] giant cavernous hemangioma, the hemolytic-uremic syndrome, cyanotic congenital heart disease, leukemia, and meningococcemia.[7] The use in cyanotic congenital heart disease, however, awaits further study.

It has already been stated that fibrinolysis which accompanies intravascular coagulation serves advantageously in the lysis of fibrin thrombi. Only where fibrinolysis is excessive, which is rare in children, is there a need to block fibrinolysis by the use of epsilon-aminocaproic acid (Amicar), an anti-fibrinolytic agent. Blocking fibrinolysis during the course of intravascular coagulation would probably result in increased fibrin deposition. Inactivation of this system is justified only if fibrinolysis is a major factor in the progression of bleeding. Streptokinase has also been administered to lyse the thrombi in addition to treatment with heparin.[252] Urokinase extractable from human urine acts directly on plasminogen and is possibly less toxic. Unfortunately, thromboplastic contaminants hamper its therapeutic use.

Rabiner and Friedman[300] have shown that infusion of hemolyzed erythrocytes (hemolysate) into dogs produces hypercoagulability frequently followed by actual intravascular coagulation as evidenced by depressed factor V and factor VIII activity, fall in fibrinogen, and demonstrable pulmonary artery thrombi. They postulated that hemolysis can be an important contributing factor in the pathogenesis of "the syndromes of disseminated intravascular coagulation." They also suggested that the thrombotic phenomena associated with the generalized Shwartzman phenomenon, thrombotic thrombocytopenic purpura, the hemolytic-uremic syndrome, paroxysmal nocturnal hemoglobinuria, and incompatible blood transfusions may be related to intravascular hemolysis. A complicating factor is the decreased reticuloendothelial activity secondary to an acute immunological reaction producing shock, as a result of which there is a slow clearance of stroma with resultant intravascular coagulation.

*Tests for anticoagulants.* A screening test for the presence of clotting inhibitors is an integral part of a complete coagulation study. Patients with circulating anticoagulants usually show prolonged clotting and recalcification times. Although normal whole blood or plasma will correct a deficiency, the presence of an anticoagulant in the patient's blood or plasma will prolong the normal clotting time. The screening test consists of mixing various amounts of the patient's blood or plasma with normal blood or plasma and determining the clotting and recalcification times of the mixtures.[332] Circulating anticoagulants can also be detected by the thromboplastin generation test by mixing either the patient's serum or adsorbed plasma with the corresponding normal reagent. With an inhibitor little or no thromboplastin is generated.[54]

*Treatment.* Attempts to overcome the refractory state in the various types of hemophilia by repeated transfusions with massive amounts of blood have been of questionable success. This measure may be necessary, however, in the face of continued bleeding although there is the risk of generating increased amounts of anticoagulant. ACTH and steroids have been of limited value. Recently, the use of other immunosuppressive agents, including cyclophosphamide, has met with variable success.[132a,225a,339a] However, the anticoagulant has been known to disappear spontaneously, or the bleeding may be minimal despite its presence. If the circulating anticoagulant is of the antifactor VIII or IX type, concentrated preparations of either factor VIII or factor IX, respectively, should be tried if the patient's life is in jeopardy.[179,317a]

## SUMMARY OF REPLACEMENT THERAPY OF COAGULATION DISORDERS

The frequency of plasma administration depends upon the life-span of the deficient factor in the patient's circulation, loss of the factors through utilization and fever, the increased requirements with active bleeding, or, possibly, by neutralization or destructive action of anticoagulants.[320] When the critical level of a particular factor in a patient with any bleeding disorder (of the first or second stage of coagulation) falls below that deemed necessary for hemostasis, fresh frozen plasma is given in initial doses of 20 ml. per kilogram of body weight. Subsequent doses of 5 ml. per kilogram of body weight are given at intervals, depending upon the survival of a particular factor.

Fibrinogen may be administered as the concentrate, available in lyophylized 1 or 2 gm. lots to be dissolved in water. Sufficient amounts for hemostasis should be given to bring the plasma concentration to 100 mg./100 ml.

For surgery in patients with a hemophilioid disorder, a priming dose of 20 ml. of fresh frozen plasma per kilogram of body weight is given 30 minutes before the procedure, sufficient to give a concentration of 20 to 30% of the deficient factor in the patient's plasma. (With the use of the new concentrates it is even possible to take the patient to surgery with 100% of the deficient factor by giving 40 units per kilogram for all AHF-containing materials.) Blood and plasma are replaced during the procedure as necessary. After the procedure, 5 ml. of fresh frozen plasma per kilogram is given every 4 hours for 48 hours, extended to 6 to 8 hours for an additional 48 to 72 hours, and then 10 ml. per kilogram every 12 hours for 72 hours. If the surgical procedure is minimal, coverage for 5 days with plasma should be sufficient. If the operation is major (abdominal or thoracic) and hemostasis has been difficult, or if drains have been left in a cavity, it is usually wise to maintain 15 to 20% levels in the patient by using the foregoing regimen for at least 8 days and to give an extra 10 ml. per kilogram at the time the drains and sutures are advanced and removed.

If the operation has been extensive, then coverage for 8 to 10 days is probably warranted.

The product of choice for treatment of bleeding in the hemophilias is fresh frozen plasma or the specific plasma factor concentrates, when anemia is not a problem. When fresh frozen plasma or the specific plasma factor concentrates are not available, the following may be used in the conditions as listed[*]:

1. Fresh whole blood or plasma
    a. Thrombocytopenic purpura (whole blood or platelet-rich plasma collected in siliconized or plastic equipment)
    b. Hemophilia A (factor VIII, AHG deficiency)
    c. Hemophilia B (factor IX, PTC deficiency, Christmas disease)
    d. Factor XI (PTA deficiency)
    e. Parahemophilia (factor V, labile factor deficiency)
    f. von Willebrand's disease
2. Fresh or stored whole blood or plasma
    a. Prothrombin deficiency
    b. Factor VII (stable factor) deficiency
    c. Factor X (Stuart-Prower factor) deficiency

Data relative to plasma requirements in deficiencies of coagulation factors are as follows:

1. Stable when stored at 20° C.
    a. Factor IX (PTC)
    b. Factor XI (PTA)
    c. Factor II (prothrombin)
    d. Factor VII (stable factor)
    e. Factor X (Stuart-Prower)
    f. Factor I (fibrinogen)
2. Labile when stored at 4° and 20° C.
    a. Factor VIII (AHG)
    b. Factor V (labile factor)
3. Survival time of clotting factors in circulation of patient[16,222]
    a. Factor I (fibrinogen), 12 to 36 hours
    b. Factor II (prothrombin), 24 hours
    c. Factor V (labile factor), 12 hours
    d. Factor VII (stable factor), 20 to 60 minutes
    e. Factor VIII (AHG), 4 to 7½ hours
    f. Factor IX (PTC), 36 hours
    g. Factor X (Stuart-Prower), 47 hours
    h. Factor XI (PTA), 12 to 14 hours

There are certain minimum hemostatic levels below which spontaneous bleeding oc-

---

[*]From Smith, C. H.: Transfusions in pediatric practice; indications and limitations, Pediatrics 17:596, 1956.

curs.[16] The following are only approximate levels as there is a fairly broad dispersion based on the particular experience of the clinic. Since the occurrence of clinical bleeding is greatly influenced by the nature and degree of stress placed upon the hemostatic mechanism, the minimum hemostatic levels for platelets and clotting factors are difficult to define except in relative terms.

Platelets, 50,000 per cubic millimeter
Fibrinogen, 100 mg. per 100 ml.
Prothrombin, 10 to 20% of normal
Factor V (labile factor), 30% of normal
Factor VII (stable factor), 25% of normal
Factor VIII (AHG), 20 to 25% of normal
Factor IX (PTC), Same as factor VIII
Factor X (Stuart-Prower), Same as factor VIII
Factor XI (PTA), 20% of normal

## EPISTAXIS

Recurrent nosebleeds constitute a common problem in pediatric practice. They usually occur spontaneously, often at night, and frequently in the course of an upper respiratory infection. They are usually controlled by simple measures such as digital pressure or cotton packs rimmed with petroleum jelly or soaked in Adrenalin, but sometimes they require cauterization and nasal packing. Bleeding, however, may be profuse, and blood loss may be substantial.

The localization and causation of nosebleeds assume importance when tonsillectomy and adenoidectomy are contemplated. As an isolated symptom, it is rare in patients with hemophilia. In those with intractable nosebleeds, von Willebrand's disease should be considered. The platelet count is usually normal in patients with idiopathic epistaxis and depressed in those in whom epistaxis accompanies leukemia, aplastic anemia, or conditions associated with hypersplenism such as Gaucher's disease. Nosebleeds infrequently constitute the sole clinical feature of either idiopathic thrombocytopenic purpura or classic (AHG-deficient) hemophilia. Epistaxis may also occur in patients during the course of measles, rheumatic fever, systemic lupus erythematosus, typhoid fever, glomerulonephritis, sickle cell anemia, and Cooley's anemia. Allergic rhinitis has been known to cause recurrent epistaxis in children without an underlying bleeding diathesis.[133]

In thalassemia major, patients who had the most severe difficulty with epistaxis had no coagulation defects.[166] A general correlation could be found between the coagulation status and hepatic function. In this series a large number showed mild to moderate defects of PTC, PTA, and the prothrombin complex.

From present evidence it appears safe for patients with epistaxis without a history of abnormal bleeding to be operated upon without further tests. This means that in neither the patient nor any member of his family is there a history of easy bruising or persistent bleeding after dental extraction, circumcision, immunization, or eruption or loss of deciduous teeth. Furthermore, physical examination should reveal no petechiae, purpura, or ecchymoses. However, if there is any suspicion of abnormality, the partial thromboplastin time should be done as a screening test.

Following are instances of pediatric bleeding emergencies:

*Disorders of hemostasis*

1. Specific coagulation defects—AHG, PTA, PTC, etc.
   a. Spontaneous
   b. Following surgical procedures—circumcision, tonsillectomy, dental extractions
2. Thrombocytopenic syndromes
   a. Idiopathic
   b. Secondary—leukemia, aplastic anemia, lupus erythematosus, hypersplenism, i.e., Gaucher's disease, Banti's disease
3. Vascular disorders
   a. Henoch-Schönlein purpura, thrombotic thrombocytopenic purpura, hereditary hemorrhagic telangiectasia, von Willebrand's disease

*Local causes*

1. Epistaxis (with and without coagulation defect)
2. Gastrointestinal—ulcers, intussusception, polyps, Meckel's diverticulum
3. Miscellaneous—trauma, pulmonary hemosiderosis, sickle cell disease, thalassemia major

## PROCEDURE FOR SCREENING POTENTIAL BLEEDERS

Adequate screening devices before surgery are especially important in infants and children since circumcision, dental extraction, and tonsillectomy are common events in pediatric practice. Prothrombin consumption and thromboplastin generation tests provide accurate information concerning basic defects in coagulation but are obviously not suited for routine use. The following tests are currently in use for screening purposes: the bleeding time, clotting time, clot retraction, platelet count, Quick prothrombin time, and partial thromboplastin time. The latter constitutes a simple, sensitive, one-stage screening test that has been found useful and reliable for hemophilia and hemophilioid disorders. This test, the partial thromboplastin time, properly adapted, will reveal deficiencies of factors VIII, IX, XI and XII. The normal partial thromboplastin time ranges from 36 to 46 seconds. Values between 46 and 55 seconds are abnormal. Assays for the specific deficient factor are undertaken with values over 50 seconds.

The most practical course is to obtain a detailed personal and family history of hemorrhage. As a general rule a hemorrhagic disorder is suspected when the degree of bleeding is out of proportion to the extent of trauma. This circumstance usually becomes apparent by the time the child is walking without protection. More complete studies are warranted in the patient with a history of severe and uncontrollable epistaxis, easy bruising, hematomas, especially in protected areas of the body, and excessive bleeding from cuts, skin prick as for blood counts and injections, and during the eruption or loss of deciduous teeth. Importance is attached to a history of prolonged bleeding or transfusions after an operative procedure in a sibling or parent. The absence of bleeding after a dental extraction of moderate severity or after tonsillectomy usually indicates the absence of congenital disease.

The clotting time is only of value in the older child in whom a vein can be entered without difficulty. Capillary tests are unreliable because of the amount of tissue juice containing thromboplastin which enters the peripheral blood sample. Since a normal clotting time will be found in patients mildly affected with hemophilia and often in those conditions with defects in prothrombin conversion, the history becomes increasingly important. Short of the use of more complicated tests, the bleeding history is the most useful means of anticipating difficulty in patients with sporadic factor VIII (AHG) and factor IX (PTC) deficiency in whom there is no family history (25 to 30% of patients with hemophilia).

In addition to the history, a complete physical examination and examination of the blood smear for platelets to rule out thrombopenic states at the time of routine preoperative hemoglobin determinations and white cell counts constitute effective screening devices. For these reasons, a careful history is essential, and it has even been suggested that because of inherently misleading results[107] routine presurgery tests of bleeding and clotting times be abandoned.

## LABORATORY INVESTIGATION OF COAGULATION DISORDERS

*General considerations.* Investigation for a hemorrhagic disorder is usually prompted by the clinical history and physical findings which also give direction to the scope of the laboratory work-up. The test consists of the routine coagulation procedures for screening and more elaborate devices for the detection of the specific causative defect.

In evaluating the results of routine coagulation tests which may be the only ones available in a laboratory, it should be remembered that patients with the mild bleeding disorders may show few or no abnormalities upon routine testing. In such instances a careful history will compel attention toward the need for more intensive investigation.

In the history of the patient or other members of his family, those episodes are important in which bleeding from minor cuts and scratches and after dental extraction and tonsillectomy is prolonged with or without the need for transfusions. In the infant, more than normal oozing of blood after circumcision and from cuts of the tongue and lips, protracted oozing of blood from the gums during the eruption of deciduous teeth, and bleeding at the site of immunization are noteworthy. The presence of extensive bruising observed during physical examination is a sign of recurrent hemorrhage. The bruising may represent a disorder in which platelets are deficient.

Both hematologic and nonhematologic disturbances may give evidence of gross bleeding and must be differentiated from a basic bleeding tendency. Severe epistaxis, a frequent occurrence in childhood, deserves a complete coagulation study only if it is associated with

Table 33. Results of routine tests in hemorrhagic states*†

| Disorder | Bleeding time | Clotting time | Clot retraction | Tourniquet test | Platelet count | Prothrombin time |
|---|---|---|---|---|---|---|
| Platelet abnormalities | | | | | | |
|     Thrombocytopenia | A | N | A | A | A | N |
|     Thrombasthenia | A | N | N or A | N or A | N | N |
| Factor VIII (AHG) deficiency | N | A‡ | N | N | N | N |
| Factor IX (PTC) deficiency | N | A‡ | N | N | N | N |
| Factor XI (PTA) deficiency | N | A‡ | N | N | N | N |
| Factor II (prothrombin) deficiency | N | N | N | N | N | A |
| Factor V (labile factor) deficiency | N | N§ | N | N | N | A |
| Factor VII (stable factor) deficiency | N | N | N | N | N | A |
| Factor I (fibrinogen) deficiency | N | N | N | N or A | N | N or A‖ |
| Factor X (Stuart-Prower factor) deficiency | N | A | N | N | N | A |
| Vascular disorders | A | N | N | N or A | N | N |

*Modified from Schulman, I., and Smith, C. H.: Coagulation disorders in infancy and childhood. In Levine, S. Z., editor: Advances in pediatrics, vol. 9, Chicago, 1957, Year Book Medical Publishers, Inc., p. 231.
†N, normal; A, abnormal.
‡May be normal in mild to moderate degrees of deficiency.
§May be prolonged with marked deficiency.
‖Abnormal with marked deficiency since no end point present.

easy bruising and a suspicious bleeding history. For all practical purposes, a patient who has undergone circumcision, tonsillectomy, or tooth extraction without evidence of abnormal bleeding may be considered not to have hemophilia or any other serious first phase coagulation defect.

*Screening tests.* The screening tests for a suspected hemorrhagic disorder include coagulation time, bleeding time, clot retraction, prothrombin time (one stage), complete blood count, including platelet count, and capillary fragility (tourniquet test). Since diagnosis, choice of therapy, and prognosis depend upon the results of laboratory methods, meticulous attention to details is necessary in these preliminary tests as in the more elaborate procedures. (See Table 33.)

*Coagulation time.* Blood is obtained by vein puncture. Capillary coagulation tests are unreliable, because blood obtained by skin puncture is mixed with tissue juice and therefore is unsuitable for determining the clotting time. If the vein puncture is not accomplished immediately and if there is any undue manipulation, the procedure is repeated with another needle and vein. The Lee and White technique is used. One milliliter of blood is transferred into each of two clean, dry, Pyrex tubes measuring 13 by 100 mm., and tests are carried out in a water bath kept at 37° C. The first tube is tilted at half-minute intervals until no blood flows when the tube is inverted. The second tube is then similarly tilted until the blood is solidified. The point at which the blood is solidified is designated as the coagulation time. The normal range of coagulation time is 5 to 12 minutes.

*Bleeding time.* Bleeding time is determined by the Duke method or by the Ivy method.

DUKE METHOD.[179] With a No. 11 Bard-Parker blade, a small cut is made in the ear lobe to a depth of 2 to 3 mm. With a round piece of filter paper, the blood is blotted off, not wiped off, every 30 seconds. The blood should be permitted to flow onto the filter paper by capillarity. The interval between the time the incision is made and the moment when bleeding stops represents the end point. The range of normal is given as 2 to 7 minutes, falling between 1 and 4 minutes in the majority of patients.

Puncture of the ear lobe should be avoided in children with suspected hemophilia, von Willebrand's disease, and severe thrombocytopenic purpura because bleeding may be so uncontrollable as to eventually require transfusions for hemostasis.

IVY METHOD.[186] A blood pressure cuff placed just above the bend of the elbow is kept at 40 mm. pressure. The surface of the forearm is cleansed with an antiseptic and then dried. With a Bard-Parker blade or a sterile spring lancet the skin is punctured to a depth of 2 to 3 mm. and a width of 2 mm. in the fleshy part of the forearm below the elbow. The drops of blood are removed with a piece of filter paper every 30 seconds, as is done in the Duke method. The bleeding time is the time which elapses between the puncture of the forearm and the cessation of bleeding.

This method has been recommended in children because persistent bleeding from the forearm can be more readily controlled by pressure than that from the ear lobe. Despite the possibility of prolonged oozing, the Duke test is still in current use and has been found reliable in most laboratories.

*Clot retraction.* The clot in one of the tubes used in determining the clotting time is used for the clot retraction test. The test should be facilitated by loosening the clot from the walls of the tube with a platinum wire or glass applicator. The tube is stoppered, placed in a water bath at 37° C., and inspected at 1, 2, 12, and 24 hours. Normal clot retraction is usually complete in 1 or 2 hours.

In the blood of patients with abnormal conditions contractility is minimal or absent after 24 hours. Clot retraction depends upon several factors: the number of platelets, the concentration of fibrinogen, and the cell volume. Adequate numbers of intact platelets are essential for clot retraction; the higher the concentration of fibrinogen, the less the contraction. Poor clot retraction is noticeable with platelet counts below 80,000 per cubic millimeter. No retraction is observed in patients with thrombocytopenia with counts below 20,000 per cubic millimeter and in those with thrombasthenia (normal number of platelets but impaired function). It is poor in patients with an excessive red cell mass. Clot retraction is inversely proportional to the fibrinogen content and red cell mass, since the more red cells and fibrinogen in the clot, the less it can contract.[179] Clot retraction will thus be more marked in anemic than in polycythemic blood. Clot retraction is difficult to measure quantitatively, although tests are available for that purpose.

*Platelet count.* The reagent used is 3.8% sodium citrate solution. For the Rees-Ecker[366a] modification brilliant cresyl blue is added. The platelets are more easily seen with the phase-contrast microscope, but may be readily counted with the standard chamber and microscope. An accurate platelet count is a prerequisite for the diagnosis of either thrombocytopenia or thrombocytosis. Thrombocythemia refers to more persistently increased platelet levels than are observed in patients with thrombocytosis after splenectomy. It is commonly seen in patients with myeloproliferative conditions such as chronic myelocytic leukemia, Hodgkin's disease, and Boeck's sarcoid. Purpuric bleeding, often with a prolonged bleeding time, has been reported in patients with an excessively high platelet count. This situation has been encountered most often in patients with polycythemia vera, chronic myeloid leukemia, and myeloid metaplasia.[187] In those with thrombocytopenic purpura, the blood smear presents a transparent appearance under the microscope due to reduced platelet numbers. As in patients with many conditions which are accompanied by thrombocytopenia, variations in platelet morphology are likely to occur.

Syndromes have been described in which abnormal bleeding has been attributed to qualitative platelet defects—the so-called thrombocytopathic purpuras or thrombasthenias. The platelets are usually normal, rarely slightly reduced in number, highly abnormal in appearance, giant sized, abnormally small, bizarre in shape, and agranular. Glanzmann's thrombasthenia[136] is cited as an example of a syndrome in which hemorrhage occurs with a normal bleeding time, platelet count, and coagulation time but with poor clot retraction and abnormal platelet morphology. With sharper separation of platelet functions it may be possible eventually to relate a bleeding disorder to a specific defect. Patients have already been described in whom there is a defect in thromboplastin formation, clot retraction, and antiheparin activity of the blood—functions of platelets necessary for maintenance of normal hemostasis.[14,374] Treatment of these patients is limited to transfusions of fresh or whole blood or platelet-rich plasma.

In thrombasthenia, known as Glanzmann's or Glanzmann-Naegeli's disease, the defect is in the platelets, which are unable to promote clot retraction. Other features are abnormalities in platelet adhesion, aggregation, or fusion. In some cases platelet fibrinogen levels are decreased. Megakaryocytes are large and normal in number. In thrombocytopathy platelet function is defective with regard to thromboplastin generation (platelet factor 3 deficiency) and the platelets are large and bizarre. In both thrombasthenia and thrombocytopathy there is a mild to moderately severe hemorrhagic diathesis with a prolonged bleeding time.

Zucker and colleagues[404] reported a child of 10 years with thrombasthenia who showed a mild to moderate hemorrhagic diathesis. The defect in the platelets was reflected in an inability to promote clot retraction. While the platelet count was normal, the liberated adenosine diphosphate (ADP) failed to cause aggregation.

Cases of hereditary and familial thrombopathic thrombasthenia have been reported in one group in thirteen patients in three families[91] and in the other in eight affected members in three generations.[206] The thrombopathy was dominantly transmitted, platelet factor 3 was deficient, the platelets were large and heavily granular, clot retraction was normal, and in one of the groups[404] the lipid content of the patient's platelets was 27 times the normal. Bleeding occurred from mucous surfaces and after operative procedures.

In patients with von Willebrand's disease, platelet factor 3 is normal and is reduced in thrombopathies.[387]

The bleeding disorder in glycogen storage disease was studied in six patients with type I and two patients each with type III and type VI.[266] The most commonly seen abnormalities were prolonged Ivy bleeding time, low values for platelet adhesiveness, increased number of platelets, and high values for prothrombin and fibrinogen. It was concluded that patients with types I and VI, and possibly also type III, may have a bleeding disorder similar to thrombasthenia. When operations are necessary or in accidental bleeding in patients with glycogen storage disease, fresh thrombocyte-rich blood or thrombocyte suspensions may be required to correct the bleeding tendency.

*Tourniquet (Rumple-Leede) test.* The tourniquet test serves as a measure of capillary resistance. It consists of obstructing venous blood flow by a constricting band on the arm (blood pressure cuff) and recording the number of petechiae in a specified area distal to the obstruction. The intracapillary pressure is increased sufficiently to demonstrate a state of latent increased permeability (capillary fragility). The test is commonly performed by maintaining the blood pressure midway between the systolic and diastolic pressures for 3 to 5 minutes. After the cuff is removed the number of petechiae in a previously marked circular area, 5 cm. in diameter, on the flexor surface of the forearm a little below the bend of the elbow is counted. A count above five is interpreted as positive. Although the capillary resistance tends to parallel other manifestations of vascular inadequacy, many exceptions are encountered so that a positive test is not always observed with a prolonged bleeding time and thrombocytopenia. On the other hand, some have claimed that the bleeding time reflects the danger of hemorrhage much more accurately than platelet numbers.[232]

*Significance of routine coagulation tests.* The screening tests thus far described provide unequivocal evidence of a single defect—i.e., an abnormality of platelets. The combined abnormalities of clot retraction, bleeding time, the tourniquet test, and, of course, a low platelet count support such a diagnosis.

Markedly prolonged coagulation time is most commonly found in patients with deficiencies of the plasma thromboplastin precursors (factors VIII, IX, and XI), with severe fibrinogen deficiency, and with circulating anticoagulants. Mild degrees of factors VIII, IX, and XI deficiencies may coexist with entirely normal whole blood clotting time. Abnormal results of the routine tests indicate the existence of a hemorrhagic state but do not give sufficient information for a specific diagnosis. On the other hand, normal results with these tests do not exclude a coagulation defect, especially when the history is suggestive. Further investigations carried out systematically are, therefore, necessary to detect minor degrees of depletion.

### Tests for phase 1 of coagulation

The tests for the first phase of coagulation are primarily designed to differentiate the three types of hemophilia: classic hemophilia (hemophilia A) due to factor VIII deficiency, Christmas disease (hemophilia B) due to factor IX deficiency, and factor XI deficiency. Platelet defects, in number or quality, can also be recognized by these tests.

In patients with each type of hemophilia, regardless of severity, the platelet count, bleeding time, clot retraction, prothrombin time, and fibrinogen content are normal. The severe grades of the hemophilias are characterized by a markedly prolonged coagulation time. In patients with milder types, however, the clotting time may be only slightly prolonged, and in those with the mildest types it may be entirely normal. With more elaborate and sensitive tests it is possible to detect lesser degrees of deficiency of the three plasma proteins (factors VIII, IX, and XI).

The tests currently employed in first phase coagulation abnormalities are the thromboplastin generation test and the prothrombin consumption test.

***Thromboplastin generation test.*** Although the prothrombin consumption test detects moderate deficiencies of thromboplastin, it is normal in patients with mild deficiencies of the factors (VIII, IX, or XI) that enter into its formation. The thromboplastin generation test described by Biggs and Douglas[50] has proved to be a more sensitive test of thromboplastin formation defects. It not only permits the detection of slight degrees of abnormality, but, more important, it differentiates one type of abnormality from another, a distinction not provided by the whole blood-clotting time or prothrombin consumption test. Specific deficiencies of antihemophilic globulin (factor VIII), plasma thromboplastin component (factor IX), and plasma thromboplastin antecedent (factor XI) can thus be ascertained. When carried out in patients with disease of varying clinical severity, the amount of thromboplastin formed bears some relation to clinical severity.

With the thromboplastin generation test, the progressive activity of plasma thromboplastin is evaluated by incubating, at 37° C., a mixture of adsorbed barium sulfate plasma containing factors V, VIII, XI, and XII, serum containing factors IX, X, XI, and XII, platelets (or substitutes), and calcium chloride. Both the plasma and serum reagents contain factors XI and XII. Fibrinogen and factor VII are present in adsorbed plasma and serum, respectively, but these factors do not influence the generation of blood prothrombinase. At regular intervals measured samples of the incubation mixture are added to normal plasma (substrate). The thromboplastin generated in this incubation mixture causes clotting of the plasma, and the speed of clotting is a measure of thromboplastin formation. When all the first stage coagulation factors are present in normal amounts, the thromboplastin produced by the generating mixture after 3 to 7 minutes' incubation is sufficiently potent to achieve a plasma clotting time of 8 to 10 seconds.

The thromboplastin generation test is similar to the prothrombin time inasmuch as both utilize the property of thromboplastin to shorten the clotting time of recalcified plasma.

*Preparation of coagulation factors for thromboplastin generation test.* Except for fibrinogen, which can be measured quantitatively, the clotting factors involved in the production of thromboplastin and of the accessory factors in prothrombin conversion can be identified by analyzing their distinctive behavior and interaction in specially devised clotting systems. With the use of minimal suspensions which selectively adsorb some factors in plasma and not others, the knowledge that certain factors are present in plasma and absent in serum, and the knowledge of the effect of storage upon plasma and serum factors, it is possible to determine the presence or absence of factors in each stage of coagulation. In testing for deficiencies in the first stage, advantage is taken of the fact that adsorption removes several factors from normal plasma but leaves factor VIII (AHG) and factor V (labile factor) intact.

PLASMA. In many coagulation studies plasma rather than whole blood is used. It is prepared with one of the anticoagulants, and when obtained from normal blood, plasma contains all the coagulant factors in each phase of coagulation.

ADSORBED PLASMA. Several adsorbing agents are available. Aluminum hydroxide is most commonly used for citrated blood. Also in use is barium sulfate or tricalcium phosphate gel for oxalated blood. In any case deprothrombinized plasma results. These adsorbing agents remove the vitamin K–dependent factors—i.e., factor II (prothrombin), factor VII (stable factor), factor IX (PTC), and factor X (Stuart-Prower factor). They leave factor V (labile factor), factor VIII (AHG), factor XI (PTA), factor XII (Hageman factor), and factor I (fibrinogen) in the adsorbed plasma. Factors XI and XII are partly adsorbed.

SERUM. If normal whole blood is allowed to clot in a test tube, prothrombin, factors V and VIII, and fibrinogen are consumed. Normal serum then contains factor VII (stable factor), factor IX (PTC), factor X (Stuart-Prower factor), factor XI (PTA), and factor XII (Hageman factor). Both plasma and serum reagents contain factors XI and XII but serum usually

Table 34. Constituents of "reagents" prepared from normal blood*

| Reagent | Phase 1 | Phase 2 | Phase 3 |
|---|---|---|---|
| Whole plasma† | Factor VIII (AHG)<br>Factor IX (PTC)<br>Factor XI (PTA)<br>Factor X (Stuart-Prower) | Prothrombin<br>Factor V<br>Factor VII<br>Factor X | Fibrinogen |
| Adsorbed plasma | Factor VIII (AHG)<br>Factor XI (PTA) | Factor V | Fibrinogen |
| Serum | Factor IX (PTC)<br>Factor XI (PTA)<br>Factor X (Stuart-Prower) | Factor VIII<br>Factor X | .......... |

*Modified from Schulman, I., and Smith, C. H.: Coagulation disorders in infancy and childhood. In Levine, S. Z., editor: Advances in pediatrics, vol. 9, Chicago, 1957, Year Book Medical Publishers, Inc., p. 231.
†While factor V (labile factor) appears in whole and adsorbed plasma and influences the thromboplastin generation tests, it is usually assayed in phase 2. Factor X (Stuart-Prower factor) deficiency also gives phase 1 and 2 abnormalities and may be assayed in both phases. However, in phase 2 it is separated from factor VII (stable factor) deficiency by the Stypven test mentioned in the text.

contains more of these factors than adsorbed plasma.

PLATELETS. In many of the tests performed with these blood products, suspensions of normal platelets are required. Platelet substitutes such as human brain, chloroform extracts of brain, soybean phosphatide (Inosithin), and platelin are stable and give satisfactory results.

CALCIUM CHLORIDE. Calcium chloride is required to institute clotting in all tests in which plasma is used; 0.025M calcium chloride is generally employed. The factors present in each of these preparations are given in Table 34.

*Platelets in thromboplastin generation test— thrombasthenia and thrombopathia.*[69,190,374] It has been taken for granted that the platelets are normal according to the screening tests, this having been previously established by normal platelet count, clot retraction, bleeding time, and tourniquet test. However, in patients with platelet dysfunction the qualitative deficiency will be reflected in an abnormal thromboplastin generation test when the patient's platelets are placed in a system with normal adsorbed plasma and normal serum. The test is corrected with normal platelets or platelet substitutes.

Thrombasthenia, also known as hereditary thrombasthenia and Glanzmann's disease, refers to a defective function of platelets in clot retraction. Platelets show a defect in adhesiveness and aggregation and are further characterized by an inability to form pseudopods.[129] A lack of spreading in plasma and sera results in a disturbance in clot retraction.[69] Electron microscopy has shown a predominance of the "round" platelets and a virtual absence of "spread" and "dendritic" forms. Gross[142] found in thrombasthenia a hereditary defect of two glycolytic enzymes—i.e., glyceraldehyde phosphate dehydrogenase and pyruvate kinase. He regarded the lack of the former enzyme as the main cause of diminished adenosine triphosphate and the reason for disturbance in viscous metamorphosis and clot retraction. While the prognosis in the mild cases of this disease appears to be excellent, two seriously involved children have been described.[129] Thrombopathia (thrombocytopathia) refers to a defect in platelets in thromboplastin formation (platelet factor 3). In thrombocytopathia pseudopod formation and spread are normal, but the platelets are giant in size and thromboplastin generation and prothrombin consumption are disturbed. Thrombopathia has often been used as an all-inclusive term for any qualitative platelet defect.

Since the bleeding tendency is based on a platelet defect, it would seem most appropriate to treat any hemorrhagic episode in either thrombasthenia or thrombopathia with fresh whole blood, platelet-rich plasma, or platelets.

An active principle has been isolated from red cells, adenosine diphosphate (ADP) (see discussion of platelet adhesiveness), which causes the rapid aggregation of platelets in citrated or oxalated plasma, causing them to adhere to foreign surfaces such as glass. Thrombasthenia has now been defined as a congenital bleeding disorder characterized by a normal platelet count, a long bleeding time, and a failure of platelet aggregation by ADP.[147] Failure of clot retraction can be accounted for purely on the basis of failure of aggregation. Since the platelets have been found to contain normal amounts of adenosine diphosphate (ADP), the failure of platelets to aggregate has been explained by a defective release of ADP due to impermeability of the platelet membrane.

Baldini and Steiner[30] have differentiated several of these confusing conditions. Thrombocytopathy represents a defect in platelet factor 3. Thrombopathia is caused by a failure of the platelets to release ADP in response to aggregating agents (collagen, epinephrine, and thrombin).[149] Cases similar to those described by Hardisty and Hutton[149] were reported by Weiss and associates[391] of six members in one family in whom bleeding was traced to impaired release of platelet ADP. Here, as in previously reported cases, aggregation by connective tissue which requires ADP release was impaired whereas primary aggregation by ADP itself was normal. The second wave of aggregation induced by epinephrine or ADP, which is also the result of ADP release, was absent in all patients. Thrombasthenia of the Glanzmann variety has become the name for a group of bleeding disorders having in common a lack of platelet aggregation that is probably due to unresponsiveness of the platelet membrane to ADP.

In terms of recent investigations of functional abnormalities, platelet disorders may be classified into five major categories.

*Thrombasthenia.*[179a,254a,404] This disorder is characterized by absent primary aggregation with ADP, poor clot retraction, and low platelet fibrinogen. Clinical symptoms vary from none to marked bleeding. Inheritance is usually by an autosomal recessive pattern.

*Giant platelet (Bernard-Soulier) syndrome.*[43a,142b] The presence of giant platelets in association with abnormal prothrombin consumption and absent platelet aggregation with bovine fibrinogen characterize this disorder. Bleeding is clinically of marked severity, and the disorder is inherited in an autosomal recessive fashion.

*Impaired ADP release with deficiency of nucleotide storage pool.*[172a] The features of this disorder are abnormal aggregation with epinephrine and collagen, absence of the second wave of aggregation, and a reduction of the nucleotide storage pool. It is usually inherited as an autosomal dominant and, when associated with albinism, as an autosomal recessive. The clinical symptoms are mild and result in minor bleeding episodes.

*Impaired ADP release with normal storage pool.*[392a] This disorder is characterized by a decreased second wave of aggregation with collagen and epinephrine in the presence of a normal pool of ADP. Minimal to few clinical symptoms are present and its mode of inheritance is unknown.

*Wiskott-Aldrich syndrome.*[29a,142a] The classic disorder is a fatal sex-linked recessive illness associated with eczema, deficiency of IgM immunoglobulin, and increased susceptibility to infections. Small platelets with a shortened life-span and impaired function are the main features of the disorder.

Thromboplastin generation tests can be modified to provide quantitative estimates of AHG activity and of other hemophilic factors[285] (Table 35). However, specific plasma factor assays have virtually replaced the thromboplastin generation test in determining plasma factor activity.

Several simplified screening tests have been devised to detect mild to moderate deficiencies of

Table 35. Effects of normal plasma, normal deprothrombinized plasma, and normal serum on coagulation abnormalities in AHG, PTC, and PTA deficiencies*

| Reagent added to patient's plasma | Deficiency | | |
| --- | --- | --- | --- |
| | Factor VIII (AHG) | Factor IX (PTC) | Factor XI (PTA) |
| Normal plasma | Corrects | Corrects | Corrects |
| Normal adsorbed plasma | Corrects | No correction | Corrects |
| Normal serum | No correction | Corrects | Corrects |

*From Schulman, I., and Smith, C. H.: Coagulation disorders in infancy and childhood. In Levine, S. Z., editor: Advances in pediatrics, vol. 9, Chicago, 1957, Year Book Medical Publishers, Inc., p. 231.

those factors required for thromboplastin generation. The principal factors are factor VIII (AHG), factor IX (PTC), and factor XI (PTA), and a deficiency of any one of these is responsible for one of the hemophilias.

One of these methods, the Hicks-Pitney test,[163] is a useful and rapid method for eliminating those specimens in which further investigation is unnecessary. The principle of the test is the recalcification of diluted whole plasma in the presence of a platelet substitute. Thromboplastin generation is determined by adding samples of the incubation mixture to high-spun, normal, recalcified plasma.

Another test, the partial thromboplastin time, is simpler than the Hicks-Pitney and has become increasingly popular.[208,270] The procedure is based on the finding that certain thromboplastins are able to compensate only partially for the lack of plasma antihemophilic activity. The test is in effect a modification of the one-stage recalcification time. It is performed in the same manner as the prothrombin time test, except for the substitution of crude "cephalin" mixtures, derived either from mammalian brain or soybeans, for tissue thromboplastin. The cephalin preparation serves as a source of platelet-like activity. The partial thromboplastin time may be defined as the clotting time of recalcified plasma in the presence of a lipid partial thromboplastin rather than complete thromboplastin of the prothrombin time test.[208,270] Various modifications have provided for constancy in the amount of platelet-like activity in the plasma and the degree of contact activation of plasma.[10] In common use is the activation of the test plasma and control by incubation with the silica compound kaolin or Celite.[236,293] The test is particularly useful in detecting deficiencies of fibrinogen, prothrombin, and factors V, VIII, IX, X, XI, and XII. The plasma thromboplastin time is known to be insensitive to factor VII. The test is a simplified means of detecting bleeding such as mild hemophilia and Christmas disease. The partial thromboplastin time normally varies from 36 to 46 seconds. The activated partial thromboplastin time (PTT) is derived from the fact that a partial thromboplastin is formed when a deficiency is present and the test sample has a prolonged clotting time. The test is performed using 0.1 ml. citrated plasma which is incubated for 4 minutes with an activating agent such as kaolin or Celite, which provides additional surface for activation, and platelet phospholipid substitute for cephalin. Then it is recalcified with 0.1 ml. 0.025M $CaCl_2$ and the clotting time is noted.

The partial thromboplastin time can be made more specific by identifying the deficient factor. If an abnormal result is obtained, the test may be repeated after the addition of known reagents. After adsorption by barium sulfate or other agents, factors V and VIII, and to a lesser extent factors XI and XII, are retained in the plasma. Factors VII, IX, X, XI, and XII are present in serum after coagulation. The correction of the partial thromboplastin time by adsorbed plasma, but not by serum, indicates that factor V or VIII is deficient. Correction by serum, but not by adsorbed plasma, indicates that factors IX and X are deficient. Correction by both test reagents indicates factor XI deficiency. Factor VII deficiency is indicated by a normal partial thromboplastin time and a prolonged prothrombin time.

*Mutual correction tests.* The various hemophilias may be differentiated simply by testing for mutual correction in mixtures of blood or plasma from the patient with the unknown defect and from patients whose defects have been identified. Blood or plasma from a patient with AHG (factor VIII) deficiency will correct abnormal coagulation in a test tube of blood from patients with PTC (factor IX) and PTA (factor XI) defects but not from another AHG deficiency. The same principle applies for correction of PTA-deficient blood and plasma by AHG or PTC but not by PTA samples and for the correction of PTC-deficient blood by AHG and PTA but not by PTC sample. The difficulties in mutual correction tests are that a panel of blood samples from patients with known deficiencies is not always available—hence the advantage of the precise diagnostic facilities of the thromboplastin generation test.

*Comparative value of laboratory tests in detecting thromboplastin deficiency.* Antihemophilic globulin is normally present in plasma in a range of 50 to 170%.[73] Intermediate degrees of bleeding occur between the almost negligible levels of AHG in patients with classic hemophilia and the lower limit of normal. The variable sensitivity of the tests enumerated for phase 1 abnormalities must therefore be considered in the diagnosis of hemophilia. Thus, as little as 1% antihemophilic globulin is sufficient to produce a normal whole blood clotting time, 3 to 5% to yield a normal prothrombin consumption, and values of more than 15 to 20% to result in a normal thromboplastin generation. Hence, abnormal tests will result only when the antihemophilic content of plasma falls below these levels.

*Prothrombin consumption test.* The prothrombin consumption test is performed on serum after clotting has occurred in a manner similar to the one-stage test for prothrombin time of plasma, with one addition. Since serum contains stable factor (factor VII) but not fibrinogen or labile factor (factor V), these must be supplemented in order to determine the residual prothrombin after clotting. The additional factors required are present in plasma which has been adsorbed with barium sulfate or tricalcium phosphate. The treated plasma contains labile factor (factor V), and fibrinogen, but it is free of prothrombin.

With a 1 ml. serologic pipette, 0.1 ml. of serum to be analyzed (residual after clotting) is blown into a mixture of 0.1 ml. of calcium chloride, 0.1 ml. of adsorbed plasma (source of labile factor [factor V] and fibrinogen), and 0.1 ml. of thromboplastin reagent (as in the test for plasma prothrombin time). The time required for the clot to form is accurately measured.

The normal prothrombin consumption time is over 25 seconds,[114] thus indicating very little residual prothrombin. The usual range of residual prothrombin in serum is given as 0 to 25%. Usually, 75% is converted to thrombin. In patients with disorders of phase 1 the serum prothrombin time is below 25 seconds and in severely affected patients it is as short as 12 to 14 seconds. In principle the prothrombin consumption test is similar to the Quick prothrombin time test inasmuch as the former measures the prothrombin remaining in serum and the latter that which is present in the plasma before coagulation.

*Interpretation of prothrombin consumption test.* The prothrombin consumption test is a quantitative determination of the residual prothrombin in serum after clotting has occurred. When normal blood in a test tube clots, sufficient thromboplastin is formed in the initial phase of coagulation to convert virtually all of the prothrombin to thrombin so that at completion of the process there is little or no prothrombin left in the serum. If all the prothrombin is utilized and little or none is left in the serum, it can be taken for granted that adequate amounts of thromboplastin have been formed and that this first phase of coagulation is relatively normal. On the other hand, abnormalities of this phase are indicated by the presence of a large amount of residual prothrombin in the serum after clotting, indicating the formation of inadequate amounts of thromboplastin required to convert prothrombin to thrombin. Prothrombin activity of the serum is determined 1 hour after coagulation since thrombin continues to be formed after the blood or plasma has clotted. After this interval practically all the prothrombin has been consumed. The prothrombin consumption test, although useful in detecting defects affecting the formation of thromboplastin, is less sensitive than the thromboplastin generation test.

*Hageman factor (factor XII) deficiency.* The Hageman factor participates in the early stages of coagulation.[308] Present in an inactive form in normal blood, Hageman factor (factor XII) is activated by contact with a foreign substance and in turn activates plasma thromboplastin antecedent (factor XI, PTA), thereby initiating thromboplastin formation. The factor appears to be concerned with the activation of blood on contact with glass. Despite the demonstrable abnormality of in vitro coagulation, individuals with this disorder do not manifest hemorrhagic tendencies.[9] In this deficiency, bleeding time, platelet count, and clot retraction are normal. The clotting time, prothrombin consumption, recalcification time, partial thromboplastin time, and the thromboplastin generation test are markedly abnormal. There are many similarities between factor XI (PTA) and factor XII (Hageman factor) and they may be difficult to separate from each other. The recalcification time of Hageman-deficient plasma is prolonged, but it is readily corrected by the addition of small amounts of normal plasma that have been adsorbed with barium sulfate and by the addition of normal serum. Complete correction is also obtained with factor XI (PTA) deficient plasma. Since the Hageman factor (factor XII) is known to be deficient in fresh chicken serum, failure to correct the thromboplastin generation test and other tests with this material helps to establish the diagnosis. Thus, the recalcification time becomes normal when the test is performed in tubes that have been coated previously with normal serum and then thoroughly rinsed. The lengthened recalcification time of Hageman-deficient human plasma is not corrected by the addition of chicken serum or by the use of glass tubes coated with chicken serum.

In the investigation of the mechanims for thrombocytopenia and of defects of platelet function in bleeding disorders a variety of special laboratory tests may be performed.[203] Two tests, platelet adhesiveness and platelet factor 3, will be described in relation to hemostasis.

The wide range of normal values for factor XII has been explained by the concept of multiple alleles at the Hageman locus.[194] A range of 63 to 196% has been reported in normal subjects.

*Platelet adhesiveness.* In the process of viscous metamorphosis platelets are clumped and fused and release granules into the surrounding plasma.[337] Platelets or products of their disintegration are essential for the formation of intrinsic thromboplastin. During their aggregation platelets manifest an ability to adhere to other platelets and to stick to solid surfaces, particularly those that promote coagulation such as the vascular endothelium.[55] Hellem and associates[160] discovered that a heat-stable extract of red cells (factor R) could induce platelet aggregation. When the vessel is injured, red cells come into contact with the wound surface and liberate factor R, which makes the platelets adhesive and leads to formation of the platelet plug. Fractionation of this extract later showed that the active agent was adenosine diphosphate (ADP).[130] When ADP is added to platelet-rich citrated plasma in minute concentration, platelet clumping occurs. Hellem and co-workers[160] postulated that it is the adhesiveness of platelets and not their total number that is decisive in hemostasis. ADP is not restricted to red cells but can be extracted from tissues and cells other than erythrocytes,[251] thus initiating platelet adhesion after cell injury.

One of the methods to assess the adhesiveness of platelets in damaged tissues is to compare the platelet count of venous blood with that from a skin wound sample. The number of platelets from a small skin incision is lower than in venous blood. The difference measures the number of platelets adhering to damaged vessel walls, wound surfaces, and those required to arrest bleeding from small blood vessels by forming a plug. The formation of such plugs depends on the ability of the platelets to adhere to the wound surface and to one another. The difference in the platelet count between a venous blood and a "capillary" blood sample from a standard wound reflects those lost in transit and is a measure of the adhered platelets.[64] Platelet adhesiveness has been investigated in a number of conditions. While a poor correlation has been found between the bleeding time and the platelet count in cases of anemia with a long bleeding time, a good inverse correlation exists between the results of the platelet adhesiveness test and bleeding time. In von Willebrand's disease reduced in vitro platelet adhesiveness has been observed, supplementing the other features of prolonged bleeding time and a reduced level of factor VIII.[271,353,403] The platelets in patients with von Willebrand's disease are nonadhesive in vivo and the prolonged bleeding time may be explained by the lack of, or delay in, platelet plug formation.[65] Paradoxic changes in optical density have been noted on the addition of adenosine diphosphate (ADP) to plasma of patients with von Willebrand's disease. When small amounts of ADP are added to normal citrated platelet-rich plasma, the modification of platelets leads to decreased optical density. In von Willebrand's disease the optical density at 610 m$\mu$ increases instead of decreases.[371] These differences may be due to the prolonged bleeding time in this disease and to the failure of platelets to adhere to the vessel wall.[65]

A subnormal percentage of adhesive platelets has also been observed in iron-deficiency anemia, especially in those children with occult blood in the stool. The return to normal platelet adhesion when the anemia was corrected suggested that the occult blood resulted from the hemostatic defect associated with decreased platelet adhesion.[8]

Other methods have been devised for measuring the ability of platelets to stick to solid surfaces so as to stimulate normal and damaged vascular endothelium. Many of the methods are based on modifications in which platelets are counted before and after exposure of a sample of blood or plasma to glass surfaces.[399] A method for estimating the platelet adhesiveness employs citrated blood.[159] Blood is forced from a graduated syringe through a glass bead column at a constant rate. The reduction in platelet count after passage through the glass bead column is taken as a measure of platelet adhesiveness. It is assumed that reduction in platelet number during the passage is caused by adhesiveness to the glass beads. Another in vitro method has also been devised which requires no anticoagulant before contact of the blood with a foreign surface, in this case a glass bead filter.[324] Under these conditions platelet adhesiveness in normal individuals is 36 to 60%. It also falls within the normal range in disorders of blood coagulation and in patients receiving heparin, but is deficient in thrombasthenia and in von Willebrand's disease. The retention of platelets in the glass bead filter required a divalent cation, probably calcium.

Caution must be exercised in interpretation of tests of platelet adhesiveness, because of the possible sources of error in counting platelets and the loss of platelets that is not due to adhesion to a surface but to disintegration or clumping without adhesion.[55]

*Aspirin and platelet function.* It has been emphasized that aspirin should be used with discretion in patients with bleeding disorders.

Quick[298] found that in a series of normal medical and college students over 50% showed a small but significant prolongation of the bleeding time upon the ingestion of 1.3 gm. of aspirin, and some even had a small increase after 0.65 gm. of the drug. The increased bleeding observed after aspirin ingestion is the result of impaired platelet aggregation due to inhibition in the release of platelet-adenosine diphosphate (ADP).[119,389,390]

Kaneshiro and associates[193] found that Ivy bleeding times before and 2 hours after 1 gm. of aspirin in fourteen patients with mild hemophilia A, two with mild hemophilia B, three with PTA deficiency, and three with established or suspected von Willebrand's disease did not differ significantly from those found earlier in normal controls. Mean bleeding times before aspirin were normal in eleven patients with severe hemophilia A and eight with severe hemophilia B. Four patients in each group had profoundly prolonged bleeding times after aspirin. Seven patients eventually required transfusion to stop the bleeding. The combination of aspirin and the severe clotting defect "paralyzed" the formation of the platelet aggregates that stop bleeding in the bleeding time test, illustrating the potential therapeutic hazard of aspirin in some patients with severe hemophilia.

In vitro, aspirin impairs aggregation of platelets by collagen but not by thrombin. Aspirin inhibits the release of ADP from platelets by collagen. In severe hemophilia the formation of thrombin is greatly impeded. Platelet plugs must, therefore, form primarily as the result of aggregation induced by collagen.

These observations have led to the conclusion that aspirin should be used with caution in the hemophiliac. Effective and safe medications for use with hemophiliacs can be established only after much study. However, preliminary studies indicate that Darvon, Tylenol, and Tempra are effective as analgesics and do not have the aspirin effect.

Another technique has been described which measures the adhesion of platelets to connective tissue fragments in platelet-rich plasma.[349] The principle of the method is measurement of the optical density in EDTA platelet-rich plasma to which connective tissue fragments have been added. A full optical density occurs as the platelets line up on connective tissue fibers. Aspirin-treated platelets adhere normally, although they show reduced aggregation in citrated platelet-rich plasma. In the presence of sufficient connective tissue, all platelets participate in the adhesion reaction.

*Platelet factor 3 deficiency.* The participation of platelets in the intrinsic pathway of blood coagulation is through their content of platelet factor 3. There is no doubt that the phospholipid liberated from lysed platelets is essential for the generation of plasma thromboplastin. It has also been postulated that the membranes of aggregated platelets in a hemostatic plug probably furnish a catalytic lipoprotein surface for the interaction of plasma coagulation factors involved in the intrinsic pathway. Despite its shortcomings as a true biochemical entity, methods have been advised for studying platelet phospholipid availability. A simple test of platelet factor 3 availability is to determine the kaolin clotting time of platelet-rich plasma.[148,348] Russell viper venom (Stypven) is also widely used as a test reagent for platelet factor 3. The venom clots plasma in the presence of "available" platelet lipoprotein.[233] The term thrombopathia has been used to designate bleeding disorders in which release of platelet factor 3 is reduced (see p. 737).

In a group of eight patients with mild bleeding disorders routine studies of hemostasis gave normal results.[392] Using a quantitative assay for platelet factor 3 (thromboplastin factor) in which platelet suspensions of constant, low concentration were employed in the thromboplastin generation test, all were found to have decreased factor 3 activity. Other platelet functions were normal. The single patient with prolonged bleeding time had the same platelet defect.

*Platelet aggregometer.* The instrument is a spectrophotometer attached to a recorder which measures the density of the platelet-rich plasma. As aggregation appears greater intensity of light is transmitted through the cuvette. The ability of the platelets to respond to additives such as ADP, epinephrine, and collagen is routinely measured when the ability of the platelets to aggregate is explored.

## Tests for phase 2 of coagulation

**Prothrombin complex deficiencies.** In carrying out in vitro tests prothrombin, factor V, factor VII, and the Stuart-Prower factor (factor X) must be present in sufficient amounts to convert prothrombin to thrombin and give a normal prothrombin time. These factors collectively are frequently designated as the prothrombin complex. A failure to effect conversion to thrombin may result from a deficiency of one or a combination of these factors. It should again be emphasized that these are in vitro tests designed to isolate defects of any one or a combination of factors in the laboratory.

**Prothrombin time (*plasma prothrombin time*).** The one-stage test of Quick[294] has been found most useful in determining disturbances of the second phase of coagulation (the conversion of prothrombin to thrombin after activation by thromboplastin). The Quick test measures the time needed for the thrombin titer of plasma to reach the clotting level in the presence of a fixed amount of thromboplastin and calcium. By adding an excess of tissue extract (thromboplastin) and optimal amounts of calcium to measured samples of citrated or oxalated plasma, prothrombin activity is measured by the time required for coagulation to occur. The one-stage prothrombin time serves as a specific indicator of phase 2 involvement and includes the entire prothrombin complex—prothrombin and the accelerator agents, factor V (labile), factor VII (stable), and factor X (Stuart-Prower factor). In our laboratory the normal prothrombin time by this method is 11 to 15 seconds. It should be remembered that no definitive prothrombin time can be stated that is the same for every laboratory. Since the value obtained depends upon the potency of the thromboplastin used, a normal control must be simultaneously determined. In terms of prothrombin activity by comparison on a curve from suitable plasma dilutions, the normal range is from 70 to 120%.

An elevated prothrombin time may reflect any single or combined deficiency of prothrombin, factor VII, factor V, factor X (Stuart-Prower factor), and fibrinogen (absence of end point). An unusually low plasma content of fibrinogen may also account for a prolonged one-stage reading, but this value can be determined chemically. A normal prothrombin time serves therefore incidentally as evidence of a normal fibrinogen content of plasma. With the help of simple correction tests a deficiency of either labile (factor V) or stable factor (factor VII) can be readily determined.

The one-stage prothrombin test is performed as follows.[332] The thromboplastin used is generally obtained from rabbit brain or rabbit lung. Many excellent, well-standardized thromboplastin preparations are commercially available. This test requires exacting technique; the patient's plasma must be obtained in a standard manner, the concentration of calcium chloride must be exact, the temperature must be controlled at 37° C., a stop watch is used for timing, and controls are carried out. With most techniques, 0.1 ml. of thromboplastin is then added. Timing is started at this point, and the clotting time is recorded. Commercial preparations are available in which the thromboplastin and calcium are already mixed in proper amounts (Simplastin). The test then requires only one step. Preparations of control plasma for testing thromboplastic reagent are also commercially available (Diagnostic Plasma, Protrol). As previously stated, with most techniques the one-stage prothrombin times are usually 12 to 14 seconds.

Differential tests can be carried out in conjunction with the one-stage prothrombin time to determine a deficiency of factor V, factor VII, prothrombin, or factor X (Stuart-Prower factor). It there is correction of the Quick prothrombin time by the addition of the patient's plasma to deprothrombinized plasma

Table 36. Differentiation of prothrombin complex deficiencies

| Deficient factor causing abnormal (prolonged) prothrombin time | Effect of addition of | | |
|---|---|---|---|
| | Normal plasma | Serum | Adsorbed plasma |
| Prothrombin | Corrects | No correction | No correction |
| Factor V (labile factor) | Corrects | No correction | Corrects |
| Factor VII (stable factor) | Corrects | Corrects | No correction |

(barium sulfate–adsorbed) the patient lacks factor V (labile factor); if there is correction of the Quick prothrombin time by the addition of serum, the patient lacks factor VII (stable factor); if there is no improvement by adding both reagents (deprothrombinized plasma and serum), the patient has a deficiency of prothrombin itself.

Normal plasma, serum, and adsorbed plasma (with barium sulfate, hence deprothrombinized) contain the following factors of the prothrombin complex: normal plasma—prothrombin and factor V (labile factor), factor VII (stable factor), and factor X (Stuart-Prower factor); normal serum—factor VII (stable factor) and factor X (Stuart-Prower factor); and adsorbed plasma—factor V (labile factor).

The differentiation of the prothrombin complex deficiencies is indicated in Table 36. Factor X (Stuart-Prower factor) deficiency, which follows the same pattern as stable factor (factor VII) deficiency, is not included in the table.

Other differential tests for factor V (labile factor) and factor VII (stable factor) deficiencies are based on the fact that when oxalated plasma is stored, factor V (labile factor) disappears rapidly, whereas factor VII (stable factor) and prothrombin remain in high concentration. A reagent for determining the factor VII (stable factor) deficiency can also be prepared by the passage of plasma through a 30% asbestos filter, which removes factor VII (stable factor) but retains prothrombin and factor V (labile factor).

**Combined prothrombin and factor VII (stable factor) deficiency.** If the patient's plasma does not correct the prolonged prothrombin time with aged plasma (contains factor VII [stable factor] but no factor V [labile factor]), factor V (labile factor) is deficient. If factor V (labile factor) is present and the addition of small amounts of serum (contains abundant factor VII [stable factor]) only partially corrects the prothrombin time, then presumably both prothrombin and factor VII (stable factor) are deficient.

**Stuart-Prower factor (factor X).** Investigation of patients with a long Quick prothrombin time led to the discovery of a defect heretofore ascribed as a deficiency of factor VII.[101,181] The Stuart-Prower factor (factor X) is present in normal plasma and is relatively heat and storage stable. This factor is now known to be essential for both normal plasma thromboplastin production and conversion of prothrombin to thrombin by its interaction with tissue extract. The Stuart-Prower factor (factor X) and factor VII are both adsorbed by tricalcium phosphate and other similar adsorbing agents. A deficiency of the Stuart-Prower factor (factor X) results in an abnormal thromboplastin generation test. It can be differentiated from factor VII when Stypven (Russell's viper venom) combined with cephalin replaces tissue thromboplastin in the prothrombin test. An abnormal prothrombin time is then obtained with Stuart-Prower factor (factor X) deficiency in contrast to a normal prothrombin time with plasma deficient in factor VII.[19] Factor VII is not needed in the thromboplastin generation test, whereas the Stuart-Prower factor (factor X) is a necessary ingredient. The clotting time in Stuart-Prower factor (factor X) deficiency is slightly prolonged. Stuart-Prower (factor X) levels were found to be low in premature newborn infants at birth, with an increase toward normal by the sixth day of life whether or not vitamin $K_1$ was given to the infants at birth.[335]

### Tests for phase 3 of coagulation

**Fibrinogen deficiencies.** With adequate thrombin formation, fibrinogen is converted to solid fibrin. Fibrinogen occurs in plasma in a concentration of approximately 180 to 400 mg. per 100 ml. A threshold concentration of at least 60 mg. per 100 ml. is necessary for clotting to be detectable.[398] Many methods are available for clinical quantitation of fibrinogen after its separation from plasma. One of the simplest methods for clinical use is to measure the turbidity of a suspension of salt-precipitated fibrinogen with a spectrophotometer.[123] A simple test for determining the presence of fibrinogen in coagulable blood is the addition of thromboplastin or thrombin. In patients with fibrinogenopenia, the blood will remain incoagulable.

With increasing attention given to fibrinolytic states and with the advent of such fibrinolytic inhibitors as epsilon-aminocaproic acid (Amicar), it has become important to have access to methods for demonstrating the presence of increased plasmin and/or plasminogen activator levels.[78,316,382] The simplest method is the use of whole blood or plasma to measure the rate of fibrinolysis. Whole blood is allowed to clot in a tube at 37° C. and is observed 24 hours later. If no clot is seen, the test is read as positive. When normal plasma is substituted for whole blood, it is clotted by the addition of thrombin or calcium and is incubated under sterile conditions at 37° C. With the whole blood or plasma abnormal bleeding cannot be ascribed to fibrinolysis, if the clot is intact 24 hours after clotting. For either test fibrinolysis is difficult to assess when fibrinogen levels are greatly diminished.

The euglobulin fraction of plasma contains plasminogen activator, plasminogen, and fibrinogen. The euglobulin fibrinolysis time test in frequent use[78] utilizes a precipitate of the euglobulin prepared from citrated plasma and brought to a pH of 5.3 by acetic acid. The precipitate is resuspended in saline solution and clotted with calcium chloride, incubated at 37° C., and inspected at intervals. Normal clots require more than 2 hours for lysis. Values under this period are abnormal.

*FI TEST.* Fibrinolysis during the course of intravascular coagulation (defibrination) may produce fibrin or fibrinogen split products in the circulation which can be detected. One drop of patient's serum is put on a slide with one drop of FI TEST Latex Anti-Human Fibrinogen reagent* and mixed with a wooden applicator stick over an area approximately 20 by 25 mm. The slide is tilted from side to side and observed for macroscopic agglutination. The time it takes for agglutination to occur is recorded. The same procedure is followed in doing a normal control, and the results are compared. If agglutination appears more rapidly with the patient's serum, several dilutions of the serum are prepared to determine quantitatively how much of the fibrin split products are present.

*Interpretation.* A positive agglutination with higher dilution indicates a greater quantity of split products present. Although the antibody is antihuman fibrinogen, agglutination will occur with fibrin split products.

Other methods to determine fibrinolysis include the thromboelastogram, which records fibrin formation and lysis, the fibrin plate method, which measures digestion zones on fibrin plates, and the Ouchterlony technique for double immunodiffusion. Alternative techniques in current use for the determination of fibrin degradation products include the tanned red cell hemagglutination immunoassay (TRCHII), the staphylococcal clumping test, the flocculation test, and the assay for anticoagulant activity.[234a] The sensitivity of each test varies since there are differences in the reactivity of each test system with undigested fibrinogen and intermediate degradation fragments. In one study in which six different techniques for detecting fibrin degradation products were used, the TRCHII test was the most reactive, but the flocculation test was found to be reliable, rapid, simple, and of greatest value in emergency clinical situations. Other investigators, employing the TRCHII, immunodiffusion, latex agglutination (FI test), and the staphylococcal clumping test, were able to detect the elevated levels of fibrin degradation product present in patients with consumption coagulopathy.[365a]

## REFERENCES

1. Aas, K. A., and Gardner, F. H.: Survival of blood platelets labeled with chromium[51], J. Clin. Invest. 37:1257, 1958.
2. Aballi, A. J., Banus, V. L., deLamerens, S., and Rozengvaig, S.: Coagulation studies in the newborn period, alterations of thromboplastin generation and effects of vitamin K in full-term infants, Amer. J. Dis. Child. 94:598, 1957.
3. Aballi, A. J., Banus, V. L., deLamerens, S., and Rozengvaig, S.: Coagulation studies in

---

*Reagents. Hyland FI TEST Rapid Slide Test for Hypofibrogenemia, list No. 050-030.

the newborn period; hemorrhagic disease of the newborn, Amer. J. Dis. Child. 97:524, 1959.
4. Aballi, A. J., Banus, V. L., deLamerens, S., and Rozengvaig, S.: Coagulation studies in the newborn period, deficiency of Stuart-Prower factor as a part of the clotting defect of the newborn, Amer. J. Dis. Child. 94:549, 1959.
5. Aballi, A. J., and deLamerens, S.: Coagulation changes in the neonatal period and in early infancy, Ped. Clin. N. Amer. 9:785, 1962.
6. Abe, T., Sato, K., Kazama, M., and Matsumara, T.: Effect of epsilon-aminocaproic acid in haemophilia, Lancet 2:405, 1962.
7. Abildgaard, C. F.: Recognition and treatment of intravascular coagulation, J. Pediat. 74:163, 1969.
8. Abildgaard, C. F., Alcalde, V., and Schulman, I.: Relationship of hematocrit, platelet count, and platelet adhesion to occult blood loss in iron deficiency anemia, Program of Society for Pediatric Research, Seattle, Wash., June 18-20, 1964.
9. Abildgaard, C. F., Cornet, J. A., Alcalde, V., and Schulman, I.: Hageman factor deficiency in a child, Pediatrics 32:280, 1963.
10. Abildgaard, C. F., Cornet, J. A., Johnson, H., and Schulman, I.: Screening tests for disorders of thromboplastin formation, Ped. Clin. N. Amer. 9:819, 1962.
11. Abildgaard, C. F., Simone, J. V., Corrigan, J. J., Seeler, R. A., Edelstine, G., and Schulman, I.: Treatment of hemophilia with glycine-precipitated factor VIII, New Eng. J. Med. 275:471, 1966.
12. Abildgaard, C. F., Simone, J. V., Honig, G. R., Forman, E. N., Johnson, P. A., and Seeler, R. A.: von Willebrand's disease; a comparative study of diagnostic tests, J. Pediat. 73:355, 1968.
13. Abildgaard, C. F., Simone, J. V., and Schulman, I.: Factor VIII (antihaemophilic factor) activity in sickle-cell anaemia, Brit. J. Haemat. 13:19, 1967.
14. Ackroyd, J. F.: Role of platelets in coagulation, thrombosis and haemostasis, with some observations on platelet dysfunction, including thrombasthenia, Brit. M. Bull. 11:21, 1955.
15. Adelson, E., Rheingold, J. J., and Crosby, W. H.: The platelets as a sponge; a review, Blood 17:767, 1961.
16. Aggeler, P. M.: Physiological basis for transfusion therapy in hemorrhagic disorders, Transfusion 1:71, 1961.
17. Aggeler, P. M., Hoag, M. S., Wallerstein, R. O., and Whissell, D.: The mild hemophilias occult deficiencies of AHF, PTC and PTA frequently responsible for unexpected surgical bleeding, Amer. J. Med. 30:84, 1961.
18. Aggeler, P. M., White, S. G., Glendening, M. B., Page, E. W., Leake, T. B., and Bates, G.: Plasma thromboplastin component (PTC) deficiency; a new disease resembling hemophilia, Proc. Soc. Exp. Biol. Med. 79:692, 1952.
19. Alexander, B.: Clotting factor VII (proconvertin); synonymy, properties, clinical and clinolaboratory aspects, New Eng. J. Med. 260:1218, 1959.
20. Alexander, B., and Goldstein, R.: Dual hemostatic defect in pseudohemophilia, J. Clin. Invest. 29:795, 1950.
21. Alexander, B., and Goldstein, R.: Parahemophilia in three siblings, Amer. J. Med. 13:255, 1952.
22. Alexander, B., Goldstein, R., Landwehr, G., and Cook, C. D.: Congenital SPCA deficiency; a hitherto unrecognized coagulation defect with hemorrhage rectified by serum and serum fractions, J. Clin. Invest. 30:596, 1951.
23. Alexander, B., Goldstein, R., Rich, L., Le Bolloc'h, A. G., Diamond, L. K., and Borges, W.: Congenital afibrinogenemia; a study of some basic aspects of coagulation, Blood 9:843, 1954.
24. Allen, D. M.: Heparin therapy of purpura fulminans, Pediatrics 38:211, 1966.
25. Angelopoulos, B., Kourepi, M., Vicatou, M., and Mourdjinis, A.: Hemophilia due to combined deficiency of AHG, PTC and PTA factors, Acta Haemat. 31:36, 1964.
26. Apt, L., and Downey, W. S., Jr.: "Melena" neonatorum: the swallowed blood syndrome; a simple test for the differentiation of adult and fetal hemoglobin in bloody stools, J. Pediat. 47:6, 1955.
27. Arnold, W. A., Granda, J., and Hilgartner, M. W.: Acid phosphatase levels in synovial fluid of patients with hemophilia, Abstract, American Society of Hematology Meeting, Dec., 1971, San Francisco.
28. Astrup, T.: Fibrinolysis in the organism, Blood 11:781, 1956.
29. Astrup, T., Brakman, P., Ollendorff, P., and Rasmussen, J.: Haemostasis in haemophilia in relation to the haemostatic balance in the normal organism and the effect of peanuts, Thromb. Diath. Haemorrhag. 5:329, 1960.
29a. Baldini, M., Kim, B., Steiner, M., Kuramoto, A., Okuma, M., and Otridge, B. W.: Metabolic defect in the Wiskott-Aldrich syndrome, Pediat. Res. 3:377, 1969.
30. Baldini, M. G., and Steiner, M.: Thrombo-

cytopathies with and without thrombocytopenia, New Eng. J. Med. 281:904, 1969.
31. Barkhan, P.: Haematuria in a haemophiliac treated with epsilon-aminocaproic acid, Lancet 2:1061, 1964.
32. Barkhan, P., and Silver, M. J.: Biological activities of human platelets; biochemical, physiological and clinical aspects. In Tocantins, L. M., editor: Progress in hemotology, vol. III, New York, 1962, Grune & Stratton, Inc.
33. Barnett, C. P.: Hemorrhagic diathesis due to factor VII deficiency, Arch. Intern. Med. 99:280, 1957.
34. Barnhart, M. I.: Cellular fibrinogen. In Koller, F., editor: Fibrinogen and fibrin turnover of clotting factors, Stuttgart, 1963, F. K. Schattauer Verlag.
35. Barrow, E. M., and Graham, J. B.: In Moore, C. V., and Brown, E. B., editors: Progress in hematology, vol. IV, New York, 1964, Grune & Stratton, Inc.
36. Barry, A., and Delage, J-M.: Congenital deficiency of fibrin-stabilizing factor; observation of a new case, New Eng. J. Med. 272:943, 1965.
37. Bayer, W. L., Curiel, D. C., Szeto, I. L. F., and Lewis, J. H.: Acquired factor X deficiency in a Negro boy, Pediatrics 44:1007, 1969.
38. Beck, E. A.: Congenital variants of human fibrinogen. In Laki, K., editor: Fibrinogen, New York, 1968, Marcel Dekker, Inc.
39. Beck, E. A., Charache, P., and Jackson, D. P.: A new coagulation disorder caused by an abnormal fibrinogen ("fibrinogen Baltimore"), Nature 208:143, 1965.
40. Bell, W. N., and Alton, H. G.: A brain extract as a substitute for platelet suspensions in the thromboplastin generation test, Nature 174:880, 1954.
41. Bennett, E., and Huehns, E. R.: Immunological differentiation of three types of haemophilia and identification of some female carriers, Lancet 2:956, 1970.
42. Bentley, H. P., and Krivit, W.: An assay of antihemophilic globulin activity in the carrier female, J. Lab. Clin. Med. 56:613, 1960.
43. Bergsagel, D. E., and Hougie, C.: Intermediate stages in the formation of blood thromboplastin, Brit. J. Haemat. 2:113, 1956.
43a. Bernard, J., and Soulier, J. P.: Sus une nouvelle varieté de dystrophie thrombocytaire hémorragipare congénitale, Sem. Hosp. Paris 24:3217, 1948.
44. Bidwell, E.: The purification of bovine antihaemophilic globulin, Brit. J. Haemat. 1:35, 1955.
45. Bidwell, E.: The purification of antihaemophilic globulin from animal plasma, Brit. J. Haemat. 1:386, 1955.
46. Biggs, R.: Inhibitory effect of haemophilic plasma, Brit. J. Haemat. 4:192, 1958.
47. Biggs, R.: The control of traumatic bleeding in patients with von Willebrand's disease. In Brinkhous, K. M., editor: The hemophilias, International Symposium Washington, Chapel Hill, N. C., 1964, University of North Carolina Press.
48. Biggs, R., and Bidwell, E.: A method for the study of antihaemophilic globulin inhibitors with reference to six cases, Brit. J. Haemat. 5:379, 1959.
49. Biggs, R., Bidwell, E., Handley, D. A., Macfarlane, R. G., Trueta, J., Elliott-Smith, A., Dike, G. W. R., and Ash, B. J.: The preparation and assay of a Christmas-factor (factor IX) concentrate and its use in the treatment of two patients, Brit. J. Haemat. 7:349, 1961.
50. Biggs, R., and Douglas, A. S.: The thromboplastin generation test, J. Clin. Path. 6:23, 1953.
51. Biggs, R., Douglas, A. S., Macfarlane, R. G., Dacie, J. V., Pitney, W. R., Merskey, C., and O'Brien, J. R.: Christmas disease; a condition previously mistaken for haemophilia, Brit. M. J. 2:1378, 1952.
52. Biggs, R., Eveling, J., and Richards, G.: Assay of antihaemophilic globulin activity, Brit. J. Haemat. 1:20, 1955.
53. Biggs, R., and Macfarlane, R. G.: Haemophilia and related conditions; a survey of 187 cases, Brit. J. Haemat. 4:1, 1958.
54. Biggs, R., and Macfarlane, R. G.: Diagnosis of the haemophiloid states, Acta Haemat. 20:118, 1958.
55. Biggs, R., and Macfarlane, R. G.: Human blood coagulation and its disorders, ed. 3, Philadelphia, 1962, F. A. Davis Co.
56. Biggs, R., and Macfarlane, R. G.: Christmas disease, Postgrad. M. J. 38:3, 1962.
57. Biggs, R., and Macfarlane, R. G.: Treatment of haemophilia and other coagulation disorders, Philadelphia, 1966, F. A. Davis Co.
58. Biggs, R., and Matthews, J. M.: The treatment of haemorrhage in von Willebrand's disease and the blood level of factor VIII (AHG), Brit. J. Haemat. 9:203, 1963.
59. Blackburn, E. K., Macfie, J. M., Monaghan, J. H., and Page, A. P. M.: Antihaemophilic factor deficiency, capillary defect of von Willebrand type and idiopathic thrombocytopenia in one family, J. Clin. Path. 14:540, 1961.
60. Blombäck, M., Blombäck, B., and Nilsson, I. M.: Response to fractions in von Willebrand's disease. In Brinkhous, K. M., editor:

The hemophilias, International Symposium Washington, Chapel Hill, N. C., 1964, University of North Carolina Press.
61. Blombäck, M., Jorpes, J. E., and Nilsson, I. M.: Von Willebrand's disease, Amer. J. Med. 34:236, 1963.
62. Bolton, F. G., and Clarke, J. E.: A method of assaying Christmas factor, its application to the study of Christmas disease (factor IX deficiency), Brit. J. Haemat. 5:396, 1959.
63. Bond, T. P., Levin, W. C., Celander, D. R., and Guest, M. M.: "Mild hemophilia" affecting both males and females, New Eng. J. Med. 266:220, 1962.
64. Borchgrevink, C. F.: A method for measuring platelet adhesiveness in vivo, Acta Med. Scandinav. 168:157, 1960.
65. Borchgrevink, C. F.: Platelet adhesion in vivo in patients with bleeding disorders, Acta Med. Scandinav. 170:231, 1961.
66. Boudreaux, H. B., and Frampton, V. L.: A peanut factor for hemostasis in haemophilia, Nature 185:469, 1960.
67. Bouhasin, J. D., and Altay, C.: Factor XIII deficiency; concentrations in relatives of patients and normal infants, J. Pediat. 72:336, 1968.
68. Brain, M. C., Dacie, J. V., and Hourihane, D. O'B.: Microangiopathic hemolytic anaemia; the possible role of vascular lesions in pathogenesis, Brit. J. Haemat. 8:358, 1962.
69. Braunsteiner, H., and Pakesch, F.: Thrombocytoasthenia and thrombocytopathia—old names and new diseases, Blood 11:965, 1956.
70. Breckenridge, R. T., and Ratnoff, O. D.: Studies on the action of a circulating anticoagulant in disseminated lupus erythematosus, Clin. Res. 11:190, 1963.
71. Brinkhous, K. M.: Physiopathology of hemophilia, Acta Haemat. 20:125, 1958.
72. Brinkhous, K. M.: Hemophilia; pathophysiologic studies and the evolution of transfusion therapy, Amer. J. Clin. Path. 41:342, 1964.
73. Brinkhous, K. M., Langdell, R. D., Penick, G. D., Graham, J. B., and Wagner, R. H.: Newer approaches to the study of hemophilia and hemophilioid states, J.A.M.A. 154:481, 1954.
74. Brinkhous, K. M., Penick, G. D., Langdell, R. D., Wagner, R. H., and Graham, J. B.: Physiologic basis of transfusion therapy in hemophilia, Arch. Path. 61:6, 1956.
75. Brinkhous, K. M., Smith, H. P., and Warner, E. D.: Plasma prothrombin level in normal infancy and in hemorrhagic disease of the newborn, Amer. J. Med. Sci. 193:475, 1939.
76. Britten, P. F. H.: Congenital deficiency of factor XIII (fibrin-stabilizing factor); report of a case and review of the literature, Amer. J. Med. 43:751, 1967.
77. Brown, D. L., Hardisty, R. M., Kosoy, M. H., and Bracken, C.: Antihaemophilic globulin; preparation by an improved cryoprecipitation method and clinical use, Brit. Med. J. 2:79, 1967.
78. Buckell, M.: The effect of citrate on euglobulin methods of estimating fibrinolytic activity, J. Clin. Path. 11:403, 1958.
79. Bull, B. S., Rutenberg, M. L., Dacie, J. V., and Brain, M. C.: Microangiopathic haemolytic anaemia; mechanisms of red-cell fragmentation, in vitro studies, Brit. J. Haemat. 14:643, 1968.
79a. Caen, J. P., Crinberg, S., Levy-Toledano, S., Kubitz, P., and Pinkhas, J. P.: New data on Glanzmann's thrombasthenia, Proc. Soc. Exp. Biol. Med. 136:1082, 1971.
80. Caffey, J.: Pediatric x-ray diagnosis, ed. 3, Chicago, 1956, Year Book Medical Publishers, Inc.
81. Canale, V. C., Hilgartner, M. W., Smith, C. H., and Lanzkowsky, P.: Effect of corticosteroids on factor VIII level, J. Pediat. 71:878, 1967.
82. Castaldi, P. A., and Caen, J.: Platelet fibrinogen, J. Clin. Path. 18:579, 1965.
83. Charytan, C., and Purtilo, D.: Glomerular capillary thrombosis and acute renal failure after epsilon-amino caproic acid therapy, New Eng. J. Med. 280:1102, 1969.
84. Chen, T. I., and Tsai, C.: The mechanism of haemostasis in peripheral vessels, J. Physiol. 107:280, 1948.
85. Clifford, S. H.: Hemorrhagic disease of the newborn, J. Pediat. 14:333, 1939.
86. Colman, R. W., and Rodriguez-Erdman, F.: Terminology of intravascular coagulation, New Eng. J. Med. 282:99, 1970.
87. Cooperberg, A. A., and Teitelbaum, J.: The concentration of antihaemophilic globulin (AHG) related to age, Brit. J. Haemat. 6:281, 1960.
88. Cornu, P., Larrieu, M. J., Caen, J., and Bernard, J.: Transfusion studies in von Willebrand's disease; effect on bleeding time and factor VIII, Brit. J. Haemat. 9:184, 1963.
89. Council on drugs: an antifibrinolytic agent, aminocaproic acid (Amicar), J.A.M.A. 191:145, 1965.
90. Crosby, W. H., and Stefanini, M.: Pathogenesis of the plasma transfusion reactions with special reference to the blood coagulation system, J. Lab. Clin. Med. 40:374, 1952.
91. Cullum, C., Cooney, D. P., and Schrier, S. L.: Familial thrombocytopenic thrombocytopathy, Brit. J. Haemat. 13:147, 1967.

92. Dallman, P. R., and Pool, J. G.: Treatment of hemophilia with factor VIII concentrates, New Eng. J. Med. 278:199, 1968.
93. Dam, H., Dyggve, H., Larsen, H., and Plum, P.: The relation of vitamin K deficiency to hemorrhagic disease of the newborn. In Levine, S. Z., editor: Advances in pediatrics, vol. 5, Chicago, 1952, Year Book Medical Publishers, Inc., p. 129.
94. Darte, D. M. M.: Defect of anti-hemophilic globulin in von Willebrand's disease, Amer. J. Dis. Child. 90:561, 1955 (abst.).
95. Davidson, C. S., Epstein, R. D., Miller, G. F., and Taylor, F. H. L.: Hemophilia; a clinical study of forty patients, Blood 4:489, 1949.
96. Davidson, E., and Tomlin, S.: The levels of plasma coagulation factors after trauma in childbirth, J. Clin. Path. 16:112, 1963.
97. Davie, E. W., and Ratnoff, O. D.: Waterfall sequence for intrinsic blood clotting, Science 145:1310, 1964.
98. De Gruchy, G. C.: Clinical haematology in medical practice, Springfield, Ill., 1958, Charles C Thomas, Publisher, p. 542.
99. De Grouchy, J., Veslot, J., Bonnette, J., and Roidot, M.: Case of ?6p-chromosomal aberration, Amer. J. Dis. Child. 115:93, 1968.
100. De la Chapelle, A., Ikkala, E., and Nevanlinna, H. R.: Haemophilia A in a girl, Lancet 2:578, 1961.
101. Denson, K. W.: Studies of the Prower-factor; a blood coagulation factor which differs from factor VII, Brit. J. Haemat. 4:313, 1958.
102. Denson, K. W. E., Biggs, R., and Mannucci, P. M.: An investigation of three patients with Christmas disease due to an abnormal type of factor IX, J. Clin. Path. 21:160, 1968.
103. De Palma, A. F.: Management of hemophilic arthropathy—hemophilia and hemophilioid diseases. International Symposium, Chapel Hill, N. C., 1957, University of North Carolina Press.
104. De Vries, A., Matoth, P., and Shamir, Z. S.: Familial congenital labile factor deficiency with syndactylism; investigation on the mode of action of the labile factor, Acta Haemat. 5:129, 1951.
105. De Vries, A., Rosenberg, T., Kochwa, S., and Boss, J. H.: Precipitating antifibrinogen antibody appearing after fibrinogen infusions in a patient with congenital afibrinogenemia, Amer. J. Med. 30:486, 1961.
106. Deykin, O.: The role of the liver in seruminduced hypercoagulability, J. Clin. Invest. 45:256, 1966.
107. Diamond, L. K., and Porter, F. S.: The inadequacies of routine bleeding and clotting times, New Eng. J. Med. 259:1025, 1958.
108. Didisheim, P., Ferguson, J. H., and Lewis, J. H.: Hemostatic data in relatives of hemophiliacs A and B, Arch. Intern. Med. 101:347, 1958.
109. Didisheim, P., and Lewis, J. H.: Congenital disorders of the mechanism for coagulation of blood, Pediatrics 22:478, 1958.
110. Dische, F. E., and Benfield, V.: Congenital factor VII deficiency; haematological and genetic aspects, Acta Haemat. 21:257, 1959.
111. Doses of water-soluble vitamin K analogues in hemorrhagic disease of the newborn, J.A.M.A. 164:1331, 1957.
112. Douglas, A. S.: Antihemophilic globulin assay following plasma infusions in hemophilia, J. Lab. Clin. Med. 51:850, 1958.
113. Douglas, A. S., and Davies, P.: Hypoprothrombinaemia in the newborn, Arch. Dis. Child. 30:509, 1955.
114. Dreskin, O. H.: Prothrombin consumption test; a simplified technique, Amer. J. Clin. Path. 22:140, 1952.
115. Duckert, F., Fluckiger, P., Matter, M., and Koller, F.: Clotting factor X; physiologic and physio-chemical properties, Proc. Soc. Exp. Biol. Med. 90:17, 1955.
116. Duckert, F., Jung, E., and Schmerling, D. H.: A hitherto undescribed congenital haemorrhagic diathesis probably due to fibrin stabilizing factor deficiency, Thromb. Diath. Haemorrhag. 5:179, 1960.
117. Editorial: Hemophilia prophylaxis, J.A.M.A. 212:2256, 1970.
118. Editorial: Management of haemophilic haemarthrosis, Lancet 1:1376, 1970.
119. Evans, G., Peckham, M. A., Nishizawa, E. E., Mustard, J. F., and Murphy, E. A.: Effect of acetylsalicylic acid on platelet function, J. Exp. Med. 128:877, 1968.
120. Feinstein, D. I., Rapaport, S. I., and Chong, M. N. Y.: Immunologic characterization of 12 factor VIII inhibitors, Blood 34:85, 1969.
121. Foley, J. R., and Stickler, G. B.: Petechiae in the newborn infant, Amer. J. Dis. Child. 102:365, 1961.
122. Forman, W. B., Boyer, M. H., and Ratnoff, O. D.: Hereditary defect in the coagulation of fibrinogen by thrombin; studies in a family with fibrinogen Cleveland, Blood 30:863, 1967.
123. Fowell, A. H.: Turbidometric method of fibrinogen assay; results with the Coleman junior spectrophotometer, Amer. J. Clin. Path. 25:340, 1955.
124. Fresh, J. W., Ferguson, J. H., Stamey, C., Morgan, F. M., and Lewis, J. H.: Blood prothrombin, proconvertin and proaccelerin in normal infancy; questionable relation-

ships to vitamin K, Pediatrics **19**:241, 1957.
125. Frick, P. G.: Hemophilia-like disease following pregnancy; with transplacental transfer of an acquired circulating anticoagulant, Blood **8**:598, 1953.
126. Frick, P. G.: The relative incidence of antihemophilic globulin (AHG), plasma thromboplastin component (PTC), and plasma thromboplastin antecedent (PTA) deficiency, J. Lab. Clin. Med. **43**:860, 1954.
127. Frick, P. G., Bachmann, F., and Duckert, F.: Vascular anomaly associated with plasma thromboplastin antecedent deficiency, J. Lab. Clin. Med. **54**:680, 1959.
128. Frick, P., and McQuarrie, I.: Congenital afibrinogenemia, Pediatrics **13**:44, 1954.
129. Friedman, L. L., Bowie, E. J. W., Thompson, J. H., Brown, A. L., and Owen, C. A.: Familial Glanzmann's thrombasthenia, Mayo Clin. Proc. **39**:308, 1964.
130. Gaarder, A., Jonsen, J., Laland, S., Hellem, A., and Owren, P. A.: Adenosine diphosphate in red cells as a factor in the adhesiveness of human blood platelets, Nature **192**:531, 1961.
131. Gans, H., and Krivit, W.: Problems in hemostasis during and after open-heart surgery. VI. Over-all changes in blood coagulation mechanism, J.A.M.A. **179**:153, 1962.
132. Gaston, L. W.: The blood-clotting factors, New Eng. J. Med. **270**:236, 290, 1964.
132a. George, J. N., Miller, G. M., and Breckenridge, R. T.: Studies on Christmas disease; investigation and treatment of a familial acquired inhibitor of factor IX, Brit. J. Haemat. **21**:333, 1971.
132b. Gilchrist, G. S., Ekert, H., Shanbrom, E., and Hammond, G. D.: Evaluation of a new concentrate for treatment of factor IX deficiency, New Eng. J. Med. **280**:291, 1969.
133. Girsch, L. S.: Allergic rhinitis, a common cause of recurrent epistaxis in children, Amer. J. Dis. Child. **99**:818, 1960.
134. Gitlin, D., and Borges, W. H.: Studies on the metabolism of fibrinogen in two patients with congenital afibrinogenemia, Blood **8**:679, 1953.
135. Gladner, J. A.: The action of thrombin on fibrinogen. In Laki, K., editor: Fibrinogen, New York, 1968, Marcel Dekker, Inc.
136. Glanzmann, E.: Hereditäre hamorrhagische thrombasthenie, Ann. Paediat. **88**:113, 1918.
137. Gokcen, M., and Yunis, E.: Fibrinogen as a part of platelet structure, Nature **200**:590, 1963.
138. Gollub, S., and Ulin, A. W.: Heparin induced thrombocytopenia in man, J. Lab. Clin. Med. **59**:430, 1962.
139. Gordon, R. R., and Dean, T.: Foetal deaths from antenatal anticoagulant therapy, Brit. M. J. **2**:719, 1955.
140. Graham, J. B., Barrow, E. M., and Hougie, C.: Stuart clotting defect; the genetic aspects of a "new" hemorrhagic state, J. Clin. Invest. **36**:497, 1957.
141. Greenberg, L. H., Schiffman, S., and Wing, Y. S. S.: Factor XIII deficiency, J.A.M.A. **209**:264, 1969.
142. Gross, R.: Metabolic aspects of normal and pathological platelets. In Johnson, S. A., editor: Blood platelets, Boston, 1961, Little, Brown Co.
142a. Gröttum, K. A., Hovig, J., Holmsen, H., Abrahamsen, A. F., Jeremic, M., and Seip, M.: Wiskott-Aldrich syndrome; qualitative platelet defects and short platelet survival, Brit. J. Haemat. **17**:373, 1969.
142b. Gröttum, K. A., and Solum, N. O.: Thrombocytopenia with giant platelets, Brit. J. Haemat. **16**:277, 1969.
143. Hall, C. A., Rapaport, S. I., Ames, S. B., and DeGroot, J. A.: A clinical and family study of hereditary proconvertin (factor VII) deficiency, Amer. J. Med. **37**:172, 1964.
144. Hammond, J. D. S., and Verel, D.: Observations on the distribution and biological half-life of human fibrinogen, Brit. J. Haemat. **5**:431, 1959.
145. Hanna, M.: Congenital deficiency of factor XIII; report of a family from Newfoundland with associated mild deficiency of factor XII, Pediatrics **46**:611, 1970.
146. Hardisty, R. M.: The reaction of blood coagulation factors with brain extract, Brit. J. Haemat. **1**:323, 1955.
147. Hardisty, R. M., Dormandy, K. M., and Hutton, R. A.: Thrombasthenia; studies on three cases, Brit. J. Haemat. **10**:371, 1964.
148. Hardisty, R. M., and Hutton, R. A.: The kaolin clotting-time of platelet-rich plasma; a test of platelet factor III availability, Brit. J. Haemat. **11**:258, 1965.
149. Hardisty, R. M., and Hutton, R. A.: Bleeding tendency associated with new abnormality of platelet behavior, Lancet **1**:983, 1967.
150. Hardisty, R. M., and Pinniger, J. L.: Congenital afibrinogenemia; further observations on the blood coagulation mechanisms, Brit. J. Haemat. **2**:139, 1956.
151. Harker, L. A.: Platelet production, New Eng. J. Med. **282**:492, 1970.
152. Harker, L. A., and Finch, C. A.: Thrombokinetics in man, J. Clin. Invest. **48**:963, 1969.
153. Hartmann, R. C.: Hemorrhagic disorder occurring in patients with cyanotic congenital heart disease, Bull. Johns Hopkins Hosp. **91**:49, 1952.
154. Hathaway, W. E.: Coagulation problems in

155. Hathaway, W. E., and Alsever, J.: The relationship of "Fletcher factor" to factors XI and XII, Brit. J. Haemat. 18:161, 1970. [Reference 154 continued: the newborn infant, Ped. Clin. N. Amer. 17:929, 1970.]
156. Hathaway, W. E., Moll, M. M., and Pechet, G. S.: Disseminated intravascular coagulation in the newborn, Pediatrics 43:233, 1969.
157. Hay, J. D., Hudson, F. P., and Rodgers, T. S.: Vitamin K in the prevention of haemorrhagic disease of the newborn, Lancet 1:423, 1951.
158. Heiner, D. C., Sears, J. W., and Kniker, W. T.: Multiple precipitins to cow's milk in chronic respiratory disease, Amer. J. Dis. Child. 103:634, 1962.
159. Hellem, A. J.: The adhesiveness of human blood platelets in vitro, Scandinav. J. Clin. Lab. Invest. (supp.) 12:51, 1960.
160. Hellem, A. J., Borchgrevink, C. F., and Ames, S. B.: The role of red cells in haemostasis; the relation between haematocrit, bleeding time and platelet adhesiveness, Brit. J. Haemat. 7:42, 1961.
161. Hemker, H. C., Hemker, P. W., and Loeliger, E. A.: Kinetic aspects of the interaction of blood clotting enzymes. I. Derivation of basic formulas, Thromb. Diath. Haemorrhag. 13:155, 1965.
162. Henry, E. I., Rosenthal, R. L., and Hoffman, I.: Spontaneous hemorrhages caused by plasma-thromboplastin-antecedent deficiency, J.A.M.A. 162:727, 1956.
163. Hicks, N. D., and Pitney, W. R.: A rapid screening test for disorders of thromboplastin generation, Brit. J. Haemat. 3:227, 1957.
164. Hilgartner, M. W.: Intrarenal obstruction in haemophilia, Lancet 1:486, 1966.
165. Hilgartner, M. W., Engle, M. A., and Redo, S. F.: Cardiac surgery in patients with plasma thromboplastin antecedent (PTA) deficiency, J. Thoracic Surg. 49:974, 1965.
166. Hilgartner, M. W., Erlandson, M. E., and Smith, C. H.: The coagulation mechanism in patients with thalassemia major, J. Pediat. 63:36, 1963.
167. Hilgartner, M. W., and Smith, C. H.: Hemorrhagic disorders. In Gellis, S. S., and Kagan, B. M., editors: Current pediatric practice, Philadelphia, 1964, W. B. Saunders Co.
168. Hilgartner, M. W., and Smith, C. H.: Plasma thromboplastin antecedent (factor XI) in the neonate, J. Pediat. 66:747, 1965.
169. Hill, J. M., and Speer, R. J.: Combined hemophilia and PTC deficiency, Blood 10:357, 1955.
170. Hjort, P., Rapaport, S. I., and Owren, P. A.: Evidence that platelet accelerator (platelet factor 1) is adsorbed plasma proaccelerin, Blood 10:1139, 1955.
171. Hoag, M. S., Johnson, F. F., Robinson, J. A., and Aggeler, P. M.: Treatment of hemophilia B with a new clotting-factor concentrate, New Eng. J. Med. 280:581, 1969.
172. Holman, C. A., and Wolf, P.: Human antihaemophilic factor; the preparation in a hospital of a concentrate for clinical use, Lancet 2:4, 1963.
172a. Holmsen, H., and Weiss, H. J.: Hereditary defect in the platelet release reaction caused by a deficiency in the storage pool of platelet adenine nucleotides, Brit. J. Haemat. 19:643, 1970.
173. Honig, G. R., Forman, E. N., Johnson, C. A., Seeler, R. A., Abildgaard, C. F., and Schulman, I.: Administration of single doses of AHF (factor VIII) concentrates in the treatment of hemophilic hemarthrosis, Pediatrics 43:26, 1969.
174. Horowitz, H. D., and Fujimoto, M. M.: Acquired hemophilia due to a circulating anticoagulant; report of two cases with review of the literature, Amer. J. Med. 33:501, 1962.
175. Horowitz, H. I., and Spaet, T. H.: Generation of coagulation product I and its interaction with platelets and phospholipids, J. Appl. Physiol. 16:112, 1961.
176. Horowitz, H. I., Wilcox, W. P., and Fujimoto, M. M.: Assay of plasma thromboplastin antecedent (PTA) with artificially depleted normal plasma, Blood 22:35, 1963.
177. Hougie, C.: Circulating anticoagulants, Brit. M. Bull. 11:16, 1955.
178. Hougie, C.: Reactions of Stuart factor and factor VII with brain and factor V, Proc. Soc. Exp. Biol. Med. 101:132, 1959.
179. Hougie, C.: Fundamentals of blood coagulation in clinical medicine, New York, 1963, McGraw-Hill Book Co.
180. Hougie, C.: Sequential reactions of factor VIII, IX and X. In Brinkhous, K. M., editor: The hemophilias, International Symposium Washington, Chapel Hill, N. C., 1964, University of North Carolina Press.
181. Hougie, C., Barrow, E. M., and Graham, J. B.: Stuart clotting defect; segregation of an hereditary hemorrhagic state from the heterogeneous group heretofore called "stable factor" (SPCA proconvertin, factor VII) deficiency, J. Clin. Invest. 36:485, 1957.
182. Hougie, C., and Twomey, J. J.: Haemophilia $B_m$; a new type of factor IX deficiency, Lancet 1:698, 1967.
183. Hoyer, L. M., and Breckenridge, R. T.: Immunologic studies of antihemophilic factor (AHF, factor VIII); cross reacting material

in a genetic variant of hemophilia A, Blood **32**:962, 1968.
184. Israels, L. G., Zipursky, A., and Sinclair, C.: Factor V levels in the neonatal period, Pediatrics **15**:180, 1955.
185. Iversen, T., and Bastrup-Madsen, P.: Congenital familial deficiency of factor V (parahaemophilia) combined with deficiency of antihaemophilic globulin, Brit. J. Haemat. **2**:265, 1956.
186. Ivy, A. C., Shapiro, P. R., and Melnick, P.: Bleeding tendency in jaundice, Surg. Gynec. Obstet. **60**:781, 1935.
187. Jackson, D. P., Hartmann, R. C., and Conley, C. L.: Clot retraction as a measure of platelet function; clinical disorders associated with qualitative platelet defects (thrombocytopathic purpura), Bull. Johns Hopkins Hosp. **93**:370, 1953.
188. Jackson, D. P., Morse, E. F., Zieve, P. D., and Conley, C. L.: Thrombocytopathic purpura associated with defective clot retraction and absence of platelet fibrinogen, Blood **22**:827, 1963.
189. Johnson, S. A., and McKenna, J. L.: An investigation of the possible role of platelet fibrinogen in thrombi formation, Thromb. Diath. Haemorrhag. **9**:102, 1963.
190. Johnson, S. A., Monto, R. W., and Caldwell, M. J.: A new approach to the thrombocytopathies; thrombocytopathy A, Thromb. Diath. Haemorrhag. **2**:279, 1958.
191. Jones, J. H., Rizza, C. R., Hardisty, R. M., Dormandy, K. M., and Macpherson, J. C.: Combined deficiency of factor V and factor VIII (antihaemophilic globulin); a report of three cases, Brit. J. Haemat. **8**:120, 1962.
192. Jordan, H. H.: Hemophilic arthropathies, Springfield, Ill., 1958, Charles C Thomas, Publisher.
193. Kaneshiro, M. M., Mielke, C. H., Jr., Kasper, C. K., and Rapaport, S. I.: Bleeding time after aspirin in disorders of intrinsic clotting, New Eng. J. Med. **281**:1039, 1969.
194. Kasper, C. K., Whissell Buechy, D. Y. E., and Aggeler, P. M.: Hageman factor (factor XII) in an affected kindred and in normal adults, Brit. J. Haemat. **14**:543, 1968.
195. Kaufman, R. M., Airo, R., Pollack, S., and Crosby, W. H.: Circulating megakaryocytes and platelet release in the lung, Blood **26**:720, 1965.
196. Kaufman, R. M., Airo, R., Pollack, S., Crosby, W. H., and Doberneck, R.: Origin of pulmonary megakaryocytes, Blood **25**:767, 1965.
197. Kellermeyer, R. W., and Graham, R. C., Jr.: Kinins—possible and pathologic roles in man, New Eng. J. Med. **279**:754, 1968.
198. Kingsley, C. S.: Familial factor V deficiency; the pattern of heredity, Quart. J. Med. **23**:323, 1954.
199. Kisker, C. T., and Burke, C.: Double-blind studies on the use of steroids in the treatment of acute hemarthrosis in patients with hemophilia, New Eng. J. Med. **282**:639, 1970.
200. Koller, F.: Symposium: What is hemophilia? Is hemophilia a nosologic entity? Blood **9**:286, 1954.
201. Koller, F., Gasser, C., Krüsi, G., and de Muralt, G.: Purpura fulminans nach Scharlach mit Factor V Mangel und Antithrombinüberschuss, Acta Haemat. **4**:33, 1950.
202. Koller, F., Loeliger, A., and Duckert, F.: Experiments on a new clotting factor (factor VII), Acta Haemat. **6**:1, 1951.
203. Krivit, W.: Purpuras; diagnosis and treatment, Ped. Clin. N. Amer. **9**:833, 1962.
204. Künzer, W., and Lütgemeier, J.: Zur entwicklungsbedingten Abhängigkeit des plasmagehaltes an fibrinstabilisierendem Factor (FSF), Ann. Paediat. **204**:232, 1965.
205. Kurkcuoglu, M., and McElfresh, A. E.: The Hageman factor; determinations of its concentration during the neonatal period and presentation of a case of Hageman factor deficiency, J. Pediat. **57**:61, 1960.
206. Kurstjens, R., Bolt, C., Vossen, M., and Haansen, C.: Familial thrombopathic thrombocytopenia, Brit. J. Haemat. **15**:305, 1968.
207. Laki, K., and Lorand, L.: On the solubility of fibrin clots, Science **108**:280, 1948.
208. Langdell, R. D., Wagner, R. H., and Brinkhous, K. M.: Effect of anti-hemophilic factor in one-stage clotting tests, J. Lab. Clin. Med. **41**:637, 1953.
209. Larkin, I. M., and Philipp, E. E.: Further experience with hypofibrinogenemia of pregnancy, J. Obstet. Gynaec. Brit. Emp. **64**:215, 1957.
210. Larrieu, M. J., and Soulier, J. P.: Déficit en facteur antihémophilique A chez une fille, associé à un trouble du saignement, Rev. Hémat. **8**:361, 1953.
211. Lascari, A. D., Hoak, J. C., and Taylor, J. C.: Christmas disease in a girl, Amer. J. Dis. Child. **117**:585, 1969.
212. Leeksma, C. H. W., and Cohen, J. A.: Determination of the life span of human blood platelets using labelled diisopropylfluorophosphate, J. Clin. Invest. **35**:964, 1956.
213. Lewis, J. H.: Synthesis of AHF in von Willebrand's disease, Blood **23**:233, 1964.
214. Lewis, J. H., Didisheim, P., Ferguson, J. H., and Li, C. C.: Genetic consideration in familial hemorrhagic disease. I. Sex-linked recessive disorders, hemophilia and PTC de-

215. Lewis, J. H., and Doyle, A. P.: Effects of epsilon-aminocaproic acid on coagulation and fibrinolytic mechanisms, J.A.M.A. 188:56, 1964.
216. Lewis, J. H., and Ferguson, J. H.: Afibrinogenemia; report of a case, Amer. J. Dis. Child. 88:711, 1954.
217. Lewis, J. H., Ferguson, J. H., and Arends, T.: Hemorrhagic disease with circulating inhibitors of blood clotting; anti-AHF and anti-PTC in eight cases, Blood 11:846, 1956.
218. Lewis, J. H., Ferguson, J. H., Spaugh, E., Fresh, J. W., and Zucker, M. B.: Acquired hypoprothrombinemia, Blood 12:84, 1957.
219. Libre, E. P., Cowan, D. H., and Shulman, N. R.: Influence of spleen and platelets on factor VIII levels, Blood 26:890, 1965.
220. Libre, E. P., Cowan, D. H., Watkins, S. P., Jr., and Shulman, N. R.: Relationships between spleen, platelets and factor VIII levels, Blood 31:358, 1968.
221. Loeliger, A., and Koller, F.: Behavior of factor VII and prothrombin in late pregnancy and in newborn, Acta Haemat. 7:157, 1952.
222. Loeliger, E. A., Van der Esch, V. D., Mattern, M. J., and Hemker, H. C.: The biological disappearance rate of prothrombin, factors VII, IX and X from plasma in hypothyroidism, hyperthyroidism, and during fever, Thromb. Diath. Haemorrhag. 10:267, 1963.
223. Lorand, L.: Properties and significance of the fibrin stabilizing factor (FSF), Thromb. Diath. Haemorrhag. 7 (supp.):238, 1962.
224. Losowsky, M. S., Hall, R., and Goldie, W.: Congenital deficiency of fibrin-stabilizing factor, Lancet 2:156, 1965.
225. Lucey, J. F., and Dolan, R. G.: Injection of a vitamin-K compound in mothers and hyperbilirubinemia in the newborn, Pediatrics 22:605, 1958.
225a. Lusher, J. M., and Evans, R. K.: Effective suppression of factor VIII antibody with cyclophosphamide, Abstract, American Society of Hematology Meeting, Dec., 1971, San Francisco.
226. Lusher, J. M., Shuster, J., Evans, R. K., and Poulik, M. D.: Antibody nature of an AHG (factor VIII) inhibitor, J. Pediat. 72:325, 1968.
227. Lusher, J. M., Staub, R. T., and Belote, J. H.: Antihemophilic globulin deficiency in a chromosomal female, Amer. J. Dis. Child. 108:309, 1964.
228. Mac Ausland, W. R., Jr., and Gartland, J. J.: The treatment of acute hemophilic hemarthrosis; a report on the use of hyaluronidase, New Eng. J. Med. 247:755, 1952.
229. Macfarlane, R. G.: The bleeder, Brit. M. J. 1:1080, 1955.
230. Macfarlane, R. G.: Purification of factor X, its activation by Russell's viper venom and also physiological factors, Thromb. Diath. Haemorrhag. 7 (supp.):222, 1961.
231. Macfarlane, R. G., Biggs, R., Ash, B. J., and Denson, K. W.: The interaction of factors VIII and IX, Brit. J. Haemat. 10:530, 1964.
232. Marchal, G., Samama, M., Dausset, J., and Prost, R. J.: La place du temps de saignement dans l'exploration actuelle des thrombopenies, Nouv. Rev. Franç. Hematol. 3:304, 1963.
233. Marcus, A. J.: Platelet function, New Eng. J. Med. 280:1213, 1969.
234. Marcus, A. J., and Zucker, M. B.: The physiology of blood platelets; recent biochemical, morphologic and clinical research, New York, 1965, Grune & Stratton, Inc.
234a. Marder, V. J., Matchett, M. D., and Sherry, S.: Detection of serum fibrinogen and fibrin degradation products; comparison of six technics using purified products and application of clinical studies, Amer. J. Med. 51:71, 1971.
235. Marder, V. J., and Shulman, N. R.: Clinical aspects of congenital factor VII deficiency, Amer. J. Med. 37:182, 1964.
236. Margolis, J.: The kaolin clotting time, J. Clin. Path. 11:506, 1958.
237. Margolis, J.: Hageman factor and capillary permeability, Australian J. Exp. Biol. Med. Sci. 37:239, 1959.
238. Matter, M., Newcomb, R. F., Melly, A., and Finch, C. A.: Vascular hemophilia; the association of a vascular deficiency with a deficiency of antihemophilic globulin, Amer. J. Med. Sci. 232:421, 1956.
239. McCracken, G. H., and Dickerman, J. D.: Septicemia and disseminated intravascular coagulation, Amer. J. Dis. Child. 118:431, 1969.
240. McElfresh, A. E.: Coagulation during the neonatal period, Amer. J. Med. Sci. 240:771, 1961.
241. McElfresh, A. E., Sharpsteen, J. R., and Akabane, T.: The generation of thromboplastin and levels of plasma thromboplastin component of the blood of infants, Pediatrics 17:870, 1956.
242. Medal, L. S., and Lisker, R.: Circulating anticoagulants in disseminated lupus erythematosus, Brit. J. Haemat. 5:284, 1959.
243. Mellman, W., Jr., Wolman, I. J., Wurzel, H. A., Moorhead, P. S., and Qualls, D. H.: A

chromosomal female with hemophilia A, Blood 17:719, 1961.
244. Merskey, C.: The occurrence of hemophilia in the human female, Quart. J. Med. 20: 299, 1951.
245. Merskey, C.: Defibrination, New Eng. J. Med. 282:688, 1970.
246. Merskey, C., Johnson, A. J., Kleiner, G. J., and Wohll, H.: The defibrination syndrome; clinical features and laboratory diagnosis, Brit. J. Haemat. 13:528, 1967.
247. Michael, S. E., and Tunnah, G. W.: The purification of factor VIII (antihaemophilic globulin), Brit. J. Haemat. 9:236, 1963.
248. Miller, D. R., Hanshaw, J. B., O'Leary, D. S., and Hnilicka, J. V.: Fatal disseminated herpes simplex virus infection and hemorrhage in the neonate; coagulation studies in a case and a review, J. Pediat. 76:409, 1970.
249. Miller, S. P.: Congenital deficiency of proconvertin; a clinical and laboratory report, Blood 14:1322, 1959.
250. Milstone, J. H.: The chain reaction of the blood clotting mechanism in relation to the theory of hemostasis and thrombosis, Blood 4:1290, 1949.
251. Mitchell, J. R. A., and Sharp, A. A.: Platelet clumping in vitro, Brit. J. Haemat. 10: 78, 1964.
252. Monnens, L., and Schretten, E.: Haemolyticuremic syndrome, Lancet 2:735, 1968.
252a. Morawitz, P.: The chemistry of blood coagulation, translation by Hartman, R. C., and Guenther, P. F., Springfield, Ill., 1958, Charles C Thomas, Publisher.
253. Mountain, K. R., Hirsch, J., and Gallus, A. S.: Neonatal coagulation defect due to anticonvulsant drug treatment in pregnancy, Lancet 1:265, 1970.
254. Nachman, R. L.: Immunologic studies of platelet protein, Blood 25:703, 1965.
254a. Nachman, R. L.: Thrombasthenia; immunologic evidence of a platelet protein abnormality, J. Lab. Clin. Med. 67:411, 1966.
255. Nachman, R. L., Marcus, A. J., and Zucker-Franklin, D.: Subcellular localization of platelet fibrinogen, Blood 24:853, 1964.
256. Naeye, R. L.: Thrombotic disorders with increased levels of antiplasmin and antiplasminogen, New Eng. J. Med. 265:867, 1961.
257. Neel, J. V., and Schull, W. J.: Human heredity, Chicago, 1954, University of Chicago Press.
258. Nemerson, Y.: The phospholipid requirement of tissue factor in blood coagulation, J. Clin. Invest. 47:72, 1968.
259. Nemerson, Y., and Spaet, T. H.: The activation of factor X by extracts of rabbit brain, Blood 23:657, 1964.
260. Nevanlinna, H. R., Ikkala, E., and Vuopio, P.: Von Willebrand's disease, Acta Haemat. 27:65, 1962.
261. Newton, W. A., Jr., Kontras, S. B., and Sirak, H. D.: Hemostatic studies in children with congenital heart disease, J. Pediat. 63: 466, 1963.
262. Nilsson, I. M., and Blombäck, M.: Von Willebrand's disease in Sweden—occurrence, pathogenesis and treatment, Thromb. Diath. Haemorrhag. 2 (supp.):103, 1963.
263. Nilsson, I. M., Blombäck, M., Jorpes, E., Blombäck, B., and Johansson, S. A.: Von Willebrand's disease and its correction with human plasma fraction I-O, Acta Med. Scandinav. 159:179, 1957.
264. Nilsson, I. M., Blombäck, M., and Ramgren, O.: Haemophilia in Sweden; the treatment of haemophilia A with the human antihaemophilic factor preparation (fraction I-O), Acta Med. Scandinav. (supp.) 379:61, 1962.
265. Nilsson, I. M., Blombäck, M., Thilen, A., and Francken, I. V.: Carriers of hemophilia A; a laboratory study, Acta Med. Scandinav. 165:357, 1959.
266. Nilsson, I. M., and Öckerman, P. A.: The bleeding disorder in hepatomegalic forms of glycogen storage disease, Acta Paediat. Scand. 59:127, 1970.
267. Norman, J. C.: Splenic homotransplantation for hemophilia, New Eng. J. Med. 283:435, 1970.
268. Norman, J. C., Lambilliotte, J. P., Kojima, Y., and Sise, H. S.: Antihemophilic factor release by perfused liver and spleen; relationship to hemophilia, Science 158:1060, 1967.
269. Nussbaum, M., and Morse, B. S.: Plasma fibrin stabilizing factor activity in various diseases, Blood 23:669, 1964.
270. Nye, S. W., Graham, J. B., and Brinkhous, K. M.: The partial thromboplastin time as a screening test for the detection of latent bleeders, Amer. J. Med. Sci. 243:279, 1962.
271. Odegaard, A. E., Skalheyg, B. A., and Hellem, A. J.: ADP-induced platelet adhesiveness as a diagnostic test in von Willebrand's disease, Thromb. Diath. Haemorrhag. 11:23, 1964.
272. Owen, C. A., Jr., Amundsen, M. A., Thompson, J. H., Jr., Spittel, J. A., Jr., Bowie, E. J. W., Stilwell, G. G., Hewlett, J. S., Mills, S. D., Sauer, W. G., and Gage, R. P.: Congenital deficiency of factor VII (hypoconvertinemia); critical review of literature and report of three cases, with extensive pedigree study and effect of transfusions, Amer. J. Med. 37:71, 1964.
273. Owen, C. A., and Cooper, T. E.: Parahemophilia, Arch. Intern. Med. 95:194, 1955.

274. Owren, P. A.: Coagulation of the blood; investigations on a new clotting factor, Acta Med. Scandinav. (supp.) 194:1, 1947.
275. Owren, P. A.: Prothrombin and accessory factors, Amer. J. Med. 14:201, 1953.
276. Owren, P. A.: Tests for control of anticoagulant therapy. In Koller, F., editor: Fibrinogen and fibrin turnover of clotting factors, Stuttgart, 1963, F. K. Schautter Verlag.
277. Pascuzzi, C. A., Thompson, J. H., Jr., Spittel, J. A., Jr., and Owen, C. A., Jr.: Simplified laboratory detection of deficiency in Hageman factor, Amer. J. Clin. Path. 35:288, 1961.
278. Paul, M. H., Currimbhoy, Z., Miller, R. A., and Schulman, I.: Thrombocytopenia in cyanotic heart disease, Amer. J. Dis. Child. 102:597, 1961.
279. Pechet, L., and Alexander, B.: Increased clotting factors in pregnancy, New Eng. J. Med. 265:1093, 1961.
280. Penick, G. D., and Brinkhous, K. M.: Relative stability of plasma antihemophilic factor (AHF) under different conditions of storage, Amer. J. Med. Sci. 232:434, 1956.
281. Perry, S., and Craddock, C. G., Jr.: Platelet adsorptive properties and platelet extracts in thromboplastin generation, Blood 8:177, 1958.
282. Perry, S., Opfell, R., and Baker, M.: Combined deficiencies of PTA and AHG with vascular fragility, Blood 16:1184, 1960.
283. Phillips, L. L., and Skrodelis, V.: The fibrinolytic enzyme system in normal, hemorrhagic and disease states, J. Clin. Invest. 37:965, 1958.
284. Pison, J., Boyan, C. P., and Cliffton, E. E.: Fibrinolytic activity in patients during operation, J.A.M.A. 191:1026, 1965.
285. Pitney, W. R.: The assay of antihaemophilic globulin (AHG) in plasma, Brit. J. Haemat. 2:250, 1956.
286. Pitney, W. R., and Arnold, B. J.: Plasma antihaemophilic factor (AHF) concentrations in families of patients with haemorrhagic states, Brit. J. Haemat. 5:184, 1959.
287. Pitney, W. R., and Arnold, B. J.: Laboratory findings of patients suffering from von Willebrand's disease, Brit. J. Haemat. 6:81, 1960.
288. Pitney, W. R., Kirk, R. L., Arnold, B. J., and Stenhouse, N. S.: Plasma antihaemophilic factor VIII concentration in normal families, Brit. J. Haemat. 8:421, 1962.
289. Pool, J. G., and Robinson, J.: Observations on plasma banking and transfusion procedures for haemophilic patients using a quantitative assay for antihaemophilic globulin (AHG), Brit. J. Haemat. 5:24, 1959.
290. Pool, J. G., and Shannon, B. S.: Production of high-potency concentrates of antihemophilic globulin in a closed-bag system, assay in vitro and in vivo, New Eng. J. Med. 273:1443, 1965.
291. Preston, A. E.: The plasma concentration of factor VIII in the normal population. I. Mothers and babies at birth, Brit. J. Haemat. 10:110, 1964.
292. Prichard, R. W., and Vann, R. L.: Congenital afibrinogenemia; report on a child without fibrinogen and review of the literature, Amer. J. Dis. Child. 88:703, 1954.
293. Proctor, R. R., and Rapaport, S. I.: The partial thromboplastin time with kaolin; a simple screening test for first stage plasma clotting factor deficiencies, Amer. J. Clin. Path. 36:212, 1961.
294. Quick, A. J.: Hemorrhagic diseases, Philadelphia, 1957, Lea & Febiger.
295. Quick, A. J.: Mild hemophilia A; probability of a variant, Amer. J. Med. Sci. 244:535, 1962.
296. Quick, A. J.: The physician's approach to the hemophiliac. In Brinkhous, K. M., editor: The hemophilias, International Symposium Washington, Chapel Hill, N. C., 1964, University of North Carolina Press.
297. Quick, A. J.: Hereditary thrombopathic thrombocytopenia and Minot–von Willebrand syndrome: probable coexistence in a family, Amer. J. Med. Sci. 250:1, 1965.
298. Quick, A. J.: Salicylates and bleeding; aspirin tolerance test, Amer. J. Med. Sci. 252:265, 1966.
299. Quick, A. J., Pisciotta, A. V., and Hussey, C. V.: Congenital hypoprothrombinemic states, Arch. Intern. Med. 95:2, 1955.
300. Rabiner, S. F., and Friedman, L. H.: The role of intravascular haemolysis and the reticulo-endothelial system in the production of the hypercoagulable state, Brit. J. Haemat. 14:105, 1968.
301. Rabiner, S. F., and Kretchmer, N.: The Stuart-Prower factor; utilization of clotting factors obtained by starch-block electrophoresis for genetic evaluation, Brit. J. Haemat. 7:99, 1961.
302. Rabiner, S. F., and Telfer, M. C.: Home transfusions for patients with hemophilia A, New Eng. J. Med. 283:1011, 1970.
303. Rabiner, S. F., Winick, M., and Smith, C. H.: Congenital deficiency of factor VII associated with hemorrhagic disease of the newborn; report of a case, Pediatrics 25:101, 1960.
304. Raccuglia, G., and Neel, J. V.: Congenital vascular defect associated with platelet abnormality and antihemophilic factor deficiency, Blood 15:807, 1960.

305. Rapaport, S. I., Ames, S. B., and Duvall, B. J.: A plasma coagulation defect in systemic lupus erythematosus arising from hypoprothrombinemia combined with antiprothrombinase activity, Blood 15:212, 1960.
306. Rapaport, S. I., Proctor, R. R., Patch, M. J., and Yettra, M.: The mode of inheritance of PTA deficiency; evidence for the existence of major PTA deficiency and minor PTA deficiency, Blood 18:149, 1961.
307. Ratnoff, O. D., Busse, R. J., Jr., and Sheon, R. P.: The demise of John Hageman, New Eng. J. Med. 279:760, 1968.
308. Ratnoff, O. D., and Colopy, J. E.: A familial hemorrhagic trait associated with deficiency of a clot-promoting fraction of plasma, J. Clin. Invest. 34:602, 1955.
309. Ratnoff, O. D., and Colopy, J. E.: PTA deficiency and Hageman trait, Scandinav. J. Haemat. (Series Haemat.) 7:29, 1965.
310. Ratnoff, O. D., and Davie, E. W.: The activation of Christmas factor (factor IX) by activated plasma thromboplastin antecedent (activated factor XI), Biochemistry 1:677, 1962.
311. Ratnoff, O. D., Davie, E. W., and Wallett, D. L.: Studies on the action of Hageman factor; evidence that activated Hageman factor in turn activates plasma thromboplastin antecedent, J. Clin. Invest. 40:803, 1961.
312. Ratnoff, O. D., and Holland, T. R.: Coagulation components in normal and abnormal pregnancies, Ann. N. Y. Acad. Sci. 75:626, 1959.
313. Ratnoff, O. D., and Rosenblum, J. M.: Role of Hageman factor in the initiation of clotting by glass; evidence that glass frees Hageman factor from inhibition, Amer. J. Med. 25:160, 1958.
314. Ratnoff, O. D., and Steinberg, A. G.: Further studies on the inheritance of Hageman trait, J. Lab. Clin. Med. 59:980, 1962.
315. Reid, W. O., Lucas, O. N., Francisco, J., Geisler, P., and Erslev, A. J.: The use of epsilon-aminocaproic acid in the management of dental extractions in the hemophiliac, Amer. J. Med. Sci. 248:184, 1964.
316. Reid, W. O., Somlyo, A. V., Somlyo, A. P., and Custer, R. P.: The role of the platelet in fibrinolysis with a sensitive test for fibrinolytic activity, Amer. J. Clin. Path. 37:561, 1962.
317. Report of Committee on Nutrition: Vitamin K, compounds and the water-soluble analogues; use in therapy and prophylaxis in pediatrics, Pediatrics 28:501, 1961.
317a. Robboy, S. J., Lewis, E. J., Schur, P. H., and Colman, R. W.: Circulating anticoagulants to factor VIII; immunochemical studies and clinical response to factor VIII concentrates, Amer. J. Med. 49:742, 1970.
318. Roberts, H. R., Scales, M. B., Madison, J. T., Webster, W. P., and Penick, G. D.: A clinical and experimental study of acquired inhibitors to factor VIII, Blood 26:805, 1965.
319. Rosenthal, M. C.: A mechanism of plasma refractoriness in hemophilia—hemophilia and hemophilioid diseases, International Symposium, Chapel Hill, N. C., 1957, University of North Carolina Press.
320. Rosenthal, M. C.: The therapy of disorders of coagulation, J. Chron. Dis. 6:383, 1957.
321. Rosenthal, R. L.: Properties of plasma thromboplastin antecedent in relation to blood coagulation, J. Lab. Clin. Med. 45:123, 1955.
322. Rosenthal, R. L., Dreskin, O. H., and Rosenthal, N.: A new hemophilia-like disease caused by deficiency of a third plasma thromboplastin factor, Proc. Soc. Exp. Biol. Med. 82:171, 1953.
323. Saidi, P., Hoag, S., and Aggeler, P. M.: Transplacental transfer of bishydroxycoumarin in the human, J.A.M.A. 191:157, 1965.
324. Salzman, E. W.: Measurement of platelet adhesiveness; a simple in vitro technique demonstrating an abnormality in von Willebrand's disease, J. Lab. Clin. Med. 62:724, 1963.
325. Sautter, R. D., Emanuel, D. A., Fletcher, F. W., Wenzel, F. J., and Matson, J. I.: Urokinase for the treatment of acute pulmonary thromboembolism, J.A.M.A. 202:215, 1967.
326. Schachter, M.: Kallikreins and kinins, Physiol. Rev. 49:509, 1969.
327. Schiffman, S., Rapaport, S. I., and Patch, M. J.: The identification and synthesis of activated plasma thromboplastin component (PTC), Blood 22:733, 1963.
328. Schmidt, P. J., Penden, J. C., Jr., Brecher, G., and Baranowsky, A.: Thrombocytopenia and bleeding tendency after extracorporeal circulation, New Eng. J. Med. 265:1181, 1961.
329. Schulman, I., and Currimbhoy, Z.: Hemorrhagic disorders, Ped. Clin. N. Amer. 4:531, 1957.
330. Schulman, I., Currimbhoy, Z., Smith, C. H., Erlandson, M. E., Schorr, J. B., Fort, E., and Wehman, J.: Phosphatides as platelet substitutes in blood coagulation, Ann. N. Y. Acad. Sci. 75:195, 1958.
331. Schulman, I., and Smith, C. H.: Hemorrhagic disease in an infant due to deficiency of a previously undescribed clotting factor, Blood 8:794, 1952.

332. Schulman, I., and Smith, C. H.: Coagulation disorders in infancy and childhood. In Levine, S. Z., editor: Advances in pediatrics, vol. 9, Chicago, 1957, Year Book Medical Publishers, Inc.
333. Schulman, I., Smith, C. H., Erlandson, M., Fort, E., and Lee, R. E.: Vascular hemophilia, a familial hemorrhagic disease in males and females characterized by combined antihemophilic globulin deficiency and vascular abnormality, Pediatrics 18:347, 1956.
334. Schulz, J., and van Creveld, S.: Stuart-Prower factor in newborn infants, Études Neonatales 7:133, 1958.
335. Schulz, J., and van Creveld, S.: Stuart-Prower factor in newborn infants. In Brinkhous, K. M., editor: Hemophilia and other hemorrhagic states, International Symposium Rome, Chapel Hill, N. C., 1959, University of North Carolina Press, p. 167.
336. Seligsohn, V., and Ramot, B.: Combined factor V and factor VIII deficiency; report of four cases, Brit. J. Haemat. 16:475, 1963.
337. Sharp, A. A.: Viscous metamorphosis of blood platelets; a study of the relationship to coagulation factors and fibrin formation, Brit. J. Haemat. 4:28, 1958.
338. Sharp, A. A.: Pathological fibrinolysis, Brit. M. Bull. 20:240, 1964.
339. Sharp, A. A.: Present status of platelet aggregation, New Eng. J. Med. 272:89, 1965.
339a. Sherman, L. A., Goldstein, M. A., and Sise, H. S.: Circulating anticoagulants (anti-factor VIII) treated with immunosuppressive drugs, Thromb. Diath. Haemorrhag. 21:249, 1970.
340. Sherry, S.: Fibrinolytic agents. In Disease-a-Month, May, 1969, Chicago, 1969, Year Book Medical Publishers, Inc.
341. Simone, J. V., Abildgaard, C. F., and Schulman, I.: Blood coagulation in thyroid dysfunction, New Eng. J. Med. 273:1057, 1965.
342. Simone, J. V., Cornet, J. A., and Abildgaard, C. F.: Acquired von Willebrand's syndrome in systemic lupus erythematosus, Blood 31:806, 1968.
343. Singer, K., and Ramot, B.: Pseudohemophilia type B; hereditary hemorrhagic diathesis characterized by prolonged bleeding time and decrease in antihemophilic factor, Arch. Intern. Med. 97:115, 1956.
344. Singh, P., Kontras, S. B., and Newton, W. A., Jr.: Hemostatic deficiency in children with congenital heart disease, Amer. J. Dis. Child. 102:601, 1961.
345. Spaet, T. H.: Editorial: Clinical implications of acquired blood coagulation abnormalities, Blood 23:839, 1964.
346. Spaet, T. H.: Hemostatic mechanisms, Blood 28:112, 1966.
347. Spaet, T. H., and Cintron, J.: Pathways to blood coagulation product I formation, Blood 21:745, 1963.
348. Spaet, T. H., and Cintron, J.: Studies on platelet factor III availability, Brit. J. Haemat. 11:269, 1965.
349. Spaet, T. H., and Lejnieks, I.: A technique for estimation of platelet-collagen adhesion, Proc. Exp. Biol. Med. 132:1038, 1969.
350. Stafford, J. L.: Fibrinolysis and intrinsic haemostasis, Brit. M. Bull. 20:179, 1964.
351. Stark, S. N., White, J. G., Langer, L., Jr., and Krivit, W.: Epsilon-aminocaproic acid therapy as a cause of intrarenal obstruction in haematuria of haemophiliacs, Scandinav. J. Haemat. 2:99, 1965.
352. Stefanini, M.: Fibrinolysis and "fibrinolytic purpura," Blood 7:1044, 1952.
353. Stefanini, M., and Dameshek, W.: The hemorrhagic disorders, ed. 2, New York, 1962, Grune & Stratton, Inc.
354. Stein, H. L., and Hilgartner, M. W.: Alteration of coagulation mechanism of blood by contrast media, Amer. J. Roentgen. 104:458, 1968.
354a. Stites, D. P., Hershgold, E. J., Perlman, J. D., and Fudenberg, H. H.: Factor VIII detection by hemagglutination inhibition; hemophilia A and von Willebrand's disease, Science 171:196, 1971.
355. Strauss, H. S.: Use of an in vitro test for platelet adhesiveness in the diagnosis of von Willebrand's disease, Program of the Society for Pediatric Research, 34th Annual Meeting, Seattle, Wash., June 18-20, 1964.
356. Strauss, H. S.: The perpetuation of hemophilia by mutation, Pediatrics 39:186, 1967.
357. Strauss, H. S.: Diagnosis and treatment of hemophilia, Boston, 1967, The Children's Hospital Medical Center.
358. Strauss, H. S., and Bloom, G. E.: Von Willebrand's disease; use of a platelet-adhesiveness test in diagnosis and family investigation, New Eng. J. Med. 273:171, 1965.
359. Strauss, H. S., and Merler, E.: Characterization and properties of an inhibitor of factor VIII in the plasma of patients with hemophilia A following repeated transfusions, Blood 30:137, 1967.
360. Strauss, H. S., and Olson, S. L.: Hemophilia B (Christmas disease) in a female, Pediatrics 44:268, 1969.
361. Surgenor, D. M., McMillan, C. W., Diamond, L. K., and Steele, B. B.: Studies with AHF-rich fibrinogen in classical hemophilia, Vox Sang. 5:80, 1960.
362. Sweny, W. M.: Aminocaproic acid, an in-

hibitor of fibrinolysis, Amer. J. Med. Sci. **249**:576, 1965.
363. Szalontai, S.: Submicroscopic morphology of the fibrinogen-fibrin transition. In Laki, K., editor: Fibrinogen, New York, 1968, Marcel Dekker, Inc.
364. Taylor, F. H. L., Davidson, C. S., Tagnon, H. J., Adams, M. A., MacDonald, A. H., and Minot, G. R.: Studies in blood coagulation; the coagulation properties of certain globulin fractions of normal human plasma in vitro, J. Clin. Invest. **24**:698, 1945.
365. Telfer, T. P., Denson, K. W., and Wright, D. R.: A "new" coagulation defect, Brit. J. Haemat. **2**:308, 1956.
365a. Thomas, D. P., Niewiarowski, S., Myers, A. R., Bloch, K. J., and Colman, R. W.: A comparative study of four methods for detecting fibrinogen degradation products in patients with various diseases, New Eng. J. Med. **283**:663, 1972.
366. Tillett, W. S., and Garner, R. L.: The fibrinolytic activity of hemolytic streptococci, J. Exp. Med. **58**:485, 1933.
366a. Tocantins, L. M.: Technical methods for the study of blood platelets, Arch. Path. **23**:850, 1937.
367. Tocantins, L. M.: Hemophilic syndromes and hemophilia, Blood **9**:281, 1954.
368. Tocantins, L. M., and Holburn, R. R.: The coagulation of blood; methods of study, New York, 1955, Grune & Stratton, Inc., p. 178.
369. Trieger, N., and McGovern, J. J.: Evaluation of corticosteroids in hemophilia A; a controlled study during oral surgery, New Eng. J. Med. **266**:432, 1962.
370. Uttley, W. S., Allan, A. G. E., and Cash, J. D.: Fibrin/fibrinogen degradation products in sera of normal infants and children, Arch. Dis. Child. **44**:761, 1969.
371. Vainer, H., and Caen, J. P.: A useful photometric test for the diagnosis of von Willebrand's disease, J. Clin. Path. **17**:191, 1964.
372. Valberg, L. S., and Brown, G. M.: Haemorrhagic capillary disorder associated with antihaemophilic globulin deficiency, Medicine **37**:181, 1958.
373. Van Creveld, S., Baker, H., Niessing, T., Sipkema, J. J., and Smits, C. A. A. M.: Thromboplastin formation in the blood of the newborn infant, Études Neonatales **3**:217, 1954.
374. Van Creveld, S., Ho, L. K., and Veder, H. A.: Thrombopathia, Acta Haemat. **19**:199, 1958.
375. Van Creveld, S., Kloosterman, G. J., Mochtar, I. A., and Koppe, J. G.: Interchange between blood of mother and fetus in vascular hemophilia, Biol. Neonat. **4**:379, 1962.
376. Van Creveld, S., and Mochtar, I. A.: Von Willebrand's disease, a plasma deficiency cause of the prolonged bleeding time, Ann. Paediat. **194**:37, 1960.
377. Van Creveld, S., Nagel, C. G. M., Nijenhuis, J. H., Miranda, S. I., and Kie, T. S.: Thromboplastin formation in the blood of the newborn, Études Neonatales **3**:135, 1954.
378. Van Creveld, S., and Paulssen, M. M. P.: Isolation and properties of a third clotting factor in blood platelets, Lancet **1**:23, 1952.
379. Vaughan, V. C., III: Management of hemolytic disease of the newborn infant, J. Pediat. **54**:586, 1959.
380. Vasquez, J. J., and Lewis, J. H.: Immunocytochemical studies on platelets; the demonstration of a common antigen in human platelets and megakaryocytes, Blood **16**:968, 1960.
381. Verel, D., Mazurkie, S. J., Blackburn, E. K., Emery, J. L., Varadi, S., and Wolman, L.: Thrombocytopenia in congenital heart disease, Brit. Heart J. **24**:92, 1962.
382. Von Kaulla, K. N., and Schultz, R. L.: Methods for the evaluation of human fibrinolysis, Amer. J. Clin. Path. **29**:104, 1958.
383. Von Willebrand, E. A.: Über hereditäre-Pseudohämophilie, Acta Med. Scandnav. **76**:521, 1931.
384. Wankin, J. J., Eyring, E. J., and Kontras, S. B.: Should haemophilic haemarthroses be aspirated? Lancet **2**:1253, 1969.
385. Webster, W. R., Roberts, H. R., and Penick, G. D.: Hemostasis in factor V deficiency, Amer. J. Med. Sci. **248**:195, 1964.
386. Wefring, K. W.: Hemorrhage in the newborn and vitamin K prophylaxis, J. Pediat. **61**:686, 1962.
387. Weiss, H. S.: Platelet aggregation, adhesion and adenosine diphosphate release in thrombopathia (platelet factor III deficiency); a comparison with Glanzmann's thrombasthenia and von Willebrand's disease, Amer. J. Med. **43**:570, 1967.
388. Weiss, H. J.: von Willebrand's disease—diagnostic criteria, Blood **32**:668, 1968.
389. Weiss, H. J.: Bleeding-time after aspirin ingestion, Lancet **1**:527, 1968.
390. Weiss, H. J., and Aledort, L. M.: Impaired platelet/connective tissue reaction in man after aspirin ingestion, Lancet **2**:495, 1967.
391. Weiss, H. J., Chervanick, P. A., Zalusky, R., and Factor, A.: Familial defect in platelet function associated with impaired release of adenosine diphosphate, New Eng. J. Med. **281**:1264, 1969.
392. Weiss, H. J., and Eichelberger, J. W.: The detection of platelet defects in patients with

mild bleeding disorders, Amer. J. Med. **32:** 872, 1962.

392a. Weiss, H. J., and Rogers, J.: Thrombocytopathia due to abnormalities in platelet release reaction—studies on six unrelated patients, Blood **39:**187, 1972.

393. White, J. G., Yanis, E., Colliander, M., and Krivit, W.: Prolonged bleeding time in a patient with plasma thromboplastin antecedent deficiency; observation on correction of the bleeding time by platelet transfusion, J. Pediat. **63:**1081, 1963.

394. Wilkinson, J. F., Nour-Eldin, F., Israels, M. C. G., and Barrett, K. E.: Hemophilia syndromes; a survey of 267 patients, Lancet **2:** 947, 1961.

395. Wilner, G. D., Nossel, H. L., and LeRoy, E. C.: Activation of Hageman factor by collagen, J. Clin. Invest. **47:**2608, 1968.

396. Wilner, G. D., Nossel, H. L., and LeRoy, E. C.: Aggregation of platelets by collagen, J. Clin. Invest. **47:**2616, 1968.

397. Witt, I., Müller, H., and Künzer, W.: Evidence for the existence of foetal fibrinogen, Thromb. Diath. Haemorrhag. **22:**101, 1969.

398. Wolman, I. J.: Laboratory applications in clinical pediatrics, New York, 1957, The Blakiston Co.

399. Wright, H. P.: The adhesiveness of blood platelets in normal subjects with varying concentrations of anticoagulants, J. Path. Bact. **53:**255, 1941.

400. Wright, I. S.: Concerning the functions and nomenclature of blood clotting factors, with a preliminary report of the profile of blood clotting factors in young males, Ann. Intern. Med. **51:**841, 1959.

400a. Zimmerman, T. S., Ratnoff, O. D., and Powell, A. E.: Immunological differentiation of classic hemophilia (factor VIII deficiency) and von Willebrand's disease, J. Clin. Invest. **50:**244, 1971.

401. Zucker, M. B.: Platelet agglutination and vasoconstriction as factors in spontaneous hemostasis in normal thrombocytopenic, heparinized and hypoprothrombinemic rats, Amer. J. Physiol. **148:**275, 1947.

402. Zucker, M. B.: In vitro abnormality of the blood in von Willebrand's disease correctable by normal plasma, Nature **197:**601, 1963.

403. Zucker, M. B.: Platelet adhesion, release and aggregation. In Hunter, R. B., Chairman; Koller, F., editor; Beck, E., associate editor: Fibrinogen and fibrin turnover of clotting factors, Stuttgart, 1963, F. K. Schattauer Verlag.

404. Zucker, M. B., Pert, J. H., and Hilgartner, M. W.: Platelet function in a patient with thrombasthenia, Blood **28:**524, 1966.

405. Zucker, M. B., and Rapport, M. M.: Identification and quantitative determination of serotonin in platelets; the source of serum serotonin, Fed. Proc. **3:**170, 1954.

406. Zucker, M. B., and Woodward, H. Q.: Elevation of serum acid glycerphosphatase activity in thrombocytosis, J. Lab. Clin. Med. **59:**760, 1962.

# 27 THE PURPURAS

The purpuras embrace a miscellaneous group of blood disorders that have in common skin hemorrhages, with or without bleeding into the mucous membranes and other sites and into internal organs. Extravasations of blood may vary from small pinpoint petechiae to large ecchymotic areas. Purpura is a variable symptom complex resulting from a diversity of etiologic agents often with thrombocytopenia and with other conditions in which there are no platelet changes but which have striking clinical features.

Purpura is the Latin derivative from the Greek word "porphyra" the designation for the purple fish *(Purpura lapillus)* from whose gills a purple dye was obtained. While the word was used for many centuries in Greek and Roman times to designate the color purple and related connotations, it did not come into use in disease until the sixteenth century or thereabouts. Epidermoid spotted fevers in the sixteenth century—either plague, typhus, or cerebrospinal fever—were called purpura fevers. Following this time, the term was used to designate any eruption of a purple color. With the discovery that the purple spots often came independent of fever, the word acquired a narrower meaning.[178]

***Classification of purpura.*** Purpuras can be classified as thrombocytopenic, in which case they are classified as either idiopathic or secondary to well-defined disorders, or as nonthrombopenic, such as Henoch-Schönlein disease.

1. With low platelet count (thrombocytopenic states)
   a. Idiopathic thrombocytopenic purpura
   b. Congenital and neonatal thrombocytopenia
   c. Symptomatic thrombocytopenic purpura
      (1) Caused by infections
          (a) Sepsis
          (b) Subacute bacterial endocarditis
          (c) Typhus
          (d) Measles
          (e) Rubella
          (f) Varicella
          (g) Scarlet fever
          (h) Hemorrhagic smallpox
          (i) Rocky Mountain spotted fever
      (2) Caused by chemicals, drugs, physical agents (x-ray, radioactive substance)
      (3) Associated with blood disorders
          (a) Secondary to marrow infiltration: leukemia, neoplasms, fibrosis
          (b) Anemias (hypoplastic and aplastic) in association with autoimmune hemolytic anemia, pernicious anemia, megaloblastic anemia of infancy.
          (c) Secondary to splenic hyperfunction in various diseases—Gaucher's disease, Banti's syndrome, Felty's syndrome, lymphomas, lupus erythematosus, hypersplenism
          (d) Miscellaneous blood disorders—thrombocytopenia associated with hemangioma, thrombotic (thrombohemolytic) thrombocytopenic purpura, infectious mononucleosis, massive blood transfusions, hemolytic uremic syndrome, Aldrich's syndrome
2. With normal platelet count (nonthrombopenic)
   a. Allergic purpura (Henoch-Schönlein purpura)
   b. Congenital vascular defects, i.e., hereditary hemorrhagic telangiectasia, Ehlers-Danlos syndrome, etc.
   c. Purpura simplex
   d. Idiopathic pulmonary hemosiderosis
   e. Infections such as meningococcemia (Waterhouse-Friderichsen syndrome) and scarlet fever (purpura fulminans)
   f. Drugs and chemical agents and avitaminosis (scurvy)
   g. Thrombasthenia and thrombopathia
   h. Auto erythrocyte sensitization
   i. DNA autosensitivity

Thrombocytopenic states may also be classified on the basis of the bone marrow content of megakaryocytes.[324]

1. With normal or increased megakaryocytes in the marrow
   a. Idiopathic thrombocytopenic purpura
   b. Congenital (neonatal) thrombocytopenic purpura
   c. Secondary to splenic hyperfunction in various diseases (Gaucher's disease, Banti's syndrome, Felty's syndrome, lymphomas, lupus erythematosus, (hypersplenism)
   d. Drug sensitization (such as caused by quinidine)
2. With decreased megakaryocytes in the marrow
   a. Secondary to marrow replacement by tumor, leukemia, fibrosis
   b. Aplastic anemia
   c. Marrow damage due to drugs, chemical agents (such as chloramphenicol), radiation, etc.
   d. Congenital (neonatal) thrombocytopenic purpura

In patients with amegakaryocytic thrombocytopenia the megakaryocytes are strikingly reduced in number. Most often, the disappearance of megakaryocytes is due to replacement and infiltration of bone marrow by abnormal cells, as occurs in patients with leukemia and lymphosarcoma and other types of neoplasms. It will be noted that congenital thrombocytopenia may be associated with either decreased or normal numbers of megakaryocytes.

*Platelet counts in normal full-term and premature infants*

Two surveys of platelet counts in normal full-term infants revealed mean values of 200,000 per cu. mm.[4a] and 251,000 per cu. mm.,[2] with ranges of 100,000 to 300,000 per cu. mm. and 117,000 to 450,000 per cu. mm., respectively. In a study of 273 healthy premature infants, Aballi and co-workers[2] found a similar mean and range of platelet counts. The incidence of platelet counts below 100,000 per cu. mm. during the first month of life in the premature infant was below 3.6%. Thus, thrombocytopenia in the newborn period may be defined as a platelet count below 100,000 per cu. mm.

*Thrombocytopenia in the newborn.* The maternal history must be screened for the diseases known to cause thrombocytopenia such as rubella, for prepregnancy disorders such as lupus or idiopathic thrombocytopenic purpura (ITP), and for drugs such as thiazides, quinine, dicumarol, anti-convulsants, etc. Also to be investigated are the hereditary disorders such as sex-linked purpura and a history of previous infants with purpura.

When the physical examination of the infant is normal with only petechiae and no other bleeding manifestations and no associated physical abnormalities, laboratory tests may be helpful.

Antibody in the infant directed against the infant's platelets may be passively acquired from previous ITP, systemic disease, or drugs in the mother, or it may represent isoimmunization in the mother against the infant's platelets (see p. 778).

Complement fixation techniques have demonstrated antibody types and have shown that the platelet antigens are shared by granulocytes and lymphocytes (see p. 778). The description of the platelet antigen systems has led to the diagnosis of incompatibility of the fetal and maternal platelets resulting in neonatal thrombocytopenia analogous to that described for red cell incompatibility leading to erythroblastosis fetalis.

Since thrombocytopenia may herald the onset of aplastic anemia, a bone marrow examination will indicate either the presence of many early megakaryocytes as seen with the immune anemias or their absence may indicate either congenital aplasia or the early onset of an aplastic anemia.

Where there are associated physical findings the approach to diagnosis is somewhat different. Hepatosplenomegaly suggests some type of infection. A bacterial sepsis must be ruled out and other infections considered such as herpes simplex, cytomegalic inclusion disease, toxoplasmosis, and syphilis. Congenital leukemia is also a probability.

Skeletal anomalies such as phocomelia, absent radius, or abnormal configuration of the extremities may be associated with thrombocytopenia, or they occur as a sequela of the rubella syndrome or in the syndrome termed TAR (thrombocytopenia and absent radii). Depleted platelets and purpura may be associated also with giant hemangioma. The liver and spleen are not usually enlarged in this condition.

# THROMBOCYTOPENIC PURPURAS

## Idiopathic thrombocytopenic purpura (ITP, Werlhof's disease, purpura hemorrhagica)

Idiopathic thrombocytopenic purpura is a disease of unknown etiology characterized by a hemorrhagic tendency resulting from a marked reduction in the number of platelets with extravasation of blood into the skin, mucous membranes and subcutaneous tissues.

**Pathogenesis.** Many theories have been suggested for the pathogenesis of idiopathic thrombocytopenic purpura to explain its central features: the thrombocytopenia, increased capillary permeability, and the role of the spleen.[326] These include the movement of platelets from the circulation to the site of injured vessels with corresponding reduction in the peripheral blood,[344] decreased platelet formation due to an abnormal humoral factor elaborated by the spleen and inhibiting megakaryocytic function,[87] and the destruction of platelets after their selective sequestration by the spleen.[103] Studies with fluorescent antiplatelet antibodies have demonstrated a great excess of reactive material, presumably platelets, in spleens of patients with idiopathic thrombocytopenic purpura.[310] While the evidence in favor of the concept of hypersplenic sequestration is well founded clinically and experimentally, there is still evidence of the existence of splenic humoral factors.[81]

More recently, interest has shifted to an immunoallergic mechanism as an etiologic factor. Information from two sources suggested the possibility that an immunologic reaction might be involved in idiopathic thrombocytopenic purpura. The observation that infants born to mothers with this disease were often purpuric was ascribed to the transmission of an immune body across the placenta. In addition, Evans and co-workers[113,114] presented evidence for the existence of a relationship between acquired hemolytic anemia and primary thrombocytopenic purpura. They noted that acquired hemolytic anemia with sensitization of the red cells is often accompanied by thrombocytopenia and that primary thrombocytopenia, in turn, was frequently accompanied by red cell sensitization with or without hemolytic anemia. Since acquired hemolytic anemia had been shown to be due to an autoantibody, Evans and associates suggested that primary thrombocytopenic purpura was due to a thrombocyte autoantibody.

Harrington and co-workers[156] have demonstrated that an immunologic mechanism is responsible for the low platelet count in many patients with idiopathic thrombocytopenic purpura. Platelet agglutinins have been demonstrated in vitro in the plasma of many patients whose thrombocytopenia was of the idiopathic variety. A factor presumably identical to this platelet agglutinin was found to be capable of inducing thrombocytopenic purpura and altering megakaryocytes in normal recipients of this plasma.[155] In terms of this concept the spleen is involved in pathogenesis by removing sensitized platelets and producing platelet agglutinin in variable amounts. Some of the antibody is made in the spleen; the major portion is made elsewhere.

In spite of evidence that idiopathic thrombocytopenic purpura is often based on an immunologic mechanism, circulating platelet antibodies have not been universally found with standard procedures.

In a case of chronic thrombocytopenic purpura, significant lymphocyte transformation could be induced with autologous platelets as a stimulant.[262] Modulation of normal platelet antigens by viral or chemical factors or adsorption of such factors on platelet membrane could explain the observed reactions.

The failure to demonstrate platelet agglutinins in so many children with thrombocytopenic purpura and the large number of remissions with minimal or no treatment suggest other mechanisms of pathogenesis. The increased evidence of a relationship to preceding infection is apparent in the collected series reported by Ferguson.[118] Of a total of 276 cases of idiopathic thrombocytopenic purpura, 172 were closely preceded by an acute infection of one kind or another. Such episodes usually occur at the height or during convalescence of a respiratory infection. It is in this group with preceding infection that the need for treatment is often questioned. The fact that many of these recover spontaneously has led to their designation as the acute group as separated from the chronic and resistant group for whom treatment is mandatory. The precise manner in which infection, presumably bacterial or viral, affects platelets is unknown. It is conceivable that these infectious agents combine with platelets to render them antigenic.

The altered platelets could lead to the formation of a specific antiplatelet antibody analogous to that postulated in drug sensitivity. The damaged platelets would be removed by the reticuloendothelial system. Whether direct platelet damage and destruction can occur without the mediation of antibody is still to be determined.

That a capillary defect undoubtedly plays a role in the etiology of the disease is reflected in the prolonged bleeding time and purpuric manifestations. On the other hand, there is no true correlation between the bleeding time or hemorrhage and the degree of thrombocytopenia. A factor in pathogenesis is the demonstration[214] that normal capillary contraction does not occur in patients with thrombocytopenic purpura and other hemorrhagic states.

The concept of a "thrombocytopoietin" for platelet formation comparable to erythropoietin for red cells is suggested by a case report of a child with chronic idiopathic thrombocytopenic purpura in whom a marked increase in the number of platelets followed transfusion with fresh or stored blood or plasma.[293] The pathogenesis of the purpura in this patient appeared to be related to a congenital deficiency of a platelet-stimulating factor present in normal plasma. The factor appears to act by stimulating megakaryocyte maturation and platelet production.[294] The existence of a human thrombopoietin system regulating thrombopoiesis was also described in thrombocythemic human serum.[186] Evidence for a humoral substance that regulates platelet production has come from additional sources.[94,245,261]

Baldini[32] has summarized the modern concept of the pathogenesis of idiopathic thrombocytopenic purpura as follows: that the thrombocytopenia is the result of increased platelet destruction, that an antiplatelet factor with the features of antibody is present in the plasma of these patients, and that the disease is not always idiopathic. It is frequently found to be secondary to drug hypersensitivity, viral infection, platelet isoimmunity, a lymphoproliferative disorder, systemic lupus erythematosus, and other conditions. With this information as a background, the criteria for the syndrome embrace these characteristics: thrombocytopenia, abundant megakaryocytes in the bone marrow, a short platelet life-span, and an immunologic pathogenesis.[32]

Observations with mice—e.g., with anti-mouse platelet serum and irradiation[110]—suggest that thrombocytopenia causes a stimulation of thrombocytopoiesis. These studies provide evidence for the existence of a feedback system by which the number of circulating platelets influences megakaryocytopoiesis. They also suggest that there may be a pool of unrecognizable megakaryocytic precursor cells which are not damaged by radiation, perhaps by virtue of being nondividing cells, and which have a maturation time of about a day. Alternatively, there may be a sequestration site, like the spleen in human beings, in which newly-found platelets are retained for about a day before being released into the peripheral blood. By analogy to erythropoiesis and erythropoietin, it is possible that the sublethally irradiated animal may prove to be more sensitive than the normal as an assay system for thrombopoietin.

A comparative study of the functional capacity of young versus old platelets from a donor with thrombopoietin deficiency showed that her thrombocytopenia was due to a lack of a plasma factor necessary for platelet production. As a result of this unusual deficiency, she responded to infusions of fresh frozen plasma with predictable and reproducible cycles of platelet production.[4,293,294] Her platelets obtained 4 days after infusion were used as young test cells and compared regarding function with platelets obtained at 18 or 21 days.[177] The young platelets were found to be associated with normal bleeding times, normal clot retraction, normal or increased platelet adhesiveness, normal aggregation to ADP and collagen, and normal platelet factor 3 availability. Old platelets were found to be associated with long bleeding times, decreased platelet adhesiveness in vivo and in vitro, and deficient platelet factor 3 availability. The clot retraction and aggregation to ADP and collagen of old platelets, however, were normal. It was of interest that toward the end of a treatment cycle (by plasma transfusion), mild hemorrhagic difficulties such as epistaxis or superficial bruising occurred apparently concomitant with the presence of the aging platelets.

The fact that platelets are rich in acid phosphatase[380] has been utilized to differentiate thrombocytopenia due to increased platelet destruction from that due to failure of production. Children with acute and chronic thrombocytopenic purpura show plasma acid phosphatase values above normal. In sharp contrast the values are below normal in those with bone marrow failure and evidence of impaired megakaryocyte production. Findings are equivocal in patients with thrombocytopenia secondary to congestive splenomegaly.[250]

In another study it was demonstrated that in congestive splenomegaly, the major factor inducing thrombocytopenia was pooling of platelets in the spleen, with their redistribution from the general circulation to the splenic vascular bed.[24] Later, transfer to the circulation could be compared to the mobilization of platelets from the spleen by infusions of epinephrine. The lowered peripheral platelet count in subjects with splenomegaly may therefore be due to increase in the splenic platelet pool and not to suppression of thrombopoiesis. When splenectomy is performed, this large pool is removed and circulating platelets commence to rise immediately.[255]

Confirmatory evidence for this concept has been observed in the rat,[278] namely, that normally the role of the spleen lies only in the distribution of the circulating platelet mass with a higher concentration of platelets in the spleen. In "hypersplenism" the thrombocytopenia occurs because of excessive pooling of the platelets in the enlarged spleen while the bone marrow provides a larger than normal number of platelets. After splenectomy the bone marrow continues to produce platelets at the same rate as before, so that removal of the splenic platelet pool would cause the platelet numbers to increase in the circulation. These data, however, neither support nor refute the possibility that in "hypersplenic" thrombocytopenia a shortened life-span may partially contribute to the low platelet count. Nor is there any explanation of the mechanism whereby thrombocytopenia can stimulate megakaryocytopoiesis and thereby increase platelet production.

The labeling of platelets with $^{51}Cr$ permits the differentiation of at least two varieties of idiopathic thrombocytopenic purpura, one caused by decreased platelet production and another by increased platelet destruction.[75] Differences in sequestration of $^{51}Cr$-labeled human platelets were noted after reaction in vivo with various amounts of isoantibody. With relatively small amounts of isoantibody, platelets were slowly destroyed in the spleen, whereas with larger quantities they were quickly destroyed in the liver.[26] Normally the labeling procedure of itself damages platelets in some way so that they are sequestered in the liver immediately after transfusion.[25] About one-half of these platelets are returned to the circulation, but are partially destroyed in the spleen so that less than one-third survive.

In several studies[75,239] it has been shown that in idiopathic thrombocytopenic purpura, the platelet life-span fluctuates in various phases of the disease. Whether due to an immune mechanism, infection, or other causes, in the active disease the life-span is sharply reduced. In the remission following splenectomy or steroid therapy or occurring spontaneously, the platelet life-span returns to normal.

It should be emphasized that the characteristic feature in all cases of acute or chronic thrombocytopenic purpura is the shortened survival time of platelets.[1] The normal survival time of human platelets labeled with $^{51}Cr$ is 8 to 10 days.[1] Using this technique the shortest survival curves were obtained in acute cases. It has further been shown that the level of platelets in the peripheral blood is determined exclusively by the rate of platelet destruction with no apparent change in the rate of platelet production by the bone marrow.[32]

The shortened life-span of platelets as a prime etiologic factor in thrombocytopenic purpura is the observation of the finding of numerous platelets and platelet fragments in the smear from the spleen of a patient post-rubella.[236] This phenomenon is probably based on the damage to platelets by circulating virus, altering their survival.

*Pathology.* The bone marrow findings will be discussed elsewhere in connection with other laboratory data. Large histiocytes containing an accumulation of lipid have been described in the spleens of patients with idiopathic thrombocytopenic purpura.[197,286] The cells vary in size from 15 to $35\mu$. The cytoplasm is clear, vacuolated, or reticulated. The nucleus is pale, small, round, or oval, and is central or eccentric in position. Histochemical and chemical analysis of the removed spleens shows that the histiocytes contain phospholipid, with a large proportion of sphingomyelin. These lipid-laden histiocytes are particularly recognizable and more frequently encountered with the aid of fluorescent methods.[107] Fat stains failed to reveal lipid in only one series; instead, foamy histiocytes were found which contained mucopolysaccharide.[82] Steroid therapy has been suggested as a factor but not the only one in the accumulation of lipid in the histiocytes. The presence of these cells cannot be related to any clinical or laboratory data. (See Fig. 99.)

In a series of autopsies on thirty-six adults with this disorder, the spleen showed no characteristic histologic findings.[160] The malpighian corpuscles were prominent as observed in young people. The sinuses of the pulp were frequently filled and distended with small groups of red cells. Megakaryocytes were occasionally seen in the sinuses of the pulp. It is of interest that in twelve of the thirty-six cases death was due to intracranial hemorrhage.

In another series the histologic findings of the spleen showed enlargement of the germinal centers, dilatation of the sinusoids of the red pulp, presence of varying numbers of

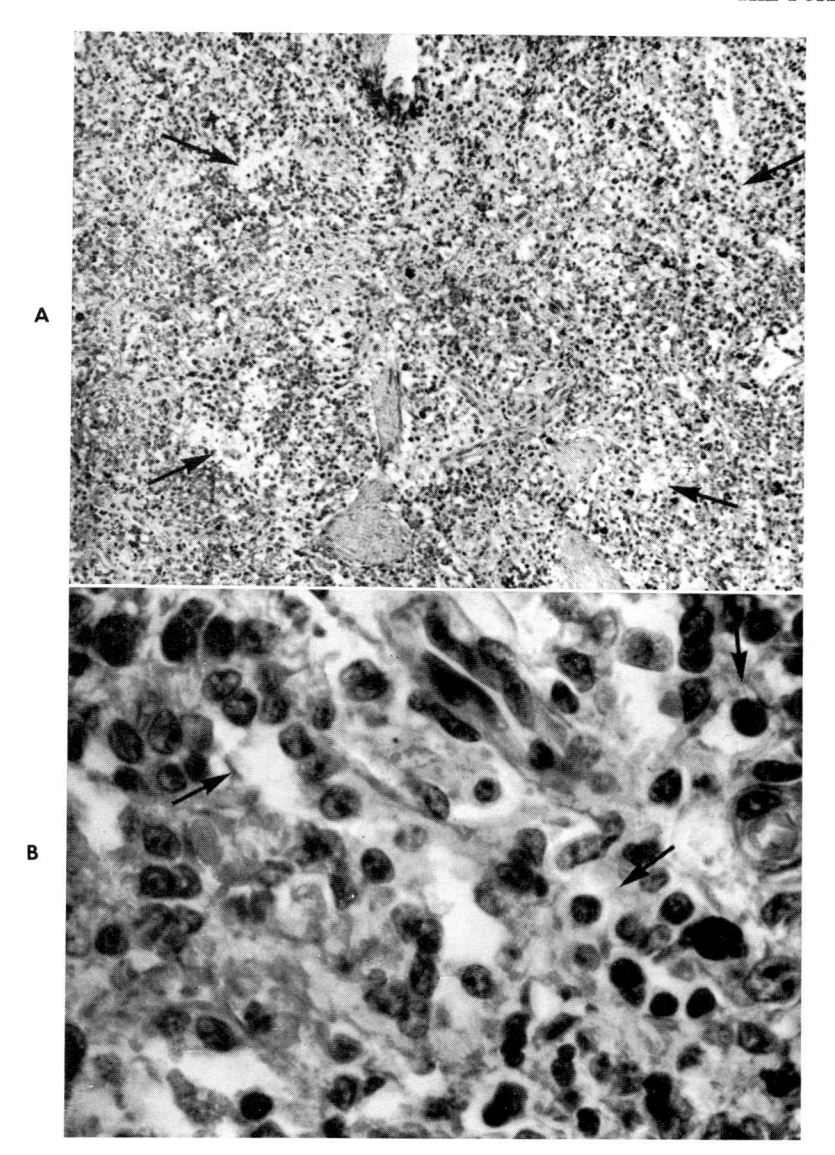

Fig. 99. Photomicrograph of spleen in a 4½-year-old girl with idiopathic thrombocytopenic purpura. Arrows point to foci of large, pale, foamy histiocytes between the sinusoids. **A**, Low power (×130). **B**, High power (×1075).

megakaryocytes, eosinophils and neutrophils, and lipid-laden histiocytes.[60]

*Clinical manifestations.* Idiopathic thrombocytopenic purpura occurs in one of two major types—an acute self-limited form or a chronic protracted disease with occasional remissions. The disease occurs most commonly in children and young adults, with the greater frequency in younger age groups and usually between 2 and 8 years of age.[242] In one series it was observed that 85% of patients were under 8 years of age.[104] In the adult the disease occurs four to five times as frequently in females as in males; in children no sex difference is noted. In a survey of 737 cases the ratio of females to males was 3.7:1 in those 16 years of age and older.[211] The disease is rare in Negroes.[169]

The acute form, which is common in children, has a sudden onset, frequently after an upper respiratory infection or following measles,[122] rubella,[5,118,323,359] chickenpox,[365] mumps,[188] or infectious mononucleosis.[18,268] Rarely, thrombocytopenic purpura occurs during the prodromal period—i.e., a day or two preceding the exanthem—of varicella and measles. The interval between the rubella rash and the onset of bleeding or purpura was between 2 and 8 days in one series, with the peak in the third day and in one case simultaneous with the rash; in another case the interval was 11 days.[118] In one series[213] it was estimated that about 83% of the cases of idiopathic thrombocytopenic purpura were associated with an antecedent infectious disease, and of these one-fifth followed an exanthem. Thrombocytopenic purpura has been reported in association with cat-scratch disease[39,47,175] and with Colorado tick fever.[217] While severe thrombocytopenia is regarded as an unusual complication of infectious mononucleosis, a large enough group of cases has been reported to justify a consideration of infectious mononucleosis in any patient who presents severe thrombocytopenia.[72] It is usually difficult to relate the disease to an infection or to a drug employed during treatment. An increased incidence of allergic manifestations has been found among relatives of patients and in about 15% of the patients.[73]

The chief complaint is easy bruising. Cutaneous purpura is either spontaneous or secondary to minor trauma. The size of the hemorrhage varies from small petechiae of pin-head size to large ecchymoses. The initial period is often marked by widely scattered petechiae with purpura, with large extravasations of blood following later. The color changes from red to purplish to brown with progressive liberation of pigments. Nosebleeds, gingival bleeding, and bleeding into and from the oral mucous membranes, gastrointestinal tract, kidneys, and vagina frequently accompany the purpura, especially at the onset. Petechiae may be found in the subconjunctivae and in the palate. The anterior surfaces of the lower extremities, the buttocks, and especially over bony prominences such as the ribs, scapulae, shoulders, legs, and pubic area are commonly affected. Hematomas form over the lower extremities. Chronic leg ulcer has been observed, perhaps due to breaking down of confluent patches of purpura.[375] Hematuria, hematemesis, melena, and hemarthroses are infrequent. Menorrhagia at or shortly after puberty may be the first indication of idiopathic thrombocytopenic purpura, with a deficiency in blood platelets and impaired capillary resistance appearing soon after.[137] This may be related to the physiologic decrease in the number of platelets in the circulating blood in the 2 weeks preceding menstruation. Intracranial hemorrhage is uncommon in children and constitutes the most serious complication of this disease, occurring usually early in its course. With the exception of purpuric manifestations there are few physical findings. The spleen is not palpable or is barely so. If significant splenomegaly is present, other diagnoses should be considered, notably leukemia, lymphosarcoma, Banti's syndrome, or other conditions associated with hypersplenism.

In a series of fifteen cases of thrombocytopenic purpura following rubella, the median interval between the onset of rash and onset of purpura was 4 days.[236] The frequency of serious hemorrhage appeared to correlate with the degree of thrombocytopenia. In one of their cases a 13-year-old boy died of intracranial bleeding 5 days after admission despite vigorous treatment with corticosteroids and splenectomy.

Prompt, transient, mild depression of the platelet count was observed in 86% of children receiving attenuated measles vaccination.[249] Although transient platelet depression was observed in all ages, the greatest degree was observed in the younger age group. In several patients in whom more frequent platelet counts were obtained it was noted that the count began to fall within 3 days of vaccination. It reached a minimum at 4 to 8 days and then gradually returned to normal. In three patients a fall in megakaryocyte count was observed by the third vaccination day. Within 3 weeks of vaccination the platelet count had returned to normal. This mild thrombocytopenia appears to be a consequence of decreased platelet production, not increased destruction. The platelet count never fell below 64,000 per cu. mm. It has been suggested, though not established, that the thrombocytic depression during the prodromal phase of an infection may be due to viral proliferation within the megakaryocytes. While no purpuric manifestations were noted in this study, a 12-month-old white girl was reported[370] who received an injection of live attenuated measles virus with the addition of gamma globulin and who had a febrile reaction 7 days later; on the tenth day petechiae appeared with a drop in platelets to 60,000/cu. mm. On the eleventh day postvaccination a hyperplasia of megakaryocytes

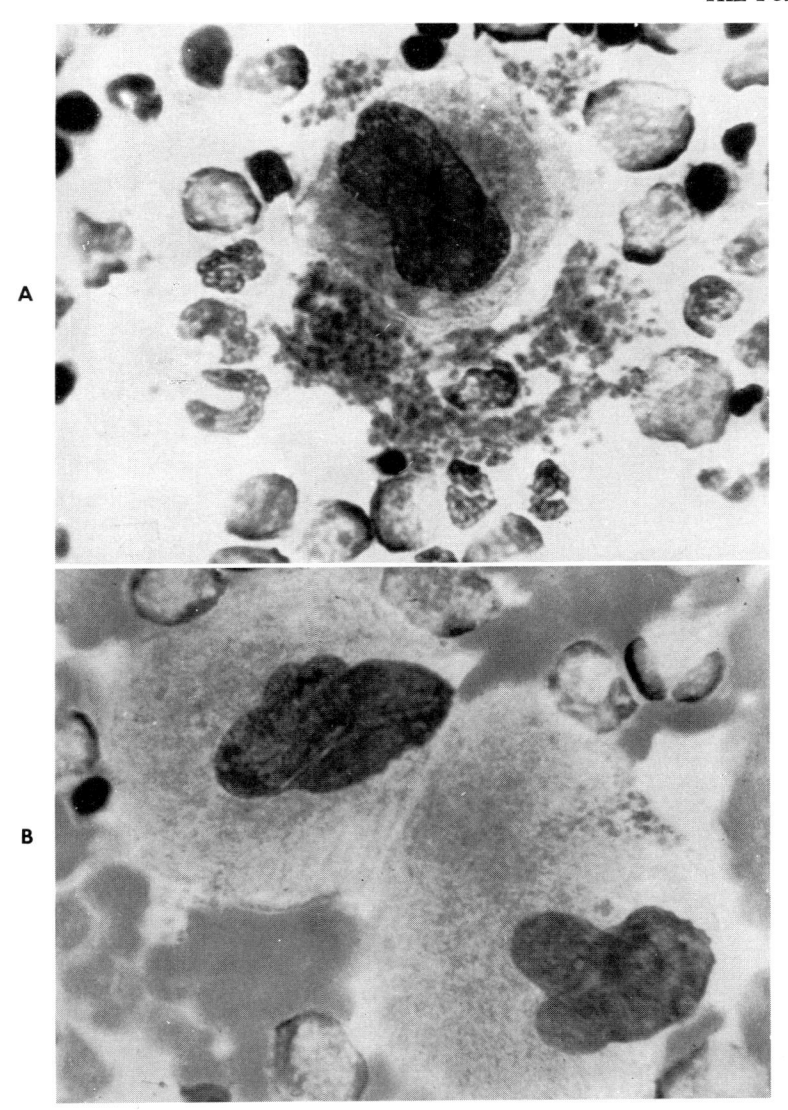

Fig. 100. A, Smear from normal bone marrow. Note mature megakaryocyte containing large lobulated nucleus. Cytoplasm is granular with platelets in the process of formation. Masses of platelets are chiefly grouped about the periphery of the cell. B, Intermediate megakaryocytes. These are usually found in increased numbers in the bone marrow of patients with idiopathic thrombocytopenic purpura. Cytoplasm is more abundant and less granular than that shown in A, and platelet differentiation is either absent (upper cell) or slight (lower cell). (Courtesy Dr. Robert L. Rosenthal, New York, N. Y.)

was noted on bone marrow aspiration. The platelet count gradually increased.

In a comparable case,[15] a 14-month-old white boy developed purpura 9 days after the administration of live attenuated measles vaccine. On the eleventh postvaccination day the platelet count dropped to 13,000/cu. mm., and the bone marrow showed a hyperplasia of megakaryocytes. The child recovered completely, with a marked platelet rise by the sixteenth postvaccination day. By contrast, the thrombocytopenia observed in naturally occurring measles does not appear until the clinical manifestation of the exanthem has been established.[165] In another series purpura occurred from 2 to 14 days (mean of 6 days) after the onset of the classical rash.

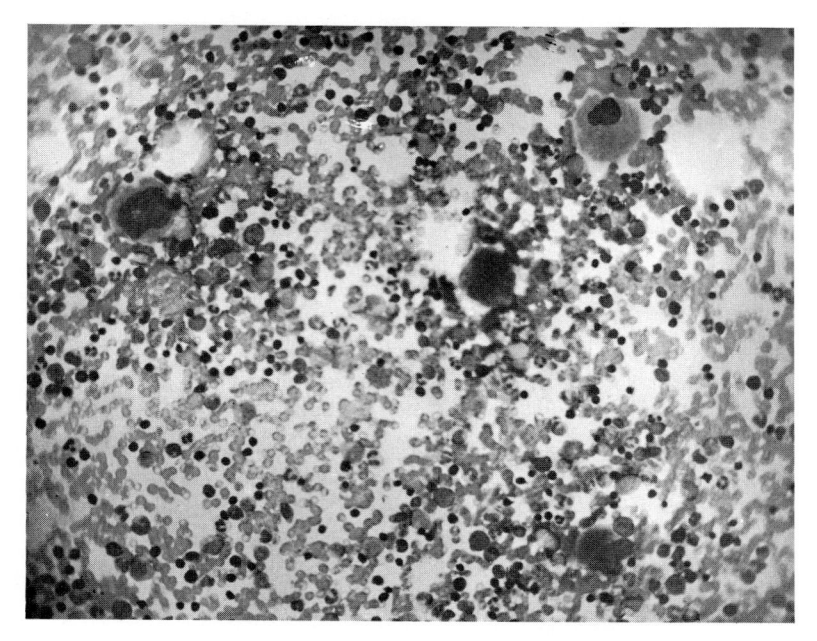

Fig. 101. Low-power view of bone marrow in idiopathic thrombocytopenic purpura. Note increased numbers of immature megakaryocytes. (×150.)

**Laboratory data.** Examination of the bone marrow and peripheral blood is usually sufficient to establish the diagnosis.

*Blood findings.* The most significant finding in the laboratory examination of the patient with thrombocytopenia is a platelet count usually below 60,000 per cubic millimeter and frequently below 20,000. This may be confirmed by the sparsity of platelets in the blood smear in which the relatively few platelets seen are often single, large, and abnormal in shape. The bleeding time is characteristically prolonged, the tourniquet test is positive, and clot retraction is poor to absent. The prothrombin time and whole blood clotting time are normal. The existence of a true disturbance in the coagulation mechanism in idiopathic thrombocytopenic purpura is demonstrated by an abnormal prothrombin consumption test which is indicative of impaired thromboplastin formation. A normochromic anemia with reticulocytosis occurs if there is epistaxis or if bleeding into the urinary tract or gastrointestinal canal is severe. A moderate leukocytosis with an increase in granulocyte forms occurs, if purpura is excessive.

In occasional cases of chronic thrombocytopenia isolated red cells appear contracted and show multiple projections similar to burr cells or pyknocytes. These cells are especially noticeable following splenectomy.[317] Also, transient neutropenia with or without leukopenia may occasionally follow splenectomy.

*Bone marrow findings.* In patients with idiopathic thrombocytopenic purpura the principal abnormality is confined to the megakaryocytes. In patients with active bleeding, normoblastic and often myeloid hyperplasia may be present. The megakaryocytes are normal or increased in number and show reduced platelet formation. The megakaryocytes vary in size, amount of cytoplasm, and lobulation of the nucleus. Agranular, vacuolated, degenerated, and immature forms are present. (See Figs. 100 and 101.)

In one study[87] platelet production was found in only 8 to 19% of all megakaryocytes and following splenectomy in 69 to 85% of all cells. As the disease enters the chronic phase, megakaryocytes, although more mature, still show a reduction in granulation and platelet formation. The massive liberation of platelets after splenectomy has been interpreted as an indication that the spleen inhibits platelet formation from the megakaryocyte and prevents their delivery in the circulating blood.[326]

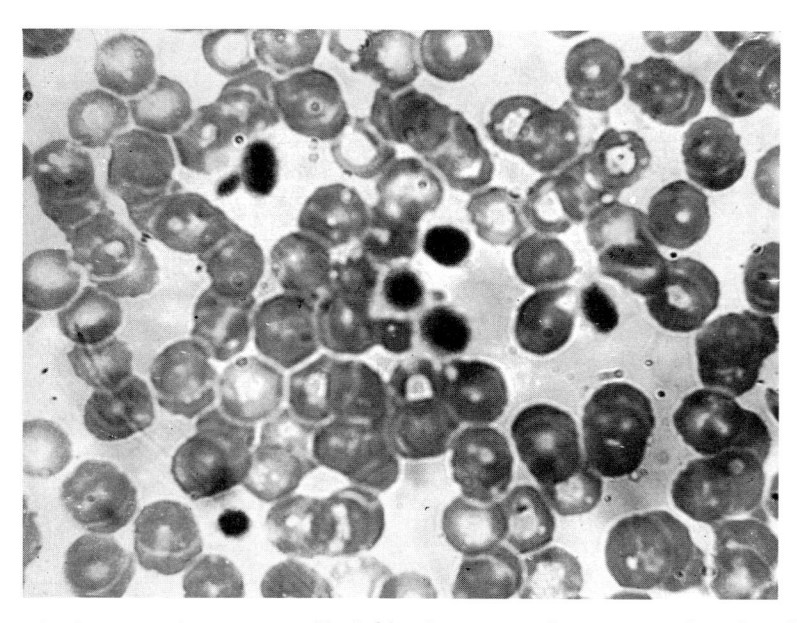

Fig. 102. Blood smear of a 13-year-old child splenectomized 4 years earlier for idiopathic thrombocytopenic purpura. The platelets are still decreased in numbers. Note enormous size. Each darkly stained body in this smear is a platelet. Classified as an atypical thrombasthenia, although in this case the bleeding time, prothrombin consumption, and clot retraction are normal. Other platelet functions were abnormal. (×1350.)

Despite these considerations, bone marrow examination cannot be regarded as diagnostic of idiopathic thrombocytopenic purpura. Its chief function lies in the exclusion of disease with which idiopathic thrombocytopenic purpura can be confused, principally aplastic anemia and leukemia and, less often, lymphosarcoma and other infiltrative diseases.

Several studies have shown that there is no consistent pattern of megakaryocytes that can be correlated with the course or prognosis of idiopathic thrombocytopenic purpura.[98,242] In patients with a complete or almost complete absence of megakaryocytes, however, splenectomy is contraindicated and an underlying condition should be sought. Bone marrow examinations should be repeated to establish the existence of decreased megakaryocytes. Eosinophilia in the bone marrow, frequently observed in this disease and regarded as a favorable prognostic sign for spontaneous recovery[297,298] has not been confirmed. Platelet functions vary greatly in patients recovering from thrombocytopenia.[348] Complete recovery of functions usually takes place slowly so that numbers may return to normal; yet not all functions are restored. In these cases, the platelets may be dustlike or greatly enlarged (Fig. 102). Purpura may be present in spite of a normal count. The tardy return in spite of normal numbers occurs with or without splenectomy.

As stated previously, it is a common finding for the megakaryocytes to be increased in number with a relative increase of immature forms revealing evidence of cytoplasmosis and nuclear degeneration, vacuolization, and deficient budding around the cytoplasmic margins.[32] These abnormalities may be viral in origin since megakaryocytes are known to harbor viruses.[102] It is possible also that the autoantibody responsible for increased platelet destruction in the peripheral blood acts to depress megakaryocytic formation in the bone marrow.[32] The megakaryocytic hyperplasia which is usually noted in the bone marrow may therefore be interpreted as ineffective rather than effective thrombocytopoiesis.[32]

*Diagnosis.* It is important initially to distinguish between nonthrombocytopenic and thrombocytopenic purpura. To establish a diagnosis of idiopathic thrombocytopenic purpura, secondary causative factors, such as chemical and physical agents, blood disorders, and infections which depress platelets, must be eliminated. Bone marrow aspiration is an aid in differentiating idiopathic thrombocytopenia from aplastic anemia and leukemia since it may resemble these conditions closely in some phase of the respective diseases. In patients with thrombocytopenia, megakaryocytes are normal or increased, and red cell and granulocytic precursors are normal. In those with aplastic anemia and leukemia all elements, including the megakaryocytes, are depressed (amegakaryocytic), and in the latter the bone marrow is infiltrated with blast forms. The thrombocytopenia of metastatic carcinoma and lymphosarcoma is also associated with an amegakaryocytic bone marrow.

In patients with idiopathic thrombocytopenia the spleen is not enlarged. Where moderate or marked splenomegaly exists in association with thrombocytopenia, other conditions such as Gaucher's disease, Banti's syndrome, and reticuloendotheliosis are to be considered. Sudden epistaxis or gastrointestinal hemorrhage together with thrombocytopenia in an infant whose spleen has become enlarged may indicate reticuloendotheliosis.

Disseminated lupus erythematosus may exist as an underlying disturbance manifesting itself solely as thrombocytopenic purpura without rash or joint manifestations. Examination for L.E. cells has therefore been recommended as a routine test in all patients with thrombocytopenic purpura, preferably before steroids are administered. The development of overt disseminated lupus erythematosus following splenectomy for idiopathic thrombocytopenic purpura has been interpreted as an indication that the intact spleen exerts an inhibitory influence in preventing the full expression of the latent disease.[88,267] Although the development of lupus erythematosus has been estimated to have occurred in as many as 25% of all patients splenectomized for thrombocytopenic purpura,[89] this sequence has not as yet been observed in our clinic nor in another children's clinic.[43] The fear that splenectomy in idiopathic thrombocytopenic purpura may contribute to dissemination of latent lupus erythematosus has been questioned in a large experience with persons of all ages.[46] Nevertheless, a lupus preparation should constitute an essential part of the routine study of all patients with thrombocytopenic purpura.

Following 2 years of typical thrombocytopenic purpura, an 8-year-old child in our experience developed an acute hemolytic anemia, positive Coombs and L.E. tests, and antinuclear antibodies.

*Course and prognosis.* A spontaneous remission occurs in 75% of infants and children as compared with 25 to 30% of adults. The disease may run its course in a few weeks without recurrence. The majority of children recover completely within 3 months, usually in the first 6 weeks, and 10 to 15% recover within 4 to 6 months. Spontaneous and permanent recovery may not occur for 6 months to 1 year, during which time purpura remits and relapses with varying degrees of thrombocytopenia with each attack. About 10% of children develop the chronic form, and of these approximately 85% recover with splenectomy. In chronically affected patients especially, a constant search must be made for an underlying disease, particularly aplastic anemia, in which the definitive features of the complete disease may not be manifest for a year or more.

*Treatment.* Fresh blood, platelet transfusions, corticosteroids, and splenectomy are used in the treatment of thrombocytopenic purpura. Early treatment consists of transfusions of fresh whole blood in the event of severe anemia from blood loss and the administration of adrenocortical steroids. Although intracranial hemorrhage is rare in children, rest or modified activity is advisable when platelet counts drop below 30,000 per cubic millimeter. Subsequent attendance at school and resumption of a normal regime depend upon cessation of cutaneous hemorrhages and an increase in the number of platelets.

It may well be that acute and chronic purpura are separate entities. Splenectomy is only of importance in the latter type because of the high incidence of spontaneous recovery in the acute form. The separation between the two types is frequently difficult, thus posing problems of therapy.

*Transfusions.* In the nonanemic patient whose bleeding is not controlled by steroids and tends to be progressive, viable platelets can be obtained either as platelet-rich plasma by sedimentation or slow centrifugation of fresh whole blood or preferably as platelet concentrates obtained from several units of blood. Transfusions of fresh platelets are effective in controlling bleeding in idiopathic thrombocytopenic purpura but their frequent administration causes the risk of reducing the platelet life-span due to the development of platelet-isoantibodies. Platelet transfusions are indicated in the event of an acute bleeding episode with marked blood loss and in preparing the patient for an operative procedure.

Following the demonstration that normal plasma may contain a platelet-stimulating factor,[293,294] fresh plasma transfusions (10 to 20 ml. per kilogram of body weight) have been given to patients with thrombocytopenic purpura. While favorable responses have been reported,[42] it is the exceptional chronic case in which a permanent remission is observed. This form of therapy is difficult to evaluate because of the tendency of the majority of pediatric cases to remit spontaneously. Plasma injections are worthy of trial before splenectomy, but complete evaluation requires more extensive experience and at present must be considered experimental.[292]

Comparing transfusions of platelet-rich plasma obtained after centrifugation of blood with platelet concentrates, it was found that the former was superior in terms of platelet increments, when given to patients with thrombocytopenia.[205] The most important single factor responsible for poor response to transfusion of concentrates is probably the direct physical injury sustained by the platelets during actual centrifugation. Concentrates have the advantage, however, in ease of handling and administration and the avoidance of large plasma volumes and minor transfusion reactions.

*Steroids.* Idiopathic thrombocytopenic purpura in children runs so variable a course that it is difficult to lay down strict guidelines of management, particularly with regard to the evaluation of therapeutic measures introduced early in the disease. The need for the use of adrenocortical steroids is moderated by the knowledge that in the era before these hormones were available a majority of children were known to recover spontaneously within a period of 3 to 6 months of onset and often in a matter of weeks. With the demonstration of the effectiveness of the adrenocortical steroids in controlling bleeding and perhaps in preventing the rare complication of intracranial hemorrhage, these agents have become an integral part of therapy.[361] It has also been shown that nearly all deaths occur in the first month of the disease.[190] Furthermore, it is possible that steroids may shorten the disease by accelerating the onset of a remission. A major objective has been to expedite a rise in the platelet count when the values persist at low levels for prolonged periods. Such a statement cannot, however, be made dogmatically because a high proportion of patients make a complete recovery often without treatment.

The disadvantages of prolonged corticosteroid therapy are manifold and include the greater susceptibility to infection, hypertension, development of peptic ulcer, osteoporosis, growth retardation, moon facies, and hirsutism. One group of investigators[213] would restrict the use of hormone therapy to cutaneous massive purpura, continued profuse epistaxis, and the presence of retinal hemorrhages as a possible indication of bleeding within the central nervous system. The clinical course of all surviving patients in their series justified the conclusion that, once begun, the continuation of steroid therapy should not be determined by the platelet count but by the duration of the bleeding tendency; in other words, the child and not the platelet count should be treated. In this series the high incidence of antecedent viral infection supports the view that acute purpura in children is infectious or postinfectious in origin and differs in etiology and pathogenesis from the chronic forms in adults.

With this background it is apparent that the course of treatment depends on an appraisal of the severity of the clinical and hematological findings at the outset. Where cutaneous hemorrhage is mild and thrombocytopenia is moderate, daily blood counts will soon demonstrate that a spontaneous remission is in progress. When the combination of findings indicates a disease of greater severity, treatment with adrenocortical steroids in small doses carries minimal hazard.

As to the choice of a drug, adrenocortical steroids and ACTH are both effective in the relief of bleeding symptoms, both by an early hemostatic effect mediated by action on the blood vessel wall[115] and by a later rise in platelets. Of the various agents, prednisone or a like substance is most useful because of ease of administration and the fact that it lends itself more readily to regulation of dosage. An increase in the number of platelets in the patient with acute idiopathic thrombocytopenic purpura with a favorable prognosis occurs within a week or 10 days after the initiation of therapy. The mechanism of the platelet increase is not apparent; one of the explanations offered is that prednisone reduces the concentration of antibody responsible for platelet destruction or megakaryocytic inhibition.[89]

The dosage of steroids is variable and is adjusted for the age of the patient, severity of the disease, and the individual tendency to develop the side effects. The dose of prednisone varies from 1 to 2 mg. per kilogram of body weight per day. A dosage of 40 mg. of prednisone is rarely exceeded in the younger patient, nor 60 mg. in the older child. Unless bleeding is severe, the smaller amount is given. Four-fifths of the dose is given for triamcinolone (Aristocort or Kenacort) and methyl prednisone (Medrol) compounds. Like all adrenocortical steroids, the drug is given in three or four divided doses at 8- or 6-hour intervals. In the infant the dose must be carefully adjusted to avoid hypertension, even in this age period.

Frequently, a normal platelet level is obtained with 3 weeks of steroid treatment, in which case the drug is tapered off during the fourth week. In the majority of patients only one course of treatment is required. Regardless of recovery, blood counts are carried out at regular intervals for several months and years to assure the permanency of the remission. Maintenance therapy with smaller doses (depending on the individual patient) has been advocated when the platelets have reached normal levels[85,89] in the hope that this will assure a permanent remission and reduce the need for later splenectomy. This plan may be followed in children with a history of relapsing purpura in whom splenectomy seems inevitable. In the few patients in whom this form of treatment has been carried out, the minimal dosage necessary to maintain adequate platelet response was 15 mg. There are several objections to maintenance therapy in children as a routine procedure: persistent and excessive hypercorticism, generalized osteoporosis, and retardation of growth. Several 3-week courses, followed by 1 week of reduced dosage, with an interval of 1 or 2 months of no treatment, are frequently necessary before a therapeutic response is achieved. If the response with the steroids in successive courses is transient or inadequate, better results are occasionally obtained by the intramuscular administration of three or four single daily doses of 60 units of corticotropin in a gelatin menstruum. In an occasional patient, after several courses of treatment with corticosteroids, the platelet count may become stabilized at levels of approximately 100,000 per cubic millimeter without maintenance therapy and without evidence of purpura. Under these conditions, splenectomy may be postponed. If at any time during its course, especially in the first weeks, purpura becomes marked and severe epistaxis occurs, the maximal dosage of prednisone, 2 mg. per kilogram and even higher, is given and, if necessary, steroid therapy is supplemented by platelet transfusions.

Prednisone therapy sustained in high dosage has been thought to inhibit platelet production by a catabolic effect on the megakaryocytes.[74] In several cases reducing the dose of prednisone permitted the platelet count to rise to significantly higher levels.

In general, ACTH gives similar results to prednisone, but it is usually not employed because of the formation of hematomas following injections. In occasional cases ACTH causes a remission when prednisone has produced no platelet response.[52] There is still no satisfactory explanation why ACTH should sometimes be therapeutically effective after corticosteroids have failed. Dosage or duration of therapy are not factors. It is, therefore, worth trying a course of ACTH for several weeks, if no response occurs with adequate prednisone dosage, before splenectomy is contemplated.

We have found it advisable to follow the platelets for at least 1 year beyond their return to normal. Occasionally, thrombocytopenia will recur with minimal skin manifestations. Eventually, platelet counts are permanently restored to normal, although sometimes not until after a lapse of 1 to 2 years. Steroids are readministered only with a drastic drop in platelets.

Despite the assurance that the acute disease in most children runs a favorable course with eventual recovery, the possibility of cerebral or other uncontrollable hemorrhage may occur not only in the early weeks of the disease, but after several years as well.[312,358] It is for this reason that, regardless of recovery with or without splenectomy, blood counts should be carried out routinely for several months and even after a year to assure the permanency of remission.

The importance of following the platelet count is illustrated in the case of an 8-year-old

Negro boy who apparently recovered completely from an initial episode of thrombocytopenic purpura. A recurrence 14 months later resulted in death from intracranial hemorrhage.[86,169] This report emphasized the possibility that even after an apparent cure a second episode of idiopathic thrombocytopenic purpura may result in death from central nervous system bleeding.

Recurrent episodes of thrombocytopenic purpura have been reported and attributed to allergic sensitivity, administration of vaccine, or viral exposure.[86] In some instances the development of thrombocytopenia was associated with a potent thrombocytolytic process which was only active during relapse. Remission periods of 3 to 18 years' duration were reported in one series.[86]

With the dose and duration of therapy carefully controlled, other schedules of treatment have been suggested. Schulman,[292] for instance, starts therapy with prednisone in a dose of 1 mg. per kilogram of body weight. Treatment at this dosage level is continued for a maximum of 3 weeks, and the corticosteroids are tapered and discontinued during the fourth week, regardless of whether the platelet count improves or not. Should thrombocytopenia persist beyond 3 months, a second course of corticosteroids is tried, again limited to 4 weeks.

Hilgartner and co-workers[161] found that patients with thrombocytopenic purpura may attain a normal platelet count, only to demonstrate functional and morphologic aberrations of platelets and become subject to recurrences. They also found another group of asymptomatic patients who had recovered following steroid therapy and showed a transient drop in platelet counts to 100,000 per cubic millimeter with infections.

*Immunosuppressive agents.* Increasing interest in the suppression of the immune response by antimetabolites stems from the successful results reported by Schwartz and Dameshek[296] in the treatment of autoimmune hemolytic anemia with mercaptopurine and thioguanine. These cytotoxic agents are known to interfere with the growth of immunocompetent cells and to minimize the immunologic response in experimental animals sensitized to foreign proteins.[17] A logical application of the concept that idiopathic thrombocytopenic purpura (ITP) is an autoimmune disorder[32] is to treat this disorder by agents capable of suppressing the immune response.[9] While corticosteroids and splenectomy are the accepted therapeutic measures for treating ITP, these methods have their shortcomings. Prolonged steroid therapy has undesirable and occasionally dangerous complications and splenectomy in children may be associated with life-threatening and occasionally fatal infections.[316] Bouroncle and Doan[54,55] introduced the use of azathioprine (Imuran) as an effective immunosuppressive agent in ITP. The drug has a less toxic effect on the bone marrow and is easier to control than the previous metabolites employed. In a series of seventeen patients (including two children) who were refractory to conventional therapy with splenectomy and corticosteroids, azathioprine was effective in inducing a complete hematologic and clinical remission in twelve patients and a partial remission in two patients. With the exception of transitory and reversible leukopenia, no toxic effects resulted after 2 years of therapy. They advise the use of small doses of prednisone with the azathioprine therapy since the corticosteroids have a synergistic effect in obtaining a remission. Sussman[337] reported clinical remissions in seven of eight patients with refractory thrombocytopenic purpura with the use of azathioprine.

Hilgartner and associates[162] treated five children with refractory ITP with azathioprine for 8 to 27 months. This drug was given in a dose of 2.0 mg./kg./day. If there was no platelet response within 4 weeks the dose was increased to 3 to 4 mg./kg./day, and if there was no response in 8 weeks a small dose of steroids (0.2 mg./kg./day) was added. Complete blood counts were carried out twice weekly for 5 weeks and thereafter every 2 to 3 weeks, depending on the degree of leukopenia and platelet count. The leukocyte count was allowed to drop to 2,000/cu. mm. and the hemoglobin was allowed to drop 2 gm./100 ml. before the dosage of the drug was decreased. Of the five children, three had an excellent result, one had a good response, whereas one unsplenectomized patient failed to respond to this therapy but made an excellent response to splenectomy.

The limited experience with azathioprine in the treatment of ITP in children and the known variability of this disorder render it difficult to assess its value or to define its precise role in therapy. On the basis of available data its greatest value appears to be in the treatment of recurring purpura following splenectomy. On the other hand, experience indicates that azathioprine is a safe and often an effective means of inducing remission in cases refractory to conventional therapy and perhaps should be considered before surgical intervention. As already stated, a small dose of corticosteroids given in conjunction with the full dose of azathioprine is more effective than the latter alone.

Another immunosuppressive drug used with varying degrees of success in the treatment of "refractory" thrombocytopenic purpura is cyclophosphamide (Cytoxan). In one series,[200] nine patients previously treated with corticosteroids (of whom seven had been splenectomized) were treated with cyclophosphamide in a daily dose of from 50 to 200 mg. The duration of immunosuppressive therapy ranged from 1.2 to 8.0 months. Of the nine patients, six had an excellent response which appeared from 2 to 10 weeks after the initiation of therapy and remained in complete hematologic remission for 5 to 30 months after discontinuation of the drug. Here, too, this agent has been advocated in cases refractory to corticosteroids for trial before splenectomy is considered.

*Splenectomy.* Splenectomy was introduced as a form of treatment in this disease by Kaznelson.[185] Splenectomy is indicated if with adequate therapy thrombocytopenia persists for 6 months or longer, especially when associated with recurrent purpura or overt bleeding provided secondary or symptomatic forms of thrombocytopenic purpura have been eliminated and megakaryocytes are present in normal or increased numbers in the bone marrow. The finding of a few or no megakaryocytes warrants a search for an underlying condition and is a contraindication to splenectomy. An expectant policy is followed beyond the 6-month period if the bleeding tendency is not manifested, despite thrombocytopenia, and the patient is asymptomatic. In such children a decision is usually reached when at the end of a year platelet levels either return to normal or are eventually associated with hemorrhagic manifestations. When platelet counts fluctuate about 100,000 per cubic millimeter or more without bleeding, the patient is followed beyond a year before the spleen is removed. Complete clinical and hematologic remissions can be expected in about 85% of children with the chronic disease in whom splenectomy is performed. In a series comprising patients of all ages, splenectomy was successful in 81% of those with idiopathic thrombocytopenic purpura, whereas corticosteroid therapy was successful in only 38%.[69] The parent is to be advised that in about 15% of patients splenectomy may be followed by several years of frequent episodes of thrombocytopenia.

In one series of nineteen patients with ITP, it was observed that in eleven no relapse occurred when the platelet count exceeded 500,000 per cu. mm. 1 week after splenectomy.[201] The difficulty in employing this criterion was shown in one of our patients in whom the spleen had been removed at 8 years of age and whose platelet count approximated 500,000 per cu. mm. and persisted at this level for several weeks after the operation. In this child, however, marked thrombocytopenia recurred over prolonged periods for the following 8 years.

Splenectomy is to be recommended after 6 months' treatment without remission in those children whose lives are restricted by the need for constant supervision and are chronically invalided, and in the girl with thrombocytopenic purpura who, having reached menarche, has recurrent severe bleeding with each menstrual period. Early splenectomy in the first weeks of illness is necessary in any child showing severe and uncontrollable generalized bleeding.

It should be clear that no method is available which can predetermine that a sustained remission will follow splenectomy, nor can one be certain that children with ITP will not recover spontaneously with a minimum of therapy given for prolonged periods. Splenectomy is recommended when ITP is severe and unremitting, relapses when corticosteroids are discontinued, persists despite this therapy, requires relatively large doses to maintain a state free of bleeding, and shows no tendency to spontaneous remission over a period of 6 to 12 months of close supervision.

Two patients with idiopathic thrombocytopenic purpura have been reported requiring urgent surgical intervention, one with massive cerebral hemorrhage necessitating cranial decompression, the other for abdominal laparotomy for intestinal obstruction. Splenectomy resulted in platelet responses and hemostasis in less than 2 hours, permitting surgical management without bleeding.[290] These are measures of desperation. When available, platelet concentrates are to be given primary consideration. There is no assurance that splenectomy will produce a platelet rise in every case.

In preparing the patient for splenectomy due consideration must be given to the stress challenge of the operative procedure in view of the preceding vigorous treatment with adrenocorticosteroids. In the unprepared patient, adrenal insufficiency may conceivably compromise the patient's ability to deal with acute stress which may develop during splenectomy. To forestall this contingency, the patient is treated with hydrocortisone in a comprehensive manner. In this case hydrocortisone is preferable to prednisone and other synthetic analogues in which side reactions are minimized. Until more extensive information is obtained as to the degree of homeostatic imbalance induced by prolonged adrenocorticosteroid therapy, the following regimen is suggested. While splenectomy is the operation usually contemplated in the patient with idiopathic thrombocytopenic purpura, other occasions of lesser or greater moment may arise for which adequate preparation and postoperative medication are required. Such schedules have accordingly been included. The preoperative use of ACTH originally advocated to control hemostasis during splenectomy awaits further confirmation.[142]

Following is an outline of the preoperative and postoperative management of pediatric patients with idiopathic thrombocytopenic purpura or other disorders who have been receiving steroids.

1. Preoperative management
   a. Twelve hours before operation, 50 mg. hydrocortisone intravenously
   b. One hour before operation, 100 mg. hydrocortisone intravenously
2. During the operation
   a. 100 mg. hydrocortisone intravenously in dextrose water (slow drip)
3. In recovery room
   a. 100 mg. hydrocortisone intravenously
4. Postoperative management
   a. 7 A.M., 50 mg. hydrocortisone intravenously
      Evening, 50 mg. hydrocortisone intravenously first and second days
   b. Third and fourth days, 10 mg. prednisone three times daily (abruptly discontinued on the fifth day)
5. For the patient currently on prednisone
   a. 50 mg. hydrocortisone intravenously before the procedure and 50 mg. on leaving the treatment room when dental extraction or other minor operation under anesthesia is required
   b. 100 mg. hydrocortisone given quickly through a drip and 100 mg. hydrocortisone in a drip (slow drip) during the operation when patient is to be subjected to emergency major surgery

Because of the excessive number of platelets known to follow splenectomy, platelet levels should be followed routinely. Anticoagulant therapy previously recommended when platelet counts rose above 1 million per cubic millimeter[145] is no longer prescribed because of the rarity of thromboembolic complications in children. The possibility of this contingency must, nevertheless, be kept in mind. In a 13-year-old patient recently splenectomized for idiopathic thrombocytopenic purpura the platelets persisted at a level of 2.5 million per cubic millimeter. An oral coumarin preparation was given during the period of thrombocytosis to avoid complications.

The use of a broad-spectrum antibiotic for 2 years following the operation[316] is advised, although overwhelming postsplenectomy infection is exceptional but has occurred.

It should be pointed out that in certain children, especially those in the preadolescent and adolescent groups, splenectomy may not provide the anticipated cure. We have encountered several children in whom thrombocytopenia with overt bleeding accompanied by a positive Coombs test with or without hemolytic anemia recurred following a remission of several months to a year. The failure of platelets to increase following splenectomy may indicate the presence of a more widespread disease and a fatal outcome. A case in point is that of a boy whose spleen was removed at 14 years of age for thrombocytopenic purpura. The platelet count following the operation remained depressed and could only be restored to normal levels by large doses of steroids. After a remission of 9 months, hemolytic anemia occurred in which the Coombs test was negative. Soon after recovery from the anemia, marked thrombocytopenia recurred which could not be controlled, and the patient eventually succumbed with a fatal hemorrhage. The Coombs test was positive in the final episode despite the absence of an anemia due to a hemolytic process. Throughout the entire course, the test for lupus erythematosus was consistently negative. Such a combination of circumstances is suggestive of the concept of Evans and co-workers[113,114] who emphasized the immunologic relationship between acquired hemolytic anemia and thrombocytopenic purpura.

Since the success of splenectomy in the treatment of idiopathic thrombocytopenic purpura is presumably due to removal of a major site of platelet destruction, it would seem possible to anticipate the success of this procedure by identifying preoperatively those patients in whom there is a predominant splenic sequestration of $^{51}$Cr-labeled platelets. Najean and his associates[240] concluded that surface scanning could be used to differentiate two distinct disease states characterized by splenic and hepatic platelet destruction, respectively. They suggested that splenectomy be withheld from patients showing hepatic sequestration. Aster and Keene[27] also found that the major site of platelet destruction was related to the severity of the disease process, splenic sequestration being seen in mild and moderately severe disease and significant hepatic destruction when the T½ is of the order of a few minutes and platelet levels are profoundly lowered. They concluded, however, that surface scanning after injection of labeled platelets, while of interest in studying the pathogenesis of ITP, may not have special value in predicting the response to splenectomy. They suggested that the decision for or against splenectomy should be based upon clinical criteria such as response to and tolerance of corticosteroids and the duration of thrombocytopenia rather than the site at which labeled platelets are destroyed at the time of a single platelet study.

Furthermore, Baldini[32] has shown that a number of patients showing predominant radioactivity over the liver after infusion of $^{51}$Cr-labeled platelets have obtained a rapid and complete response to splenectomy. On the other hand, there are patients with a pattern of predominant uptake by the spleen who may not respond to the surgical removal of the spleen.

### Hereditary thrombocytopenic purpura

A genetic basis for the occurrence of multiple cases of thrombocytopenic purpura in one family has been the subject of controversy. Several families have been reported, however, in which a hereditary or congenital disposition toward primary thrombocytopenic purpura appeared unequivocal. In some cases bleeding is noted from birth; in others, the disease becomes manifest later in childhood. Roberts and Smith[275] described one family in which three of the children showing thrombocytopenic purpura died between 3 and 7 years of age. One died of identical symptoms without ever having been studied. Seip[300] reported another family in which a mother and two sons showed purpura, ecchymoses, and thrombocytopenia from early childhood. Quick and Hussey[266] described a bleeding disorder in eight members of one family. The platelets were only moderately reduced and defective in quality. The condition was described as a hereditary thrombocytopathic thrombocytopenia.

Vestermark and Vestermark[354] described a family of five children with thrombocytopenia in two generations, occurring solely in boys. One of the patients became symptom free spontaneously at about the time of puberty, while the other responded to splenectomy at 18 years of age. The overlapping with Aldrich's (Wiskott-Aldrich) syndrome was apparent in the other three patients who, in addition to the hemorrhagic diathesis, showed a mild tendency to infection and eczema. Chronic idiopathic purpura in four boys of a family of nine children was reported by Schaar.[289] In each boy purpura appeared in early infancy and continued from 1 to 3 years, until controlled by splenectomy. In another family of five generations with forty-seven members, eight of ten members had undue bleeding shown to be due to thrombocytopenia.[28] The authors regard this disorder to be different from ordinary idiopathic thrombocytopenia in its male preponderance and poor response to steroids and as being clearly distinct from congenital thrombocytopenia and Aldrich's syndrome. They concluded that this disease is probably due to a sex-linked mendelian dominant gene, with incomplete penetrance in the female.

Bithell and associates[48] reported a family of eight members of a kindred in which four generations have been afflicted with a mild hemorrhagic diathesis that appears to be the result of mild thrombocytopenia inherited as an autosomal dominant trait. They state that, with few exceptions, neither splenectomy nor corticosteroid therapy appears to be of value in the treatment of inherited thrombocytopenia. Harms and Sachs[153] reported a family with chronic idiopathic thrombocytopenia and platelet autoantibodies (three sisters, the mother, and the grandmother on the mother's side) associated with a diminution of the clotting factor X.

Murphy and associates[238] reported a family in which thrombocytopenia was present in three generations of a kindred and was transmitted as a dominant trait. The clinical picture was quite similar to that of idiopathic thrombocytopenic purpura but thrombokinetic studies clearly distinguished the two diseases. Platelet-survival studies after labeling with $^{51}$Cr demonstrate shortened life-spans of the patients' platelets, both in themselves and in normal volunteers. Platelets from healthy volunteers, however, survived normally in these patients, indicating that the accelerated destruction resulted from an intrinsic platelet defect and not one extrinsic to the cell. Splenectomy in two patients was followed by improvement in the thrombocytopenia, but the postoperative platelet survival remained short. Normal numbers of morphologically normal megakarocytes were observed in smears of marrow of the propositus (a 5-year-old boy). Patients with hereditary thrombocytopenia have rarely responded to corticosteroid therapy and only in specific circumstances to splenectomy. The bleeding tendency is mild and resembles the clinical picture of idiopathic thrombocytopenic purpura.

Sheth and Prankerd[304] reported a family with congenital thrombocytopenia through four generations where the mode of inheritance appeared to be an autosomal dominant. Spontaneous bruising of varying severity, menorrhagia, and profuse bleeding at operation necessitating transfusion were predominant in the history. Platelet function tests were performed on the various patients. Platelet aggregation by adenosine diphosphate (ADP) was found to be defective. Investigations of platelet function in affected members of the family showed no deficiency in their thromboplastin generating activity but an abnormality of their adhesive qualities—thus fitting into the category of thrombasthenia. Platelet survival was not studied. A deficiency of megakaryocytes indicates that the lack of platelets was probably due to a failure in production rather than to increased destruction.

Gutenberger and colleagues[149] examined forty-five members of a kindred in which thrombocytopenia, an elevated level of serum immunoglobulin A (IgA), and hematuria were frequent. Thrombocytopenia was present in twelve members, of whom ten were male. It appeared that the thrombocytopenia was inherited as an X-linked trait. An abnormal rate of production rather than an increased destruction accounted for the thrombocytopenia. Eight of the thrombocytopenic members of the kindred had elevated serum IgA levels, whereas only one nonthrombocytopenic member had a significantly increased serum IgA level. None had decreased resistance to infection. Renal biopsies in three thrombocytopenic brothers with hematuria showed varying degrees of glomerulonephritis. This disorder differs from the Wiskott-Aldrich syndrome, which is also an X-linked condition associated with thrombocytopenia and elevated serum IgA levels but which is characterized by eczema, an increased susceptibility to infections, and early death. Renal manifestations have been reported from kindreds of familial thrombocytopenia. The hematuria in these have not been explained.

These syndromes should be differentiated from thrombocytopathic thrombocytopenic purpura in which there is a decreased platelet factor 3 activity and abnormal platelet morphology. The Wiskott-Aldrich syndrome is transmitted as a classic sex-linked recessive trait in which both normal and short platelet life-spans have been reported. In this disorder, all platelet functions requiring energy are defective—aggregation, phagocytosis, and survival.[195]

*Congenital thrombocytopenic purpura*

Congenital thrombocytopenic purpura occurs infrequently, but the literature contains many case reports and studies bearing on its pathogenesis.* It appears in infants born of mothers with idiopathic thrombocytopenic purpura who either have had a splenectomy or are symptomless and unaware of a lowered content of platelets, of normal mothers, or of mothers with drug-induced thrombocytopenic purpura such as follows the ingestion of quinine.

*Etiology.* Current concepts implicate an immunoallergic mechanism in the causation of the disease in the infant.[181] According to Harrington,[154] one-third of the patients do not have any demonstrable autoantibodies for platelets and are assumed to have a defect of platelet formation from megakaryocytes as the sole factor causing thrombocytopenia. Mothers of this type of idiopathic thrombocytopenia give birth to normal infants. On the other hand, patients with autoimmune idiopathic thrombocytopenic purpura possess a circulating antibody which damages both

---

*See references 180, 220, 234, 276, and 291.

platelets and megakaryocytes. Mothers with this variety of thrombocytopenia give birth to infants with purpura. The antibodies which cross the placenta into the fetal circulation consist of autoagglutinins as well as isoagglutinins for the platelets of the mother and infant.

In the case of normal mothers it has been postulated that the mother develops isoagglutinins for the baby's platelets, presumably on the basis of platelet incompatibility between mother and infant in a manner analogous to Rh sensitization in infants with erythroblastosis. She may also have been sensitized to platelet antigen in a previous transfusion or to fetal platelets of a different antigenic composition during pregnancy. The precise nature of the immune substance is not always obvious.

Fetal-maternal platelet incompatibility has been serologically proved as a cause of neonatal purpura in otherwise normal infants by the production in the mother of isoantibodies to fetal platelet antigen. Three infants, born to normal mothers who gave no history or laboratory evidence of purpura, developed purpura and thrombocytopenia within the first few hour after birth.[295] They also showed marked diminution of megakaryocytes. Platelets in normal numbers returned in 2 weeks. Studies in the third pregnancy revealed antibodies in the postpartum plasma which agglutinated the platelets of the husband, infant, and a group of normal controls.

In nine infants, Pearson and co-workers[253] also affirmed the pathogenesis of the isoimmune disease which involved fetal-maternal incompatibility of platelet antigen and the destruction of fetal platelets by a transplacental transfer of maternal antibody. Three different platelet antigens were implicated, none corresponding to known erythrocyte antigens, but two of the antigens were shared by granulocytes and lymphocytes. Platelet counts were less than 30,000 per cubic millimeter in all nine infants but returned to normal (with treatment) in 3 weeks. The disease occurred in otherwise normal children of mothers who were hematologically normal. Intracranial hemorrhage was documented in two cases. Petechiae were common, melena and hematuria uncommon. In their cases megakaryocytes were normal, increased, or absent.

Other causes of thrombocytopenic purpura may be those due to infection—i.e., septicemia, syphilis, cytomegalic inclusion disease, toxoplasmosis, and maternal rubella acquired in the first trimester of pregnancy. Congenital leukemia, osteopetrosis, and congenital absence of megakaryocytes may also produce a depletion of platelets and purpura. Hemolytic disease due to Rh sensitization is a common cause of thrombocytopenia in the newborn infant. Congenital purpura may result from mechanical causes during birth and is often nonthrombocytopenic. Petechiae at birth, due to thrombocytopenia, must be differentiated from benign petechiae that appear in the first day or two of life and are aggravated by cyanosis in the newborn infant.[19,264] In a series of 250 newborn infants 44% were found to have petechiae of a localized nature, due to local or regional increase in venous pressure resulting from temporary compression of superficial veins.

Quinine-induced thrombocytopenic purpura in a mother and her newborn infant has been observed[219] with in vitro evidence of quinine-platelet "antibodies" in the plasma of the mother and of the infant just after delivery. The administration of quinine before delivery resulted in thrombocytopenia and purpura due to the presence of preformed antibody from maternal sensitization to the drug originally given in childhood.

Thrombocytopenia caused by decreased megakaryocyte production has been reported in newborn infants whose mothers received one of the thiazides during the antepartum period.[277] One of the thiazides had been given for variable periods up to the day of delivery. Neither drug antibody nor isoantibody was found in any of the cases. One neonatal death occurred. The remaining patients recovered completely. Pancytopenia was also present in one case and leukopenia in another. The inconsistency of this association is the report of a small series[227] in which the therapeutic administration of thiazides to the pregnant women had no predictable or common effect on the platelets of their infants.

In a report of two other cases, the administration of maternally ingested chlorothiazide resulted in Heinz body hemolysis in the newborn infant. In one infant an exchange transfusion was done for hyperbilirubinemia; in the other a purpuric rash was also present. It is noteworthy that erythrocytic glucose-6-phosphate dehydrogenase deficiency was found in neither infant.[152]

The syndrome of thrombocytopenia and intestinal bleeding observed in a nursery in Baltimore affected more than 10% of the infant population.[182] Thrombocytopenia did not invariably accompany the bleeding. Bone marrow aspirates revealed megakaryocytes of normal morphology and number. The affected infants were not otherwise ill and complete recovery was the rule. The etiologic agent is obscure.

*Prognosis.* In our experience the prognosis in the infant is usually good, with the restoration of a normal number of platelets within the first 2 or 3 weeks of life and usually not beyond 3 months. Frequently, the baby appears normal at birth but develops purpura several hours after delivery. The course may not be benign, especially when the pregnancy is associated with overt purpura. In one report consecutive infants born of a mother who had been splenectomized for idiopathic thrombocytopenic purpura succumbed on the first day of life.[367] Megakaryocytes are increased in patients with primary thrombocytopenic purpura and, when markedly decreased or absent, signify the presence of an underlying condition. In patients with congenital thrombocytopenic purpura, however, megakaryocytes may be normal in number or frequently depressed. The persistence of an amegakaryocytic condition beyond the first months of life carries a poor prognosis.

The variability of prognosis given in different series must be based on factors still unknown, and, therefore, requires judicious scrutiny of the individual case as to the advisability of treatment. Anthony and Krivit[19] cite fourteen newborn infants in seven families who recovered without sequelae, in contrast to mortality ranging from 25 to 30% in various reviews and death in 12% of untreated cases given by Pearson and associates.[253]

*Treatment.* In families in which a severe case of thrombocytopenia has occurred, subsequent siblings should be carefully followed and, when platelets are reduced, therapy immediately instituted. Treatment consists of corticosteroids or fresh blood or platelet transfusions. In the seriously ill infant hydrocortisone is administered intravenously during the first 2 to 5 days in a dosage of 10 to 15 mg. per kg. per day in four divided doses. Prednisone may be substituted in a dosage of 2 to 3 mg. per kg. per day. The dosage is reduced to half that amount in the second week and tapered gradually during the third week. The maintenance of steroid therapy beyond these periods depends upon the severity of the disease. Milder cases may be treated with prednisone in a dosage of 1 to 2 mg. per kg. of body weight. As in patients with idiopathic thrombocytopenic purpura, individual adjustment of dosage is necessary.[61] Exchange transfusion has been advocated in severely affected infants to remove circulating antibody.[253] Antepartum steroids to the mother has also been suggested in cases in which neonatal purpura is anticipated on the basis of previous purpuric infants and/or measurement of antibody in maternal serum.[253] With severe bleeding or purpura transfusion of fresh blood for its content of viable platelets or platelet transfusions are indicated. The use of exchange transfusion followed by compatible washed maternal platelet concentrates has been effective in controlling severe hemorrhage.[8]

It is difficult to evaluate critically the effectiveness of therapy in neonatal thrombocytopenia because of the variations in clinical severity which are probably conditioned by a multiplicity of antigen-antibody systems. In one series the mean duration of thrombocytopenia was 20.8 days in thirty-four patients not treated or given only simple transfusions, compared with 10.2 days in twelve infants given ACTH or corticosteroids.[253]

### Thrombocytopenia in fetal rubella

Neonatal thrombocytopenia has been reported with increasing frequency in the offspring of mothers who have acquired rubella during the first trimester of pregnancy. In the majority of cases it is associated with malformations such as cataracts (rarely glaucoma), hazy corneas, congenital heart lesions, skeletal defects, deafness, encephalitis, renal anomalies, full fontanels, and intrauterine growth retardation.[41,167,212] Many of the newborn infants are premature. Transient hepatosplenomegaly may be noted. Megakaryocytes are scanty, rarely normal in number, and also immature.[76,269,270] The purpura seems to be an integral part of the embryopathy. In the rubella syndrome neonatal purpura often appears as widespread infiltrative skin lesions. Intravascular obstruction in the liver, brain, spleen, and other organs has been found.[36] Persistent, prolonged fetal-neonatal infection, associated with thrombosis, may explain the varied lesions in congenital rubella. Thrombocytopenia may persist from 1 to 8 weeks, and recovery usually takes place without treatment. In a series of twenty-five infants with clinical manifestations of the rubella syndrome, thrombocytopenia was present in eighteen infants during the first week of life.[284] Platelet counts ranged from 6,000 to 130,000 per cubic millimeter, with a mean of 47,000 per cubic millimeter. In this series roentgenograms of the long bones revealed irregularity of the trabecular pattern, consisting of small longitudinal areas of radiolucency in the metaphysis of the long bones in more than one-half of the patients studied. Platelet transfusions and, possibly, adrenocorticosteroids[167] may be given for excessive bleeding. Rubella has been isolated from a mother in the first month of pregnancy and from viable fetal tissue delivered by uterine curettage 57 days after onset of the maternal exanthem.[158]

Alford and co-workers[11] recovered the virus from placental and fetal tissues and from amniotic fluid after a prolonged period, following subsidence of infection in the mother. Furthermore, virus was also isolated from three infants with the congenital rubella syndrome for periods up to 4½ months after birth. In another series[259] virological studies were carried out on 600 specimens, collected from 85 infants born during an epidemic of congenital rubella syndrome. Thirty-six of these infants (42%) yielded rubella virus from at least one specimen. In the first month of life, virus could be recovered readily from the throat and cerebrospinal fluid and in decreasing order of frequency from the urine, peripheral blood, and bone marrow.

It is possible that cases of congenital thrombocytopenic purpura in the past may have resulted from unrecognized rubella in the mother in the first trimester of pregnancy. The need for quarantine is evident from the number of cases contracted by exposure to fetal rubella.

In twenty-one cases of fetal rubella Zinkham and associates[379] noted the frequent occurrence of anemia, leukopenia, and thrombocytopenia. The anemic babies exhibited persistent reticulocytosis, intermittent normoblastemia, and abnormal red cell morphology. Bone marrow aspirates during the first 4 weeks of life showed reduction in the number of megakaryocytes in the thrombopenic infants. In five babies reticulum cells in the bone marrow had ingested a variety of blood cells, notably polynuclear neutrophils and red blood cells. Cultures for rubella virus in the bone marrow were positive in nine infants and correlated with the severity of the infection (Fig. 103).

Thrombocytopenia, as seen in association with congenital rubella, cytomegalic inclusion disease, and toxoplasmosis should be verified with a bone marrow examination and followed closely. Steroid therapy is probably contraindicated in fetal rubella. Platelet and fresh whole blood transfusions should be used to control bleeding. The thrombocytopenia is usually self-limited, recovery taking place within 2 to 3 weeks.

*Thrombocytopenia in miscellaneous infections*

Thrombocytopenia may accompany hemorrhagic phenomena in a number of infections. In the newborn period it is particularly common in sepsis, cytomegalic inclusion disease, disseminated herpes simplex infection, and congenital syphilis.[124] At any age in children it may occur in measles,[165] varicella, mumps, whooping cough, tuberculosis (especially miliary), typhoid fever, scarlet fever, vaccinia, cat-scratch disease,[39] infectious mononucleosis (see Chapter 21), and many viral diseases. In Rocky Mountain spotted fever[283] it is related to a vasculitis with proliferation of vascular endothelium, and platelet clumping with intravascular thrombosis. In many of these cases the mechanism by which infection with any of these agents produces thrombocytopenia is obscure. Where reported, megakaryocytic abnormalities are infrequent.

*Thrombocytopenia with renal vein thrombosis*

Thrombocytopenia in association with renal vein thrombosis was reported in two newborn infants of diabetic mothers.[29,179] It was suggested that the thrombocytopenia might be due to deposition of platelets in the thrombin or in the hemorrhagic kidney. In the infant described by Jones and Reed,[179] maternal thiazide may have been a factor in producing the thrombocytopenia. Following nephrectomy the platelet count rose from 33,000/cu. mm. preoperatively to 422,000/cu. mm. on the fourth postoperative day. At 6 months of age the infant appeared healthy and vigorous.

*Thrombocytopenia induced by drugs*

Thrombocytopenia induced by drugs may be either amegakaryocytic or megakaryocytic.[326] In the former group are the myelosuppressive chemical and physical agents such as x-ray radiation that involves the other bone marrow elements as well as the platelets to produce hypoplastic and aplastic anemia. A variety of drugs have been incriminated as

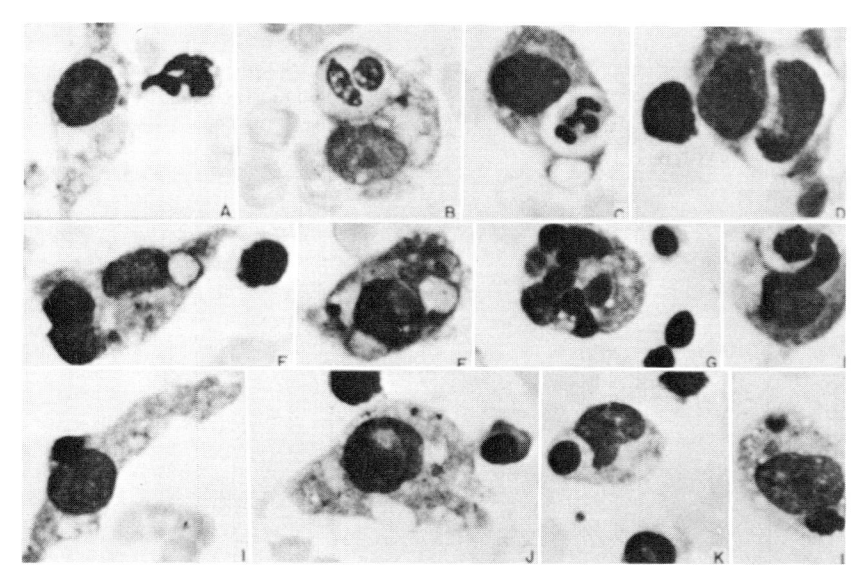

Fig. 103. Phagocytic reticulum cells in the bone marrow (A to K) and peripheral blood (L) of infants with congenital rubella. A, A reticulum cell beginning to ingest a polymorphonuclear neutrophil. B, A recently ingested polymorphonuclear neutrophil. C, An ingested polymorphonuclear neutrophil which is being digested. D, A reticulum cell that has ingested another reticulum cell. E, F, and G, Reticulum cells that have phagocytized red cells, red cell precursors, and lymphocytes. H, A phagocytic complex (reticulum cell plus ingested material) that has been phagocytized by a reticulum cell. I, J, and K, Reticulum cells ingesting red cells and nuclear material. L, A reticulum cell from the peripheral blood that has ingested cellular material. (Original magnification ×1750.) (From Zinkham, W. H., and others: Blood and bone marrow findings in congenital rubella, J. Pediat. 71:512-524, 1967.)

being among those producing thrombocytopenia. These include, among others, Mesantoin, thyroid-depressing drugs, sulfonamides, benzol, arsenic, and chloramphenicol. Here, the effect on the bone marrow is due either to individual idiosyncrasy or to overdosage and emphasizes the need for routine blood studies as a check on toxicity. Drugs used currently in the treatment of patients with leukemia, Hodgkin's disease, and other disorders of the lymphoma group are capable of producing thrombocytopenia by megakaryocytic aplasia.

Megakaryocytic thrombocytopenia may result from sensitization produced in the patient by previous administration of the drug as in the case of Sedormid, quinine, and quinidine. It has been shown that the addition of Sedormid to platelets suspended in the serum of a sensitized patient causes the agglutination without complement and lysis with it.[6] Patients who have recovered from purpura caused by Sedormid possess an antiplatelet antibody in the circulating blood which is capable of destroying platelets. The fact that normal serum had no such effect indicates that the abnormality in the blood of such a person lies in the serum and not in the platelets.

In patients with thrombocytopenic purpura due to Sedormid and probably other drugs, the antibody acts on megakaryocytes, platelets, and capillary endothelium. In those with nonthrombocytopenic purpura the platelets, for some unknown reason, escape injury. The drug presumably combines with vascular endothelium rendered antigenic and therefore is capable of uniting with the antibody. Thrombocytopenia due to quinine presents a similar mechanism—i.e., an antibody combined with antigen consisting of the drug and platelets.[334]

The diagnosis of drug purpura producing thrombocytopenia has been subjected to a variety of techniques.[164] Antibody activity is demonstrated by in vitro mixtures of platelets, immune serum, drug, and complement. Tests based on platelet damage include clot retraction inhibition (one of the oldest and best tests for drug hypersensitivity), platelet factor 3 release, alpha amino-nitrogen generation from platelets, and inhibition of serotonin uptake. Drugs may lead to purpura with and without thrombocytopenia. The mechanism of the latter is unknown but is presumed to result from an antiendothelial cell effect of the drug and immune serum.[164]

## Aplastic anemia with onset as congenital thrombocytopenic purpura

A newborn infant was observed who had what appeared to be congenital thrombocytopenic purpura. After the first weeks of life, however, anemia and subsequently granulocytopenia became associated with the depletion of platelets. Although a normal bone marrow was present at the end of the first month, by the seventh month the blood, bone marrow, and clinical findings were consistent with aplastic anemia. Although this sequence so early in life is exceptional, it is significant, nevertheless, that congenital thrombocytopenia, usually benign, may represent the initial stage of aplastic anemia.

## Chronic hypoplastic thrombocytopenia with depression of megakaryocytes

Chronic hypoplastic thrombocytopenia with depression of megakaryocytes is occasionally observed in pediatric practice in patients without congenital anomalies and consists of persistent thrombocytopenia with a depletion of megakaryocytes and periodic attacks of epistaxis, purpura, or both. There is no involvement of red or white cell elements nor any coagulation defect. These patients must be observed for the possible ultimate development of the total picture of aplastic anemia or for evidence of secondary thrombocytopenia due to causes such as infection, drugs, and leukemia or other infiltrative disorders.

For treatment of this condition successive monthly courses of prednisone or substitutes are administered, especially if bleeding or purpura is excessive. If there is difficulty in maintaining platelet levels to prevent bleeding, maintenance therapy may be attempted on a dosage of 2.5 to 15 mg. daily. Continuous therapy, even with minimal dosage, necessitates alertness for the development of hyperadrenocorticism. When the administration of steroids has proved ineffective in patients with severe and recurrent nosebleeds, large doses of ascorbic acid (1,000 mg. daily) have occasionally resulted in improvement. The value of removing the spleen is debatable, especially since this organ is not enlarged.

## Thrombocytopenia with absent radius (congenital hypoplastic thrombocytopenia, primary amegakaryocytic thrombocytopenia, phocomelia and congenital hypoplastic thrombocytopenia, myeloid leukemoid reaction, TAR)

This syndrome of unknown etiology consists of a congenital absence or a marked reduction in the number of megakaryocytes without a reduction in the other elements of the bone marrow coexisting with multiple somatic deformities.[198,243] Among the first cases to be described was that reported by Greenwald and Sherman,[143] in which defective formation of megakaryocytes was associated with anomalies of the heart and thymus gland.

The association with skeletal abnormalities was recorded in another patient first observed at 3 months of age, in whom thrombocytopenic purpura was present with congenital dislocation of the hip and bilateral absence of the radii.[326] After mild improvement with ACTH and cortisone therapy, splenectomy was performed at 10 months of age. Bleeding stopped, the number of platelets increased, and 1 year later the platelets numbered 350,000 per cu. mm. Other reports also emphasized the coexistence of congenital skeletal anomalies with bleeding manifestation from birth, an amegakaryocytic bone marrow, and a leukemoid reaction.[40,112,303]

Hall and her associates[150] described a group of cases under the title of "thrombocytopenia with absent radius (TAR)," which in many respects resembles the condition previously described as "congenital hypoplastic thrombocytopenia"[315] and also corresponds to the cases reported by Dignan and his associates as "phocomelia with thrombocytopenia and myeloid leukemia."[99] The cases included in Hall's series were nine affected individuals in three families, four unrelated affected individuals, and twenty-seven previously reported cases. Skeletal deformities of the arms often involved bones other than the radius. The ulnae were absent in eleven of the forty cases; in their cases the limbs were more severely affected than the trunks, the arms more than the legs. Five fingers were present on both hands in all cases collected. Cardiac anomalies were present in one-third of the cases such as tetralogy of Fallot, atrial septal defects, patent foramen ovale, and dextrocardia. The onset of hematologic complication usually occurred at birth or during early infancy. Thrombocytopenia might be episodic and sometimes was accompanied by leukemoid reaction and eosinophilia. More than half the cases had leukemoid reactions with a shift to the left and leukocytosis greater than 35,000 WBC/cu. mm. These leukemoid reactions were usually confined to the first 6 months of life, rarely occurred later. Bone marrow examinations revealed decreased and/or abnormal megakaryocytes with normal myeloid and erythroid precursors. Splenic enlargement often coexisted in those with leukemoid reactions. Thrombocytopenia was always present during the leukemoid reaction, constituting a critical period for those patients since it was during such episodes that the disease was fatal.

Anemia was present in most cases at some time during their course, possibly secondary to blood loss. Polychromatophilia and moderate anisocytosis and poikilocytosis were occasionally present. In some of these cases red cell survival was shortened and persisted in the older patient. The absence of anemia and a reticulocytosis reflect a compensating bone marrow. Erythrocyte osmotic fragility was occasionally abnormal.

Therapy includes blood and/or platelet transfusions, steroids, and splenectomy. In one case[40] of primary aplasia of megakaryocytes and absence of both radii, splenectomy resulted in a transitory increase in the number of platelets. Improvement was not maintained and the infant died with cerebral hemorrhage. Many patients succumb in the first weeks and months of life, despite transfusions and splenectomy.[191] With adequate treatment, however, patients survive but the results of therapy are difficult to evaluate because of the variable course and the occurrence of spontaneous improvement.

Orthopedic treatment is well tolerated, but preoperative platelet transfusions may be necessary.

In general, the prognosis is good if the patient survives to 1 year of age. The exception is a small group of patients who progress to aplastic anemia. Large follow-up studies have not, however, become available.

From a broad point of view these cases of thrombocytopenia and absent radii might be classified as the neonatal equivalent of the Fanconi syndrome. The latter, however, is associated with pancytopenia and death occurs within 2 to 3 years of the onset. In the syndrome under discussion apparent survival with intermittent thrombocytopenia and fairly good health are common after episodes of severe thrombocytopenia in the first year of life. In thalidomide embryopathy similar effects were encountered but no hematologic abnormalities were present.

Dignan and his associates[99] reported five patients with phocomelia of the upper extremities and associated blood cell abnormalities. The skeletal anomalies consisted of absent radii and ulnae and hypoplastic humeri. In a typical patient, five-fingered hands arose directly from the shoulder and the shoulder girdle was poorly formed. Petechiae were seen at birth or within the first few days in three patients and at age 5 and 6 weeks in the others. Episodes of anemia, thrombocytopenia, leukocytosis, and splenomegaly lasted for a week or longer. Marrow study in three patients showed no megakaryocytes in an otherwise hyperplastic sample at the time of crises. Most platelet counts were in the abnormally low ranges. The thrombocytopenia was most profound in the early months of life and tended to improve with age. In each patient there was a persistent hypoplastic thrombocytopenia. Each patient also had episodes of leukemoid reaction.

O'Gorman-Hughes classifies amegakaryocytic thrombocytopenia as types with and without congenital abnormalities.[247] He also described a group in which amegakaryocytic thrombocytopenia preceded aplastic anemia. Anomalies were rare in this group and often an interval of several years elapsed between the recognition of thrombocytopenia and the development of overt pancytopenia. Eisenstein[109] described twenty-two cases and found that a leukemoid reaction predominated in children with absent radii.

### Thrombotic (thrombohemolytic) thrombocytopenic purpura

Thrombotic thrombocytopenic purpura, originally described by Moschcowitz,[237] is an acute febrile disease characterized by thrombocytopenic purpura, severe hemolytic anemia, and transitory focal neurologic signs and symptoms. The varied clinical features are due to widespread intracapillary and intra-arteriolar thrombi affecting most frequently the brain, kidneys, heart, and spleen. Diffuse involvement of the gray matter is shown by aphasia, cortical blindness, seizures, restlessness, delirium, stupor, or coma. Hemiparesis is occasionally seen.[244] The possibility of thrombotic thrombocytopenic purpura should be considered whenever an unusually severe or fulminating purpura associated with thrombopenia is encountered.[369]

*Pathogenesis.* It had originally been postulated that thrombotic thrombocytopenic purpura represents an immunohematologic disorder in which the autoimmune process is set in motion against the red cell, platelets, megakaryocyte, and vessel wall.[7] The association with marked eosinophilia in the occasional patient[121] tends further to support this concept. The hypersensitive basis of the histologic picture is analogous to other collagen diseases, particularly periarteritis nodosa and lupus erythematosus, and to the necrotizing vascular lesion produced in experimental animals[272] by a variety of agents such as foreign proteins, sulfonamides, and iodine.

It has recently been demonstrated, however, that the occlusions in this disease are not due to agglutinated platelets as was first thought, but instead to hyaline thrombi which appear to be wholly or largely composed of fibrinogen or fibrin and devoid of platelets.[79] In a 14-year-old boy with this disease the fibrinogen level was reduced,[64] suggesting the possibility of widespread intravascular coagulation. These and other data[173] led to the concept that thrombohemolytic thrombocytopenic purpura possesses many aspects that can be explained on the basis of intravascular coagulation.[341] The presence of precipitated fibrin in blood vessels has been regarded as an indication that intravascular coagulation has occurred comparable to the generalized Shwartzman reaction in experimental animals in which the consumption of clotting factors also occurs.[139] Hemolysis and the peculiar red cell alterations (fragmented and triangular cells) have been ascribed to the impact of the red cells upon the altered caliber of the vessel and texture of the endothelial surface, due to fibrin deposits.[58] Thrombocytopenia, another component of the syndrome, has also been related to the presence of intravascular thrombi which are released during the coagulation process. Since the injured platelets have not been observed in histologic lesions, they are probably rapidly removed by the spleen. Thrombotic thrombocytopenic purpura also has many features resembling those of the hemolytic uremic syndrome.[215]

The generalized Shwartzman phenomenon was originally produced in rabbits by the intravenous administration of two properly spaced doses of bacterial endotoxin. The phenomenon is associated with severe intravascular clotting and widespread fibrin deposition resulting in bilateral cortical necrosis in the rabbit.[78] This reaction is frequently applied to explain the pathogenesis of the hemolytic-uremic syndrome and thrombotic thrombocytopenic purpura and purpura fulminans.

Intravascular coagulation with fibrin deposition characterizes both the hemolytic-uremic syndrome and thrombotic thrombocytopenic purpuras. Red cell fragmentation results from this "microangiopathic hemolytic anemia" and is produced by the interaction of rapidly moving red cells with fibrin strands. Brain and Hourihane[59] regard the clinical and hematologic findings in thrombotic thrombocytopenic purpura as secondary consequences of the fibrinoid necrosis and hyaline occlusion of arterioles and capillaries. Experimental support of this hypothesis was observed and provided further evidence that changes in small blood vessels may lead to hemolytic anemia.

In the differential diagnosis, Amorosi and Ultmann[16] enumerate a number of disorders for consideration. They include idiopathic thrombocytopenic purpura, Evan's syndrome (coexistence of autoimmune hemolytic anemia and thrombocytopenia), systemic lupus erythematosus, periarteritis nodosa, eclampsia, drug reaction, toxin exposure, sepsis, aplastic anemia, paroxysmal nocturnal hemoglobinuria, and leukemia. The marked neurologic abnormalities, hemolysis with a negative Coombs test, and the evidence of renal disease set thrombotic thrombocytopenic purpura apart from other diseases.

*Clinical course and laboratory findings.* The course is usually rapidly progressive, terminating fatally within a few days to several weeks from the onset. In a few patients the illness is more prolonged and of a relapsing nature. Petechiae and ecchymoses are few or numerous; enlargement of the spleen and liver occurs in many of the patients. The blood shows the evidence of a hemolytic anemia with jaundice in one-half of the patients. In the peripheral blood the smear shows fragmented, triangular, and helmet shaped or "burred" erythrocytes. Anemia, reticulocytosis, microspherocytosis, leukocytosis, thrombocytopenia, and erythroid hyperplasia of the bone marrow are present. The Coombs test is ordinarily negative, occasionally positive.[355] In a case that followed four months after measles, $^{51}$Cr studies revealed a marked extracorpuscular and a moderate intracorpuscular hemolytic effect.[339]

A case has been reported in a 9-month-old infant in whom the diagnosis of hemolytic-uremic syndrome was considered unlikely because of a normal level of blood urea.[230] In an extensive review of thrombotic thrombocytopenic purpura, clinical evidence of kidney involvement was present in the majority (88%) but not all cases.[16] In this series also while the majority of cases ranged from 10 to 39 years of age, the peak age incidence was in the third decade. It is obvious that borderline cases in the pediatric age group may be difficult to differentiate from the hemolytic-uremic syndrome.

*Treatment.* Large doses of adrenocortical steroids have been proposed alone or in combination with splenectomy. Instances of either complete or incomplete recovery are described, however, following treatment with massive doses of ACTH (up to 1,000 units) and prednisone (up to 1,000 mg.), followed quickly by splenectomy.[341] Blood and platelet transfusions are supportive only. Other forms of therapy include exchange transfusion on the basis of a possible relationship to an autoimmune disorder. The use of heparin is still under investigation with a view that this agent may prevent progression of intravascular thrombosis. Anticoagulants such as heparin had been previously regarded without effect since the occlusions were thought to be caused by a primary pathologic reaction of the vascular wall to a damaging agent in the absence of fibrin in the thrombi.[313] While the nature of the occluding material is still in doubt, there is some evidence that the material is either fibrin or both platelet and fibrin material.

Cahalane and Horn[68] reported an adult with a course of at least 3 years' duration. They found in the literature that eight of eighteen patients with thrombotic thrombocytopenic purpura subjected to splenectomy had a protracted course. Two were living in complete remission 32 months following surgery. They pointed out that endocardial vegetations and occlusion of large blood vessels occur in cases of prolonged disease and that platelet-derived fibrinogen may form the occlusive material in the arterioles and capillaries.

In the large series reported by Amorosi and Ultmann,[16] thirteen reported cases of the classic disease were still alive. Therapy in these cases varied and included blood transfusion, heparin, corticosteroids, testosterone and adrenal steroids, exchange transfusion, and, in six cases, adrenal steroids and splenectomy. In another report a patient who did not respond to large doses of steroids and massive blood transfusions had a dramatic remission following splenectomy.[231] The patient remains well 3 years after the operation. Similar experiences are apparently not uncommon.[101]

### Wiskott-Aldrich syndrome

The triad of thrombocytopenic purpura, eczema, and recurrent infections has been the subject of many reports.* Bloody diarrhea, anemia, epistaxis, recurrent otitis media, marked susceptibility to infection, and a fatal outcome are additional features. Most children die in the early years of life. More recently longer survivals in the sex-linked variety of the disease have been reported, and in one instance a 24-year-old adult with the clinical and laboratory findings compatible with the Wiskott-Aldrich syndrome is still alive.[226]

Hepatosplenomegaly is occasionally present. Subperiosteal hemorrhage,[274] bronchopneumonia, and pansinusitis[30] have been reported. Infections may be mild or severe ranging from recurrent skin sepsis and otitis media to septicemia and meningitis often caused by the pneumococcus. Fulminating septicemia and bilateral adrenal hemorrhage are frequently terminal events.

Persistent thrombocytopenia is present despite the usual findings of normal numbers and morphology of megakaryocytes.[194] Others have described bizarre nuclear abnormalities of megakaryocytes[254] and platelets of reduced size and shape.[147,148] Both normal[254] and shortened life-span of platelets have been reported.[147,148] Plasma cells are normal. Lymphocytes are usually low and decline progressively. The pattern is that of a sex-linked recessive disease with transmission by unaffected fe-

---

*See references 10, 77, 141, 168, 187, 274, 279, 285, 374, 376, and 377.

males to male members. There is a frequent development of lymphoreticular malignancy. A characteristic feature is the low titer of anti-A and anti-B (blood group) antibodies.

Malignancy of the reticuloendothelial system developed in two of four brothers with the Wiskott-Aldrich syndrome.[342] Both died with multiple metastatic tumors of the brain. Five other instances of development of malignancy in this syndrome were included in this report. The diagnosis of the various tumors included reticulum cell sarcoma and malignant lymphoma. The occurrence of neoplasia was explained as influenced by the chronic stimulatory effect of infections on the reticuloendothelial system or perhaps directly from the immunological deficiencies present.

The etiology of this disease is unknown, but it has been attributed to a disease of hypersensitivity, a reticuloendotheliosis, and a chronic infectious disease.[279] Milk allergy was strongly suspected as a major factor in producing the eczema in one series.[168] The presence of circulating antibodies to cow's milk[159,279] and the clinical observation that patients have been sensitive to milk, eggs, and other foods have aroused suspicion of an allergic etiology. Many patients show a lack of natural blood group isoagglutinins. Primary herpetic gingivostomatitis in three children with this syndrome was attributed to a defect in cellular resistance. It was postulated that this defect allowed the virus to persist in the tissues with the induction of partial to complete immunologic tolerance.[285] An impressive feature common to the children in the latter group was the rapidity with which they developed fulminating infections after splenectomy.[168] The outcome is fatal despite ACTH and steroid therapy. Although there is a clinical resemblance to Letterer-Siwe disease, the genetic pattern and combination of symptoms differentiate this condition from reticuloendotheliosis and other conditions in which either eczema or purpura is present. Viruses, bacteria both of high and low grade virulence, fungi, and *Pneumocystis carinii* all have represented life-threatening infections in these children.

Therapy in this disease is extremely limited. Severe bleeding episodes due to thrombocytopenia require platelet transfusions. A trial of topical steroids may be cautiously employed for the eczema. Stiehm and co-workers[335] obtained encouraging results in keeping two patients with this syndrome free from infection by administering plasma (10 ml./kg.) from hepatitis-free donors since these patients cannot form antibodies of the IgM class.

*Immunological consideration.* The total gamma globulin levels have been consistently normal mainly because the IgG has always been normal. A low IgM and an elevated IgA are frequent. The patient's ability to form antibodies to several polysaccharide antigens, including blood groups A and B, and Forssman antigens is deficient. The genetic fault in Wiskott-Aldrich syndrome results in a primary inability to process certain polysaccharide antigens as required for normal induction of the immune process.[49,77] Lymphopenia is a fairly consistent feature of this syndrome. Examination of lymph nodes reveals a depletion of lymphocytes in the thymus-dependent paracortical areas. The small lymphocyte deficiency is the major component of the circulating lymphopenia of the Wiskott-Aldrich syndrome.[77] This cell system may function early in the life of the patient with this syndrome. With time, there is a progressive depletion of thymus-dependent small lymphocytes concomitant with the development of a general decrease in cellular immunity.

There have been various views as to platelet survival. In one study[234] it was claimed that the characteristic thrombocytopenia in the Wiskott-Aldrich syndrome did not result from increased peripheral destruction of platelets but from decreased, defective production or faulty maturation related to megakaryocyte structural abnormalities. In another study[147,148] it was demonstrated that the platelets possessed abnormal morphology with reduced size and shape. Labeling autologous platelets showed a marked shortening of platelet survival. It was suggested that the platelets produced in the bone marrow are qualitatively deficient and therefore disappear from the circulation. Increased platelet destruction by phagocytosis of platelets takes place in the reticuloendothelial system. Platelet aggregation induced by collagen and ADP are deficient, and these pathological platelets are handled as foreign particles in the reticuloendothelial system.

Kuramoto and colleagues[195] have demonstrated various qualitative platelet defects in the Wiskott-Aldrich syndrome. Most striking was the lack of aggregation with ADP, collagen, and particularly, epinephrine. Platelets also showed a depression in citric acid cycle activity. The failure to release the citric acid cycle–stimulating factor was postulated as the primary defect in this syndrome. These defects may contribute to the thrombocytolysis noted in this disease.

## Thrombocytopenia following transfusions

A tendency to bleed based on platelet depletion has been described in patients receiving large amounts of compatible banked blood.[193] Several reasons have been cited for thrombocytopenia resulting from transfusions. When bleeding is excessive, the patient loses both platelets and substances required in the coagulation process. In blood collected by ordinary blood bank procedures, the agglutination and destruction of platelets are considerable so that the donor contributes inadequate amounts of viable platelets during transfusion. No significant thrombocytopenia results in patients receiving small amounts of blood over a period of days or weeks.

Another factor contributing to thrombocytopenia is the possible depressive effect of transfusions on platelet formation, as is known to occur with erythropoiesis. A factor which reduces platelets has also been described in normal plasma which, acting alone or with the recipient's diluted platelets, operates to produce thrombocytopenia.[325] A combination of these factors has been shown to reduce the number of platelets in infants with erythroblastosis receiving replacement transfusions, although overt bleeding is rare.[193]

Abnormal bleeding may complicate blood transfusion in other ways—from incompatible as well as large compatible transfusions.[171] The mechanism of the bleeding tendency following incompatible transfusions seems to be that of the defibrination syndrome due to intravascular clotting. Posttransfusion purpura may result from an isoantibody provoked by a mismatched platelet antigen which has the capacity to destroy platelets in sensitized individuals.[306] This concept stems from differences in types of antigens on platelets with the introduction by transfusion of a different type of platelet antigen than that of the recipient. The antibody is complexed with the foreign antigen (from platelets) and is absorbed by autologous platelets. The disease is self-limited.

Posttransfusion purpura has been reported as occurring in a middle-aged multiparous woman.[234] Severe purpura developed in a patient about 6 days after a blood transfusion. A potent platelet isoantibody appeared in her plasma which persisted for 6 weeks, the period of the thrombocytopenia. Morse[235] pointed out that the sudden onset of purpura approximately 7 days after transfusion was due to an antibody formed from a foreign platelet antigen. Remaining in the patient's circulation after transfusion it might be adsorbed to the patient's platelets nonspecifically and lead to the destruction of the antigen-negative platelets. The treatment suggested for this type of posttransfusion thrombocytopenic purpura is the use of corticosteroids or exchange transfusion.

## Hemolytic-uremic syndrome

This is an acute disease of infancy and childhood (most often 3 months to 3 years of age) characterized by signs and symptoms of acquired hemolytic anemia, thrombopenia, glomerulonephritis, and cerebral symptoms. Because of the presence of irregularly contracted, distorted, and fragmented red cells in the blood smear, it has also been termed the "red cell fragmentation syndrome." This syndrome constitutes one of the established conditions in which disseminated intravascular coagulation (DIC) occurs and is responsible for the progressive pathologic damages in this disease. A familial occurrence is rare but has been reported in sibs. In two such cases the onset was in the first 2 months of life.[20]

In 1955, Gasser and colleagues[127] described a syndrome which was termed the hemolyticuremic syndrome, consisting of hemolytic anemia, thrombocytopenia, and renal failure clinically resembling acute glomerulonephritis with hematuria and proteinuria (Figs. 104 and 105). The patients were children from 2 months to 7 years of age, and each patient at postmortem examination revealed bilateral renal cortical necrosis. In time it was noted that "irregularly contracted" red cells (burr, triangular, helmet red cells), previously described in the blood of patients suffering from uremia or carcinomatosis,[83,299] were an integral part of this syndrome.[14]

*Clinical features.* In the younger age group the initial manifestations are often those of an acute febrile illness with an insidious onset characterized by mild gastrointestinal symptoms (vomiting and diarrhea), followed in 2 to 5 days by hematuria, anemia, thrombocytopenia, acute renal failure, and often central nervous system abnormalities (irritability, drowsiness, restlessness, stupor, convulsions, coma). On admission, hypertension, gastro-

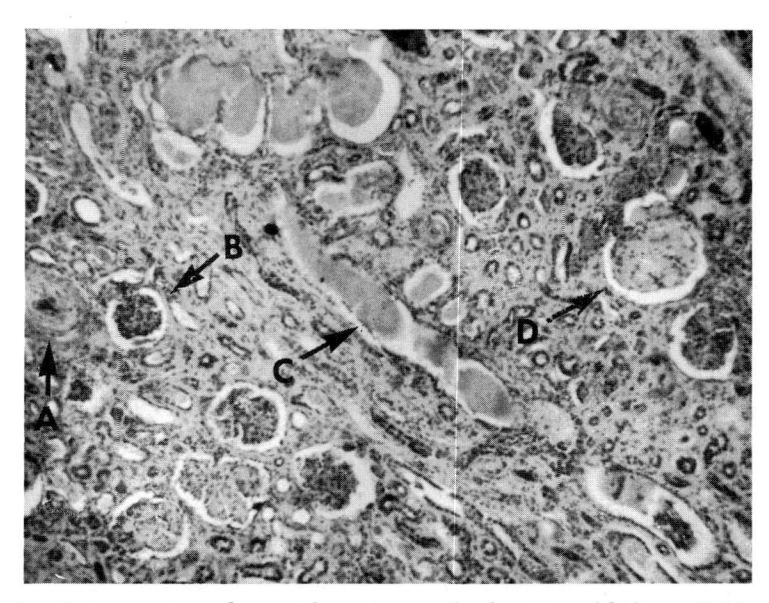

Fig. 104. Hemolytic-uremic syndrome. Photomicrograph of section of kidney. Child was almost 5 years of age at time of death. Illness lasted 3 months with periods of marked anuria and oliguria. **A,** Small artery with markedly thickened wall; **B,** shrunken hypercellular glomerulus with two similar glomeruli nearby; **C,** cast of proteinaceous precipitate in a dilated tubule; **D,** necrotic glomerulus with disappearance of all cellular elements. (×120.)

intestinal and cutaneous hemorrhages, and hyperkalemia are often present. The acute stage of the disease is characterized by profound anemia, repeated hemolytic crises, thrombocytopenia, azotemia, and prolonged renal failure. Oliguria is common and anemia may ensue. Moderate splenomegaly may be present. In addition to the anemia, leukocytosis, thrombocytopenia, and altered red cells (burr cells) are present. Bone marrow shows an increase in all erythrocyte precursors, megakaryocytes are present in normal or increased numbers, and platelet formation is active.[287,308,309] Characteristic microangiopathic lesions have been found in paraffin sections of aspirated marrow.[50] Fibrinogen, prothrombin, factor V and factor VIII, and platelets are usually decreased. These deficiencies characterize the syndrome of disseminated intravascular coagulation, a condition which is suspected when low levels of the coagulation factors, fibrin-split products, and thrombocytopenia are found. Red cell fragmentation, hemolysis, and hemoglobinemia result when a rapidly moving stream of blood interacts with fibrin attached to the endothelial surface of blood vessels during the process of disseminated intravascular coagulation.[31,59,65,282] Patients who do not have thrombocytopenia when initially examined may eventually show a decrease in platelet count as the disease progresses. There is evidence of rapid red cell destruction and regeneration so that reticulocytes are elevated. In addition to the anemia, leukocytosis and distorted triangular and irregularly contracted fragmented and crenated red cells are common. Spherocytes are noted in small numbers. These alterations in red cell structure reflect the presence of intravascular hemolysis. In the event of severe intravascular hemolysis, the concentration of hemoglobin in the plasma is elevated and, with this degree of destruction, hemoglobinuria and hematuria result. This syndrome is separated from autoimmune hemolytic disease by the negative Coombs test and the unusual red cell morphology. In many aspects it resembles a form of hypersensitivity and has been regarded as related to thrombotic thrombocytopenic purpura.

This illness may be rapidly fatal[127] or marked by recurrence,[307] or the patient may recover spontaneously after a single episode.[14] In the group of patients who recovered spontaneously renal damage did not persist. In-

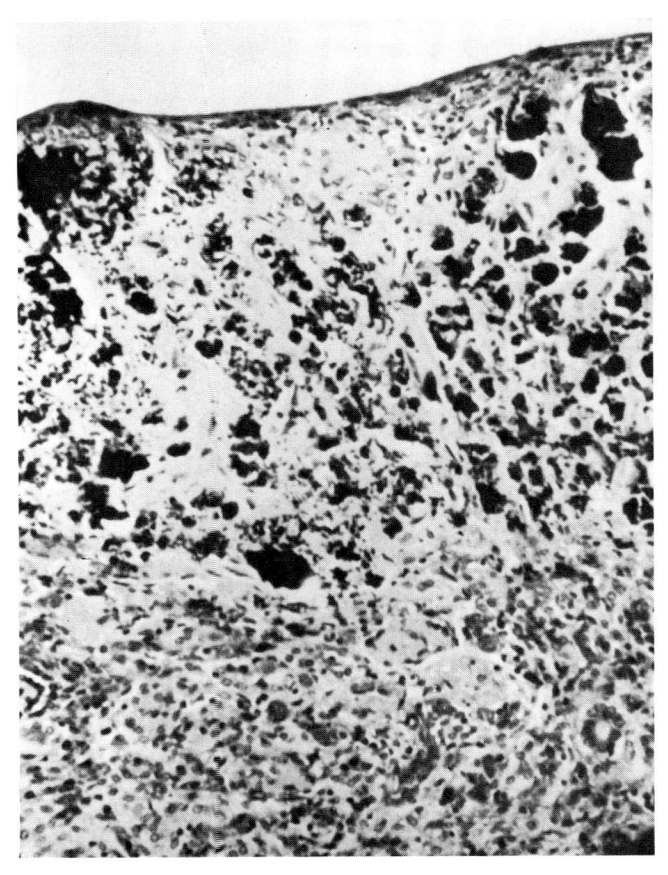

Fig. 105. Hemolytic-uremic syndrome. Photomicrograph of kidney of 20-month-old child with this syndrome. Note widespread necrosis of outer three-fourths of renal cortex with degenerative calcification. Heavily pigmented masses of finely granular basophilic material staining as calcium are scattered through the cortex. A zone of less severely affected cortex is observed in the lower portion of the section. Course of illness was progressive, lasting 3 months.

creasing numbers of reports of the occurrence of acute hemolytic anemia associated with renal failure, thrombocytopenia, and poikilocytosis continue to appear.* The disease can occur in epidemic form as in the series of fifty-eight cases from Buenos Aires in infants from 4.5 to 36 months of age (mean age of 12.6 months),[132] or in an outbreak of ten cases occurring within a short period in a small area in North Wales.[224]

*Pathogenesis.* A number of theories have been postulated to explain the pathogenesis of the hemolytic-uremic syndrome. Among those listed are the following:[108] that the pathologic process is based on an immunologic mechanism, that it is related to the Shwartzman-Sanarelli reaction and to vasculitis with destruction of erythrocytes and depletion of platelets, that primary vascular damage is either generalized or limited to the kidney producing fibrin deposition and to initial erythrocyte destruction and platelet agglutination followed by activation of coagulation factors and deposition of fibrin in the glomerular capillaries. Lanzkowsky and McCrory[199] postulated that fibrin is rapidly generated when intravascular coagulation is incited by some viral or bacterial endotoxic chemical. As fibrin is formed and deposited on the surface of the vascular tree, the microcirculation is obstructed especially in the kidney, producing a condition known as thrombotic microangiopathy. As the

---

*See references 130, 131, 144, 174, 196, 206, 209, 224, 225, 232, 260, and 280.

erythrocytes pass through the diseased small thrombotic blood vessel, interaction with the deposited fibrin causes their distortion and fragmentation.[56,57] In the kidney a severe glomerulitis, cortical necrosis, and acute necrotizing glomerulonephritis result. Endothelial damage of small blood vessels provides sites for the agglutination of platelets and destruction of erythrocytes, releasing coagulant material in the process. This in turn causes the release of thrombin so that more fibrin is progressively deposited. During this process many blood factors are consumed, among them fibrinogen, platelets, prothrombin, and factor V and factor VIII. Endogenous fibrinolytic mechanisms are then activated to dispose of the accumulation of fibrin. Activation of the fibrinolytic enzyme system results in the dissolution of fibrin and fibrinogen and the release of fibrin-split products into the plasma. Some[364] regard hemolysis as the primary event in the pathogenesis of the hemolytic-uremic syndrome. Liberation of thromboplastin-like substances from the erythrocyte stroma initiates intravascular coagulation causing fibrin deposition in the glomerular tufts of the kidneys. The reticuloendothelial system usually removes thromboplastin-fibrin aggregates from the circulation, protecting against intravascular clotting. According to this concept this function is depressed and intravascular clotting results.

*Etiology.* In the series of Gianantonio and associates[132] a viral agent was isolated from the blood during the acute phases of the disease but was not specifically identified. Mettler[228] has recently isolated from two patients with hemolytic-uremic syndrome and from another with thrombotic thrombocytopenic purpura an agent provisionally classified as a *Microtatobiote*, order *Rickettsiales*, family *Bartonellaceae*. The same organism was recovered from mites collected in the bedroom of one of the children with the hemolytic-uremic syndrome. The organism was seen as dark-blue formations on the outside margins of red cells when Wright's stain was used. The organism was found not only on red cells but also on platelets, lymphocytes, and immature red cells that appeared in considerable numbers in infected mice.

*Pathology.* No consistent picture is found on pathologic examination. Bilateral cortical necrosis, glomerular lesions of hyaline thrombosis, occlusion of isolated capillary loops with areas of fibrinoid necrosis, and acute and chronic glomerulonephritis have been observed (Figs. 104 and 105). The thrombi in the hemolytic-uremic syndrome are predominantly located in the renal glomerular capillaries, whereas in thrombohemolytic thrombocytopenic purpura the thrombi are ubiquitous. Definitive changes in the central nervous system are infrequent.

The difficulties of classifying this syndrome are illustrated by an early case of a 21-month-old child described as having the hemolytic-uremic syndrome[307] who, after many exacerbations of the disease, came to autopsy at 13½ years of age with the typical lesions of thrombotic thrombocytopenic purpura.[215]

Brain and associates[58] postulate that the distorted red cells, hemolytic anemia, and thrombocytopenia in acute renal failure are related to pathologic changes affecting small blood vessels (necrotizing arteritis, intraluminal hyaline thrombi, fibrinoid necrosis of arterioles). This type of hemolytic anemia they termed "microangiopathic haemolytic anemia," in which the causation is comparable to the anemia produced by a regurgitant jet of blood impinging on a bare area of Teflon in repair of an atrial septal defect.

Shumway and Terplan[308] have pointed out that thrombotic thrombocytopenic purpura, eclampsia, renal cortical necrosis, and disseminated lupus erythematosus have in common the presence of "fibrinoid" material within the lumina and/or walls of the small arterioles and/or capillaries. The presence of this material has led to the suggestion that the hemolytic-uremic syndrome may represent a hypersensitivity state analogous to the generalized Sanarelli-Shwartzman[287,309] phenomenon in experimental animals. In rabbits this reaction is characterized by the occurrence of bilateral renal cortical necrosis, following the intravenous administration of two properly spaced injections of endotoxin prepared from gram-negative bacteria. With the onset of the generalized Sanarelli-Shwartzman reaction there is thrombocytopenia, hemolytic anemia, and deposition of fibrinoid material within the glomerular capillaries of the rabbit. Others[305] have thought it unlikely that a single etiologic agent could account for all cases. It is more likely that the syndrome is a response to a variety of sensitizing antigens in a constitutionally predisposed individual.

Pathologic and immunopathologic studies were done on four patients with hemolytic-uremic syndrome. The principal lesions involved the endothelial and subendothelial region of the renal arterioles and of the glomerular capillaries. The endothelial cells were smaller and, in the case of the glomerular capillary loops, separated from the basement membrane by an accumulation of material in the subendothelial space. In contrast to the glomerular capillaries, the endothelial changes in the renal arterioles were associated with a striking deposition of fibrinogen or its derivative. The principal lesion is confined to the kidney and involves the endothelial and subendothelial regions of the arterioles and glomeruli. Increase in plasma renin accounts for the marked hypertension. The absence of immune globulin or complement deposition at the site of these lesions make an immune mechanism of the types known to be associated with vascular injury unlikely.[129]

*Prognosis.* In the large series described by Gianantonio, the most significant prognostic factor has been the severity of the acute phase of the disease, reflected in the impaired renal function and in the degree of renal glomerular damage observed in renal biopsies. In his original series of fifty-eight affected infants and children, Gianantonio and his associates found an overall mortality of 29%.[132] Later, in a series of 250 cases, they found that the overall mortality rate fell from 23% in the first 150 patients to 5% in the last 100 cases.[130] It was pointed out, however, that the improvement was in part due to the inclusion of mild forms of the disease and also improvements which had taken place in the management of acute renal failure in infants during the past 10 years of the study.

A prolonged period of anuria usually carries a grave prognosis, as does extensive glomerular damage.[56]

*Treatment.* The most important element in treatment is the prompt recognition of the disease. Treatment is symptomatic and depends on awareness of the daily fluctuation in the extent of renal disease. It is claimed that the fall in mortality reflects the improvements in the care of the uremic child.[56] The therapeutic agents employed are peritoneal dialysis, transfusions of packed cells or platelets or both, exchange transfusion, corticosteroids, heparin, and, at times, fibrinolytic agents.

Peritoneal dialysis has enabled children to recover renal function after periods of 2 or more weeks of anuria.[56] This procedure should be undertaken early in the disease to prevent marked azotemia. Blood transfusion to maintain a reasonable hemoglobin level, the administration of platelets to combat thrombocytopenia, and measures to control hypertension have contributed to improved prognosis. Corticosteroids (prednisone, 2 mg. per kg. of body weight per day) have proved beneficial in some cases and ineffective in others. Exchange transfusions have been occasionally employed with moderate success.

The analogies between the hemolytic-uremic syndrome and generalized Shwartzman-Sanarelli reaction, the presence of fibrin-like material in renal glomeruli, and the more recent evidence of systemic intravascular coagulation have prompted the use of heparin in treatment.[56] Furthermore, heparin interferes with induction of the Shwartzman phenomenon if given prior to the inciting agent.[260] The treatment is difficult to evaluate in patients who receive several forms of treatment simultaneously. The efficacy of heparin therapy is most pronounced when it is used early in the disease before extensive tissue damage has occurred. Not all reports document the depletion of coagulation factors, and in one group of cases[133] heparin was effective in reducing mortality despite high levels of fibrinogen, factor V, and factor VIII which may occur as a "rebound" phenomenon following intravascular clotting.[288] Heparin appeared to be of value in preventing the formation of new thrombi and further consumption of platelets and coagulation factors. All patients received heparin intravenously as soon as the hemolytic-uremic syndrome was diagnosed. Its use has been difficult to assess, especially in patients who go into spontaneous remission. (For dosage of heparin and management, consult Chapter 26, the section on disseminated intravascular coagulation.)

With the discovery of specific agents responsible for the hemolytic-uremic syndrome it is hoped that more specific therapy will be available for this disease.

In summary, the hemolytic-uremic syndrome is an unusual form of acute renal failure associated with hemolytic anemia and thrombocytopenia. Clinical features include mild diarrhea and vomiting; pallor, listlessness, lethargy; azotemia, marked oliguria (anuria); petechiae, frequent ecchymoses; convulsions, hypertension, and cardiac failure. Usually infants 12 months of age or younger are affected, but occasionally the condition may be noted up to 10 years of age. Blood findings include anemia, thrombocytopenia, and red cell fragmentation. The pathologic changes are glomerulonephritis, renal cortical necrosis, and thrombotic thrombocytopenic purpura.

Shapiro and colleagues[302] reported two adults with the syndrome of acute microangiopathic hemolytic anemia and severe oliguric renal failure. Therapy consisted of prednisone, careful attention to fluid balance, and in one patient peritoneal dialysis. Both patients recovered. Because of the presence of severe renal failure at the outset, the diagnosis of hemolytic-uremic syndrome was favored rather than thrombotic thrombocytopenic purpura. The clinical distinction was regarded as important since the former has a more favorable prognosis whereas the latter is almost uniformly fatal.

## Cyclic thrombocytopenic purpura related to the menstrual cycle

A physiologic decrease in the number of platelets occurs in the 2 weeks before menstruation in the majority of women, reaching the lowest levels during the first day of menstruation. Easy bruising is a reflection of this alteration. A gradual increase in the number of platelets takes place during the following 2 weeks.[263] Intermittent thrombocytopenic purpura has been described which was confined to the menstrual period and was followed by a spontaneous remission.[229] In patients with idiopathic thrombocytopenic purpura the platelet count may be lowest during menstruation and highest during ovulation.[256] Severe menorrhagia may be an indication of this change and sometimes the sole clinical manifestation of this disease.

## Hemangioma and thrombopenia (Kasabach-Merritt syndrome)

Thrombocytopenic purpura has been reported in association with hemangioma in infancy.[184] A hemorrhagic tendency and bleeding into the hemangiomatous site may occur. The lesions may be so extensive as to result in a fatal outcome as thrombopenia develops.[311] With the use of $^{51}$Cr-tagged platelets the thrombocytopenia in a case of giant hemangioma was traced to platelet sequestration in the tumor.[62] Here irradiation was the essential therapeutic factor, resulting in the gradual disappearance of petechiae and return of platelet numbers to normal. On the other hand, spontaneous involution of a huge cavernous hemangioma of the leg in the first 6 months of life was associated with regression of thrombocytopenic purpura.[360] The thrombopenia-hemangioma syndrome may or may not show an increased number of young and agranular megakaryocytes in the bone marrow. The occurrence of platelet thromboses within the vessels of the hemangioma conceivably results in their sequestration in the tumor with peripheral depletion of platelets.[140] The mechanism of the syndrome has also been attributed to a reaction in the endothelium of the tumor vessels which stimulates the production of an antiplatelet antibody, destroying platelets and exerting an effect on megakaryocytes within the marrow.[338] In seven of nineteen reported cases, the bone marrow revealed an increased number of megakaryocytes which were described as immature and not producing platelets. Elimination of the hemangioma results in return of the platelet count to normal, whereas splenectomy is without effect on the blood dyscrasia unless the spleen is the site of the hemangioma.[51,62,90,140] Multiple hemangiomas and thrombocytopenia have also been reported. Surgical excision resulted in severe bleeding.[135] A huge hemangioma in the neck with accompanying thrombocytopenia, hemorrhage, and anemia reacted well with x-ray treatment.[95]

It has been demonstrated in recent years that thrombocytopenia, which was considered the distinguishing feature of the Kasabach-Merritt syndrome, is associated with the depletion of other clotting factors.[163,343,353,356] Extensive studies have now shown that thrombocytopenia occurs with depression of clotting factors II, V, and VIII and fibrinogen as well as the presence of fibrin-split products. It appears that the occurrence of intravascular coagulation within the sinusoids of a hemangioma may lead to decreased levels of coagulation factors resulting in excessive bleeding. While the majority of hemangiomas can occur in almost any location (usually the skin), those reported with thrombocytopenia and hypofibrinogenemia have usually been of the large cavernous variety situated within soft tissue, muscle, or organs.[343] Splenic tumors are uncommon but hemangiomas should be suspected in benign tumors of this organ. When splenic hemangiomas are removed by splenectomy, the platelets and other coagulation factors are restored to normal.

Several cases may be cited to illustrate that disseminated intravascular coagulation accounts for the bleeding in the Kasabach-Merritt syndrome. A newborn girl with giant hemangioma and diffuse bleeding[353] was too critically ill and the hemangioma too large for radiotherapy or surgery. Heparin therapy followed immediately by transfusion of small amounts of heparinized plasma and packed cells resulted in a rise in fibrinogen level. In another case a 16-month-old boy presented with bleeding, an abdominal mass, thrombocytopenia, and afibrinogenemia.[343] Preoperative coagulation studies revealed low platelet levels, absent fibrinogen, and near normal levels of factors V and VIII, all of which returned to normal after splenectomy. The half-life of $^{131}$I-labeled fibrinogen was 36 hours preoperatively and 72 hours postoperatively.

When intravascular coagulation is definitely established in the Kasabach-Merritt syndrome, treatment with heparin is indicated (see Chapter 26 for dosage). Platelet concentrates and packed red cells can be used in conjunction with heparin therapy. Unless these vascular tumors subsequently regress spontaneously, with improvement after heparin therapy efforts should be made toward excision of the involved site or radiation therapy. Splenectomy has been ineffective in raising the platelet count unless the hemangioma was present within this organ. Corticosteroids do not affect the thrombocytopenia. On the other hand, patients with extensive hemangiomas without thrombocytopenia have frequently shown regression of the tumor following the use of corticosteroids.[123,216]

## NONTHROMBOCYTOPENIC PURPURAS

### Allergic purpura (anaphylactoid purpura, Henoch-Schönlein or Schönlein-Henoch purpura)

Allergic purpura refers to a type of nonthrombocytopenic purpura accompanied by a pleomorphic urticaria-like and purpuric type of cutaneous eruption in combination with gastrointestinal symptoms (Henoch's purpura), painful swelling of the joints (Schönlein's purpura rheumatica), and a tendency toward renal involvement. These features are grouped together as the Henoch-Schönlein syndrome (also referred to as the Schönlein-Henoch purpura), with the realization that these symptom complexes can occur individually, in combination, or in sequence.

*Etiology and pathogenesis.* The relationship of the purpuric state to allergy is suggested by the symptoms of urticaria, diffuse erythema, and subcutaneous and submucous extravasations of blood and lymph. Although hypersensitivity is generally considered to underlie the Henoch-Schönlein syndrome, a definite allergen is only rarely identified. Food and, less frequently, bacterial infection and drugs, including antibiotics, are suspected as the exciting factors. A large variety of foods have been chiefly implicated—eggs, milk, chocolate, wheat, nuts, and beans and, to a lesser extent, fish, pork, lamb, chicken, and a variety of fruits.[6] In one patient an insect bite led to joint swelling, blood-tinged stools, and hematuria.[66] Acute vascular purpura has also been reported following immunization with Asiatic influenza vaccine.[329] Although a relationship is suggested clinically, skin tests are generally negative, and more is gained by eliminating the suspected foods from the diet and observing for the subsidence of symptoms.

The high incidence of preceding upper-respiratory infections, often with beta hemolytic streptococci, and the similarity between the latent period of 1 to 3 weeks until the appearance of the hemorrhagic manifestations have suggested both a close association between Henoch-Schönlein purpura and acute nephritis and the hyperimmune nature of both diseases. On the other hand, Bywaters and co-workers[67] found in a series of sixty-four cases that although Henoch-Schönlein purpura was preceded by an upper respiratory infection in 72% of their patients, group A beta hemolytic streptococci were isolated in only one-fourth of the patients investigated. This evidence was intermediate between that found in patients with rheumatic fever and in a control series of children admitted for nonrheumatic carditis. Thus, there is no clear evidence that this type of specific infection is an invariable causative factor. It may well be that the increasing use of the sulfonamide drugs and antibiotics in connection with the treatment of acute upper respiratory infections may be responsible for the apparent increasing incidence of the Henoch-Schönlein syndrome.[136] This disorder has been reported following smallpox vaccination.[176]

A disturbance of the vascular endothelium resulting in increased capillary fragility and permeability is a basic factor in the symptomatology. Osler[251] was among the first to call attention to the association between arthritis and intestinal symptoms and the erythema group of skin diseases and to emphasize the renal complication. The erythematous exanthem of the Henoch-Schönlein syndrome has been differentiated from true purpura in which the surrounding skin is normal.[6] However, the two conditions are not always separable, and true purpura in the sense of this definition is often observed in children in conjunction with other features of Henoch-Schönlein purpura.

The Henoch-Schönlein syndrome has been linked[96,126] with acute nephritis, rheumatic fever, and polyarteritis nodosa and other collagen diseases. They have overlapping clinical characteristics and a similar pathogenesis based on an antigen-antibody reaction involving the endothelium of blood vessels. Henoch-Schönlein purpura can be classified as an immunovascular disorder resulting in a generalized blood vessel disturbance, an acute perivasculitis or angiitis affecting the skin, joints, intestinal tract, and renal glomeruli.[84] Kreidberg and associates[192] postulated a latent period between the remission of a preceding infection and the appearance of purpura during which an immunologic mechanism develops. The resulting antigen-antibody reaction at the vascular level would explain the generalized vascular damage. The histopathologic features of acute necrotic involvement of vessel walls and hemorrhage, which are prime features, have led to the designation of this disease as allergic angiitis.[372] The pathologic lesion in skin and kidney biopsies consists of fibrinoid thrombi in capillaries and an associated endothelial and perivascular reaction.[350] The syndrome has also been described as the visceral form of necrotizing or allergic vasculitis showing, pathologically, a marked perivascular localization, homogenization, necrosis of periadventitial connective tissues, and vascular and perivascular accumulation of inflammatory infiltrate.[373]

An antiserum made experimentally from vascular endothelium has been found to produce diffuse hemorrhagic purpura in the skin and internal organs. Following the direction of previous Japanese investigators, Clark and Jacobs,[71] using suspensions of dog vascular endothelium from the aorta and vena cava, produced a rabbit antiserum which, when injected in dogs, produced a generalized nonthrombocytopenic hemorrhagic purpura. The resulting lesions corresponded to the diffuse vasculitis involving small blood vessels with perivascular collections of polymorphonuclear cells, lymphocytes, and macrophages observed in Henoch-Schönlein disease, changes which provide a basis for the increased permeability of small blood vessels.

An infectious agent (a drug or toxin, for example) may supposedly form a complex with capillary endothelium or platelets along the lines suggested by Ackroyd[6] with Sedormid therapy, thus initiating active immunization. A further confirmation of the concept of Henoch-Schönlein purpura as a hyperimmune disease was the application of a precipitin test, using a preparation of the aorta of newborn infants. A positive precipitin test with decalcified serum was obtained in six of eight patients with allergic purpura and three of four patients with periarteritis nodosa.[328]

*Clinical features.* Henoch-Schönlein purpura occurs more commonly in males than in females, is slightly more frequent in children and adolescents, and has a peak incidence in children from 2 to 15 years of age. The average duration of the disease is about 4 weeks. The disease is marked by a tendency toward recurrences. In a series of 131 pediatric patients with allergic purpura, Allen and associates[13] reported an age range of 6 months to 16 years, with a median of 4 years. Three-fourths of these patients were under 7 years of age and about one-third were either 2 or 3 years old. Within 6 weeks of the onset of the disease, 40% of these patients had one or more recurrences after a period of well-being. Recurrences were more common in patients over 2 years of age than in younger patients. The occurrence of the disease in several siblings in one family is rare, but it has been reported.[345] The disease is ushered in by headaches, anorexia, and abdominal pain. Fever is rarely over 101° F. The onset is variable, and early in the course symptoms from the skin, gastrointestinal tract, or joints or any combination may predominate. Localized edema occurs on the backs of the hands and around the eyes, face, scalp, and lips.[92] Subconjunctival hemorrhage may be present. Although skin lesions usually occur initially, colicky abdominal pain and gastrointestinal bleeding or joint symptoms may precede any type of skin rash for prolonged periods. Younger patients tend to show more frequent edema of the soft tissue of the scalp, face, eyes, hands, and feet, and older

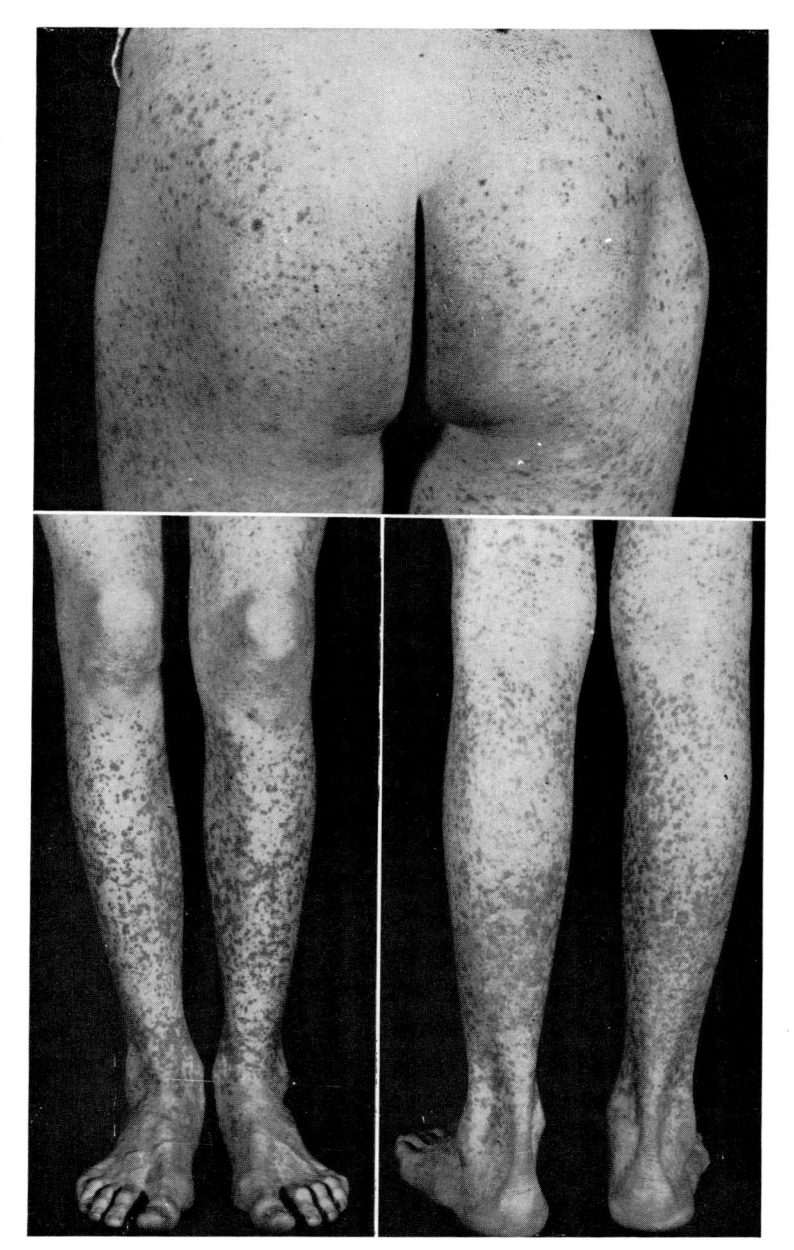

Fig. 106. Henoch-Schönlein purpura in a 13-year-old boy, occurring 2 weeks after an acute upper respiratory infection. The hemorrhagic and erythematous lesions are characteristically shown on some of the most commonly affected sites—buttocks and lower extremities.

children are more prone to gastrointestinal and renal manifestations.[13] (See Fig. 106.)

*Skin.* The specific skin lesion progresses from recurrent crops of urticarial lesions to maculopapules which are at first pink and then red. Petechial hemorrhages occur in a zone of erythema with new lesions appearing every few days. Ecchymoses, urticarial wheals, and edema are common. The lesions tend to spread, forming larger patches, often with a hemorrhagic component as a later development. The most commonly affected sites are the buttocks, lower back, extensor surfaces of the elbows and arms, and the back of the

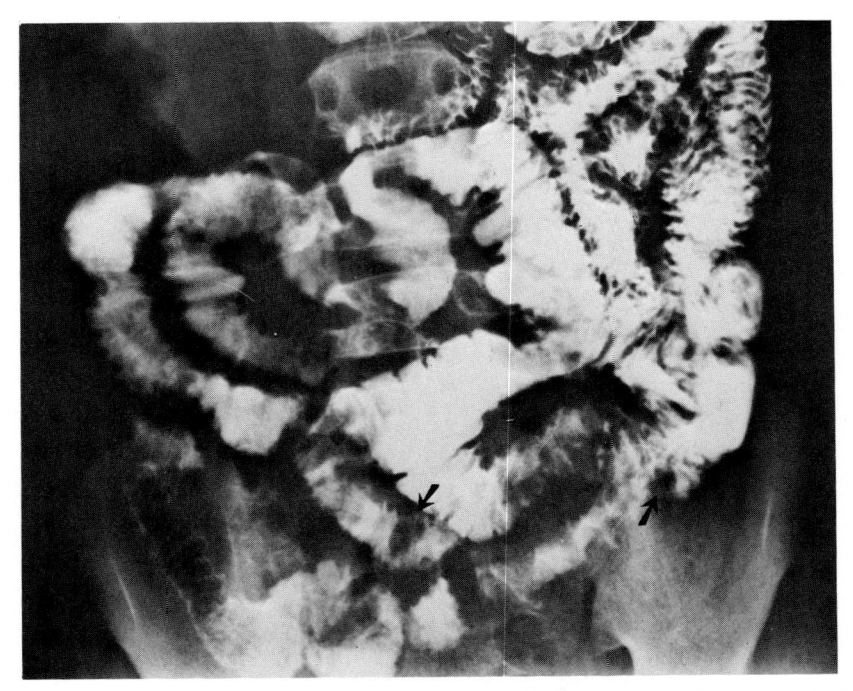

**Fig. 107.** Small intestinal series in Henoch-Schönlein purpura. The small bowel, filled with nonflocculating barium, shows separation of loops, coarse mucosal folds, with polyploid ileal filling defects (arrows). The pattern resembles nonstenotic diffuse ileitis. (From Grossman, H., Berdon, W. E., and Baker, D. H.: Abdominal pain in Schönlein-Henoch syndrome, Amer. J. Dis. Child. **108:**67, 1964.)

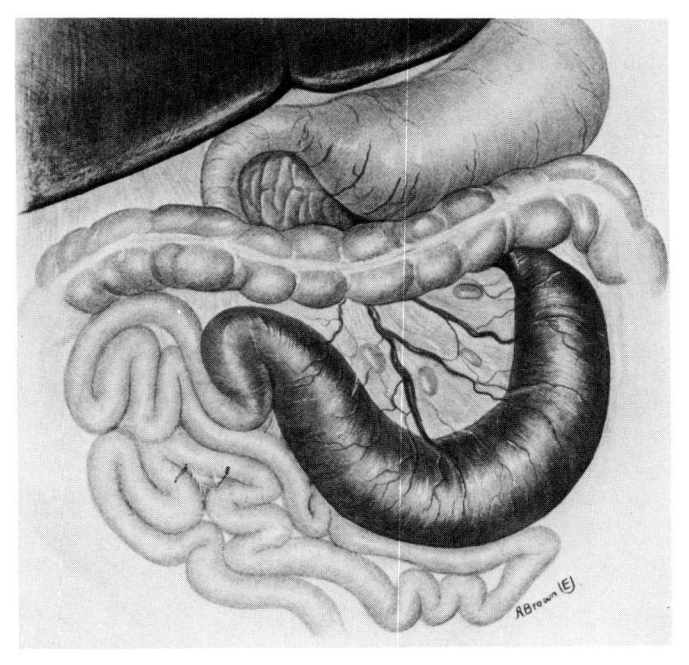

**Fig. 108.** Artist's rendition of edematous, distended, purpuric segment of small intestine in a patient with Henoch-Schönlein purpura. (From Balf, C. L.: The alimentary lesion in anaphylactoid purpura, Arch. Dis. Child. **26:**20, 1951. Reprinted from Archives of Disease in Childhood, 1951, Volume 26, Page 20, by permission of the Publishers.)

lower leg, ankle, and foot. Rash on the calves and thighs has been prominent in some patients. A petechial and purpuric eruption simulating the embolic phenomena of meningococcal sepsis may occur. Epistaxis and bleeding from the gums are rare. Histologic changes are restricted to the small vessels of the corium which are surrounded by an acute inflammatory exudate.[126] Tissue eosinophilia suggests a local hypersensitivity reaction.

*Abdominal symptoms.* Abdominal pain frequently referred to the umbilical region is common. Recurrent colicky pain is the most striking symptom of the disease. The attacks are associated with vomiting, often with melena consisting of the passage of blood and mucus. The lower ileum is usually involved, although both the stomach and jejunum may be affected (Fig. 107). Colic, when severe, may suggest intestinal obstruction, intussusception, and acute appendicitis. These symptoms may precede or accompany the purpuric rash. Perforation is a rare occurrence.[35]

Laparotomy is occasionally undertaken to eliminate these possibilities, although at operation no remedial surgery is usually required. Exception is taken in the case of the patient with intussusception, a rare complication of Henoch-Schönlein purpura in which operation is urgently indicated.[333] The abdominal symptoms are related to edema or extravasations of blood or serosanguineous fluid into the wall of the intestine (Fig. 108). Despite the fact that the alimentary lesions have been compared to the skin purpura, they have also been interpreted as local vasospasms secondary to damage to the arterioles.[33] With atypical abdominal symptoms surgical intervention should not be undertaken without questioning as to previous attacks of purpura.[6] The tip of the spleen is occasionally palpable.

Barium studies may show the small bowel filled with nonflocculating barium, separation of loops, coarse mucosal folds, with polypoid ileal filling defects resembling nonstenotic diffuse ileitis.[23,146] The separation of loops of bowel is due to thickening of the walls of the intestine. With improvement, the small intestinal pattern returns to normal. Similar radiographic changes are found secondary to other bleeding disturbances such as hemophilia and leukemia. The marked abnormalities of the small bowel caused by hemorrhage and edema of both wall and mesentery probably account for the severe abdominal pain.

Colicky abdominal pain, vomiting, fresh blood in the stool, and often a palpable mass occurring in Henoch-Schönlein purpura are suspicious signs of intussusception, and such a patient deserves surgical exploration.[111] In one series nine children had exploratory operations and intussusception was found in four.[117] A tumor mass is not always felt. Roentgenographic examination is sometimes of value in establishing a diagnosis. Delayed operation may result in intestinal gangrene, perforation, and peritonitis. Many patients with nephritis in this disease complain of some abdominal pain.

*Joint involvement.* Joint symptoms vary from transient puffiness of a single joint to recurrent warm and painful swelling of many joints often associated with a limp. The knees and ankles are most commonly affected. The swelling is due to periarticular involvement rather than intra-articular bleeding or effusion. There is no permanent damage to the joints.

*Renal complications.* Renal involvement has been estimated to occur in as high as one-half of the children with Henoch-Schönlein purpura[248] and constitutes by far the most serious complication of the disease. Glomerulonephritis is manifested by gross and microscopic hematuria, cylindruria and proteinuria. Although the majority of children make a complete recovery, some may develop a latent chronic nephritis and eventual renal failure.[97,363] The prognosis must be guarded in those with prolonged hematuria.

The pathology of the kidneys in allergic purpura has been subject to close analysis and varied interpretation. Renal biopsy has made it possible to correlate the clinical and laboratory findings with the actual pathologic status of the kidney.[44,45,350] It is realized that the severity and chronicity of the glomerulonephritis vary from case to case in this disease. According to Vernier and associates,[351] the acute glomerular lesion is characterized by segmental glomerular proliferation and occlusion of capillaries by Schiff-positive fibrinoid material with organized hyaline material or segmental scars in the older lesions. Focal lesions of fibrinoid deposition and endothelial proliferation within scattered glomeruli are most common.[352] Skin biopsy also showed perivascular infiltration of the small dermal vessels with polynuclears and lymphocytes. These authors, therefore, regard the kidney lesion as one not similar to acute glomerular nephritis but rather as part of a diffuse vascular disease with lesions resembling those seen in patients with disseminated lupus erythematosus. Bergstrand and associates[44] interpret the renal lesions as remnants of an inflammatory process similar to glomerulonephritis with the histologic changes favoring a good prognosis even in patients with persistent hematuria.

Glomerulonephritis coincident with or following anaphylactoid purpura may be insidious and in some cases fatal.[166] It is noteworthy that absence of clinical signs of renal involvement during the acute illness does not give assurance that severe and even progressive nephritis may not develop later. From renal biopsy findings it has been estimated that as many as 83% of children with anaphylactoid purpura will have renal involvement, although a much smaller percentage will have clinical evidences of nephritis.[166] Absence of clinical signs of renal involvement during the acute illness does not preclude the possibility of severe or even progressive nephritis developing. Clinical signs of nephritis may persist for up to 2 years, to be followed by apparent complete recovery. Follow-up of children with Henoch-Schönlein purpura should include not only multiple urinalyses during the initial stages of the disease but also determinations at that time of serum urea nitrogen, 24-hour creatinine clearance, Addis count, and quantitative protein excretion. Subsequent follow-up examinations are predicated on the results of the various tests.

Henoch-Schönlein purpura was studied in a group of fourteen adults in whom the disorder was accompanied by renal disease.[34] The renal lesion was found to be a form of glomerulonephritis in some cases focal and likely to heal, in others diffuse and likely to terminate in uremia, as happened in about one-fourth of the cases in this series. The renal manifestations mimic those of poststreptococcal glomerulonephritis, but hypertension and circulatory failure were prominent. Although the clinical findings were unreliable prognostic indicators, there appeared a good correlation between the diffuse glomerular lesion with crescent formation and a fatal outcome.

*Neurologic complications.* Serious neurologic complications are rare. In two children the exanthem, intestinal colic, vomiting, arthralgia, and nephritis were accompanied by subarachnoid hemorrhage which was fatal in one patient.[205] In another patient swelling of an ankle joint preceded the purpuric rash and was followed by colic and fatal cerebral hemorrhage.

*Laboratory findings.* The bleeding time, coagulation studies, and clot retraction are normal. Platelets are normal in number. Anemia and leukocytosis occur only in patients with severe blood loss, and eosinophilia is rare. The tourniquet test is positive in only 25% of patients.[92]

In one series, sixteen of forty-five patients (36%) had evidence of streptococcal infection prior to the onset of anaphylactoid purpura.[352] Using positive antistreptolysin (ASO) titers alone as evidence of recent streptococcal infection, the percentage was 33%. Renal involvement as determined by serial Addis counts was found in 62% of patients.

A rising leukocyte count accompanied by distressing abdominal pain often prompts a consideration of surgical intervention. In a 5½-year-old boy the white blood count rose from 23,400 to 36,700/cu.mm. and the polynuclear count rose to 96%. Throughout this episode severe and persistent generalized abdominal pain was present. No evidence of intussusception could be demonstrated. Anemia was moderate (hemoglobin 9.8 gm./100 ml., hematocrit 31%). Steroids were continued in moderate amount—2 mg./kg./day. The abdominal pain subsided gradually and the white count returned to normal within about 4 weeks.

*Diagnosis.* The typical purpuric erythematosus eruption, colic, and articular and periarticular swelling in a patient with a normal platelet count differentiates the Henoch-Schönlein syndrome from the thrombocytopenic purpuras. The normal coagulation studies serve further to separate this condition from established bleeding disorders.

*Course and prognosis.* The disease is variable in its manifestations and duration. In the majority of patients there is only a single acute episode which clears up spontaneously in a month. Recurrences are common. In its mildest form the disease runs its course in a few days, with transient purpura on the extremities and lower trunk and fleeting abdominal or joint pain or both.

At the other extreme are the serious and fatal forms, often with an insidious onset with progressive purpura, severe arthralgia, gastrointestinal hemorrhages, abdominal pain, hypertension, and kidney and cerebral hemorrhage. In patients with recurrent abdominal pain there is constant concern over the need for surgical intervention.

A chronic course with exacerbations over a period of years is not uncommon. In some patients successive seasonal attacks often occur in the spring with complete remissions in the intervening months. Rarely, the disease progresses with the eventual clinical picture of rheumatoid arthritis and transient purpura. The prognosis for the outcome of a single attack is good, and ultimate recovery, even with repeated attacks, is generally good.

Chronic renal disease constitutes the most serious aspect, and the persistence of proteinuria and red cells in the urine necessitates close supervision. Abnormal urinary findings, i.e., gross and microscopic hematuria and/or proteinuria, have been reported by various investigators to occur in 40 to 50% of the cases during the acute attack. These findings persist as chronic nephritis in about 25% of cases and are confirmed by biopsy evidence.[106] Prognosis is especially guarded when there is nervous system involvement or when abdominal symptoms are sufficiently urgent to require surgical exploration.

*Treatment.* The treatment is essentially symtomatic. Bed rest is required during an attack. In cases which appear to be related to upper respiratory infections, either acute or chronic in nature, foci of infection should be investigated. Only when pathogenic organisms are definitely isolated should antibacterial therapy be instituted. Antibiotics may be of value, although infrequently in our experience; when given, they should be used with discrimination and caution to avoid provoking or aggravating already existing purpura. Occasionally, in patients with Henoch-Schönlein purpura associated with hemolytic streptococci, tonsillectomy has been effective in preventing recurrences.

Antihistamine drugs, vitamins C and K, rutin, and hesperidin have been of questionable value. The most favorable results have been obtained by the detection of an offending food and its elimination from the diet. Suspected foods should, therefore, be systematically investigated for their possible role in etiology, although this is usually not too successful. Chocolate, nuts, fish, tomatoes, and other foods mentioned previously should be investigated for their effect on recurrence of attacks of purpura.

The adrenocortical steroids are commonly employed but with only fair results. It might be expected that the allergic type of hypersensitivity as exemplified by Henoch-Schönlein purpura should respond because of the beneficial effect of the steroids in other members of the collagen group of diseases to which it is related. Although these drugs do not prevent relapses nor modify the course of nephritis, they are worthy of trial.[327] In patients with moderately severe allergic purpura, steroids (prednisone or substitutes) are given orally, according to age. The dose ranges from 1 to 2 mg. per kilogram of body weight (usually 30 to 60 mg. daily) in divided doses four times daily for brief periods of time. Thus treatment should be supervised, especially for the effect on blood pressure elevation and aggravation of abdominal signs. In patients with severe and uncontrollable disease, ACTH or hydrocortisone is given intravenously by drip over an 8-hour period in a dosage of 25 mg. and 100 mg. respectively. ACTH is given intramuscularly when oral administration of steroids has been ineffective.

In the series of Allen and associates[13] corticosteroids were of no value in the management of the skin manifestations or renal involvement. They were found to be useful in arthralgia, soft tissue swelling, and scalp edema. These authors emphasize the need for corticosteroids in sufficient dosage for the relief of abdominal pain. The steroids did not, however, alter the frequency of recurrences nor the duration of illness.

As has already been mentioned, clinical signs indicating abdominal involvement usually do not necessitate surgical intervention. An exception is made for the patient with severe colic, suggesting intussusception. The latter has been ascribed to intramural hematomas of the intestinal tract serving as a leading point for peristaltic invagination.[333] Reduction or resection of the gangrenous segment is usually successful. Some investigators, however, feel that with severe abdominal colic steroids may help prevent the development of intussusception by decreasing the edema in the bowel. Since the patient's life may be in jeopardy by internal hemorrhage, obstruction, or perforation, constant clinical scrutiny is necessary.

Children with acute renal failure should be treated like those with acute glomerulonephritis. Intensive therapy with corticosteroids and immunosuppressive therapy would be indicated on the same grounds that would apply to other acute glomerulonephritides. There is reason to believe that combined therapy holds more promise of a beneficial effect on renal lesions than corticosteroids alone. This awaits documentation of clinical trial. Studies at the present time do not indicate that this form of nephritis has the same benign outlook as poststreptococcal nephritis, in which recovery can be expected in 90 to 95% of children.[221] Prognosis is to be guarded.

### Congenital vascular defects

**Von Willebrand's disease (pseudohemophilia).** Von Willebrand's disease has been described in connection with coagulation disorders (Chapter 26). It was held that this syndrome could be classified into two distinct groups, both possessing a capillary defect with prolonged bleeding time. One group was demonstrated to be associated with marked deficiency in antihemophilic globulin (pseudohemophilia B); in the other the abnormality was confined to the vascular defect (pseudohemophilia A) with no abnormality of coagulation. Von Willebrand's disease is currently regarded as a congenital bleeding disorder with a dominant inheritance and characterized by a prolonged bleeding time and low levels of antihemophilic globulin (factor VIII). It is questionable whether there is a type such as pseudohemophilia A since in most cases some deficiency of factor VIII can be found.

**Hereditary hemorrhagic telangiectasia (Rendu-Osler-Weber disease).** Rendu-Osler-Weber disease is a hereditary condition characterized by the presence of telangiectases, either localized or generalized, and by a tendency to bleed from these lesions. It is transmitted as a simple dominant affecting both sexes, although a generation may be skipped. The individual lesions are slightly raised, are 1 to 4 mm. in size, have a bright red and violaceous appearance, and consist of localized dilatations of capillaries and venules in the skin and mucous membrane. Because of their exposed nature they give rise to profuse hemorrhage either spontaneously or as a result of trauma. The onset is typically in childhood, with epistaxis due to a localized lesion in the nasal mucous membrane. The telangiectases increase in number and become widespread in adult life.[318]

Quick[265] offers several explanations for the basic pathology of this disorder. One is a structural weakness of the minute blood vessels, particularly of the capillaries and venules; the other is a developmental defect of the mesenchymal tissue in which the microcirculation is imbedded, and which normally contributes to the structural maintenance of these microvessels having little or no contractile power of their own. As a result of this lack of mesenchymal tissue support, dilatation of capillaries and venules occurs. Abnormal bleeding in this disease is secondary and usually results from traumatization of a telangiectasis. Quick[265] also encountered one patient in whom both telangiectasia and the von Willebrand syndrome were combined.

Recurrent and severe epistaxis in childhood and in older persons justifies nasopharyngoscopic examination for possible demonstration of telangiectases. The lesions are located most commonly in the nasal mucous membrane and less often on the palate, tongue, conjunctivae, lips, scalp, ears, and face and under the fingernails. Visceral lesions account for gastrointestinal,[371] genitourinary, and pulmonary bleeding and less often for bleeding in other organs. In patients with von Willebrand's disease in whom nosebleed is also severe, the bleeding time is prolonged in contrast to normal findings in patients with hereditary telangiectases. Borderline cases occur.[366]

Therapy consists of protection against local trauma and topical and hemostatic agents, including thermocautery, transfusions, and iron for severe hypochromic anemia when the loss of blood is severe. The disease is rarely fatal since patients rarely die from hemorrhage.

In differential diagnosis, hereditary hemorrhagic telangiectasia is to be distinguished from ataxia-telangiectasia.[210] The latter is a clinical syndrome characterized by progressive cerebellar ataxia, oculocutaneous telangiectasia, and frequent sinopulmonary infection beginning in infancy and early childhood.[188] While bleeding is common in the Rendu-Osler-Weber syndrome, it is rare in ataxia-telangiectasia. In the latter, ataxia is noted when the child starts walking. The cerebellar and extrapyramidal systems are seriously affected. The telangiectasias have a later onset, usually from 4 to 6 years of age, and involve the bulbar conjunctivae, the butterfly area of the face, external ears, palate, creases of the neck, the antecubital and popliteal fossae, and the hands and feet. These patients also show immunologic abnormalities associated with changes in their thymicolymphoid systems. Affected individuals have decreased levels of serum immunoglobulin, usually a selective absence of IgA (gamma-A-globulin) as determined by electrophoresis, and decreased blast formation when the lymphocytes are cultured in vitro with phytohemagglutinin.[203] There is a variable but

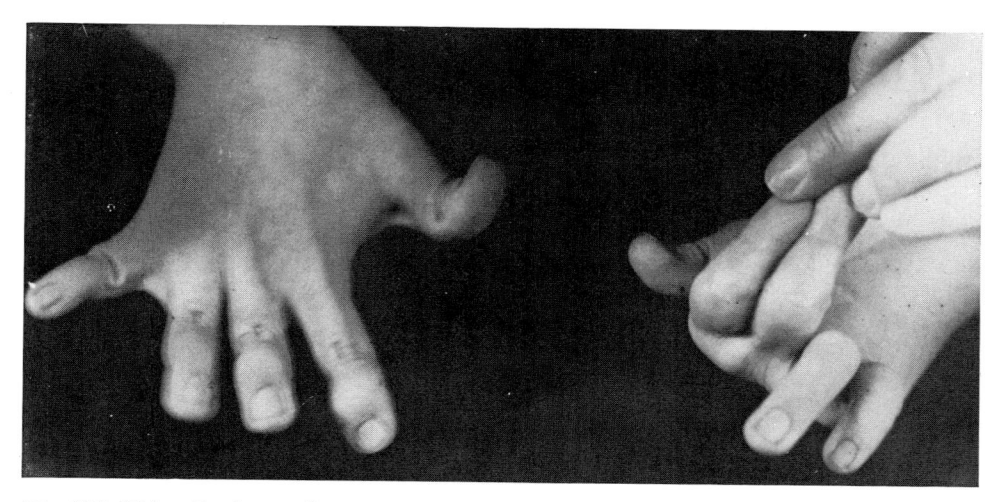

Fig. 109. Ehlers-Danlos syndrome. Hyperlaxity of the joints is especially prominent in the fingers. (From Smith, C. H.: Dermatorrhexis [Ehlers-Danlos syndrome], J. Pediat. 14:632, 1939.)

generally decreased ability for delayed hypersensitivity to develop, and inability to reject a skin homograft.[281] Another feature is an increased incidence of a fatal outcome with a lymphoreticular malignancy.[257] Histologic examination reveals thymic dysplasia with very few thymic lymphocytes, abnormal lymphoid tissue, with decided diminution in Hassall's corpuscles.[258] Inconsistent but frequent lymphopenia may be present. A case associated with granulocytopenia has been reported. Death followed in this patient at 30 months of age with the development of reticulum cell sarcoma.[116] An autosomal recessive type of inheritance has been postulated.[340] As in two other autosomal recessive disorders—Bloom's syndrome and Fanconi's anemia with thrombocytopenia—chromosomal breakage has been described.

Most patients die in their early teens. The conspicous neuropathologic finding is cerebellar cortical degeneration with meningeal telangiectasias. Treatment is symptomatic.

*Ehlers-Danlos syndrome.* The Ehlers-Danlos syndrome is due to a constitutional and congenital dysplasia of the mesenchyme and comprises the following clinical features: friability of the skin (dermatorrhexia) and of the blood vessels, overextensibility of the joints (arthrochalasis), hyperplasticity of the skin, pseudotumors, and freely movable subcutaneous nodules (Fig. 109).[314,336] These pea-sized nodules consist of subcutaneous fat. With the onset of walking, injuries sustained by the infant result in gaping, incised wounds with bleeding due to tearing of the adjacent blood vessels. Spontaneous rupture of large arteries such as the popliteal and subclavian have been reported[222] as well as dissecting aneurysm of the aorta.[223] A number of cardiac defects have been observed more frequently in recent years and may eventually constitute a part of the syndrome.[301,346] The pathologic background is represented by scanty subcutaneous tissue, thinning of collagenous fibers, and an increase of the elastic tissue in the corium which is arranged in irregular and coarse bundles. With the reduced subcutaneous tissue and friability of the skin, the blood vessels are susceptible to trauma. McKusick[223] believes that the Ehlers-Danlos syndrome is a disorder of collagen. The histopathologic picture of the skin reveals normal morphology for the blood vessels, but a diminution and fragmentation of the collagen fibers in the dermis.[125] With defective collagen tissue, the skin stretches excessively (Fig. 110) and lacerates easily on local trauma. Others believe that the basic disorder is the increased number of elastic fibers in the dermis. There is no bleeding tendency. Bleeding and coagulation tests are usually normal.[93] In three patients all tests of hemostasis were within normal limits except for a consistently positive tourniquet test.[125] There is no epistaxis, oozing from mucous surfaces, nor undue bleeding from wounds. Bleeding from the gums may occasionally occur with brushing of the teeth and from tooth sockets after dental extractions. This syndrome is re-

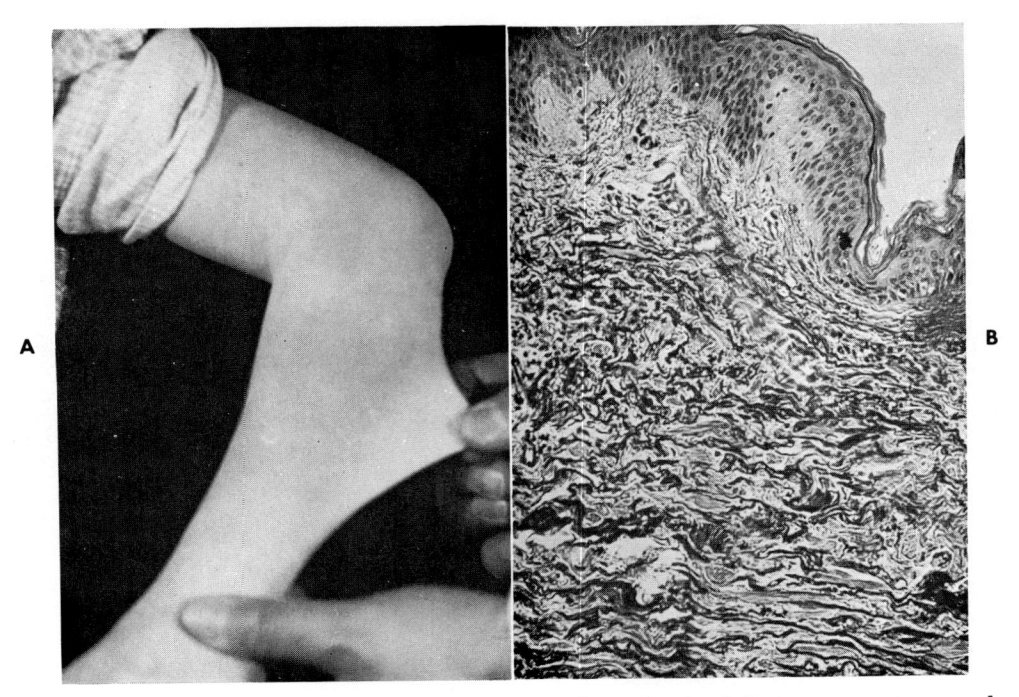

Fig. 110. A, Loose and hyperelastic skin, stretched beyond normal limits, returns to normal position when released. B, High-power photomicrograph of skin. Note that the malpighian layer of the epidermis is reduced in cellular content. The dense reticulum of coarse elastic elements in the corium and the diminution of collagen fibers are important factors in the production of the gaping incised wounds characteritsic of the syndrome. (×260.) (From Smith, C. H.: Dermatorrhexis [Ehlers-Danlos syndrome], J. Pediat. 14:632, 1939.)

garded as a hereditary disease with dominant transmission (simple autosomal dominant)[223] occurring in both sexes, but not in all patients is there a familial incidence.[314]

A child with Ehlers-Danlos syndrome has been described who, in addition to hyperelastic skin and increased mobility of joints, had many tortuous systemic arteries and widespread severe peripheral pulmonary arterial stenosis.[202] Pulmonary artery and skin biopsies showed changes consistent with Ehlers-Danlos syndrome. The findings suggested that the collagen defect thought to be responsible for this syndrome may be present in pulmonary and systemic arteries.

Two families have been described in whom the Ehlers-Danlos syndrome was apparently transmitted as an X-linked recessive character.[37] The results of tests for the Xg blood groups and for color vision show that the locus for the Ehlers-Danlos syndrome is not close to that for the Xg groups nor very close to the locus for deutan color-blindness. The clinical features of this variety of the Ehlers-Danlos syndrome include considerable hyperextensibility of the skin and a bruising tendency.

There is no specific treatment that can alter the fundamental abnormalities of this condition. Therapy consists of the attempt to increase the deposition of fat in the subcutaneous layer to act as a buffer against trauma.

Many of the features of this syndrome can make surgical procedures difficult in these patients. Skin lacerations resulting from minor trauma do not bleed extensively, but the margins of these lesions tend to retract and often heal slowly. The extreme tissue friability encountered at operations makes it difficult to judge the size of an incision; the tissues tear when cutting is attempted and the wound may widen spontaneously.[38]

Factor IX (plasma thromboplastin component) deficiency was observed in a mother and her daughter with the Ehlers-Danlos syndrome.[207] Since the abnormal gene is carried on the X chro-

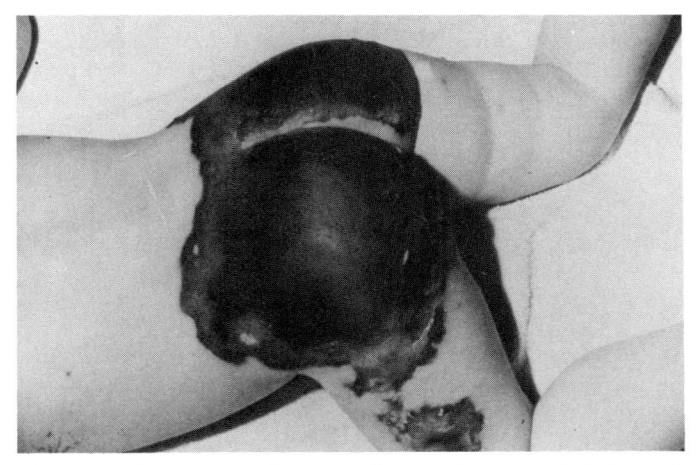

Fig. 111. Well-demarcated, symmetrical necrotic lesion of purpura fulminans in a 2-year-old child. Treatment consisted of heparin and later skin grafting; improvement followed treatment. (Courtesy Dr. Denis R. Miller, New York, N.Y.)

mosome, the disease (factor IX deficiency) can only be fully expressed in the male. No clinical significance can therefore be attached to this deficiency occurring in Ehlers-Danlos syndrome in these cases. It is of interest, however, that a male member of the family with the Ehlers-Danlos syndrome was a bleeder. Apparently, the thromboplastin generation test which had brought to light the defect in the two patients was not used to test the male bleeder.

In another patient 14 months of age with the Ehlers-Danlos syndrome, an acquired encephalocele was not surgically removed because of easy bruisability.[105] No coagulation defect was found, however, although the authors state that a number of hematologic defects have been reported in this condition. These include factor IX (PTC) deficiency, platelet thromboplastin defect with clot retraction abnormality, factor XII (Hageman factor) deficiency, and reduced capillary resistance.

In three cases of this syndrome easy bruising could be attributed to ultrastructural abnormalities of the platelets and their increased tendency to aggregate, forming numerous complex structures.[273] Platelet counts were normal, while prothrombin consumption was abnormal in each case. Platelet thromboplastin generation ranged from normal to defective in this group.

A case of Ehlers-Danlos syndrome of the severe arterial type has been reported in an adult[170] characterized by formation of multiple aneurysms and rupture of medium-sized arteries. The vascular episodes occurred over several years. Death occurred with acute rupture of a splenic vein aneurysm. In this paper the Ehlers-Danlos syndrome is subdivided into three groups—the classical group, mild varicose group, and arterial type.

## Purpura fulminans

Purpura fulminans is a rare form of nonthrombocytopenic purpura characterized by anemia, fever, shock, and sudden and rapidly spreading skin hemorrhages usually occurring symmetrically in the lower extremities[322] (Fig. 111). Marked prostration occurs almost exclusively in young children and follows an infectious disease. The course is usually rapidly fatal within a few days. Of the diseases of childhood, purpura fulminans follows scarlet fever most often[70,362] but it may also be associated with varicella,[322] measles, and upper respiratory infections.[100] Food has also been incriminated as a causative agent. The basic lesion consists of extensive vasculitis which leads to necrosis of tissues and intravascular thrombosis. Because it resembles a hypersensitivity reaction, it is often regarded as a variant of Henoch-Schönlein purpura,[100] although the cardinal features of the latter (mucous membrane bleeding and joint, intestinal, and renal symptoms) are absent. Necrotizing vasculitis in purpura fulminans may be so extensive as to require amputation of the lower legs. The similarity between pathology of the lesion (circumscribed epidermal and dermal necrosis and intravascular thrombosis) and the local Sanarelli-Shwartzman phenomenon is noteworthy. Here, too fibrinogenopenia is attributed to depletion of fibrinogen by coagulation in the thrombotic process.[208] Little reported that striking clinical recovery followed heparinization in the patient whose condition had deteriorated on treatment with fibrinogen and corticosteroids.[208] Contributing to the clinical picture of purpura fulminans is the diminution in clotting factors such as labile factor (factor V)[189] and fibrinogen[157] due to depletion of fibrinogen by coagulation in the thrombotic process. Rarely, the platelet count is decreased.[80] On the other hand, purpura fulminans has been reported in a newborn infant who died on the eighth day after birth[349] in whom hemorrhage was associated with thrombocytopenia and hypofibrinogenemia. In this case the evidence pointed to an onset in utero. In another case[53] the fibrinolysin was so rapidly active and strong that the whole blood-clotting time was greatly prolonged. Treatment with fibrinogen alone was successful.

Recent observations[12] indicate that, while mild cases subside spontaneously, the severe and frequently fatal cases are associated with laboratory evidence of consumption coagulopathy (disseminated intravascular coagulation). When recognized early the findings reveal lowered levels of platelets, prothrombin, factors V and VIII, and fibrinogen. At a later stage it is not always possible to demonstrate all of these deficiencies.

*Treatment.* A variety of therapeutic agents have been employed, on occasion with success. These are adrenocortical steroids, dextran,[252] and hyperbaric oxygenation.[357] Intravenous fluids and antibiotics are given when indicated. However, when there is evidence of intravascular coagulation by laboratory findings of complete or incomplete consumption coagulopathy as outlined above, aqueous heparin is administered in a dose of 50 to 100 units per kilogram every 4 hours. Appropriate coagulation tests are carried out preceding each dose of heparin to determine when the intravascular process has terminated. If the patient is bleeding, transfusion is required after the heparin injection. Hyperfibrinolysis is infrequently associated with this syndrome; when certain of this finding, intravenous epsilon-aminocaproic acid is given. In the absence of definitive and marked fibrinolysis, the administration of this agent potentiates the thrombosis.

A recent concept relating the pathogenesis of purpura fulminans to the Sanarelli-Shwartzman phenomenon and intravascular coagulation suggested treatment of this condition with heparin. In a 3½-year-old child heparin was administered in a dosage of 100 units (1 mg.) per kilogram of body weight every 4 hours. Treatment terminated on the eighth day when the platelet count and all other measurements had stabilized at normal levels.[21]

### Waterhouse-Friderichsen syndrome

Waterhouse-Friderichsen syndrome is a rapidly fatal form of severe purpura associated with adrenal hemorrhage during the course of meningococcemia or other severe septicemias. Fever, shock, prostration, vascular collapse, and widespread hemorrhages are prominent features. The disease usually affects infants from 2 to 15 months of age, and in 90% of all cases it occurs in children under 9 years old. Therapy must be prompt and vigorous. Besides appropriate antimicrobial therapy, heparin[3] and adrenocortical steroids are used in treatment and have occasionally been helpful.[241] Intravenous hydrocortisone is particularly useful.

### Idiopathic pulmonary hemosiderosis

Idiopathic pulmonary hemosiderosis has been described as immunoallergic purpura and by Virchow as brown lung induration.[218] It is a disease occurring most frequently in childhood and in young adults and is characterized by dyspnea, cyanosis, fever, cough, blood-streaked sputum, and pallor, with laboratory evidence of iron-deficiency anemia. These features are associated with the basic pathologic process in which blood is extravasated in the pulmonary alveoli by repeated hemorrhages.

*Clinical course.* The diagnosis of idiopathic pulmonary hemosiderosis should be considered in patients with severe cough, dyspnea, dullness, rales, bronchial breathing, and anemia. The course is one of remissions and exacerbations with intermittent hemoptysis and hematemesis. Acute episodes last 2 to 10 days but occasionally persist for several weeks.[*] Mild jaundice appears after a few days. Occasionally, the disease occurs with a rapidly fatal outcome without recurrent manifestations.[319] Physical examination during an acute attack may not be striking. The roentgenogram of the chest shows a variety of findings: diffuse homogenous opacities, bilateral perihilar patchy

---

[*]See references 63, 151, 172, 271, 319, 320, 368, and 378.

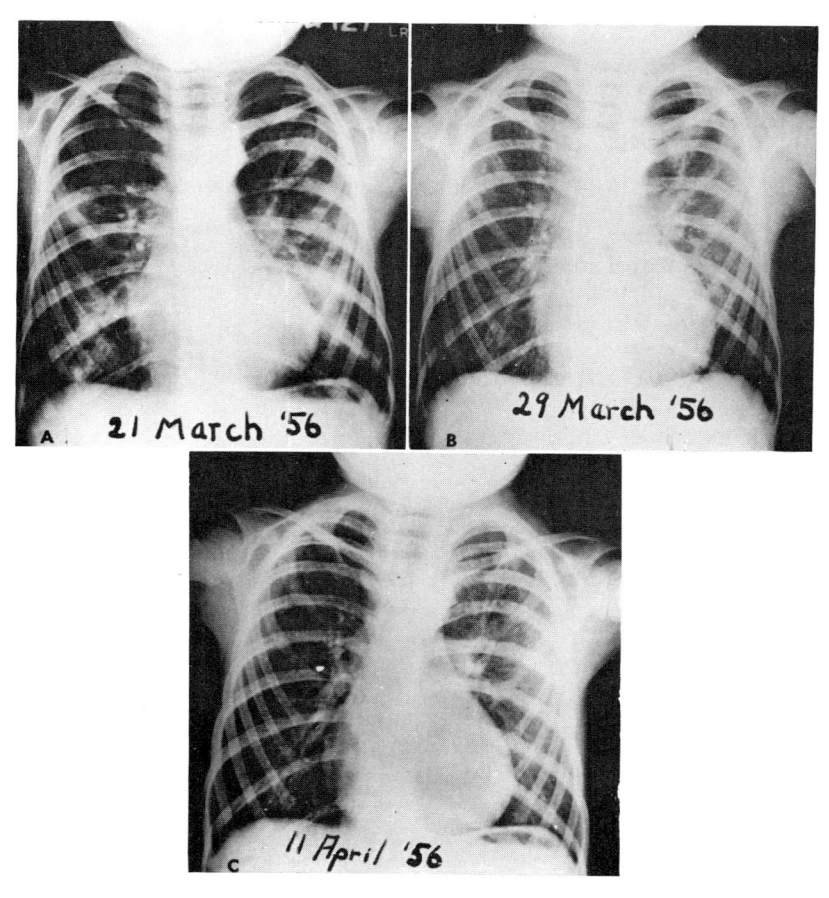

Fig. 112. Roentgenograms of a 4-year-old girl with pulmonary hemosiderosis. A and B, Note perihilar and pulmonary infiltration due to extravasation of blood into the alveoli by repeated hemorrhages. C, The attacks are recurrent, with substantial clearing during convalescence.

infiltration, or diffuse pulmonary infiltrations with increase in bronchial markings extending from the hilar region (Fig. 112). Clearing of the pulmonary fields occurs subsequently but roentgenographic examination shows a residual flecked reticular pattern or a persistent miliary type of infiltration radiating from the hilus. At the onset the disease resembles virus pneumonia or a severe upper respiratory infection. The most frequent peaks of incidence are at 1 to 2 years of age and at 13 to 15 years of age.[320] An apical systolic murmur may be present, the spleen may be palpable, and in children in whom the disease has become chronic the liver is enlarged. The disease must be differentiated from pulmonary hemosiderosis secondary to mitral stenosis, diffuse vasculitis as in polyarteritis nodosa, and other collagen diseases. Readmission to the hospital is sought for respiratory distress, fever, and hemoptysis.

Sputum, gastric washings, and aspiration from lung puncture[128] reveal macrophages laden with granules of hemosiderin stained deep blue with the Prussian blue reaction. Intra-alveolar pulmonary blood loss accounts for a hypochromic microcytic iron-deficiency anemia with reticulocytosis. In two children 3 and 8 years of age under observation, evidence of the iron-deficiency anemia was further confirmed by a low serum iron content of the blood and a moderate increase in latent iron-binding capacity. Studies of the anemia and iron distribution in patients with idiopathic pulmonary hemosiderosis[22] revealed that during the acute phase there was an excessive plasma iron turnover and an iron kinetic pattern characteristic of an iron-deficiency anemia and hemorrhage and not of hemolysis. Erythrocytes labeled with chromium have a shortened survival, and sequestration in the lung is demonstrable by in vivo surface counting using a scintillation counter. The tuberculin and Coombs tests are negative; the platelet and coagulation factors are normal. The transient jaundice and elevation of indirect-reacting bilirubin in the serum following acute or subacute episodes indicate the degradation of intra-alveolar blood. Purpura may occur, although platelet counts have been normal. A rapidly progressive form of diffuse glomerulonephritis and a high incidence of specific renal lesions have been noted and may dominate the clinical picture.[246]

Gilman and Zinkham[134] reported the case of a 9-year-old child with idiopathic pulmonary hemosiderosis without respiratory difficulty, hemoptysis, or radiologic evidence of pulmonary pathology. The major clue to diagnosis was severe, recurrent iron-deficiency anemia which could not be attributed to blood loss from the gastrointestinal or urinary tract. Gastric material obtained in a fasting state showed a few macrophages containing hemosiderin. Subsequently a transthoracic needle pulmonary aspirate revealed a large number of hemosiderin-laden macrophages. The authors conclude that "idiopathic pulmonary hemosiderosis should be considered especially in the child in whom attempts to demonstrate a source of gastrointestinal bleeding are unrevealing."

*Prognosis.* After a course of several years, the disease usually ends with an acute fatal exacerbation. Terminal cardiorespiratory failure results from the effects of recurrent pulmonary bleeding. In a review by Soergel[320] the average duration was 2.9 years, the shortest 5 weeks, and the longest 10 years. Of thirty-two patients, nine had died, ten were still active, five showed no progression of the disease, and eight had become symptom free.

*Pathology.* The basic pathologic process is repeated intra-alveolar hemorrhages, massive in patients with acute attacks and of variable amounts in those with subacute or chronic phases. There is no hemosiderosis of other organs. The pulmonary findings in a 4-year-old child with a 14-month history of several exacerbations typify the usual fatal case. There was a diffuse fibrous thickening of the alveolar septa, which showed broken, thin, and sparse strands of elastic tissue, clumps of golden pigment-laden macrophages in numerous alveolvar spaces, and extensive hemorrhages into alveolar spaces, bronchioles, and small bronchi. When a special stain is employed, the pigment in the macrophages stains blue, indicating the presence of iron or evidence of old hemorrhage. Hyaline membrane formation was

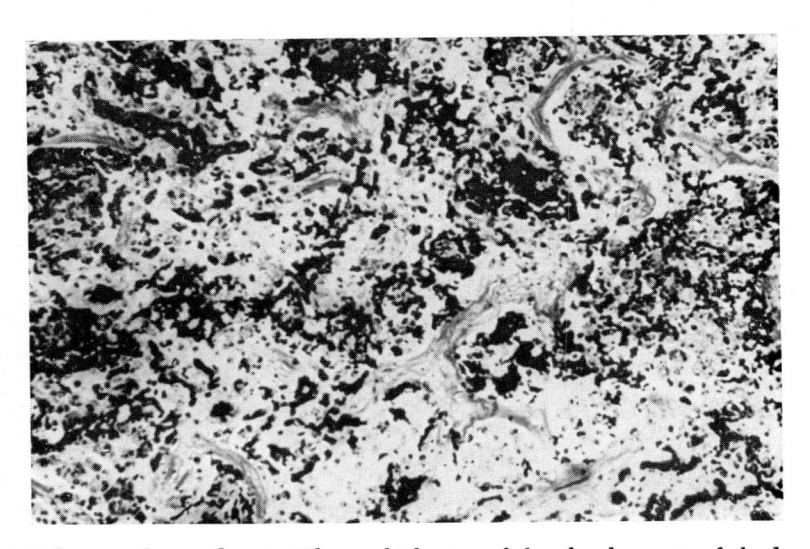

Fig. 113. Pulmonary hemosiderosis. Fibrous thickening of the alveolar septa of the lung showing broken, thin, and sparse strands of elastic tissue. Extensive hemorrhage into alveolar spaces, bronchioles, and small bronchi is evidenced by the presence of diffuse hemosiderosis. (Heavily stained areas are indicative of iron deposition.) (×150.)

also found in many alveoli and in some bronchioles (Fig. 113).

*Pathogenesis.* The etiology of this disease has been ascribed to a primary developmental defect of the elastic fibers, with their fragmentation resulting in stasis within capillary vessels and hemorrhages. The failure to find destruction of elastic tissue in all patients led Steiner[330] to regard essential pulmonary hemosiderosis as an antigen-antibody reaction caused by a still unknown sensitizing agent inducing the production of autoantibodies. With the lungs as a shock organ the antigen-antibody reaction produces capillary dilatation, stasis, diapedesis, rhexis, and increased destruction of red corpuscles and deposits of hemosiderin.

Soergel and Sommers,[321] in reviewing various theories of pathogenesis, conclude that idiopathic pulmonary hemosiderosis is an isolated disease of the pulmonary alveolar epithelial cells that leads to widespread alveolar capillary hemorrhages of variable intensity. Since the normal air-blood barrier consists only of thin layers of endothelium, basement membrane, and an attenuated alveolar epithelial cytoplasm, a disease of the alveolar epithelial cells may, therefore, critically affect the mechanical stability of the alveolar capillaries.

Heiner and co-workers[159] report a syndrome occurring in young children accompanied by precipitins in their serum to one or more of the milk proteins. The symptoms were predominantly of the respiratory tract, consisting of chronic rhinitis, cough, recurrent pneumonia, and sometimes hemoptysis, hemosiderosis, and iron-deficiency anemia. Several patients were shown to have iron-laden macrophages in bronchial or gastric aspirates, suggesting a similarity or identical likeness of their illness with idiopathic pulmonary hemosiderosis. Symptoms disappeared on removal of cow's milk from the diet. They suggest that all patients with a diagnosis of idiopathic pulmonary hemosiderosis, especially in infancy, should be given the benefit of a trial diet devoid of cow's milk and milk products regardless of the results of precipitin tests.

*Treatment.* For the effects of acute and chronic blood loss into the lungs, almost continuous iron therapy, transfusions, bed rest, and oxygen are required. Iron from the extravasated blood in the pulmonary alveoli is available for hemoglobin formation following each episode.[119] Antibiotics are employed for superimposed infection. Based on these immunoallergic hypotheses, prednisone (2 mg. per kilogram per day, orally) has been advocated to be continued until the acute episode has completely subsided. A smaller effective dose may be employed as necessary. On reviewing the combined experience with twenty-eight patients, Soergel and Sommers[321] found that the short-term use of steroid therapy during bleeding episodes speeds recovery and perhaps improves the patient's immediate prognosis, but that long-term steroid therapy does not alter the course or prognosis of the disease. Favorable reports with this treatment require further evaluation because of the great variations in the frequency and severity of attacks. Similarly, splenectomy designed to reduce the severity of the bleeding episodes needs to be subjected to more prolonged trial. It had been originally advocated because pulmonary hemosiderosis had been considered as an immunohematologic problem. Available evidence[321] does not as yet suggest that splenectomy favorably influences the course of this disease. While chelating agents have been effective in increasing urinary iron excretion from iron liberated during alveolar hemorrhages,[331] they are not effective therapeutic agents. Steiner and Nabrady[332] used azathioprine (Imuran) with good results in the treatment of a boy 16 years of age when steroids caused side effects without controlling the disease. A dose of 2.5 mg. per kilogram per day (of the azathioprine) was used for approximately 6 weeks, followed by 1.25 mg. per kilogram per day until all signs and symptoms subsided. Further experience with immunosuppressive therapy is awaited.

### Miscellaneous purpuric disorders (nonthrombocytopenic)

Valberg and Brown[347] reviewed a number of syndromes consisting of capillary disorders with and without coagulation defects. Purpura simplex refers to mild skin purpura unassociated with specific blood disorders. Hereditary familial purpura simplex is a condition in which spontaneous cutaneous purpura occurs on a transmissable basis involving several generations.[91] The bleeding time is normal; the tourniquet test is positive. This type of purpura occurring in association with congenital ptosis of the eyelids has been described in eleven members of a family representing four generations.[120] Still unclassified is the report of thrombocytopenia in asociation with immunoglobulin abnormalities (hypo-IgG with hyper-IgM) and with intestinal lymphoid hyperplasia in a 2-year-old girl.[138]

A discussion of purpura associated with "autoerythrocytic sensitization" will be found in Chapter 11.

## REFERENCES

1. Aas, K. A., and Gardner, F. H.: Survival of blood platelets labeled with chromium[51], J. Clin. Invest. 37:1257, 1958.
2. Aballi, A. J., Puapondh, Y., and Desposito, F.: Platelet counts in thriving premature infants, Pediatrics 42:685, 1968.
3. Abildgaard, C. F.: Recognition and treatment of intravascular coagulation, J. Pediat. 74:163, 1969.
4. Abildgaard, C. F., Simone, J. V., Seeler, R. A., and Schulman, I.: Chronic thrombocytopenia due to "thrombopoietin" deficiency, a progress report, Blood 30:546, 1967.
4a. Ablin, A. R., Kushner, J. H., Murphy, A., and Zippin, C.: Platelet enumeration in the newborn period, Pediatrics 28:822, 1961.
5. Ackroyd, J. F.: Three cases of thrombocytopenic purpura occurring after rubella; with a review of purpura associated with infections, Quart. J. Med. 18:299, 1949.
6. Ackroyd, J. F.: Allergic purpura, including purpura due to foods, drugs and infections, Amer. J. Med. 14:605, 1953.
7. Adelson, E., Heitzman, E. J., and Fennessey, J. F.: Thrombohemolytic thrombocytopenic purpura, Arch. Intern. Med. 94:42, 1954.
8. Adner, M. M., Fisch, G. R., Starobin, S. G., and Aster, R. H.: Use of "compatible" platelet transfusions in treatment of congenital isoimmune thrombocytopenic purpura, New Eng. J. Med. 280:244, 1969.
9. Aisenberg, A. C.: Current concepts; drugs employed for suppression of immunologic responsiveness, New Eng. J. Med. 272:1114, 1965.
10. Aldrich, R. A., Steinberg, A. G., and Campbell, D. C.: Pedigree demonstrating a sex-linked recessive condition characterized by draining ears, eczematoid dermatitis and bloody diarrhea, Pediatrics 13:133, 1954.
11. Alford, C. A., Jr., Neva, F. A., and Weller, T. H.: Virologic and serologic studies on human products of conception after maternal rubella, New Eng. J. Med. 271:1275, 1964.
12. Allen, D. M.: Heparin therapy of purpura fulminans, Pediatrics 38(part 1):211, 1966.
13. Allen, D. M., Diamond, L. K., and Howell, D. A.: Anaphylactoid purpura in children (Schönlein-Henoch syndrome); review with a follow-up of the renal complications, Amer. J. Dis. Child. 99:833, 1960.
14. Allison, A. C.: Acute haemolytic anaemia with distortion and fragmentation of erythrocytes in children, Brit. J. Haemat. 3:1, 1957.
15. Alter, H. J., Scanlon, R. T., and Schechter, G. P.: Thrombocytopenic purpura following vaccination with attenuated measles virus, Amer. J. Dis. Child. 115:111, 1968.
16. Amorosi, E. L., and Ultmann, J. E.: Thrombotic thrombocytopenic purpura; report of 16 cases and review of the literature, Medicine 45:139, 1966.
17. Andre, J. A., Schwartz, R. S., Mitus, W. J., and Dameshek, W.: Morphologic responses of lymphoid system to homografts. II. Effect of antimetabolites, Blood 19:334, 1962.
18. Angle, R. M., and Alt, H. L.: Thrombocytopenic purpura complicating infectious mononucleosis; report of a case and serial platelet counts during the course of infectious mononucleosis, Blood 5:449, 1950.
19. Anthony, B., and Krivit, W.: Neonatal thrombocytopenic purpura, Pediatrics 30:776, 1962.
20. Anthony, P. P., and Kaplan, A. B.: Haemolytic-uraemic syndrome in two sibs, Arch. Dis. Child. 43:316, 1968.
21. Antley, R. M., and McMillan, C. W.: Sequential coagulation studies in purpura fulminans, New Eng. J. Med. 276:1287, 1967.
22. Apt, L., Pollycove, M., and Ross. J. F.: Idiopathic pulmonary hemosiderosis; study of anemia and iron distribution using radio-iron and radiochromium, J. Clin. Invest. 36:1150, 1957.
23. Arcomano, J. P., and Eskes, P. W. H.: Schönlein-Henoch syndrome, roentgen changes in the upper gastrointestinal tract, Amer. J. Dis. Child. 114:674, 1967.
24. Aster, R. H.: Studies of mechanism of "hypersplenic" thrombocytopenia in rat and man, Blood 26:890, 1965.
25. Aster, R. H., and Jandl, J. H.: Platelet sequestration in man. I. Methods, J. Clin. Invest. 43:843, 1964.
26. Aster, R. H., and Jandl, J. H.: Platelet sequestration in man. II. Immunological and clinical studies, J. Clin. Invest. 43:856, 1964.
27. Aster, R. H., and Keene, W. R.: Sites of platelet destruction in idiopathic thrombocytopenic purpura, Brit. J. Haemat. 16:61, 1969.
28. Ata, M., Fisher, O. D., and Holman, C. A.:

Inherited thrombocytopenia, Lancet 1:119, 1965.
29. Avery, M. E., Oppenheimer, E. H., and Gordon, H. H.: Renal vein thrombosis in the newborn infants of diabetic mothers, New Eng. J. Med. 256:1134, 1957.
30. Baker, D. H., Parmer, E. A., and Wolff, J. A.: Roentgen manifestations of the Aldrich syndrome, Amer. J. Roentgen. 88:458, 1962.
31. Baker, L. R., Rubenberg, M. L., Dacie, J. V., and Brain, M. C.: Fibrinogen catabolism in microangiopathic haemolytic anaemia, Brit. J. Haemat. 14:617, 1968.
32. Baldini, M.: Idiopathic thrombocytopenic purpura, New Eng. J. Med. 274:1245, 1966.
33. Balf, C. L.: The alimentary lesion in anaphylactoid purpura, Arch. Dis. Child. 26:20, 1951.
34. Ballard, H. S., Eisinger, R. P., and Gallo, G.: Renal manifestations of the Henoch-Schoenlein syndrome in adults, Amer. J. Med. 49:328, 1970.
35. Basu, R.: Perforation of the bowel in Henoch-Schönlein purpura, Arch. Dis. Child. 34:342, 1959.
36. Bayer, W. L., Sherman, F. E., Michaels, R. H., Szeto, I. L. F., and Lewis, J. H.: Purpura in congenital and acquired rubella, New Eng. J. Med. 273:1362, 1965.
37. Beighton, P.: X-linked recessive inheritance in the Ehlers-Danlos syndrome, Brit. Med. J. 3:409, 1968.
38. Beighton, P., and Horan, F. T.: Surgical aspects of the Ehlers-Danlos syndrome, Brit. J. Surg. 56:255, 1969.
39. Belber, J. P., Davis, A. E., and Epstein, E. A.: Thrombocytopenic purpura associated with cat-scratch disease, Arch. Intern. Med. 94:321, 1954.
40. Bell, A. D., Mold, J. W., Oliver, R. A. M., and Shaw, S.: Study of transfused platelets in a case of congenital hypoplastic thrombocytopenia, Brit. M. J. 2:629, 1956.
41. Berge, T., Brunnhage, F., and Nilsson, L. R.: Congenital hypoplastic thrombocytopenia in rubella embryopathy, Acta Paediat. 52:349, 1963.
42. Berglund, G.: Plasma transfusion treatment of six children with idiopathic thrombocytopenic purpura, Acta Paediat. 52:523, 1962.
43. Berglund, G., and Broberger, O.: Treatment of idiopathic thrombocytopenic purpura in childhood, Acta Paediat. (supp. 117) 48:7, 1959.
44. Bergstrand, A., Bergstrand, C. G., and Bucht, H.: Kidney lesions associated with anaphylactoid purpura in children, Acta Paediat. 49:57, 1960.
45. Bergstrand, C. G., and Bucht, H.: Renal biopsy in children, Acta Paediat. (supp. 117) 48:126, 1959.
46. Best, W. R., and Darling, D. R. A.: A critical look at the splenectomy—S.L.E. controversy, Med. Clin. N. Amer. 46:19, 1962.
47. Billo, O. E., and Wolff, J. A.: Thrombocytopenic purpura due to cat-scratch disease, J.A.M.A. 174:1824, 1960.
48. Bithell, T. C., Didisheim, G. E., and Wintrobe, M. M.: Thrombocytopenia inherited as an autosomal dominant trait, Blood 25:231, 1965.
49. Blaese, R. M., Strober, W., Brown, R. S., and Wardmann, T. A.: The Wiscott-Aldrich syndrome; a disorder with a possible defect in antigen processing or recognition, Lancet 1:1056, 1968.
50. Blecher, T. E., and Raper, A. B.: Early diagnosis of thrombotic microangiopathy by paraffin sections of aspirated bone-marrow, Arch. Dis. Child. 42:158, 1967.
51. Bogin, M., and Thurmond, J.: Hemangioma with purpura, thrombocytopenia and erythrocytopenia, Amer. J. Dis. Child. 81:675, 1951.
52. Bonnin, S. A.: The management of thrombocytopenic states with particular reference to platelet thromboplastic function. I. Idiopathic and secondary thrombocytopenic purpura, Brit. J. Haemat. 7:250, 1961.
53. Bouhasin, J. D.: Purpura fulminans, Pediatrics 34:264, 1964.
54. Bouroncle, B. A., and Doan, C. A.: Refractory idiopathic thrombocytopenic purpura treated with azathioprine, New Eng. J. Med. 275:630, 1966.
55. Bouroncle, B. A., and Doan, C. A.: Treatment of refractory idiopathic thrombocytopenic purpura, J.A.M.A. 207:2049, 1969.
56. Brain, M. C.: The haemolytic-uraemic syndrome, Seminars Hemat. 6:162, 1969.
57. Brain, M. C.: Microangiopathic hemolytic anemia, New Eng. J. Med. 281:833, 1969.
58. Brain, M. C., Dacie, J. V., and Hourihane, D. O'B.: Microangiopathic haemolytic anaemia; the possible role of vascular lesions in pathogenesis, Brit. J. Haemat. 8:358, 1962.
59. Brain, M. C., and Hourihane, D. O'B.: Microangiopathic haemolytic anaemia; the occurrence of haemolysis in experimentally produced vascular disease, Brit. J. Haemat. 13:135, 1967.
60. Breckenridge, R. T., Moore, R. D., and Ratnoff, O. D.: A study of thrombocytopenia; new histologic criteria for the differentiation of idiopathic thrombocytopenia and thrombocytopenia associated with dis-

seminated lupus erythematosus, Blood **30**:39, 1967.
61. Bridges, J. M., and Carré, I. J.: Congenital thrombocytopenic purpura treated by exchange transfusion, Arch. Dis. Child. **36**:210, 1961.
62. Brizel, H. E., and Raccuglia, G.: Giant hemangioma with thrombocytopenia: radioisotopic demonstration of platelet sequestration, Blood **26**:751, 1965.
63. Browning, J. R., and Houghton, J. D.: Idiopathic pulmonary hemosiderosis, Amer. J. Med. **20**:374, 1956.
64. Bukowski, M. J., and Koblenzer, P. T.: Thrombotic thrombocytopenic purpura; report of a case with the unusual features of hypofibrinogenemia and leukopenia, J. Pediat. **60**:84, 1962.
65. Bull, B. S., Rubenberg, M. L., Dacie J. V., and Brain, M. C.: Microangiopathic haemolytic anaemia; mechanism of red cell fragmentation; in vitro studies, Brit. J. Haemat. **14**:643, 1968.
66. Burke, D. M., and Jellinek, H. L.: Nearly fatal case of Schoenlein-Henoch syndrome following insect bite, Amer. J. Dis. Child. **88**:772, 1954.
67. Bywaters, E. G. L., Isdale, I., and Kempton, J. J.: Schönlein-Henoch purpura; evidence for a group A beta haemolytic streptococcal aetiology, Quart. J. Med. **26**:161, 1957.
68. Cahalane, S. F., and Horn, R. C.: Thrombotic thrombocytopenic purpura of long duration, Amer. J. Med. **27**:333, 1959.
69. Carpenter, A. G., Wintrobe, M. M., Fuller, E. A., Haut, A., and Cartwright, G. E.: Treatment of idiopathic thrombocytopenic purpura, J.A.M.A. **171**:1911, 1959.
70. Chambers, W. N., Holyoke, J. B., and Wilson, R. F.: Purpura fulminans; report of two cases following scarlet fever, New Eng. J. Med. **247**:933, 1952.
71. Clark, W. G., and Jacobs, E.: Experimental non-thrombocytopenic vascular purpura; a review of the Japanese literature with preliminary confirmatory report, Blood **5**:320, 1950.
72. Clarke, B. F., and Davies, S. H.: Severe thrombocytopenia in infectious mononucleosis, Amer. J. Med. Sci. **248**:703, 1964.
73. Clement, D. H., and Diamond, L. K.: Purpura in infants and children, Amer. J. Dis. Child. **85**:259, 1953.
74. Cohen, P., and Gardner, F. H.: The thrombocytopenic effect of sustained high-dosage prednisone therapy in thrombocytopenic purpura, New Eng. J. Med. **265**:613, 1961.
75. Cohen, P., Gardner, F. H., and Barnett, G. O.: Reclassification of the thrombocytopenias by the $Cr^{51}$-labeling method for measuring platelet life span, New Eng. J. Med. **264**:1284, 1961.
76. Cooper, L. Z., Green, K. H., Krugman, S., Giles, J. P., and Mirick, G. S.: Neonatal thrombocytopenic purpura and other manifestations of rubella contracted in utero, Amer. J. Dis. Child. **110**:416, 1965.
77. Cooper, M. D., Chase, H. P., Lowman, J. T., Krivit, W., and Good, R. A.: Wiscott-Aldrich syndrome, an immunologic deficiency disease involving the afferent limb of immunity, Amer. J. Med. **44**:499, 1968.
78. Corrigan, J. J., Abildgaard, C. F., Vandesherchen, J. F., and Schulman, I.: Quantitative aspects of blood coagulation in the generalized Shwartzman reaction. I. Effects of variation of preparative and provocative doses of E. coli endotoxin, Pediat. Res. **1**:39, 1967.
79. Craig, J. M., and Gitlin, D.: The nature of the hyaline thrombi and thrombotic thrombocytopenic purpura, Amer. J. Path. **33**:251, 1957.
80. Crawford, S. E., and Riddler, J. G.: Purpura fulminans, Amer. J. Dis. Child. **97**:198, 1959.
81. Crosby, W. H.: Is hypersplenism a dead issue? Blood **20**:94, 1962.
82. Czernobilaky, B., Freedman, H. H., and Frumin, A. M.: Foamy histiocytes in spleens removed for chronic idiopathic thrombocytopenic purpura, Blood **19**:99, 1962.
83. Dacie, J. V.: The haemolytic anaemias, New York, 1954, Grune & Stratton, Inc.
84. Dameshek, W.: Acute vascular purpura, an immuno-vascular disorder, Blood **8**:382, 1953.
85. Dameshek, W.: Controversy in idiopathic thrombocytopenic purpura, J.A.M.A. **173**:1025, 1960.
86. Dameshek, W., Ebbe, S., Greenberg, L., and Baldini, M.: Recurrent acute idiopathic thrombocytopenic purpura, New Eng. J. Med. **269**:647, 1963.
87. Dameshek, W., and Miller, E. B.: The megakaryocytes in idiopathic thrombocytopenic purpura, a form of hypersplenism, Blood **1**:27, 1946.
88. Dameshek, W., and Reeves, W. H.: Exacerbation of lupus erythematosus following splenectomy in "idiopathic" thrombocytopenic purpura and autoimmune hemolytic anemia, Amer. J. Med. **21**:560, 1956.
89. Dameshek, W., Rubio, F., Jr., Mahoney, J. P., and Reeves, W. H.: Treatment of idiopathic thrombocytopenic purpura (ITP) with prednisone, J.A.M.A. **166**:1805, 1958.
90. Dargeon, H. W., Adiao, A. C., and Pack, G.

T.: Hemangioma and thrombocytopenia, J. Pediat. 54:285, 1959.
91. Davis, E.: Hereditary familial purpura simplex; review of 27 families, Lancet 1:145, 1941.
92. Davis, E.: The Schönlein-Henoch syndrome of vascular purpura, Blood 3:129, 1948.
93. Day, H. J., and Zarafonetis, C. J. D.: Coagulation studies in four patients with Ehlers-Danlos syndrome, Amer. J. Med. Sci. 242:565, 1961.
94. de Gabriele, G., and Penington, D. G.: Regulation of platelet production; "thrombopoietin," Brit. J. Haemat. 13:210, 1967.
95. DePree, M. J.: A case of giant hemangioma with thrombocytopenia, Acta Paediat. 52:410, 1963.
96. Derham, R. J., and Rogerson, M. M.: The Schönlein-Henoch syndrome and collagen disease, Arch. Dis. Child. 27:139, 1952.
97. Derham, R. J., and Rogerson, M. M.: The Schönlein-Henoch syndrome with particular reference to renal sequelae, Arch. Dis. Child. 31:364, 1956.
98. Diggs, L. W., and Hewlett, J. S.: A study of the bone marrow from thirty-six patients with idiopathic hemorrhagic (thrombopenic) purpura, Blood 3:1090, 1948.
99. Dignan, P. St. J., Mauer, A. M., and Frantz, C.: Phocomelia with congenital hypoplastic thrombocytopenia and myeloid leukemoid reactions, J. Pediat. 70:561, 1967.
100. Dingman, R. O., and Grabb, W. C.: Postinfectious intravascular thrombosis with gangrene, Plast. Reconstr. Surg. 31:58, 1963.
101. Distenfeld, A., and Oppenheim, E.: Treatment of acute thrombotic thrombocytopenic purpura with corticosteroids and splenectomy, Ann. Intern. Med. 65:245, 1966.
102. Dmochowski, L.: Viruses and tumors in light of electron microscope studies; review, Cancer Res. 20:977, 1960.
103. Doan, C. A.: Hypersplenism, Bull. N. Y. Acad. Med. 25:625, 1949.
104. Doan, C. A., Bouroncle, B. A., and Wiseman, B. K.: Idiopathic and secondary thrombocytopenic purpura; clinical study and evaluation of 381 cases over a period of 28 years, Ann. Intern. Med. 53:861, 1960.
105. Dodge, J. A., and Shillito, J., Jr.: Ehlers-Danlos syndrome associated with acquired encephalocele, J. Pediat. 66:1061, 1965.
106. Dodge, W. F., Daeschner, C. W., Jr., Brennan, J. C., Rosenberg, H. S., Travis, L. B., and Hopps, H. C.: Percutaneous renal biopsy in children. II. Acute glomerulonephritis, chronic glomerulonephritis and nephritis of anaphylactoid purpura, Pediatrics 30:297, 1962.
107. Dollberg, L., Casper, J., Djaldetti, M., Klibansky, C., and DeVries, A.: Lipid-laden histiocytes in the spleen in thrombocytopenic purpura, Amer. J. Clin. Path. 43:16, 1965.
108. Edelman, C. H., Jr.: The hemolytic-uremic syndrome (editorial), New Eng. J. Med. 281:1072, 1969.
109. Eisenstein, E. M.: Congenital amegakaryocytic thrombocytopenic purpura, Clin. Pediat. 5:143, 1966.
110. Elbe, S., and Stohlman, F., Jr.: Stimulation of thrombocytopoiesis in irradiated mice, Blood 35:783, 1970.
111. Emanuel, B., and Lieberman, A. D.: Intussusception due to Henoch-Schönlein purpura; case reports and review of the literature, Illinois M. J. 122:162, 1962.
112. Emery, J. L., Gordon, R. R., Rendle-Short, J., Varadi, S., and Warrach, A. J. M.: Congenital amegagaryocytic thrombocytopenia with congenital deformities and a leukemoid blood picture in the newborn, Blood 12:567, 1957.
113. Evans, R. S., and Duane, R. T.: Acquired hemolytic anemia; the relation of erythrocyte antibody production to activity of the disease; the significance of thrombocytopenia and leucopenia, Blood 4:1196, 1949.
114. Evans, R. S., Takahashi, K., Duane, A. B., Payne, R., and Iiu, C.: Primary thrombocytopenic purpura and acquired hemolytic anemia; evidence for a common etiology, Arch. Intern. Med. 87:48, 1951.
115. Faloon, W. W., Greene, R. W., and Lozner, E. L.: Hemostatic defect in thrombocytopenia as studied by use of ACTH and cortisone, Amer. J. Med. 13:12, 1952.
116. Feigin, R. D., Vietti, T. J., and Wyatt, R. G., Kaufman, D. G., and Smith, C. H., Jr.: Ataxia telangiectasia with granulocytopenia, J. Pediat. 77:431, 1970.
117. Feldt, R. H., and Stickler, G. B.: The gastrointestinal manifestations of anaphylactoid purpura in children, Proc. Staff Meet. Mayo Clin. 37:465, 1962.
118. Ferguson, A. W.: Rubella as a cause of thrombocytopenic purpura, Pediatrics 25:400, 1960.
119. Finch, S. C., and Finch, C. A.: Idiopathic hemochromatosis, an iron storage disease; iron metabolism in hemochromatosis, Medicine 34:381, 1955.
120. Fisher, B., Zuckerman, G. H., and Douglass, R. C.: Combined inheritance of purpura simplex and ptosis in four generations of one family, Blood 9:1199, 1954.
121. Fisher, E. R., and Creed, D. L.: Thrombotic thrombocytopenic purpura; report of

a case with discussion of its tinctorial features, Amer. J. Clin. Path. **25**:620, 1955.
122. Fisher, O. D., and Kraszewski, T. M.: Thrombocytopenic purpura following measles, Arch. Dis. Child. **27**:144, 1952.
123. Fost, N. C., and Esterly, N. B.: Successful treatment of juvenile hemangiomas with prednisone, J. Pediat. **72**:351, 1968.
124. Freiman, I., and Super, M.: Thrombocytopenia and congenital syphilis in South African Bantu infants, Arch. Dis. Child. **41**:87, 1966.
125. Frick, P. G., and Krafchuk, J. D.: Studies of hemostasis in the Ehlers-Danlos syndrome, J. Invest. Dermat. **26**:453, 1956.
126. Gairdner, D.: The Schönlein-Henoch syndrome (anaphylactoid purpura), Quart. J. Med. **17**:95, 1948.
127. Gasser, C., Gautier, E., Steck, A., Siebenmann, R. E., and Oeschlin, E.: Hämolytisch-urämische Syndrome; bilateral Nierenrindennekrosen bei akuten erwobenen hämolytisehen Anämien, Schweiz. med. Wchnschr. **85**:905, 1955.
128. Gellis, S. S., Reinhold, J. D. L., and Green, S.: Use of aspiration lung puncture in the diagnosis of idiopathic pulmonary hemosiderosis, Amer. J. Dis. Child. **85**:303, 1953.
129. Gervais, M., Richardson, J. B., Chiu, J., and Drummond, K. N.: Immunofluorescent and histologic findings in the hemolytic uremic syndrome, Pediatrics **47**:352, 1971.
130. Gianantonio, C. A., Vitacco, M., Fernando, M., and Gallo, G.: The hemolytic-uremic syndrome; renal status of 76 patients at long-term follow-up, J. Pediat. **72**:757, 1968.
131. Gianantonio, C. A., Vitacco, M., Mendilaharzu, J., Mendilaharzu, F., and Rutty, A.: Acute renal failure in infancy and childhood, J. Pediat. **61**:660, 1962.
132. Gianantonio, C., Vitacco, M., Mendilaharzu, F., Rutty, A., and Mendilaharzu, J.: The hemolytic-uremic syndrome, J. Pediat. **64**:478,1964.
133. Gilchrist, G. S., Lieberman, E., Ekert, H., Fine, R. N., and Grushkin, C.: Heparin therapy in the haemolytic-uraemic syndrome, Lancet **1**:1123, 1969.
134. Gilman, P. A., and Zinkham, W. H.: Severe idiopathic pulmonary hemosiderosis in the absence of clinical or radiologic evidence of pulmonary disease, J. Pediat. **75**:118, 1969.
135. Gilon, E., Ramot, B., and Sheba, C.: Multiple hemangiomata associated with thrombocytopenia; remarks on the pathogenesis of the thrombocytopenia in this syndrome, Blood **14**:74, 1959.
136. Glaser, J.: Letter to editor, Pediatrics **19**:1152, 1957.
137. Goldburgh, H. L., and Gouley, B. A.: Postpubertal menorrhagia and its possible relations to thrombocytopenic purpura hemorrhagica, Amer. J. Med. Sci. **200**:499, 1940.
138. Goldstein, G. W., Krivit, W. J., and Hong, R.: Hypoimmunoglobulin G, hyperimmunoglobulin M, intestinal nodular hyperplasia and thrombocytopenia, Arch. Dis. Child. **44**:621, 1969.
139. Good, R. A., and Thomas, L.: Studies of the generalized Shwartzman reaction. IV. Prevention of the local and generalized Shwartzman reaction with heparin, J. Exp. Med. **97**:871, 1953.
140. Good, T. A., Carnazzo, S. F., and Good, R. A.: Thrombocytopenia and giant hemangioma in infants, Amer. J. Dis. Child. **90**:260, 1955.
141. Gordon, R. R.: Aldrich's syndrome; familial thrombocytopenia, eczema and infection, Arch. Dis. Child. **35**:259, 1960.
142. Greene, R. W., Faloon, W. W., and Lozner, E. L.: The use of ACTH in preparing patients with idiopathic thrombocytopenic purpura for splenectomy, Amer. J. Med. Sci. **226**:203, 1953.
143. Greenwald, H. M., and Sherman, I.: Congenital essential thrombocytopenia, Amer. J. Dis. Child. **38**:1245, 1929.
144. Griffiths, J., and Irving, K. C.: Haemolytic uraemic syndrome in infants, Arch. Dis. Child. **36**:500, 1961.
145. Gross, R. E.: The surgery of infancy and childhood; its principles and techniques, Philadelphia, 1953, W. B. Saunders Co.
146. Grossman, H., Berdon, W., and Baker, D.: Abdominal pain in Schönlein-Henoch syndrome, Amer. J. Dis. Child. **108**:67, 1964.
147. Gröttum, K. A., Hovig, T., Holmsen, H., Abrahamsen, A. F., Jeremic, M., and Seip, M.: Wiskott-Aldrich syndrome; qualitative platelet defects and short platelet survival, Brit. J. Haemat. **17**:373, 1969.
148. Gröttum, K. A., Hovig, T., Holmsen, H., and Nordøy, A.: Wiskott-Aldrich syndrome; qualitative platelet defects and short platelet survival, Blood **34**:542, 1969.
149. Gutenberger, J., Trygstad, C. W., Stiehm, E. R., Opitz, J. M., Thatcher, L. G., Bloodworth, J. M. B., Jr., and Setzkorn, R.: Familial thrombocytopenia, elevated serum IgA levels and renal disease; a report of a kindred, Amer. J. Med. **49**:729, 1970.
150. Hall, J. G., Levin, J., Kuhn, J. P., Ottenheimer, E. J., von Berkum, K. A. P., and McKusick, V. A.: Thrombocytopenia with absent radius (TAR), Medicine **48**:411, 1969.
151. Halvorsen, S.: Cortisone treatment of idio-

pathic pulmonary hemosiderosis, Acta Paediat. 45:139, 1956.
152. Harley, J. D., Robin, H., and Robertson, S. E. J.: Thiazide-induced neonatal haemolysis? Brit. M. J. 1:696, 1964.
153. Harms, D., and Sachs, V.: Familial chronic thrombocytopenia with platelet autoantibodies, Acta Haemat. 34:30, 1965.
154. Harrington, W. J.: The clinical significance of antibodies for platelets, Sang 25:712, 1954.
155. Harrington, W. J., Hollingsworth, J. W., Minnich, V., and Moore, C. V.: Demonstration of thrombocytopenic factor in blood of patients with idiopathic thrombocytopenic purpura, J. Clin. Invest. 30:646, 1951.
156. Harrington, W. J., Sprague, C. C., Minnich, V., Moore, C. V., Ahlvin, R. C., and Dubach, R.: Immunologic mechanisms in idiopathic and neonatal thrombocytopenic purpura, Ann. Intern. Med. 38:433, 1953.
157. Heal, F. C., and Kent, G.: Purpura fulminans with afibrinogenemia, Canad. M.A.J. 69:367, 1953.
158. Heggie, A. D., and Weir, W. C.: Isolation of rubella virus from a mother and fetus, Pediatrics 34:278, 1964.
159. Heiner, D. C., Sears, J. W., and Kniker, W. T.: Multiple precipitins to cow's milk in chronic respiratory disease, Amer. J. Dis. Child. 103:634, 1962.
160. Hertzog, A. J.: Essential thrombocytopenic purpura; autopsy findings in thirty-six cases, J. Lab. Clin. Med. 32:618, 1947.
161. Hilgartner, M., Halvorson, E., and Smith, C. H.: Prognosis for idiopathic thrombocytopenic purpura in childhood, Program of the Society for Pediatric Research, 35th Annual Meeting, Philadelphia, May 4-6, 1965, p. 79.
162. Hilgartner, M. W., Lanzkowsky, P., and Smith, C. H.: The use of azathioprine in refractory idiopathic thrombocytopenic purpura in children, Acta Paediat. Scand. 59:409, 1970.
163. Hillman, R. S., and Phillips, L. L.: Clotting-fibrinolysis in a cavernous hemangioma, Amer. J. Dis. Child. 113:649, 1967.
164. Horowitz, H. I., and Nachman, R. L.: Drug purpura, Seminars Hemat. 2:287, 1965.
165. Hudson, J. B., Weinstein, L., and Chang, T. W.: Thrombocytopenic purpura in measles, J. Pediat. 48:48, 1956.
166. Hughes, L. A., and Wenzl, J. E.: Anaphylactoid purpura nephritis in children, Clin. Pediat. 8:594, 1969.
167. Hugh-Jones, K., Manfield, P. A., and Brewer, H. F.: Congenital thrombocytopenic purpura, Arch. Dis. Child. 35:146, 1960.
168. Huntley, C. C., and Dees, S. C.: Eczema associated with thrombocytopenic purpura and purulent otitis media, Pediatrics 19:351, 1957.
169. Hyatt, H. W., Jr.: Fatal recurrence of acute thrombocytopenic purpura in an 8-year-old Negro child, J. Pediat. 65:456, 1964.
170. Imahori, S., Bannerman, R. M., Graf, C. J., and Brennan, J. C.: Ehlers-Danlos syndrome with multiple arterial lesions, Amer. J. Med. 47:967, 1969.
171. Ingram, G. I. C.: Editorial review: the bleeding complication of blood transfusion, Transfusion 5:1, 1965.
172. Irvin, J. M., and Snowden, P. W.: Idiopathic pulmonary hemosiderosis, Amer. J. Dis. Child. 93:182, 1957.
173. Jacobson, B. M., and Vickery, A. L.: Hemolytic anemia and thrombopenia in an 84 year old woman; case record, New Eng. J. Med. 278:36, 1968.
174. Javett, S. N., and Senior, B.: Syndrome of hemolysis, thrombocytopenia, and nephropathy in infancy, Pediatrics 29:209, 1962.
175. Jim, R. T. S.: Thrombocytopenic purpura in cat-scratch disease, J.A.M.A. 176:1036, 1961.
176. Jiménez, E. L., and Dorrington, H. S.: Vaccination and Henoch-Schönlein purpura; correspondence, New Eng. J. Med. 279:1171, 1968.
177. Johnson, C. A., Abildgaard, C. F., and Schulman, I.: Functional studies of young versus old platelets in a patient with chronic thrombocytopenia, Blood 37:163, 1971.
178. Jones, H. W., and Tocantins, L. M.: The history of purpura hemorrhagica, Ann. Med. Hist. 5:349, 1933.
179. Jones, J. E., and Reed, J. F., Jr.: Renal vein thrombosis and thrombocytopenia in a newborn infant, J. Pediat. 67:681, 1965.
180. Jones, T. G., Goldsmith, K. L. G., and Anderson, I. M.: Maternal and neonatal platelet antibodies in a case of congenital thrombocytopenia, Lancet 2:1008, 1962.
181. Kaplan, E. Congenital and neonatal thrombocytopenic purpura, J. Pediat. 54:644, 1959.
182. Kaplan, E., and Klein, S. W.: Thrombocytopenia and intestinal bleeding in premature infants, J. Pediat. 61:17, 1962.
183. Karpati, G., Eissen, A. H., Andermann, F., Bacal, H. L., and Robb, P.: Ataxia telangiectasia; further observations and report of eight cases, Amer. J. Dis. Child. 110:51, 1965.
184. Kasabach, H. H., and Merritt, K. K.: Capillary hemangioma with extensive purpura; report of a case, Amer. J. Dis. Child. 59:1063, 1940.
185. Kaznelson, P.: Verschwinden der hämor-

rhagischen Diathese bei einem Falle von essentieller Thrombopenie (Frank) nach Milzextirpation, Wein, klin. Wchnschr. 29:1451, 1916.
186. Kelemen, E., Cserhati, I., and Tanos, B.: Demonstration and some properties of human thrombopoietin in thrombocythaemic sera, Acta Haemat. 20:350, 1958.
187. Kildeberg, P.: The Aldrich syndrome; report of a case and discussion of pathogenesis, Pediatrics 27:362, 1961.
188. Kolars, C. P., and Spink, W. W.: Thrombopenic purpura as a complication of mumps, J.A.M.A. 168:2213, 1958.
189. Koller, F., Gasser, C., Krüsi, G., and Muralt, G. de: Purpura fulminans nach Scharlach mit Factor V; Mangel und antithrombin Überschuss, Acta Haemat. 4:33, 1950.
190. Komrower, G. M., and Watson, G. H.: Prognosis in idiopathic thrombocytopenic purpura of childhood, Arch. Dis. Child. 29:502, 1954.
191. Korn, D.: Congenital hypoplastic thrombocytopenia; report of a case and review of the literature, Amer. J. Clin. Path. 37:405, 1962.
192. Kreidberg, M. B., Dameshek, W., and Latorraca, R.: Acute vascular (Schönlein-Henoch) purpura, an immunologic disorder? New Eng. J. Med. 253:1014, 1955.
193. Krevans, J. R., and Jackson, D. P.: Hemorrhagic disorder following massive whole blood transfusions, J.A.M.A. 159:171, 1955.
194. Krivit, W., and Good, R. A.: Aldrich's syndrome (thrombocytopenia, eczema and infection in infants); studies of the defense mechanisms, Amer. J. Dis. Child. 97:137, 1959.
195. Kuramoto, A., Steiner, M., and Baldini, M.: Lack of platelet response to stimulation in the Wiskott-Aldrich syndrome, New Eng. J. Med. 282:475, 1970.
196. Lamvik, J.: Acute glomerulonephritis with hemolytic anemia in infants; report of three fatal cases, Pediatrics 29:220, 1962.
197. Landing, B. H., Strauss, L., Crocker, A. C., Braunstein, H., Henley, W. L., Will, J. R., and Sanders, M.: Thrombocytopenic purpura with histiocytosis of the spleen, New Eng. J. Med. 265:572, 1961.
198. Landolt, R. F.: Kongenitale (neonatale) thrombopenien, Helvet. Paediat. Acta 3:3, 1948.
199. Lanzkowsky, P., and McCrory, W. W.: Disseminated intravascular coagulation as a possible factor in the pathogenesis of thrombotic microangiopathy (hemolytic-uremic syndrome), J. Pediat. 70:460, 1967.
200. Laros, R. K., Jr., and Penner, J. A.: "Refractory" thrombocytopenic purpura treated successfully with cyclophosphamide, J.A.M.A. 215:445, 1971.
201. Larrieu, M. J., Meshaka, G., Caen, J., and Bernard, J.: Traitement des purpura thrombopénique idiopathique, Sem. Hôp. Paris 40:403, 1964.
202. Lees, M. H., Menashe, V. D., Sunderland, C. O., Morgan, C. L., and Dawson, P. J.: Ehlers-Danlos syndrome associated with multiple pulmonary artery stenoses and tortuous system arteries, J. Pediat. 75:1031, 1969.
203. Leikin, S. L., Bazelon, M., and Park, K. H.: In vitro lymphocyte transformation in ataxia telangiectasia, J. Pediat. 68:477, 1966.
204. Levin, R. H., Pert, J. H., and Freireich, E. F.: Response to transfusion of platelets pooled from multiple donors and the effects of various technics of concentrating platelets, Transfusion 5:54, 1965.
205. Lewis, I. C., and Philpott, M. G.: Neurological complications in the Schönlein-Henoch syndrome, Arch. Dis. Child. 31:369, 1956.
206. Lieberman, E., Heuser, E., Donnell, G. N., Landing, B. H., and Hammond, G. D.: Hemolytic-uremic syndrome; clinical and pathological considerations, New Eng. J. Med 275:227, 1966.
207. Lisker, R., Nogueron, A., and Sanchez-Medal, L.: Plasma thromboplastin component deficiency in the Ehlers-Danlos syndrome, Ann. Intern. Med. 53:388, 1960.
208. Little, J. R.: Purpura fulminans treated successfully with anticoagulation; report of a case, J.A.M.A. 169:104, 1959.
209. Lock, S. P., and Dormandy, K. M.: Red cell fragmentation syndrome; a condition of multiple aetiology? Lancet 1:1020, 1961.
210. Louis-Bar, D.: Sur un syndrome progressit comprenant des telangiectasies capillaires cutanees et conjunctivales symetriques adisposition naevoide et des troubles cerebelleurs, Confin. Neurol. 4:32, 1941.
211. Lozner, E. L.: The thrombocytopenic purpuras, Bull. N. Y. Acad. Med. 30:184, 1954.
212. Lundstrom, R.: Rubella during pregnancy, Acta Paediat., supp. 133, 1962.
213. Lusher, J. M., and Zuelzer, W. W.: Idiopathic thrombocytopenic purpura in childhood, J. Pediat. 68:971, 1966.
214. MacFarlane, R. G.: The mechanism of haemostasis, Quart. J. Med. 10:1, 1941.
215. MacWhinney, J. B., Packer, J. T., Miller, G., and Greendyke, R. M.: Thrombotic thrombocytopenic purpura in childhood, Blood 19:181, 1962.
216. Margileth, A. M., and Museles, M.: Cutaneous hemangiomas in children, J.A.M.A. 194:523, 1965.

217. Markovitz, A.: Thrombocytopenia in Colorado tick fever, Arch. Intern. Med. 111:307, 1963.
218. Matsaniotis, N., Karpouzas, J., Apostolopoulou, E., and Messaritakis, J.: Idiopathic pulmonary haemosiderosis in children, Arch. Dis. Child. 43:307, 1968.
219. Mauer, A. M., DeVaux, L. O., and Lahey, M. E.: Neonatal and maternal thrombocytopenic purpura due to quinine, Pediatrics 19:84, 1957.
220. McAllenney, P. F., and Kristan, J. J.: Thrombopenic purpura in the newborn, Amer. J. Dis. Child. 78:401, 1949.
221. McCrory, W. W., and Shibuya, M.: Acute glomerulonephritis in childhood; long-term follow-up, N. Y. State J. Med. 68:2416, 1968.
222. McFarland, W., and Fuller, D. E.: Mortality in Ehlers-Danlos syndrome due to spontaneous rupture of large arteries, New Eng. J. Med. 271:1309, 1964.
223. McKusick, V. A.: Heritable disorders of connective tissue, ed. 3, St. Louis, 1966, The C. V. Mosby Co.
224. McLean, M. M., Jones, C. H., and Sutherland, D. A.: Haemolytic-uraemic syndrome; a report of an outbreak, Arch. Dis. Child. 41:76, 1966.
225. McQuiggan, M. C., Oliver, W. J.: Littler, E. R., and Cerny, J. C.: Hemolytic uremic syndrome, J.A.M.A. 191:787, 1965.
226. Meadl, M. A., Watson, J. I., and Rose, B.: The Wiscott-Aldrich syndrome; immunopathologic mechanisms and a long-term survival, Ann. Intern. Med. 68:1050, 1968.
227. Merenstein, G. B., O'Loughlin, E. P., and Plunket, D. C.: Effects of maternal thiazides on platelet counts of newborn infants, J. Pediat. 76:766, 1970.
228. Mettler, N. E.: Isolation of a microtatobiote from patients with hemolytic-uremic syndrome and thrombotic thrombocytopenic purpura and from mites in the United States. New Eng. J. Med. 281:1023, 1969.
229. Minot, G. R.: Purpura hemorrhagica with lymphocytosis; acute type and intermittent menstrual type, Amer. J. Med. Sci. 192:445, 1936.
230. Monnens, L. A. H., and Retera, R. J. M.: Thrombotic thrombocytopenic purpura in a neonatal infant, J. Pediat. 71:118, 1967.
231. Moorhead, J. F.: Thrombotic thrombocytopenic purpura; recovery after splenectomy, Arch. Intern. Med. 117:284, 1966.
232. Moorhead, J. F., Edwards, E. C., and Goldsmith, H. J.: Hemodialysis of three children and one infant with a haemolytic-uraemic syndrome, Lancet 1:570, 1965.
233. Morris, M. B.: Thrombocytopenic purpura in the newborn, Arch. Dis. Child. 29:75, 1954.
234. Morrison, F. S., and Mollison, P. L.: Post-transfusion purpura, New Eng. J. Med. 275:243, 1966.
235. Morse E. E.: Topics in internal medicine; post-transfusion thrombocytopenic purpura, Johns Hopkins Med. J. 121:365, 1967.
236. Morse, E. E., Zinkham, W. H., and Jackson, D. P.: Thrombocytopenic purpura following rubella infection in children and adults, Arch. Intern. Med. 117:573, 1966.
237. Moschcowitz, E.: An acute febrile pleiochromic anemia with hyaline thrombosis of the terminal arterioles and capillaries, Arch. Intern. Med. 36:89, 1925.
238. Murphy, S., Oski, F. A., and Gardner, F. H.: Hereditary thrombocytopenia with an intrinsic platelet defect, New Eng. J. Med. 281:857, 1969.
239. Najean, Y., Ardaillou, N., Caen, J., Larrieu, M-J., and Bernard, J.: Survival of radio-chromium-labeled platelets in thrombocytopenias, Blood 22:718, 1963.
240. Najean, Y., Ardaillou, N., Dresch, C., and Bernard, J.: The platelet destruction site in thrombocytopenic purpuras, Brit. J. Haemat. 13:409, 1967.
241. Nelson, J., and Goldstein, N.: Nature of Waterhouse-Friderichsen syndrome; report of case with successful treatment with cortisone, J.A.M.A. 146:1193, 1951.
242. Newton, W. A., Jr., and Zuelzer, W. W.: Idiopathic thrombopenic purpura in childhood, New Eng. J. Med. 245:879, 1951.
243. Nilsson, L. R., and Landholm, G.: Congenital thrombocytopenia associated with aplasia of the radius, Acta Paediat. 49:29, 1960.
244. O'Brien, L. J., and Sibley, W. A.: Neurologic manifestations of thrombotic thrombocytopenic purpura, Neurology 8:55, 1958.
245. Odell, T. T., and Kniseley, R. M.: The origin, lifespan, regulation, and fate of blood platelets. In Tocantins, L. M., editor: Progress in hematology, vol. 3, New York, 1962, Grune & Stratton, Inc.
246. Ognibene, A. J., and Johnson, D. E.: Idiopathic pulmonary hemosiderosis in adults; report of case and review of literature, Arch. Intern. Med. 111:503, 1963.
247. O'Gorman-Hughes, D. W.: Neonatal thrombocytopenia; assessment of aetiology and prognosis, Aust. Paediat. J. 3:276, 1967.
248. Oliver, T. K., Jr., and Barnett, H. L.: The incidence and prognosis of nephritis associated with anaphylactoid (Schönlein-Henoch) purpura in children, Amer. J. Dis. Child. 90:544, 1955.

249. Oski, F. A., and Naiman, J. L.: Effect of live measles vaccine on the platelet count, New Eng. J. Med. 275:352, 1966.
250. Oski, F. A., Naiman, J. L., and Diamond, L. K.: Use of the plasma acid phosphatase value in the differentiation of thrombocytopenic states, New Eng. J. Med. 268:1423, 1963.
251. Osler, W.: On the visceral manifestations of the erythema group of skin diseases, Amer. J. Med. Sci. 127:1, 1904.
252. Patterson, J. H., Pierce, R. B., Amerson, J. R., and Watkins, W. L.: Dextran therapy of purpura fulminans, New Eng. J. Med. 273:734, 1965.
253. Pearson, H. A., Shulman, N. R., Marder, V. J., and Cone, T. E.: Isoimmune neonatal thrombocytopenic purpura; clinical and therapeutic consideration, Blood 23:154, 1964.
254. Pearson, H. A., Shulman, N. R., Oski, F. A., and Eitzman, D. V.: Platelet survival in Wiskott-Aldrich syndrome, J. Pediat. 68:754, 1966.
255. Penny, R., Rozenberg, M. C., and Firkin, B. G.: The splenic platelet pool, Blood 27:1, 1966.
256. Pepper, H., Liebowitz, D., and Lindsay, S.: Cyclical thrombocytopenic purpura related to the menstrual cycle, Arch. Path. 61:1, 1956.
257. Peterson, R., Cooper, M., and Good, R.: The pathogenesis of immunologic deficiency diseases, Amer. J. Med. 38:579, 1965.
258. Peterson, R. D. A., Kelly, W. O., and Good, R. A.: Ataxia telangiectasia; its association with a defective thymus, immunological-deficiency disease and malignancy, Lancet 1:1189, 1964.
259. Phillips, C. A., Melnick, J. L., Yow, M. D., Bayatpour, M., and Burkhardt, M.: Persistence of virus in infants with congenital rubella and in normal infants with a history of maternal rubella, J.A.M.A. 193:1027, 1965.
260. Piel, C. F., and Phibbs, R. H.: The hemolytic-uremic syndrome, Ped. Clin. N. Amer. 13:295, 1966.
261. Pierre, R., and Linman, J. W.: Studies on thrombopoiesis—promoting activity of normal urine, Proc. Soc. Exp. Biol. Med. 113:398, 1963.
262. Piessens, W. F., Wybran, J., Manaster, J., and Strijckmans, P. A.: Lymphocyte transformation induced by autologous platelets in a case of thrombocytopenic purpura, Blood 36:421, 1970.
263. Pohle, F. J.: Blood platelet count in relation to menstrual cycle in normal women, Amer. J. Med. Sci. 197:40, 1939.
264. Poley, J. R., and Stickler, G. B.: Petechiae in the newborn infant, Amer. J. Dis. Child. 102:365, 1961.
265. Quick, A. J.: Telangiectasia; its relationship to the Minot–von Willebrand syndrome, Amer. J. Med. Sci. 254:585, 1967.
266. Quick, A. J., and Hussey, C. V.: Hereditary thrombopathic thrombocytopenia, Amer. J. Med. Sci. 245:643, 1963.
267. Rabinowitz, Y., and Dameshek, W.: Systemic lupus erythematosus after "idiopathic" thrombocytopenic purpura; review, Ann. Intern Med. 52:1, 1960.
268. Radel, E. G., and Schorr, J. B.: Thrombocytopenic purpura with infectious mononucleosis, J. Pediat. 63:46, 1963.
269. Rausen, A. R., London, R. D., Mizrahi, A., and Cooper, L. Z.: Generalized bone changes and thrombocytopenic purpura in association with intrauterine rubella, Pediatrics 36:264, 1965.
270. Rausen, A. R., Richter, P., Tallal, L., and Cooper, L. Z.: Hematologic effect of intrauterine rubella, J.A.M.A. 199:75, 1967.
271. Repetto, G., Lisboa, C., Emparanza, E., Ferretti, R., Neira, M., Etchart, M., and Meneghello, J.: Idiopathic pulmonary hemosiderosis; clinical, radiological and respiratory function studies, Pediatrics 40:24, 1967.
272. Rich, A. R.: Hypersensitivity in diseases, Harvey Lect. 42:106, 1946-1947.
273. Riddle, J. M., Kashiwagi, H., Abraham, J. P., and Frame, B.: Ultrastructural platelet abnormalities in Ehlers-Danlos syndrome, J. Lab. Clin. Med. 64:998, 1964.
274. Rivera, A. M., and Brehusen, F. C.: Aldrich's syndrome; a report of a case with subperiosteal hemorrhage, J. Pediat. 57:86, 1960.
275. Roberts, M. H., and Smith, M. H.: Thrombocytopenic purpura; report of four cases in one family, Amer. J. Dis. Child. 79:820, 1950.
276. Robson, H. N., and Walker, C. H. M.: Congenital and neonatal thrombocytopenic purpura, Arch. Dis. Child. 26:175, 1951.
277. Rodriguez, S. U., Leikin, S. L., and Hiller, M. C.: Neonatal thrombocytopenia associated with antepartum administration of thiazide drugs, New Eng. J. Med. 270:881, 1964.
278. Rolovic, Z., and Baldini, M.: Megakaryocytopoiesis in splenectomized and "hypersplenic" rats, Brit. J. Haemat. 18:257, 1970.
279. Root, A. W., and Speicher, C. E.: The triad of thrombocytopenia, eczema and recurrent infections (Wiskott-Aldrich syndrome) associated with milk antibodies, giant-cell pneumonia, and cytomegalic inclusion disease, Pediatrics 31:444, 1963.

280. Rosenthal, D., Schwartz, H. C., Yaffe, S. J., and Kretchmer, N.: The syndrome of hemolytic anemia, thrombocytopenia, and uremia, Amer. J. Dis. Child. 104:473, 1962.
281. Rosenthal, I. M., Markowitz, A. S., and Medenis, R.: Immunologic incompetence in ataxia-telangiectasia, Amer. J. Dis. Child. 110:69, 1965.
282. Rubenberg, M. L., Regoeczi, E., Bull, B. S., Dacie, J. V., and Brain, M. C.: Microangiopathic haemolytic anaemia; the experimental production of haemolysis and red-cell fragmentation by defibrination in vivo, Brit. J. Haemat. 14:627, 1968.
283. Rubio, T., Riley, H. D., Jr., Nida, J. R., Brooksaler, F., and Nelson, J. D.: Thrombocytopenia in Rocky Mountain spotted fever, Amer. J. Dis. Child. 116:88, 1968.
284. Rudolph, A. J., Yow, M. D., Phillips, C. A., Desmond, M. M., Blattner, R. J., and Melnick, J. L.: Transplacental rubella infection in newly born infants, J.A.M.A. 191:843, 1965.
285. St. Geme, J. W., Jr., Prince, J. T., Burke, B. A., Good, R. A., and Krivit, W.: Impaired cellular resistance to herpes-simplex virus in Wiskott-Aldrich syndrome, New Eng. J. Med. 273:229, 1965.
286. Saltzstein, S. L.: Phospholipid accumulation in histiocytes of splenic pulp associated with thrombocytopenic purpura, Blood 18:73, 1961.
287. Sanarelli, G.: De la pathogénie du choléra expérimental, Ann. Inst. Pasteur 38:11, 1924.
288. Sanchez-Avalos, J., Vitacco, M., Molinas, F., Penalver, J., and Gianantonio, C.: Coagulation studies in the hemolytic-uremic syndrome, J. Pediat. 76:538, 1970.
289. Schaar, F. E.: Familial idiopathic thrombocytopenic purpura, J. Pediat. 62:546, 1963.
290. Scharfman, W. A., Tartaglia, A. P., and Propp, S.: Splenectomy preceding surgical intervention in idiopathic thrombocytopenic purpura, Arch. Intern. Med. 116:406, 1965.
291. Schoen, E. J., King, A. L., and Duane, R. T.: Neonatal thrombocytopenic purpura, Pediatrics 17:72, 1956.
292. Schulman, I.: Diagnosis and treatment; management of idiopathic thrombocytopenic purpura, Pediatrics 33:979, 1964.
293. Schulman, I., Pierce, M., Lukens, A., Currimbhoy, Z., and Fort, E.: A factor in normal human plasma which stimulates platelet production; chronic thrombocytopenic purpura due to its deficiency, Amer. J. Dis. Child. 98:633, 1959.
294. Schulman, I., Pierce, M., Lukens, A., and Currimbhoy, Z.: Studies on thrombopoiesis. I. A factor in normal human plasma required for platelet production; chronic thrombocytopenia due to its deficiency, Blood 16:943, 1960.
295. Schulman, I., Smith, C. H., and Ando, R. E.: Congenital thrombocytopenic purpura; observations in three infants of a nonaffected mother; demonstration of platelet agglutinin and evidence for platelet isoimmunization, Amer. J. Dis. Child. 88:784, 1954.
296. Schwartz, R., and Dameshek, W.: Treatment of autoimmune hemolytic anemia with 6-mercaptopurine and thioguanine, Blood 19:483, 1962.
297. Schwartz, S. O.: Prognostic value of marrow eosinophils in thrombocytopenic purpura, Amer. J. Med. Sci. 209:579, 1945.
298. Schwartz, S. O., and Kaplan, S. R.: Thrombocytopenic purpura; the prognostic and therapeutic value of the eosinophil index; an analysis of 100 cases, Amer. J. Med. Sci. 219:528, 1950.
299. Schwartz, S. O., and Motto, S. A.: The diagnostic significance of "burr red cells," Amer. J. Med. Sci. 218:563, 1949.
300. Seip, M.: Hereditary, hypoplastic thrombocytopenia, Acta Paediat. 52:370, 1963.
301. Sestak, Z.: Ehlers-Danlos syndrome and cutis laxa; an account of families in the Oxford area, Ann. Human Genet. 25:313, 1962.
302. Shapiro, C. M., Kanter, A., Lopas, H., and Rabiner, S. F.: Hemolytic-uremic syndrome in adults, J.A.M.A. 213:567, 1970.
303. Shaw, S., and Oliver, R. A. M.: Congenital hypoplastic thrombocytopenia with skeletal deformities, Blood 14:374, 1959.
304. Sheth, N. K., and Prankerd, T. A. J.: Inherited thrombocytopenia with thrombasthenia, J. Clin. Path. 21:154, 1968.
305. Shinton, N. K., Galpine, J. F., Kendall, A. C., and Williams, H. P.: Haemolytic anaemia with acute renal disease, Arch. Dis. Child. 39:455, 1964.
306. Shulman, N. R., Aster, R. H., Leitner, A., and Hiller, M. C.: Immunoreactions involving platelets; post-transfusion purpura due to a complement-fixing antibody against a genetically controlled platelet antigen; a proposed mechanism for thrombocytopenia and its relevance in "autoimmunity," J. Clin. Invest. 40:1597, 1961.
307. Shumway, C. N., Jr., and Miller, G.: An unusual syndrome of hemolytic anemia, thrombocytopenic purpura and renal disease, Blood 12:1045, 1957.
308. Shumway, C. N., and Terplan, K. L.: Hemolytic anemia, thrombocytopenia, and renal disease in childhood; the hemolytic-uremic syndrome, Ped. Clin. N. Amer. 11:577, 1964.

309. Shwartzman, G.: Phenomenon of local tissue reactivity and its immunological, pathological and clinical significance, New York, 1937, Paul B. Hoeber, Inc.
310. Silber, R., Benitez, R., Ereland, W. C., Akeroyd, J. H., and Dunne, C. J.: The application of fluorescent antibody methods to the study of platelets, Blood 16:958, 1960.
311. Silver, H. K., Aggeler, P. M., and Crane, J. T.: Hemangioma (capillary and cavernous) with thrombocytopenic purpura; report of a case with observations at autopsy, Amer. J. Dis. Child. 76:513, 1948.
312. Simpkiss, M. J., and Cathie, I. A. B.: Splenectomy for idiopathic thrombocytopenic purpura, Great Ormond St. J. 7:9, 1954.
313. Singer, K.: Thrombotic thrombocytopenic purpura. In Snapper, I., and Dock, W., editors: Advances in internal medicine, vol. 6, Chicago, 1954, Year Book Medical Publishers, Inc., p. 195.
314. Smith, C. H.: Dermatorrhexis (Ehlers-Danlos syndrome), J. Pediat. 14:632, 1939.
315. Smith, C. H.: Blood diseases of infancy and childhood, ed. 2, St. Louis, 1969, The C. V. Mosby Co., pp. 714-715.
316. Smith, C. H., Erlandson, M., Schulman, I., and Stern, G.: Hazard of severe infections in splenectomized infants and children, Amer. J. Med. 22:390, 1957.
317. Smith, C. H., and Khakoo, Y.: Burr cells; classification and effect of splenectomy, J. Pediat. 76:99, 1970.
318. Smith, J. L., and Lineback, M. I.: Hereditary hemorrhagic telangiectasia; nine cases in one Negro family with special reference to hepatic lesions, Amer. J. Med. 17:41, 1954.
319. Smith, W. E., and Fienberg, R.: Early nonrecurrent idiopathic pulmonary hemosiderosis in an adult; report of a case, New Eng. J. Med. 259:808, 1958.
320. Soergel, K. H.: Idiopathic pulmonary hemosiderosis; review and report of two cases, Pediatrics 19:1101, 1957.
321. Soergel, K. H., and Sommers, S. C.: Idiopathic pulmonary hemosiderosis and related syndromes, Amer. J. Med. 32:499, 1962.
322. Stamey, C. C., Mauley, J. H., and London, A. H.: Purpura fulminans following chickenpox, North Carolina M. J. 17:115, 1956.
323. Steen, E., and Torp, K. H.: Encephalitis and thrombocytopenic purpura after rubella, Arch. Dis. Child. 31:470, 1956.
324. Stefanini, M.: Management of thrombocytopenic states, Arch. Intern. Med. 95:543, 1955.
325. Stefanini, M., and Chatterjea, J. B.: Studies on platelets IV, Proc. Soc. Exp. Biol. Med. 79:623, 1952.
326. Stefanini, M., and Dameshek, W.: The hemorrhagic disorders; a clinical and therapeutic approach, New York, 1955, Grune & Stratton, Inc.
327. Stefanini, M., Roy, C. A., Zannos, L., and Dameshek, W.: Therapeutic effect of pituitary adrenocorticotropic hormone (ACTH) in case of Henoch-Schönlein vascular (anaphylactoid) purpura, J.A.M.A. 144:1372, 1950.
328. Stefanini, M., and Mednicoff, I.: Demonstration of antivessel agents in serum of patients with anaphylactoid purpura and periarteritis nodosa, J. Clin. Invest. 33:967, 1954.
329. Stefanini, M., Piomelli, S., Mele, R., Ostroski, J. T., and Colpoys, W. P.: Acute vascular purpura following immunization with Asiatic-influenza vaccine, New Eng. J. Med. 259:9, 1958.
330. Steiner, B.: Essential pulmonary haemosiderosis as an immuno-haematological problem, Arch. Dis. Child. 29:391, 1954.
331. Steiner, B.: Ethylenediaminetetraacetic acid (EDTA) in treatment of essential pulmonary haemosiderosis, Helvet. Paediat. Acta 16:97, 1961.
332. Steiner, B., and Nabrady, J.: Immunoallergic lung purpura treated with azathioprine, Lancet 1:140, 1965.
333. Steinhardt, I. D., and Jonas, A. F.: Coexistence of intussusception and Henoch's purpura, New Eng. J. Med. 257:553, 1957.
334. Steinkamp, R., Moore, C. V., and Doubeck, W. G.: Thrombocytopenic purpura caused by hypersensitivity to quinine, J. Lab. Clin. Med. 45:18, 1955.
335. Stiehm, E. R., Vaerman, J-P., and Fudenberg, H. H.: Plasma infusions in immunologic deficiency states; metabolic and therapeutic studies, Blood 28:918, 1966.
336. Summer, G. K.: The Ehlers-Danlos syndrome, Amer. J. Dis. Child. 91:419, 1956.
337. Susman, L. N.: Azathioprine in refractory idiopathic thrombocytopenic purpura, J.A.M.A. 202:259, 1967.
338. Sutherland, D. A., and Clark, H.: Hemangioma associated with thrombocytopenia; report of a case and review of the literature, Amer. J. Med. 33:150, 1962.
339. Swaiman, K., Schaffhausen, M., and Krivit, W.: Thrombotic thrombocytopenic purpura; report of an unusual clinical case and chromium[51] red cell survival studies, J. Pediat. 60:823, 1962.
340. Tadjoedin, M. K., and Fraser, F. C.: Heredity of ataxia-telangiectasia (Louis-Bar syndrome), Amer. J. Dis. Child. 110:64, 1965.
341. Taub, R. M., Rodriguez-Erdmann, F., and Dameshek, W.: Intravascular coagulation,

the Shwartzman reaction and the pathogenesis of I.T.P., Blood **24**:775, 1964.
342. ten Bensel, R. W., Stadlan, E. M., and Krivit, W.: The development of malignancy in the course of the Aldrich syndrome, J. Pediat. **68**:761, 1966.
343. Thatcher, L. G., Clatanoff, D. V., and Stiehm, E. R.: Splenic hemangioma with thrombocyotpenia and afibrinogenemia, J. Pediat. **73**:345, 1968.
344. Tidy, H. L.: Haemorrhagic diathesis; angiostaxis, Lancet **2**:365, 1926.
345. Towner, C. H.: Familial incidence of the Henoch-Schönlein syndrome, Brit. M. J. **2**:1385, 1959.
346. Tucker, D. H., Miller, D. E., and Jacoby, W. J., Jr.: Ehlers-Danlos syndrome with sinus of Valsalva aneurysm and aortic insufficiency simulating rheumatic heart disease, Amer. J. Med. **35**:715, 1963.
347. Valberg, L. S., and Brown, G. M.: Haemorrhagic capillary disorder associated with antihaemophilic globulin deficiency, Medicine **37**:181, 1958.
348. Van Creveld, S., Ho, L. K., and Veder, H. A.: Thrombopathia, Acta Haemat. **19**:199, 1958.
349. Van der Horst, R. L.: Purpura fulminans in a newborn infant, Arch. Dis. Child. **37**:436, 1962.
350. Vernier, R. L.: Kidney biopsy in the study of renal disease. In Kelley, V. C., editor: Symposium on recent clinical advances, Ped. Clin. N. Amer. **7**:353, 1960.
351. Vernier, R. L., Farquhar, M. G., Brunson, J. G., and Good, R. A.: Chronic renal disease in children; correlation of clinical findings with morphologic characteristics seen by light and electron microscopy, Amer. J. Dis. Child. **96**:306, 1958.
352. Vernier, R. L., Worthen, H. G., Peterson, R. D., Colle, E., and Good, R. A.: Anaphylactoid purpura. I. Pathology of the skin and kidney and frequency of streptococcal infection, Pediatrics **27**:181, 1961.
353. Verstraete, M., Vermylen, C., Vermylen, J., and Vandenbroucke J.: Excessive consumption of blood coagulation components as cause of hemorrhagic diathesis, Amer. J. Med. **38**:899, 1965.
354. Vestermark, B., and Vestermark, S.: Familial sex-linked thrombocytopenia, Acta Paediat. **53**:365, 1964.
355. Villasenor, J. B., and Ambrosius, K.: Thrombotic thrombocytopenic purpura; report of a case with some unusual characteristics, Ann. Intern. Med. **46**:378, 1957.
356. Wacksman, S. J., Flessa, H. C., Glueck, H. I., and Will, J. J.: Coagulation defects and giant cavernous hemangioma; a case study in infancy, Amer. J. Dis. Child. **111**:71, 1966.
357. Waddell, W. B., Saltzman, H. A., Fuson, R. I., and Harris, J.: Purpura gangrenosa treated with hyperbaric oxygenation, J.A.M.A. **191**:971, 1965.
358. Walker, J. H., and Walker, W.: Idiopathic thrombocytopenic purpura in childhood, Arch. Dis. Child. **36**:649, 1961.
359. Wallace, S.: Thrombocytopenic purpura after rubella, Lancet **1**:139, 1963.
360. Wallerstein, R. O.: Spontaneous involution of giant hemangioma, Amer. J. Dis. Child. **102**:111, 1961.
361. Watson-Williams, E. J., Macpherson, A. I. S., and Davidson, S.: The treatment of idiopathic thrombocytopenic purpura; a review of ninety-three cases, Lancet **2**:221, 1958.
362. Webb, B. D., Dubs, E. J., and Conrad, E.: Postscarlatinal gangrene with prolonged prothrombin time, J. Pediat. **30**:76, 1947.
363. Wedgewood, R. J. P., and Klaus, M. H.: Anaphylactoid purpura (Schönlein-Henoch syndrome); a long term followup study with special reference to renal involvement, Pediatrics **16**:196, 1955.
364. Wehninger, H., and Künzer, W.: Haemolytic-uraemic syndrome, Lancet **2**:1085, 1968.
365. Welch, R. G.: Thrombocytopenic purpura and chicken-pox, Arch. Dis. Child. **31**:38, 1956.
366. Wells, E. B.: Hereditary hemorrhagic telangiectasia, Amer. J. Med. Sci. **211**:577, 1946.
367. Whitney, L. H., and Barritt, A. S., Jr.: Spontaneous and hereditary thrombopenic purpura in a mother and two sons, Amer. J. Dis. Child. **64**:705, 1942.
368. Wigod, M.: Idiopathic pulmonary hemosiderosis; report of a case in early childhood with severe anemia, New Eng. J. Med. **253**:413, 1955.
369. Wile, S. A., and Sturgeon, P.: Thrombotic thrombocytopenic purpura; review of the subject with a report of three cases in children, Pediatrics **17**:882, 1956.
370. Wilhelm, D. J., and Paegle, R. E.: Thrombocytopenic purpura and pneumonia following measles vaccination, Amer. J. Dis. Child. **113**:534, 1967.
371. Williams, G. A., and Brick, I. B.: Gastrointestinal bleeding in hereditary hemorrhagic telangiectasia, Arch. Intern. Med. **95**:41, 1955.
372. Winkelman, R. K.: Clinical and pathologic findings in the skin in anaphylactoid purpura (allergic angiitis), Proc. Staff Meet. Mayo Clin. **33**:277, 1958.
373. Winkelman, R. K., and Ditto, W. B.: Cutaneous and visceral syndromes of necrotizing

or "allergic" angiities; a study of 38 cases, Medicine 43:59, 1964.
374. Wiskott, A.: Familiarer angeborener Morbus Werlhofii, Monatsschr. Kinderh. 68:212, 1937.
375. Witt, L. J.: Chronic leg ulcer in purpura hemorrhagica; report of two cases, Brit. M. J. 2:309, 1942.
376. Wolff, J. A.: Wiskott-Aldrich syndrome; clinical, immunologic and pathologic observations, J. Pediat. 70:221, 1967.
377. Wolff, J. A., and Bertucio, M.: A sex-linked genetic syndrome in a Negro family manifested by thrombocytopenia, eczema, bloody diarrhea, recurrent infection, anemia and epistaxis, Amer. J. Dis. Child. 93:74, 1957.
378. Wyllie, W. G., Sheldon, W., Bodian, M., and Barlow, A.: Idiopathic pulmonary haemosiderosis, Quart. J. Med. 17:25, 1948.
379. Zinkham, W. H., Medearis, D. N., Jr., and Osborn, J. E.: Blood and bone marrow in congenital rubella, J. Pediat. 71:512, 1967.
380. Zucker, M. B., and Woodward, H. Q.: Elevation of serum acid glycerophosphatase activity in thrombocytosis, J. Lab. Clin. Med. 59:760, 1962.

# Author index

**A**

Aach, R., 431
Aagenæes, Ø, 124
Aarskog, D., 520
Aase, J. M., 284
Aballi, A., 19, 20, 717
Abbatt, J. D., 588
Abbott, R. R., 510
Abbuhl, J. W., 649
Abe, T., 746
Abelson, N. M., 147, 173, 177
Abernathy, M. R., 501
Abildgaard, C. F., 284, 464, 746, 751, 757, 808, 810, 813
Ablin, A. R., 20, 622, 808
Abraham, J. P., 464, 816
Abrahamov, A., 6, 10, 444
Abrahams, C., 234
Abrahamsen, A. F., 750, 812
Abrams, G. D., 586
Abrams, I., 238
Abt, A. F., 284, 674
Acevedo, G., 674
Achong, B. G., 548
Ackerman, B. D., 71, 147
Ackerman, G. A., 501, 586
Ackerman, L. V., 649, 674
Ackroyd, J. F., 338, 746, 794, 808
Adam, A., 348, 350, 508
Adams, D. W., 150
Adams, E. B., 256, 520
Adams, F. H., 58, 464
Adams, J. T., 173
Adams, M. A., 758
Adams, W. S., 522, 535
Adamson, J., 467
Adelson, E., 339, 550, 746, 808
Adinolfi, M., 433
Adner, M. M., 522, 808
Afifi, A. M., 216, 234
Aftahi, F., 174
Agathopoulos, A., 87, 441
Ager, E. A., 593
Ager, J. A. M., 431, 435, 436, 441, 448
Aggeler, P. M., 288, 327, 350, 464, 587, 746, 751, 752, 756, 818
Agle, D. P., 203
Ahern, E. J., 679
Aherne, W. A., 71
Ahlvin, R. C., 813
Ahnquist, G., 674
Ahrens, E. H., Jr., 124
Aidin, R., 147
Ainger, L. E., 71, 675
Airo, R., 751
Aisenberg, A. C., 641, 647, 808
Aisner, M., 586
Akabane, T., 442, 753
Akatsaka, J., 284
Akerblom, O., 431
Akeroyd, J. H., 58, 59, 291, 341, 818

Akerren, Y., 124
Aksoy, M., 234, 431
Aladag, T., 431
Alavi, I., 443
Albright, C. D., 348
Albritton, E. C., 20
Alcalde, V., 746
Alcayaga, R., 468
Aldrich, C. A., 348
Aldrich, R. A., 234, 338, 808
Aldridge, J. E., 443
Aledort, L. M., 758
Alexander, B., 746, 755
Alexander, F., 464
Alexander, M. J., 488, 627, 650
Alexander, S., 675
Alford, C. A., 30, 33, 780, 808
Alfrey, C. P., Jr., 284, 464, 466
Alison, F., 14, 20
Alki, A. A., 588
Allan, A. G. E., 758
Allansmith, M., 31, 33
Allen, D. M., 177, 284, 285, 507, 623, 678, 746, 794, 799, 808
Allen, D. W., 10, 58, 237
Allen, E. L., 129
Allen, F. A., 675
Allen, F. H., Jr., 85, 87, 101, 127, 147, 148, 150, 174, 507, 547
Allen, J. C., 85, 431
Allen, R. A., 586
Allen, T. D., 431
Allen, V. R., 547
Allen, W. M., 21, 237
Allison, A. A., 339
Allison, A. C., 124, 147, 284, 431, 432, 675, 808
Allmeling, A., 15, 21
Almeida, J. D., 586
Almklov, J. R., 586
Alper, T., 234
Alperin, J. B., 432
Alpert, L. I., 110, 124
Alpert, M. E., 675
Al-Rashid, R. A., 586
Alsever, J., 751
Alt, A. L., 20
Alt, H. L., 547, 808
Altay, C., 748
Alter, A. A., 285, 534
Alter, H. J., 101, 102, 433, 587, 808
Alterman, K., 124
Altman, A. A., 149
Altman, K. I., 284, 351
Altman, K. L., 348
Altman, S. J., 625
Alton, H. G., 747
Alvarado, J., 101, 622
Alving, A. S., 339, 340, 342, 350

Ambrosius, K., 819
Ambrus, C. N., 502
Ambrus, J. C., 502
Ambuel, J. P., 154, 178
Amerman, E. E., 174
Amerson, J. R., 816
Ames, S. B., 750, 751, 756
Amiel, J. L., 103, 287, 541, 626
Amorosi, E., 73, 785, 808
Amundsen, M. A., 754
Andelman, M. B., 234
Andermann, F., 813
Andersen, D. H., 150
Anderson, A. F., 234
Anderson, C. M., 256
Anderson, D. H., 127, 590
Anderson, E. E., 129
Anderson, H. M., 350, 509
Anderson, I. M., 813
Anderson, J. W., 442, 443
Anderson, L. M., 256
Anderson, O. W., 202
Anderson, R., 432
Anderson, R. C., 586
Anderson, R. E., 85, 502, 647
Anderson, R. L., 339
Anderson, S. B., 284
Anderson, W. A. D., 647
Anderson, W. F., 443
Ando, R. E., 62, 103, 177, 288, 447, 817
Andre, J. A., 808
Andreeva, M., 435
Andresen, M. I., 21
Andrews, J. R., 520
Angella, J. J., 174
Angelopoulos, B., 11, 746
Angle, C. R., 464
Angle, R. M., 547, 808
Angus, J., 128, 149
Anjou, H., 523
Anrode, H. G., 174
Anstall, H. B., 102
Anthony, B., 128, 808
Anthony, P. P., 808
Antley, R. M., 808
Apell, G., 439
Apostolopoulou, E., 815
Applewhaite, F., 440
ap Rees, W., 339
Apt, L., 5, 10, 130, 235, 510, 746, 808
Arcomano, J. P., 808
Ardaillou, N., 815
Ardeman, S., 502
Ardner, F. C., 548
Arends, T., 432, 753
Arey, J. B., 176, 203
Arey, L. B., 10
Arias, D., 20
Arias, I. M., 125, 126, 128
Armbruster, R., 149
Armstrong, D. H., 10
Arnason, B. G., 284, 502
Arnason, G., 520
Arnold, B. J., 755

Arnold, C. A., 445
Arnold, W. A., 746
Aronson, S. F., 586
Arrowsmith, W. R., 238, 259
Arterberry, J. D., 502
Arthurton, M., 101
Asboe-Hansen, G., 647
Ash, B. J., 747, 753
Ashburn, L. L., 648
Ashby, W., 58
Ashenbrucker, H., 464, 502, 506, 520
Asher, Y., 350
Ashley, D. J. B., 502
Ask-Upmark, E., 586
Astaldi, G., 432, 502
Aster, R. H., 776, 808, 817
Astrup, T., 587, 746
Ata, M., 808
Athens, J. W., 502, 503, 506, 520
Atkins, L., 149, 624
Atkinson, J. B., 622
Atwater, J., 432
Aub, J. C., 464
Auditore, J. V., 339
Auerbach, M. L., 464
Auld, P. A. M., 21, 127
Aur, R. J., 626
Austin, R. F., 339
Avellera, R. M., 175
Avery, M. A., 28, 35
Avery, M. E., 344, 432, 675, 809
Avioli, L. U., 675
Awai, M., 234
Axelrod, A. R., 447
Axelrod, J., 129
Aydelotte, J. V., 87
Ayeni, O., 339
Ayers, V. E., 236
Ayers, W. W., 483, 502
Ayvazian, J. H., 234
Azevedo, M., 508, 522

**B**

Bacal, H. L., 813
Bachmann, F., 750
Back, N., 502
Backman, A., 177
Baehner, R. L., 288, 346, 502
Baer, R. L., 344
Baglioni, C., 427, 432, 446
Baikie, A. G., 11, 34, 62, 342, 351, 522, 534, 586, 623
Baile, M. D., 339
Bailey, I. S., 432
Bain, A. D., 125
Bain, B., 289
Bain, H. W., 345, 504
Bain, J. A., 258, 468
Bainton, D. F., 234
Baird, R. L., 339, 432, 439
Bakay, L., 147
Bakemeier, R. F., 339

821

# AUTHOR INDEX

Baker, D., 809, 812
Baker, H., 257, 758
Baker, H. J., 350
Baker, L. A., 237, 434
Baker, L. R., 809
Baker, M., 755
Baker, R. D., 586
Baker, R. J., 101
Baker, S. J., 259
Bako, F., 289
Bakst, H., 547
Baldini, M., 101, 447, 738, 746, 763, 776, 809, 810, 815, 816
Bale, W. F., 238
Balf, C. L., 809
Balfour, W. M., 238
Baliah, T., 130
Balis, M. E., 59
Ballard, H. S., 809
Ballard, M. S., 432
Baltimore, D., 586
Banatvala, J. E., 547
Bancroft, I. M., 73
Bancroft, P. M., 351
Bang, O., 563, 588
Bank, A., 391, 432, 433, 437, 589
Banker, B. Q., 675
Banks, L. O., 432, 445
Bannatyme, R. M., 502
Banner, E. A., 127
Bannerman, R. M., 60, 339, 432, 437, 813
Banov, C. H., 445
Banti, G., 658, 675
Banus, V. L., 745, 746
Banwell, G. S., 234
Baranovsky, A., 177, 756
Barber, R., 594
Barbor, P. R. H., 445
Barcroft, J., 6, 10
Bard, H., 10
Barker, W. H., 287
Barkhan, P., 284, 427, 432, 474
Barlow, A., 820
Barltrop, D., 207, 234
Barnes, G. R., Jr., 534
Barnes, R. D. S., 284
Barness, L. A., 71, 173, 467
Barnett, C. P., 747
Barnett, D. R., 433
Barnett, E. V., 87, 351, 502, 509
Barnett, G. O., 810
Barnett, H. L., 432, 815
Barnett, L., 59
Barnhart, M. I., 747
Barnum, C. P., 345
Barondess, J. A., 547, 549
Barr, D. P., 20, 339
Barr, M. L., 33
Barr, Y. M., 548
Barreras, L., 432
Barrett, A. M., 71, 432
Barrett, C. T., 160, 174, 177
Barrett, K. E., 759
Barrett-Connor, E., 432
Barrie, J., 177
Barritt, A. S., Jr., 819
Barrow, E. M., 747, 750, 751
Barry, A., 747
Barry, M., 305, 339
Barth, R. F., 676
Barton, C. J., 432
Barton, E. G., 586
Barton, H. R., 548
Basa, B. H., 547
Bashors, R., 145, 149
Bass, J. C., 347
Bass, M., 33

Bass, M. H., 464, 485, 502, 675
Bassen, F. A., 14, 22, 71, 72, 289, 506, 522, 550, 586
Basson, V., 547
Basten, A., 502
Bastrup-Madsen, P., 752
Basu, R., 809
Bates, G. C., 339, 746
Batson, R., 502
Battaglia, F. C., 6, 10
Battle, C. U., 586
Baty, J. M., 432, 586
Bauer, S., 549
Baughan, M. A., 339, 347, 350, 351, 507, 509
Baum, J., 627
Baxter, E., 343
Bayatpour, M., 816
Bayer, W. L., 474, 809
Bayrd, E. D., 506, 590, 647, 677
Bazelon, M., 814
Beadle, G. W., 23
Beal, G. A., 593
Beal, R. W., 339, 444
Beal, V. A., 234
Beale, D., 464
Beam, A. S., 236
Beard, M. E. J., 410, 432
Beard, M. F., 259
Bearn, A. G., 234, 499, 502, 503
Beasley, J., 343
Beattie, C. P., 125, 548
Beattie, K. M., 88
Beatty, E. C., Jr., 127, 589, 626
Beaudry, P. H., 36
Beaven, G. H., 10, 11, 435, 438, 449
Beaver, P. C., 509
Beck, E. A., 747
Beck, W. S., 256, 348, 594
Becker, A. H., 29
Becker, C. E., 651
Beckers, T., 348
Becroft, D. M. O., 71, 256
Bedell, R. F., 35
Bedizel, M., 677
Bedo, A. V., 447
Bedwell, G. A., 586
Beeson, P. B., 548, 675
Beet, E. A., 370, 432
Begg, C. F., 677
Behar, M., 259
Behrend, T. V., 342
Behrman, R. E., 10, 110, 112, 125, 128, 129, 147, 149, 572, 587
Beier, F. R., 590, 675
Beighton, P., 809
Belber, J. P., 809
Belcher, E. H., 256
Belkin, A., 288
Bell, A. D., 809
Bell, H. E., 203
Bell, R. E., 71
Bell, W. N., 439, 747
Bell, W. R., 627
Bellanti, J. A., 284, 503
Beloff, J. S., 534
Belote, J. H., 753
Belsky, H., 650
Bemiller, C. R., 550
Benante, C., 535
Ben-Bassat, I., 678
Bender, C. E., 548
Bender, R. A., 440
Benditt, E. P., 508
Benesch, R., 7, 10, 58
Benesch, R. E., 10, 58, 432, 433
Benfield, V., 749

Ben-Ishay, D., 587
Benitez, R., 818
Benjamin, B., 256
Bennett, D. C., 345
Bennett, D. E., 121, 125
Bennett, E., 747
Bennett, I. L., Jr., 675
Bennett, J. M., 467, 502, 647
Bennett, M. C., 256, 340
Bennison, R. J., 234
Benson, T. E., 678
Bentley, H. P., 174, 587, 747
Bentzel, C. J., 624, 626
Benvenisti, D. S., 559, 587
Benz, E. J., Jr., 391, 433
Benzer, S., 433
Berard, C. W., 647
Bercher, G., 177
Berdon, W., 812
Berendes, H., 472, 502, 507, 522
Berg, P., 548
Berge, T., 809
Berger, M., 177
Berggord, I., 502
Berglund, G., 809
Bergot, F., 434
Bergren, W. R., 73, 439, 447
Bergsagel, D. E., 747
Bergstrand, A., 809
Bergstrand, C. G., 339, 809
Beritic, T., 71
Berk, L., 433, 464
Berkel, I., 650
Berlin, L. I., 466
Berlin, N. I., 340, 587
Berlyne, G. M., 33
Berman, L., 502
Bernard, C., 624
Bernard, J., 349, 622, 623, 747, 748, 814, 815
Bernardelli, E., 432
Bernhard, W. G., 587
Bernini, L., 433
Bernstein, J., 344, 432, 433
Bernstock, L., 432
Berry, D. H., 627
Berry, V., 256
Berthong, W., 437
Bertino, J. R., 548
Bertles, J. F., 433
Bertram, E. G., 33
Bertucio, M., 820
Bessis, M. C., 234, 433, 466, 502
Besson, P. B., 502
Best, W. R., 227, 284, 626, 809
Bethard, W. F., 587
Bethell, F., 60, 535, 627
Betke, K., 11, 343, 354, 437, 440, 443
Betke, L., 236
Bettex, M., 202
Beutler, E., 58, 319, 339, 342, 343
Bevan, G. H., 71
Bevans, M., 289
Beverly, J. K. A., 125, 548
Bevis, D. C. A., 147
Bezan, A. J., 258
Bhardwaj, B., 237
Bhatia, H. M., 85
Bhende, Y. M., 85
Bianchini, E., 343
Bianco, I., 433, 446
Bickers, J. N., 461, 464
Bidwell, E., 700, 747
Bienzle, U., 339

Bierman, H. R., 502, 587, 675
Biessle, J. J., 285
Biggs, R., 696, 700, 708, 736, 747, 749, 753
Bigler, J. A., 173, 521, 676
Bilello, F. P., 73, 448
Billing, B. H., 58, 125, 129
Billo, O. E., 809
Binder, R. A., 433
Binger, C. M., 622
Bini, L., 444
Birchard, E. L., 130
Bird, G. W. G., 433
Bird, O. D., 627
Birge, R. F., 587
Birkhill, F. R., 58, 101
Bisgard, J. D., 467
Bishop, J. E., 586
Biswer, G. J., 340
Bithell, T. C., 284, 776, 809
Bitter, T., 507
Bjore, J., 521
Bjorkman, S. E., 675
Black, E., 258
Black, O., 128
Blackburn, C. R. B., 444
Blackburn, E. K., 339, 747, 758
Blackburn, W. R., 203
Blackfan, K. D., 285, 432
Blackman, A., 287
Blaese, R. M., 809
Blaisdell, R. K., 339
Blaksmore, A. H., 680
Blanc, W. A., 148, 150, 176
Blanchard, M. C., 130
Bland, W. H., 348
Blankenship, W. J., 33
Blattner, R. J., 627, 817
Blecher, T. E., 809
Bloch, K. J., 758
Block, J., 624
Block, M., 392, 433, 587
Blomback, B., 747, 754
Blomback, M., 708, 747, 748, 754
Blomfield, J., 10
Bloodworth, J. M. B., Jr., 812
Bloom, A. D., 587
Bloom, G. E., 259, 284, 548, 568, 587, 757
Bloom, W., 677
Bloomberg, H. H., 436
Blum, L., 348
Blum, S. F., 347
Blumberg, B. S., 86, 97, 101, 102, 433, 587
Blumberg, W. E., 62
Blume, R. S., 502
Blumenfeld, N., 258
Blumenschein, S. D., 125
Blumgart, H. L., 343
Bodansky, O., 464
Bodey, G. P., 587, 590, 593, 623, 626
Bodian, M., 126, 820
Bogart, F. B., 647
Boggs, D. R., 502, 587, 623
Boggs, J. D., 127
Boggs, T. R., 147, 150, 154, 156, 168, 174
Bogin, M., 809
Bogle, J. M., 590, 625
Boiron, M., 622, 623
Boitnott, J. K., 626
Bolande, R. P., 58
Boley, J. O., 121, 125
Bollman, J. L., 127
Bolt, C., 752
Bolton, F. G., 748
Bomford, R. R., 284, 464

## AUTHOR INDEX

Bonadonna, G., 623
Bond, T. P., 748
Bond, U. P., 504
Bond, V. P., 548, 588
Bondy, P. K., 548
Bonfiglio, T. A., 586
Bonnette, J., 749
Bonnin, J. A., 456, 464, 502
Bonnin, S. A., 809
Bono, V., 647
Bookchin, R. M., 433
Booker, C., 445, 449
Boon, W. H., 125
Booth, P. B., 86
Boothby, K., 234
Borchgrevink, C. F., 748, 751
Borda, E., 625
Borella, L., 590, 624
Borges, W. H., 239, 467, 587, 589, 592, 726, 746, 750
Borthwick, R. A., 568, 589
Borum, A., 33
Boshea, B., 72
Boss, J. H., 749
Bostanci, N., 431
Botha, M. C., 464
Bothwell, T. H., 202, 223, 234, 235, 238, 433, 464
Boudreaux, H. B., 748
Bouhasin, J. D., 748, 809
Bound, J. P., 125
Bouroncle, B. A., 339, 347, 647, 679, 773, 809, 811
Boushey, H., 651
Bowdler, A. J., 339, 433
Bowen, W. R., 174
Bowie, E. J. W., 534, 750, 754
Bowie, J. H., 125
Bowie, J. W., 234
Bowman, B. H., 433, 448
Bowman, H. A., 314, 339
Bowman, H. S., 234
Bowman, J. M., 129, 145, 147, 174
Bowman, J. W., 339
Bowman, W. D., 148, 174
Boxton, C. L., 35
Boyan, C. P., 755
Boyd, D. A., 102
Boyd, E. M., 439
Boyer, A., 174, 177
Boyer, M. H., 502, 749
Boyer, S. H., 58
Boyett, J. D., 234, 464
Boylston, B. F., 591
Brabec, V., 347
Bracken, C., 748
Bradford, W. L., 385, 391, 449
Bradley, C., 649
Bradley, J., 174
Bradley, T. B., Jr., 433, 444
Bradlow, B. O., 234, 464
Brady, R. O., 502, 675, 679
Bragg, K. V., 202
Brain, M. C., 58, 71, 439, 449, 748, 790, 809, 810, 817
Brainton, D. F., 227
Brakman, P., 587, 746
Bramson, M., 535
Brancato, G. J., 178
Branche, G. C., Jr., 441
Brandbury, J. T., 12
Brandes, W. W., 86
Brandt, I. K., 518, 522
Brangle, R. W., 203
Braun, E. H., 502, 521
Braun, H., 11, 440
Braunstein, H., 648, 814
Braunsteiner, H., 748

Braunwald, E., 240
Braverman, A. J., 432, 433
Braverman, N., 34
Brawner, J. N., III, 433
Bray, W. E., 86
Breakey, V. K. St. G., 464
Breau, G., 12
Brecher, G., 238, 548, 594, 626, 627
Breckenridge, A., 340
Breckenridge, R. T., 748, 750, 751, 809
Brecker, G., 62, 548, 756
Brecy, H., 503
Breener, S., 59
Breg, W. R., 33, 587
Bregani, P., 587
Brehusen, F. C., 816
Breitenbucher, R. P., 435
Brennan, J. C., 811, 813
Brennenmann, J., 521
Brent, R. L., 125
Brescia, M. A., 174, 587
Breton-Gorius, J., 234, 433
Brewer, G. J., 59, 339, 340, 350
Brewer, H. F., 813
Brewster, H. H., 438
Brick, I. B., 436, 819
Bricka, M., 502
Brickley, W. J., 591
Bridge, R. G., 33
Bridgeforth, E. P., 241
Bridgen, W., 550
Bridgers, W. H., 433
Bridges, J. M., 102, 587, 810
Bridges, R., 150, 472
Bridges, R. A., 34, 284, 502, 503
Brieger, H., 467
Brigandi, E., 21
Brigety, R. E., 234
Briggs, O., 86
Bright, N. H., 130
Brill, A. B., 587
Brilliant, R., 436
Brimhall, B., 467
Brinkhous, K. M., 102, 696, 748, 752, 754, 755
Brinkman, R., 354, 433
Brise, H., 234
Britten, P. F. H., 691, 748
Brittingham, T. E., 102, 503
Britton, C. J. C., 204, 468
Britton, H. A., 234
Brizel, H. E., 810
Broberger, O., 809
Brock, N., 623
Brodey, M., 506
Brodie, H. R., 10
Brodine, C. R., 443
Brodribb, H. S., 340
Brodsky, I., 521
Brody, J., 433, 447
Brok, F., 678
Broman, B., 129, 147
Bromberg, M., 10
Bronson, W. R., 231, 239, 623
Bronte-Stewart, B., 464
Brook, C. G. D., 410, 433
Brooksaler, F., 817
Broome, J. D., 603, 623
Bross, I. D. J., 589
Brough, A. J., 240, 352
Brough, A. S., 130
Broughton, P. M., 111, 125, 161, 174
Broun, G. O., 587, 678
Brounstein, O., 60
Brown, A. K., 73, 125, 130, 174, 342
Brown, A. L., 750
Brown, D. L., 748

Brown, E. B., 234, 236, 439
Brown, E. R., 589, 593
Brown, E. W., 21, 203, 205, 236
Brown, G. M., 587, 758, 807, 819
Brown, H. W., 441
Brown, J. A., 624
Brown, J. W., 289
Brown, R. R., 288
Brown, R. S., 127, 809
Browne, E. A., 340, 521
Browning, J. R., 810
Brubaker, C. A., 240, 590, 613, 615, 623, 625, 628, 648
Brunetti, P., 340
Brunnhage, F., 809
Brunson, J. G., 819
Brus, I., 340
Bruton, O. C., 125, 259, 340
Bryan, W. B., 176
Bryan, W. R., 534
Buchanan, J. G., 503
Bucht, H., 809
Buckell, M., 748
Buckley, M., 587
Buckner, C. D., 287, 619, 623, 627, 629
Buckton, K., 88, 586, 587
Buckwold, A. E., 502, 521
Buechler, S., 521
Buhr, J. L., 433
Bukowski, M. J., 810
Bull, B. S., 748, 810, 817
Bullock, W. H., 445
Bumbalo, T. S., 503
Bunnell, W. W., 586, 549
Bunting, H., 58, 433
Burch, G. E., 449
Burchenal, J. H., 433, 464, 550, 587, 593, 594, 610, 615, 623, 625
Burgert, E. O., Jr., 284, 591, 592, 676
Burgess, D., 438
Burka, E. R., 389, 441
Burke, B. A., 817
Burke, C., 752
Burke, D. M., 810
Burke, F. G., 35
Burkhardt, J., 346
Burkhardt, M., 816
Burkitt, D., 647
Burko, H., 433, 488
Burman, D., 58, 256, 340
Burn, G. P., 675
Burnet, E. M., 202
Burnet, F. M., 284, 331, 340, 504
Burney, S. W., 202
Burnham, L., 35, 86, 149
Burnie, K. L., 71
Burny, A., 594
Burrell, S. B., 648
Burrows, B. A., 465
Burt, D., 148
Buschke, W., 468
Bush, J. A., 71, 464, 675
Busse, R. J., Jr., 756
Butler, E. A., 439
Butler, J. J., 521
Butler, L. J., 11
Butler, S. S., 636, 638, 649
Butt, H. R., 126, 127, 129
Butterworth, C. E., 464
Butterworth, M., 33
Buttimer, R. J., 87
Byrd, R. B., 234
Byron, R. L., Jr., 502
Bywaters, E. G. L., 793, 810

**C**

Cabannes, R., 433
Cade, J. F., 34
Caen, J. P., 748, 758, 814, 815
Caffey J., 202, 394, 433, 675, 748
Cahalane, S. F., 785, 810
Cahan, A., 86, 87, 591
Calder, B., 650
Caldwell, M. J., 464, 752
Callen, I. R., 464
Callender, S. T., 234, 235, 256, 432, 443
Calvin, J., 466
Cameron, A. H., 73
Cameron, C., 34
Cameron, D. G., 256
Camli, N., 234
Camp, F. R., Jr., 443
Camp, W. A., 345
Campbell, B., 504
Campbell, C. G., 438
Campbell, D. C., 808
Campbell, H., 237
Campbell, J. A., 590
Campbell, J. S., 350
Campbell, S., 464
Campbell, W. G., 586
Canale, V., 435, 437, 448, 647, 748
Canales, L., 548, 549
Canby, J. P., 234
Canham, P. A. S., 236
Cannon, R. O., 236
Cantrow, A., 464
Caplan, J., 464
Cappell, D. F., 434
Capps, R. B., 60
Caraway, C. T., 467
Carbone, P. P., 508, 587, 589, 594, 627, 647
Carew, J. P., 522
Caris, T. N., 548
Carleton, A., 237
Carlisle, H. N., 675
Carlsen, E., 47, 59
Carlson, A., 237
Carmel, W. J., 587
Carnazzo, S. F., 812
Carnehan, C. E., 591
Carnes, W. H., 237
Carnot, P., 48, 59
Carothers, E. L., 236
Carpenter, A. G., 810
Carpenter, D. G., 503
Carpenter, P. L., 86
Carper, J. S. M., 587
Carr, D. H., 36, 593
Carr, M. H., 675
Carre, I. J., 810
Carrell, R. W., 59, 434, 439, 440
Carretero, R., 467
Carrington, H. T., 434, 436
Carroll, I. N., 238
Carson, P. E., 60, 311, 340, 350
Carstairs, K. C., 340, 351
Carter, B. B., 174
Carter, C., 147
Carter, C. H., 503
Carter, C. O., 287
Cartwright, G. E., 62, 202, 225, 234, 237, 239, 241, 287, 288, 340, 345, 348, 435, 464, 466, 467, 468, 506, 520, 587, 588, 592, 593, 623, 625, 626, 627, 647, 648, 678, 810
Carvalho, G., 522
Carvallo, G., 508
Cary, W., 147

# AUTHOR INDEX

Cash, J. D., 758
Casper, J., 811
Cassady, G., 125
Cassell, M., 432
Casserd, F., 678
Cassidy, G., 33
Castaldi, P. A., 748
Castle, W. B., 60, 175, 244, 249, 256, 257, 342, 343, 344, 433, 438, 446, 464, 465, 548, 588
Castor, W. R., 174
Cathcart, R., 445
Cathey, W. J., 623
Cathie, I. A. B., 102, 284, 818
Cattan, A., 103, 626
Catz, C. S., 125, 130
Caviles, A. P., 287
Cecil, R. L., 125
Celander, D. R., 748
Celano, M. J., 86
Cella, L. J., Jr., 648
Ceppelini, R., 434, 440
Cerami, A., 383, 434, 435, 437
Cerny, J. C., 815
Cetingil, A. I., 431
Chadwick, B., 258
Chadwick, D. L., 506, 677
Chambers, J. W., 86
Chambers, W. N., 810
Chan, A. C., 147
Chanarin, I., 256, 257, 259, 284, 340, 502
Chandler, D., 202
Chandler, J. G., 505
Chang, T. W., 813
Chanutin, A., 10
Chaplin, H., 102, 339, 432, 434, 464, 503
Chapman, A. Z., 237, 434, 438, 446
Chapman, R. G., 340
Charache, P., 747
Charache, S., 10, 340, 431, 434, 464
Charley, P. J., 235
Charlton, R. W., 234, 235
Charmot, G., 434
Charney, E., 381, 434
Charytan, C., 748
Chase, H. P., 810
Chase, J., 86
Chatten, J., 202
Chatterjea, J. B., 445, 675, 818
Chatterji, A., 445
Cheatham, W. J., 588
Chediak, M. M., 503
Chen, T. I., 748
Chen, Y-C., 240
Cheney, K., 456, 464
Chernick, W. S., 502
Chernoff, A. I., 10, 340, 434, 443, 446, 648
Chernoff, P. R., 434
Cherry, R. B., 127
Chertkow, G., 340
Chervanick, P. A., 758
Cheung, M. W., 440
Chew, W. B., 588
Chikkappa, G., 521
Child, C. G., III, 675
Child, J. A., 255, 257
Childs, B., 36, 125, 130, 340, 352
Chilgren, R. A., 507
Ching, R. E., 435
Chisolm, J. J., Jr., 340, 463, 465
Chiu, J., 812
Choay, J., 287
Chodoff, P., 624

Chodorkoff, J., 434
Chodos, R. B., 235
Chong, M. N. Y., 749
Chongchareonsuk, S., 442
Choremis, C., 434
Chown, B., 12, 26, 34, 36, 148, 150, 174, 178, 235
Christensen, N. A., 505
Christenson, W. N., 340, 341, 588
Christian, J. R., 240
Christie, A., 502
Christy, R. A., 121, 125
Chung, F., 147
Chunn, C. F., 465
Chute, A. L., 504
Cintron, J., 757
Cirksena, W. J., 284
Claireaux, A. E., 647, 675
Clark, A. C. L., 623
Clark, D., 591
Clark, D. R., 288
Clark, H., 445, 818
Clark, P. A., 623
Clark, W. G., 794, 810
Clark, W. M., Jr., 235
Clarke, B. F., 810
Clarke, B. S., 674, 675
Clarke, C. A., 174, 175, 178
Clarke, J. E., 748
Clarke, R. R., 624
Clarkson, B., 284, 624, 625
Clarkson, D. D., 648
Clarysse, A. M., 623
Clatanoff, D. V., 452, 467, 648, 819
Clausen, S. W., 61, 102
Clay, B., 217, 235
Clayton, C., 548
Clayton, E. M., 434
Clayton, R. J., 125
Clegg, J., 434, 464
Clein, G. P., 588
Cleland, W. P., 349
Clemens, T., 235
Clement, D. H., 284, 534, 810
Cleveland, O., 466
Clifford, G. O., 448
Clifford, J. H., 148
Clifford, P., 647
Clifford, S. H., 35, 748
Cliftton, E. E., 755
Clift, R. A., 102, 623, 647
Cline, M. J., 340, 503
Clink, H. M., 346
Close, H. P., 445
Cochran, W., 174
Cock, T. C., 125
Cockburn, F., 286
Cockshott, W. P., 432
Coddon, D. R., 345
Coe, J., 87
Coen, R., 503
Cohen, A., 286
Cohen, B. M., 647, 650
Cohen, F., 17, 20, 26, 34, 162, 169, 174, 434
Cohen, G., 72
Cohen, H., 348
Cohen, I., 88
Cohen, J. A., 102, 752
Cohen, L. S., 240
Cohen, M. H., 647
Cohen, M. M., 125, 588
Cohen, P., 810
Cohen, S. N., 176
Cohen, T., 588
Cohlan, S. Q., 34
Cohn, I., 467
Cohn, Z. A., 503
Cole, D. R., 675
Cole, P. G., 125

Cole, R. B., 21
Cole, R. D., 11
Colebatch, J. H., 623, 676
Coleman, D. H., 59, 235, 239, 465
Collard, P., 438
Colle, E., 819
Collen, W. H., 593
Colliander, M., 759
Collins, W., 347
Colman, R. W., 748, 756, 758
Colombani, J., 329, 342, 503, 521
Colombani, M., 503, 521
Colopy, J. E., 756
Colpoys, W. P., 818
Coltman, C. A., 208, 235
Colucci, D. D., 103
Colussi, P., 506
Comer, P. B., 434
Comfort, M. W., 257
Commerford, L., 624
Compston, N., 626
Comroe, J. H., 47, 59
Con, I., 284
Conchu, T. L., 679
Condie, R., 34, 503, 507
Condit, P. K., 289
Cone, T. E., Jr., 287, 443, 592, 816
Conley, C. L., 10, 258, 360, 433, 434, 437, 438, 446, 447, 465, 467, 648, 752
Conley, D. D., 510
Conn, H. O., 340, 434
Connell, G. E., 340, 347
Conney, A. H., 128
Conrad, E., 819
Conrad, F. G., 223, 341
Conrad, M. E., Jr., 235, 240, 625
Conrad, W. E., 341
Conte, F. A., 36
Contopoulos, A., 508
Contrera, J. T., 59
Cook, C. D., 3, 9, 10, 746
Cook, J. E., 647
Cook, W. L., Jr., 587
Cooke, J. V., 561, 563, 588, 647
Cooke, W. T., 257
Cooley, J. C., 385, 434
Cooley, T. B., 434, 435
Coombs, R. R. A., 138, 148
Cooney, D. P., 748
Cooper, B., 257
Cooper, B. A., 244, 257
Cooper, C. D., 435
Cooper, E. L., 340
Cooper, G. R., 438
Cooper, H. L., 489, 503
Cooper, L. Z., 129, 340, 348, 810, 816
Cooper, M., 810, 816
Cooper, R. A., 65, 71, 340
Cooper, T., 234, 647, 754
Cooperberg, A. A., 588, 748
Cooperman, J. M., 258, 441
Coopland, A. T., 588
Corallo, L. A., 678
Corcino, J., 521
Cordes, F. L., 502, 587
Cordonnier, J. K., 61, 442
Cordova, F. A., 444
Corkery, J. J., 174
Cormick, J., 62
Cornblath, M., 62, 465
Cornelius, E. A., 443
Corner, B., 147
Cornet, J. A., 464, 746, 757
Cornu, P., 709, 748
Corr, W. P., Jr., 534
Correa, J. M., 508, 522

Corrigan, J. J., 746, 810
Costea, N., 101
Costello, J. M., 71
Cotlove, E., 626
Cottom, D. G., 6, 10
Cottone, D. G., 627
Couchman, K. G., 260
Court-Brown, W. M., 34, 586, 587, 588
Coventry, W. D., 340
Cowan, D. H., 753
Cowger, M. L., 343
Cox, F. H., 549
Craddock, C. G., 503, 508, 588, 649, 755
Craig, J. M., 126. 129, 130, 503, 506, 521, 677, 810
Craig, L. C., 60
Cramblett, H. G., 588, 623, 625
Crane, J. F., 677, 818
Craver, L. F., 593, 647, 649, 650, 677
Cravioto, J., 257
Crawford, A., 174
Crawford, H., 86, 342
Crawford, J. D., 128
Crawford, R. P., 73, 445
Crawford, S. E., 810
Cree, I. C., 287
Creed, D. L., 811
Creger, W. P., 28, 34, 588
Cremer, R. J., 111, 126
Crepaldi, G., 508
Crick, F. H. C., 59
Crigler, J. F., Jr., 61, 122, 123, 126, 148
Crile, M., 587
Crinberg, S., 748
Crisalli, M., 534
Crocker, A. C., 675, 678, 814
Crockett, C. L., Jr., 446, 593
Crockett, E. J., 438
Crofton, J. W., 485, 503
Crome, L., 11
Cronkite, E. P., 503, 504, 548, 588
Crookston, J. H., 71, 341
Crookston, M. C., 71, 86, 437
Crosby, M. E., 223, 224
Crosby, W. H., 58, 59, 71, 72, 125, 235, 240, 241, 285, 286, 291, 338, 340, 341, 342, 346, 347, 351, 435, 675, 678, 746, 748, 752, 810
Cross, E. R., 236
Cross, R. S., 588
Crosse, V. M., 148, 167, 174
Crossen, P. E., 589
Crowder, J. G., 503
Crowley, J. H., 508, 678
Crozier, D. N., 150
Cruchaud, A., 503
Cserhati, I., 814
Cullum, C., 748
Cumings, J. N., 346
Cummer, C. L., 435
Cummins, J. F., 285
Cunningham, J. E., 433
Cunningham, M. D., 126
Cunningham, R. S., 491, 503
Cunningham, S. C., 58, 464
Curiel, D. C., 747
Curnish, R. R., 10
Currarino, G., 435, 436
Currimbhoy, Z., 755, 756, 817
Curtis, C. D., 235
Curtis, E. M., 446
Curwen, W. L., 341
Custer, R. P., 10, 534, 548, 647, 756

# AUTHOR INDEX

Cutbush, M., 16, 21, 85, 86, 142, 149, 174, 176, 341, 441
Cutting, H. O., 341, 517, 521, 522
Czar, B., 339
Czernobilaky, B., 810

## D

Dacie, J. V., 62, 66, 71, 85, 86, 102, 202, 256, 257, 274, 284, 300, 301, 311, 313, 323, 324, 340, 341, 343, 345, 349, 351, 435, 437, 439, 465, 503, 521, 522, 747, 748, 809, 810, 817
Daeschner, C. W., Jr., 811
Daft, F. S., 521
Dagg, J. H., 238
Dagovitz, L., 87
Daiber, A., 284
Daland, G. A., 465
Daland, G. E., 677
Dale, J. H., Jr., 588
Dales, M., 285
Dallman, P. R., 235, 257, 749
Daly, M., 508
Dam, H., 713, 719, 749
Dameshek, W., 101, 103, 116, 126, 150, 202, 203, 235, 257, 270, 284, 285, 287, 289, 332, 341, 342, 349, 350, 435, 447, 465, 503, 521, 522, 548, 564, 588, 589, 623, 626, 634, 647, 650, 675, 679, 757, 773, 808, 810, 814, 816, 817, 818
Dammin, G. J., 624
Dance, N., 11, 438
Dancis, J., 30, 34, 59
Danes, B. S., 499, 502, 503
D'Angio, G. J., 204, 441, 588, 624, 627
Daniel, E. C., 536, 550
Danks, D., 126, 435
Danoff, S., 59, 174
Danon, D., 427, 444, 504
D'Antonio, J., 465
Darby, W. J., 236
Dargeon, H. W., 593, 627, 647, 649, 650, 677, 810
Darling, D. R. A., 809
Darling, R. C., 465
Darragh, J. H., 549
Darrow, D., 130
Darte, D. M. M., 749
Darte, J. M., 503, 648
Das, M. R., 594
Datta, P., 339
Daughaday, W. H., 465
Dausset, J., 329, 342, 503, 521, 753
Davey, M. G., 102
Davidsohn, I., 102, 177, 342, 548
Davidson, C. S., 749, 758
Davidson, E., 749
Davidson, J. D., 240
Davidson, L. T., 21
Davidson, R. G., 34
Davidson, S., 819
Davidson, W. M., 86, 503
Davie, E. W., 749, 756
Davie, J., 548
Davies, B. S., 148
Davies, J. N. P., 649
Davies, P., 749
Davies, S. H., 810
Davis, A. E., 809
Davis, B. C., 438
Davis, E., 811

Davis, J. A., 71, 175
Davis, L. J., 342, 466
Davis, P. S., 235, 237
Davis, S. K., 587
Davison, K. B., 507
Dawber, N. H., 129
Dawson, A. M., 586
Dawson, J. P., 126, 284, 342, 465
Dawson, P. J., 674, 675, 814
Day, H. J., 811
Day, R., 148, 176
Day, R. L., 127, 148, 175
Dean, T., 34, 750
Deane, H. W., 504
De Bernardinis, C. T., 522
de Capoa, A., 589
Decker, E., 468
DeConti, R. C., 647
Dees, S. C., 813
Deflandre, C., 48, 59
de Furia, F. G., 384, 435
de Gabriele, G., 811
DeGowin, R. L., 588
DeGroot, J. A., 750
De Grouchy, J., 749
DeGruchy, G. C., 61, 257, 311, 314, 318, 341, 342, 348, 465, 675, 749
Deiss, A., 345
Deiss, W. P., Jr., 648
DeJong, W. W., 442
de Konig, J., 448
De la Chapelle, A., 749
Delafresnaye, J. E., 440
De La Fuente, V., 647
Delage, J-M., 747
deLamerens, S., 745, 746
DeLawder, A. M., 10
deLeeuw, N. K. M., 235
De Lena, M., 623
Delivoria-Papadopoulos, M., 443, 468
Deller, D. J., 235, 237
Deller, J. J., 272, 284
deLorimier, A. A., 202
Delta, B. G., 202, 588
DeMarsh, Q. B., 16, 20, 339
Demis, J. D., 342
Dempsey, E., 21, 237
Dempsey, H., 241, 350
de Muralt, 752
Denborough, M. A., 256
Denenholz, E. J., 674
Denko, C. W., 623
Dennis, L. H., 521
Densen, P. M., 236
Denson, K. W., 749, 753, 758
Dent, C. E., 647
Denton, R. L., 177
Deo, M. G., 236
De Palma, A. F., 749
DePree, M. J., 811
Derbey, P., 288
Derham, R. J., 811
Dern, R. J., 339, 342
Desai, R. G., 28, 34
De Sanctis, A. G., 680
Descovich, C., 534
Desforges, J. F., 72, 126, 143, 148, 315, 339, 342, 445, 465, 467, 593
Desmond, M. M., 817
Despande, C. K., 85
Desposito, F., 20, 284, 808
Destine, M. L., 176, 203
De Torregrosa, M. V., 435
de Vassal, F., 591, 626
DeVaux, L. O., 815
DeVaux, W., 35
deVerdier, C. H., 431
DeVita, V. T., 647, 650
De Vries, A., 749, 811

de Vries, J. A., 259
Dewey, K. W., 435
Deykin, D., 749
DeYoung, V. R., 175
Dherte, P., 435
Diamond, E. F., 175
Diamond, H. D., 647, 649, 650, 677
Diamond, I., 135, 148
Diamond, L. K., 11, 12, 35, 61, 72, 73, 85, 101, 127, 129, 147, 148, 150, 174, 175, 177, 203, 235, 238, 239, 257, 259, 266, 284, 285, 288, 343, 346, 347, 348, 349, 350, 352, 432, 437, 442, 443, 446, 507, 510, 522, 587, 588, 592, 624, 675, 678, 746, 749, 757, 808, 810, 816
Dickerman, J. D., 677, 753
Dickie, W. K., 260
Dickstein, B., 14, 22
Didisheim, G. E., 309
Didisheim, P., 588, 749, 752
Diehl, V., 536, 549
Dienet, G., 675
Dietrich, E. B., 102
Dietz, A. A., 72
Diggs, L. W., 432, 435, 436, 439, 811
Dignan, P. St.J., 782, 783, 811
Di Guglielmo, G., 634, 647
Dike, G. W. R., 747
Dillon, H., 284
Dillon, H. C., 175
Di Marco, A., 623
Dimson, S. B., 257
Dingle, J. H., 344, 594
Dingman, R. O., 811
Dinning, J. S., 59, 467
Di Sant'Agnese, P. A., 676
Dische, F. E., 749
Dische, M. R., 71, 437
Dische, R., 127
Discombe, G., 647
Distenfeld, A., 811
Disthasongchan, P., 448
Dittman, W. A., 435
Ditto, W. B., 819
Diwany, M., 435
Dixon, W. F., 340
Djaldetti, M., 811
Djerassi, I., 101, 102, 622, 623
Dmochowski, L., 623, 811
Doan, C. A., 503, 504, 523, 647, 658, 676, 679, 680, 773, 809, 811
Doan, J. K., 548
Dobbins, W. T., 447
Dobkin, G., 534
Dod, K. S., 587, 675
Dodge, H. T., 465
Dodge, J. A., 811
Dodge, J. T., 72
Dodge, W. F., 811
Doenges, J. P., 435
Doig, R. K., 292
Dolan, R. G., 35, 128, 753
Dolery, P. T., 340
Dolgopol, V. B., 548
Doll, R., 505, 587, 588
Dollberg, L., 811
Doloff, M. J., 350
Donahue, D. D., 11
Donald, W. C., 464
Donath, J., 334, 342
Donegan, C. C., Jr., 102, 435
Doniach, D., 259, 260
Donnell, G. N., 814
Donnelly, W. J., 72

Donohoe, W. T. A., 174, 175, 178
Donohue, D. M., 59, 234, 548
Donohue, W. L., 504, 521
Donoso, A., 284
Donowho, E. M., Jr., 440
Doorenbos, D. E., 12
Dorfman, A., 504
Dorfman, R. F., 647
Dormandy, K. M., 435, 750, 752, 814
Dormell, G. N., 126
Dorr, A. D., 504
Dorrington, H. S., 813
Dosik, H., 285, 588
Doubeck, W. G., 818
Dougan, L., 594
Doughtery, T. F., 504, 623
Douglas, A. S., 736, 747, 749
Douglas, D. M., 647
Douglas, H., 34
Douglas, S. D., 504, 505
Douglass, R. C., 811
Dowben, R. M., 127, 128
Dowd, J. E., 589
Dowdy, A. H., 286
Downey, H., 10, 536, 548
Downey, W. S., 5, 10, 746
Doxiadis, S. A., 126, 130, 313, 342, 345
Doyle, A. P., 753
Doyle, E. F., 259
Dozy, A. M., 439
Drachman, R. H., 376, 449
Drake, W. L., Jr., 594
Drance, N., 432
Draznin, S. Z., 676
Dresbach, M., 342
Dresch, C., 815
Dresdale, D. T., 548
Dreskin, O. H., 508, 650, 749, 756
Drevets, C. G., 650
Drexler, E., 502
Driscoll, R., 35
Driscoll, S. G., 34, 127, 132, 148, 150, 160, 175, 203
Driscoll, T. S., 108, 111, 128
Drorbaugh, J. F., 127
Druez, G., 72
Drummond, K. N., 812
Duane, A. B., 811
Duane, R. T., 36, 342, 811, 817
Duarte, L., 288
Dubach, R., 235, 238, 287, 444, 465, 813
Dubin, I. N., 102, 126
Dubois, E. L., 502
Dubowitz, V., 174
Dubs, E. J., 819
Duckert, F., 749, 750, 752
Ducrov, W., 309, 342
Duerst, M. L., 507
Duma, H., 435
Dumermuth, G., 676
Dumitriscu-Pirvu, D., 592
Duncan, C. N., 534
Duncan, P. A., 534
Dunea, G., 443
Dunn, P. M., 175
Dunn, S. C., 259
Dunne, C. J., 818
Dunning, E. K., 34
Dunsford, I., 34
Dunsky, I., 342
Durkin, C. M., 34, 178
Durrum, E. L., 442
Dusholm, K., 549
Dutcher, T. F., 240
Duthie, H. L., 235
Duthie, J. J. R., 287, 626
DuToit, C. H., 35

# AUTHOR INDEX

Dutton, G. J., 126
Duvall, B. J., 756
Dworkin, D., 440
Dyer, G. Y., 147
Dyggve, H., 749
Dyment, P. G., 648
Dystra, O. H., 465

## E

Eades, S. M., 177
Ealeins, J. D., 237
Easrman, N. J., 6, 10
Eaton, J. W., 59
Eaton, O. M., 548
Ebaugh, F. G., 209, 235, 504, 521, 677
Ebbe, S., 810
Ebbs, J. H., 35
Ebert, R. V., 676
Edelman, C. H., Jr., 811
Edelstine, G., 746
Eden, E. G., 61
Eder, H. A., 465
Edington, G. M., 10, 435
Edwards, E. C., 815
Edwards, J. E., 72
Edwards, M. J., 467
Efrati, P., 504, 648
Efremov, G., 435
Efron, M. L., 437
Egan, B., 252, 258
Egdahl, R. H., 435
Egozcue, J., 588
Ehrlich, J. C., 678
Ehrlich, P., 285
Eichelberger, J. W., 758
Eichenwald, H. F., 126, 679
Eichman, M. F., 346
Eichwald, E. J., 678
Eisenmann, G., 285, 342
Eisenstein, E. M., 811
Eisentraut, A., 506
Eisinger, R. P., 809
Eisner, A., 349
Eissen, A. H., 813
Eitzman, D. V., 588, 816
Ekelund, H., 550
Ekert, H., 750, 812
Ekman, C. A., 676
El-Alfi, O. S., 285
Elbe, S., 811
Elderkin, J., 441
Elegant, L. D., 466
El Hefni, A., 435
Elion, G. B., 589, 625
Elizondo, J., 467
Elks, C. A., 677
Ellefson, R. D., 679
Ellerman, V., 563, 588
Elliott, S. M., 587
Elliott, W. D., 235
Elliott-Smith, A., 747
Ellis, E. F., 676
Ellis, J. M., 629, 648
Ellis, J. T., 102, 235, 435
Ellis, M. J., 10, 432
Ellison, R. R., 680
Elson, G., 174
Elveback, L. R., 590
Elvehjem, C. A., 467
Elves, M. W., 504
Elwood, P. C., 235
Emanuel, B., 811
Emanuel, D. A., 756
Embil, J. A., 97, 102
Emerson, C. P., 342, 465, 593
Emery, A. E. H., 148
Emery, J. L., 14, 21, 648, 758, 811
Emlinger, P. J., 59, 102
Emparanza, E., 816
Emson, H. E., 502, 521
Ende, N., 236

Endenburg, P. M., 436
Enders, J. F., 588, 591
Endicott, K. M., 521
Eng, G. D., 504
Eng, L. L., 235
Eng, L-I. L., 361, 435, 436
Engel, R. R., 588
Engle, C. E., 434
Engle, M. A., 436, 441, 445, 549, 751
Engle, R. L., Jr., 86, 345
Engleman, K., 203
English, C. T., 86
Epstein, E. A., 809
Epstein, I. S., 594
Epstein, J. H., 348
Epstein, L. B., 548
Epstein, R. B., 102, 287, 623, 627
Epstein, R. D., 749
Epstein, W. L., 504
Erdem, S., 234
Ereland, W. C., 818
Erf, L. A., 289, 590, 648
Erickson, W. D., 676
Erikson, N., 442
Erlandson, M. E., 59, 101, 102, 148, 175, 235, 258, 342, 350, 433, 435, 436, 438, 442, 446, 447, 679, 751, 756, 757, 818
Erle, H., 547
Erman, S., 436
Ernster, L., 150
Erslev, A. J., 48, 59, 235, 285, 432, 436, 465, 756
Ertel, I. J., 286
Esbaughpoor, E., 126
Eschbach, J. W., Jr., 627
Eskes, P. W. H., 808
Essellier, A. F., 504
Estborn, B., 676
Esterly, N. B., 812
Estes, J. E., 436
Estren, S., 270, 285, 675
Etchart, M., 816
Etcubanas, E., 509
Etteldorf, J. N., 436, 447, 465
Ettinger, R. H., 60
Evans, A. E., 102, 588, 591, 623
Evans, A. F., 624
Evans, A. S., 537, 548
Evans, F. A., 550
Evans, G., 749
Evans, H. E., 59
Evans, M. M., 174
Evans, R. K., 753
Evans, R. S., 331, 342, 343, 762, 775, 811
Evans, T. S., 405, 504, 589
Eveling, J., 747
Everett, C. R., 589
Evin, D. M., 351
Ewing, M. C., 465
Excardo, F. E., 129
Eyring, E. J., 758
Eyster, E., 103, 342

## F

Factor, A., 758
Fadem, R. S., 72, 343
Fahey, J., 258
Fahey, J. L., 340, 436
Fahraeus, R., 59
Faigel, H. C., 445
Fainstat, T. D., 34
Fairbanks, V. F., 343, 466
Fairchild, J. P., 548
Fairhall, L. T., 464
Fairley, N. F., 343
Fairweather, D. V. I., 148
Falco, D. J., 625

Falkinburg, L., 86
Falkowski, F., 86
Falls, H. F., 73, 239
Faloon, W. W., 811, 812
Fanconi, G., 269, 285, 521
Fanger, H., 648
Fantoni, A., 343
Farber, E. M., 436
Farber, H. K., 676
Farber, S., 101, 102, 203, 623, 624, 625, 676
Fargasoya, I., 176
Farhangi, M., 507, 592
Farmer, M. B., 436
Farquhar, J. D., 130
Farquhar, J. W., 486, 504
Farquhar, M. G., 819
Farrar, J. F., 10
Farrell, F. J., 127
Fashena, G. J., 677
Faucett, R. L., 465
Faver, J. G., 259
Fear, R. E., 34
Fedorka, M. E., 504
Feichtmeir, T. V., 257
Feigin, R. D., 811
Feinberg, A. W., 343
Feinstein, D. I., 749
Feldhaus, W. D., 434
Feldman, B. H., 589
Feldman, F., 535
Feldman, F., 616, 624
Feldman, J., 88
Feldt, R. H., 811
Felson, B., 680
Fennell, R. H., Jr., 504
Fennessey, J. F., 808
Fenninger, W. D., 10
Ferguson, A., 339, 432, 438
Ferguson, A. D., 434, 436, 439, 445
Ferguson, A. W., 762, 811
Ferguson, J. H., 749, 753
Ferguson, J. J., 752
Ferguson-Smith, M. A., 72
Fernando, M., 812
Fernbach, D. J., 204, 238, 624, 627, 650
Ferrebee, J. W., 619, 624, 627
Ferretti, R., 816
Ferriro, M., 128, 176
Fertman, M. A., 72
Fertman, M. H., 72
Fessas, P. H., 126, 342, 402, 436, 437, 441, 447, 504
Fetterman, G. H., 203
Feuerstein, R. C., 622
Fichter, E. G., 465
Fiedler, A. J., 434
Field, L., 286
Field, R. E., 648
Feinberg, R., 126, 818
Fieschi, A., 504
Figley, M. M., 676
Figueroa, E., 176
Figueroa, W. G., 549, 649
Filatov, N. F., 536, 548
Finch, C. A., 59, 60, 202, 227, 228, 234, 235, 236, 238, 239, 288, 343, 346, 433, 436, 447, 465, 625, 647, 678, 750, 753, 811
Finch, J., 258
Finch, S. C., 203, 228, 235, 288, 343, 436, 504, 508, 592, 811
Finch, S. S., 521
Findley, L., 126
Fine, M. H., 284
Fine, R. N., 624, 812
Finegold, S. M., 288
Fink, H., 437
Finkel, H. E., 241, 443, 623

Finkel, K., 589, 624
Finn, R., 34, 162, 175, 178, 437
Finne, P. H., 59, 60
Finster, M., 128
Finucane, D. L., 534
Fiorentino, R., 625
Firkin, B. G., 59, 339, 351, 589, 816
Fisch, G. R., 808
Fischer, D. S., 203
Fischer, E., 59
Fischer, G. A., 624
Fish, M. B., 257, 349, 508, 548
Fisher, B., 73, 446, 626, 811
Fisher, E. R., 676, 680, 811
Fisher, J., 62
Fisher, J. H., 121, 130
Fisher, J. W., 465
Fisher, N., 87
Fisher, O. D., 808, 812
Fisher, O. E., 110, 125
Fisher, S., 348, 508
Fitch, C. D., 467
Fitch, L. I., 347
Fite, F. K., 594
Fitzgerald, P. H., 566, 589
Fitzpatrick, T. B., 346
Flanagan, C. L., 340
Flatow, F. A., 282, 285
Flatz, G., 628
Fleischer, A. S., 344
Fleman, S. R. J., 521
Flemans, R. J., 505, 588
Fleming, A., 504
Fleming, E. M., 342, 343, 446
Flessa, H. C., 819
Fletcher, F. W., 756
Flexner, J. M., 257
Fliedner, T. M., 503, 504, 548
Flint, W. F., 125
Florentin, I., 129
Florman, A. L., 286, 343
Fluckiger, P., 749
Fluharty, R. G., 465
Flume, J. B., 627
Flynn, F. V., 439
Foconi, S., 59
Foerster, R. F., 437
Fogel, B. I., 174
Fogel, B. J., 19, 20
Foley, J. R., 749
Foley, F. E., 33
Folkins, D. F., 102
Follette, J. H., 285
Folley, J. H., 589
Follis, R. H., Jr., 468
Fong, S. W., 166, 175
Forbes, R. E., 235
Ford, D. D., 589
Forget, B. G., 391, 433
Forman, E. N., 349, 746, 751
Forman, W. B., 722, 749
Fornaini, G., 343
Forrester, R. M., 148, 351
Forsham, P. H., 509, 625
Forshaw, J. W. B., 61, 259
Forssman, H., 544, 548
Forsyth, C. C., 72
Forsythe, W. I., 676
Fort, E., 756, 757, 817
Fosbrooke, A. S., 72, 73
Fossati-Bellani, F., 623
Fost, N. C., 812
Foster, K. M., 547, 548
Foster, W. D., 594
Fostripoulos, G., 436
Foulk, W. T., 126, 129
Fountain, J. R., 285, 624
Fowell, A. H., 749

# AUTHOR INDEX

Fowler, J. F., 86
Fowler, W. M., 647
Foy, H., 257, 258, 285, 465
Fox, M., 88
Fraad, L. M., 125
Frajola, W. J., 339
Frame, B., 816
Frampton, V. L., 748
France, M. E., 11
Francis, H. C., 680
Francisco, J., 756
Francken, F. V., 754
Francone, W. H., 71
Frank, O., 257
Frankel, E. P., 548
Frankland, A. W., 502
Franklin, E. G., 86
Franklin, J. W., 647
Frantz, C., 811
Fraser, F. C., 34, 818
Fraser, I. D., 11
Fraumeni, J. F., Jr., 203, 561, 589, 648, 676
Frayer, Z., 444
Frazer, A. C., 256, 257
Frech, R. S., 626
Fred, H. L., 434
Freda, V. J., 148, 163, 175
Fredericks, R. E., 62, 350, 535
Frederickson, D. S., 239
Freed, B. A., 522
Freedman, H. H., 810
Freedman, M. H., 545, 548
Freeman, G., 625
Freeman, J. A., 504
Frei, E., III, 587, 593, 594, 624, 625, 626, 627, 647
Freiman, D. G., 648
Freiman, I., 812
Freireich, E. J., 282, 285, 587, 590, 591, 592, 593, 623, 624, 625, 626, 814
French, I. M., 256
French, J., 339, 432
Frenkel, E. P., 510
Frenkel, M., 510, 550, 680
Frenkel-Tietz, H., 351
Fresh, J. W., 749, 753
Freud, P., 676
Freund, M., 587
Freundlich, E., 441
Freymann, J. G., 465, 648
Frezal, J., 72
Frick, P. G., 343, 437, 749, 812
Fried, W., 59, 60, 236, 285, 466
Friedman, A. B., 175
Friedman, B. I., 289, 648
Friedman, I. A., 434
Friedman, J. L., 588
Friedman, L. H., 729, 755
Friedman, L. L., 750
Friedman, R., 258
Friedman, S. B., 624
Friedman, V., 148
Friesen, R. F., 174
Friesen, W. J., 588
Frischer, H., 340
Frosch, W. A., 588
Fruhling, L., 34
Frumin, A. M., 349, 810
Fuchs, F., 148
Fudenberg, H. H., 36, 85, 86, 87, 250, 257, 348, 505, 508, 647, 650, 757, 818
Fuhr, J., 391, 437
Fujimoto, M. M., 751
Fukutake, K., 647
Fulginiti, V., 203
Fuller, D. E., 815
Fuller, E. A., 810
Fuller, L. M., 593

Fundi, M., 349
Funk, D. D., 236
Furlow, L. T., Jr., 440
Furman, M., 125
Furtado, D., 592
Furtado, V., deP., 234
Furth, F., 551, 589
Fuson, R. I., 819

## G

Gaarder, A., 750
Gabr, M., 435
Gabriele, O. F., 437
Gabrio, B. W., 59, 346
Gabuzda, T. G., 437
Gaetani, M., 623
Gaffney, P. C., 203, 649
Gafni, D., 348, 444, 508
Gage, R. P., 754
Gairdner, D., 11, 13, 14, 15, 20, 21, 208, 236, 343, 812
Galbraith, P. A., 588
Galen, R. S., 175
Gall, E., 548, 591
Gallagher, N. I., 466
Gallardo, F. O., 149
Gallardo, J. T., 467
Gallo, G., 809, 812
Gallo, R. C., 589
Gallus, A. S., 34, 754
Galpine, J. F., 817
Galton, D. A. G., 589, 624
Galvan, R. R., 257
Gamsu, H., 648
Gang, K. M., 534
Gans, H., 750
Garbode, F., 87
Garby, L., 236, 431
Garcia, J. F., 240
Garcia, M. L., 176
Gardiner, C. C., 548
Gardner, F. H., 61, 72, 102, 203, 236, 259, 343, 346, 347, 437, 465, 745, 808, 810, 815
Gardner, L. I., 203, 204
Gardner, L. J., 679
Gardner, R. H., 534
Garner, R. L., 758
Garnett, T. J., 344
Garrey, W. E., 534
Garriga, S., 285
Garrison, M., Jr., 440
Garry, P. J., 238
Garson, O. M., 509
Gartland, J. J., 753
Gartner, L. M., 125, 126
Gasser, C., 72, 126, 267, 285, 343, 456, 465, 499, 521, 676, 752, 787, 812, 814
Gasser, G., 504
Gasster, M., 257
Gaston, E. O., 676
Gaston, L. W., 750
Gath, S., 510
Gatt, S., 680
Gatti, R. A., 17, 18, 21
Gaucher, E., 662, 676
Gautier, E., 465, 812
Gautier, M., 35, 591
Gavis, G., 446
Gavosto, F., 548
Gawronska, M., 176
Gayle, E., 434
Gaynor, E., 650, 677
Gechman, E., 34
Gecht, E. A., 535
Geddes, A. K., 676
Gee, T. S., 624
Geeraets, W. J., 441
Geiling, E. M. K., 10
Geiser, C. F., 203
Geisler, P., 756
Gelb, A. G., 87

Gellhorn, A., 626
Gellis, S. S., 121, 122, 126, 127, 129, 130, 148, 176, 437, 548, 549, 676, 812
Gelman, S., 506, 522
Gelpi, A. P., 236, 348
Gens, R. D., 102
George, J. N., 750
George, P., 624, 648
Gerald, P. S., 11, 12, 284, 288, 348, 357, 420, 437, 443, 587
Gerbie, A. B., 146, 149
Gerrard, J. W., 148
Gervais, M., 812
Gerver, J. M., 148
Ghai, O. P., 236
Ghavimi, F., 628
Ghitis, J., 285, 589
Gianantonio, C. A., 790, 791, 812, 817
Gibbel, N., 87
Giblett, E. R., 59, 86, 240, 287, 343, 437, 678
Gibson, A., 534
Gibson, G. W., 240
Gibson, J. G., II, 465
Gibson, J. M., 388, 443
Gibson, Q. H., 464, 465
Gibson, R. W., 566, 589
Gibson, S., 342
Gie, L. H., 436
Giedion, A., 522
Gilbert, A., 126
Gilbert, E. F., 589, 677
Gilbert, E. S., 592, 624
Gilbert, H. S., 468
Gilbraith, P., 548
Gilchrist, G. S., 548, 623, 626, 750, 812
Giles, D., 594
Giles, J. P., 102, 810
Giles, S. P., 340
Gilles, H. M., 437
Gillespie, C. E., 439
Gillespie, E. B., 438
Gillette, P., 383, 437
Gilliam, A. G., 589
Gilligan, D. R., 343
Gilliland, B. C., 343
Gillis, E. M., 534
Gillman, J., 236
Gillman, T., 236
Gilman, P. A., 806, 812
Gilmour, J. R., 11
Gilon, E., 812
Ginn, H. E., 442
Ginsberg, U., 440
Ginsberg, V., 441
Ginsburg, S. M., 285
Girdany, B. R., 589
Girdwood, R. H., 59, 257
Girsch, L. S., 750
Giselson, N., 457, 466
Githens, J. H., 72, 203, 285, 343, 437, 466, 649
Gitlin, D., 34, 148, 503, 505, 508, 521, 624, 676, 726, 750, 810
Gittler, C., 467
Giunta, F., 111, 127
Gladner, J. A., 750
Gladstein, E., 648
Glagov, S., 34
Glanzmann, E., 734, 750
Glaser, J., 103, 812
Glaser, K., 14, 21
Glass, A. G., 203, 562, 589
Glass, B., 258
Glass, H., 20
Glass, L., 59
Glassford, G. H., 175
Glauser, E. M., 129

Glauser, S. C., 129
Glendening, M. B., 746
Glenn, W. W. L., 679
Glidewell, O., 625
Glueck, H. I., 819
Glynn, K., 466, 467
Godwin, H. A., 521, 676
Gofstein, R., 148, 437
Gokcen, M., 750
Gold, A. P., 466
Gold, N. J., 109, 126
Goldberg, A., 234, 236, 238
Goldberg, A. F., 466, 504, 534
Goldberg, L. S., 250, 257
Goldberg, M. A., 437
Goldberg, S. R., 446
Goldbloom, A., 59
Goldbloom, R. B., 127
Goldburgh, H. L., 812
Goldenberg, H., 650
Goldenburg, E. W., 339
Goldie, W., 753
Goldman, J. M., 648
Goldman, M. C., 677
Goldring, D., 203
Goldsmith, E. I., 549
Goldsmith, H. J., 815
Goldsmith, K. L. G., 813
Goldsmith, M. H., 433
Goldsmith, Y., 550, 594
Goldstein, B. D., 467
Goldstein, F., 349
Goldstein, G. W., 812
Goldstein, M. A., 757
Goldstein, M. L., 650
Goldstein, N., 815
Goldstein, R., 746
Goldwasser, E., 59, 60, 236, 285, 466
Gollerkeri, M., 548
Gollub, S., 750
Goluboff, N., 466
Golubow, J., 436
Gomez, F., 257
Gomez-Leal, A., 288
Good, M., 240
Good, R. A., 21, 34, 129, 284, 345, 472, 488, 493, 502, 503, 504, 505, 507, 508, 510, 522, 571, 590, 649, 679, 810, 812, 814, 816, 817, 819
Good, T. A., 812
Goodall, H., 34, 343
Goodman, H., 129, 177
Goodman, M. L., 73
Goodman, R. M., 446
Goodwin, J. F., 240
Gordin, F., 257
Gordin, R., 260, 504
Gordon, A. S., 59, 61, 466
Gordon, E. B., 88, 150
Gordon, F. H., 285
Gordon, H. H., 809
Gordon, H. W., 572, 589
Gordon, R. R., 34, 750, 811, 812
Gordon, R. S., 236, 240
Gordon, S., 467
Gore, I., 587
Gorios-Breton, J., 502
Gorman, J. G., 148, 175, 505
Gorodischer, R., 126
Gorten, M. K., 215, 236
Gotoff, S. P., 505
Gottfried, E. L., 344, 677
Gottlieb, A., 343
Gottlieb, C., 288
Gottlieb, R., 59
Gottman, A. W., 127, 589
Gould, W. R., 589
Gouley, B. A., 812
Goulis, G., 125, 174

## AUTHOR INDEX

Gouttas, A., 437
Gowans, J. L., 527, 534
Grabstald, H., 62
Graf, C. J., 813
Graham, F. S., 34
Graham, J. B., 467, 747, 748, 750, 751, 754
Graham, R. C., Jr., 752
Grahn, E. P., 69, 72
Granda, J., 746
Granick, S., 59, 221, 224, 236
Grant, W. C., 60
Grantz, C., 174
Granville, N., 257, 287
Grasbeck, R., 257
Grassi, M. A., 548
Graves, D., 11, 12, 594
Graw, R. G., Jr., 589, 624
Gray, J. D., 589
Gray, L. W., 550
Gray, M. P., 346
Green, K. H., 810
Green, M., 618, 624
Green, O. C., 173
Green, R. H., 340
Green, S., 236, 237, 812
Green, T. W., 437, 648, 676
Greenberg, G. R., 257
Greenberg, L., 750, 810
Greenberg, M. S., 60, 258, 286, 343, 344, 437, 439
Greenberg, R. E., 203
Greenberg, S. D., 550
Greendyke, R. M., 814
Greene, J. B., 438
Greene, M. A., 548
Greene, R. W., 811, 812
Greene, S. A., 591
Greene, W. J. W., 235
Greenfield, J. B., 259
Greengard, J., 238
Greenspan, I., 589, 593
Greenwald, H. M., 782, 812
Greenwalt, T. J., 236
Greer, D., Jr., 177
Greer, M., 204
Gregory, C. H., 127
Gregory, K. O., 35
Greig, H. B. W., 505, 521
Grello, F. W., 592
Gren, A., 347
Grey, R., 442
Grieder, H. R., 130
Griffin, S., 87
Griffith, K. M., 627
Griffiths, J., 812
Griffiths, P. D., 234
Griggs, R. C., 437
Grimes, A. J., 311, 343, 435, 437, 440, 594
Grinstein, M., 60, 338, 432, 437
Grisolia, S., 434
Griswold, H. E., 348
Groat, W. A., 648
Grobbelaar, B. G., 34
Groce, E. J., 594
Groch, G. S., 203
Groen, J., 587, 666, 676, 680
Groover, R. V., 592
Gross, L., 563, 564, 589
Gross, R., 737, 750
Gross, R. E., 203, 676, 812
Gross, R. T., 60, 237, 312, 343, 346, 437, 506
Gross, S., 129, 236, 239, 349, 443, 591, 626
Grossbard, L., 589
Grossman, A., 127
Grossman, H., 435, 437, 549, 812
Grossowicz, N., 258
Grottum, K. A., 750, 812

Grove, W. J., 679
Grove-Rasmussen, M., 35, 102
Grubb, R., 86
Gruenstein, M., 650
Gruham, S., 589
Grumbach, M. M., 36
Grumet, F. C., 285
Grundbacher, F. J., 86
Grush, O., 503
Grushkin, C., 812
Gubler, C. J., 237, 241
Guernsey, J. M., 648
Guerry, D., III, 441
Guest, G. M., 21, 203, 205, 236
Guest, M. M., 748
Guggenheim, K., 521
Guha, D. K., 209, 236
Guichirit, I., 441
Guidotti, G., 60
Guild, H. G., 675
Gunn, C. K., 148
Gunn, R., 72, 401, 443
Gunson, H. H., 34, 175, 345
Gunz, F. W., 564, 566, 568, 588, 589, 647
Gurney, C. W., 49, 60, 508
Gussoff, B. D., 285
Gustafson, D. C., 34, 174
Gutenberger, J., 812
Guyda, H., 60
Guzman, S. V., 548
Gyland, S. P., 238

## H

Haab, O., 502, 520
Haansen, C., 752
Haber, A., 328, 348
Haber, J. M., 102, 148, 175
Haberman, S., 148
Haddow, A., 624
Haddy, T. B., 589, 627
Hadorn, B., 522
Haeger-Aronson, B., 343
Haggard, M. E., 437, 445, 589, 627
Haghbin, M., 621, 624
Hagitte, C., 592
Hagstrom, J. W. C., 445
Hahn, D. A., 238
Hahn, E. V., 438
Hahn, K., 129
Hahn, P. F., 236, 238
Hahn, R., 258
Haidas, S., 440
Haining, R. G., 343
Halbert, M. L., 21
Halbertsma, T., 465
Halbrecht, I., 175, 438
Haldane, E. V., 102
Halkett, J. A. E., 235
Hall, B. E., 509
Hall, B. D., 548
Hall, C. A., 257, 750
Hall, D. O., 60
Hall, E. W., 676
Hall, J. G., 782, 812
Hall, R., 723
Hall, S. W., 505
Hall, T. C., 625
Hallberg, L., 234
Hallenbeck, G. A., 287
Hallman, N., 177
Halpern, J., 649
Halstead, J. A., 238, 257
Haltalin, K. C., 438
Halterman, R. H., 624
Halvorsen, K., 505
Halvorsen, S., 60, 239, 812
Halvorson, E., 813
Ham, A. W., 586
Ham, T. H., 342, 343, 438, 449

Hamberg, D. A., 624
Hamilton, A., 258
Hamilton, H. B., 466
Hamilton, H. E., 509, 650
Hamilton, L., 589, 625
Hamm, C. W., 587
Hammaker, L., 129
Hammond, G. D., 60, 236, 285, 548, 588, 590, 623, 625, 627, 750, 814
Hammond, J. D. S., 750
Hammond, J. H., 549
Hamper, J., 87
Hamperl, H., 657
Hampson, R., 467
Hamrick, J. G., 649
Hananian, J., 650
Hand, A. M., 177
Handler, P., 468
Handley, D. A., 349, 747
Hanel, K. H., 344
Hanford, R. B., 343
Hanlon, D. G., 72, 505
Hanna, M., 149, 347, 750
Hansen, A. E., 649
Hansen, H. M., 285
Hansen, J. D. L., 259
Hanshaw, J. B., 127, 130, 535, 589, 754
Hansman, C. F., 589
Hanson, T. A., 35
Hanstein, A., 149, 344, 347
Harber, L. C., 344, 346
Harboe, M., 86
Harden, A. S., 438
Hardisty, R. M., 72, 432, 556, 578, 590, 738, 748, 750, 752
Hardy, N., 129
Hargraves, M. M., 475, 477, 505, 647
Hargreaves, T., 127, 344, 505
Harker, L. A., 228, 236, 682, 683, 750
Harkins, H. N., 465
Harley, E. L., 345
Harley, J. D., 34, 72, 127, 813
Harms, D., 813
Harnden, D. G., 586
Harnred, R. K., 586
Harper, D. T., 175, 437
Harrald, B., 344
Harrington, W. J., 289, 762, 777, 813
Harris, H., 60
Harris, I. M., 676
Harris, J., 819
Harris, J. S., 591, 650
Harris, J. W., 60, 72, 257, 437, 438, 449, 466
Harris, L. C., 285
Harris, L. E., 127
Harris, R. C., 124, 127, 129, 148
Harris, S., 505
Harris, T. N., 505
Harrison, D. C., 464
Harrison, E., 442
Harrison, H. E., 465
Harrison, J. F., 86
Harrison, J. W. E., 502
Harrison, T. R., 466, 548
Harrison, W. E., Jr., 676
Harrow, B. R., 438
Hart, E. B., 467
Hartfall, S. J., 344
Hartigak, J. D., 344
Hartman, J., 439, 625, 649
Hartmann, A. F., 465
Hartmann, J. R., 347

Hartmann, R. C., 257, 339, 344, 750, 752
Harvard, E., 676
Harvey, C. C., 467
Hasekura, H., 82, 86
Haselhorst, G., 15, 21
Haserick, J. R., 505
Hasselback, R. C., 586
Hasterlik, R. J., 590
Hathaway, W. E., 34, 72, 202, 203, 285, 343, 437, 591, 750, 751
Hathorn, M., 236
Hatoff, A., 586
Hattori, M., 349, 508
Haupt, H., 344
Haurani, F. I., 203, 625
Hauschka, T. S., 593
Hauser, A. D., 441
Hauser, G. H., 467
Hausman, C. F., 203
Haut, A., 435, 467, 625, 810
Havard, C. W. H., 285, 286
Havens, W. P., 677
Haverback, B. J., 127
Havrani, F., 349
Hawkins, C. F., 256, 550
Hawkins, V. R., 289
Hawkinson, V., 338
Hay, J. D., 751
Hayashi, T. T., 149
Hayati, M., 287
Hayatt, M., 591, 626
Hayes, D. M., 505, 676
Hayhoe, F. G. J., 505, 521, 649
Hazeltine, F. G., 160, 175
Heal, F. C., 813
Heath, C. W., Jr., 257, 590, 591
Heaton, L. D., 286
Hebenstreit, W., 442
Hecht, F., 11
Heck, F. J., 346
Hedenberg, F., 438, 521
Hedenstedt, S., 34, 72, 148
Hedenstrom, G., 648
Heemstra, J. G., 549
Hefmeyer, N. G., 287
Heggie, A. D., 813
Hegsted, D. M., 236
Heide, K., 344
Heilmeyer, L., 236, 344
Heimlich, E. M., 240
Heinegard, D., 466
Heinemann, H. O., 507, 592
Heinenberg, S., 467
Heiner, D. C., 241, 505, 751, 807, 813
Heinle, R. W., 244, 260
Heins, H. L., Jr., 349, 351, 508, 509
Heitzman, E. J., 808
Hellegers, A. E., 10, 434
Hellem, A. J., 741, 750, 751, 754
Heller, P., 287, 443, 446, 510, 535
Hellman, L. M., 35, 149
Hellstrom, I., 590
Hellstrom, K. E., 590
Helman, R. S., 60
Helmholz, H. F., Jr., 72
Helz, M. K., 344
Hemingway, E., 129
Hemker, H. C., 751, 753
Hemker, P. W., 751
Hempelmann, L. H., 593
Hemsted, E. H., 435
Henchman, D. C., 127
Henderson, A. B., 438
Henderson, E. S., 587, 593, 610, 624, 625

Henderson, F., 236
Henderson, L., 468
Henderson, P., 508
Hendrickse, R. G., 260, 438
Hendry, D. W. W., 343
Henkin, W. A., 438
Henle, G., 549
Henle, W., 549
Henley, W. L., 814
Hennessy, I. V., 342
Henricks, F. D., 286
Henry, E. I., 751
Henry, J. R. K., 522
Henry, M. D., 438
Henry, R. L., 442, 443
Henry, W. L., 439
Hepner, R., 236
Heppard, P. M., 175
Herbet, V., 60, 242, 243, 245, 257, 258, 521
Herbut, P. A., 590, 648
Heremans, J. F., 29, 34
Herman, E. C., 438
Hermann, H. E., 586
Hernandez, J. R., 203
Hernandez, K., 624
Herres, P., 506
Herrick, J. B., 371, 438
Hersh, E. M., 590, 625
Hershgold, E. J., 757
Hertzog, A. J., 813
Hertzog, K. P., 439
Herve, L., 284
Herz, F., 176, 345
Herzig, G. P., 624
Hesch, J. A., 622
Hesse, deV., 286
Heuser, H., 814
Hewitt, J., 128, 176
Hewlett, J. S., 72, 346, 754, 811
Hewlitt, D., 594
Heyn, R. M., 281, 286, 592, 625
Heyssel, R. M., 587
Heywood, J. D., 438
Hibbard, E., 147, 149
Hicks, N. D., 751
Higgins, G., 126
Higmans, W., 550
Hijmans, W., 36
Hildebrand, F. L., 505
Hilgartner, M. W., 235, 286, 342, 436, 438, 446, 679, 746, 748, 751, 757, 759, 773, 813
Hilkovitz, G., 435, 438
Hill, A. B., 588
Hill, F. S., 438
Hill, H. A., 589
Hill, J. E., 128
Hill, J. H., 506
Hill, J. M., 534, 625, 751
Hill, R. J., 60
Hill, R. W., 345
Hillborg, P. O., 676
Hiller, M. C., 35, 816, 817
Hillestead, L. K., 590
Hillman, R. S., 344, 813
Hills, A. G., 509, 625
Hilts, S. V., 534
Hin, P. S., 436
Hippe, E., 258
Hirasa, J., 340
Hird, A. J., 590
Hirschhorn, K., 124, 129, 285, 588
Hirsh, J., 34, 503, 504, 505, 754
Hitchings, G. H., 625
Hitzig, W. H., 343, 344, 437, 521, 522
Hjelt, L., 177
Hjort, P., 751

Hnilicka, J. V., 754
Ho, L. K., 758, 819
Hoag, M., 217, 236, 240, 746, 751
Hoag, S., 464, 756
Hoagland, R. J., 540, 549
Hoak, J. C., 752
Hodapp, R. V., 21
Hodes, H. L., 675
Hodgman, J. E., 286
Hoeprich, P. D., 592, 626
Hoff, G., 549
Hoffenberg, R., 258
Hoffman, I., 751
Hoffman, J. F., 344
Hoffmann, H. N., II, 127
Hoga, T., 505, 625
Hogg, G. R., 175
Höhgman, C., 431
Hohorst, H. J., 623
Hoja, W. A., 676
Holburn, R. R., 758
Holden, D., 344
Holder, T. H., 62, 127, 130
Holland, J. F., 590, 625
Holland, P., 347, 507, 534
Holland, T. R., 756
Hollingsworth, J. W., 11, 60, 127, 236, 813
Holloway, A., 591
Holman, C. A., 175, 751, 808
Holman, G. H., 148, 167, 175, 345
Holman, H., 505
Holman, S., 260
Holmberg, L-G., 466
Holmes, B., 472, 505
Holmsen, H., 750, 751, 812
Holroyde, C. P., 72
Holswade, G. R., 549
Holt, L. E., Jr., 174, 258, 467
Holt, M., 270, 286
Holton, C. P., 590, 624
Holton, J. B., 127
Holtzman, N. A., 444
Holyoke, J. B., 674, 810
Homan, C. A., 87
Hong, R., 812
Honig, G. R., 746, 751
Hook, E. W., 438, 506
Hopkinson, D. A., 60
Hopps, H. C., 811
Horan, F. T., 809
Horan, M., 21, 676
Horger, E. O., III, 148
Hörlein, H., 420, 438
Horn, R. C., 785, 810
Hornstein, S., 36
Horonick, A., 506
Horowitz, H., 438
Horowitz, H. D., 751
Horowitz, H. I., 813
Horowitz, M. S., 534
Horrigan, D. L., 466
Horsfall, W. R., 286
Horton, B. F., 648
Hoshino, T., 647
Hoskins, D. W., 258
Houck, A. H., 549
Houghton, J. D., 810
Hougie, C., 747, 750, 751
Houx, V. N., 549
Hourihane, D. O. B., 71, 748, 809
House, E., 62
Hovig, J., 750
Hovig, T., 812
Howard, P. F., 439
Howarth, B. E., 466
Howell, D. A., 650, 808
Howell, J., 236, 438

Howell, W. H., 11
Howqua, J., 505, 648
Hoxie, T. B., 586
Hoyer, L. M., 751
Hsia, D. Y-Y., 59, 112, 116, 121, 125, 126, 127, 128, 148, 168, 175, 176, 286, 438, 549, 676
Hsia, H. H., 148
Hsia, Y. E., 623
Hsieh, Y-S., 235, 350, 509
Hsu, K. S., 60, 176, 345
Hsu, L. Y., 285, 588
Hsu, T. H. J., 174
Huang, N. N., 522
Hubbell, J. P., Jr., 127
Hubble, D., 73, 286
Huber, H., 505
Hudson, F. P., 751
Hudson, J. B., 813
Huehns, E. R., 11, 361, 433, 438, 439, 505, 747
Huennekens, F. M., 59
Huff, R. L., 59, 102
Hughes, A. A., 236
Hughes, D. W. O'G., 286
Hughes, G., 438, 439
Hughes, L. A., 813
Hughes, W. L., 624
Hughes-Jones, N. C., 174, 175, 344
Hugh-Jones, K., 813
Huguley, C. M., Jr., 258, 521, 625
Huisman, T. H. J., 11, 354, 439, 440, 441, 442, 448
Humble, J. G., 286, 489, 505
Humphreys, E. W., 442
Humphreys, G. H., II, 286
Humphreys, S., 464, 468
Hung, W., 259
Hungerford, D. A., 590, 592
Hungerford, G. F., 505
Hunt, J. A., 439
Hunt, J. S., 549
Hunt, M. L., 149, 176
Hunt, V. M., 535
Hunter, O. B., Jr., 86
Huntley, C. C., 439, 813
Hunton, D. B., 129
Huntsman, R. G., 11, 60, 234, 441, 623
Hurdle, D. A. F., 175
Hurley, T. H., 72, 449
Hurtado, A. V., 234
Hurwitt, E. S., 286
Hurwitz, R. E., 60, 343, 506
Hurworth, E., 130
Hussey, C. V., 755, 776, 816
Husson, G. S., 548
Hustu, H. O., 624, 626, 648
Hutaff, R. J., 676
Hutchinson, H. E., 72, 236, 434, 466
Hutchinson, W. D., 448
Hutt, M. S. R., 466
Hutton, R. A., 738, 750
Hwang, Y. F., 439
Hyatt, H. W., Jr., 812
Hyman, C. B., 163, 175, 590, 614, 621, 623, 625
Hyman, G. A., 590, 650, 679
Hyman, J. B., 679

**I**

Iber, F. L., 125
Ickes, C. E., 340
Ignatov, V. G., 449
Iiu, C., 811
Ikin, E. W., 86
Ikkala, E., 749, 754
Ikura, Y., 350

Imach, D., 127
Imahori, S., 813
Imerslund, O., 258
Ingall, D., 259, 286
Ingalls, T. H., 590
Inglefinger, F. J., 548
Ingram, G. I. C., 813
Ingram, V. M., 11, 41, 60, 357, 366, 416, 433, 437, 439
Inman, J. K., 237
Innes, J., 589
Irvin, J. M., 813
Irving, K. C., 812
Irwin, S., 588
Isaacs, R., 648
Isacs, W. A., 464
Isdale, I., 810
Isenberg, H., 509
Ishihara, T., 593
Ishikawa, A., 60
Ishimori, T., 82
Israels, L. G., 11, 12, 36, 60, 62, 150, 163, 178, 507, 522, 752
Israels, M. C. G., 286, 466, 504, 759
Isselbacher, K. J., 127
Itano, H. A., 73, 439, 440, 443, 447, 448, 449
Iuchi, I., 466
Ivemark, B. I., 676
Iversen, T., 752
Iverson, T., 590
Ivy, A. C., 752
Ivy, R. E., 439
Izzo, M. J., 351, 679

**J**

Jablonski, W. J., 168, 175
Jack, I., 547, 548
Jack, J. A., 86
Jackson, D. P., 747, 752, 814, 815
Jackson, J. F., 439
Jackson, L. O., 236
Jackson, R. L., 238
Jackson, S. H., 504, 678
Jacob, F., 8, 11, 439
Jacob, G. F., 439
Jacob, H. S., 344, 439, 677
Jacobs, A., 223, 237, 304
Jacobs, A. S., 61, 444
Jacobs, E., 794, 810
Jacobs, K., 467
Jacobs, P., 464
Jacobs, P. A., 34, 586, 590, 648
Jacobs, P. M., 88
Jacobs, P. S., 587
Jacobson, A., 438
Jacobson, B. M., 813
Jacobson, L. O., 50, 60, 285, 466, 587, 676, 677
Jacobson, W. A., 550
Jacoby, M. D., 506, 677
Jacoby, W. J., Jr., 819
Jacquillat, C., 623
Jaenicke, L., 257
Jaffé, E. R., 60, 344, 350, 509
Jaffe, H. L., 677
Jaffe, N., 590
Jager, B. V., 344
Jahsman, D. P., 286
James, D. H., Jr., 648
James, J., 627
James, J. D., 86
Jandl, J. H., 10, 58, 60, 65, 71, 172, 175, 237, 258, 296, 340, 344, 346, 439, 677, 808

# AUTHOR INDEX

Janeway, C. A., 34, 473, 503, 505, 508, 521, 676
Janković, B. D., 284, 502, 520
Janssen, W., 592
Jarrett, A., 346
Jarrold, J., 591
Jarrold, T., 289
Jaslowitz, B., 649, 650
Jasmin, C., 287, 626
Javert, C. T., 34
Javett, S. N., 813
Javid, J., 149, 344
Jeanneret, R. L., 504
Jefferson, R. N., 446
Jeffries, G. H., 258
Jeliu, G., 176
Jellinek, H. L., 810
Jenkin, R. D. T., 643, 648
Jenkins, D. E., 344
Jenkins, G. C., 234
Jenkins, M., 73
Jenkins, M. E., 439, 445
Jenkins, W. J., 86, 87, 344
Jenks, A. L., Jr., 587
Jennison, R. F., 148
Jensen, G. R., 589
Jensen, W. N., 345, 346, 445, 463, 466
Jensson, O., 344
Jepson, J. H., 286
Jeremic, M., 750, 812
Jernigan, J. P., 434
Jiji, R. M., 259
Jim, R. T. S., 439, 813
Jimenez, C. T., 439
Jimenez, E. L., 813
Jobard, P., 34
Johansson, S. A., 754
John, G. G., 127
Johns, D., 127
Johnson, A. J., 754
Johnson, B. F., 237
Johnson, C. A., 751, 813
Johnson, D. E., 815
Johnson, F. B., 126, 129
Johnson, F. F., 751
Johnson, G. C., 502
Johnson, H., 746
Johnson, H. D., 590, 592
Johnson, L., 148, 176
Johnson, P., 150, 175
Johnson, P. A., 746
Johnson, S., 464
Johnson, S. A., 347, 752
Johnson, W. W., 590, 592, 593, 626
Johnston, C. C., Jr., 633, 648
Johnston, F. E., 439
Johnston, R. B., Jr., 473, 502, 505
Joleff, C. R., 441
Jonas, A. F., 818
Jonas, W., 504
Jonasson, T. H., 344
Jones, A. R., 175, 344, 624
Jones, B., 21, 237, 439, 646, 648, 677
Jones, C. H., 815
Jones, C. R., 677
Jones, D. L., 623
Jones, H. W., 813
Jones, J. E., 780, 813
Jones, J. H., 752
Jones, N. C., 60
Jones, N. F., 466
Jones, P. N., 60
Jones, R. T., 62, 442, 447, 467
Jones, R. V., 440
Jones, R. W., 449
Jones, S. R., 433, 440
Jones, T. G., 813
Jonsen, J., 750

Jonsson, U., 286, 440
Jonxis, J. H. P., 61, 354, 361, 433, 440
Joos, H. A., 61, 102
Jordan, A., 339
Jordan, H. H., 752
Jordan, W. S., Jr., 344
Jordans, G. H. W., 505
Jorpes, E., 754
Jorpes, J. E., 748
Josephs, H. W., 214, 237, 286, 344, 466
Josephson, A. M., 340, 349, 440, 446
Joske, R. A., 259
Joske, R. G., 466
Joubert, S. M., 351
Jowett, M., 434
Judisch, J. M., 237
Juhlin, L., 508
Jung, E., 349, 508, 749
Jurkiewicz, M. J., 440
Jurow, S. S., 235

## K

Kaalund-Jorgensen, O., 647
Kääriäinen, L., 549
Kabat, E. A., 86
Kabins, S. A., 376, 440
Kach, V. D., 594
Kach, Y. D., 12
Kagan, B. M., 466
Kahle, L. L., 505
Kaiser, E., 466
Kalayjian, B. S., 590
Kalderon, A. E., 344
Kallen, R. J., 125
Kalpaktsoglou, P. K., 14, 21
Kan, Y. W., 440
Kane, C. A., 73
Kanero, I., 257
Kanfer, J. N., 149
Kann, H. E., 346
Kanter, A., 817
Kao, V., 286
Kaplan, A. B., 808
Kaplan, E., 11, 21, 60, 72, 176, 178, 237, 345, 440, 449, 813
Kaplan, H. G., 506
Kaplan, H. S., 590, 642, 648
Kaplan, M. E., 549
Kaplan, S. R., 817
Kaplan, S. S., 508, 592
Kaplow, L. S., 505, 521
Karaklis, A., 126, 345, 436
Karanas, A., 555, 590
Kark, R. W., 237
Karnicki, J., 175
Karnofsky, D. A., 625, 643, 648
Karnovsky, M. L., 344, 471, 502
Karon, M., 127, 438, 623, 624, 625, 627
Karpati, G., 813
Karpinski, F. E., Jr., 549
Karpouzas, J., 441, 815
Karson, E. F., 505
Kasabach, H. H., 813
Kasai, M., 127
Käser, H., 202
Kashemsant, C., 434
Kashiwagi, C., 548, 816
Kasper, C. K., 752
Kasper, C. N., 289
Kass, C., 651
Kass, E. H., 346, 437
Kastenbaum, M. A., 591
Kaster, J. D., 535
Kato, K., 21, 203
Kato, R., 674
Kattamis, C., 73, 410, 440

Kattlove, H. E., 666, 677
Katz, J. H., 237
Katz, S., 258
Katzin, E. M., 149
Katzin, F. M., 35, 86
Kauder, E., 176, 503, 505, 520, 521, 627, 677
Kauffman, A., 349
Kaufman, D. G., 811
Kaufman, M., 440
Kaufman, R. E., 549
Kaufman, R. M., 752
Kaufman, S. F., 445
Kaufmann, R. W., 345
Kaump, D. H., 535
Kaupp, H. A., 286
Kay, E. H. M., 11
Kayden, J. H., 72, 73
Kaye, D., 679
Kazama, M., 746
Kaznelson, P., 774, 813
Keats, T. E., 677
Keefer, V., 236
Keeley, K., 464
Keen, R., 443
Keene, W. R., 776, 808
Keidan, S. E., 679
Keideling, W., 236
Keighley, G., 285
Keil, J. V., 11, 439
Keimowitz, R., 72
Keitel, H. G., 147, 434, 440
Keith, H. M., 590
Keith, J. D., 504
Keitt, A. S., 345
Kekwick, R. A., 86
Kelemen, E., 814
Keller, R. W., 339
Keller, W., 236
Keller, W. M., 130
Kellermeyer, R. W., 350, 752
Kellman, L., 466
Kellner, A., 103, 547
Kelly, J. J., III, 345
Kelly, K. H., 502, 587, 675
Kelly, V. J., 236
Kelly, W. O., 649, 816
Kelsey, W. M., 590
Kemp, J. A., 447
Kemp, N. H., 590
Kempe, C. H., 203
Kempton, J. J., 810
Kendell, A. C., 817
Kennedy, A. C., 342, 448
Kennedy, B. J., 286, 648
Kennedy, R. L. J., 284
Kent, E., 505, 813
Kerber, I. J., 34
Kerlan, I., 286
Kessler, B. J., 678
Keusch, G., 432
Kevy, S. V., 102, 505, 677
Keydar, J., 594
Khakoo, Y., 73
Khanna, N. N., 127
Khattak, B. Z., 257
Khaw, K. O., 288
Khaw, K. T., 522
Kho, L. K., 258, 286
Kidd, J. G., 603, 625
Kie, T. S., 758
Kiely, J. M., 506
Kikawa, Y., 344
Kilby, R. A., 587
Kildeberg, P., 814
Killander, A., 168, 176
Killman, S. A., 504, 521
Kim, B., 746
Kim, B. S., 590
Kimball, H. R., 521, 523, 676
Kimball, R. S., 651
Kimber, C., 237

Kimber, R. J., 309, 342
Kimbro, E. L., 340
Kimmelstiel, P., 440
Kindwall, J. A., 503
King, A. L., 36, 817
King, E. R., 443
King, H., 440
King, J. C., 435, 446
King, M. J., 534
King, O., 509
Kingma, S., 442
Kingsley, C. S., 752
Kinney, T. D., 236
Kinsolving, C. R., 348
Kiossoglov, K. A., 440
Kirchbaum, A., 590
Kirk, R. L., 87, 755
Kirkman, D., 535, 594
Kirkman, H. N., 34, 35, 203, 345
Kirkpatrick, C. I. F., 286, 440
Kirshbaum, I. D., 590
Kirsner, J. B., 592
Kisker, C. T., 752
Kissane, J., 431
Kistenmacher, M. L., 509
Kjeldsen, J., 21
Klajman, A., 648
Klatskin, G., 56, 60, 128, 679
Klatte, E. C., 590
Klaus, M. H., 819
Klebanoff, S. J., 472, 505
Kleckner, M. S., Jr., 237
Kleihauer, E., 11, 440
Klein, E., 625
Klein, H., 62, 448
Klein, R., 286
Klein, S. J., 21
Klein, S. W., 813
Kleiner, G. J., 754
Kleinman, L. I., 21
Klemola, E., 549
Klibansky, C., 811
Kline, A., 345
Klinefelter, H. F., 440
Klingberg, W. G., 21, 237, 439, 646, 648
Klingman, A. W., 504
Klinman, A., 102
Klion, F. M., 440
Klipstein, F. A., 254, 258, 441
Kloosterman, G. J., 758
Klotz, A. P., 675
Kniker, W. T., 751, 813
Kniseley, R. M., 815
Knisely, M. H., 677
Knoblich, R., 440
Knock, H. K., 437
Knock, H. L., 466
Knoedler, J. P., 587
Knoll, W., 11
Knospe, W. H., 625
Knowles, J. P., 257
Knox, W. E., 286
Knudtson, K. P., 127
Koblenzer, P. T., 810
Kocabalkan, N., 431
Koch, B., 448
Koch, C. A., 176
Koch, E. A., 86
Kochaseni, S., 442
Kochwa, S., 87, 176, 749
Kohler, C. M., 234
Kohler, H. G., 35
Kohn, J. L., 586
Kojima, Y., 754
Kolars, C. P., 814
Koler, R. D., 288, 444, 467, 534, 590
Koller, F., 749, 752, 753, 814

## AUTHOR INDEX

Kolmeier, K. H., 590
Kolodny, E. H., 149
Komninos, Z. D., 258, 341, 650
Komrower, G. M., 814
Kondi, A., 253, 257, 258, 285, 465
Kong, K. L., 436
Konigberg, W., 60
Konotey-Ahulu, F. I. D., 440
Kontos, H. A., 345
Kontras, S. B., 754, 757, 758
Koop, C. E., 127, 203
Kooptzoff, O., 86
Kopelman, A. E., 112, 127
Koppe, J. G., 758
Korber, E., 353, 440
Korein, J., 345
Korn, D., 814
Kornberg, A. J., 521
Kornzweig, A. L., 71, 72
Korst, D. R., 467, 648
Kosan, N., 286
Kosinksi, A. A., 235
Koskelai, S-L., 594
Kosower, N., 346
Kosoy, M. H., 748
Kossman, R. J., 345
Kostmann, R., 518, 521
Koszewski, B. J., 258
Kough, R. H., 441
Kourepi, M., 746
Kove, S., 127, 128
Kowal, J., 465
Kozak, M., 505
Kracke, R. R., 521
Krafchuk, J. D., 812
Krafft, C. J., 148
Krakoff, I. H., 625
Kramer, L. I., 133, 149
Kramer, S., 464
Krammer, A., 466
Krantz, S. B., 286
Krasner, I., 127
Kraszewski, T. M., 812
Krauss, A. P., 35, 345, 435
Kraut, J. M., 346
Kravitz, H., 466
Kreidberg, M. B., 794, 814
Kreimer-Birnbaum, M., 432
Kretschmer, N., 720, 755, 817
Krevans, J. R., 12, 175, 447, 449, 814
Krill, C. E., Jr., 521
Kriss, J. P., 237, 437
Kristan, J. J., 815
Kritzler, R. A., 506
Krivans, J. R., 437
Krivit, W., 174, 175, 204, 240, 345, 571, 587, 588, 590, 612, 615, 625, 626, 627, 650, 747, 750, 752, 757, 759, 808, 810, 812, 814, 817, 818, 819
Kronenberg, H., 86, 339
Kronfield, S. T., 590
Krüger, G., 624
Krugman, S., 102, 340, 810
Krumbhaar, E. B., 535
Krusi, G., 751, 814
Kubitz, P., 748
Kühlback, R., 257
Kuhn, J. P., 812
Kuhns, M., 522
Kulke, W., 175, 178
Kung, F., 20
Kunkel, H. G., 11, 85, 86, 237, 431, 440, 502, 505, 507
Kunstling, T. R., 345
Kuntzman, R., 128
Kunz, H. W., 440

Künzer, W., 752, 759, 819
Kuramoto, A., 746, 786, 814
Kurkcuoglu, M., 149, 752
Kurland, L. T., 590
Kurstjens, R., 752
Kurth, D., 345
Kushner, J. H., 20, 622, 808
Kuwabara, T., 129
Kyle, R. A., 287, 345, 517, 521 534, 561, 563, 590, 600, 620

L

Labbe, R. F., 343
LaBree, R. H., 340
LaCelle, P. L., 346, 351, 677
Lackey, R. W., 677
Lacson, P. S., 509, 650
Ladefoged, J., 284
Laforet, M. T., 443
Lagergren, J., 535
Lahey, M. E., 35, 229, 237, 239, 241, 258, 506, 590, 675, 677, 815
Laki, K., 690, 752
LaLand, S., 750
Lalezari, P., 506, 522
Lambilliotte, J. P., 754
Lambotte, C., 440
Lamont, N. Mc. E., 236
Lampkin, B. C., 258, 549, 626
Lamvik, J., 814
Lamy, F., 72
Lander, H., 102
Landholm, G., 815
Landing, B. H., 126, 128, 472, 506, 675, 677, 814
Landolt, R. F., 535, 814
Landsberg, J. W., 62
Landsteiner, K., 79, 86, 334, 342
Landwehr, G., 746
Lane, M., 284, 464, 466
Lang, D. J., 549
Lang, D. L., 547
Lang, J. E., 517, 521, 522
Langdell, R. D., 452, 748
Lange, R. D., 466, 591
Langer, L., Jr., 757
Langley, F. A., 237
Langley, F. H., 678
Langston, M. F., Jr., 345
Lanman, J. T., 675
Lann, S. H., 126
Lanz, H., 506
Lanzkowsky, P., 15, 21, 203, 207, 237, 258, 286, 448, 506, 748, 789, 813, 814
Lapey, J. D., 522
Lapidus, P. H., 550
Lapin, J., 506
Larkin, I. M., 752
LaRocco, C. G., 435
Laros, R. K., Jr., 814
Larrieu, M. J., 748, 752, 814, 815
Larsen, H., 749
Larson, A., 345
Lascari, A. D., 752
Laserohn, J. T., 675
Laski, B., 345, 504
Laster, L., 240
Laszlo, J., 440, 505, 625
Lathe, G. H., 58, 125, 128, 176
Lathem, W., 345
Latorraca, R., 814
Latte, B., 433
Laurence, J. H., 240
Laurendeau, T., 128
Laurie, H. C., 627
Lavietes, P. H., 48, 59

Lavy, N., 648
Law, L. W., 284
Lawler, S. D., 86, 343, 503
Lawlor, D. P., 474, 507
Lawrence, J. H., 464, 466, 587
Lawrence, J. S., 285, 286, 288, 506, 508, 522, 535
Lawson, N. S., 440
Layrisse, M., 240, 258, 432
Lazar, H. P., 549
Leake, T. B., 746
Lear, A. A., 465
Leavell, B. S., 102, 435, 441, 446, 448, 535
Leaver, F. Y., 677
Lechaux, P. A., 589
Leddy, J. F., 339, 345, 351
Lederer, M., 345
Lee, B. J., 648
Lee, C. L., 548
Lee, C. W., 623
Lee, G. R., 237, 259
Lee, H. C., 587
Lee, J. A. H., 591
Lee, P., 434, 435
Lee, R. C., 385, 441, 757
Lee, S. K., 550
Lee, S. L., 285, 534, 588, 591
Leeksma, C. H. W., 102, 752
Lees, M. H., 814
Lefkowitz, E., 508
Lehane, D., 174, 175, 178
Lehman, W. L., 593
Lehmann, H., 10, 11, 59, 60, 386, 431, 433, 434, 435, 436, 439, 440, 441, 443, 448, 464
Lehndorff, H., 385, 506
Lehrer, R. I., 503
Leichsenring, J. M., 21
Leikin, S. L., 35, 238, 240, 258, 259, 345, 444, 445, 446, 504, 626, 814, 816
Leitner, A., 817
Leitner, S., 506
Lejeune, J., 35, 591
Lejnieks, I., 650, 757
Lembert, G. L., 535
Lemire, R. J., 11
Lemon, B. K., 535
Lenert, T. F., 535
Lenhard, R. E., Jr., 352
Lenman, J. A. R., 59, 257
Lennard-Jones, J. E., 286
Leonard, B. J., 466, 591
Leonard, S., 128
Leonardi, G., 442
Leoncini, G., 343
Lepow, I. H., 348
Lereboullet, P., 126
Lerner, A. B., 286, 345, 441
Lerner, C., 376, 440
LeRoy, E. C., 759
Leroy, P., 586
Lescher, F. G., 286
Lesi, F., 437
Lesses, M. F., 102
Lessmann, E. M., 36
Lester, R., 61, 128
Levenson, S. M., 58, 101
Leventhal, B., 212, 237
Leventhal, B. G., 624
Levi, A. J., 346
Levin, J., 812
Levin, M. B., 203
Levin, M. L., 589
Levin, R. H., 814
Levin, W. C., 289, 348, 349, 441, 589, 649, 748
Levine, P., 35, 79, 82, 86, 87, 149, 176, 550
Levine, R. A., 128
Levinson, B., 648

Levitan, R., 649, 677
Levitt, M. F., 441
Levy, G., 127, 130
Levy, S. J., 85, 521
Levy, M. A., 591
Levy, M. S., 441
Levy, R. N., 272, 286
Levy-Toledano, S., 748
Lewin Smith, R. G., 234
Lewis, C. N., 274, 286, 323, 324
Lewis, E. B., 591
Lewis, E. J., 756
Lewis, F., 149, 203
Lewis, I. C., 623, 675, 814
Lewis, J. H., 747, 749, 752, 753, 758, 809
Lewis, P. M., 257
Lewis, S. J., 85, 521
Lewis, S. M., 71, 257, 284, 286, 340, 341, 345, 349, 503
Leydorf, M. M., 147
Lhowe, J., 73
Li, C. C., 752
Li, J. G., 507
Liachowitz, C., 441
Liakakos, D., 434, 441
Libre, E. P., 753
Lichtenstein, A., 14, 21
Lichtenstein, L., 506, 669, 677
Lichtman, H. G., 284, 344, 441, 446, 448, 468, 680
Lichtman, M. A., 346, 442, 466
Lidsky, I., 175
Lieb, W. A., 441
Lieberman, A. D., 811
Lieberman, E., 812, 814
Lieberman, J., 236
Lieberman, P., 62, 509, 669, 677
Lieberman, R., 534
Liebman, J., 347
Liebman, N. C., 438
Liebowitz, D., 816
Liebowitz, J., 547
Liebowitz, S., 549
Liegler, D. G., 508
Liem, H. H., 149, 347
Lien-Keng, K., 258
Lightwood, R., 287
Liley, A. W., 149, 166, 176
Lilienfeld, A. M., 589
Limarzi, L. R., 21, 464, 592, 626
Limentani, D., 350
Lind, J., 22, 34
Linden, G., 202
Lindenbaum, J., 254, 258, 441, 506
Lindsay, S., 149, 816
Lindstedt, E., 466
Lindstedt, G., 466
Lineback, M. I., 818
Lingley, J. F., 203
Linman, J. W., 60, 203, 517, 521, 649, 816
Lippman, H. S., 21
Lipschutz, F., 468
Lipscomb, J. M., 348
Lipton, E. E., 593
Lipton, E. L., 72, 128, 346, 677
Liquori, A. M., 441
Lisboa, E., 816
Lischner, H. W., 176, 203
Lisker, R., 441, 753, 814
Lister, J., 174
Litchman, H., 648
Little, A. S., 203
Little, B., 34
Little, J. R., 803, 814
Little, S. C., 548

Littlefield, J. W., 149
Littler, E. R., 815
Liu, C., 342
Livingstone, F. B., 445
Livingstone, J. L., 503
Lloyd, H. O., 33, 591
Lloyd, J. K., 72
Lloyd, P. C., 549
Lloyd, S. K., 73
LoBuglio, A. F., 259, 346
Lochte, H. L., Jr., 624, 627
Lock, S. P., 64, 72, 435, 814
Loder, P. B., 61, 342, 348
Loeb, R. F., 125
Loeb, V., Jr., 287, 647
Loeliger, E. A., 751
Loeliger, A., 752, 753
Loge, J. P., 466
Lohmuller, H. W., 442
Lokietz, H., 128
London, A. H., 818
London, I. M., 56, 60, 61, 125
London, R. D., 348, 816
London, W. T., 102
Lonergan, E. T., 73
Long, W. K., 340
Longcope, W. T., 549
Lonn, L., 442
Loos, J. A., 347, 348
Loos, M. C., 178
Lopas, H., 817
LoPresti, J. M., 444, 675
Lorand, L., 690, 752, 753
Lorber, J., 648
Lord, P. S., 174
Lord, T., 648
Lorenz, E., 286
Loria, A., 441
Lorincz, A. E., 499, 508
Lorkin, P. A., 443
Losowsky, M. S., 753
Louis, H. S., 676
Louis, J., 626
Louis-Bar, D., 814
Loukopoulos, D., 436, 441
Lousuebsakul, B., 150
Love, F. M., 677
Lovell, G. R., 468
Lowe, B. A., 348
Lowe, C. V., 258
Lowenbraun, S., 650
Lowenstein, L., 235, 286, 289
Lowman, J. T., 810
Lowrey, G. H., 680
Lozner, E. L., 811, 814, 912
Lubert, M., 175
Lubin, B. H., 346, 442
Lucas, A. O., 339
Lucas, O. N., 756
Luce, J., 626
Lucey, J. F., 35, 108, 111, 125, 128, 143, 148, 149, 161, 176, 723
Lucia, S. P., 149, 176
Ludman, H., 649
Luecke, P. E., Jr., 148
Lufti Vural, I., 522
Luhby, A. L., 35, 61, 258, 441, 518, 522, 588
Luke, C. G., 235, 237
Lukens, A., 817
Lukes, R. J., 549, 636, 638, 649
Lund, C. J., 22, 239, 240
Lundeen, E., 466
Lundh, B., 293, 346
Lundstrom, R., 814
Lusher, J. M., 442, 443, 649, 693, 753, 814
Lutgemeier, J., 752
Lutz, V., 508
Lutz, W. B., 507

Lutzner, M., 505
Luzzatto, L., 339, 370, 441
Lyle, W. H., 346
Lynch, B. L., 345
Lynn, H. B., 676
Lynn, R., 677
Lyon, M. F., 24, 35
Lyons, W. S., 72
Lytle, W. J., 339

**M**

Maass, A. R., 467
Mabarro, S. N., 349
Macauley, D., 128, 346
Macauley, J. C., 130
MacAusland, W. R., Jr., 753
MacCarthy, J. D., 343, 344, 626
MacDonald, A. H., 758
MacDonald, W. P., 466
MacDougall, L., 212, 216, 237, 257, 258, 285
Mace, J. W., 126
Macfarlane, R. G., 453, 696, 747, 814
Macfie, J. M., 747
MacGibbon, B. M., 256
MacGillivray, M. H., 128, 517, 522
MacIlroy, M., 87
MacIlwaine, W. A., 102, 435
MacIver, J. E., 258, 449
MacKay, E. V., 149
MacKay, I. R., 240, 505, 648
MacKay, R. B., 9, 11
MacKenzie, I., 589, 649
MacKinney, A. A., 346, 543, 549
Mackinnon, N. L., 259
Maclachlan, M. J., 504
MacLean, J. R., 148
MacMahon, B., 591, 593
MacMahon, H. E., 124, 677
Macpherson, A. I. S., 819
Macpherson, J. C., 752
Macris, N. T., 35, 149
MacWhinney, J. B., 72, 346, 814
Madenlioglu, M., 258
Madison, J. T., 756
Magee, J. H., 345
Magidson, J., 506
Magill, F. B., 260, 285, 289
Magnus, A., 297
Magnus, I. A., 346
Mahoney, F. J., 622
Mahoney, J. P., 810
Maillard, J. A., 467
Maisel, J. E., 535
Makowski, E. L., 10
Malaka, K., 350
Malcolm, D., 61
Maldonado, J. E., 506
Malina, R. M., 439
Malinin, T. I., 677
Mallett, B. J., 433
Mallory, T. B., 506, 591
Maloney, J. R., 33
Maloney, M. A., 58, 101
Maloney, W. C., 583
Malter, I. J., 591
Manahan, L., 129
Manaster, J., 816
Mandel, H. G., 626
Mandel, G. L., 506
Manfield, P. A., 813
Manfredi, R., 549
Mangalik, A., 238
Manganaro, J. S., 591
Manganelli, G., 444
Mangel, T. K., 550
Mangkornkanok, M., 150
Mangum, J. F., 442
Manion, W. C., 678

Mann, J. D., 87
Mann, T., 101
Manning, J. M., 383, 434, 435, 437
Manning, M. D., 203, 441
Mannings, G. B., 128
Mannucci, P. M., 749
Manyan, D. R., 287
March, H. C., 591
Marchal, G., 753
Marchasin, S., 237
Marcurelli, J., 284
Marcus, A. J., 521, 753, 754
Marcus, D. M., 77, 87
Marden, P. M., 11
Marder, V. J., 753, 816
Margaretta, W., 129
Margileth, A. M., 128, 814
Margolies, M. P., 383, 441
Margolis, A. J., 175
Margolis, J., 753
Marianni, G., 548, 661
Marinetti, G. V., 61
Markovitz, A., 815
Markowitz, A. S., 817
Markowitz, H., 241
Marks, E. K., 676, 677
Marks, J., 8, 9, 11, 20, 21, 236
Marks, P. A., 35, 312, 343, 346, 389, 432, 437, 441, 506
Markum, A. J., 258, 286
Marler, E. A., 648
Marlow, A. A., 239, 341, 466
Marmorston, J., 678
Marsaglia, G., 627
Marsh, C. L., 441
Marsh, G. W., 346
Marsh, J. A., 506
Marsh, J. C., 677
Marsh, W., 86, 87, 344
Marshall, G. J., 625
Marshall, R., 86
Marshall, S. R., 238
Marshall, W. C., 433
Martelo, O. J., 287
Marten, R. A., 509
Martensson, J., 522
Marti, H. R., 354, 433
Martin, F. I. R., 447
Martin, H. F., 128
Martin, J., 626
Martin, J. D., 467
Martin, J. W., 128
Martin, L. W., 203
Martin, M., 236
Martin, N., 61, 176
Martin, R. R., 503
Martin, W. J., 346, 522
Martin, W. W., 435, 438, 441
Martin du Pan, R., 35
Martine, R. M., 467
Martinez-Maldonado, M., 535
Martino, N. B., 627
Martland, H. S., 287
Maruffo, C. A., 588
Marvin, F., 345
Masartis, L., 177
Mase, K. B., 535
Masek, B., 594
Mason, H. L., 61, 126
Mason, J. W., 624
Masri, M. S., 440
Massimo, L., 344, 502
Master, J., 441
Masters, P., 432
Mastrangelo, R., 352, 651
Mastrokalos, N., 436
Matalon, R., 504
Matchett, M. D., 753
Mathal, C. K., 339

Mathe, G., 103, 287, 591, 603, 626
Mathews, P., 148
Mathews-Roth, M. M., 346
Mathieson, D. R., 127
Mathis, H. B., 506
Matioli, G., 441
Matoth, P., 749
Matoth, Y., 258, 441, 506
Matsaniotis, N., 87, 440, 815
Matson, G. A., 87
Matson, J. I., 756
Matsuda, G., 442
Matsumara, T., 746
Matsuzawa, T., 130
Mattern, M. J., 753
Matthews, D. M., 359
Matthews, J. M., 747
Mauer, A. M., 21, 35, 72, 149, 176, 269, 287, 502, 506, 520, 521, 522, 534, 549, 591, 626, 627, 674, 677, 811, 815
Mauger, D. C., 677
Mauley, J. H., 818
Maurer, H. M., 109, 128
Mauzerall, D., 61
Maximow, A. A., 677
May, C. D., 258, 260
Mayak, N. C., 678
Mayer, J., 239
Mayer, K., 342
Mayon-White, R. M., 465
Mazia, O., 344
Mazur, A., 221, 236, 237
Mazurkie, S. J., 758
Mazzitello, W. F., 677
Mbaya, V., 258
McAfee, J. G., 675
McAlister, J. M., 466, 676
McAllenney, P. F., 815
McAllister, R. M., 591
McAllister, W., 649
McBryde, R. R., 72, 346
McCall, M. S., 506
McCammon, R. W., 234
McCarthy, E. A., 127
McCarthy, E. F., 11
McCarthy, J. T., 549
McCarthy, K., 588
McCausland, D. J. M., 649
McClellan, B. H., 33
McClellan, G. S., 236
McClellan, J. T., 520
McCollum, R. W., 102, 548, 549
McConnell, R. B., 175, 178
McCoord, A. B., 61, 102
McCormick, W. F., 442
McCoy, K., 444
McCracken, G. H., 677, 753
McCrory, W. W., 789, 814, 815
McCullough, N. B., 593
McCune, D. J., 649
McCurdy, P. R., 287, 442, 444
McCutcheon, E., 34
McDonald, B. L., 350
McDonald, D. B., 649
McDonald, R., 238, 442
McDougal, R. A., 346
McElfresh, A. E., 149, 442, 445, 522, 752
McEmery, J. T., 238
McFadzean, A. J. S., 466
McFarland, R. B., 624
McFarland, W., 287, 345, 443, 549, 815
McFarlane, D. B., 238
McFeely, A. E., 550
McGill, D. B., 129
McGinley, J. M., 445
McGinniss, M. H., 102, 623

McGoldrick, K. E., 203
McGolvray, E., 589
McGovern, J. J., 35, 120, 758
McGovern, R., 128
McHugh, W. J., 341
McIlvanie, S. K., 626
McInnes, I. W. S., 444
McIntire, M. S., 464
McIntosh, A. J., 127
McIntosh, J., 234
McIntyre, N., 346
McIntyre, O. R., 258, 347, 677
McIntyre, P. A., 22, 250, 258
McKay, E., 287
McKay, R. J., 125, 128, 149, 168, 176, 815
McKee, R. W., 465
McKelvey, E., 623
McKenna, J. L., 752
McKenzie, D., 258, 506
McKenzie, S., 342
McKeown, E. F., 676
McKinlay, C. A., 536, 548
McKusick, V. A., 125, 348, 801, 812, 815
McLean, M. M., 522, 815
McMaster, J. D., 449
McMichael, J., 677
McMillan, C. W., 592, 757, 808
McMullen, G. P., 128
McMullin, G. P., 109
McNicholl, B., 252, 258
McPeak, C. N., 649
McPhedran, P., 591
McPhee, W. R., 346
McQuarrie, I., 750
McQuiggan, M. C., 815
McQuiston, D. T., 87
McSorley, J. G. A., 503
Meachen, G. C., 591
Meade, R. H., III, 549
Meadl, M. A., 815
Meadows, R. W., 648
Meadows, S. R., 72
Medal, L. S., 467, 753
Medearis, D. N., Jr., 128, 820
Medenis, R., 817
Medici, P. T., 61
Mednicoff, I., 818
Medoff, A. S., 677
Medoff, H. S., 21
Megas, J., 448
Mehta, S., 258, 346
Meisler, A., 343, 435, 457
Mele, R. H., 36, 523, 818
Melhorn, D. K., 626
Mellin, G. W., 440
Mellman, W. Jr., 509, 753
Melly, A., 753
Melly, M. A., 678
Melnick, J. L., 816, 817
Melnick, P., 752
Melnyk, K. J., 648
Melton, J., 650
Menashe, V. D., 814
Mendel, G. A., 238
Mendes de Leon, D. E., 351
Mendilaharzu, F., 812
Meneghello, J., 816
Menendez-Corrada, R., 535
Mengel, C. S., 346
Menken, V., 506
Menten, M. L., 649
Mentzer, W. C., 442
Mercado, C., 59
Mercer, R. D., 624
Merenstein, G. B., 815
Meriwether, W. D., 346
Merler, E., 757
Merman, A. C., 677
Merrill, S. W., 351

Merrit, D. H., 591
Merritt, A. D., 509, 648
Merritt, C. R., 348
Merritt, K. K., 21, 813
Merskey, C., 259, 727, 728, 749, 754
Mesa Arrau, C., 675
Meschia, G., 10
Meshaka, G., 814
Messaritakis, J., 815
Messite, J., 446
Metcalf, J., 467
Mettier, S., 464, 534
Mettler, N. E., 790, 815
Metts, J. C., 447
Meuten, M. L., 344
Meyer, H., 507
Meyer, L. M., 259, 535, 649
Meyer, O., 588, 649
Meyer, T. C., 128, 148, 149, 167, 176
Meyers, A. J., 234
Meyerson, R. M., 677
Miale, J. B., 61, 81, 87, 535
Mibashan, R. S., 588
Michael, A. F., Jr., 21, 149, 466
Michael, S. E., 754
Michael, S. R., 506, 522
Michaels, J. P., 35
Michaels, R. H., 449, 809
Michaëlsson, M., 176
Michaud, L., 467
Michels, N. A., 506
Middleman, E., 626
Mielke, C. H., Jr., 752
Mier, M., 72
Miesch, D. C., 649
Miescher, P., 346, 506
Migliorini, E., 340
Mijer, F., 35
Mikkelsen, C., 622
Miles, W., 102
Milgrom, F., 203
Millard, R. E., 506
Miller, A. A., 467
Miller, C., 442
Miller, D. E., 819
Miller, D. G., 648, 649
Miller, D. R., 251, 259, 287, 346, 347, 435, 442, 466, 506, 510, 522, 586, 591, 678, 754
Miller, E. B., 679, 810
Miller, E. R., 675
Miller, F. R., 591
Miller, G., 61, 72, 102, 177, 284, 346, 351, 381, 434, 535, 814, 817
Miller, G. F., 749
Miller, G. L., 506
Miller, G. M., 750
Miller, H. C., 35, 465
Miller, I. F., 259
Miller, J., 148, 572
Miller, J. F. A. P., 506, 522, 535
Miller, J. L., 506
Miller, J. McC., 591
Miller, J. Q., 675
Miller, M. D., 34
Miller, M. E., 506
Miller, M. H., 468
Miller, M. J., 35, 445
Miller, O., 589
Miller, O. J., 33, 587
Miller, R. A., 755
Miller, R. W., 558, 561, 566, 589, 591, 647, 648
Miller, S. P., 591, 650, 754
Millichap, J. G., 346
Mills, G. C., 347
Mills, L. C., 591

Mills, S. D., 61, 287, 591, 754
Milner, G., 259
Milner, P. F., 434, 442, 445
Milner, R. D. G., 503
Milstone, J. H., 754
Milnusky, A., 149
Minarikova, E., 176
Minick, O. T., 505
Minnich, V., 61, 238, 361, 434, 442, 443, 465, 813
Minno, A. M., 587
Minogue, W. F., 258
Minot, A. S., 464
Minot, G. R., 758, 815
Minton, S. A., 346
Mintz, A. A., 176
Miranda, S. I., 758
Mirčevová, L., 347
Mirick, G. S., 102, 340, 810
Mirman, B., 466
Mirsa, D. K., 287
Mistry, S. P., 237
Mitani, M., 592
Mitchell, B., 506
Mitchell, D. W., 535
Mitchell, J. R. A., 754
Mitchell, W. A., 678
Mitchison, J. M., 73, 444
Mitchner, J. W., 11, 442, 448
Mittwoch, U., 507, 591
Mitus, W. J., 287, 548, 588, 591, 623, 624, 808
Miwa, S., 350, 351
Miwa, T., 593
Miyaji, T., 466
Mizrahi, A., 348, 816
Mizutani, S., 594
Mladenovski, B., 435
Mobley, J. E., 444
Mochtar, I. A., 758
Modell, W., 287, 346
Modest, E. J., 678
Moe, P. J., 238
Moeschlin, S., 238, 442, 478, 507, 522
Mohabbat, O. M., 594
Mohberg, N. R., 623
Mohos, S. C., 588
Moinichen, S. L., 101
Mokhtar, N., 435
Mold, J. W., 809
Molinas, F., 817
Moll, M. M., 751
Mollin, D. L., 66, 71, 229, 238, 245, 256, 257, 259, 260
Mollison, P. L., 11, 16, 21, 61, 77, 86, 87, 90, 91, 102, 128, 149, 152, 174, 175, 176, 178, 346, 433, 464, 815
Moloney, W. C., 504, 535, 588, 590, 591, 594
Molthan, L., 149, 346, 449
Monaghan, J. H., 747
Moncrieff, A., 522
Monfardini, S., 623
Monge, C., 467
Monk-Jones, M. E., 259
Monnens, L., 754, 815
Monod, J., 8, 11, 357, 439
Monroe, J. H., 587
Montfort, J., 678
Montgomery, C. M., 87
Montgomery, T. L., 432
Monto, R. W., 286, 752
Mooallem, F., 258
Moon, R. L., 288
Moore, A., 260

Moore, C. V., 60, 61, 235, 238, 287, 432, 433, 434, 437, 442, 444, 465, 466, 589, 647, 818
Moore, D. H., 35, 591
Moore, E. W., 591, 593
Moore, G. T., 534, 535
Moore, J. E., 507
Moore, R. D., 809
Moore, S., 11, 676
Moore, T. D., 507, 591, 678
Moores, P., 86
Moores, R. R., 62, 238
Moorhead, J. F., 815
Moorhead, P. S., 753
Moosa, A., 174
Mora, J., 678
Morandi, L., 504
Morawitz, P., 684, 754
Moreland, H. J., 448
Moreno, G. D., 466
Moreno, H., 505
Mores, A., 176
Morgan, A. F., 239
Morgan, C. L., 814
Morgan, F. M., 749
Morgan, W. T. J., 85, 87
Morgenthau, J. E., 239, 288, 447
Mori, P. G., 502
Morley, A. A., 516, 522
Morris, B., 679
Morris, M. B., 815
Morrison, A. B., 125
Morrison, D. B., 435
Morrison, F. R., 289
Morrison, F. S., 815
Morrison, M., 468, 508, 649, 650
Morse, B. S., 754
Morse, E. E., 623
Morse, E. F., 707, 752
Morse, J. H., 507
Morton, J. A., 149
Morton, N. E., 346
Morton, R., 505
Moschcowitz, E., 783, 815
Moschovakis, C., 434
Moseley, J. E., 442, 678
Moser, K. M., 442
Moskowitz, R. M., 346
Moss, W. T., 649
Motamedy, F. F., 175
Motteram, R., 260
Mottironi, V. D., 509
Motto, S. A., 73, 817
Motulsky, A. G., 11, 59, 61, 72, 125, 340, 346, 347, 350, 439, 442, 447, 448, 678
Mountain, K. R., 714, 754
Mourant, A. E., 148
Mourdjinis, A., 746
Mouriquand, C., 72, 237
Moutalenti, G., 433
Movassaghi, N., 238
Movitt, E. R., 442
Mowrey, F. H., 345
Moyer, J. H., 591
Mudgett, R. T., 150
Mueller, J. F., 289
Muggia, F. M., 507, 592
Mugrage, E. R., 21
Muir, A. R., 238
Muir, C. S., 678
Muir, H., 507
Muir, W. A., 446
Mukherjee, A. M., 445
Mull, M. M., 34
Muller, C. J., 61, 442
Muller, H., 759
Müller-Eberhard, U., 145, 149, 176, 293, 344, 347, 438, 440, 442, 507
Mullinax, G. L., 432

Mumford, D. M., 594, 627
Munsey, F. A., 468
Muralt, G., 814
Murayama, M., 368, 442
Muro, P. D., 442
Murphy, A., 20, 236, 808
Murphy, E. A., 749
Murphy, J. R., 347
Murphy, J. W., 678
Murphy, M. E. B., 249, 260
Murphy, M. L., 509, 587, 615, 623, 625, 626, 628, 649
Murphy, S., 102, 776, 815
Murphy, W. H., 592
Murray, S., 148, 150
Muschel, L. H., 549
Muschenheim, C., 548
Museles, M., 814
Mustard, J. F., 749
Mustard, W. T., 679
Muster, A. J., 21
Musto, D. F., 347
Mychaljiro, O., 342
Myers, A. R., 758
Myerson, R. M., 238, 442
Myrik, Q. N., 87, 204

## N

Nabrady, J., 807, 818
Nachman, R. L., 286, 684, 754, 813
Nadas, A. S., 238, 239, 467
Nadimi, M., 238
Nadler, E. B., 146, 149, 467
Naeslund, J., 34, 148, 149
Naets, J. P., 467
Nago, T., 274, 287, 615, 626
Nagao, T., 274, 287, 615, 626
Nagel, C. G. M., 758
Nagel, R. L., 433
Nagi, N. A., 593, 627
Naiman, J. L., 21, 61, 176, 182, 202, 203, 238, 259, 347, 351, 442, 507, 816
Najean, Y., 349, 776, 815
Najjar, V. A., 61, 122, 123, 125, 126, 148, 588
Nakai, H., 128, 129, 649
Nakamura, K., 240
Nalbandian, R. M., 202, 442, 443
Na-Nakorn, S., 434, 442, 443, 448
Nance, W. E., 347, 443
Nappi, R., 150
Nasralla, M., 176
Nathan, D. G., 61, 67, 72, 73, 236, 239, 259, 285, 347, 352, 388, 391, 401, 437, 440, 442, 443, 502
Nathan, D. J., 592
Nathanson, I. T., 286
Natta, C., 437
Natzschka, J. C., 125
Naughton, M. A., 444
Naylor, J., 676
Neblett, R. T., 347
Necheles, T. E., 62, 284, 384, 387, 443, 449, 623
Need, D. J., 347, 649
Neel, J. V., 11, 61, 385, 434, 440, 443, 445, 449, 754, 755
Neelands, P. J., 12, 36, 150, 178
Neerhout, R. C., 13, 21, 61, 347, 592
Nefzeger, D., 592
Neil, J. V., 72
Neill, C. A., 349
Neill, D. W., 676
Neiman, G. M. A., 588

Neira, M., 816
Nelson, C. E., 238
Nelson, E. N., 258
Nelson, J., 815
Nelson, J. D., 176, 438, 817
Nelson, J. H., 648
Nelson, L. R., 521
Nelson, M. G., 102, 347, 587
Nelson, M. M., 148
Nelson, P., 678
Nelson, R. S., 129, 549
Nelson, T. L., 203
Nemerson, Y., 754
Nenci, G., 340
Nenna, A., 503
Nesbit, M. E., 627
Nesbit, R. R., 504, 589
Nestadt, A., 260, 289
Neuhauser, E. B. O., 675
Neumark, E., 287, 506
Neva, F. A., 808
Nevanlinna, H. R., 749, 754
New, M., 436
Newcomb, R., 347, 753
Newman, A. J., 129, 236, 443, 626
Newman, C. G. H., 102
Newman, N. M., 623
Newns, G. H., 167, 176
Newstead, G. J., 591
Newton, W. A., Jr., 204, 347, 593, 627, 754, 757, 815
Niccum, W. L., 238
Nicholas, J. W., 87
Nichols, B. M., 443
Nichols, D. R., 522
Nicklas, J. W., 587
Nickle, J. F., 433
Nickol, K., 647
Nida, J. R., 817
Niederman, J. C., 548, 549
Niedziela, B., 85
Nienhuis, A. W., 391, 443
Nies, B. A., 584, 590, 592, 623, 626
Niessing, T., 758
Nievi, R. L., 592
Nieweg, H. O., 259
Niewiarowski, S., 758
Nijenhuis, J. H., 758
Nilsson, I. M., 708, 747, 748, 754
Nilsson, L. R., 809, 815
Nishikawa, M., 350
Nishizawa, E. E., 749
Nist, R. T., 237
Nixon, D. D., 650
Nixon, R. K., 467
Noades, J., 86, 87
Noble, L., 21
Nobrega, F. T., 590
Nogueron, A., 814
Noll, J. B., 443
Nomura, T., 444
Nondasuta, A., 150
Nordenson, N. G., 14, 21
Nordøy, A., 812
Norman, J. C., 754
Norris, H. J., 592
Norris, L. M., 21
Norron, K. R., 167, 176
Norton, P. M., 258
Nossel, H. L., 759
Nour-Eldin, F., 759
Novy, M. J., 467
Nowell, P. C., 488, 507, 592
Noyes, W. D., 202, 238, 443
Nusbacher, J., 129
Nussbaum, M., 506, 522, 754
Nwachuko-Jarrett, E. S., 441
Nye, S. W., 754
Nyhus, L. M., 101
Nyman, M., 11, 345

## O

Oalaes, T., 176
Obenour, W., Jr., 440
Oberman, H. A., 669, 678
Oberman, J. W., 35
O'Brien, D., 101
O'Brien, J. R., 747
O'Brien, J. S., 678
O'Brien, L. J., 815
Obrinsky, W., 129
Ockerman, P. A., 754
O'Connell, L. G., 143, 148
O'Conner, J. F., 676
O'Connor, W. J., 35
O'Conor, G. T., 649
Oda, J. M., 59, 102
Odang, O., 258, 286
Odegaard, A. E., 754
Odell, G. B., 125, 127, 145, 149, 154, 176, 178
Odell, T. T., 815
Odom, J. L., 439
O'Donnell, W. M., 587
O'Donohue, N. V., 129, 448
Odultoa, A., 437
Oechslin, R. K., 465
Oehme, J., 592
Oeschlin, E., 812
Ogawa, S., 62
Ogden, F. H., 260, 649
Ognibene, A. J., 815
O'Gorman, P., 284
O'Gorman-Hughes, D. W., 783, 815
Oguro, M., 467
Oh, M-H. K., 507
Ohno, S., 339
Oikawa, Y., 129
Okada, S., 678
Okcuoglu, A., 129
Okita, G. T., 340
Okuma, M., 746
Okuno, K., 350
Olafsson, O., 344
Oldfield, M. G., 550
O'Leary, D. S., 754
Oleinick, A., 594
Oleinick, M. M., 572
Oliner, H., 202, 287, 342, 443, 626
Oliver, C. P., 433
Oliver, M., 350
Oliver, R. A. M., 809, 817
Oliver, T. K., Jr., 160, 174, 177, 815
Oliver, W. J., 815
Ollendorff, P., 746
O'Loughlin, E. P., 815
Olsen, R. N., 35
Olshin, I., 443
Olson, C., 346
Olson, L. C., 535
Olson, R. L., 678
Olson, S. L., 757
Omenn, G. S., 678
O'Neill, D., 12
O'Neill, P., 203
Oort, M., 315, 347, 348
Opfell, R., 443, 755
Opitz, J. M., 812
Oppé, T. E., 176
Oppenheim, E., 811
Oppenheim, E. G., 626
Oppenheimer, E. H., 809
Oram, S., 270, 286
Orchard, N. P., 507, 678
Orfer, E., 505
Orgeron, J. D., 467
Origenes, M. L., Jr., 347, 649
Orlandini, O., 35
Orme, R. L. E., 177

O'Rourke, W., 467
Ortiz, A., 435
Osathanondh, V., 467
Osborn, J. E., 820
Osborne, W. P., 285
Osgood, E. E., 444, 507, 534, 590
Oski, F. A., 20, 21, 61, 62, 71, 72, 73, 126, 149, 177, 182, 203, 238, 259, 288, 309, 346, 347, 351, 352, 442, 443, 447, 467, 468, 507, 522, 678, 815, 816
Osler, W., 794, 816
Osofsky, M., 259
Osserman, E. F., 474, 507, 592
Osterland, C. K., 86
Ostroski, J. T., 818
O'Sullivan, E. F., 34
O'Sullivan, M. A., 535, 592
O'Sullivan, W. J., 256
Oswald, N. C., 503
Otani, S., 678
Otridge, B. W., 746
Ott, M., 521
Ottenheimer, E. J., 527, 812
Ottesen, J., 507, 535
Overland, E. S., 344
Owen, C. A., 750
Owen, C. A., Jr., 126, 754, 755
Owen, D. M., 443
Owen, G. M., 206, 238
Owen, R. D., 87
Owren, P. A., 267, 287, 302, 347, 714, 750, 751, 755
Ozaeta, P. B., Jr., 349
Ozer, F. L., 649
Ozer, L., 347

## P

Pablete, E., 21
Pachter, M. R., 347
Packer, J. T., 814
Packman, E. W., 502
Padawer, J., 507
Pader, E., 549
Paegle, R. E., 819
Paeth, G. W., 442
Page, A. P. M., 747
Page, A. R., 505, 507, 522, 649
Page, D. L., 434
Page, E. B., 445
Page, E. W., 746
Page, R. H., 130, 352, 651
Paglia, D. E., 339, 347, 350, 351, 507, 509
Paidoucis, M., 73
Paik, C. H., 443
Pakesch, F., 748
Palek, J., 347
Palmen, K., 287
Palmer, C., 346
Palmer, H. D., 148
Palmer, J. G., 678
Palmer, J. M., 60
Panich, V., 448
Pansky, B., 61
Pantelakis, S. N., 345
Pantuck, K. E., 128
Papayannopoulou, T., 447
Pappenheimer, A. M., 73
Papps, J. P., 550
Parer, J. T., 447
Parffit, A. M., 230, 238
Parish, A., 285
Park, B. H., 507
Park, K. H., 814
Park, S. K., 433
Parker, D. D., 73
Parker, F. P., 521
Parker, W. C., 234

# AUTHOR INDEX 835

Parkin, D., 148
Parlic, G. J., 347
Parmer, E. A., 809
Parr, C. W., 347
Parry, T. E., 259
Parson, I. C., 342
Partin, J. C., 505
Pascher, F., 443
Pascuzzi, C. A., 755
Pascher, I., 257
Patch, M. J., 756
Patchefsky, A. S., 587
Patel, D. A., 129
Paterson, J. C. S., 447, 589
Pathak, M. A., 341, 346
Patterson, J. H., 816
Patterson, P., 127, 129
Patterson, R. B., 259
Paul, J. R., 536, 549
Paul, M. H., 21, 442, 755
Paulik, M. D., 352
Pauling, L., 73, 353, 366, 443, 444
Paulson, G. S., 647
Paulssen, M. M. P., 758
Payne, L. C., 441
Payne, M. A., 680
Payne, R., 35, 342, 478, 507, 522, 811
Paz, A., 258
Peach, R. O., 148
Peacock, M., 284
Peacock, W. C., 465
Pearce, L., 503
Pears, M. A., 351
Pears, M. Q., 260
Pearsall, N. N., 87, 204
Pearse, A. G. E., 507
Pearson, C. M., 348
Pearson, H. A., 9, 11, 21, 35, 57, 61, 206, 234, 238, 259, 287, 348, 372, 440, 443, 445, 499, 508, 588, 592, 778, 816
Pease, G. L., 284, 287, 345
Pechet, G. S., 34, 751
Pechet, L., 755
Peckham, M. A., 749
Peden, J. C., 177
Pederson, J., 21
Peeney, A. L. P., 257
Peisach, S., 62
Peltonen, T., 651
Pena, C. E., 680
Penalver, R., 817
Penden, J. C., Jr., 756
Penfold, J. B., 348
Pengelly, C. D. R., 592
Penick, G. D., 102, 748, 755, 756, 758
Penington, D. C., 467
Penington, D. G., 811
Penner, J. A., 466, 814, 816
Pennybacker, W., 594
Pepper, H., 816
Perera, D. R., 592
Perez, C., 259
Perez, R. T., 592
Perez-Tamayo, R., 678
Perillie, P. E., 508, 592
Perkins, H. A., 87
Perkins, K. W., 444
Perkoff, G. T., 348
Perla, D., 678
Perlman, J. D., 757
Perlow, A., 35
Perlstein, M., 73, 150
Perosa, L., 444
Perrin, J. C. S., 626
Perrine, R. P., 348
Perrotta, P., 587
Perry, J., 257
Perry, R., 128, 177

Perry, S., 506, 508, 521, 522, 523, 535, 592, 626, 676, 677, 755
Perryman, F. W., 126
Pert, J. H., 347, 759, 814
Perutz, M. F., 44, 61, 73, 444
Pestaner, L. C., 349, 508
Petering, H. G., 21
Peterman, M. G., 535
Peters, D. K., 237
Peters, E. R., 126
Peters, H. R., 88, 648
Peters, M. V., 648, 649
Peterson, E. T., 549
Peterson, J. C., 236, 259
Peterson, R., 816, 819
Peterson, R. D. A., 649, 679
Peterson, R. E., 235, 434
Peterson, W. L., 434
Petmezaki, S., 130
Petrakis, N. L., 587
Petz, L. D., 348
Pew, W. L., 177
Pfeiffer, E., 536, 549
Phibbs, R. H., 816
Philipp, E. E., 752
Philips, F. S., 627
Philips, R. S., 534
Philipsborn, H. D., 177
Philipsborn, H. F., Jr., 58
Phillips, C. A., 816, 817
Phillips, C. L., 149
Phillips, G. B., 72, 73, 506
Phillips, J. H., 288
Phillips, L. I., 256
Phillips, L. L., 755, 813
Phillips, R. F., 648
Philpott, M. G., 814
Phipps, R. H., 133, 150
Phythyon, J. M., 434
Pick, L., 678
Pickles, M. M., 103, 149, 150
Piel, C. F., 816
Pierce, L. E., 259, 444
Pierce, M., 592, 625, 626, 628, 817
Pierce, M. I., 60
Pierce, P. P., 348
Pierce, R. B., 816
Pierre, R., 590, 816
Pierson, W. E., 160, 177
Piessens, W. F., 816
Pildes, R. S., 129
Pileri, A., 548
Piliero, S. J., 61
Pillemer, L., 348
Pillow, R. P., 287
Pinedo-Veels, C., 448
Pingitore, N. E., 675
Pinkas, A., 258
Pinkel, D., 202, 203, 284, 588, 592, 593, 624, 626, 648, 650
Pinker, G., 432
Pinkerton, P. H., 238
Pinkhas, J. P., 748
Pinksy, L., 150
Pinkus, H., 203
Pinniger, J. L., 750
Piomelli, S., 61, 285, 433, 818
Piper, D. R., 549
Pirofsky, B., 348
Pirzio-Biroli, G., 59, 234, 433
Pisciotta, A. V., 239, 508, 649, 650, 755
Pison, J., 755
Pitney, W. R., 259, 348, 747, 751, 755
Pizzuto, J., 288
Plachta, A., 444
Plata, E., 592
Platou, E. S., 129, 522

Platzer, R. F., 351
Plaut, G., 86
Playfair, J. H. L., 1, 11
Plentl, A. A., 150
Plum, C. M., 521
Plum, P., 749
Plunket, D. C., 444, 815
Plzak, L., 59, 60, 236, 285, 466
Pohle, F. J., 816
Poley, J. R., 816
Polhemus, D. W., 678
Polhemus, J. A., 502
Polimeros, D., 441
Pollack, J. M., 147
Pollack, S., 752
Pollack, W., 150, 175
Pollak, V. E., 508
Pollock, J., 12, 36, 145, 150, 178
Pollycove, A., 464
Pollycove, M., 235, 236, 238, 240, 257, 808
Polonovski, J., 72
Pommerenke, W. T., 238
Poncher, H. G., 21, 592
Ponder, E., 287
Pool, J. G., 701, 749, 755
Pootrakol, K., 448
Poppers, P. J., 128
Pornpatkul, M., 448
Porro, R. S., 71
Porteous, D. D., 465
Porter, E., 150, 157, 174, 177, 178
Porter, F. S., 259, 348, 444, 467, 649, 749
Porter, R., 351
Porter, W. R., 442
Porters, S. F., 259
Porto, S. O., 112, 129
Post, R. L., 348
Potter, E., 150, 467
Potts, E. B., 438
Poulik, M. D., 651
Pourfar, M., 534
Powars, D., 11, 287
Powell, A. E., 759
Powell, E. O., 434
Powell, L. H., 123, 129
Powers, W. T., 549, 550
Powles, C. P., 589
Prader, A., 522
Prager, D., 627
Praising, R., 506
Prankerd, T. A. J., 61, 287, 339, 346, 348, 432, 466, 676, 678, 777, 817
Prasad, A. S., 207, 238
Pratt, C. B., 626
Pratt, E. I., 440
Pravit, W., 442
Preston, A. E., 755
Prestin, F. W., 286
Pretlow, T. G., 592
Pretty, H. M., 87
Preuss, F. S., 590
Prevot-Pignede, J., 14, 20
Pribilla, W., 238
Price, J. M., 288, 466
Price-Jones, C., 203
Prichard, R. W., 755
Pridie, G., 592
Priest, R. E., 339
Prieto, E. N., 174
Primikirios, N., 649
Prince, A. E., 438
Prince, A. M., 97, 103
Prince, J. T., 817
Princiotto, I., 436
Prindle, K. H., 444
Prins, H. K., 347, 348
Prockop, D. J., 284
Procopio, F., 314, 339

Proctor, R. R., 755, 756
Proiano, G., 348
Prolla, J. C., 592
Propp, S., 594, 817
Prospero, J. D., 508, 522
Prost, R. J., 753
Prouty, R. L., 344
Prunty, F. T. G., 509
Pryles, C. V., 535, 592
Pryor, D. S., 348
Puapondh, Y., 20, 808
Pulliam, H. N., 435
Punnett, H. H., 176, 203, 509
Punt, K., 439
Purcell, M. K., 445
Purfar, M., 592
Purtilo, D., 748
Purugganan, G., 238, 240
Putnam, L. E., 286
Putnam, S. M., 535
Putschar, W. G. J., 678
Puxeddu, A., 340

**Q**

Qayum, O., 234
Quagliana, J. M., 287, 348
Quaglino, D., 505, 521, 649
Quaisser, K., 287
Qualls, D. H., 753
Queenan, J. T., 5, 11, 34, 150, 177
Quick, A. J., 696, 706, 742, 755, 776, 800, 816
Quie, P. G., 505, 507, 508
Quinto, M. G., 259

**R**

Raab, S. A., 626
Raab, S. O., 467, 502, 520, 592
Rabiner, S. F., 720, 729, 755, 817
Rabinowitz, Y., 816
Raccuglia, G., 755, 810
Race, R. R., 85, 86, 87, 148
Radel, E., 432, 549, 816
Rafsum, S., 124
Ragab, A. A., 626
Raine, D. N., 436
Ralston, L. S., 549
Ramboer, C., 109, 129
Ramgren, O., 754
Ramos, J., 239
Ramot, B., 11, 312, 348, 444, 508, 678, 757, 812
Ramsay, D. H. E., 467
Ramunni, M., 444
Randell, D. L., 649
Raney, R. B., 592
Rankin, R. E., 349, 508
Ranney, H. M., 61, 433, 441, 444, 626
Ransome-Kuti, S., 437
Rapaport, S. E., 749, 750, 751, 752, 755, 756
Rape, C. E., 447
Raper, A. B., 11, 439, 444, 448, 809
Rapmund, G., 129
Rappaport, H., 341, 346
Rappaport, S., 502
Rapport, M. M., 759
Rasmussen, J., 746
Rath, C. E., 259, 436, 444, 467
Rath, J., 127
Rather, L. J., 238, 676
Ratnoff, O. D., 203, 748, 749, 756, 759, 809
Rau, S. M., 259
Rauner, T. A., 87
Rausen, A., 21, 129, 348, 816
Rawson, A. J., 177

## AUTHOR INDEX

Reacy, M., 150
Read, R., 345
Reader, G. G., 339
Reardon, A. E., 507
Rebuck, J. W., 286, 473, 508, 678
Reddy, S., 441
Redeker, A., 348
Redman, J. F., 444
Redmond, A. J., 550
Redo, S. F., 549, 751
Reed, C. F., 53, 55, 62, 294, 297, 347, 348, 351
Reed, C. L., 61
Reed, J. F., Jr., 780, 813
Reed, W. B., 348
Reeder, P .S., 434
Reeds, C. S., 467
Reeves, W. H., 503, 810
Regas, D. A., 507
Regoeczi, E., 817
Reich, C., 678
Reich, R. S., 333
Reid, H. A., 437
Reid, W. O., 756
Reidbord, H., 676
Reidenberg, M. M., 346
Reiff, R. H., 59
Reilly, W. A., 508
Reimann, H. A., 521, 522
Reinhard, E., 444, 647
Reinhart, H. L., 647
Reinhold, J., 59, 287, 467, 812
Reiquam, C. W., 148, 649
Reisman, L. E., 555, 566, 592
Reisman, L. I., 88
Reismann, K. R., 61
Reisner, E. H., Jr., 53, 61, 259
Reiss, A. M., 150
Reiss, C., 34
Reissmann, K. R., 444
Remenchik, A. P., 679
Remington, J. S., 35
Rendle-Short, J., 648, 811
Renwick, J. H., 339
Repetto, G., 816
Repplinger, E., 625
Restrepo, E., 289
Retera, R. J. M., 815
Retief, F. P., 287
Rey, J., 72
Reyersbach, G., 535
Reyes, G. R., 592
Reynafarje, C., 239
Reynaud, R., 434
Reynolds, E. H., 259
Reynolds, J., 285, 444, 508, 522
Reynolds, T. B., 590
Reznikoff, P., 464
Rheingold, J. J., 338, 746
Rhinesmith, H., 61, 444
Rhoads, C. P., 284, 287
Rhodes, J., 237
Ribas-Mundo, M., 488, 508
Rice, E. C., 35, 589
Rich, A., 444, 816
Rich, L., 746
Richards, A. G., 103
Richards, D. H., 126
Richards, G., 747
Richards, R., 445
Richardson, C., 34
Richardson, J., 176, 812
Richardson, S. N., 10, 434
Richmond, H., 505
Richmond, J. B., 468
Richmond, M. D., 176
Richter, M. N., 680
Richter, P., 348, 816
Ricketts, W. E., 348

Rickles, F. R., 346
Rico, M. G., 288
Riddell, N. M., 101, 433
Riddle, J. M., 816
Riddler, J. G., 810
Rider, T. L., 649
Rieder, R. F., 407, 444
Rieders, F., 467
Rieselbach, R. E., 626
Rifkind, R. A., 444
Rigas, D. A., 444
Rigby, P. G., 28, 35
Riley, H. D., 34, 35, 203, 345, 502, 817
Riley, J. F., 508
Rimington, C., 61
Rimington, G., 346
Rincon, A. R., 432
Ripstein, C. B., 548
Rittenberg, D., 61
Ritz, N. D., 328, 348, 592
Ritzmann, S. E., 348
River, G. L., 444
Rivera, A. M., 816
Rivera de Sala, A., 535
Rivers, S. L., 258
Rizza, C. R., 752
Roath, O. S., 286, 440
Roath, S., 504
Robb, P., 813
Robbins, A. B., 444
Robbins, J. B., 35, 445
Robbins, S. L., 240
Robboy, S. J., 756
Robb-Smith, A. H. T., 673, 679
Roberts, A. T. M., 503
Roberts, H. R., 756, 758
Roberts, M. H., 776, 816
Roberts, P. M., 246, 259
Roberts, W. C., 508, 593
Robertson, O. H., 103
Robertson, S. E., 34, 177, 813
Robey, J. S., 128
Robin, H., 34, 127, 813
Robin, S., 446
Robins, M. M., 287
Robinson, A., 174, 177, 434, 445, 449, 649
Robinson, J., 86, 439
Robinson, J., 550, 751, 755
Robinson, M., 433, 448
Robinson, M. A., 61, 348
Robinson, M. G., 259, 348, 376, 445
Robinson, S., 56, 61, 445
Robinson, T. W., 678
Robscheit-Robbins, F. S., 239
Robson, H. N., 287, 589, 626, 816
Robson, M. E., 677
Robson, M. J., 676
Roche, M., 258
Rodey, G. E., 507
Rodgers, C. L., 678
Rodgers, T. S., 751
Rodman, T., 445
Rodnan, G., 235, 504
Rodriguez, S., 35, 445, 816
Rodriguez-Erdmann, F., 748, 818
Roeckel, I. E., 203
Rogentine, G. N., 624
Roger, S., 34
Rogers, D. E., 678
Rogers, H. M., 678
Rogers, J., 759
Rogers, L. E., 259
Rogerson, M. M., 811
Rogoway, W., 203, 508, 592
Rohde, R., 11
Rohn, R., 590
Rohr, K., 287

Roidot, M., 749
Roitman, E., 258
Roitt, I. M., 260
Roland, A. S., 287
Roland, M., 62
Rolfs, M., 507
Rolfs, M. R., 35, 522
Rolleston, G. L., 568, 589
Rolovic, Z., 816
Ronanelli, E. G., 432
Rook. A. J., 338
Root, A. W., 816
Root, W. S., 60
Rooth, G. W., 9, 11
Roscoe, J. D., 11, 20, 21, 236
Rose, B., 349, 815
Roselbach, R., 624
Roselle, H. A., 239
Roseman, J. M., 439
Rosen, D., 589
Rosen, F. S., 34, 503, 508, 521, 676, 677
Rosen, G., 628
Rosen, P. J., 676
Rosen, R., 339
Rosenbach, L. M., 287
Rosenbaum, S., 535
Rosenberg, A., 550
Rosenberg, B., 235
Rosenberg, D. H., 678
Rosenberg, H. S., 649, 811
Rosenberg, N. J., 444
Rosenberg, S. A., 648, 649, 650
Rosenberg, S. J., 467
Rosenberg, T., 749
Rosenblatt, P., 447
Rosenblum, J. M., 756
Rosenblum, S. A., 446
Rosenfeld, A. B., 593
Rosenfeld, S., 508
Rosenfield, R. E., 81, 87, 149, 176
Rosenstein, B. J., 203
Rosensweig, L., 259
Rosenthal, D., 817
Rosenthal, I. M., 129, 817
Rosenthal, K., 508
Rosenthal, L. L., 593
Rosenthal, M. C., 350, 650, 756
Rosenthal, N., 289, 350, 594, 650, 756
Rosenthal, R. L., 287, 751, 756
Rosowsky, A., 675, 678
Ross, A. H., 627
Ross, C. A. C., 256
Ross, C. F., 339
Ross, J., 343
Ross, J. D., 61, 349, 467, 593, 594
Ross, J. F., 235, 288, 504, 521, 593, 808
Ross, O. A., 348
Ross, R. R., 650
Ross, S., 35
Ross, S. W., 508
Rosse, W. F., 345, 349, 508
Rossi, J. P., 518, 522
Rossiter, E. J., 125, 174
Ross Russel, I., 234
Rosten, S., 350
Roth, J., 111
Roth, K. L., 349
Rothberg, H., 678
Rothchild, J., 342
Rothenberg, M. B., 627
Rothman, D., 257
Rothstein, G., 239
Rotor, A. B., 129
Roughton, F. J. W., 465
Rous, P., 61

Rousselot, L. M., 678
Rousso, C., 88, 351
Rowe, A. W., 102, 103
Rowe, S., 28, 35
Rowland, R. S., 679
Rowley, D. A., 508, 679
Roy, C. A., 818
Roy, S., III, 593
Royston, N. J. W., 259
Rozenberg, M. C., 816
Rozengvaig, S., 349, 745, 746
Rubenberg, M. L., 809, 810, 817
Rubenstein, E., 445
Rubenstein, H. M., 446
Rubin, A. D., 503
Rubin, D., 288
Rubin, E., 212, 286, 489
Rubin, M., 436
Rubin, R., 650
Rubini, J. R., 548
Rubio, F., Jr., 810
Rubio, T., 817
Ruby, A., 344
Rucknagel, D. L., 445, 466, 467
Rudnicki, R. P. T., 435
Rudolph, A. J., 127, 817
Rudolph, A. M., 239, 467
Rudolph, N., 349
Rudolph, R. D., 623
Ruebner, B., 125
Ruggiero, S., 440
Ruiz-Reyer, G., 441
Rundles, R. W., 73, 239
Russel, A., 11
Russell, A. V., 502, 521
Russell, L. B., 36
Russell, P. A., 351
Russell, P. S., 288, 445
Russell, R. P., 467
Russell, S. H., 178
Rutenberg, M. L., 748
Ruth, W. E., 444
Rutty, A., 812
Rutzky, J., 260
Ryan, G. M. S., 61, 259
Ryan, J., 130
Ryder, R. J. W., 535

S

Sabin, F. R., 503
Sabine, J. E., 349
Sabine, J. C., 508
Sacchetti, C., 504
Sachs, V., 813
Sacker, L. S., 522
Sacks, H. J., 435
Sacks, M. O., 87
Sacks, M. S., 259
Sadikario, A., 435
Sadusk, J. F., 550
Sagerman, R. H., 203
Saha, A., 237
Saidi, P., 288, 756
Saifi, M. F., 467
Saiki, A. K., 549
St. Geme, J. W., Jr., 817
Sakhadeo, S., 432
Salen, G., 349
Sallings, S. A., 437
Salmon, R. J., 258
Salmonsen, L., 522
Salt, H. B., 73
Saltzman, H. A., 440, 819
Saltzman, P., 235
Saltzstein, S. L., 817
Salvaggio, J. E., 445
Salzberger, M., 10
Salzman, E. W., 756
Samaha, R. J., 625
Samama, M., 753

# AUTHOR INDEX

Sammay, J., 594
Sammons, H. G., 256, 257
Sampson, C. C., 87, 438
Sampson, N., 235
Samuels, L., 239, 627
Samuels, S. I., 235
Sanarelli, G., 817
Sanchez-Avalos, J., 817
Sanchez-Medal, L., 288, 814
Sandberg, A. A., 593, 627, 649
Sandella, J. E., 522
Sanders, M., 592, 814
Sanger, R., 85, 86, 87
Sansais, L., 87
Santamaria, A., 678
Santamaria, J. N., 342
Santarsierg, M., 534
Santora, E., 587
Santos, A. S., 239
Santulli, T. V., 203
Sapin, S. O., 675
Saraiva, L. G., 508, 522
Sarjeant, B. E., 445
Sarles, H. E., 349
Sarmiento, F., 148, 176
Sarnatora, V. F., 587
Sartain, P., 351, 449
Sarvajic-Dottor, J., 258
Saslaw, S., 675, 679
Sass-Kirtsak, A., 35
Sathe, Y. S., 587
Sato, K., 746
Sauer, W. G., 754
Saunders, E. F., 627
Sautter, R. D., 756
Savage, D. V., 234
Sawitsky, A., 286, 349, 443, 550, 666, 679
Saxena, V. H., 445
Say, B., 650
Sayed, H. M., 337, 349
Scales, M. B., 756
Scalettar, H. E., 535
Scanlon, R. T., 808
Scannell, J. G., 550
Scarpinato, B., 623
Schaad, J. D. G., 439
Schaar, F., 260, 776, 817
Schabel, F. M., Jr., 627
Schachter, M., 756
Schade, H., 593
Schaefer, J., 33
Schaefer, L., 506
Schafer, W. B., 129, 678
Schaffhausen, M., 818
Schaffner, F., 440
Scharfman, W. A., 817
Scharfman, W. B., 594
Schechter, G. P., 345, 808
Scheinberg, I. H., 239
Schell, N. B., 445
Schellhammer, P. F., 445
Schenker, S., 129
Schersten, B., 466
Schettini, F., 445
Scheuer, P. J., 339
Schiff, L., 129, 680
Schiffman, G., 87
Schiffman, F., 750, 756
Schilling, R. F., 252, 259, 346, 648
Schirger, O., 522
Schleicher, E. M., 73
Schlicht, I., 354, 433
Schlom, J., 594
Schloss, O. M., 234
Schlumberger, J. R., 103, 287, 591, 626
Schmerling, D. H., 749
Schmickel, R. D., 33, 587
Schmid, E., 522
Schmid, R., 62, 128, 129, 176, 177, 297, 349, 445

Schmidt, F. H., 234
Schmidt, P. J., 177, 756
Schmidt, P. S., 102
Schmidt, R., 350
Schneider, A. S., 349, 351, 508, 509
Schneider, G. F., 343
Schneider, M., 103, 287, 591, 626
Schneider, R. G., 433, 435, 437, 445, 448
Schneiderman, M. A., 593
Schnider, U., 238, 442
Schnitzer, B., 440, 445
Schoeck, V. W., 679
Schoeller, L., 593
Schoen, E. J., 36, 817
Schoenfield, L. J., 129
Scholl, M. L. L., 150
Schollman, H. M., 563, 593
Schore, P., 548
Schorr, J. B., 125, 432, 549, 756, 816
Schreiner, G. E., 467
Schretten, E., 754
Schrier, L., 748
Schrier, S. E., 60
Schrimshaw, N. S., 259
Schroeder, E. A., 60
Schroeder, L. R., 623
Schroeder, W., 10, 61
Schroeder, W. A., 12, 62, 439, 444, 447, 448, 594
Schubert, W. K., 229, 237, 239
Schuckmell, N., 679
Schulaner, F. A., 589
Schulhoff, C., 174
Schull, W. J., 754
Schulman, H., 149
Schulman, I., 22, 59, 62, 102, 103, 150, 177, 235, 239, 288, 342, 350, 435, 436, 445, 446, 447, 464, 679, 746, 751, 756, 757, 808, 810, 813, 817, 818
Schulman, L., 755
Schultz, C., 87
Schultz, G., 443
Schultz, J., 650
Schultz, L. E., 550
Schultz, M. G., 592
Schultz, R. L., 758
Schultze, H. E., 236, 344
Schultze, K. W. D., 593
Schulz, J., 239, 757
Schulze, H. V., 239
Schumacher, H. R., 542, 550
Schumacher, J. J., 679
Schuman, L. M., 589, 593
Schunk, G. J., 593
Schur, P. H., 756
Schuyler, K., 35
Schvit, H., 36
Schwab, M., 177
Schwab, R. B., 593
Schwachman, H., 238
Schwartz, A., 127
Schwartz, A. D., 443
Schwartz, E., 445, 593
Schwartz, G., 648
Schwartz, H., 388, 445
Schwartz, H. C., 62, 235, 445, 817
Schwartz, L., 502, 650
Schwartz, M., 279
Schwartz, R., 202, 287, 342, 349, 432, 622, 817
Scharwtz, R. S., 203, 588, 626, 808
Schwartz, S., 479
Schwartz, S. O., 72, 73, 342, 437, 444, 561, 563, 589, 593, 817

Schwarz, E., 272, 238, 650
Schwarz, G., 650
Schwarzenberg, L., 103, 287, 591, 616
Scialom, C., 349
Scoggins, R. B., 258
Scott, C. H., 520
Scott, J. L., 288
Scott, J. T., 507
Scott, P. J., 71
Scott, R., 339, 432
Scott, R. B., 73, 286, 349, 432, 434, 436, 439, 445, 673, 679
Scrimgeour, J. B., 148
Seakins, M., 442
Seaman, A. J., 288, 349, 507, 534, 550, 590
Sears, D. A., 293, 349
Sears, J. W., 751, 813
Sebrell, W. H., 521
Secer, F., 431
Sednick, E. M., 549
Seeds, A. F., 10
Seeler, R. A., 129, 675, 746, 751, 808
Seftel, H., 464
Segar, W. E., 349
Seife, M., 678
Seifter, S., 125
Seip, M., 22, 203, 239, 288, 508, 750, 776, 812, 817
Seitanidis, B., 550
Selawry, O. S., 650
Seki, M., 21
Seligmann, M., 508
Seligsohn, V., 757
Selirio, E. S., 285, 588
Seltzer, C. C., 239
Selwyn, J. G., 62, 73, 300, 301, 313, 349
Sen Gupta, P. C., 445
Senior, B., 813
Sered, B. R., 234
Sergovich, F. R., 36, 593
Serjeant, G. R., 372, 445
Serpick, A. A., 510, 610, 647
Sestak, Z., 817
Sestakof, D., 431
Setzkorn, J., 812
Severo, N., 628
Sevette, J., 36
Sfikakis, P., 446
Sha'afi, R., 73, 352
Shafer, A. W., 239
Shafer, W. A., 349
Shaheedy, M., 351, 627
Shahidi, N. T., 11, 61, 239, 288, 347, 349, 446, 452, 467
Shahin, N., 446
Shaldon, C., 680
Shaldon, S., 679
Shalet, M. F., 62
Shamir, Z., 441, 749
Shanbrom, E., 591, 750
Shanklin, D. R., 443
Shannon, B. S., 755
Shapiro, C. M., 349, 792, 817
Shapiro, H., 441
Shapiro, H. D., 448, 680
Shapiro, J., 502
Shapiro, L. M., 14, 22
Shapiro, P. R., 752
Shapiro, S. R., 676
Shapland, C., 260
Shapleigh, J. B., 434
Sharnoff, J. G., 650
Sharp, A. A., 260, 351, 547, 754, 757
Sharp, H. L., 627
Sharpe, J. C., 467

Sharpsteen, J. R., 442, 753
Shaw, C. C., 534
Shaw, E. B., 535
Shaw, R., 127, 591, 593
Shaw, S., 589, 809, 817
Shay, T. L., 650
Shea, J. G., 442
Sheagren, J. N., 647
Sheba, C., 348, 350, 446, 508, 812
Sheehy, T. W., 235
Sheets, J. A., 676
Sheets, R. F., 509, 650
Sheldon, W., 820
Shelley, W. B., 508
Shelley, W. M., 446
Shelton, J. B., 62
Shelton, J. R., 439
Shelton, S., 176
Shelton, T. R., 62
Shemin, D., 61
Shen, S. C., 342, 343, 446, 467
Sheon, R. P., 756
Shepard, M. K., 10, 434, 446
Shepard, T. E., 11
Shephard, M., 22
Sheppard, C. W., 236
Sheppard, P. M., 178
Sherlock, S., 129, 339, 346, 679
Sherman, F. E., 809
Sherman, I., 812
Sherman, J. D., 286, 522
Sherman, L. A., 757
Sherman, S. D., 259
Sherrill, J. G., 591
Sherry, S., 753, 757
Sherwood, J. B., 349
Sheth, N. K., 777, 817
Shibata, S., 466
Shibuya, M., 815
Shields, G., 35, 446
Shields, M. J., 260, 351
Shih, V. E., 149
Shiller, J. G., 36, 168, 177
Shillito, J., Jr., 811
Shimizu, K., 448
Shimkin, M. B., 587, 593, 650, 675
Shinefield, H. R., 654, 679
Shinton, N. K., 550, 817
Shirkey, H. S., 472, 506
Shively, J. A., 346
Shiver, C. B., Jr., 548, 550
Shmerling, D. H., 522
Shoden, A., 239
Shohet, S. B., 73, 347, 352
Shojania, A. M., 62, 239, 347, 349
Shore, E., 235
Shore, N. A., 258, 623, 624
Short, I. A., 33
Shorter, R. G., 127
Shortleff, D. B., 343
Shotton, D., 446
Shugarman, P. M., 285
Shuiti, H. R., 550
Shulman, L. E., 507
Shulman, N. R., 349, 753, 816, 817
Shulman, R. G., 62
Shumacker, H. B., Jr., 440
Shumway, C. N., 177, 345, 790, 817
Shuster, J., 753
Shwachman, H., 288, 522
Shwartzman, G., 818
Sibley, W. A., 815
Sidbury, J. B., Jr., 62, 259
Sidel, V. W., 72, 73, 347
Siebenmann, R. E., 465, 812
Siebenthal, B. L., 128

# AUTHOR INDEX

Siegelman, S., 594
Sigler, A. T., 349, 550, 587
Silber, R., 72, 73, 467, 818
Silberstein, E. B., 259
Silpisornkosol, S., 150
Silver, H. K., 446, 508, 818
Silver, H. M., 548
Silver, M. J., 747
Silver, R. H., 258
Silver, R. T., 555, 590, 593, 594, 627
Silverberg, M., 129
Silverman, F. N., 506, 593, 677
Silverman, W. A., 129, 150, 168, 177
Silverstein, M. N., 666, 679
Silverstein, S., 508
Silverthorne, N., 504
Silvester, F., 257
Silvestroni, E., 433, 446
Simmons, B. M., 548
Simmons, R. L., 237
Simon, E. R., 339
Simone, J. V., 626, 746, 757, 808
Simons, E. L., 676
Simonson, R. J., 348
Simovitch, H., 62
Simpkiss, M. J., 818
Simpson, C. L., 593
Sinclair, C., 752
Singer, K., 35, 72, 73, 104, 116, 126, 347, 350, 353, 440, 446, 647, 676, 679, 757, 818
Singer, L., 440, 446
Singer, S. J., 73, 443
Singh, P., 757
Siniscalco, M., 433
Sinks, L. F., 593, 627
Sipkema, J. J., 758
Sirak, H. D., 754
Sise, H. S., 754, 757
Sisson, T. R. C., 22, 112, 129, 177, 231, 239, 240
Sitt, C., 235
Siwe, S. A., 679
Sjoberg, W. E., Jr., 234
Sjolin, S., 59, 176, 236, 288, 438
Sjostedt, S., 9, 11
Skalheyg, B. A., 754
Skanderberg, J., 60
Skeel, R. T., 589, 593
Skinner, D., 36, 523
Skipper, H. E., 610, 627
Sklavurw-Zurukzoglu, S., 350
Skolling, R., 11
Skowron, P. N., 502
Skrodelis, V., 755
Slater, L. M., 446
Slater, R. J., 502
Slaughter, D. P., 650
Sleisinger, M. H., 258
Sloane, J. A., 438
Slobody, L. B., 35, 518, 522
Slocum, G. J. C., 593
Slotkowski, E. L., 177
Smellie, J. M., 647
Smetana, A. F., 650
Smetana, H. F., 129, 647
Smiley, R. K., 350
Smith, C., 21
Smith, C. A., 10, 35, 127
Smith, C. H., 22, 36, 59, 73, 87, 102, 103, 129, 150, 177, 183, 203, 226, 235, 237, 239, 288, 342, 350, 435, 436, 438, 441, 442, 445, 446, 447, 467, 508, 509, 535, 593, 627, 679, 748, 755, 756, 757, 813, 817, 818

Smith, C. H., Jr., 811
Smith, D. R., 86, 503, 550
Smith, D. W., 284
Smith, E., 447
Smith, E. B., 440, 445, 548, 590
Smith, E. L., 62, 468
Smith, E. W., 435, 447
Smith, F., 342
Smith, G. M., 433
Smith, G. W., 448
Smith, H. D., 509, 521
Smith, H. P., 748
Smith, I., 447
Smith, J., 467
Smith, J. A., 73
Smith, J. D., 436
Smith, J. E., 339
Smith, J. L., 818
Smith, K. E., 73
Smith, L., 177
Smith, M. D., 204
Smith, M. G., 115, 129
Smith, M. H., 776, 816
Smith, N. J., 239, 240, 284, 288, 509, 679
Smith, P. M., 285
Smith, R. J., 35
Smith, R. L., 593
Smith, R. S., 72, 432, 447
Smith, R. T., 36, 129, 259, 345, 518, 522, 676
Smith, T., 162, 177
Smith, U. S., 287, 289
Smith, V., 72, 347
Smith, W. E., 818
Smithers, D. W., 638, 650
Smithies, O., 340, 350, 356, 447
Smits, C. A. A. M., 758
Smits, H. L., 381, 447
Sneath, J. S., 87
Sneath, P. H. A., 87
Snelling, C. E., 504
Snodgrass, G. J. A., 7, 11
Snowden, P. W., 813
Snyder, J., 587
Snyder, R. A., 679
Snyderman, S. E., 258, 467
Sobotka, H., 257
Sobrevilla, L. A., 73
Soderstrom, M., 648
Soeiro, R., 36
Soergel, K. H., 806, 807, 818
Sohn, D., 650
Sokal, J. E., 36
Soloff, L. A., 550
Solomon, A., 340
Solomon, J., 87, 627, 650
Solomon, J. D., 523
Soltan, H. C., 36, 593
Soltys, R. D., 433
Solum, N. O., 750
Somlyo, A. P., 756
Somlyo, A. V., 756
Sommers, S. C., 807, 818
Song, Y. S., 447
Sonley, M. J., 550, 623, 627
Sookanek, M., 448
Soster, G., 447
Soulier, J. P., 747, 752
Southam, C. M., 550, 593, 594
Southworth, H., 286
Spach, M. A., 650
Spackman, D. H., 11
Spada, U., 433
Spaet, T. H., 350, 437, 445, 447, 506, 522, 650, 751, 754, 757
Sparkes, R., 87
Spaugh, E., 753
Spear, P. W., 649
Spector, H., 467

Speed, D. E., 590
Speer, R. J., 751
Speicher, C. E., 816
Speirs, R. S., 509
Spencer, N., 60
Spencer, R. P., 443
Spier, R. D., 444
Spies, T. D., 468
Spink, W. W., 505, 814
Spittel, J. A., Jr., 754, 755
Spitz, H., 648
Spivack, M., 677
Sprague, C., 447, 464, 813
Spray, C. M., 206, 240
Spray, G. H., 259
Sprinz, H., 129
Sporfkin, B. F., 680
Sproul, A., 177
Sprunt, T. P., 550
Spurling, C. L., 62, 259, 448
Spurr, C. L., 489, 505, 676
Spurrell, J. R., 434
Staatsma, B. R., 586
Stadlan, E. M., 650, 819
Stafford, J. L., 590, 757
Stahl, W. C., 350
Stahman, A. W., 73, 448
Stallings, S. A., 175
Stamatoyannopoulos, G., 436, 439, 442, 446, 447, 467
Stamey, C. C., 129, 150, 350, 749, 818
Stamos, H. F., 260
Stamp, T. C. B., 284
Stanage, W. F., 549
Stanbury, J. B., 239
Stanfield, J. B., 447
Stanier, W., 126
Stapleton, T., 432
Stark, A., 174
Stark, J. M., 466
Stark, S. N., 757
Starkey, N. M., 483, 502
Starobin, S. G., 808
Starr, A., 348, 349, 550
Stasney, J., 548
Stats, D., 350, 650
Staub, R. T., 753
Stauffer, U., 343
Stavrakakis, D., 126
Stead, E. A., Jr., 676
Stearns, G., 238
Steck, O., 465, 812
Stedman, E., 509
Steele, B. B., 757
Steen, C. E., 818
Stefani, S. S., 72
Stefanini, M., 36, 103, 150, 523, 550, 627, 675, 748, 757, 818
Steier, W., 440
Steiger, W. A., 449
Stein, A. A., 649
Stein, H. J., 468
Stein, H. L., 757
Stein, M., 679
Stein, W. H., 11
Steinberg, A. G., 87, 343, 564, 594, 756, 808
Steinberg, B., 509
Steiner, B., 818
Steiner, H., 11
Steiner, M., 447, 738, 746, 807, 814
Steinfel, J. L., 650
Steinfield, J. L., 240, 627
Steinhardt, I. D., 818
Steinkamp, R., 818
Steinke, I., 160, 175
Stempel, R., 150
Stempfel, R., 129
Stenfert Kroese, W. F., 259
Stenhouse, N. S., 755
Stephen, S. A., 343
Stephenson, A. G., 649

Sterk, V. V., 510
Sterle, V. V., 680
Sterling, K., 73
Sterling, T. D., 626
Stern, G. S., 22, 59, 62, 103, 177, 235, 239, 288, 350, 436, 441, 445, 446, 447, 679, 818
Stern, K., 102, 172, 177, 342, 548
Stern, L., 127, 130, 177
Sternlieb, I., 239
Stetson, C. A., Jr., 447
Stetson, R., 79, 86
Stevens, A. R., Jr., 235, 239, 465
Stevens, B. L., 432
Stevens, D. A., 542, 550
Stevens, H., 548
Stevenson, I. H., 126
Stevenson, J. D., 448
Stevenson, M. E., 432
Stevenson, T. D., 350, 593, 627
Stewart, A., 594
Stewart, C. T., 258
Stewart, J. M., 679
Stewart, M. J., 344
Stewart, R. A., 236
Stewart, W. B., 679
Stich, M. H., 650
Stickler, G. B., 650, 749, 811
Stickney, J. M., 436
Stiehm, E. R., 130, 812, 818, 819
Stiehm, S. R., 36
Stilwell, G. G., 754
Stites, D. P., 757
Stocks, A. E., 447
Stohlman, F., Jr., 62, 212, 237, 238, 288, 811
Stokes, J., Jr., 120, 130
Stolberg, C. S., 352
Stone, B., 87
Stone, G., 502
Storb, R., 623
Storey, B., 125
Storiko, K., 344
Stossel, T. B., 443
Stout, H. A., 548
Stout, R., 677
Straessle, R., 346
Stransky, E., 594, 679
Straumfjord, J. V., 33
Strauss, H. S., 693, 757
Strauss, L., 21, 124, 150, 203, 814
Strauss, M. B., 240
Strauss, R., 550
Street, R. B., Jr., 288
Streiff, R. R., 259
Streitmatter, D. E., 509
Stretton, A. O. W., 416, 439
Strickland, B., 679
Strickler, G. B., 816
Strieder, J. M., 288
Strijckmans, P. A., 816
Strindberg, B., 352
Strober, W., 230, 240, 809
Strong, J. A., 34
Strosselli, E., 432
Stroup, M., 87
Strouth, J. C., 509
Strumia, M. M., 103
Stulberg, C. S., 651
Stulling, C. S., 130
Sturgeon, P., 14, 22, 73, 78, 87, 163, 175, 215, 239, 240, 288, 350, 439, 447, 678, 819
Sturgis, C. C., 523, 535, 594, 650
Stutzman, L., 649
Suda, M., 350

# AUTHOR INDEX

Suderman, H. J., 11
Suess, J., 350
Sugiyama, S., 503
Sui, M., 343
Suires, R., 344
Suksta, A., 468
Sullivan, L. W., 258
Sullivan, M. P., 204, 594, 621, 627, 650
Summer, G. K., 818
Sundberg, R. D., 260, 349, 505
Sunderland, C. O., 814
Sunshine, P. J., 35
Super, M., 812
Surgenor, D. M., 757
Sussman, L. N., 87, 818
Suterland, J. M., 21
Sutherland, D. A., 506, 815, 818
Sutherland, D. W., 348
Sutherland, J. M., 130
Sutnick, A. I., 102
Sutow, W. W., 204, 594, 624, 627, 650
Swaiman, K., 818
Swan, H. T., 339
Swanson, S., 87
Sweeney, M. J., 447
Sweeny, W. M., 757
Swenseid, M. E., 627
Swenson, O., 121, 130
Swift, M. R., 270, 288
Swiller, A. I., 508, 650
Swisher, S. N., 61, 87, 345, 348, 351, 502, 594
Sydenstricker, V. P., 447
Sylvester, R. F., Jr., 624
Syverton, J. T., 594
Szalontai, S., 758
Szeinberg, A., 250, 348, 508
Szeto, I. L. F., 747, 809
Szulman, A. E., 177
Szur, L., 60, 204, 344

## T

Tabuis, J., 502
Taddeini, L., 296, 350
Tadjoedin, M. K., 818
Tagnon, H. J., 758
Takahashi, K., 342, 811
Talbot, T. R., Jr., 33
Tallal, L., 176, 348, 816
Tan, C., 509, 549, 587, 616, 623, 624, 628
Tanaka, K. R., 62, 87, 236, 311, 350, 351, 448, 535
Tandon, B. N., 236
Tanner, R., 590
Tanos, B., 814
Tarlov, A. R., 339, 340, 350
Tarokosk, P. H., 339
Tarr-Gloor, E., 507, 522
Tartaglia, A. P., 594, 817
Tarui, S., 350
Tatum, E. L., 23, 33
Taub, R. M., 818
Tauxe, W. N., 234
Taylor, A. I., 509
Taylor, F. L. H., 749, 758
Taylor, F. M., 649
Taylor, G., 465
Taylor, J. C., 752
Taylor, J. E. D., 260, 289
Taylor, J. F., 132, 150
Taylor, K. B., 260
Taylor, L., 350
Taylor, P. M., 130
Tavsi, K., 499, 509
Tefft, M., 628, 677
Teitelbaum, J., 748
Telek, A., 177
Telfer, M. C., 755
Telfer, T. P., 125, 758
Temin, H. M., 594

ten Bensel, R. W., 650, 819
Tenczar, F. J., 509
Teodosijev, D., 435
Terasaki, P. I., 479, 509
Terce, T. M., 591
Terner, J. Y., 506
Terplan, K. L., 503, 817
Terragna, A., 534
Terry, R. D., 677
Teruya, J., 130, 174, 353
Thajeb, S., 258, 286
Thaler, M. M., 122, 130
Thannhauser, S. J., 679
Thatcher, L. G., 284, 509, 625, 627, 675, 679, 812, 819
Thayer, W. W., 126, 342
Theime, W. T., 346
Thelander, H., 535, 587
Thibeault, D. W., 21
Thiery, J. P., 509
Thilen, A., 754
Thirayothin, P., 240
Thomaidis, T., 77, 87
Thomas, C., 87
Thomas, D. B., 11
Thomas, D. P., 758
Thomas, E. D., 102, 287, 288, 488, 619, 623, 627
Thomas, L., 204, 812
Thomas, L. B., 591, 592, 593, 624, 626
Thompson, D., 440
Thompson, E. N., 433
Thompson, H., 677
Thompson, J., 240
Thompson, J. H., Jr., 750, 754, 755
Thompson, K. P., 73
Thompson, M. D., 257
Thompson, O. L., 448
Thompson, R. B., 11, 260, 442, 443, 448, 504
Thompson, R. I., 352, 651
Thompson, R. P. H., 129
Thorell, B., 441
Thorn, G. W., 509
Thorup, O. A., 448
Thumasathit, B., 150
Thurm, R. H., 348, 550
Thurman, W. G., 50, 62, 204, 444, 624, 650
Thurmond, J., 809
Tidy, H. L., 536, 550, 819
Till, M., 578, 590, 624
Tillett, W. S., 758
Tilley, R. F., 627
Tills, D., 341
Timmis, G. M., 624
Ting, R. C., 589
Tippett, P., 87
Tipput, P., 86
Tisdale, W. A., 679
Tiselius, A., 29, 36
Tisman, W., 129
Tivey, H., 507, 627
Tizard, J. P. M., 522
Tjio, J. H., 568, 587, 594, 627
Tocantins, L. M., 22, 203, 432, 625, 758, 813
Toch, R., 625
Todaro, G. J., 285, 588
Todd, E. W., 348, 679
Todd, R. McL., 288, 448
Toghill, P. J., 679
Tomlin, S., 749
Tomlinson, W. J., 448
Tomonaga, M., 587
Tompkins, E. H., 503
Tooley, W. H., 150
Topley, E., 509
Torbert, J. V., 340, 447
Torp, K. H., 818
Torre-Lopez, E., 288

Tough, I. M., 586, 590, 648
Touliatos, N., 440
Tovey, C. H., 87
Tovey, G., 147, 177
Towner, C. H., 819
Townes, P. L., 72, 346, 468
Traft-Jensen, J., 344
Traisman, H. S., 58, 177
Trasler, D. G., 34
Travis, L. B., 811
Travnicek, M., 594
Treacy, N., 175
Trieger, N., 758
Tripp, N., 507
Tritus, D. H., 678
Trolard, P., 287
Trolle, D., 109, 130, 168, 177
Trombold, J. S., 538
Troup, S. B., 594
Trowell, H. C., 443
Trsuting, W. L., 589
Truant, J. P., 347
Truax, W. E., 348, 649
Trubowitz, S., 535, 594
Trueta, J., 747
Trujillo, J. M., 555, 592
Trumper, M., 464
Trusler, G. A., 259
Trygstad, C. W., 812
Tsai, C., 748
Tsai, S. Y., 289
Tseghi, C., 434
Tsevrenis, H., 437
Tsong, M., 61
Tubergen, D. G., 286
Tuchinda, S., 434, 442
Tucker, D. H., 819
Tudhope, G. R., 339, 468
Tuffy, P., 73
Tullis, J. L., 62, 509, 523
Tunnah, G. W., 754
Turnbull, A., 240, 468
Turnbull, E. P. N., 8, 9, 11, 12
Turner, D. L., 591
Turner, J. D., 550
Turpin, R., 35, 591
Tuttle, A. H., 292, 350, 436, 448
Tveteras, E., 550
Twomey, J. J., 535, 751
Tyuma, I., 448

## U

Ugoretz, R. J., 434
Ulin, A. W., 750
Ullrich, A., 509
Ulstrom, R. A., 240
Ultmann, J. E., 559, 587, 588, 650, 785, 808
Ulutin, O. N., 464
Umpierre, G., 240
Unchalipongse, P., 150
Underitz, E., 509
Unger, L. J., 88
Ungley, C. C., 260
Usher, R., 15, 22
Utterback, J. G., 149
Uttley, W. S., 758
Utz, J. P., 593
Uzman, L. L., 680
Uzsoy, N. K., 448

## V

Vaananen, I., 594
Vaerman, J. P., 36, 818
Vahlquist, B., 36, 236, 266, 287, 523, 543, 550
Vainer, H., 758
Valaes, T., 126, 130, 342, 345
Valberg, L. S., 758, 807, 819
Valensi, Q., 650
Valentine, G. H., 177

Valentine, W. N., 62, 285, 286, 311, 313, 339, 347, 349, 350, 351, 385, 443, 507, 508, 509, 522, 535, 593, 594
Vallbana, C., 176
Valtis, D. J., 11, 62, 351, 448
Vanbellinghen, P., 534, 590
Vance, V. K., 432
van Creveld, S., 680, 757, 758, 819
Van de Hagen, C. B., 124
Van de Kamer, J. H., 260
Vandenbroucke, J., 819
Vandepitte, J., 435
Van der Esch, V. D., 753
Van der Hart, M., 351
Van der Hauwaert, L. G., 178
Van der Horst, R. L., 819
Van der Sar, A., 509
Vandervoot, R., 588
Vandesherchen, J. F., 810
VanDyke, D. C., 240
Vanecko, M., 87
VanEps, L. W. S., 373, 448
van Furth, R., 36, 543, 550
Vanier, T., 445
VanLeewwen, G., 128
Van Loghem, J. J., Jr., 351
van Loon, E. J., 259
Vann, R. L., 755
Van Praagh, R., 178
VanRood, J. J., 289
van Roogen, C. E., 102
Van Slyck, E. J., 550
Varadi, S., 130, 351, 650, 758, 811
Varga, C., 680
Vargas, D., 435
Vas, M. R., 289
Vasquez, J. J., 758
Vathianathan, T., 178, 448
Vats, T., 448
Vaughan, J., 345, 351, 467, 502, 550
Vaughan, S., 432
Vaughan, V. C., III, 149, 150, 178, 758
Vavra, J. D., 60, 437
Vawter, G. F., 238, 675, 677
Veall, N., 178
Veder, H. A., 758, 819
Veiga, S., 448
Vella, F., 436, 448
Vellios, F., 648
Venn, R. J., 286
Verdon, T. A., Jr., 351
Verel, D., 468, 750, 758
Verga, S., 178
Verhaeghe, L. K., 178
Verloop, M. C., 468
Vermylen, C., 819
Vermylen, J., 819
Vernick, J., 625, 627
Vernier, R. L., 797, 819
Verstraete, M., 819
Vertries, K. M., 443
Veslot, J., 749
Vest, M. F., 130
Vestermark, B., 776, 819
Vestermark, S., 776, 819
Vicatou, M., 746
Vickers, C. F. H., 33
Vickery, A. L., 813
Videbaek, A., 564, 594
Vietti, T. J., 236, 449, 468, 624, 626, 627, 811
Vikbladh, I., 522
Villasenor, J. B., 819
Villeneuve, P., 350
Vilter, R. W., 289, 468
Vinograd, J. R., 448
Vinson, R., 259
Viranuvatti, V., 59

Virchow, R., 551, 594, 804
Visnich, S., 102, 587
Vitacco, M., 812, 817
Viteri, F., 259
Vivell, O., 236
Vlaski, R., 435
Vogel, C. L., 647
Vogel, J. M., 523
Vogel, P., 35, 86, 87, 149, 288, 289
Vogler, W. R., 234
Vogt, E. C., 586
Voline, F. I., 505
von Berkum, K. A. P., 812
Von Bonsdorff, B., 260
Von Hofe, F. H., 73, 449
Von Kaulla, K. N., 758
Von Willebrand, E. A., 706, 758
Voorhess, M. L., 202, 204
Vorhees, A. B., Jr., 680
Vos, D., 87
Vos, G. H., 87
Vossen, M., 752
Vossough, P., 240
Vowles, K. D. J., 680
Voyce, M. A., 289
Vries, G. H., 448
Vuopio, P., 754
Vural, I. L., 506, 508, 650

W

Wachter, H. E., 203
Wacker, W. E. C., 435
Wacksman, S. J., 819
Waddell, W. B., 819
Wade, L. J., 444, 448
Waggoner, D. E., 550
Wagner, K., 478, 507, 522
Wagner, R. H., 748, 752
Waisman, H. A., 468
Waite, M. E., 103
Wake, E. J., 345
Waksman, B. H., 284, 502, 520
Walden, B., 436, 438
Waldenstrom, J., 351
Waldman, B., 235
Waldmann, T. A., 240
Walford, R. L., 85, 235, 502, 523, 549
Walin, B. N. S., 236
Walker, A. G., 175
Walker, A. H. C., 148, 150
Walker, B. E., 34
Walker, C. H. M., 816
Walker, F. A., 127
Walker, J., 8, 9, 11, 12
Walker, J. H., 819
Walker, M., 128
Walker, N. F., 350
Walker, R., 87, 680
Walker, W., 148, 150, 819
Walknowska, J., 36
Wall, R. L., 679
Wallace, H. M., 593
Wallace, S., 819
Wallace, W. S., 680
Wallaeger, E. E., 257
Wallenius, G., 237, 440
Wallerstein, R., 236, 237, 240, 288, 289, 351, 746, 819
Walles, G. P., 174
Wallett, D. L., 756
Wallgren, A., 680
Wallis, L. A., 86
Walsh, A. M., 174
Walsh, J. R., 86, 87, 468, 509, 510
Walt, F., 260, 289
Walter, B. A., 648
Walters, D. H., 448
Walters, T. R., 62

Walzer, S., 7, 11, 12, 437
Wan, A. T., 503
Wantz, G. E., 680
Ward, A., 257
Ward, C. E., 550
Ward, F. A., 88
Ward, R., 102
Wardlew, A. C., 348
Wardmann, T. A., 809
Warford, L. R., 259
Warkany, J., 23, 35, 36
Warner, E. D., 748
Warner, J., 36, 507, 522
Warner, S., 284
Warr, O. S., III, 34
Warrach, A. J. M., 811
Warren, A. M., 626
Warren, C. B., 125, 174
Warren, S., 289
Warshow, A. L., 128
Warthen, R. O., 235
Washburn, A. H., 22
Wasi, P., 448
Wasserman, A. J., 345
Wasserman, H. P., 287
Wasserman, L. R., 176, 257, 350, 468, 650
Wassmuth, D. R., 509
Water, A. H., 260
Waterhouse, B. E., 550
Waterhouse, J. A. H., 148
Waters, W. E., 235
Waters, W. J., 150, 157, 174, 177, 509, 650
Watkin, D. M., 260
Watkins, C. H., 509, 647
Watkins, S. P., Jr., 753
Watkins, W., 627, 816
Watkins, W. M., 85, 87
Watson, C. J., 62, 296, 339, 345, 350
Watson, D., 130, 149, 351
Watson, E. H., 680
Watson, G. H., 814
Watson, G. M., 256
Watson, J., 73, 343, 433, 448, 815
Watson, K., 594
Watson, L., 647
Watson, R. J., 35, 149, 259, 376, 441, 445, 446, 448, 468, 680
Watson-Williams, E. J., 819
Watt-Tobin, R. J., 59
Waugh, D. F., 434
Ways, P. O., 339
Weatherall, D. J., 10, 22, 434, 444, 446, 448, 464
Webb, B. D., 819
Webb, J., 594
Weber, G., 420, 438
Weber, J. L., 502
Webster, W. P., 756
Webster, W. R., 758
Wedgewood, R. J. P., 819
Weech, A. A., 130
Weech, L. A., 522
Weed, R. I., 53, 55, 62, 346, 351, 442, 446, 677
Weens, H. S., 438, 448
Wefring, K. W., 758
Wegelius, R., 22, 572, 594, 651
Wehman, J., 235, 436, 756
Wehninger, H., 819
Weidemann, H. R., 509
Weiden, S., 260
Weigle, J., 507
Weijer, H. A., 260
Weil, M., 623
Weiler, R. J., 238
Weinberger, M. M., 572, 594
Weiner, A. S., 88, 159
Weiner, I., 443

Weiner, M. J., 440
Weiner, W., 509
Weinstein, A., 680
Weinstein, I. M., 60, 62, 448, 508
Weinstein, J. B., 260
Weinstein, L., 813
Weintraub, L. R., 235, 237, 240, 241
Weir, H. G., 592
Weir, W. C., 813
Weisberger, A. J., 548
Weisberger, A. S., 288, 591, 651
Weiser, R. S., 87, 204
Weisman, R., Jr., 72, 346, 449, 466
Weiss, D., 339, 432
Weiss, H. J., 738, 751, 759
Weiss, H. S., 758
Weiss, I. H., 351
Weiss, L., 679, 680
Weiss, S., 593
Weissberg, J., 468
Weissman, G., 509
Weissman, S., 260, 438
Weksler, M. B., 286
Welbourn, H. F., 448
Welch, A. D., 260, 612, 627
Welch, C. S., 680
Welch, H., 286
Welch, J., 238
Welch, R. G., 819
Weldon, V. V., 178
Welford, N. T., 651
Weliky, N., 442
Weller, T. H., 127, 130, 589, 808
Wellman, W. E., 522
Wells, B. B., 508
Wells, C. E., 594
Wells, E. B., 819
Wells, I. C., 449
Wells, J. C., 73, 443
Wells, R. H. C., 448
Welsh, J. S., 130
Welsh, R. A., 509
Wendmiller, J., 650
Wennberg, E., 680
Wennersten, G., 520
Went, L. N., 442, 449
Wenzel, B. J., 239
Wenzel, F. J., 756
Wenzl, J. E., 813
Wertlake, P. T., 593
West, M., 535
West, R., 61
Westberg, J. A., 175
Western, K. A., 592
Wetherall, J. H., 550
Wetherley-Mein, G., 503, 594, 627
Wethers, D., 446
Wett, I., 759
Wexler, I. B., 79, 88, 150, 178
Whalen, L. E., 177
Whang, J., 587, 594, 627
Whang-Peng, J., 624
Whaun, J. M., 62, 347, 468
Wheaton, R., 466
Wheby, M. S., 240, 448
Wheeler, C. H., 339
Wheeler, E. O., 550
Wheeler, H. E., 623
Wheeler, J. T., 12, 449
Wheeler, W. E., 150, 154, 178
Wheelock, E. F., 594
Whipple, A. O., 680
Whipple, G. H., 22, 239, 240, 385, 449
Whissell, D., 746

Whissell Buechy, D. Y. E., 752
Whitaker, J. A., 351, 449, 468, 627
Whitby, L. E. H., 204, 468
Whitcomb, F. F., Jr., 126, 127
White, A., 468, 503, 504, 509, 623
White, C. A., 12
White, L. R., 11, 438
White, J. C., 10, 71, 368, 432, 435, 449
White, J. G., 449, 509, 757, 759
White, L. P., 587
White, L. R., 505
White, S. G., 746
White, W. E., 130
Whitehouse, R. H., 433
Whiteside, J. A., 627
Whitney, L. H., 819
Whittaker, J. N., 234
Whitten, C. F., 240, 351, 433, 434
Whittington, R. M., 466
Wickes, I. G., 260
Wickster, G. Z., 240
Widdowson, E. M., 206, 240
Wiener, A. S., 26, 36, 76, 79, 81, 83, 86, 103, 137, 150, 172, 178
Wiener, J., 592
Wiener, L. M., 550
Wiernick, P. H., 510
Wigod, M., 819
Wilbur, J. R., 594, 627
Wilcox, W. P., 751
Wilcox, W. S., 627
Wile, S. A., 350, 819
Wiley, J. S., 59, 351
Wilhelm, D. J., 819
Wilkinson, J. F., 592, 759
Will, J. J., 289, 648, 819
Will, J. R., 814
Willerson, D., 637, 651
Willerson, J. T., 549
Willi, H., 72, 521, 676
Williams, C. M., 204
Williams, D. L., 432
Williams, G. A., 819
Williams, H. P., 817
Williams, K., 590, 623, 625
Williams, M., 126, 594
Williams, R., 129, 339, 465, 506
Williams, W. J., 61, 442
Willis, L., 260
Willoughby, M. L. N., 260, 351, 627
Wilmers, M. J., 351
Wilner, G. D., 759
Wilson, G. M., 468
Wilson, J. F., 241, 258, 590
Wilson, J. L., 35
Wilson, J. T., 130
Wilson, M. G., 7, 12, 571, 594
Wilson, R. F., 810
Wilson, R. M., 510
Wilson, S. J., 550
Wiltshaw, E., 535, 594
Winchester, P. H., 437
Windhorst, D. B., 505, 510
Windle, W. F., 12, 18, 20, 22, 149
Windmiller, J., 449
Wing, M., 21
Wing, Y. S. S., 750
Winick, M., 755
Winkelman, R. K., 819
Winkelstein, J. A., 449
Winn, H. J., 288, 445
Winship, T. O., 73, 351

# AUTHOR INDEX

Winsor, T., 449
Winter, A., 148
Winterhalter, K., 439
Wintrobe, M. M., 12, 62, 204, 225, 234, 237, 241, 284, 285, 287, 288, 289, 343, 348, 435, 464, 466, 467, 468, 502, 503, 504, 506, 520, 550, 587, 592, 593, 623, 625, 626, 627, 628, 648, 678, 809
Wirth, P., 130
Wirts, C. W., 349
Wirtschafter, S. K., 127
Wirtshafter, Z. T., 468
Wisch, N., 343
Wise, S. P., 435
Wiseman, B. K., 504, 523, 550, 680, 811
Wiskott, A., 820
Witebsky, E., 178, 203, 204, 351
Witt, L. J., 820
Witts, L. J., 62, 256, 259, 260, 520
Witwer, E. R., 435
Witzleben, C. L., 449, 594
Wnakin, J. J., 758
Wochner, R. D., 240
Wohler, F., 236, 449
Wohll, H., 754
Wohlman, I. J., 130
Wolf, J., 440
Wolf, P. L., 443
Wolfendale, M. R., 11
Wolff, J. A., 73, 128, 203, 204, 259, 268, 289, 449, 464, 468, 592, 624, 625, 628, 809, 820
Wolff, O. H., 73
Wolff, S. M., 502, 521, 523, 676
Wolfson, I. N., 594
Wolfson, J. H., 130
Wolfson, S., 125, 443
Wollner, N., 628
Wolman, B., 510

Wolman, I., 14, 22, 204, 440, 449, 468, 594, 759
Wolman, L., 758
Wolman, M., 510, 680
Wolnisty, C., 550
Wong, H., 343
Wong, P. Y. C., 467
Wong, V. G., 625
Woo, T. A., 510
Wood, D. D., 596
Wood, I. J., 260
Wood, J. L., 22, 468
Woodliff, H. J., 562, 594
Woodrow, J. C., 162, 178
Woodruff, C. W., 205, 241
Woodruff, M. F. A., 88
Woods, D. D., 628
Woodward, D. J., 523
Woodward, H. Q., 759, 820
Woolford, R. M., 468
Woolley, D. W., 628
Woprssam, A. R. H., 340
Workman, J. B., 236
Workman, W. G., 102
Worlledge, S. M., 88, 340, 351
Worthen, H. G., 819
Wranne, L., 288, 438
Wrenn, E. L., 648
Wright, C. H., 438, 658, 676
Wright, D. H., 590, 647, 648, 651
Wright, D. O., 680
Wright, D. R., 758
Wright, H. P., 759
Wright, I. S., 759
Wroblewski, F., 127, 128
Wuepper, K. D., 348
Wuthrick, K., 62
Wvandt, H., 73, 351
Wyatt, J. P., 236, 438, 449
Wyatt, R. G., 811
Wyatt, T. C., 648
Wybran, J., 816
Wyllie, W. G., 820
Wyman, J., Jr., 10
Wyngaarden, J. B., 239

## X

Xefteri, E., 437

## Y

Yaffe, S. J., 109, 125, 127, 130, 817
Yaguda, A., 594
Yakavac, W. C., 127
Yam, L. T., 241
Yamaguchi, M. Y., 234
Yamamoto, R., 647
Yamane, T., 62
Yamawaki, T., 589
Yang, S. S., 589
Yanis, E., 759
Yankee, R. A., 285, 502, 523, 593, 624
Yannet, H., 35, 534
Yarbro, M. T., 439
Yardley, J., 590
Yettra, M., 339, 756
Yingling, W., 344
Yoffey, J. M., 11
Yonemoto, R. H., 60, 344
York, W. H., 550
Yoshida, A., 439, 442, 467
Young, L. E., 62, 177, 346, 348, 351, 594, 679
Young, L. W., 591
Young, W. A., 587
Yow, M. D., 816, 817
Yu, C. D., 432
Yu, K-P., 624
Yunis, A. A., 289
Yunis, E., 150, 750
Yunis, J. J., 11

## Z

Zabriskie, J., 59
Zail, S., 351, 464
Zak, S. J., 34, 503, 508, 650
Zalusky, R., 243, 245, 258, 352, 758
Zamir, R., 258
Zandstra, R., 624
Zannos, L., 449, 818
Zannos-Mariolea, L., 73
Zarafonetis, C. J. D., 449, 811

Zarkowsky, H. S., 73, 308, 347, 352, 443
Zatuchni, J., 550
Zawadzki, Z. A., 680
Zawisch, C., 651
Zee, P., 626
Zeffren, J. F., 651
Zeid, S. S., 680
Zelickson, A. S., 510
Zelson, J. H., 443
Zeltmacher, K., 289
Zeman, W., 509
Zetterstrom, R., 129, 150, 352, 651
Ziegler, J. L., 647
Ziegler, N. R., 174
Zieve, P. D., 752
Zimmer, S. M., 648
Zimmerman, H. J., 129, 446, 509, 510
Zimmerman, H. S., 535
Zimmerman, T. S., 521, 676, 759
Zinkham, W., 36, 62, 130, 340, 349, 352, 444, 510, 780, 806, 812, 815, 820
Zippin, C., 20, 808
Zipursky, A., 12, 36, 60, 62, 131, 150, 162, 163, 178, 241, 352, 752
Zlotnick, A., 666, 680
Zoger, S., 622
Zucker, M. B., 735, 753, 759, 820
Zucker-Franklin, D., 754
Zuckerman, G. H., 811
Zuelzer, W. W., 17, 20, 34, 72, 73, 88, 115, 125, 130, 150, 174, 178, 237, 260, 331, 345, 352, 434, 440, 445, 449, 510, 523, 566, 592, 594, 612, 621, 624, 628, 651
Zugibe, F. T., 677
Zuigg, W., 60
Zulik, R., 289
Zurcher, C., 348

# Subject index

**A**

$A_2$ hemoglobin in thalassemia, 407-408
$A_2$ thalassemia, 402
Abdomen in lymphocytosis, 529
Abdominal symptoms in allergic purpura, 797
Abnormal hemoglobin; *see* Hemoglobins, abnormal; Hemoglobinopathy
Abnormal hemolysis, tests for, 299-302
Abnormal maturation of erythrocytes, 52-53
Abnormalities, morphologic, of erythrocytes; *see* Erythrocytes, morphologic abnormalities of
A-B-O agglutinogens, 74
A-B-O blood groups
  distribution of, 76
  inheritance of, 76
  system of, 76-79
A-B-O compatibility and Rh-Hr immunization, 172
A-B-O erythroblastosis, 169-173
A-B-O incompatibility, carboxyhemoglobin levels in, 142; *see also* Erythroblastosis fetalis
Absorption tests for infectious mononucleosis, 544
Acanthocytosis, 68-71
Acholuric jaundice, chronic, 303-309
Acid-citrate-dextrose for blood preservation, 99-100
Acid phosphatase in platelets, 684
Acid-serum test, Ham, 324
Aciduria, hereditary orotic, and megaloblastic anemia, 245
Acquired anticoagulants, 726-727
Acquired aplastic anemia, 270-273
Acquired fibrinogen deficiency, 722
Acquired hemolytic anemias; *see* Hemolytic anemias, acquired
ACTH for leukemia, 604
Acute anemia
  hemolytic, acquired, 336-337
  hemoglobin and hematocrit levels in, 90-91
  and naphthalene, as cause of jaundice, 114
Acute blast cell crisis, 601
Acute erythroblastopenias, 267
Acute hemorrhage, anemia of, 459
Acute infantile form of Gaucher's disease, 663
Acute infectious lymphocytosis, 527-532
  differentiated from leukemia, 585
Acute iron intoxication, 231-232
Acute leukemia; *see also* Leukemias
  drug therapy in, 610-612
  lymphoblastic, 531-533

Acute leukemia—cont'd
  lymphocytic, infectious mononucleosis in, 542, 545-546
  megakaryocytic, 633
  monocytic, 490-491
  myeloblastic, treatment of, 616-619
  myelocytic, 553
  remissions in, 615-616
  stem cell, 551
Acute renal failure in allergic purpura, 799-800
Adenosine diphosphate
  impaired release of, in blood coagulation, 738
  in platelets, 683
Adenosine triphosphatase deficiency and hemolytic anemia, 315
Adenosine triphosphate in erythrocyte metabolism, 39
Adenovirus type 12 in lymphocytosis, 528
Adrenaline test in hypersplenic syndromes, 655
Adrenocortical steroids; *see also* Steroids
  in autoimmune hemolytic anemia, 332
  in leukemia, 606
    acute, 611-612
Adriamycin for leukemia, 602
Adult versus fetal hemoglobin, 4-5
Adult hemoglobin, switch mechanism, 7-8
Afibrinogenemia, congenital, 721-722
Agammaglobulinemia
  in alymphocytosis, 519
  plasma cell in, 493
Agglutination
  of leukocytes, 478
  tests of, differential, 543-545
Agglutinins
  cold, 84
    in hemolytic anemia, 330-331
  incomplete, 138
  leukocyte, 478-479, 513
Agglutinogens, 74
Aggregometer, platelet, 743
Agnogenic myeloid metaplasia, 630-631
Agranulocytosis, 514
  infantile genetic, 517-518
  neonatal, 518-519
  transient, 32
Air embolism in transfusion, 99
Albers-Schonberg disease, 631-633
  bone and joint manifestations of, 196

# INDEX

Albumin
    binding capacity of, 157
    concentrated serum, in exchange transfusion, 156-157
Alder's anomaly, 496
Alkali denaturation method for fetal hemoglobin, 353-354
Alkaline phosphatase
    in differentiation of leukemia and leukemoid reactions, 525-526
    serum, in infectious mononucleosis, 543
Alleles, definition of, 24, 74-75
Allelomorphs, definition of, 24, 74-75
Allergic purpura; see Purpura, nonthrombocytopenic, allergic
Allergic reactions in transfusions, 99
Alpha-thalassemia, 413-414
    homozygous, hydrops fetalis from, 361-362
Alymphocytosis, 519
Amato bodies, 493, 495
Amaurotic familial idiocy, infantile, 500
Amethopterin for leukemia, 596-598
Amino acids in hemoglobins, 41
Aminocaproic acid for fibrinolysis, 724
Aminopterin for leukemia, 596-598
Amniocentesis in erythroblastosis fetalis, 143-145
Amniotic fluid, examination of, 145-147
Anaphylactoid purpura, 793-800
Androgen-corticosteroid therapy for aplastic anemia, 279-281
Anemia(s)
    acute and chronic, hemoglobin and hematocrit levels in, 90-91
    of acute hemorrhage, 459
    age incidence in relation to, 181-182
    aplastic; see Aplastic anemia
    bone marrow examination in, 186-188
    chronic hemorrhagic, 459-460
    chronic, outpatient transfusion clinic for, 94
    of chronic renal insufficiency, 455-457
    classification of, 179
    congenital nonspherocytic, 310-311
    Cooley's; see Thalassemia
    definition of, 179
    diagnosis of, 180-188
    diagnostic features of blood smear, 197-199
    erythroblastic; see Thalassemia
    in erythroblastosis fetalis, 163-164
    erythropoiesis and, 189-194
    Fanconi, 268-270
    ferrokinetics and erythrokinetics and, 188-189
    in Gaucher's disease, 666
    general considerations, 179-204
    Heinz body, in newborn, 114
    hemolytic; see Erythroblastosis fetalis; Hemolytic anemias
    hereditary factors of, 197
    heredity, Heinz body, 428-431
    history and physical examination, 181
    hypochromic, refractory, 232-234

Anemia(s)—cont'd
    hypoplastic
        acquired, 267
        aplastic crisis in, 267
        classification of, 261-262
        general considerations, 261
        and leukopenia, 515
        pathologic findings, 264
        pure red cells; see Anemia, pure red cell
    of hypothyroidism, 462
    of infection, 457-459
    from insect bites, 326
    iron-deficiency; see Iron-deficiency anemia
    Lederer's, 336-337
    of leukemia, 577-578
    Mediterranean; see Thalassemia
    megaloblastic; see Megaloblastic anemia
    microdrepanocytic, 421-422
    from multiple transfusions, 267
    in newborn, diagnosis of, 181-182
    normoblastic macrocytic, 256
    pernicious, juvenile, 248-253
    physiologic, of newborn, 14
        and iron-deficiency anemia, 208-209
    preceding leukemia, 569-570
    in premature infant, 219-220
    principles of treatment, 199
    "pseudoleucaemia," 385
    pure red cell, 262-267
        clinical features of, 263-264
        definition of, 262
        diagnosis of, 264-265
        laboratory findings, 264
        pathogenesis of, 262-263
        prognosis of, 266-267
        treatment of, 265-266
    and red cell count, hemoglobin, and volume of packed red cells, 184-186
    refractory; see Aplastic anemia
    reticulocyte count and stain in, 184
    sickle cell, 371-384
        blood picture in, 378
        bone and joint manifestations of, 196
        clinical features of, 374-377
        crises of, 378-382
        diagnosis of, 382
        hand-foot syndrome of, 375-376
        pathology of, 371-374
        prognosis of, 384
        skeletal changes in, 377-378
        treatment of, 382-384
    sideroachrestic, 323-324
    sideroblastic, 323-324
        and monocytic, 558-559
    spherocytic, 303-309
    splenic, 658-661
    in twin-to-twin transfusion, 17
    and vitamin deficiencies, 460-462
Aneuploidy in leukemia, 566
Anisocytosis, 63

Anoxia, bone marrow, and erythropoiesis, 48
Antagonists in treatment of leukemia, 596-600
Antibiotics in acute myeloblastic leukemia, 617-618
Antibody(ies)
 anti-Rh, 161-162
 "blocking," 138
 cold, in hemolytic anemia, 330
 formation of, 470-471
  multiple transfusions and, 543
 Forssman, 544
 heterophil, in infectious mononucleosis, 543
 and isoagglutinins, placental transmission of, 28-29
 leukocyte, 513-514
 maternal
  in A-B-O erythroblastosis, 170-171
  prenatal testing for, 136
 neutralization of, 161
 plasmatic theory of synthesis of, 493
 tests for, 138-140
 transmission of, 138
Anticoagulant drugs in pregnancy, 33, 714
Anticoagulants
 circulating, 726-730
  acquired, 726-727
 heparin as, in exchange transfusion, 160
 for stored blood, 100-101
 tests for, 729
Anticonvulsant therapy and megaloblastic anemia, 253
Antigens; *see also* Blood groups
 anti Kp, 83
 anti Le, 83
 anti Jk$^a$, 84
 anti Xg$^a$, 84
 Australia, 97
  in leukemia sera, 586
 i, in thalassemia major, 402
 I, 84
 Js, 83
 low incidence, 84
Antiglobulin reactions in acquired hemolytic disease, 330
Antiglobulin test, 138-139
Antihemophilic factor (globulin), 688
 concentrates of, for hemophilia, 700-701
 deficiency of, 692-705
  bleeding in, treatment of
   local, 695
   transfusions, 695-703
  clinical aspects of, 694
  dental extractions in, 704
  hemarthrosis in, 694-695
   treatment of, 704-705
  hematuria in, treatment of, 703
  hereditary aspects of, 692-694
  management of, 695
Antimicrobial agents causing aplastic anemia, 270-271
Anti-Rh antibody, 161-162

Anti-Rh titer, maternal, 136-137
Antithromboplastin, 726
Aplastic anemia, 267-284
 acquired, 270-273
 androgen-corticosteroid therapy for, 279-281
 bone marrow transplantation for, 283
 clinical features of, 273-274
 cobalt for, 282
 congenital or constitutional, 268-270
 and congenital thrombocytopenic purpura, 782
 course and prognosis, 283-284
 definition of, 267-268
 differential diagnosis, 276
 from leukemia, 585
 erythopoietin in, 275-276
 etiology of, 268
 infection in, control of, 278-279
 laboratory findings in, 274-276
 leukopenia in, 514
 pathology of, 273
 phytohemagglutinin for, 282-283
 prevention of, 276-278
 splenectomy for, 282
 transfusions for, 278
Aplastic crisis
 in hemolytic anemia, 302
 and hemolytic crisis in sickle cell anemia, 380-381
 in hypoplastic anemia, 267
 in thalassemia major, 401
Aregenerative crisis in sickle cell anemia, 380-381
Arsenic poisoning, anemia in, 326
Arthritis, rheumatoid, differentiated from leukemia, 585-586
Aspiration
 bone marrow, 193-194
 splenic, 655
Aspirin and platelet function, 742
Asplenia, functional, in sickle cell anemia, 372
Ataxia-telangiectasia, differentiated from hereditary hemorrhagic telangiectasia. 800-801
Atresia
 of bile ducts, as cause of jaundice, 118-119
 biliary
  cirrhosis in, 122
  distinguished from neonatal hepatitis, 121-122
 of extrahepatic ducts as cause of jaundice, 118-119
 of intrahepatic ducts as cause of jaundice, 119
Auer bodies, 493
Australia antigen, 97
 in leukemia sera, 586
Autoantibodies
 in acquired hemolytic anemia, 331
 in autoimmune hemolytic anemia, 329
 in blood disorders, 200
Autoerythrocytic sensitization, 201
Autohemolysis test, 300-301
Autoimmune hemolytic anemia, 328-334
Autoimmune hemolytic disease, chronic idiopathic, 328-344

Autoimmune mechanisms in pernicious anemia, 250
Autoimmunization in blood disorders, 199
Autoleukocyte antibodies, 513-514
Autophagic vacuoles, 474
Autosensitivity, DNA, 201
Azaserine for leukemia, 599-600
Azathioprine
  in autoimmune hemolytic anemia, 333
  for idiopathic thrombocytopenic purpura, 773-774

## B

$B_2$ hemoglobin in thalassemia, 408
Bacteremia, incidence of, in exchange transfusion, 159
Banti's syndrome, 658-661
Bart's hemoglobin, 361
  in alpha-thalassemia, 413-414
Basophilia
  in maturation of red cells, 51
  punctate, and siderocytes, differentiation of, 66-67
Basophilic leukemia, 629
Basophilic megaloblast, 53
Basophilic normoblast, 52
Basophilic stippling of erythrocytes, 66
Basophils, 486-487
  and eosinophils, changes in, during growth, 19
Bassen-Kornzweig syndrome, 68-71
Benign familial polycythemia, 450-451
Benign granulocytopenia, chronic, 516-517
Bernard-Soulier syndrome, 738
Beta-thalassemia minor, 404
Bile
  excretion of, 56-57
  inspissated, syndrome of, in erythroblastosis fetalis, 117-118
Bile ducts, atresia of, 118-119
Biliary atresia
  cirrhosis in, 122
  and neonatal hepatitis, 121-122
Biliary obstruction in erythroblastosis fetalis, 117-118
Bilirubin; *see also* Hyperbilirubinemia
  binding of, by erythrocytes, 46
  conversion of, in newborn, 108
  in cord blood, 143
  direct and indirect, 56
  in erythroblastosis fetalis, 143
  formation of, 55-56
    in neonate, 57
  indirect
    enzymatic conversion of, 104-105, 107
    and kernicterus, 133
    inhibition of oxidative phosphorylation by, 134
  levels of
    in cord blood, 143
    as indication for exchange transfusion, 152-154
    in newborn, effect of novobiocin on, 109
    serum, in full-term infant, 107-108

Bilirubin—cont'd
  in sickle cell anemia, 378
  types of, 104
Bilirubin encephalopathy, 133-134
Bilirubinemia, nonhemolytic unconjugated, 111
Biopsy of liver in obstructive jaundice, 121
Bishydroxycoumarin, effect of, on infant, 714
Bites, insect, anemia and, 326
Blast cell crisis acute, in chronic myelocytic leukemia, 601
Bleeders, potential, screening of, 731-732
Bleeding; *see also* Hemorrhage
  fetal, into maternal circulation, 26-27
  in glycogen storage disease, 735
  in hemophilia, treatment of, 695-704
  in newborn, 716-717
  from placental surface, 27-28
  in renal disease, 456
Bleeding emergencies, pediatric, 731
Bleeding time, 733-734
Blood
  in anemia of acute hemorrhage, 459
  in autoimmune hemolytic anemia, 329
  cellular component of, life-span of, 89
  citrated, 99-100
  cord
    bilirubin levels in, 143
    erythrocytes of, 13-14
    haptoglobins in, 292-293
    hemoglobin in, 15-16, 142
      and fetal oxygen saturation, 8-9
    hemoglobinopathies of, 361
    immunoglobulin in, 30-31
    membrane lipid of red cell in, 37
  destruction of
    excessive; *see* Hemolytic anemias
    by spleen, 654
  dosage of, for simple transfusion, 91-92
  fetal, and oxygen dissociation, 6-7
  in Gaucher's disease, 666
  heparinized, for exchange transfusion, 160
  in idiopathic thrombocytopenic purpura, 768
  in infectious mononucleosis, 540, 542-543
  in iron-deficiency anemia, 210-211
  in Letterer-Siwe disease, 671
  in lymphocytosis, 529
  in Niemann-Pick disease, 668
  in placental vessels, 15-16
  of premature infant, 20
  preservation of, 100-101
  in sickle cell anemia, 378
  storage and preservation of, 99-100
  stored, potassium in, 45-46
  swallowed, by newborn, 5-9
  in thalassemia major, 397-402
  whole
    choice and dosage of, 91
    or plasma, in classic hemophilia, 695
    versus sedimented red cells for exchange transfusion, 156

Blood-brain barrier in kernicterus, 134
Blood cells
  and bone marrow, disorders affecting, 196
  fragmentation of, 53-58
  origin and development of, 1-12
    bone marrow at birth, infancy, and childhood, 9-10
    embryonic hemoglobin, 2-3
    fetal hemoglobin, 3-5
    in fetus, 1-2
    theories of, 2
  primitive, 50-51
  red; see Erythrocytes
  white; see Leukocytes
Blood changes during growth, 13-22
Blood chimeras, 78
Blood coagulation, 681-759
  anticoagulants, circulating, 726-730
  bone and joint manifestations of, 196
  disorders of
    laboratory investigation of, 732-745
    replacement therapy for, 730-731
  disseminated intravascular, 727-729
  dynamics of, 691
  epistaxis and, 731
  factors of; see Factors, blood coagulation
  mechanisms of, 684-691
  natural inhibitors of, 691-692
  in newborn, 717
  normal hemostatic mechanisms, 681-692
  phase 1, 687-689
    disorders of, 692-712
      Christmas disease, 709-711
      hemophilia, 692-705
      plasma thromboplastin antecedent deficiency, 711-712
      von Willebrand's disease, 706, 708-709
    tests for, 735-743
  phase 2, 689-690
    disorders of, 712-721
      factor V, congenital deficiency of, 714-715
      factor VII, congenital deficiency of, 715-716
      factor X, deficiency of, 720
      factor XII, deficency of, 720-721
      multiple defects, 721
      of newborn, 716-720
      vitamin K deficiency, 713-714
    tests for, 743-744
  phase 3, 690-691
    disorders of, 721-726
      acquired fibrinogen deficiency, 722
      congenital afibrinogenemia, 721-722
      dysfibrinogenemias, 722
      fibrinolysis, 723-725
      laboratory findings in, 725
      treatment of, 725-726
    tests for, 744-745
  platelets and, 681-684
  screening procedures for potential bleeders, 731-732

Blood coagulation—cont'd
  tests, significance of, 735
  vascular factors, role of, 681
Blood count, red
  hemoglobin, and volume of packed red cells, in anemia, 184-186
  in premature infant, 20
Blood disorders
  diagnostic features of, 23
    of bone marrow in, 186-188
  hereditary basis of, 23
  immunoallergic implications of, 199-201
  and porphyrins, 44
  role of spleen in, 642
Blood dyscrasias
  drug-induced, 319-321
    prevention of, 277
  and maternal-fetal interaction, 23-36
    biochemical and genetic aspects, 23-24
    bleeding from placental surface, 27-28
    and congenital anomalies, 24-25
    fetal-maternal transfusion, 26-27
    gamma globulins, 29
    hereditary basis of blood diseases, 23
    immunologic relationships, 31-32
    passage of leukocytes and platelets, 28
    placental physiology and defects, 25-26
    placental transmission
      of antibiotics and isoagglutinins, 28-29
      of drugs, 32-33
      of L.E. factor, 29
    plasma protein, 29-31
    roentgenographic examination in, 195-196
Blood elements, appearance of, in fetus, 1-2
Blood factors; see Blood groups; Factors, blood coagulation
Blood formation in fetus, 1-2
Blood glucose levels in erythroblastosis fetalis, 160-161
Blood groups, 74-88
  A-B-O system, 76-79
  antigens, 74
    I, 84
    private, 84
  Bombay, 77
  C-D-E, notations for, 79
  chimeras, 78
  cross-matching, 74
  definition of terms, 74-76
  Duffy, 83
  and erythroblastosis, frequency of, 140
  factor U, 82-83
  Gm system, 84-85
  Kell, 83
  Kidd, 84
  Lewis, 83
  low incidence antigens, 84
  Lutheran, 83
  M-N-Ss and P system, 82-83
  mosaicism, 78-79

# INDEX

Blood groups—cont'd
  Rh-hr system, 79-82
  sex-linked Xg$^a$ system, 84
  substances in secretions, 78
  Sutter, 83
  universal donor and recipient, 78
Blood loss; see Hemorrhage
Blood pressure, umbilical arterial, 25-26
Blood production; see also Erythropoiesis
  by spleen, 652-653
  suppression of, transfusions and, 97-98
Blood smear
  in anemia, 197-199
    sickle cell, with splenomegaly, 372
  in sickle cell–thalassemia disease, 421-422
Blood storage by spleen, 653-654
Blood typing, definition of, 74
Blood values, normal, 182-183
Blood volume, 90
  in newborn, 15
Bohr effect and oxygen affinity, 365
Bombay blood type, 77
Bone changes
  in leukemia, 575-576
  in thalassemia, 394-397
Bone marrow
  in agranulocytosis, 514
  in anemia
    with erythroblastosis fetalis, 164
    hemolytic, 295-296
    iron-deficiency, 211
  anoxia, and erythropoiesis, 48
  aspiration of, 193-194
  at birth, infancy, and childhood, 9-10
  changes of
    in lymphoma, 642
    in newborn, 14-15
  in chronic benign granulocytopenia, 516-517
  diagnostic features of, in blood disorders, 186-188
  dysfunction, in pancreatic insufficiency, 514-515
  examination of, 186-188
  failure of; see also Aplastic anemia
    in paroxysmal nocturnal hemoglobinuria, 323
  in idiopathic thrombocytopenic purpura, 768
  invasion of, by foreign cells, 189-190
  iron in immature erythrocytes in, 220-221
  in leukopenia, 511-512
  in lymphocytosis, 529
  normal values of, 186
  osteoblasts and osteoclasts in, 194
  overgrowth of, in thalassemia, 394-395
  in renal disease, 456-457
  replacement of, and leukoerythroblastosis, 630
  in thalassemia, 392
    minor, 404
  transplantation of
    in aplastic anemia, 283
    for leukemia, 619-620
Bony masses in hereditary spherocytosis, 205

Brain, changes in, in erythroblastosis fetalis, 133-136
Breast feeding and hyperbilirubinemia, 110-111
Brill-Symmer's disease, 640
Bruising in thrombocytopenic purpura, 766
Burkitt's tumor, 640
Burr cells, 68
Busulfan for chronic leukocytic leukemia, 600-601
Byler's disease, 120

## C

Cabot rings, 67
Cancer chemotherapeutic drugs, effect of, on fetus, 33
Capillary defect in idiopathic thrombocytopenic purpura, 763
Carbonic anhydrase activity in respiratory distress, 13-14
Carboxyhemoglobin levels in erythroblastosis fetalis, 142
Cardiac failure in erythroblastosis fetalis, 165-166
Cardiac involvement in thalassemia, 409
Carotenemia and jaundice, 123-124
Catecholamine production in neuroblastoma, 190
C-D-E notation for blood groups, 79
Celiac disease, 255-256
Cell(s)
  blood; see Erythrocytes; Leukocytes
  burr, 68
  Downey, in infectious mononucleosis, 540, 542
  Gaucher, 663
    in leukemia, 553
  immunocompetent, 201
  L.E., 475-476
  megaloblastic, 53
  mononuclear, in infectious mononucleosis, 540
  Niemann-Pick, 667
  plasma, 492-493
    and antibody formation, 471
    changes in, during growth, 19
  red blood; see Erythrocytes
  Reed-Sternberg, in Hodgkin's disease, 641-642
  Rieder, 493
  target, 65
    and abnormal hemoglobins, 363-364
  tissue mast, 487
  trypsinized, tests with, for antibodies, 139-140
  Türk's 493
  white; see Leukocytes
Cell stains, 500-501
Cellano factor, 83
Cellular components of blood, life-span of, 89
Cellular development, nucleic acid and, 51-52
Cellular elements, blood, and placenta size, 1-2
Cellular metachromasia, 499
Central nervous system, changes in
  in leukemia, 582
  in sickle cell anemia, 374
Cephalhematoma and jaundice, 124
Charcot-Leyden crystals, 483-485

Chediak-Higashi anomaly of leukocytes, 496-498
Chelating agents
   for hematochromatosis, 229
   in thalassemia, 411
Chemotactic factors of leukocytes, 469-470
Chemotaxis and opsonins, 471-472
Chemotherapeutic agents
   causing anemia, 270-271
   cancer, effect of, on fetus, 33
   for leukemia, 596-600
      choice of, 607-610
      cyclic use of, 612-613
Chickenpox, exposure to, in leukemia, 606
Chimeras, blood, 78
Chlorambucil for lymphomas, 644
Chloramphenicol as cause of aplastic anemia, 277-278
Chloroleukemia and chloroma, 634-635
Chloroma and chloroleukemia, 634-635
Chlorothiazide as cause of congenital thrombocytopenic purpura, 778
Cholelithiasis in sickle cell anemia, 373
Christmas disease, 709-711
   factor IX in, 693-694
Chromosomal abnormalities, leukemia and, 566
Chromosomal terminology, glossary of, 567-568
Chromosomes
   human, 23-24
   and leukemia, 566-568
   Philadelphia, 555-556
      in leukemia, 567
Chronic acholuric jaundice, 303-309
Chronic anemia
   acquired hemolytic, 328-334
   hemoglobin and hematocrit levels in, 90-91
   hemorrhagic, 459-460
   outpatient transfusion clinic for, 94
Chronic benign granulocytopenia, 516-517
Chronic congestive splenomegaly, 658-661
Chronic eosinophilia, 486
Chronic familial jaundice, 303-309
Chronic Gaucher's disease, 663, 665-666
Chronic granulocytic leukemia, 553, 555
Chronic granulomatous disease, 472-473
Chronic hypoplastic neutropenia, 516
Chronic hypoplastic thrombocytopenia with depression of megakaryocytes, 782
Chronic idiopathic autoimmune hemolytic disease, 328-334
Chronic idiopathic jaundice, 116
Chronic infection, anemia of, 457-459
Chronic lymphadenopathy, 640
Chronic lymphocytic leukemia, differentiated from lymphocytosis, 532
Chronic myelocytic leukemia, 553, 555-558
   busulfan for, 600-601
Chronic nonspecific infectious lymphocytosis, 532-534
Chronic portal hypertension, 658-661
Chronic renal insufficiency, anemia of, 455-457

Circulating anticoagulants, 726-730
Circulation, maternal, fetal hemorrhage into, 26-27
Circulatory overload in transfusions, 97
Cirrhosis
   in biliary atresia, 122
   idiopathic, in newborn, 120
Citrated blood, possible harmful effects of, 99-100
Citrovorum factor, 596
Clot retraction, 734
Clotting factors, vitamin K–dependent, 713; see also Blood coagulation
Coagulopathy, consumption, 727-729
Coagulation, blood; see Blood coagulation
Coagulation factors; see Factors, blood coagulation
Coagulation tests, routine, significance of, 735
Coagulation time, 733
Cobalt
   in aplastic anemia, 282
   effect of, in erythropoiesis, 49
   in iron-deficiency anemia, 218
Cohn's fraction 1 for hemophilia, 702
Cold agglutinins, 84
   in hemolytic anemias, 330-331
Cold antibodies in hemolytic anemia, 330
Cold hemogloburinuria, paroxysmal, 334-335
Colonic perforation and peritonitis after exchange transfusion, 161
Compensated hemolytic disease, 58
Congenital afibrinogenemia, 721-722
Congenital anomalies
   and aplastic anemia, 268-270
   and blood dyscrasias, 24-25
   and leukemia, 570-571
Congenital aplastic anemia, 268-270
Congenital atresia of bile ducts, 119
Congenital cytomegalic inclusion disease, 115
Congenital dyserythropoietic multinuclearity, 71
Congenital factor V deficiency, 714-715
Congenital factor VII deficiency, 715-716
Congenital familial nonhemolytic jaundice with kernicterus, 122-123
Congenital heart disease, cyanotic
   hypofibrinogenemia in, 722-723
   iron-deficiency anemia in, 232
   polycythemia in, 451
Congenital hemolytic jaundice, 303-309
Congenital hemolytic syndromes; see Hemolytic anemia, congenital
Congenital hypoconvertinemia, 715-716
Congenital hypofibrinogenemia, 722
Congenital hypoplastic thrombocytopenia, sporadic congenital spherocytosis with, 309-310
Congenital hypoprothrombinemia, 714
Congenital leukemia, 570-571
   chronic granulocytic, 555
Congenital methemoglobinemia, 453
   with hemoglobin M, 453
Congenital nonspherocytic anemia, 310-311
Congenital obliteration of bile ducts, 118-119
Congenital porphyria, 297

Congenital rubella, anemia of, 326
Congenital spherocytosis, sporadic, with hypoplastic thrombocytopenia and malformations, 309-310
Congenital syphilis, anemia of, 326
Congenital thrombocytopenic purpura, 777-779
　and aplastic anemia, 782
Congenital toxoplasmosis, 115-116
Congenital vascular defects, 800-803
Conglutation, 171
Conjugated bilirubin, 104
Consumption coagulopathy, 727-729
Contrast microscopy, 501
Cooley's anemia; see Thalassemia
Coombs test, 138-139
　in A-B-O erythroblastosis, 170
　positive, in erythroblastosis fetalis, 154
Copper in iron-deficiency anemia, 218
Copper deficiency in infants, 229
Coproporphyrin
　in anemia of infection, 458
　and protoporphyrin, erythrocyte, 296
Cord, clamping of, in erythroblastosis fetalis, 164
Cord blood
　bilirubin levels in, 143
　erythrocytes of, 13-14
　haptoglobins in, 292-293
　hemoglobin in, 15-16, 142
　　and oxygen saturation, 8-9
　hemoglobinopathies, 361
　immunoglobulin in, 30-31
　red cell membrane lipid of, 37
Corpuscular hemoglobin concentration, mean, 185-186
Corpuscular volume, mean, 185
Corticosteroid-androgen therapy for aplastic anemia, 279-281
Corticosteroids; see also Steroids
　for hemophilia, 703
　in pure red cell anemia, 265
Cortisone for leukemia, 604
Coumadin, effect of, on fetus, 33
Courtland antihemophilic factor, 701-702
Crenation of erythrocytes, 68
Crigler-Najjar syndrome
　as cause of jaundice, 122-123
　phenobarbital therapy for, 109
Crisis
　acute blast cell, in chronic myelocytic leukemia, 601
　aplastic
　　in hemolytic anemia, 302
　　and hemolytic crisis in sickle cell anemia, 380-381
　　in hypoplastic anemia, 267
　　in thalassemia major, 401
　　in sickle cell anemia, 378-382
Cross-matching, 74
Cryofibrinogenemia, 335-336
Cryoglobulinemia, 335

Cryoprecipitate for hemophilia, 701
Cyanosis and hemoglobin, 43
Cyanotic heart disease, congenital
　hypofibrinogenemia in, 722-723
　iron-deficiency anemia in, 232
　polycythemia in, 451
　and transfusion, 94
Cyclic thrombocytopenic purpura, 792
Cyclophosphamide
　for idiopathic thrombocytopenic purpura, 774
　for leukemia, 601
　for lymphomas, 644
Cystic disease, medullary, 457
Cytomegalic inclusion disease
　as cause of jaundice, 115
　in leukemia, 579
Cytomegalovirus pneumonia in leukemia, 579
Cytoplasmic changes in leukocytes, 493-500
Cytosine arabinoside for leukemia, 602-603
Cytotoxic agents
　in autoimmune hemolytic anemia, 332-333
　for leukemia, 600-602
Cytoxan for leukemia, 601

**D**

$D_1$ trisomy syndrome, hematologic changes in, 7
Daunorubicin for leukemia, 602
Desferroxamine
　for iron intoxication, 231
　in thalassemia, 411-412
Defibrination syndrome, 727-729
Deformability of erythrocytes, 55
Deoxyribonucleic acid
　autosensitivity of, 201
　in cellular development, 51
　and protein synthesis, 23-24
　synthesis of, in lymphocytes, 488-489
Dextran, iron-, for iron-deficiency anemia, 217-218
Di Guglielmo's disease, 634
2,3-Diphosphoglycerate
　and oxygen affinity, 365
　　of maternal and fetal blood, 6-7
　in oxygen dissociation, 41
2,3-Diphosphoglycerate mutase, deficiency of, and hemolytic anemia, 316
Direct bilirubin, 56
　enzymatic conversion of indirect to, 104-105, 107
Direct Coombs test, 138-139
Disseminated intravascular coagulation, 727-729
Disseminated lupus erythematosus, 475-477
　and thrombocytopenic purpura, 770
Dissociation, oxygen
　and 2,3-diphosphoglyceride, 41
　and fetal blood, 6-7
　and thickness of red cells, 47
DNA; see Deoxyribonucleic acid
Dohle bodies, 496
Downey cells in infectious mononucleosis, 540, 542
Down's syndrome
　chromosomal abnormality in, 24

Down's syndrome—cont'd
  hematologic changes in, 7
  and leukemia, 571-572
DPG; see 2,3-diphosphoglycerate
Drepanocytes, 64
Drepanocytic anemia; see Sickle cell anemia
Drug-induced blood dyscrasias, 319-321
  prevention of, 277-278
Drug-induced hemolytic anemias, 327-328
Drug-induced methemoglobinemia, 453-454
Drug-induced thrombocytopenia, 780-782
Drugs
  as cause of leukopenia, 513
  transplacental passage of, 32-33
Dubin-Johnson type jaundice, 116
Dubin-Sprinz disease, 116
Duffy blood groups, 83
Duodenum and absorption of iron, 222-224
Dyscrasias, blood
  drug-induced, 319-321
    prevention of, 277
  and maternal-fetal interaction, 23-36
    biochemical and genetic aspects, 23-24
    bleeding from placental surface, 27-28
    and congenital anomalies, 24-25
    fetal-maternal transfusion, 26-27
    gamma globulins, 29
    hereditary basis of blood diseases, 23
    immunologic relationships, 31-32
    passage of leukocytes and platelets, 28
    placental physiology and defects, 25-26
    placental transmission
      of antibodies and isoaggultinins, 28-29
      of drugs, 32-33
      of L.E. factor, 29
    plasma proteins, 29-31
  roentgenographic examination in, 195-196
Dyserythropoietic multinuclearity, congenital, 71
Dysfibrinogenemias, 722
Dysproteinemias, 335-336
  transient, 229

### E

Ehlers-Danlos syndrome, 801-803
Electrolyte composition of red cells, 45-47
Electrolyte disturbances from transfusions, 99-100
Electrophoresis, 354-356
  starch block, in thalassemia, 407-408
Electrophoretic determination of serum proteins, 358
Electrophoretic mobility of hemoglobin, 357-358
Elliptocytes, average survival of, 64
Elliptocytic hemolytic anemia, 114
Elliptocytosis of erythrocytes, 64
  hereditary
    and hemoglobin C trait, 417
    with hemolytic anemia, 317-319
Elution test
  acid, for fetal hemoglobin, 354
  for antibodies, 139-140

Embolism, air, in transfusion, 99
Embryo, blood formation in, 1-2
Embryonic hemoglobin, 2-3
Enanthem in infectious mononucleosis, 538
Encephalopathy, bilirubin, 133-134
Endocardial fibroelastosis, 165-166
Endotoxin, effect of, on hematopoietic tissue, 480
Enteropathy, exudative, 229-231
Enterovirus as cause of lymphocytosis, 528
Enuresis in sickle cell anemia, 374
Enzymatic conversion of bilirubin, 104-105, 107
Enzyme deficiency, hemolytic anemia and, 319-321
Enzymes in erythrocyte metabolism, 39
Enzymopathies, 311-316
Eosinopenia, 486
Eosinophilia, 484-486
Eosinophilic granuloma, 673
Eosinophilic leukemia, 485-486, 559-560
Eosinophilic lung, 485
Eosinophils, 483-486
  and basophils, changes in during growth, 19
Epistaxis
  and blood coagulation, 731
  in thalassemia major, 402
Epsilon-aminocaproic acid
  for fibrinolysis, 724
  for hemophilia, 703
Epstein-Barr virus in infectious mononucleosis, 536-537
Erythematosus, disseminated lupus, 475-477
  and thrombocytopenic purpura, 770
Erythremia, 450
Erythremic myelosis, 634
Erythroblast, 52
  in fetus, 2
Erythroblastic anemia; see Thalassemia
Erythroblastopenias, 267
Erythroblastosis fetalis, 131-150
  A-B-O incompatibility, 169-173
  amniocentesis in, 143-145
  anemia in, 163-164
  antibodies and, 138
  blood group factors causing, 140-141
  and cardiac failure, 165-166
  clinical features of, 132-133
  definition of, 131
  differential diagnosis of, 173
    toxoplasmosis, congenital, 115
  early jaundice in, 133
  extravascular bilirubin pool in, 151
  family severity, patterns of, 141
  and heterozygous or homozygous father, 137-138
  and immunization in Rh-positive mother and infant, 137
  kernicterus and, 133-136
  laboratory findings in, 141-143
  management of, 164-165
  and maternal anti-Rh titer, 136-137
  obstructive jaundice in, 117-118
  pathogenesis, 131-132

Erythroblastosis fetalis—cont'd
  pathology of, 136
  prenatal testing for maternal antibodies, 136
  prevention of, 161-162
  and previous transfusions, 137
  prognosis of, 141
  rebound bilirubin in, 151
  and rupture of spleen, 164
  tests for antibodies in, 138-140
  treatment of, 151-178
    exchange transfusions, 151-161
      age at time of, 154-155
      blood, amount to be used, 157
      complications of, 160-161
      concentrated serum albumin for, 160
      heparinized blood for, 160
      indications for, 152-154
      and prematurity, 155
      procedure for, 157-159
      rationale for, 151-152
      saphenous vein method of, 159-160
      whole blood versus sedimented red cells for, 156
    glucuronic acid, 161
    induction of labor, 155-156
    intraperitoneal transfusion of fetus, 166-167
    objectives of, 151
    overall results of, 163
    photherapy, 161
Erythrocyte(s)
  abnormal autoantibodies against, in hemolytic anemia, 331
  abnormal maturation of, 52-53
  absorption by surface of, 46
  acetylcholinesterase activity of, in A-B-O erythroblastosis, 172
  acid phosphatase in, 40
  altered phospholipid composition of, in hereditary nonspherocytic hemolytic anemia, 316
  appearance of in fetus, 2
  autoantibodies affecting, 329
  binding of bilirubin by, 46
  color index of, 184-185
  of cord blood, 13-14
  deformability of, and life-span, 55
  determination of destruction of, 188
  electrolyte considerations, 45-47
  in erythroblastosis fetalis, 141
  erythron, 37
  fetal, survival time of, 9
  fetal hemoglobin in, demonstration of, 354
  fragmentation of, 53-58
    syndrome of, 787-792
  freezing of, 101
  H substance in, 76-77
  heme-heme interaction, 43-44
  hemoglobin components of, 41-42
    structure and function of, 40-41
  in hereditary spherocytosis, 303-305
  immature, iron in, 220-221

Erythrocyte (s)—cont'd
  indices of, 185-186
  integrity of, glutathione and, 320
  iron content of, and oxygen capacity, 42-43
  in iron-deficiency anemia, 211, 212
  life-span of, 54
    and erythrocyte deformability, 55
    in hemolytic disorders, tests for, 301-302
    in iron-deficiency anemia, 212
    in newborn, 54-55
    in thalassemia, 405-406
  mass, volume of, 51-52
  maturation of, 51-52
  mechanical fragility of, 47
  membrane of, 37-38
  metabolism of, 38-40
    and nonspherocytic hemolytic anemia, 310-311
  morphologic abnormalities of, 63-73
    acanthocytosis, 68-71
    basophilic stippling, 66
    burr cells, 68
    Cabot rings, 67
    crenation of, 68
    familial erythroid multinuclearity, 71
    Heinz bodies, 67
    Howell-Jolly bodies, 67
    hypochromia and hyperchromia, 66
    Pappenheimer bodies, 67
    pocked, 67
    pyknocytes and infantile pyknocytosis, 68
    of shape, 64-66
    siderocytes, 66-67
    of size, 63-64
  of newborn, 13-14, 16-17
  normal destruction of, 53, 55
  nucleated, in thalassemia major, 399
  osmotic fragility of, 46-47
  packed, volume of
    in anemia, 183-184
    during growth, 118
  porphyrins and blood disorders, 44
  potassium in, 45
  of premature infant, 20
  production of, 47-53
    factors required for, 47-48
    humoral regulation of, 48-50
    ineffective, 50
    maturation, 52-53
    primitive blood cells, 50-51
    retardation of, by transfusion, 97
    stages of, 51-52
  properties of, 37-41
  protoporphyrin and coproporphyrin in, 296
  rouleaux formation in, 44-45
  sensitized, in hemolytic anemia, 332
  sickling of, 367-368; *see also* Sickle cell anemia; Sickle cell disease
  size of, and hemoglobin concentration, 18
  stippling of, in lead poisoning, 463-464

Erythrocyte (s)—cont'd
  in thalassemia major, 397
    nucleated, 399
    survival of, 405-406
  in thalassemia minor, 403-404
  thickness of, and oxygen dissociation, 47
  volume of, 40
Erythrocythemia, 451-452
Erythrocytosis, 451-452
Erythrogenesis in newborn, 13
Erythrogones, 52-53
Erythroid multinuclearity, familial, 71
Erythroid:myeloid ratio, 195
Erythrokinetics and ferrokinetics, 188-189
Erythroleukemia, 634
Erythron, definition of, 37
Erythrophagocytosis, 474-475
  in hemolytic anemia, 294
Erythropoiesis, 51-52
  depression of, by transfusion, 98
  effect of multiple transfusions on, 267
  effective and ineffective, 50
  iron-deficient, and iron-deficiency anemia, 227
  in newborn, 49-50
  by spleen, 652-653
  suppression of, transfusions and, 97-98
Erythropoietic porphyrias, 297
Erythropoietic protoporphyrias, 297-298
Erythropoietic uroporphyrias, 297
Erythropoietin, 48-50
  in aplastic anemia, 275-276
  in renal tumors, 50
  and uremia, 455
Esophagus, changes in, in leukemia, 573
Etiocholanolone as test for bone marrow function, 512
Exanthem in infectious mononucleosis, 538
Exchange transfusion
  for erythroblastosis fetalis
    age at time of treatment, 154-155
    blood, amount to be used, 157
    complications of, 160-161
    concentrated serum albumin for, 156-157
    heparinized blood for, 160
    indications for, 152-153
    and prematurity, 155
    procedure for, 157-159
    rationale for, 151-152
    saphenous vein method of, 159-160
    whole blood versus sedimented red cells for, 156
  incidence of bacteremia in, 159
  partial, in iron-deficiency anemia, 219
  in physiologic hyperbilirubinemia, 167-169
  platelet levels following, 143
  potassium excess and, 45-46
  in premature infant, 153
  as treatment for poisonings, 169

Excretion
  of bile, 56-57
  of urobilinogen as index of hemolysis, 57
Extrahepatic ducts, atresia of, 118-119
Extramedullary megakaryocytosis and megakaryocytic leukemia, 633
Exudative enteropathy, 229-231

## F

Factors
  blood; *see* Blood groups
  blood coagulation, 686-691
    factor I (fibrinogen), deficiency of, 721-726; *see also* Fibrinogen
    factor II (prothrombin), 689
      conversion of, to thrombin, disorders of, 712-721
      tests for, 743-745
    factor IV (calcium), 689
    factor V (labile factor), 689-690
      deficiency of, 714-715
      in leukemia, 553
    factor VII (proconvertin, stable factor), 689-690
      deficiency of, 715-716
      tests for, 744
    factor VIII, 688
      concentrates of, for hemophilia, 700-701
      deficiency of, 692-705; *see also* Hemophilia, classic
      in von Willebrand's disease, 706, 708-709
    factor IX (plasma thromboplastin component)
      in Christmas disease, 693-694
      deficiency of, 709-711
      in Ehlers-Danlos syndrome, 802-803
    factor X (Stuart-Prower), 688
      deficiency of, 720
      tests for, 744
    factor XI (plasma thromboplastin antecedent), deficiency of, 711-712
    factor XII (Hageman)
      deficiency of, 687-688, 720-721
      tests for, 740-741
    factor XIII (fibrin-stabilizing), 690-691
    multiple deficiencies of, 721
    preparation of, for thromboplastin generation test, 736
    vitamin K–dependent, 713
  platelet factor 3, 742-743
Familial erythroid multinuclearity, 71
Familial idiocy, infantile amaurotic, 500
Familial jaundice, chronic, 303-309
Familial megaloblastic anemia, 249
Familial methemoglobinemia, 453
Familial myeloproliferative disease, 631
Familial neonatal hyperbilirubinemia, 105
  transient, 111
Familial nonhemolytic jaundice, 123
  congenital, with kernicterus, 122-123
Familial polycythemia, benign, 450-451

Familial xanthomatosis, primary, 668-669
Fanconi anemia, 268-270
Fanconi syndrome, bone and joint manifestations of, 196
Favism, 319
Felty's syndrome, 658
Ferrokinetics and erythrokinetics, 188-189
Fetal hemoglobin, 3-5, 359
 acid elution method for determining, 354
 versus adult, 4-5
 content of, and maturity, 6
 in Down's syndrome, 7
 in erythroblastosis fetalis, 142
 in granulocytic leukemia, 557-558
 hereditary persistence of, 3-4, 359-361
  and hemoglobin C, 417
  and thalassemia, 426
 in pathologic conditions, 7
 in sickle cell disease, 360
 in thalassemia, 388-389
  minor, 402
  turnover rate of, 406
Fetal hemorrhage into maternal circulation, 26-27
Fetal gene, high, 359-361
Fetal-maternal interaction and blood dyscrasias; see Blood dyscrasias
Fetal-maternal leukocyte incompatibility, 478-479
 in congenital thrombocytopenic purpura, 778
 immunologic relationships of, 32
Fetal-maternal transfusion, 26-27
Fetal myoglobin, 9
Fetal oxygen saturation and cord blood hemoglobin, 7-8
Fetal red cells, survival time of, 9
Fetal rubella, thrombocytopenia in, 779-780
Fetus
 appearance of erythrocytes in, 2
 appearance of granulocytes and lymphocytes in, 2
 blood formation in, 1-2
 effect of chemotherapeutic drugs on, 33
 immunoglobulin synthesis by, 29-31
 iron transfer to, 206
 plasma proteins in, 29-31
FI TEST, 745
Fibrin, conversion of fibrinogen to, 690-691
Fibrin stabilizing factor, 690-691
Fibrinogen
 conversion of, to fibrin, 690-691
 deficiency of
  acquired, 722
  congenital, 721-722
  dysfibrinogenemias, 722-723
  and heart disease, 722-723
  laboratory findings in, 725
  tests for, 681-684
  treatment of, 744-745
 platelet, 684
Fibrinolysis, 723-725
 tests for, 744-745

Fibroelastosis, endocardial, 165-166
Fibrolytic purpura, 723-725
Fibrosis in thalassemia, 391-392
Fisher-Race concept, 79, 80
Folic acid, 242-244
 antagonists of, for leukemia, 596-598
 deficiency of, 243-244
  in hemolytic anemia, 294-295
  in thalassemia
   major, 401-402
   treatment of, 412
 in erythrocyte production, 47-48
 gastrointestinal absorption of, 244
 and vitamin $B_{12}$, 244
Follicular lymphoblastoma, giant, 640
Follicular lymphosarcoma, 640
Formiminoglutamic acid, 243
Forssman antibodies, 544
Fragility of erythrocytes
 mechanical, 47
 osmotic, 46-47
  test of, 299-300
  in thalassemia major, 402
Fragmentation of erythrocytes, 53-58
Fragmentation syndrome, red cell, 787-792
F-thalassemia, 402
Full-term infant
 iron deficiency in, 207
 platelet count in, 761
 serum bilirubin levels in, 107-108
Functional asplenia in sickle cell anemia, 372

G
Galactosemia as cause of jaundice, 122
Gallstones
 in hereditary spherocytosis, 305
 in sickle cell anemia, 373
Gamma globulins, 29
 in fetus, 29-30
 hereditary, in man, 84-85
Gangliosidosis, generalized, 668
Gargoylism, inclusion bodies in, 498-499
Gastroferrin, 224
Gastrointestinal absorption
 of folic acid and vitamin $B_{12}$, 244
 of iron, 222-224
Gastrointestinal disturbances
 in iron-deficiency anemia, 209
 in leukemia, 579-580
Gaucher's cells, 663
 in leukemia, 553
Gaucher's disease, 662-667
Genetic defects, examination of amniotic fluid for, 145-147
Genetics of Rh-Hr blood types, 79-81
Genotypes, definition of, 75
Giant cell hepatitis as cause of jaundice, 117, 119-120
Giant follicular lymphoblastoma, 640
Giant platelet syndrome, 738

Gilbert's disease as cause of jaundice, 123
Glanzmann's disease; *see* Thrombasthenia
Globulin
    antihemophilic (factor VIII), 688
    gamma, 29
        hereditary, in man, 84-85
Glomerulonephritis in allergic purpura, 797-798
Glucose, blood, levels of, in erythroblastosis fetalis, 160-161
Glucose-6-phosphate dehydrogenase
    deficiency of
        and hemolytic anemia, 311-313
            agents causing, 319-321
        and hyperbilirubinemia, 113
        in sickle cell anemia, 381
        in leukocytes, 470
Glucosephosphate isomerase deficiency, 315-316
Glucuronic acid for erythroblastosis fetalis, 161
Glucuronyl transferase, deficiency of, and hyperbilirubinemia, 105
Glutathione
    deficiency of, and hemolytic anemia, 315
    and maintenance of red cell integrity, 320
    stability of, in newborn, 112-113
Glutathione reductase, deficiency of, and hemolytic anemia, 315
Glycine, heme synthesis from, 40
Glycogen in erythrocytes, 44
Glycogen storage disease, bleeding in, 735
Glycolysis in cells of neonates, 20
Gm system, 84-85
Gower hemoglobins, 2-3
Graft-versus-host reaction, 201-202
Granulocytes
    and lymphocytes, appearance of, in fetus, 2
    Pelger-Hüet phenomenon of, 495-496
    polymorphonuclear, 482-487
Granulocytic leukemia
    chronic, 553, 555
    types of, 551, 553, 555-558
Granulocytic leukocytes; *see* Leukocytes
Granulocytopenia
    chronic, benign, in childhood, 516-517
    leukocyte antibodies and, 513-514
Granuloma, eosinophilic, 673
Granulomatous disease, chronic, of childhood, 472-473
Granulopoiesis maturation compartments, 479-480
Growth, blood changes during, 13-22

# H

H substance in red cells, 76-77
Hageman factor, deficiency of, 687-688, 720-721
    tests for, 740-741
Ham acid-serum test, 324
Hand-foot syndrome in sickle cell anemia, 375-376
Hand-Schüller-Christian disease, 491-492, 672-673
Haptens to prevent erythroblastosis fetalis, 161

Haptoglobin
    disappearance of, after exchange, 151-152
    in relation to hemoglobinemia, 291-293
Heart
    in infectious mononucleosis, 539-540
    infiltration of, in leukemia, 580-581
Heart disease, congenital
    cyanotic
        iron-deficiency anemia in, 232
        polycythemia in, 451
        transfusion for, 94
    hypofibrinogenemia and coagulation defects in, 722-723
Heart failure in thalassemia, 404-405
    treatment of, 411
Heart murmur in anemia, 181
Heat elution test for antibodies, 140
Heinz bodies, 67
    in hemolytic anemia, 294
    hereditary anemia, 428-431
    in newborn, 114
Heinz-Ehrlich bodies, 67
Hemangioma and thrombopenia, 792
Hemarthrosis in hemophilia, 694-695
    treatment of, 704-705
Hematoblast, 1-2
Hematocrit
    in anemia, 183-184
    effect of iron supplementation on, 206
    and hemoglobin levels in anemia, 90-91
    growth and, 18
Hematogones, 496
Hematologic aspects of maternal-fetal interaction, 25-26
Hematologic changes in $D_1$ trisomy syndrome, 7
Hematomas as cause of jaundice, 124
Hematopoiesis, prenatal, 1-2
Hematopoietic factors, deficiency of, 52-53
Hematuria
    in hemophilia, treatment of, 703
    in sickle cell anemia, 373-374
Heme, synthesis of, 40
    defect of, in thalassemia, 390
Heme-heme interaction, 43-44
    and oxygen affinity, 365
Hemochromatosis
    acquired, in thalassemia, 409
    and hemosiderosis, 227-229
        in thalassemia, 404-405
    megalobastic anemia with, 254
Hemofil for hemophilia, 702
Hemoglobin
    abnormal; *see also* Hemoglobinopathies
        geographic distribution of, 364-365
        miscellaneous, 420-421
        structure of, 356-357
        syndromes associated with, 364
    alkali-resistant, in aplastic anemia, 281
    amount of, and cyanosis, 43
    components of, 41-42

Hemoglobin—cont'd
  concentration of, 15-16
    mean corpuscular, 185-186
    in newborn, 15-16
    in sickle cell anemia, 378
    and size of red blood cells during growth, 18
  in cord blood, 15-16, 142
    and fetal oxygen saturation, 8-9
  effects of thalassemia gene of, 387
  electrophoretic mobility of, 357-358
  embryonic, 2-3
  in erythroblastosis fetalis, 141-142
  fetal, 3-5, 359
    versus adult, 4-5
    content of, and maturity, 6
    determination of, 353-354
    in Down's syndrome, 7
    in erythroblastosis fetalis, 142
    in granulocytic leukemia, 557-558
    hereditary persistence of, 3-4
      and hemoglobin C, 417
      and thalassemia, 426
    in pathologic conditions, 7
    in sickle cell disease, 360
    switch mechanism in, 7-8
    in thalassemia, 388-389
      minor, 402
    turnover rate of, 406
  formation of, retardation of, by transfusion, 98
  Gower, 2-3
  and hematocrit levels in anemia, 90-91
  heme-heme interaction in, 43-44
  hybridization of, 366-367
  iron in, 40-41
  and oxygen capacity, 42-43
  levels of
    in premature infant, 20
    in thalassemia, effect on growth, 410-411
    transfusion and, 91
  in newborn, 13
  primitive, 361
  production of, during puberty, 452
  red cell count and volume of packed red cells, in anemia, 184-186
  starch block electrophoresis of, in thalassemia, 407-408
  structure and function of, 40-41
  structure of molecule, 356
  synthesis of
    defect of, in thalassemia, 390
    in lead poisoning, 463
    metabolism of iron for, 221
  total circulating volume of, 90
  types of, methods for determining, 353-356
  unstable, in hemolytic anemias, 428-431
  variants of, and altered oxygen affinity, 431
Hemoglobin $A_2$, in thalassemia, 407-408
  major, 399
  minor, 402
Hemoglobin Alexandra, 362

Hemoglobin $B_2$ in thalassemia, 408
Hemoglobin Bart's, 361
  in alpha-thalassemia major, 413-414
Hemoglobin C
  and hereditary elliptocytosis, 417
  and hereditary persistence of fetal hemoglobin, 417
  thalassemia–, 424, 426
Hemoglobin C disease
  homozygous, 416-417
  sickle cell–, 422-424
Hemoglobin C trait, 417
Hemoglobin C variant with sickling properties, 417
Hemoglobin D, 417-418
  –sickle cell disease, 424
Hemoglobin E disease, 418
  thalassemia–, 426
Hemoglobin E trait, 418
Hemoglobin F; *see also* Hemoglobin, fetal
  –thalassemia, 416
Hemoglobin G, 418-419
  –sickle cell disease, 419
  –thalassemia, 419
Hemoglobin H, 414-416
  –thalassemia, 414-415
Hemoglobin I, 419
Hemoglobin J, 419-420
Hemoglobin Köln disease, 430
Hemoglobin Lepore, thalassemia–, 426-427
Hemoglobin M, 420
  congenital methemoglobinemia with, 453
Hemoglobin S; *see* Sickle cell disease; Sickle cell anemia
Hemoglobin Seattle, 430-431
Hemoglobin Zürich, 429-430
Hemoglobinemia
  haptoglobin in relation to, 291-293
  and hemoglobinuria, 291
  hereditary, hemoglobin variants, and altered oxygen affinity, 431
Hemoglobinopathies, hereditary, 353-449
  cord blood, 361
  Heinz body anemias, 428-431
  hereditary aspects of, 362
  sickle cell anemia; *see* Sickle cell anemia
  sickle cell disease; *see* Sickle cell disease
  sickle cell variants, 421-424
  thalassemia; *see* Thalassemia
  thalassemia variants, 424-428
Hemoglobinuria, 337
  and hemoglobinemia, 291
  paroxysmal
    cold, 334-335
    nocturnal, 46, 321-325
Hemolysis
  abnormal, tests for, 299-302
  increased, features of, 291-294
  intravascular, following open heart surgery, 337-338

Hemolysis—cont'd
  normal, 55
  urobilinogen excretion as index of, 57
Hemolytic anemia (s), 290-352
  abnormal hemolysis in, detection of, 299-302
  acquired, 325-338
    acute, 336-337
    autoimmune, 328-334
    dysproteinemias, 335-336
    intravascular hemolysis following open heart surgery, 337-338
    March hemoglobinuria, 337
    paroxysmal cold hemoglobinuria, 334-335
  acute, and naphthalene, as cause of jaundice, 114
  aplastic crisis in, 302
  classification of, 290-291
  congenital, 302-319
    hereditary elliptocytosis and, 317-319
    hereditary nonspherocytic, 310-317
    hereditary spherocytosis, 303-309
    spherocytosis, sporadic, 309-310
    with stomatocytes, 308
  definition of, 290
  elliptocytic, as cause of jaundice, 114
  enzyme deficiency and, 319-321
  and folic acid deficiency, 294-295
  hereditary
    bone and joint manifestations of, 196
    nonspherocytic, 310-311
      with altered phospholipid composition of erythrocytes, 316
  hereditary elliptocytosis with, 317
  increased hemolysis in, 291-294
  in infectious mononucleosis, 543
  marrow activity in, 295-296
  megaloblastic anemia with, 254, 294-295
  of newborn; see Erythroblastosis fetalis
  nonhereditary, 321-325
  paroxysmal nocturnal hemoglobinuria and, 321-325
  relation of vitamin K to, 112-113
  unstable hemoglobin in, 428-431
Hemolytic and aplastic crisis in sickle cell anemia, 380-381
Hemolytic disease
  compensated, 58
  Rh-Hr, phenobarbital therapy for, 109-110
Hemolytic effects of vitamin K, 112
Hemolytic jaundice, congenital, 303-309
Hemolytic syndromes, congenital, 310-311
Hemolytic transfusion reactions, 95-96
Hemolytic-uremic syndrome, 787-792
Hemopexin, 293
Hemophilia (s), 692-706
  A; see Hemophilia, classic
  B, 709-711
  bleeding in, treatment of, 695-703
  bone and joint manifestations of, 196-197
  C, 711-712

Hemophilia (s)—cont'd
  classic, 692-705
    bleeding in, treatment of
      local, 695
      transfusions, 695-703
    clinical aspects of, 694
    dental extractions in, 704
    hemarthrosis, 694-695
      treatment of, 704-705
    hematuria in, treatment of, 703
    hereditary aspects of, 692-694
    management of, 695
  general considerations, 692
  mild, 705-706
  mutual correction tests in, 739
  prophylaxis, 711
  vascular, 706, 708-709
Hemorrhage
  acute, anemia of, 459
  fetal, into maternal circulation, 26-27
  in leukemia, 573, 577
    in acute myeloblastic, 616-617
    infection and, 578
  in newborn, 716-717
  pulmonary, 27-28
Hemorrhagic anemia, chronic, 459-460
Hemorrhagic disease, of newborn, 717-720; see also Hemophilia
Hemorrhagic disorders
  screening tests for, 733-735
  transfusion therapy in, 100
Hemorrhagic telangiectasia, hereditary, 800-801
Hemosiderin deposits in thalassemia, 392
Hemosiderosis
  and hemochromatosis, 227-229
    in thalassemia, 404-405
  idiopathic pulmonary, 804-807
  transfusion and, 98-99
Hemostatic mechanisms, 681-692; see also Blood coagulation
Henoch-Schönlein purpura, 793-800
Heparin for intravascular coagulation, 729
Heparinized blood for exchange transfusion, 160
Hepatic destruction of platelets in idiopathic thrombocytopenic purpura, 776
Hepatic porphyria, 298-299
Hepatitis
  aplastic anemia following, 272-273
  giant cell, as cause of jaundice, 117, 119-120
  homologous serum, 96-97
  incidence of, in pooled plasma transfusion, 93-94
  neonatal
    as cause of jaundice, 117, 119-120
    distinguished from biliary atresia, 121-122
  plasma cell, 493
Hereditary anemia
  bone and joint manifestations of, 196
  nonspherocytic, 310-311

# INDEX

Hereditary anemia—cont'd
  nonspherocytic—cont'd
    with altered phospholipid composition of erythrocytes, 316
Hereditary basis of blood diseases, 23
Hereditary elliptocytosis
  and hemoglobin C trait, 417
  with hemolytic anemia, 317-319
Hereditary eosinophilia, 485
Hereditary factors in anemia, 197
Hereditary gamma globulins, 84-85
Hereditary Heinz body anemia, 428-431
Hereditary hemoglobinopathies
  cord blood, 361
    Heinz body anemias, 428-431
    hereditary aspects of, 362
    sickle cell anemia; *see* Sickle cell anemia
    sickle cell disease; *see* Sickle cell disease
    sickle cell variants, 421-424
    thalassemia; *see* Thalassemia
    thalassemia variants, 424-428
Hereditary hemorrhagic telangiectasia, 800-801
Hereditary leptocytosis; *see* Thalassemia
Hereditary metabolic disorders, detection of, 147
Hereditary nonspherocytic hemolytic anemia, 310-311
  with altered phospholipid composition of erythrocytes, 316
Hereditary nonspherocytic hemolytic disease as cause of jaundice, 113
Hereditary orotic aciduria and megaloblastic anemia, 245
Hereditary persistence of fetal hemoglobin, 3-4, 359-361
Hereditary spherocytosis, 303-309
  bone and joint manifestations of, 196
  as cause of jaundice, 113
  clinical features of, 305-306
  diagnosis of, 307-308
  etiology of, 303-305
  growth and, 306
  inheritance and race, 303
  laboratory data, 306-307
  in newborn, 307
  pathogenesis of, 303-305
  sickle cell–, 424
  sickling, and thalassemia, 424
  treatment of, 308
Hereditary thrombocytopenic purpura, 776-777
Heredity
  and leukemia, 564-566
  in Gaucher's disease, 666
  in Niemann-Pick disease, 668
Heteroimmunization, definition of, 74
Heterophil antibody test, 543
Heterospecific pregnancy, definition of, 75
Heterozygous, definition of, 75
Hexokinase deficiency and hemolytic anemia, 315
High fetal gene, 359-361
High hemoglobin F–thalassemia, 416

Histiocytes, 491-492
  in idiopathic thrombocytopenic purpura, 764
  sea-blue, syndrome of, 666-667
Histiocytic medullary reticulosis, 673-674
Histiocytosis X, 669-673
Hodgkin's disease, 635-638
  treatment of, 642-643
Homologous serum hepatitis, transfusions and, 96-97
Homovannilic acid in neuroblastoma, 190
Homozygous alpha-thalassemia, hydrops fetalis and, 361-362
Homozygous, definition of, 75
Homozygous hemoglobin C disease, 416-417
Hormone therapy in leukemia, 604-606
Howell-Jolly bodies, 67
Humoral regulation of erythropoiesis, 48-50
Hurler's syndrome, inclusion bodies in, 498-499
Hybridization of hemoglobin, 366-367
Hydrocortisone for leukemia, 604-605
Hydrops fetalis, 132-133
  from homozygous alpha-thalassemia, 361-362
Hyperbilirubinemia
  in breast-fed infants, 110-111
  and glucose-6-phosphate dehydrogenase deficiency, 113
  familial neonatal, as cause of jaundice, 105
  and jaundice in hemolytic anemia, 293-294
  jaundice in, in newborn, 133
  of newborn, unrelated to isoimmunization, 108-109
  nonerythroblastotic, 108-109
  phototherapy for, 111-112
  physiologic, exchange transfusion in, 167-169
  relation of vitamin K to, 112
  transient familial neonatal, as cause of jaundice, 111
  unconjugated, 105
Hyperchromia, 66
Hypergammaglobulinemia, plasma cell in, 493
Hyperinsulinemia in erythroblastosis fetalis, 160-161
Hyperkalemia during transfusion, 99-100
Hyperleukocytosis
  myeloid type, 525-526
  and severity of leukemia, 578
Hyperphagia in leukemia, 582
Hypersplenic syndromes, adrenaline test for, 655
Hypersplenism, 656-657
Hyperuricemia following antileukemia drugs, 611-612
Hypochromia, 66
Hypochromic anemia, refractory, 232-234
Hypochromic macrocytes, 63
Hypoconvertinemia, congenital, 715-716
Hypocupremia, 229
Hypofibrinogenemia
  clotting time in, 725
  as complication of obstetric conditions, 723

Hypofibrinogenemia—cont'd
  congenital, 722
  and other coagulation defects in heart disease, 722-723
Hypoglycemia in erythroblastosis fetalis, 160-161
Hypoplastic anemia, 262-267
  acquired, 267
  aplastic crisis in, 267
  classification of, 261-262
  general considerations, 261
  and leukopenia, 515
  pathologic findings, 264
  pure red cell, 262-267
    clinical features of, 263-264
    definition of, 262
    diagnosis of, 264-265
    laboratory findings, 264
    pathogenesis, 262-263
    prognosis, 266-267
    treatment of, 265-266
Hypoplastic crisis in sickle cell anemia, 381
Hypoplastic neutropenia, chronic, 516
Hypoplastic thrombocytopenia
  chronic, 782
  congenital, with malformations and sporadic spherocytosis, 309-310
Hypoprothombinemia
  idiopathic, 714
  in newborn, 717-720
Hypothyroidism
  anemia of, 462
  and jaundice, 124

# I

Icterus
  and infections, 114-115
  neonatorum, 107-108
  praecox, 170
Idiocy, infantile familial amaurotic, 500
Idiopathic autoimmune hemolytic disease, 328-334
Idiopathic cirrhosis in newborn, 120
Idiopathic hypoprothrombinemia, 714
Idiopathic jaundice, chronic, 116
Idiopathic paroxysmal myoglobinuria, 336-337
Idiopathic pulmonary hemosiderosis, 804-807
Idiopathic steatorrhea, 255-256
Idiopathic thrombocytopenic purpura; see Purpura, thrombocytopenic, idiopathic
Immune system, lymphocytes and, 487
Immunization in Rh-positive mother and infant, 137
Immunoallergic implications of blood disorders, 199-201
Immunoallergic mechanism in idiopathic thrombocytopenic purpura, 762
Immunocompetent cell, 201
Immunoglobulin
  levels of, in infants, 31
  synthesis of, by fetus, 29-31
Immunologic relationships in blood dyscrasias, 31-32
Immunologic tolerance in blood disorders, 199-200
Immunoneutropenia, 513
Immunosuppressive agents
  for idiopathic thrombocytopenic purpura, 773-774
  in autoimmune hemolytic anemia, 333
Immunotherapy for leukemia, 603-604
Inclusion bodies, 496-500
  in thalassemia major, 399-400
Inclusion disease, cytomegalic
  as cause of jaundice, 115
  in leukemia, 579
Incompatibility; see also Erythroblastosis fetalis
  fetal-maternal leukocyte, 32
  Rh and A-B-O, carboxyhemoglobin levels in, 142
Indirect bilirubin, 56
  enzymatic conversion of, 104-105, 107
  and kernicterus, 133
Indirect Coombs test, 139
Induction of labor in erythroblastosis fetalis, 155-156
Infantile agranulocytosis, 517-518
Infantile amaurotic familial idiocy, 500
Infantile pyknocytosis and pyknocytes, 68
Infection
  in acute myeloblastic leukemia, treatment of, 617-618
  anemia of, 457-459
  as cause of leukemia, 563
  as cause of leukopenia, 512-513
  control of, in aplastic anemia, 278-279
  following splenectomy in thalassemia, 412-413
  hemolytic anemia and, 326, 327
  in leukemia, 578-579
  leukocytosis caused by, 524-525
  and lymphocytosis, 532
  in newborn, as cause of jaundice, 114-115
  protection against, by spleen, 654
  thrombocytopenia in, 765-766, 780
  *Toxacara*, eosinophilia in, 484-485
  transmission of, by transfusion, 96-97
Infectious lymphocytosis
  acute, 527-532
    differentiated from leukemia, 585
  chronic, 532-534
Infectious mononucleosis, 536-550
  acute hemolytic anemia during, 543
  in acute lymphocytic leukemia, 542, 545-546
  clinical features of, 537-540
  definition of, 536
  differential diagnosis, 545-546
    leukemia, 585
    lymphocytosis, 531
      chronic nonspecific infectious, 533
  Epstein-Barr virus and, 536-537
  laboratory findings in, 540, 542-545
  pathology of, 537
  prognosis of, 546
  recurrences of, 547

Infectious mononucleosis—cont'd
  tests for, 543-545
  thrombocytopenia in, 543
  transmission of, by transfusion, 96
  treatment of, 546-547
Insect bites, anemia and, 326
Inspissated bile syndrome as cause of jaundice, 117-118
Insulin levels in erythroblastosis fetalis, 160-161
Intoxication, iron, acute, 231-232
Intrahepatic duct atresia as cause of jaundice, 119
Intraperitoneal transfusion, 100
  of fetus, 166-167
Intrauterine transfusion, 166-167
Intravascular coagulation, disseminated, 727-729
Intravascular hemolysis following open heart surgery, 337-338
Intrinsic factor in erythrocyte production, 48
Iron
  in hemoglobin, 40-41
  in immature erythrocytes in bone marrow, 220-221
  needs in infancy, 214-215
  normal metabolism of, 221
  normal values of, 205-206
  in stool, detection of, 216
  total body, of infant, 206
  transfer of, to fetus, 206
Iron absorption, 221-224
Iron-binding capacity, 220-221
  of plasma, 224-227
Iron content and oxygen capacity of hemoglobin, 42-43
Iron-deficiency anemia, 205-241
  blood picture in, 210-211
  bone marrow in, 211
  clinical features of, 209
  in cyanotic congenital heart disease, 232
  diagnosis of, 211-214
  etiology of, 205-208
  in full-term infant, 207
  gastroferrin and, 224
  iron absorption and, 221-224
  iron-binding capacity of plasma, 224-227
  iron transport, 220-221
  laboratory data, 209-211
  and occult blood loss, 209
  and physiologic anemia of newborn, 208-209
  from pica, 207
  plasma in, 211
  in premature infant, 219-221
  prenatal factors in, 205-207
  treatment of, 214-219
    cobalt, 218
    copper, 218-219
    iron-dextran, 217-218
    iron therapy, 215-217
      oral, response to, 218
    transfusions, 219
Iron deficiency and pagophagia, 208
Iron deposition in thalassemia, 404-405
Iron depletion, 225
Iron-dextran in iron-deficiency anemia, 217-218
Iron intoxication, acute, 231-232
Iron-loading anemia, hypochromic, 232-234
Iron overload and transfusions, 98-99
Iron pool, plasma, 188
Iron supplementation, effect of, on hematocrit, 206
Iron therapy, 215-218
Iron-transferrin complex, 220-221
Iron transport, 220-221
Iron turnover, plasma, calculation of, 188-189
Irradiation
  aplastic anemia caused by, 272
  and leukemia, 566, 568-569
  and leukopenia, 513
Isoagglutinins, placental transmission of, 28-29
Isoimmunization
  definition of, 74
  prevention of, 162-163
Isoleukocyte antibodies, 513-514

## J

Janus green for cell staining, 500
Jaundice
  in A-B-O erythroblastosis fetalis, 173
  chronic acholuric, 303-309
  chronic familial, 303-309
  congenital hemolytic, 303-309
  detection of, in erythroblastosis fetalis, 133
  in early neonatal period
    acute hemolytic anemia and naphthalene ingestion, 114
    causes of, 107
    chronic idiopathic, 116
    and congenital toxoplasmosis, 115-116
    and cytomegalic inclusion disease, 115
    diagnostic features of, 106
    and elliptocytic hemolytic anemia, 114
    and Heinz body anemia, 114
    and hereditary nonspherocytic hemolytic disease, 113
    and hereditary spherocytosis, 113
    and hyperbilirubinemia
      in breast-fed infants, 110-111
      unrelated to isoimmunization, 108-109
    infections and, 114-115
    phenobarbital therapy for, 111-112
    physiologic, 107-108
    transient, 111
    vitamin K and, 112-113
  and hyperbilirubinemia in hemolytic anemia, 293-294
  in late neonatal period, 116-124
    and atresia of bile ducts, 118-119
    and carotenemia, 123-124
    congenital familial nonhemolytic, with kernicterus, 122-123
    familial nonhemolytic, 123
    and hematomas, 124

Jaundice—cont'd
  in late neonatal period—cont'd
    and hypothyroidism, 124
    and inspissated bile syndrome, 117-118
    and neonatal hepatitis, 119-120
    obstructive
      and erythroblastosis, 117-118
      prolonged, 116-117, 120-122
    from pyloric stenosis, 124
  physiologic, and lack of carbohydrate, 108-109
  in sickle cell anemia, 373
Joint involvement in allergic purpura, 797
Juvenile pernicious anemia, 248-253

K

Kasabach-Merritt syndrome, 792-793
Kell blood groups, 83
Kell genes, 83
Kernicterus
  and bilirubin level in erythroblastosis, 153
  blood-brain barrier in, 134
  caused by sulfisoxazole, 135
  congenital familial nonhemolytic jaundice with, 122-123
  in erythroblastosis fetalis, 133-136
  in hyperbilirubinemia, 168
  relation of vitamin K to, 112
Kidd blood group, 84
Kidney, changes in
  in allergic purpura, 797-798
  in leukemia, 581
  in sickle cell anemia, 373-374
Kleihauer-Betke stain for fetal hemoglobin, 5, 27
Konȳne for Christmas disease, 710-711

L

Labile factor deficiency, 714-715
Labor, induction of, in erythroblastosis fetalis, 155-156
Laparotomy in obstructive jaundice, 121
L-asparaginase for leukemia, 603
L.E. phenomenon, 475-477
L.E. factor, placental transmission of, 29
Lead poisoning, blood changes in, 462-464
Lederer's anemia, 336-337
Lepore hemoglobin, thalassemia-, 426-427
Leptocytes, 65
Leptocytosis, hereditary; see Thalassemia
Letterer-Siwe disease, 491, 669-672
Leukemia, 551-594
  acute
    drug therapy in, 610-612
    lymphoblastic, differentiation of
      from chronic nonspecific infectious lymphocytosis, 533
      from lymphocytosis, 531-532
    lymphocytic, infectious mononucleosis in, 542, 545-546
    megakaryocytic, 633
    monocytic, 490-491

Leukemia—cont'd
  acute—cont'd
    myeloblastic, 553
      treatment of, 616-619
    myelocytic, 553
    promyelocytic, 553
    remissions in, 615-616
  age distribution of, 560-561
  basophilic, 629
  bone and joint manifestations of, 196
  chromosomes and, 566-568
  chronic lymphocytic, differentiated from lymphocytosis, 532
  chronic myelocytic, 553, 555-558
  classification of, 551, 553, 555-558
  congenital, 570-571
  course of, 576-577
  differential diagnosis of, 584-586
  eosinophilic, 485-486, 559-560
  epidemiology of, 561-562
  etiology of, 562-566
    heredity, 564-566
    infections, 563
    virus, 563-564
  fever in, 578-579
  frequency of types of, 560-561
  gastrointestinal disturbances in, 579-580
  granulocytic types of, 551, 553, 555-558
    acute myeloblastic, 553
    myelocytic, 553, 555-558
  heart, infiltration of, 580-581
  hemorrhage in, 577
    and infection, 578
  heredity and, 564-566
  hyperleukocytosis and severity of, 578
  incidence of, 560
  infections in, 578-579
  kidney, changes in, 581
  and leukemoid reactions, differentiation of, 525
  leukopenia in, 514
  liver, changes in, 580
  lungs, changes in, 581
  lymphoblastic
    current treatment of, 614-615
    drug therapy for, 610-612
  mast cell, 629
  meningeal, treatment of, 621
  mongolism-, 571
  monocytic, 558-559
  muramidase in, 560
  myeloblastic, acute, 553
  myelocytic, 553, 555-558
  myelogenous, 553, 555-558
  myeloid, chronic, 553, 555-558
  in newborn, 565, 570-571
  organ changes in, 580-584
  Philadelphia chromosome in, 555-556
  physical findings in, 573, 575
  plasma cell, 629-630
  pneumonia in, 581

Leukemia—cont'd
  pregnancy in, 565
  preleukemic stage, 569-570
  promyelocytic, acute, 553
  radiation and, 568-569
  remission in
    criteria for, 606-607
    spontaneous, 571-572
  renal function in, 581-582
  sex of patients, 560-561
  spleen, changes in, 580
  stem cell
    acute, 551
    current treatment of, 614-615
    differentiated from lymphocytosis, 531-532, 533
    drug therapy in, 610-612
  symptomatology, 572-573
  transformation to, from lymphosarcoma, 539
  treatment of, 595-628
    antimetabolites, 596-600
      antagonists, principles of, 596
      folic acid antagonists, 596-598
      purine antagonists, 598-600
    bone marrow transplantation, 619-620
    cytotoxic agents, 600
    detailed program for, 607-616
    hormone therapy, 604-606
    immunotherapy, 603-604
    laboratory determinations in, 620
    of nervous system involvement, 620-622
    radiation therapy, 600
    results of, 622
Leukemic meningitis, 583
Leukemoid reactions, 525-526
  differentiated from leukemia, 586
  differentiated from lymphocytosis, 532
Leukoagglutinins, 478-479
Leukocyte(s), 469-510
  agglutinins, 513
  antibodies, 513-514
  cell stains for, 500-501
  changes in, during growth, 19-20
  chemotactic factors, 469-470
  chemotaxis and opsonins, 471-472
  degenerative and toxic cytoplasmic changes, 493-500
  in erythroblastosis fetalis, 143
  erythrophagocytosis by, 474-475
  glucose-6-phosphate dehydrogenase in, 470
  growth and multiplication of, 469
  inclusion bodies of, 496-500
  incompatibility, fetal-maternal, 32
  L.E. phenomenon, 475-477
  leukoagglutinins, 478-479
  life-span of, 478
  lupus erythematosus, 477
  in lymphomas, 641
  muramidase in, 474
  neutrophilic, changes in, during growth, 19
  phagocytosis and antibody formation, 470-471

Leukocyte(s)—cont'd
  and platelets, maternal-fetal passage of, 28
  Rebuck window for study of, 473-474
  in sickle cell anemia, 378
  types of, 479-493
    granulocytic or myeloid series, 479-487
      basophils, 486-487
      eosinophils, 483-486
      granulopoiesis maturation compartments, 479-480
      metamyelocyte, 482
      myeloblast, differentiation of, from lymphoblast, 480-481
      neutrophils, 482-483
      polymorphonuclear granulocytes, 482-487
      promyelocytes and myelocytes, 481-482
    histiocytic, 491-492
    lymphocytic, 487-489
    monocytic, 489-491
    plasma cell, 492-493
Leukocyte alkaline phosphatase, 525
Leukocyte transfusion, 94
Leukocytic changes, normal, 584
Leukocytosis, 524-525
Leukoerythroblastosis and bone marrow replacement, 630
Leukokinetics, 479-480
Leukopenia, 511-523
  bone marrow in, 511-512
  causes of
    agranulocytosis, 514
      infantile genetic, 517-518
      neonatal, 518-519
    alymphocytosis, 519
    aplastic anemia, 514
    chemicals, 513
    drugs, 513
    granulocytopenia, chronic benign, 516-517
    hypoplastic anemia, 515
    immunoneutropenia, 513-514
    infection, 512-513
    irradiation, 513
    leukemia, 514
    neutropenia
      chronic hypoplastic, 516
      periodic, 515-516
      splenic, 519
    nutritional deficiencies, 519-520
    pancreatic insufficiency and bone marrow dysfunction, 514-515
  pathogenesis, 511-512
  treatment of, 520
Lewis blood group, 83
Lipid in cord blood red cell membrane, 37
Lipidoses, 500
Lipochondrodystrophy, inclusion bodies in, 498-499
Liver
  biopsy of, in obstructive jaundice, 121
  in erythroblastosis fetalis, 136
  idiopathic cirrhosis of, in newborn, 120

# 862 INDEX

Liver—cont'd
  in infectious mononucleosis, 539
  in leukemia, 573, 580
  of newborn, conversion of bilirubin by, 108
  parenchymal coagulation changes in disease, 727
  in sickle cell anemia, 372-373
  in thalassemia, 391-392
Löfflers syndrome, eosinophilia in, 485
Low-grade fever syndrome, 532-534
Low incidence antigens, 84
Lucey-Driscoll syndrome, 111
Lupus erythematosus, 477
  disseminated, 475-477
    thrombocytopenic purpura in, 770
  systemic, and L.E. phenomenon in newborn, 29
Lutheran blood group, 83
Lymph nodes
  in leukemia, 573
  in lymphocytosis, 529
Lymphadenitis in cytomegalic inclusion disease, 115
Lymphadenopathy, chronic, 640
Lymphoblast, 489
  differentiation from myeloblast, 480-481
Lymphoblastic leukemia
  acute, differentiated from lymphocytosis, 531-532
  current treatment of, 614-615
  drug therapy in, 610-612
Lymphoblastoma, giant follicular, 640
Lymphocytes, 487-489
  changes in, during growth, 19
  and granulocytes, appearance of, in fetus, 2
  mononucleosis, 542
Lymphocytic fever, 534
Lymphocytic leukemia
  acute, infectious mononucleosis in, 542, 545-546
  chronic, differentiated from lymphocytosis, 532
Lymphocytic splenomegaly, febrile postcardiotomy, 547
Lymphocytosis, 526-534
  acute infectious, 527-532
    differential diagnosis, 529, 531-532
    differentiated from leukemia, 585
  chronic nonspecific infectious, 532-534
Lymphoid tissue, neoplasia of; see Lymphomas, malignant
Lymphomas, malignant, 635-646
  blood changes in, 641-642
  bone marrow changes in, 642
  Burkitt's tumor, 640
  chlorambucil for, 644
  combination therapy for, 645-646
  cyclophosphamide for, 644
  Hodgkin's disease, 635-638
    treatment of, 642-646
  hyperthyroidism in, 635
  hypogammaglobulinemia in, 635
  lymphosarcoma, 638-640
    in childhood, roentgen-ray therapy for, 643
    treatment of, 645
  nitrogen mustard for, 644

Lymphomas, malignant—cont'd
  prognosis of, 646
  roentgen-ray therapy for, 643
  treatment of, 642-646
  triethylene melamine for, 644
  vincristine for, 645
Lymphopenia in Wiscott-Aldrich syndrome, 786
Lymphosarcoma, 638-640
  in childhood, roentgen-ray therapy for, 643
  treatment of, 646
Lysozyme, 474
  in leukemia, 560

## M

Macrocytes, 53, 63
  hypochromic, 63
  nonspecific, in thalassemia major, 397-399
Macrocytic anemias, normoblastic, 256
Macrocytosis and hemolytic anemia, 296
Macroglobulinemia of Waldenstrom, 335
Malabsorption syndrome, 255-256
Malaria and sickling of erythrocytes, 370-371
Malarial infection, anemia of, 326
Malignant lymphomas, 625-646
  blood changes in, 641-642
  bone marrow changes in, 642
  Burkitt's tumor, 640
  chlorambucil for, 644
  combination therapy for, 645-646
  cyclophosphamide for, 644
  Hodgkin's disease, 635-638
    treatment of, 642-646
  hyperthyroidism in, 635
  hypogammaglobulinemia in, 635
  lymphosarcoma, 638-640
    in childhood, roentgen-ray therapy for, 643
    treatment of, 645
  nitrogen mustard for, 644
  prognosis of, 646
  roentgen-ray therapy for, 643
  treatment of, 642-646
  triethylene melamine for, 644
  vincristine for, 645
Malignancy, megaloblastic anemia with, 254
Mannitol for hemolytic transfusion reactions, 96
Marble-bone disease, 631-633
  bone and joint manifestations of, 196
March hemoglobinuria, 337
Massive transfusions, 99
Mast cell leukemia, 629
Mast cells, tissue, 487
Maternal antibodies, testing for, 136
Maternal anti-Rh titer, 136-137
Maternal circulation, fetal hemorrhage into, 26-27
Maternal-fetal interaction and blood dyscrasias, 23-36
  biochemical and genetic aspects of, 23-24
  bleeding from placental surface, 27-28
  and congenital anomalies, 24-25
  fetal-maternal transfusion, 26-27

Maternal-fetal interaction—cont'd
  gamma globulins, 29
  hereditary basis of blood diseases, 23
  immunologic relationships, 31-32
  passage of leukocytes and platelets, 25-26
  placental physiology and defects, 25-26
  plasma proteins, 29-31
  transmission, placental
    of antibodies and isoagglutinins, 28-29
    of L.E. factor, 29
    of drugs, 32-33
Maternal-fetal passage of leukocytes and platelets, 28
Maturation of erythrocytes, 51-53
May-Hegglin anomaly, 499-500
Mean corpuscular hemoglobin concentration, 185-186
Mean corpuscular volume, 185
Measles in leukemia, 579
Measles vaccination, thrombocytopenia following, 766
Mechanical fragility of red cells, 47
Mediastinum in leukemia, 573
Mediterranean anemia; *see* Thalassemia
Medullary cystic disease, 457
Medullary reticulosis, histiocytic, 673-674
Megakaryocytes, 682-683
  in fetus, 2
  depression of, with chronic hypoplastic thrombocytopenia, 782
  in idiopathic thrombocytopenic purpura, 768
Megakaryocytic leukemia, acute, 633
Megakaryocytic thrombocytopenia, drug-induced, 781
Megakaryocytosis, extramedullary, 633
Megaloblast, 53
Megaloblastic anemia, 242-260
  causes of, 242
    anticonvulsants, 255
  familial, 249
  with fish tapeworms, 254-255
  with hemochromatosis, 254
  with hemolytic anemia, 254, 294-295
  and hereditary orotic aciduria, 245
  of infancy, 246-248
  juvenile pernicious anemia, 248-253
    clinical manifestations of, 250
    etiology of, 248-250
    laboratory findings, 250-253
  with malignancies, 254
  nutritional, 253-254
  of pregnancy, 254
  and sickle cell anemia, 381
Megaloblastoid changes in iron-deficiency anemia, 211
Meningeal leukemia, 583-584
  methotrexate for, 621
  radiation therapy for, 621
6-Mercaptopurine
  in autoimmune hemolytic anemia, 332-333
  for leukemia, 598-600

Mesenchyme in blood formation in fetus, 1
Metabolic disorders, detection of, from amniotic fluid, 147
Metabolism
  of erythrocyte, 38-40
  of iron for hemoglobin synthesis, 221
Metachromasia, cellular, 499
Metamyelocyte, 482
Metaplasia, agnogenic myeloid, 630-631
Metastasis in neuroblastoma, 190-193
Methandrostenolone for aplastic anemia, 280
Methemalbumin
  in cord blood, 292
  and methemalbuminemia, 293
Methemoglobin, 420
Methemoglobinemia, 452-454
Methotrexate for leukemia, 596-598
  meningeal, 621
Microcytes, 63
Microdrepanocytic anemia, 421-422
Microscopy, phase contrast, 501
Microspherocytes, 63-64
Microspherocytosis
  in A-B-O erythroblastosis, 170
  as cause of jaundice, 113
Mitochondria in erythrocytes, 39
M-N-Ss and P blood group system, 82-83
Mongolism; *see* Down's syndrome
Mongolism-leukemia, 571
Monocytes, 489-491
  appearance of, in fetus, 2
  changes in, during growth, 19
Monocytic anemia and sideroblastic anemia, 558-559
Monocytic leukemia, acute, 490-491
Monocytosis, 491
  in acute monocytic leukemia, 558
  in cyclic neutropenia, 516
Mononuclear cells, 540
Mononucleosis
  infectious
    acute hemolytic anemia during, 543
    in acute lymphocytic leukemia, 542, 545-546
    clinical features of, 537-540
    definition of, 536
    differential diagnosis, 545-546
      and chronic nonspecific infectious lymphocytosis, 533
      and leukemia, 585
      and lymphocytosis, 531
    Epstein-Barr virus and, 536-537
    laboratory findings, 540, 542-545
    pathology of, 537
    prognosis of, 546
    tests for, 543-545
    thrombocytopenia in, 543
    transmission of, by transfusion, 96
    treatment of, 546-547
  lymphocytes, 542
  posttransfusion, 547

**864    INDEX**

Mosaicism
  blood group, 78
  definition of, 568
Mucosal block theory of iron transport, 221
Multinuclearity, familial erythroid, 71
Multiple myeloma, 629-630
Muramidase, 474
  in leukemia, 560
Murmur, heart, in anemia, 181
Mutual correction tests in hemophilia, 739
Myeloblast, differentiation from lymphoblast, 480-481
Myeloblastic leukemia, 553
  acute, treatment of, 616-619
Myelocytes, 481-482
Myelocytic leukemia, 553, 555-558
  acute, 553
  chronic, 553, 555-558
    busulfan for, 600-601
Myelofibrosis, 630-631
Myelogenous leukemia, 553, 555-558
Myeloid:erythroid ratio, 195
Myeloid or granulocytic series of leukocytes; see Leukocytes, types of, granulocytic or myeloid series
Myeloid leukemia, chronic, 553, 555-558
Myeloid metaplasia, agnogenic, 630-631
Myeloid type of hyperleukocytosis, 525-526
Myelokathexis, 517
Myeloma, multiple, 629-630
Myeloproliferative disease, familial, 631
Myelosis, erythremic, 634
Myleran for leukemia, 600-601
Myoglobin, fetal, 9
Myoglobinuria, idiopathic paroxysmal, 336-337

**N**

Naphthalene and acute hemolytic anemia, 114
Nasopharynx in lymphocytosis, 528
Neonatal granulocytosis, 518-519
Neonatal hepatitis
  as cause of jaundice, 117, 119-120
  distinguished from biliary atresia, 121-122
Neonatal hyperbilirubinemia, familial, 105
  transient, 111
Neonatal period
  early, causes of jaundice in, 107-116
    acute hemolytic anemia and naphthalene, 114
    chronic idiopathic jaundice, 116
    congenital toxoplasmosis, 115-116
    cytomegalic inclusion disease, 115
    elliptocytic hemolytic anemia, 114
    Heinz body anemia, 114
    hereditary nonspherocytic hemolytic disease, 113
    hereditary spherocytosis, 113
    hyperbilirubinemia
      in breast-fed infants, 110-111
      unrelated to isoimmunization, 108-109
    infections, 114-115

Neonatal period—cont'd
  early, causes of jaundice in—cont'd
    phenobarbital therapy for, 109-110
    phototherapy for, 111-112
    physiologic jaundice, 107-108
    transient, from familial hyperbilirubinemia, 111
    vitamin K and, 112-113
  late, causes of jaundice in, 116-124
    atresia of bile ducts, 118-119
    carotenemia and, 123-124
    congenital familial nonhemolytic jaundice with kernicterus, 122-123
    hematomas, 124
    hypothyroidism, 124
    inspissated bile syndrome, 117-118
    neonatal hepatitis, 119-120
    obstruction and erythroblastosis, 117-118
    prolonged obstruction, 116-117
      management of, 120-122
    pyloric stenosis, 124
  platelets in, 18-19
Neonate; see also Newborn
  blood changes in, 13-14
  formation of bilirubin in, 57
  glycolysis in cells of, 20
Neoplasia of lymphoid tissue
  blood changes in, 641-642
  bone marrow changes, 642
  Burkitt's tumor, 640
  chlorambucil for, 644
  combination therapy for, 645-646
  cyclophosphamide for, 644
  Hodgkin's disease, 635-638
    treatment of, 642-646
  hyperthyroidism in, 635
  hypogammaglobulinemia in, 635
  lymphosarcoma, 638-640
    in childhood, roentgen-ray therapy for, 643
    treatment of, 645
  nitrogen mustard for, 644
  prognosis of, 646
  roentgen-ray therapy for, 643
  treatment of, 642-646
  triethylene melamine for, 644
  vincristine for, 645
Nephropathy, uric acid, in leukemia, 611
Nervous system, central, changes in
  in infectious mononucleosis, 539
  in leukemia, treatment of, 620-622
  in lymphocytosis, 528-529
  in sickle cell anemia, 374
Neuroblastoma, 190-193
  differentiated from leukemia, 585
  disseminated, treatment of, 644-645
Neurologic complications in allergic purpura, 798
Neutropenia
  in childhood, 520
  hypoplastic, 516
  neonatal, 518-519
  periodic, 515-516

Neutropenia—cont'd
  primary, splenic, 658
  severe, chronic, 517
  splenic, 519
  transitory, 32
Neutrophilia, 524-525
Neutrophilic leukocytes, changes in, during growth, 19
Neutrophilic leukocytosis, 524
Neutrophils, 482-483
Newborn
  anemia in, differential diagnosis, 181-182
  bleeding in, 716-717
  blood changes in, 13-14
  bone marrow changes in, 14-15
  conversion of bilirubin by, 108
  defect in glutathione stability, 112-113
  erythrocytes in, 16-17
    enzyme activity of, 39-40
    life-span of, 54-55
  erythropoiesis in, 49-50
  Heinz body anemia in, 114
  hemoglobin concentration in, 15-16
  hemolytic anemia of; see Erythroblastosis fetalis
  hemorrhagic disease of, 717-720
  hereditary spherocytosis in, 307
  hyperbilirubinemia in, 133; see also Jaundice in early neonatal period
    in breast-fed infants, 110-111
    familial
      neonatal, 105
      transient, 111
    phenobarbital therapy for, 109-110
    phototherapy for, 111-112
    physiologic, 167-169
    unrelated to isoimmunization, 108-109
  hypoprothrombinemia in, 717-720
  idiopathic cirrhosis in, 120
  jaundice in; see Jaundice in early neonatal period
  L.E. phenomenon in, 29
  leukemia in, 565, 570-571
  leukocytosis of, 524
  physiologic anemia of, 14
    and iron-deficiency anemia, 208-209
  plasma proteins in, 29-31
  platelet count in, 761
  pulmonary hemorrhage in, 27-28
  thrombocytopenia in, 761
  transient agranulocytosis in, 32
  transitory neutropenia in, 32
  transplacental passage of drugs affecting, 32-33
Niacin, deficiency of, and anemia, 460
Nicotinic acid, deficiency of, and anemia, 460
Niemann-Pick disease, 667-668
Nitrogen mustard for lymphomas, 644
Nocturnal hemoglobinuria, 46, 321-325
Nonerythroblastotic hyperbilirubinemia, 108-109
Nonhemolytic jaundice, familial, 122-123
Nonhemolytic transfusion reactions, 96

Nonhemolytic unconjugated hyperbilirubinemia, 111
Nonhereditary hemolytic anemia, 321-325
Nonspherocytic hemolytic anemia, hereditary, 310-311
  with altered phospholipid composition of erythrocytes, 316
Nonspherocytic hemolytic disease, 113
Nonthrombocytopenic purpura; see Purpura, nonthrombocytopenic
Nontropical sprue, 255-256
Normoblast
  basophilic, 52
  changes in during growth, 18
  orthochromatic, 52
  polychromatic, 52
Normoblastemia in hemolytic anemia, 295
Normoblastic macrocytic anemias, 256
Normoblastic response in iron-deficiency anemia, 211
Novobiocin, effect on bilirubin levels in newborn, 109
Nucleic acid and cellular development, 51-52
Nucleolysis in L.E. phenomenon, 476-477
Nucleophagocytosis distinguished from nucleolysis in L.E. phenomenon, 476-477
Nutritional deficiencies and leukopenia, 519-520
Nutritional megaloblastic anemia, 253-254

## O

Obstructive jaundice
  in erythroblastosis fetalis, 117-118
  prolonged, 116-117
    management of, 120-122
Oncogenic virus, RNA, and leukemia, 564
Oncovin for leukemia, 601-602
Opsonins and chemotaxis, 471-472
Orotic aciduria, hereditary, and megaloblastic anemia, 245
Orthochromatic megaloblast, 53
Orthochromatic normoblast, 52
Osmotic fragility of red cells, 46-47
  test for, 299-300
  in thalassemia major, 402
Osteoblasts in bone marrow, 194
Osteoclasts in bone marrow, 194
Osteopetrosis, 631-633
  bone and joint manifestations of, 196
Osteosclerosis in Gaucher's disease, 665
Outpatient transfusion clinic for chronic anemias, 94
Ovalocytic hemolytic anemia as cause of jaundice, 114
Ovalocytosis of erythrocytes, 64
Overload
  circulatory, in transfusion, 97
  iron, in transfusions, 98-99
Owren's disease, 714-715
Oxidative phosphorylation and bilirubin, 134

Oxygen affinity
    alteration of, 365
        and hemoglobin variants, 431
    of hemoglobin, 44
Oxygen capacity and iron content of hemoglobin, 42-43
Oxygen dissociation
    and 2,3-diphosphoglyceride, 41
    and fetal blood, 6-7
    and thickness of red cells, 47
Oxygen saturation, fetal, and cord blood hemoglobin, 7-8
Oxygen therapy for sickle cell anemia, 382-383
Oxymetholone for aplastic anemia, 280

P

Packed red blood cells, volume of
    in anemia, 184-186
    during growth, 18
Pagophagia and iron deficiency, 208
Pancreas, changes in, in thalassemia, 391-392
Pancreatic insufficiency and bone marrow dysfunction, 514-515
Pancytopenia, fatal, following hepatitis, 272
Panhematopenia, primary splenic, 658
Paper electrophoresis, 354-356
Pappenheimer bodies, 67
Parahemophilia, 714-715
Parenchymal liver disease, coagulation changes in, 727
Paroxysmal hemoglobinuria
    cold, 334-335
    nocturnal, 46, 321-325
Paroxysmal myoglobinuria, idiopathic, 336-337
Partial thromboplastin time, 739
Paul-Bunnell test, 543
Pelger-Hüet phenomenon of granulocytes, 495-496
Perforation, colonic, following exchange, 161
Peritonitis following exchange transfusion, 161
Pernicious anemia, juvenile, 248-253
    clinical manifestations of, 250
    etiology of, 248-250
    laboratory findings in, 250-253
    Schilling count, 482-483
Peroxidase stain for cells, 501
Pertussis, lymphocytosis in, 532
Phagocyte, 470
Phagocytosis, 470-471
Phase contrast microscopy, 501
Phenobarbital therapy for neonatal jaundice, 109-110
Phenotypes, definition of, 75
Phenylbutazone, leukemia and, 562
Philadelphia chromosome, 555-556
    in leukemia, 567
Phosphatase, acid, in red cell, 40
6-Phosphogluconate dehydrogenase deficiency and hemolytic anemia, 315
Phosphoglycerate kinase deficiency and hemolytic anemia, 316

Phosphorylation, oxidative, bilirubin and, 134
Phototherapy
    for erythroblastosis fetalis, 161
    for hyperbilirubinemia, 111-112
Physiologic anemia of newborn, 14
    and iron-deficiency anemia, 208-209
Physiologic hyperbilirubinemia, exchange transfusion in, 167-169
Physiologic jaundice, 107-108
    and lack of carbohydrate, 108-109
Physiologic leukocytosis, 524-525
Phytohemagglutinin
    for aplastic anemia, 282-283
    effect of, on lymphocytes, 488
Phytonadione for hemorrhagic disease in newborn, 719-720
Pica and iron-deficiency anemia, 207
Placenta
    bleeding from surface of, 27-28
    physiology and defects of, 25-26
    size of, and blood cellular elements, 1-2
Placental transmission
    of antibodies and isoagglutinins, 28-29
    of L.E. factor, 29, 476
Placental vessels, blood in, 15-16
Plasma
    choice and dosage of, in transfusions, 91
    for Christmas disease, 710-711
    cord, haptoglobins in, 292-293
    iron in, 220
    iron-binding capacity of, 224-227
    in iron-deficiency anemia, 211
    iron turnover in, calculation of, 188-189
    pooled, and incidence of hepatitis, 93-94
    for transfusions in classic hemophilia, 695-700
    volume of, 90
Plasma cell, 492-493
    and antibody formation, 471
    changes in during growth, 19
    hepatitis, 493
    leukemia, 629-630
Plasma proteins
    in fetus and newborn, 29-31
    loss of, and iron-deficiency anemia, 209
Plasma prothrombin time, 743-744
Plasma thromboplastin, in blood coagulation, 684, 686
Plasma thromboplastin antecedent deficiency, 711-712
Plasma thromboplastin component deficiency, 709-711
    and Ehlers-Danlos syndrome, 802-803
Plasmaphoresis, 163
Plasminogen activator, 724
Plasmocyte, 492-493
Platelet
    adhesiveness of, 741-742
    aggregometer, 743
    appearance of, in fetus, 2
    changes in, during growth, 18-19

Platelet—cont'd
   in erythroblastosis fetalis, 143
   hepatic destruction of, in idiopathic thrombocytopenic purpura, 776
   impaired function of
      by aspirin, 742
      in renal disease, 456
   incompatibility of, fetal-maternal, in congenital thrombocytopenic purpura, 778
   infusion of, in thrombocytopenia, 93
   and leukocytes, maternal-fetal passage of, 28
   levels of, following exchange transfusion, 143
   life-span of, 93
   in lymphomas, 641
   in neonatal period, 18-19
   role of, in hemostasis, 681-684
   in thromboplastic generation test, 737-738
   transfusion of, 92-94
   in Wiscott-Aldrich syndrome, 786-787
Platelet count, 734-735
   in infants, normal, 761
   in premature infant, 20
Platelet factor 3 deficiency, 742-743
Platelet syndrome, giant, 738
Pleural effusion in leukemia, 581
*Pneumocystis carinii* pneumonia in leukemia, 579
Pneumonia in leukemia, 579, 581
Pocked erythrocytes, 66
Poikilocytosis, 63
Poisoning
   arsenic, anemia in, 326
   exchange transfusion for, 169
   iron, 231-232
   lead, 462-464
Polychromasia and stippling in red cells, 51
Polychromatic megaloblast, 53
Polychromatic normoblast, 52
Polycythemia, 450-452
   in premature infants, 20
   in twin-to-twin transfusion, 17
Polymorphism, definition of, 75-76
Polymorphonuclear granulocytes, 482-487
Pooled plasma and incidence of hepatitis, 93
Porphyria, 296-299
   hepatic, 298-299
Porphyrins and blood disorders, 44
Porphyrinuria, 296
Portal hypertension, 658-661
Postcardiotomy syndrome, febrile, 547
Postnatal period, blood changes during, 13-22
Postsplenectomy thrombocytosis, 653
Posttransfusion purpura, 787
Potassium
   in stored blood, 45-46, 99-100
   and sodium in red cells, 45
Prednisolone
   for hemarthrosis in hemophilia, 704-705
   for leukemia, 605

Prednisone
   in autoimmune hemolytic anemia, 332
   for hemarthrosis in hemophilia, 704-705
   for leukemia, 605
Pregnancy
   in acute leukemia, 565
   duration of, and fetal hemoglobin, 6
   heterospecific, definition of, 75
   megaloblastic anemia of, 254
Pregnanediol in breast milk, 110
Preleukemic stage, 569-570
Premature infant
   blood of, 20
   exchange transfusion in, 154
   iron-deficiency anemia in, 219-220
   platelet count in, 761
   serum bilirubin levels in, 107-108
   transfusions in, 94-95
Prenatal blood development, 1-2
Prenatal factors in iron-deficiency anemia, 205-207
Prenatal hematopoiesis, 1-2
Prenatal testing for maternal antibodies, 136
Preservation of blood, 100-101
   with acid-citrate-dextrose, 99-100
Priapism in leukemia, 573, 575
Price-Jones curve, 185
Primary familial xanthomatosis, 668-669
Primary polycythemia, 450
Primary splenic neutropenia, 658
Primary splenic panhematopenia, 658
Primitive blood cells, 50-61
Primitive hemoglobin, 361
Private blood group antigens, 84
Proband, definition of, 75
Procarbazine for lymphomas, 645
Proconvertin deficiency, 715-716
Proerythroblast, 52
Progranulocytes, 481-482
Prolymphocytes, 489
Promegaloblasts, 52-53
Promonocyte, 490
Promyelocyte, 481-482
Promyelocytic leukemia, 553
Pronormoblast, 52
Propositus, definition of, 75
Protein-losing enteropathy, 230-231
Proteins
   plasma
      in fetus and newborn, 29-31
      loss of, in iron-deficiency anemia, 209
   serum
      electrophoresis of, 358
      as indication for exchange transfusion, 154
   synthesis of, 23-24
      defect of, in thalassemia, 389
Prothrombin, conversion of, to thrombin, 689-690
   disorders of, 712-721
      factor V deficiency, 714-715
      factor VII deficiency, 715-716
      factor X deficiency, 720-721

## 868 INDEX

Prothrombin, conversion of to thrombin—cont'd
  disorders of—cont'd
    multiple defects, 721
    of newborn, 716-717
      hemorrhagic disease of, 717-720
      vitamin K deficiency, 713-714
    tests for, 743-744
Prothrombin complex deficiency, tests for, 743
Prothrombin consumption test, 740
Prothrombin time, plasma, 743-744
Protoporphyria, erythropoietic, 297-298
Protoporphyrin
  in anemia of infection, 458
  and coproporphyrin, erythrocyte, increased, 296
Pseudohemophilia, 706, 708-709
  and vascular defects, 800
Pseudoneutropenia, 520
Pulmonary eosinophilia, 485
Pulmonary hemorrhage in newborn, 27-28
Pulmonary hemosiderosis, 804-807
Pure red cell anemia, 262-267
  clinical features of, 263-264
  definition of, 262
  diagnosis of, 264-265
  laboratory findings, 264
  pathogenesis, 262-263
  prognosis of, 266-267
  treatment of, 265-266
Purine antagonists in leukemia, 596-600
Purpura(s), 760-820
  anaphylactoid, 793-800
  classification of, 760-761
  fibrolytic, 723-725
  fulminans, 803-804
  hemorrhagic; see Purpura, thrombocytopenic, idiopathic
  Henoch-Schönlein, 793-800
  nonthrombocytopenic, 793-808
    allergic, 793-800
      abdominal symptoms in, 797
      clinical features of, 794-798
      course and prognosis of, 798-799
      diagnosis of, 798
      etiology of, 793-794
      joint involvement in, 797
      laboratory findings, 798
      neurologic complications, 798
      pathogenesis, 793-794
      renal complications, 797-798
      skin changes in, 795, 797
      steroids for, 799
      treatment of, 799-800
    congenital vascular defects, 800-803
    fulminans, 803-804
    idiopathic pulmonary hemosiderosis, 804-807
    Waterhouse-Friderichsen syndrome, 804
  thrombocytopenic, 762-793
    congenital, 777-779
      and aplastic anemia, 782
    cyclic, 792

Purpura(s)—cont'd
  thrombocytopenic—cont'd
    with eczema and infections, 785-787
    hemangioma and thrombopenia, 792
    hemolytic-uremic syndrome, 787-792
    hereditary, 776-777
    idiopathic, 762-776
      blood findings in, 768
      bone marrow in, 768-769
      clinical manifestations of, 765-767
      course and prognosis of, 770
      diagnosis of, 769-770
      differentiated from leukemia, 584
      immunosuppressive agents for, 773-774
      laboratory data, 768-769
      pathogenesis, 762-764
      pathology of, 764-765
      splenectomy for, 774-776
      steroids for, 771-773
      transfusions for, 770-771
    in newborn, 32
    thrombocytopenia; see also Thrombocytopenia
      with absent radius, 782-783
      chronic hypoplastic, 782
      drug-induced, 780-782
      in fetal rubella, 779-780
      in infection, 780
      with renal vein thrombosis, 780
      following transfusions, 737
    thrombotic, 783-784
    Wiscott-Aldrich syndrome, 785-787
Pyknocytes and infantile pyknocytosis, 68
Pyloric stenosis as cause of jaundice, 124
Pyridoxine deficiency and anemia, 460-461
Pyruvate kinase deficiency and anemia, 313-315

## Q

Quick test, one-stage, 743
Quinine-induced thrombocytopenic purpura, 778

## R

Radiation
  aplastic anemia caused by, 272
  and leukemia, 566, 568-569
  and leukopenia, 513
  as therapy
    for Hodgkin's disease, 643
    for leukemia, 600
    meningeal, 621
Rebuck window, 473-474
Red blood cells; see Erythrocytes
Red blood cell count
  and hemoglobin and volume of packed red cells in anemia, 184-186
  in premature infant, 20
Reed-Sternberg cells in Hodgkin's disease, 637, 641-642
Reilly bodies in gargoylism, 498-499
Remissions in leukemia
  acute, 615-616

Remissions in leukemia—cont'd
  criteria for, 606-607
  spontaneous, 571-572
Renal complications in allergic purpura, 797-798
Renal failure
  in allergic purpura, 799-800
  in leukemia, 611
Renal function in leukemia, 581-582
Renal insufficiency, chronic, anemia of, 455-457
Renal tumors and erythropoietin, 50
Renal vein thrombosis, 780
Rendu-Osler-Weber disease, 800-801
Reticulocyte, 52
  in erythroblastosis fetalis, 142-143
  changes in, during growth, 18
  metabolism of, 38
  in newborn, 13
  shift, 52
Reticulocyte count
  in A-B-O erythroblastosis, 170
  in anemia, 184
Reticulocytosis in hemolytic anemia, 295
Reticulosis, histiocytic medullary, 673-674
Reticulum cell sarcoma, 638-640
Reticuloendothelial system, diseases of, 661-674
  eosinophilic granuloma, 673
  Gaucher's disease, 662-667
  generalized gangliosidosis, 668
  Hand-Schüller-Christian disease, 672-673
  histiocytic medullary reticulocytosis, 673-674
  histiocytosis X, 669-673
  Letterer-Siwe disease, 669-672
  Niemann-Pick disease, 667-668
  Wolman's disease, 668-669
Reticuloendotheliosis
  differentiated from leukemia, 584
  nonlipid, 669-672
Rh incompatibility, carboxyhemoglobin in, 142
Rh₀ immune globulin, 162-163
Rh-Hr agglutinogens, 74
Rh-Hr blood group system, 79-82
Rh-Hr hemolytic disease, phenobarbital therapy for, 109-110
Rh-Hr immunization and A-B-O incompatibility, 172
Rh-positive mother and infant, immunization in, 137
Rheumatic fever
  acute, differentiated from chronic infectious lymphocytosis, 535-534
  differentiated from leukemia, 585-586
Rheumatoid arthritis differentiated from leukemia, 585-586
RHoGAM, 162-163
Riboflavin deficiency and anemia, 460
Rieder cells, 493
RNA oncogenic virus and leukemia, 564
Roentgenographic examination in blood dyscrasias, 195-196

Romanowsky stains, 500
Rose bengal in diagnosis of biliary obstruction, 121
Rouleaux formation of red cells, 44-45
Rubella
  congenital, anemia of, 326
  fetal, thrombocytopenia in, 779-780
  thrombocytopenic purpura following, 766
Rumple-Leede test, 735
Runt disease, 201-202
Rupture of spleen
  in erythroblastosis fetalis, 164
  in infectious mononucleosis, 540
Russell bodies, 496

S

Salmonella infection in sickle cell anemia, 377
Saphenous vein method of exchange transfusion, 159-160
Sarcoma, reticulum cell, 638-640
Schilling count, 482-483
Schistocytes in hemolytic anemia, 294
Schönlein-Henoch purpura, 793-800
Screening tests for hemorrhagic disorders, 733-735
Scurvy, anemia of, 461-462
Secondary polycythemia, 451-452
Sedimentation of red cells, 44-45
Sedimented red cell versus whole blood for exchange transfusion, 56
Sedormid as cause of megakaryocytic thrombocytopenia, 781
Sensitization, autoerythrocytic, 201
Serotonin in platelets, 681-682
Serum, in thromboplastic generation test, 736-737
Serum albumin for exchange transfusion, 156-157
Serum bilirubin
  in full-term infant, 107-108
  and novobiocin, effect of, 109
Serum hepatitis, homologous, from transfusion, 96
Serum iron, 220-221
Serum proteins
  electrophoresis of, 358
  level of, as indication for exchange, 154
Serum transaminase in obstructive jaundice, 121
Shift reticulocytes, 52
Sickle cell, 64
Sickle cell anemia, 371-384
  blood picture in, 378
  bone and joint manifestations of, 196
  clinical features of, 374-377
  crisis of, 378-382
  diagnosis of, 382
  hand-foot syndrome of, 375-376
  pathology of, 371-374
  prognosis of, 384
  skeletal changes in, 377-378
  treatment of, 382-384
Sickle cell disease, 365-384
  fetal hemoglobin in, 360
  –hemoglobin C, 422-424
  –hemoglobin D, 424

Sickle cell disease—cont'd
   —hemoglobin G, 419
   —hereditary spherocytosis, 424
   pathogenesis, 368-369
   sickle cell anemia; see Sickle cell anemia
   sickle cell trait, 369-371
   sickling phenomenon, 366-368
   —thalassemia, 421-422
Sickle cell trait, 369-371
Sickle hemoglobin, 360
Sickling of erythrocytes
   and hemoglobin C, 417
   hereditary spherocytosis and thalassemia, 424
   and malaria, 370-371
   phenomenon of, 366-368
Sideroachrestic anemia, 232-234
Sideroblast, 66
   in hemolytic anemia, 296
Sideroblastic anemia, 232-234
   and monocytic anemia, 558-559
Siderocytes, 66-67
   in hemolytic anemia, 295-296
   and punctate basophilia, 66-67
Siderophilin in iron transport, 220
Siderosis
   and thalassemia, 391-392
   tissue, 227-228
Skin
   in allergic purpura, 795, 797
   in leukemia, 573
   in lymphocytosis, 529
Sodium in red cells, 45
Spherocyte, 63-64
   in hemolytic anemia, 294
Spherocytic anemia, 303-309
Spherocytosis
   congenital, sporadic, with hypoplastic thrombocytopenia and malformations, 309-310
   hereditary, 303-309
     bone and joint manifestations of, 196
     as cause of jaundice, 113
     clinical features of, 305-306
     diagnosis of, 307-308
     etiology of, 303-305
     growth and, 306
     inheritance and race, 303
     laboratory data, 306-307
     in newborn, 307
     pathogenesis of, 303-305
     sickle cell–, 424
     and sickling and thalassemia, 424
     treatment of, 308
Spleen
   aspiration of, 655
   changes in, in erythroblastosis fetalis, 135
   congenital absence of, 657
   disorders of, 656-661
     congenital absence of, 657
     Felty's syndrome, 658
     hypersplenism, 656-657

Spleen—cont'd
   disorders of—cont'd
     primary splenic neutropenia, 658
     primary splenic panhematopenia, 658
     splenomegaly, 656; see also Splenomegaly
   functions of, 652-655
   in leukemia, 573, 580
   in lymphocytosis, 529
   in protection against infection, 654-655
   role of, in blood disorders, 652
   rupture of
     in erythroblastosis fetalis, 163
     in infectious mononucleosis, 540
   in sickle cell anemia, 371-372
   structure of, 652
Splenectomy
   for aplastic anemia, 282
   for autoimmune hemolytic anemia, 333-334
   for hemoglobin H disease, 415
   in hereditary Heinz body anemia, 428
   for hereditary spherocytosis, 308
   for idiopathic thrombocytopenic purpura, 774-776
   indications for, 655-656
   for myelofibrosis, 631
   for pure red cell anemia, 265-266
   for sickle cell anemia, 383
   susceptibility to infection following, 654-655
   for thalassemia, 412-413
   thrombocytosis following, 653
Splenic anemia, 658-661
Splenic neutropenia, 519
   primary, 658
Splenic panhematopenia, primary, 658
Splenic sequestration crisis, 381-382
Splenomegaly, 656
   in anemia, 181
   chronic congestive, 658-661
   congestive, thrombocytopenia in, 763-764
   and crisis of sickle cell anemia, 381-382
   febrile postcardiotomy lymphocytic, 547
   in sickle cell anemia, 371-372
Sprue, 255-256
Stable factor
   deficiency of, 715-716
   and prothrombin deficiency, tests for, 744
Starch block electrophoresis, 356
   in thalassemia, 407-408
Starch gel electrophoresis, 356
Steatorrhea, idiopathic, 255-256
Stem cell leukemia
   acute, 551
   current treatment of, 614-616
   differentiated from lymphocytosis, 531-532
     chronic nonspecific, 533
   drug therapy in, 610-612
Stenosis, pyloric, as cause of jaundice, 124
Steroids
   in allergic purpura, 799
   in autoimmune hemolytic anemia, 332

Steroids—cont'd
  for idiopathic thrombocytopenic purpura, 771-773
  for leukemia, cyclic use of, 612-613
Stippling of erythrocytes.
  basophilic, 66
  in lead poisoning, 463-464
  and polychromasia in maturation, 51
Stomatocytes in congenital hemolytic anemia, 308-309
Stomatocytosis, 64-65
Stroma of erythrocytes, 37
Stuart-Prower factor, 688
  deficiency of, 720
  tests for, 744
Succinate, heme synthesis from, 40
Sulfhemoglobinemia, 454-455
Sulfisoxazole and kernicterus, 135
Supravital staining of cells, 500-501
Sutter blood groups, 83
Swallowed blood syndrome, 5-9
Syphilis
  congenital, anemia of, 326
  transmission of, by transfusion, 96
Systemic lupus erythematosus and L.E. phenomenon in newborn, 29

# T

Tapeworms, fish, megaloblastic anemia with, 254-255
Target cells, 65
  and abnormal hemoglobins, 363-364
  in thalassemia major, 397-399
Tay-Sach's disease, 500
Telangiectasia, hereditary hemorrhagic, 800-801
Test(s)
  for abnormal hemolysis, 299-302
  acid-serum, Ham, 324
  adrenaline, for hypersplenic syndromes, 655
  for anticoagulants, 729
  autohemolysis, 300-301
  blood coagulation
    phase 1, 735-743
    phase 2, 743-744
    phase 3, 744-745
    routine, significance of, 735
  for bone marrow function, 512
  for chronic granulomatous disease, 473
  Coombs, 138-139
    in A-B-O erythroblastosis, 170
    positive, in erythroblastosis fetalis, 154
  differential agglutination, 543-545
  FI, 745
  for fibrinogen deficiencies, 744-745
  for Hageman factor (XII) deficiency, 740-741
  for hemoglobin S, 366
  in leukemia, 582
  for lupus erythematosus, 477
  mutual correction, in hemophilia, 739
  osmotic fragility, 299-300

Test(s)—cont'd
  prenatal, for maternal antibodies, 136
  prothrombin consumption, 740
  for prothrombin and factor VII deficiency, 744
  screening, for coagulation disorders, 733-735
  for Stuart-Prower factor, 744
  thromboplastic generation, 736-739
Testosterone for aplastic anemia, 279-280
Tetralogy of Fallot, polycythemia in, 451
Thalassemia, 384-421
  alpha-, 413-414
    homozygous, hydrops fetalis and, 361-362
  bone and joint manifestations of, 196
  cardiac involvement in, 409
  classification of, 384-385
  clinical types of, 387
  course of, 408-409
  diagnosis of, 406-408
  distinguished from iron-deficiency anemia, 213-214
  effect of gene on other hemoglobins, 387
  fetal hemoglobin in, 388-389
    persistent, 426
    turnover rate of, 406
  folic acid deficiency in, 412
  genetic transmission of, 386-387
  growth and maturation in, 394
  heart failure in, 404-405
    treatment of, 411
  hemochromatosis in, acquired, 409
  hemoglobin $A_2$ in, 407-408
  hemoglobin $B_2$ in, 408
  –hemoglobin C disease, 424-426
  –hemoglobin E disease, 426
  –hemoglobin G disease, 419
  hemoglobin H–, 414-415
  hemoglobin levels in, growth and, 410-411
  hemosiderosis and hemochromatosis in, 404-405
  hereditary spherocytosis, and sickling, 424
  high hemoglobin F in, 416
  history of, 385
  intermedia, 387-388
    bony masses in, 396-397
  -Lepore hemoglobin, 426-427
  major
    blood picture in, 397-402
    clinical features of, 392
    defect in protein synthesis in, 389
  minor
    beta, 404
    blood picture in, 402-404
    clinical features of, 394
  nomenclature, 385
  pathogenesis, 389-391
  pathology of, 391
  prognosis of, 408-409
  race and incidence, 385-386
  sickle cell disease–, 421-422
  skeletal changes in, 394-397

Thalassemia—cont'd
  treatment of, 410-413
    splenectomy, 412-413
    transfusions, 410-412
Thalassemia trait with $A_2$ and F thalassemia genes, 427-428
Thiazides and congenital thrombocytopenic purpura, 778
Thrombasthemia, 737-738
  Glanzmann's, 734-735
Thrombin
  conversion of prothrombin to, 689-690
  and platelets, 684
Thrombocythemia, 633-634
Thrombocytopenia
  with absent radius, 782-783
  chronic, hypoplastic, with depression of megakaryocytes, 782
  congenital hypoplastic and malformations, 309-310
  in cyanotic heart disease, 722-723
  drug-induced, 780-782
  in fetal rubella, 779-780
  in infections, 780
  in infectious mononucleosis, 543
  megakaryocytic, drug-induced, 781
  in newborn, 761
  platelet infusion in, 93
  with renal thrombosis, 780
  following transfusions, 787
Thrombocytopenic purpura
  congenital, 777-779
    and aplastic anemia, 782
  cyclic, 792
  with eczema and infection, 785-787
  hemangioma and thrombocytopenia, 792
  hemolytic-uremic syndrome, 787-792
  hereditary, 776-777
  idiopathic, 762-776
    blood findings in, 768
    bone marrow in, 768-769
    clinical manifestation of, 765-767
    course and prognosis, 770
    diagnosis, 769-770
    differentiated from leukemia, 584
    immunologic relationships of, 32
    immunosuppressive agents for, 773-774
    laboratory data, 768-769
    pathogenesis, 762-764
    pathology of, 764-765
    splenectomy for, 774-776
    steroids for, 771-773
    transfusions for, 770-771
  in newborn, 32
  thrombotic, 783-785
Thrombocytopoietin for platelet formation, 763
Thrombocytosis
  postsplenectomy, 653
  primary, 633-634

Thrombohemolytic thrombocytopenic purpura, 783-785
Thrombopathia, 737-738
Thrombopenia and hemangioma, 792-793
Thromboplastin
  deficiency of, value of tests for, 739-740
  formation of, disorders of, 692-712
    Christmas disease, 709-711
    hemophilia, 692-705
    plasma thromboplastin antecedent deficiency, 711-712
    von Willebrand's disease, 706, 708-709
  plasma, 684, 686
Thromboplastin antecedent deficiency, 711-712
Thromboplastin component deficiency, 709-711
  in Ehlers-Danlos syndrome, 802-803
Thromboplastin generation test, 736-739
Thromboplastin time, partial, 739
Thrombosis, renal vein, thrombocytopenia with, 780
Thrombotic thrombocytopenic purpura, 783-785
Thymectomy for autoimmune hemolytic anemia, 334
Thymoma with pure red cell anemia, 263-264
Thymus-independent immune system, 487
Tissue basophils, 487
Tissue mast cells, 487
Tissue siderosis, 227-228
Titer
  definition of, 75
  maternal anti-Rh, 136-137
Tourniquet test, 735
Toxacara infection, eosinophilia in, 484-485
Transaminase, serum, in obstructive jaundice, 121
Transferrin in iron transport, 220-221
Transfusion
  in acute and chronic anemia, 90-91
  for acute myeloblastic leukemia, 606-617
  air embolism in, 99
  allergic reactions in, 99
  in aplastic anemia, 278-279
  for autoimmune hemolytic anemia, 333
  choice and dosage of, 91-92
  circulatory overload in, 97
  clinic for, outpatient, 94
  in cyanotic heart disease, 94
  dosage for, 89
  electrolyte disturbances in, 99-100
  exchange
    for A-B-O erythroblastosis, 172-173
    for erythroblastosis fetalis
      age at time of transfusion, 154-155
      blood, amount to be used, 157
      complications of, 160-161
      concentrated serum albumin for, 156-157
      heparinized blood for, 160
      indications for, 152-153
      and prematurity, 155
      procedure for, 157-159
      rationale for, 151-152

Transfusion—cont'd
  exchange—cont'd
    for erythroblastosis fetalis—cont'd
      saphenous vein method of, 159-160
      whole blood versus sedimented red cells for, 156
    incidence of bacteremia in, 159
    in physiologic hyperbilirubinemia, 167-169
    platelet levels following, 143
    potassium in blood for, 45-46
    in premature infant, 153
    as treatment for poisoning, 169
  fetal-maternal, 26-27
  hemoglobin levels and, 91
  hemolytic reactions to, 95-96
  in hemophilia, classic, 695-703
  in hemorrhagic disorders, 100
  and hemosiderosis, 98-99
  at home, for hemophilia, 702-703
  hyperkalemia and, 99-100
  for idiopathic thrombocytopenic purpura, 770-771
  indications for, 90
  intraperitoneal, 100
    of fetus, 166-167
  intrauterine, 166-167
  in iron-deficiency anemia, 219
  leukocyte, 94
  limitations and hazards of, 95-100
  massive, 99
  mononucleosis following, 547
  multiple
    and anemia, 267
    antibody formation and, 99
  nonhemolytic reactions to, 96
  in pediatric practice, 89-103
  platelet, 92-94
  potassium excess in donor blood, 99-100
  in premature infant, 94-95
  previous, effect of, on mother, 137
  in pure red cell anemia, 265
  for sickle cell anemia, 382
  significant factors in therapy, 89-90
  simple, dosage for, 91-92
  storing of blood for, 100-101
  suppression of blood production by, 97-98
  technique of, 100, 101
  for thalassemia, 410-412
  thrombocytopenia following, 787
  transmission of infection by, 96-97
  twin-to-twin, 17-18
Transient agranulocytosis and fetal-maternal leukocyte incompatibility, 32
Transient dysproteinemia, 229
Transient familial neonatal hyperbilirubinemia, 111
Transitory neutropenia in newborn, 32
Transplacental bleeding from fetus, 26-27
Transplacental passage of drugs, 32-33
Transplacental viral transmission of neonatal hepatitis, 120
Transplantation, bone marrow, in aplastic anemia, 283
Triethylene melamine for lymphomas, 644
Triosephosphate isomerase deficiency and hemolytic anemia, 315
Trisomy $D_1$ syndrome, 7
Tropical eosinophilia, 485
Tropical sprue, 255-256
Trypsinized cells, tests with, for antibodies, 139
Tumor
  Burkitt's, 640
  renal, and erythropoietin, 50
  thymic, and pure red cell anemia, 263-264
  Wilms', 50
Türk's cells, 493
Twin-to-twin transfusion, 17-18

## U

U factor, 82-83
Ulcers, leg, in sickle cell anemia, 374
Umbilical arterial blood pressure, 25-26
Umbilical cord; see also Cord
  immunoglobulin in blood, 30-31
Unconjugated bilirubin, 104
  as indication for exchange transfusion, 154
Unconjugated hyperbilirubinemia, 105
  in breast-fed infants, 110-111
  nonhemolytic, 111
Universal donor and recipient, 78
Unstable hemoglobin, 428-431
Urea therapy for sickle cell anemia, 383-384
Uremia, anemia in, 455-457
Uric acid and antileukemic therapy, 611-612
Urobilinogen excretion as index of hemolysis, 57
Uroporphyrias, erythropoietic, 297

## V

Vacuoles, autophagic, 474
van den Bergh test, 56
Vanillyl-mandelic acid in neuroblastoma, 190
van Jaksch's anemia, 385
Varicella in leukemia, 579
Vascular defects, congenital, 800-803
Vascular factors in hemostatic mechanism, 681
Vascular hemophilia, 706, 708-709
Vasquez-Osler disease, 450
Venous pressure during exchange transfusion, 152
Vincristine
  for leukemia, 601-602
  for lymphoma, 645
Viral transmission, transplacental, of hepatitis, 120
Virocytes, 542
Virus as cause of leukemia, 563-564
Vitamin A, deficiency of, and anemia, 460
Vitamin B factors for aplastic anemia, 282
Vitamin $B_{12}$, 242
  causes of deficiency of, 244
  in erythrocyte production, 47-49
  and folic acid, 244
  gastrointestinal absorption of, 244

Vitamin C and anemia of scurvy, 461-462
Vitamin deficiencies and anemia, 460-462
Vitamin E deficiency and acanthocytosis, 71
Vitamin K
    antagonists of, effect on fetus, 33
    deficiency of, 713-714
        coagulation changes in, 727
        for hemorrhagic disease of newborn, 719-720
        relation to hyperbilirubinemia, kernicterus, and hemolytic anemia, 112-113
Vitamin K–dependent clotting factors, 713
    deficiency of, in newborn, 717-720
Von Willebrand's disease, 706, 708-709
    and vascular defects, 800

## W

Waldenstrom's syndrome, 335
Waring Blendor syndrome (intravascular hemolysis), 337-338
Waterhouse-Friderichsen syndrome, 804
Werlhof's disease; *see* Purpura, thrombocytopenic idiopathic
White blood cells; *see* Leukocytes
Whole blood versus sedimented red cells in exchange transfusion, 156
Wilms' tumor, 193
    and erythropoietin, 50
Wilson's disease, hemolysis in, 326
Wiscott-Aldrich syndrome
    thrombocytopenia in, 785-787
    thromboplastic generation tests in, 738-739
Wolman's disease, 668-669

## X

Xanthomatosis, primary familial, 668-669
X chromosome, 24

## Z

Zone electrophoresis, 355-356